D0078931

Handbook of Clinical Child Neuropsychology

Second Edition

A Continuation Order Plan is available for this series. A continuation order will bring delivery of each new volume immediately upon publication. Volumes are billed only upon actual shipment. For further information please contact the publisher.

Handbook of Clinical Child Neuropsychology

Second Edition

Edited by

Cecil R. Reynolds
Texas A&M University
College Station, Texas

and

Elaine Fletcher-Janzen
The Brown Schools of West Texas
Midland, Texas

Plenum Press • New York and London

Library of Congress Cataloging-in-Publication Data

Handbook of clinical child neuropsychology / edited by Cecil R.
  Reynolds and Elaine Fletcher-Janzen. -- 2nd ed.
        p.   cm. -- (Critical issues in neuropsychology)
    Includes bibliographical references and index.
    ISBN 0-306-45257-X
    1. Pediatric neuropsychology.   I. Reynolds, Cecil R., 1952-
  II. Fletcher-Janzen, Elaine.   III. Series.
    [DNLM: 1. Developmental Disabilities--diagnosis. 2. Developmental
  Disabilities--therapy. 3. Brain--growth & development. 4. Child
  Behavior. 5. Neuropsychological Tests--in infancy & childhood.
  6. Neuropsychology.   WS 350.6 H2364 1997]
  RJ486.5.H26 1997
  618.92'89--dc21
  DNLM/DLC
  for Library of Congress   96-52991
                                                                        CIP

ISBN 0-306-45257-X

© 1997, 1989 Plenum Press, New York
A Division of Plenum Publishing Corporation
233 Spring Street, New York, N. Y. 10013

http://www.plenum.com

10 9 8 7 6 5 4

Printed in the United States of America

Contributors

Russell M. Bauer • Department of Clinical and Health Psychology, University of Florida, Gainesville, Florida 32610

Thomas L. Bennett • Department of Psychology, Colorado State University, Ft. Collins, Colorado 80523

Richard A. Berg • Wilmington Health Associates, Wilmington, North Carolina 28401

Erin D. Bigler • Department of Psychology, Brigham Young University, Provo, Utah 84602; and LDS Hospital, Salt Lake City, Utah 84143

Carol A. Boliek • National Center for Neurogenic Communication Disorders, University of Arizona, Tucson, Arizona 85721

Thomas J. Boll • Department of Psychology, University of Alabama at Birmingham, Birmingham, Alabama 35294

Richard S. Boyer • Department of Radiology, Primary Children's Medical Center, Salt Lake City, Utah 84113

Ronald T. Brown • Departments of Psychiatry and Behavioral Sciences and Pediatrics, Emory University, Atlanta, Georgia 30322

Robert B. Burr • Neurology, Learning and Behavior Center, and Department of Neurosurgery, University of Utah Medical Center, Salt Lake City, Utah 84102

Manuel L. Cepeda • Department of Psychiatry, College of Medicine, University of South Alabama, Mobile, Alabama 36693-3327

Rik Carl D'Amato • Division of Professional Psychology, University of Northern Colorado, Greeley, Colorado 80639-0001

Raymond S. Dean • Neuropsychology Laboratory, Ball State University, Muncie, Indiana 47306

Arden D. Dingle • Departments of Psychiatry and Behavioral Sciences and Pediatrics, Emory University, Atlanta, Georgia 30322

Elizabeth Dreelin • Department of Psychiatry and Behavioral Sciences, Emory University, Atlanta, Georgia 30322

Robert William Elliott • Department of Student Services, Redondo Beach Unified School District, Redondo Beach, California 90277

Bryan Fantie • Department of Psychology, American University, Washington, DC 20016-8062

Eileen B. Fennell • Department of Clinical and Health Psychology, University of Florida, Gainesville, Florida 32610

Elaine Fletcher-Janzen • The Brown Schools of West Texas, Midland, Texas 79706

Heather A. Foley • Department of Psychology, Brigham Young University, Provo, Utah 84602

Barbara C. Gelder • Neuropsychology Laboratory, Ball State University, Muncie, Indiana 47306

Charles J. Golden • Center for Psychological Services, Nova Southeastern University, Fort Lauderdale, Florida 33314

Ruth Adlof Haak • Eanes Independent School District, Austin, Texas 78746

Thalía Harmony • Neurosciences Research Program, ENEP Iztacala, National University of Mexico, Mexico City 03710, Mexico

Lawrence C. Hartlage • Augusta Neuropsychology Center, Evans, Georgia 30809

Patricia L. Hartlage • Section of Child Neurology, Medical College of Georgia, Augusta, Georgia 30912

Jennifer R. Hiemenz • Department of Educational Psychology, University of Georgia, Athens, Georgia 30602

Maile R. Ho • Department of Psychology, Colorado State University, Ft. Collins, Colorado 80523

Robert L. Hodes • Department of Neurology, University of Wisconsin–Madison, Madison, Wisconsin 53792-6180

Stephen R. Hooper • Department of Psychiatry and the Clinical Center for the Study of Development and Learning, University of North Carolina, Chapel Hill, North Carolina 27599

Arthur MacNeill Horton, Jr. • Psych Associates, Towson, Maryland 21214

George W. Hynd • Center for Clinical and Developmental Neuropsychology, University of Georgia, Athens, Georgia 30602

Elizabeth Murdoch James • Department of Educational Psychology, Texas A&M University, College Station, Texas 77843

H. Dennis Kade • Psychology Department, Cumberland Hospital for Children and Adolescents, New Kent, Virginia 23124

Randy W. Kamphaus • Department of Educational Psychology, University of Georgia, Athens, Georgia 30602

Marcel Kinsbourne • New School for Social Research, New York, New York 10011

Bryan Kolb • Department of Psychology, University of Lethbridge, Lethbridge, Alberta T1K 3M4, Canada

John C. Linton • Department of Behavioral Medicine and Psychiatry, West Virginia University Health Sciences Center, Charleston, West Virginia 25326

Ronald B. Livingston • Department of Psychology, University of Texas at Tyler, Tyler, Texas 75701

Antolin M. Llorente • Department of Pediatrics, Baylor College of Medicine, and Texas Children's Hospital, Houston, Texas 77030

Charles J. Long • Psychology Department, The University of Memphis, Memphis, Tennessee 38152

Christine M. LoPresti • Department of Psychiatry and Biobehavioral Sciences, University of California, Los Angeles, Los Angeles, California 90024

Lawrence V. Majovski • Department of Psychiatry and Behavioral Sciences, University of Washington School of Medicine, Harbor View Medical Center, Seattle, Washington 98104-2499

Kenneth D. McCoy • Neuropsychology Laboratory, Ball State University, Muncie, Indiana 47306

Allison E. Morgan • Center for Clinical and Developmental Neuropsychology, University of Georgia, Athens, Georgia 30602

Juan Manuel Munoz-Cespedes • Departamento de Psicologia Basica (Procesos Cognitivas), Universidad Complutense de Madrid, 28223 Madrid, Spain

David E. Nilsson • Neurology, Learning and Behavior Center, Salt Lake City, Utah 84102; and Primary Children's Hospital, Provo, Utah 84113

Nancy L. Nussbaum • Austin Neurological Clinic, Austin, Texas 78705

John E. Obrzut • Department of Educational Psychology, College of Education, University of Arizona, Tucson, Arizona 85721

Antonio E. Puente • Department of Psychology, University of North Carolina at Wilmington, Wilmington, North Carolina 28406

Cecil R. Reynolds • Department of Educational Psychology, Texas A&M University, College Station, Texas 77843

Robert L. Rhodes • School Psychology Program, Special Education/Communication Disorders Department, New Mexico State University, Las Cruces, New Mexico 88003-8001

Becky L. Rosenthal • Intermediate Educational Cooperative, Du Page, Illinois 60510

Barbara A. Rothlisberg • Department of Educational Psychology, Ball State University, Muncie, Indiana 47306

Paul Satz • Department of Psychiatry and Biobehavioral Sciences, University of California, Los Angeles, Los Angeles, California 90024

Marion Selz • Carondelet Rehabilitation Services of Arizona, Tucson, Arizona 85716-5228

Margaret Semrud-Clikeman • Department of Neurology, University of Minnesota Medical School, Minneapolis, Minnesota 55455

Maria Sol Mora • University of North Carolina at Wilmington, Wilmington, North Carolina 28406; and Universidad de San Francisco, Quito, Ecuador

Lisa Stanford • Department of Psychiatry and Psychology, Cleveland Clinic Foundation, Cleveland, OH 44195

Phyllis Anne Teeter • Department of Educational Psychology, University of Wisconsin–Milwaukee, Milwaukee, Wisconsin 53201

Michael G. Tramontana • Division of Child and Adolescent Psychiatry, Vanderbilt University, Nashville, Tennessee 37212-3133

Renee E. VanHorn • Neuropsychology Laboratory, Ball State University, Muncie, Indiana 47306

Melanie Vaughn • Department of Educational Psychology, University of Georgia, Athens, Georgia 30602

Marie L. Walker • Austin Neurological Clinic, Austin, Texas 78705

Timothy B. Whelan • Department of Psychiatry, Baystate Medical Center, Springfield, Massachusetts 01199

Austin R. Woodard • Department of Neurology, University of Wisconsin–Madison, Madison, Wisconsin 53792-6180

Robert Henley Woody • Department of Psychology, University of Nebraska at Omaha, Omaha, Nebraska 68182-0272

Preface to the Second Edition

The first edition of the *Handbook of Clinical Child Neuropsychology* was printed in 1989. At that time, we thought that the concept of experts in the field coming together to mine the depths of child neuropsychology was appealing and necessary. The success of the first edition of the *Handbook* proved that others thought the same. Indeed, it appeared that the field of child neuropsychology was thirsty for seminal works that pushed our knowledge about the neuropsychology of these "moving targets" called children forward. We waited for a rush of criticism about some of the more extreme views expressed in the first edition: None came. We waited for other volumes to appear: None appeared. Hence, we introduce the second edition of the *Handbook of Clinical Child Neuropsychology*.

In general, the reader who is familiar with the first edition will note that we requested updates of approximately two-thirds of the original chapters. Most of those chapters retain much of the original material with later developments and current data woven into the text. On the other hand, other authors ran a bit amok and completely revised their chapters because they had reviewed previous conceptualizations and decided that newer formats would better address the topic at hand. Thalía Harmony, for example, stretched the psychophysiological examination of neuropsychological disorders and delved into the arena of subclinical seizures and transient cognitive impairment. Erin Bigler and colleagues' chapter on neuroimaging reflects the exciting changes in imaging in the past few years, and Thomas Bennett and Maile Ho's inclusion of the ketogenic diet for seizure disorders suggests a new treatment choice for those with intractible seizures. On the whole, the authors used the opportunity to take a serious look at the content and organization of their chapters and applied the benefits of their learning from the past half-dozen years.

As for new chapters, the reader will note that we have included several chapters on pediatric traumatic brain injury that clearly document the continuum of care from trauma to school reentry. Tom Boll and Lisa Stanford address the mechanisms of brain injury; Elaine Fletcher-Janzen and Dennis Kade address inpatient treatment of children with traumatic brain injury; Kenneth McCoy, Barbara Gelder, Renee VanHorn, and Raymond Dean expand their ideas about cognitive rehabilitation; and Ruth Haak and Ron Livingston complete the cycle of treatment with an examination of school reentry and management of traumatic brain injury now that it is an "official" handicapping condition in the public schools. Attention deficit hyperactivity disorder is addressed in a comprehensive forum by Carol Boliek and Jack Obrzut, and George Hynd, Allison Morgan, and Melanie Vaughn make an important addition with their chapter on neurodevelopmental anomalies and malformations. A sad commentary on our time but an exciting array of clinically relevant research findings is reflected in a new chapter about neuropsychological and neurobehavioral sequelae associated with pediatric HIV infection written by Antolin Llorente, Christine LoPresti, and Paul Satz. In addition, a welcome topic that was not addressed in the past edition is the assessment of memory in childhood by Cecil Reynolds and Erin Bigler. We also came to the conclusion that any book about children and brain–behavior relationships could not go forward without addressing the multicultural aspects of assessment and treatment. Antonio Puente, Maria Sol Mora, and Juan Munoz-Cespedes review the neuropsychological assessment of Spanish-speaking children and youth in this volume. We hope that this is the beginning of our conscious commitment to the appreciation of cultural diversity within our profession and charge others in the field to do the same: There is much work for neuropsychology to do in this area.

We have kept the format of the book essentially the same as the first edition. Part I addresses Foundations and Current Issues and gives an overview of the history and development of the field and introduces foundations such as hemispheric specialization and neuroanatomy. Part II addresses Neuropsychological Diagnosis and includes information about subjects from diagnostic imaging to interpretation of common educational tests. Part III, Techniques of Intervention, focuses on subjects such as cognitive rehabilitation, biofeedback, and the pharmacology of seizure disorders. Part IV has been changed from New Aspects of Neuropsychology to Special Topics in Clinical Child Neuropsychology to describe more accurately the breadth of topics in this section.

As usual, there are many individuals to thank. Of course, we are indebted greatly to the chapter authors for this edition. The dedication and brilliance of all of the authors are acknowledged and appreciated. Elaine wishes to thank David, Emma, and Leif for their support and encouragement. To Julia, Cecil continues to owe his unending gratitude for her confidence and support but most of all her love and companionship which keep him centered. Our new Plenum Editor, Mariclaire Cloutier, deserves our appreciation for her support, humor, and tenacity in seeing us through the production process. To Eliot Werner, original Plenum Editor, we express our thanks for encouraging us to do this second edition.

Cecil R. Reynolds
Elaine Fletcher-Janzen

Preface to the First Edition

Alexandra Luria sometimes would use one or two tests with a child and other times ten or fifteen tests. His diagnostic ability was unpredictable, irretrievable, and sometimes appeared magical. Attempts to copy his genius in assessment instruments or clinical methods have varied in success, and years later he still stands out as a unique and imaginative pioneer in clinical neuropsychology. Today we have come much further in our ability to assess children uniformly. We have a plethora of informal assessment instruments that can be given in clinics and in the schools to screen children, saving countless hours and money for parents, children, and the medical community. We have the latest sophisticated equipment that can scan the brain for pathology, giving precise localization of problems in a moment.

This is certainly a time to celebrate in the development of the field of child neuropsychology. Although a relatively young field, clinical neuropsychology has moved far and fast and is now recognized as a necessity in most medical schools and in professional preparation programs in clinical, pediatric, and school psychology. Neuropsychology is also clearly present in the public schools and, although most prominent in the area of learning disabilities, contributes to all areas of handicapping conditions. Children with severe head injuries are no longer relegated to special schools or institutional settings. The child neuropsychologist, then, works in liaison with schools, not just in purely clinical settings. Never before has science worked *in* the schools. Thousands of school personnel actively assess soft neurological signs (that may or may not affect learning) and they communicate directly with child neurologists and neuropsychologists who evaluate the hard neuropsychological signs. This is definitely a field *at work.*

The practice of clinical child neuropsychology remains an enigma in many ways. Children are growing and developing physically, neurologically, behaviorally, and emotionally, albeit in lawful if not well-understood ways, in uneven spurts, and not at all in concert across dimensions. Difficult problems such as localization, prognostication, and differential diagnosis of emotional versus brain–behavior problems with adults become geometrically more abstruse with the interactions present in the course of the child's development. This volume thus tries to take a developmental view in examining neuropsychological function and development that is both normal and abnormal. We also try to take a stand on the necessity of principles of scientific inquiry, psychometric methods, and clinical acumen as central to clinical aspects of child neuropsychology. None can stand alone; the volume presents diverse approaches ranging from the heavily clinical to the near actuarial. Ideally, this work will foster a melding of such ideas, practices, and concepts into stronger clinical practice. The work is eclectic in the theoretical approaches touted as well. There is no more complex problem in *all* of the sciences than understanding developing brain–behavior relations, and we have far to go. We also have much to offer, a good deal of which is reviewed and discussed—along with its limitations—in this *Handbook.*

There is another side of the coin, however. There are many quasi-professionals with perhaps a weekend of training using neuropsychological assessment, overinterpreting the results, and scaring parents with pseudoscientific neurological interpretations. Clinical neuropsychology is young and popular and too many people fail to recognize appropriate educational standards or even the need for years of training and supervision. This *Handbook* also addresses these highly controversial issues. There are also heavy criticisms of neuropsychological assessment instruments, rehabilitative therapies, and the inferential level of neuropsychological research studies; there are even some who negate any objective involvement at all.

This book is intended to serve the children who need neuropsychological services in several ways; (1) as a text for undergraduate and graduate courses in clinical child neuropsychology; (2) in a more general way, as a text that crosses *all* aspects of this rapidly growing field; (3) as a reference source to practitioners and professors in the discipline; and (4) as a potential "idea book" for researchers in the field. We feel that it is important to include varied aspects of opinion on proper clinical practice to represent the field faithfully. Clinical neuropsychology is too young for a consolidation of opinion that would give it a singular approach to practice. Knowledge is developing too rapidly as well to allow us such luxury. Unfortunately, this has led to a polemic—at times vitriolic—division of the field into divergent theory-driven camps. It is too easy, with a subject this size, to use reductionist tactics to forward a cause or ideology that may not be in the best interests of children. The radical behaviorist position, which seems to deny us the convenience of metaphor and the use of inferential constructs we see as so essential to the scientific process, is represented in a chapter by Reschly and Gresham. Although we find the views in the chapter myopic at best, it is an accurate portrayal of the behaviorist view of clinical neuropsychology and its application to disorders of learning. We have presented this disagreeable view to help provide balance and to show the contrasting stance of other theoretical positions. They are particularly harsh on the use of neuropsychology in educational settings, which seems appropriate because—in the remainder of the volume—we have included information not only on clinical applications in the schools but also on developing neuropsychology services in the public schools. For those who are in the field, we hope to have provided some exciting arguments from chapter to chapter. For those new to the field, we hope to have provided a grand but no less than gentle understanding of the entire scope of the field.

Part I—Foundations and Current Issues—gives an overview of the history and development of the field and introduces basic foundations such as measurement theory, neuropsychological frameworks such as hemispheric specialization, and bases for psychopathology. Part II addresses neuropsychological diagnosis. Part III focuses on techniques of intervention, and Part IV speaks to new aspects such as the neuropsychologist in private practice and establishing neuropsychological assessment and principles in the schools.

We hope that the inclusion of so many applications to the public schools will not offend those in the field: After all, *that is where the children are.*

We would like to express our appreciation to several people who aided us in the completion of this work. Angela Bailey, who performs superbly as our administrative editor on a variety of projects, was instrumental in coordinating our own work and keeping track of many of the details of the project. Mike Ash and Victor Willson of the Department of Educational Psychology at Texas A&M University deserve appreciation for their moral support and the precious places they always find to house our special projects. To each of our families, we express our thanks for your patience in our hours away. C.R.R. would like to extend a special note of gratitude to Julia; E.F.J. expresses her appreciation to David, Emma, and C.R.R. We also extend appreciation to Lawrence Hartlage for the demonstration of his remarkable clinical acumen, which continues to interest us in this field. Eliot Werner, Senior Editor at Plenum, as always proved a valuable ally and supporter in the entire development of the work. Last, we are grateful to our authors, for without their hard work this *Handbook* would not exist.

Cecil R. Reynolds
Elaine Fletcher-Janzen

Contents

III. Techniques of Intervention

IV. Special Topics in Clinical Child Neuropsychology

Handbook of Clinical Child Neuropsychology

Second Edition

I

Foundations and Current Issues

1

Development of Neuropsychology as a Professional Psychological Specialty

History, Training, and Credentialing

LAWRENCE C. HARTLAGE AND CHARLES J. LONG

Background

Although neuropsychology as a scientific field of inquiry has origins dating at least as far back as the late 19th century, it is only during the past quarter century that neuropsychology has enjoyed widespread recognition and acceptance as a formal applied professional specialty area. Until recently, neuropsychology was primarily identified with diagnostic testing of adults with verified brain injury. With the increasing recognition of neuropsychological substrates of learning and adaptive behavior problems in adults with brain injury, there developed a progressive interest in some possible central processing dysfunctions as being etiologic in a wide variety of children's learning problems (e.g., Chalfant & Scheffelin, 1969). Given impetus and support by the focus of "The Great Society" programs on identification, description, and treatment of childhood learning problems, neuropsychology increasingly was involved with the assessment of exceptional children.

The growing involvement of neuropsychology with children's problems raised a number of scientific and professional questions and issues.

As the body of research relating known brain damage to specific learning and behavior problems had for the most part involved adults, one obvious scientific question involves the extent to which this research could be applied to children. Stemming from this scientific question arose a professional issue, namely, which tests or diagnostic approaches are appropriate for use with children? If findings from adults could be applied directly to children, then presumably a downward extension of a battery appropriate for use with adults might be adequate for this purpose. Conversely, if findings from adult neuropsychology could not be applied to children, it would be necessary to develop a new data base for application to child neuropsychology.

Another specific question dealt with whether findings from individuals with known brain damage verified on neurological, neurosurgical, or neuro-radiological criterion measures could be applied to children who were presumed to have neuropsychological impairments on the basis of neuropsychological assessment, but for whom there was no definitive evidence of structural or physiological damage. This scientific question translated into obvious professional issues. Because for many children whose neuropsychological examination findings suggested a clear central nervous system dysfunction, there was no external criterion that could validate such an impression, the misclassification of such children as "brain in-

LAWRENCE C. HARTLAGE • Augusta Neuropsychology Center, Evans, Georgia 30809. CHARLES J. LONG • Psychology Department, The University of Memphis, Memphis, Tennessee 38152.

jured" could adversely influence their educational programming and management.

Assessment Approaches

In response to the demand for neuropsychological services for children, and in attempts to address the scientific and professional issues raised by this demand, two diverse approaches to provision of neuropsychological services to children emerged. One approach involved modified versions of traditional neuropsychological batteries such as the Halstead–Reitan Neuropsychological Battery (Reitan, 1955; Reitan & Davison, 1974; Selz, 1981) and the Luria–Nebraska Neuropsychological Battery (Golden, 1981; Golden, Hammeke, & Purisch, 1980; Plaisted, Gustavson, Wilkening, & Golden, 1983), which standardized the adult battery items on a child sample. For the most part, this standardization took the form of deleting from the adult battery those items that were too difficult for children. There is reportedly good congruence between the adult and child batteries on classificatory accuracy, and also between the Reitan–Indiana Children's Battery and the Luria–Nebraska Neuropsychological Battery for Children (Berg et al., 1984; Geary, Schultz, Jennings, & Alper, 1984; Golden et al., 1981). Even among proponents of a standardized battery approach, there is disagreement concerning which battery is best for which population of patients (e.g., Adams, 1980a,b; Spiers, 1981). The second emphasis is on interpretation of standard psychometric tests from a neuropsychological perspective, augmented by some measures of sensory and motor function, using relevant age-appropriate tests for children of given ages, ranging from preschool through adolescent ages (Hartlage, 1981, 1984; Hartlage & Telzrow, 1983; Telzrow & Hartlage, 1984). This approach uses standardized behavioral tests and interprets them according to the individual's strengths and weaknesses and in some cases makes inferences regarding neurological integrity. Such an approach is popular with psychologists working in school settings, and in many cases may be adequate for child neuropsychological assessment. Although there is little evidence that one approach is clearly superior, "turf skirmishes" often center on the issue of qualifications. Psychologists who have developed expertise in the use of a given neuropsychological test battery tend to support the view that the only legitimate neuropsychologists are those with a similar background and expertise. Psychologists who espoused diagnostic approaches involving traditional psychometric tests counter by

questioning the relevance of a standardized battery developed for adults with known brain lesions for assessing children who often do not have evidence of brain lesions. They also question the redundancy involved in adding a standard neuropsychological battery to the array of psychometric instruments required by most school districts for psychoeducational assessment. The second approach appears to be preferred by most professionals. A survey of internship training programs suggests that most professionals prefer the second approach (interpretation of standard psychometric tests from a neuropsychological perspective) (Goldberg & McNamara, 1984). In such settings, 78% employ nonstandardized assessment strategies, 63% the Halstead–Reitan, and 35% the Luria–Nebraska. Even those individuals employing a neuropsychological battery frequently augment the battery with common psychological tests.

Recently, there has evolved a small following of practitioners who attempt to modify subparts of existing neuropsychological batteries, such as a fairly recent publication of a "revised" children's young adolescent's version of the Category Test (Boll, 1993); or modify administration of a standardized test commonly used as part of a neuropsychological battery (e.g., Kaplan, 1991). As there is nothing conceptually new or different in such modifications of existing text or procedures, such approaches can be classified, according to use, in one of these two schemata.

Professional Context of Child Neuropsychology

With the advent of the CAT scan, NMR, and other instruments, neuropsychological assessment has shifted away from simple yes/no "organic" diagnosis as a primary endeavor and has moved toward comprehensive assessment of cognitive skills. The focus is on cognitive strengths and weaknesses and their relationship to academic performance and/or intervention strategies. Neurological integrity is only indirectly inferred as a contributing factor and the utility of such inferences is questioned. It continues to be argued that neuropsychodiagnosis has little or no relevance to education and/or rehabilitation, although it may be relevant to planning for intervention. While the data at present do not indicate that neuropsychological assessments are essential, it is often the case that this is the only assessment whereby a comprehensive investigation of a broad range of cognitive skills is evaluated in the context of emotional and situational factors.

Current interest in neuropsychological assessment has begun to focus on the ecological validity of neuropsychological tests. While relating test scores to vocational performance and real-world behaviors is difficult because of the variability across jobs and across social situations, the academic environment affords a much more stable environment. Future research in this area may well hold substantial promise for understanding the relationship between neuropsychological performance in children and effective treatment strategies.

Levels of Inference

An important issue in training and credentialing in child neuropsychology involves the purposes for which neuropsychologically relevant data are to be used. A comparatively low level of inference involves a conclusion that impaired brain function may be etiologic or at least contributory to a given problem. An example of this level of inference might be a conclusion reached by a school psychologist that a child's failure to acquire a given academic skill is likely related to brain damage or dysfunction. At a considerably higher level of inference are diagnostic statements indicating specific localizing and etiologic phenomena. An example of this level of inference might be a statement, reached by a clinical child neuropsychologist working in a neurological setting, that a child appears to have an astrocytoma confined to anterior portions of the nondominant cerebral hemisphere. Perhaps the highest level of inference involves statements concerning some irreversible intervention. An example of this type of inference might involve a clinical child neuropsychologist working in conjunction with a pediatric neurosurgeon, who concludes that removal of a major portion of a child's hippocampus will not impair memory or other mental function. Between these low and high levels of inference occur many intermediate levels involving such matters as optimal instructional mode, referral to a neurological specialist, prognostic statements based on inferred level of cortical integrity, or conclusions concerning whether (or the extent to which) a child's impaired cognitive performance may be related to an injury for which legal action is pending.

It is possible that a well-trained clinical child psychologist or school psychologist, with only moderate training (or credentials) in child neu-

ropsychology, may make appropriate lower-level inference concerning brain–behavior relationships. For example, a school psychologist may, by training, experience, and clinical skill, be quite adequately prepared to develop perfectly appropriate academic intervention programs for a child with a chronic or acquired neurological impairment, and precluding such individuals from such practice on the grounds that they are not sophisticated in brain–behavior relationships may serve to deprive a child of a valuable professional resource. Conversely, it is not reasonable to expect such a professional to detect manifestations of an early stage neurodevelopmental disorder or a neoplasm of some slowly progressive type. On the one hand, it can be argued that, until the proper diagnosis is made, it is not possible to determine what level of inference may be required: This might suggest that all questions concerning possible brain involvement in children require the involvement of a qualified child neuropsychologist. On the other hand, in a typical school population, the base rate of neurodegenerative or slowly progressive neoplastic disorders is sufficiently low that such a requirement may be considered to be unrealistic.

Interactive with the level of inference is the issue of potential harm to the child. Some chronic neurological conditions, such as might be represented by chronic cerebral hemispheric functional asymmetry, can conceivably be overlooked without necessarily causing major problems. In cases where appropriate educational and counseling services are provided, overlooking the neurological substrates of uneven levels of academic performance may be only minimally handicapping to the child. Conversely, labeling the child "brain damaged" may deprive the child of needed educational support. Similarly, the mismatch between a child's neuropsychologically mediated abilities and deficits in an ongoing educational program that does not take these factors into account may cause harm to the child, both in terms of frustration and failure to achieve academically at ability levels. Obviously, higher-order inferences regarding brain–behavior relationships should only be made by individuals whose training, experience, and clinical skills qualify them for such inferences. Although guidelines concerning training and credentialing can and should address these issues, at the present time they have not been effectively addressed. Even if they are addressed in the future, it is not reasonable to hope that such guidelines can resolve them all.

Credentialing of Psychologists

Although the study of developmental brain–behavior relationships is a relatively recent endeavor in neuropsychology (Dean, 1982), it has already been argued that there is a need for some type of credentialing and certainly for more specialized training if one is to provide appropriate neuropsychological services to children.

Clinical psychologists have traditionally tended to function as generalists—setting few limits regarding credentialing and developing no formal method for identifying a particular area of expertise. They tend not to limit their practice to a specific problem area or specific age group (VandenBos, Stapp, & Kilburg, 1981). This state of affairs no longer appears appropriate for the current practice of psychology because of the dramatic change in the knowledge base. Certainly it is clear that neuropsychological assessment requires specific knowledge not generally obtained in traditional clinical psychology training programs. Furthermore, the techniques and issues in child psychology cannot simply be deduced from knowledge of adults. Specialty training in school psychology and specialization in child psychology also speak to the changes in training promoted to meet the needs of the child.

Although only four specialty areas initially were recognized by the American Psychological Association, a review in credentialing activities by Sales (1985) identified 31 specialty credentialing boards; and at the time of this writing the American Board of Professional Psychology has added several more boards and is negotiating with others for inclusion under its umbrella approach to credentialing. The overall credentialing process is continuing to undergo review. In February 1994 the APA Council of Representatives voted to establish an APA College of Professional Psychology that will function as a credentialing body (APA Practice Directorate, 1994). Also in 1994, APA formed the Joint Interim Committee for the Recognition and Identification of Specialties and Proficiencies. These activities point out APA's awareness of organizing and clarifying the credentialing process. Even though psychologists are identifying areas of specialization and devising procedures for membership inclusion, clinical psychologists seem reluctant to limit their practice by establishing formal specialties within clinical psy-

chology and such activities are not likely to be readily endorsed. Indeed, clinical psychologists have been able to push legislation to enact state licensing and to specifically define diagnoses of brain damage, and the practice of neuropsychology, as within the specific purview of clinical psychology.

In the absence of credentialing, control is left to licensing activities, done at the state levels, resulting in a wide variety of requirements for practice in a specified area such as neuropsychology, and a tendency to rely on the individual practitioner with respect to not making professional judgments at levels of inference for which the practitioner is not qualified. As has just been noted, however, in cases involving some neuropsychological problems, an otherwise well-trained clinician may not recognize the neuropsychological nature of the problem, and at the same time feel justified by avoiding any inferential statements concerning CNS involvement. Although it could be argued that, in such a case, making no inferential statement concerning CNS deficit may in fact be inferring something about CNS integrity, such activities are extremely difficult to control within limitations of generic state licensing laws. Few states attempt to designate specialty training within psychology although recently Louisiana has identified a subspecialty in neuropsychology with inclusion contingent on satisfying the requirements of either the American Board of Professional Neuropsychology or the American Board of Clinical Neuropsychology.

A national credentialing board, not limited by legislators who enact and amend licensing laws at the state level, is an accepted approach toward ensuring some level or degree of competence among practitioners who have met the requirements of that board. With credentialing requirements set by professionals, this obviously represents an approach with considerable potential for helping ensure such competence. As participation in the activities required for credentialing is entirely voluntary (and can entail a fair amount of energy, frustration, and money), there is no assurance that the *only* qualified neuropsychology practitioners are those who are board certified. As with generic state licensure, board certification in neuropsychology does not necessarily guarantee expertise in all areas of neuropsychology. Unlike the American Board of Neurology and Psychiatry, which adds "with special competence in child neurology" (or psychiatry) for practitioners who satisfy the required training and experience for this endorsement, neuropsychology issues only generic endorsement.

At the present time there are two boards in neuropsychology: the American Board of Professional Neuropsychology and the American Board of Clinical Neuropsychology. Although both boards are attempting to comprehensively evaluate professionals and award the diplomate status to those who are judged to be qualified, the number of individuals who can be evaluated by this comprehensive process is limited. Even though both credentialing boards have been in varying states of activity since 1984, it is estimated that only about 450 individuals have successfully completed the oral examination and have been awarded the diplomate in neuropsychology. Furthermore, both boards can only comprehensively evaluate 40 to 50 per year. The result is that it will be quite some time before the majority of qualified neuropsychologists can be identified. An even greater problem relates to the fact that both boards evaluate neuropsychologists as a broad category. While the individual outlines specific areas of competency within neuropsychology such as interest in children, there is no formal designation as to those who are specifically qualified in child neuropsychology.

The awareness of a lack of understanding of the specialty practices by third-party payers led the National Academy of Neuropsychology and the APA's Division of Clinical Neuropsychology to form a Joint Task Force in 1991. After numerous discussions several guidelines were proposed. This included the formation of new neuropsychological assessment codes and a definition of a neuropsychologist.

Definition of a Clinical Neuropsychologist
A. Level I
   Certification by examination by either the American Board of Clinical Neuropsychology or the American Board of Professional Neuropsychology
B. Level II
   1. Education
      Doctorate degree in psychology from a regionally accredited institution with a program in psychology
   2. Experience
      Three years (minimum of 500 hours per-year) of clinical neuropsychological experience at either pre- or postdoctoral levels
   3. Supervision
      Two years supervision in clinical neuropsychology satisfied by one or more of the following:

a. two years postdoctoral supervision
b. one year predoctoral and one year postdoctoral supervision
c. successful completion of a postdoctoral fellowship
   4. License
      State or province licensure at the level of independent practice
   5. Definition
      Clinical neuropsychology is defined as the study of brain–behavior relationships based on a combination of knowledge from basic neurosciences, functional neuroanatomy, neuropathology, clinical neurology, psychological assessment, psychopathology, and psychological interventions

This was followed by a letter of October 1994 from Carl B. Dodrill, Ph.D., Division 40 president, in which he indicated that the above definition was in error and that the only definition of a clinical neuropsychologist approved by Division 40 was published in *The Clinical Neuropsychologist,* 1989, volume 3, p. 22 [see Appendix for guidelines for doctoral training in clinical neuropsychology], which is as follows:

A Clinical Neuropsychologist is a professional psychologist who applies principles of assessment and intervention based upon the scientific study of human behavior as it relates to normal and abnormal functioning of the central nervous system. The Clinical Neuropsychologist is a doctoral-level psychology provider of diagnostic and intervention services who has demonstrated competence in the application of such principles for human welfare following:

   A. Successful completion of systematic didactic and experiential training in neuropsychology and neuroscience at a regionally accredited university;
   B. Two or more years of appropriate supervised training applying neuropsychological services in a clinical setting;
   C. Licensing and certification to provide psychological services to the public by the laws of the state or province in which he or she practices;
   D. Review by one's peers as a test of these competencies.
   Attainment of the ABCN/ABPP Diploma in Clinical Neuropsychology is the clearest evidence of competence as a Clinical Neuropsychologist, assuring that all these criteria have been met.

As can be seen from the confusion in definitions, the issues are far from resolved regarding clinical neuropsychology in general, and the issue of specialization in child neuropsychology has not been addressed.

Further complicating the issue of board certification, usually designated as "diplomate" status, is the pervasive level of inference issue. Because only the best neuropsychological clinicians—for instance, those qualified to make the highest levels of neuropsychological inference—are likely to receive "diplomate" status, who is to do the lower level of inference work? As has been mentioned, whereas it might be considered optimal practice to have all children with any problem seen by a skilled child neuropsychologist, to ensure that problems of a neurological nature are not overlooked, this is obviously not realistic.

These problems raise the question of the use of technicians in neuropsychology. The Division 40 Task Force on Education, Accreditation, and Credentialing concluded that "the use of . . . technicians is a common and accepted practice when the supervising psychologist maintains and monitors high standards of quality assurance" (APA Task Force, 1989, p. 25). Surveys of practicing neuropsychologists indicate that 53% use technicians. It would appear that neuropsychologists can make effective use of technicians to provide more cost-effective services. Such use would not preclude the neuropsychologist spending time with the patient in obtaining the history, reevaluating questionable areas of weakness by the use of additional tests, or clarifying test findings during the debriefing with the patient.

It appears that specialty credentialing is unlikely to be accepted in the near future by the vast majority of clinical psychologists. Therefore, training must be designed and offered to best prepare these individuals for their designated area of clinical service. Such needs are being met by universities offering specialty training in school psychology, child psychology, and/or neuropsychology.

General Issues in Child Clinical Training

With respect to educational context, clinical child neuropsychology can be viewed as a subarea of clinical child psychology, and it is relevant to preface a review of issues in clinical child neuropsychology training with an overview of training issues in clinical child psychology. Presently, although there are seven formal predoctoral training programs in neuropsychology (Lubin & Sokoloff, 1983), few are specifically designed for child neuropsychology. In some programs students are required to satisfy the requirements of the child clinical and neuropsychology training programs to be designated as trained in child neuropsychology. Without such arrangements, much of the specialty training in clinical child neuropsychology currently is provided by postdoctoral positions.

The report of the task force from Division 40 recommends that in the absence of formal accredited educational programs:

> (1) The entry level credentials for the practice of clinical neuropsychology shall be predicated on the license to practice at the independent professional level in the state or province in which the practitioner resides; (2) In addition, 1600 hours of clinical neuropsychological experience, supervised by a clinical neuropsychologist at the pre- or post-doctoral level, shall be required; (3) Persons receiving a doctoral degree in psychology before 1981 may substitute 4800 hours of post-doctoral experience in a neuropsychology setting involving a minimum of 2400 hours of direct clinical service. (*Newsletter 40*, 1984)

In the absence of formal training programs in child neuropsychology, specialization in child neuropsychology must either combine two existing areas or seek further postdoctoral training.

Because of the changing nature of the nervous system in the child and the impact of nonneurological factors on the child's behavior, the child neuropsychologist needs to be trained in basic psychological, developmental, and neuropsychological issues. In addition, the role of psychological assessment in clinical child neuropsychology needs to be well understood.

The reliance on standardized tests increases with decreasing experience of professionals in any discipline. Of primary importance is the issue to be addressed or the question to be answered. If the primary question relates to whether there is cerebral dysfunction, then regardless of the test employed, the evaluators' effectiveness depends on their training in brain–behavior relationships and their understanding of the nervous system and its contributions to behavior. Without such training, effective interpretation of behavior leading to decisions regarding brain dysfunction cannot be reached. If learning disability is of primary interest, then the evaluator needs to understand the relationship between test behavior and learning disability. The same argument holds for developmental delays, emotional disorders, retardation, and so on.

New graduates, individuals shifting their area of basic training, or researchers tend to depend on a fixed battery or evaluation strategy and rigorously defend it against all others. They thus exhibit a strong tendency to become method oriented, rather than problem oriented. With further education on the part of the professional and understanding of the relationship between areas of primary importance, less reliance is made on a specific test battery and a broad range of assessment devices may be employed in order to effectively assay the behaviors in question and outline an effective treatment plan.

Clinical neuropsychology as a specialty within psychology is a fairly new area that is continuing to undergo change and self-analysis in order to outline clinical courses most appropriate to the practice of neuropsychology. The data base on neuropsychology has also served to shift psychologists into a designated specialty area as the knowledge base required to pursue neuropsychological assessment is sufficiently broad to make it difficult for traditionally trained psychologists to pursue effectively such clinical activities without extensive training or experience.

In 1977 it was recognized that a conference dealing with training in clinical child psychology was needed, and a preliminary working conference was held in 1983 with the principal conference held in May 1985. In general, the recommendations included three features involving general clinical psychology training, involving requirements for training in normal development; experience with normal children; and minimal competencies in assessment, psychopathology, and intervention with children (Johnson & Tuma, 1986; Tuma, 1986). Specific to clinical child psychology graduate training were seven recommendations, the first of which endorsed the Boulder Model for clinical child psychology. Another recommendation endorsed the APA Division 27 task force-documented Guidelines for Training Psychologists to Work with Children, Youth and Families (Roberts, Erickson, & Tuma, 1985). In general, the other recommendations specific to clinical child psychology training dealt with such issues as recognizing cultural diversity and the multiple contexts in which psychologists working with children, youth, and families must function. Internship training was recommended as involving at least two-thirds of the training experience in child clinical activity, with research incorporated into the internship program. Postdoctoral and continuing education training in clinical child psychology was recommended, although specific guidelines concerning required background prerequisites or context areas were not proposed.

With respect to recognition of proficiencies and specialty areas in psychology, the APA Board of Professional Affairs (BPA) appointed a Committee on Specialty Practice from 1970 to 1980 to explore such issues. Specialty guidelines for clinical, counseling, industrial/organizational, and school psychology were approved by the APA Council in 1980, making APA's first detailed public statement concerning service provisions in specialty areas. The BPA appointed a Subcommittee on Specialization in 1980 to address the issues involved in criteria for specialty areas not covered by these four major areas, and in 1983 a second draft manual for the identification and continued recognition of proficiencies and new specialty areas in psychology was published (Sales, Bricklin, & Hall, 1983). Differentiation was made between proficiencies and specialties, on the basis of several major criteria. A specialty was recommended as involving a body of knowledge with (1) unique client populations, (2) specific techniques and technologies, (3) problems addressed, and (4) settings wherein the knowledge applied. A proficiency, on the other hand, would involve a body of knowledge and skills that provide the basis for services in one of these four parameters.

The requirements for the identification of a specialty area involved (1) a formal organization, recognized in the field, that is responsible for managing the development of a specialty; (2) a definition of the specialty, including knowledge and skills required; and (3) an educational sequence of training and experience. Requirements for the identification of a proficiency involved (1) a formal organization, (2) a definition, (3) evidence of need and parameters of practice, (4) demonstrated efficiency, and (5) uniqueness. In this context, neuropsychology could be viewed as representing either a specialty or an area of proficiency, with clinical child neuropsychology a subarea of either a specialty or a proficiency.

In a related and somewhat parallel area, the APA Task Force on Education and Credentialing (1985) published a recommendation concerned with educational content required for designation as a psychology program. Although related in only a tangential way to clinical child neuropsychology, the designation system tends to discourage the graduate education of clinical child neuropsychologists in academic settings without a clear identification as part of a psychology program (e.g., freestanding clinical child neuropsychology programs in medical schools or professional schools would have difficulty meeting the designation criteria).

Focus on Training in Clinical Child Neuropsychology

Where does training in clinical child neuropsychology fit into this broader context? Training in clinical child neuropsychology is generally provided in one of three ways: graduate coursework, internship/practicum training, and postdoctoral training fellowships.

Graduate course offerings show considerable variability. Approximately seven programs offer a terminal degree in neuropsychology, usually as a subspecialty of clinical psychology; 40 clinical programs offer some coursework in neuropsychology; and some half-dozen clinical programs offer lectures on neuropsychology but no formal coursework (Golden & Kuperman, 1980). Thus, among the 60 or more APA-approved clinical programs that indicate they provide offerings in neuropsychology, these offerings may range from formal coursework to practica or even possible work placements.

Division 40 of the APA (Neuropsychology), aware of the need for establishing guidelines for neuropsychology training, has formed a task force to develop such guidelines (see Appendix). A preliminary report of their efforts was published in *Newsletter 40* (1984). According to those guidelines the major function of the clinical neuropsychologist is to assess current behavioral disturbances associated with neurological impairment. The report suggested that neuropsychological assessment should include measures of (1) abstract reasoning and categorical thinking, (2) cognitive flexibility and planning, (3) language communication, (4) learning and memory, (5) sensation and perception, (6) fine and gross motor functions, (7) initiation and attention, (8) affect and mood, and (9) psychosocial adaptation.

In order to effectively pursue these assessment goals, the diagnostician needs training in (1) functional neuroanatomy, (2) clinical diseases, (3) child development, (4) changes in behavior as a function of aging, (5) behavioral psychopharmacology, (6) psychophysiological principles underlying pathologies, (7) sociocultural factors, (8) personality assessment and interviewing skills, (9) principles of test construction and validation, and (10) test administration and interpretation. Properly trained neuropsychologists should be able to outline treatment plans and consult with

family members, educators, employers, and so on, in order to assist in improving the behavioral adjustment of the individual in specific situations. Remediation by a clinical neuropsychologist focuses primarily on disability associated with cerebral dysfunction and secondarily on emotional or other maladaptive behaviors that are a consequence of the individual's primary disability.

The *Newsletter* outlined the needs of the child neuropsychology training to include much of the above with adjustment in training suggested to incorporate bodies of knowledge as well as techniques and resources specific to clinical child neuropsychology. Major issues such as child development, CNS plasticity, and the nature of the referral questions are seen as primary additional areas of competence. One of the primary distinctions between child and adult neuropsychology is the emphasis on description of processes in children, because the focus on process helps delineate specific treatment plans. More so than with adults, children are often evaluated by a multidisciplinary team; thus, child neuropsychologists must have knowledge of related professions so that they may effectively interface their findings in developing the final treatment plan.

Among practicum offerings that include child neuropsychology as an area of training, these offerings in many cases exist as ancillary options, such as being available on a limited basis within a child therapy practicum. Even in practicum or internship settings wherein neuropsychology is mentioned as an area of training emphasis, there is considerable variability. This variability appears to reflect both the differing concepts of neuropsychology as a specialty area within clinical neuropsychology, and the unique backgrounds of the faculty who provide such training. In one grouping of 28 graduate settings that offered neuropsychology training, Golden and Kuperman (1980) found that the tests used most frequently were the Wechsler and Bender Gestalt.

Postdoctoral training programs in clinical child psychology are relatively rare. However, a number of postdoctoral programs in clinical neuropsychology offer some exposure to child neuropsychology, and a few provide some segment of the program devoted to work for children. Informal surveys of postdoctoral trainees who have had at least some postdoctoral training in clinical neuropsychology reveal a rather wide range of backgrounds. Some "retread" postdoctoral fellows, whose doctoral training is in nonclinical areas such as physiological psychology, have very little background in either child development or the special skills needed to evaluate children. Others with backgrounds in areas like school psychology may have excellent skills in child assessment and good knowledge of developmental phenomena, but little expertise in functional neuroanatomy or basic brain–behavior relationships. Yet others enter postdoctoral child neuropsychology training programs with good assessment skills involving both children and adults, with coursework in neuroanatomy and physiology, and prior exposure to neurologically impaired children from practicum or work experiences. Thus, the content of the "ideal" postdoctoral experience in clinical child neuropsychology may relate to the unique backgrounds that such postdoctoral fellows bring to the program.

Professional Context of Clinical Child Neuropsychology

Neuropsychologists assume that understanding brain–behavior relationships is necessary for both diagnosis and treatment planning. Such knowledge is not, however, sufficient, and therefore few neuropsychologists focus on the brain as the only contributing variable. Child neuropsychological assessment must include measures of personality/emotional well-being and identification of environmental influences. Given such a broad "systems" analysis, the child neuropsychologist can provide information of benefit to a number of other disciplines. For example, the interpretation of neurological dysfunction in the context of situational, learning, emotional, and other important dimensions provides the neurosurgeon with a more comprehensive picture of the role that a lesion or area of damage might exert on a child's behavior. This can assist teachers in the classroom and parents at home by identifying strengths and weaknesses and identifying those factors that appear to be most amenable to modification. The assumption is that one needs to identify factors that contribute to aberrant behaviors and prioritize them regarding those that would appear to require primary assistance as well as those that are most likely to change with remediation.

Unlike the adult brain, which is assumed to be developmentally static with fixed effects associated with injury, the child's brain is characterized by growth and differentiation that extends from conception up to young adulthood (Renis & Goldman, 1980; Rourke, Bakker, Fisk, & Strang, 1983). The

effects of neurological damage are influenced by age, the locus of the injury, the nature of the damage, the sex and socioeconomic status of the individual, as well as the emotional adjustment, coping, and adaptive skills of the individual (Bolter & Long, 1985). Thus, even our limited understanding of chronogenetic localization can improve the assessment and remediation of neurologically impaired children. Neurological damage during the developmental years may produce permanent deficits, temporary deficits, and/or delayed-onset deficits (Teuber & Rudel, 1962). Understanding the neurological contribution to the overall behavioral complex is necessary to effectively identify barriers and plan for remediation.

Professional Relationships

Although all psychologists view behavior from a systems perspective, problems are viewed somewhat differently depending on the specialization. School psychologists focus primarily on academic problems and secondarily on how nonacademic factors influence school performance (e.g., emotional, situational, neurological, genetic, developmental). Child psychologists focus primarily on emotional/behavioral problems with secondary focus on other areas. The child neuropsychologist focuses primarily on brain–behavior relationships with other factors being viewed as secondary.

The approach of child neuropsychologists has been challenged by professionals in other specialties. School psychologists have argued that understanding neurological systems is not important for effective treatment (Senf, 1979). It is further argued that neurological labeling connotes irreversibility and mitigates responsibility for remediation (Sandoval & Haapanen, 1981). In fact, Hynd (1982) suggested that the neuropsychological evaluation may provide information that reduces the need for referral for expensive and nonproductive neurological evaluations.

There remain many unresolved issues regarding training and practice of clinical child neuropsychology. As outlined in this chapter, the clinical child neuropsychologist must possess a knowledge base that cuts across many existing areas of specialization. Perhaps for this reason, individuals from a number of specialty areas may function in the assessment and treatment of children with neurological dysfunction in the future. Hopefully, with improved awareness and education, effectiveness of communication will be enhanced across these specialties. This may lead us to recognize the requisite combination of broad skills in general child clinical areas and specific skills in child neuropsychology as constituting clinical child neuropsychology, both a specialty and an area of proficiency.

References

Adams, K. M. (1980a). In search of Luria's battery: A false start. *Journal of Consulting and Clinical Psychology, 48,* 511–516.

Adams, K. M. (1980b). An end of innocence for behavioral neurology? Adams replies. *Journal of Consulting and Clinical Psychology, 48,* 522–523.

American Psychological Association Task Force on Education and Recommendations for a Designation System. (1985). Washington, DC: American Psychological Association.

APA Practice Directorate. (1994). College gets green light from APA Council, 2(1), 3–4.

Berg, R. A., Bolter, J. F., Ch'ien, L. T., Williams, S. J., Lancaster, W., & Cumming, J. (1984). Comparative diagnostic accuracy of the Halstead–Reitan and Luria–Nebraska Neuropsychological Adult and Children's Batteries. *International Journal of Clinical Neuropsychology, 6*(3), 200–204.

Boll, T. J. (1993). *Children's Category Test.* San Antonio, TX: The Psychological Corporation.

Bolter, J. F., & Long, C. J. (1985). Methodological issues in research in developmental neuropsychology. In L. C. Hartlage & C. F. Telzrow (Eds.), *Neuropsychology of individual differences: A developmental perspective* (pp. 41–59). New York: Plenum Press.

Chalfant, J. C., & Scheffelin, M. A. (1969). *Central processing dysfunction in children: A review of research.* Bethesda: U.S. Department of Health, Education and Welfare.

Dean, R. S. (1982). Focus on child neuropsychology. *The National Academy of Neuropsychologists Bulletin, 2*(2), 5.

Geary, D. C., Schultz, D. D., Jennings, S. M., & Alper, T. G. (1984). The diagnostic accuracy of the Luria–Nebraska Neuropsychological Battery—Children's Revision for 9 to 12 year old learning disabled children. *School Psychology Review, 13*(3), 375–380.

Goldberg, A. L., & McNamara, K. M. (1984). Internship training in neuropsychology. *Professional Psychology: Research and Practice, 15*(4), 509–514.

Golden, C. J. (1981). The Luria–Nebraska Children's Battery: Theory and formulation. In G. W. Hynd & J. E. Obrzut (Eds.), *Neuropsychological assessment and the school-age child: Issues and procedures* (pp. 277–302). New York: Grune & Stratton.

Golden, C. J., Hammeke, T. A., & Purisch, A. D. (1980). *The Luria–Nebraska Neuropsychological Battery.* Los Angeles: Western Psychological Services.

Golden, C. J., Kane, R., Sweet, J., Moses, J. A., Cardelino, J. P., Templeton, R., Vicente, P., & Graber, B. (1981). Relationships of the Halstead–Reitan Neuropsychological Battery to the Luria–Nebraska Neuropsychological Battery. *Journal of Consulting and Clinical Psychology, 49*(3), 410–417.

Golden, C. J., & Kuperman, S. K. (1980). Graduate training in clinical neuropsychology. *Professional Psychology, 11*(1), 55–63.

Hartlage, L. C. (1981). Clinical application of neuropsychological data. *School Psychology Review, 10*(3), 362–366.

Hartlage, L. C. (1984). Neuropsychological assessment of children. In P. Keller & L. Ritt (Eds.), *Innovations in clinical practice* (Vol. III, pp. 153–165). Sarasota, FL: Professional Resources Exchange.

Hartlage, L. C., & Telzrow, C. F. (1983). Assessment of neurological functioning. In B. Bracken & F. Paget (Eds.), *Psychoeducational assessment of preschool and primary aged children* (pp. 1–68). New York: Grune & Stratton.

Hynd, G. W. (1982). Neuropsychological consultation in the schools. *The National Academy of Neuropsychologists Bulletin, 2*(2), 11.

Johnson, J. H., & Tuma, J. M. (1986). The Hilton Head conference: Recommendations for clinical child psychology training. *The Clinical Psychologist, 39*(1), 9–11.

Kaplan, E. (1991). *WAIS-R as a neuropsychological instrument.* San Antonio, TX: The Psychological Corporation.

Lubin, B., & Sokoloff, R. M. (1983). An update of the survey of training and internship programs in clinical neuropsychology. *Journal of Clinical Psychology, 39*(1), 149–152.

Newsletter 40. (1984). American Psychological Association, Division of Clinical Neuropsychology, Vol. II(2).

Plaisted, J. R., Gustavson, J. W., Wilkening, J. G. N., & Golden, C. J. (1983). The Luria–Nebraska Neuropsychological Battery—Children's Revision. Theory and current research findings. *Journal of Clinical Child Psychology, 12,* 13–21.

Reitan, R. M. (1955). An investigation of the validity of Halstead's measures of biological intelligence. *AMA Archives of Neurological Psychiatry, 73,* 28–35.

Reitan, R. M., & Davison, L. (1974). *Clinical neuropsychology: Current status and applications.* Washington, DC: Winston.

Renis, S., & Goldman, J. M. (1980). *The development of the brain.* Springfield, IL: Thomas.

Roberts, M. C., Erickson, M. T., & Tuma, J. M. (1985). Addressing the needs: Guidelines for training psychologists to work with children, youth and families. *Journal of Clinical Child Psychology, 14,* 70–79.

Rourke, B. P., Bakker, D. J., Fisk, J. L., & Strang, J. O. (1983). *Child neuropsychology: An introduction to theory, research, and clinical practice.* New York: Guilford Press.

Sales, B. (1985). Specialization: Past history and future alternatives. *The Clinical Psychologist, 38,* 48–52.

Sales, B., Bricklin, P., & Hall, J. (1983). *Second draft: Manual for the identification and continued recognition of proficiencies and new areas in psychology.* Washington, DC: American Psychological Association.

Sandoval, J., & Haapanen, R. M. (1981). A critical commentary on neuropsychology in the schools: Are we ready? *School Psychology Review, 10,* 381–388.

Selz, M. (1981). Halstead–Reitan neuropsychological test batteries for children. In G. W. Hynd & J. E. Obrzut (Eds.),

Neuropsychological assessment and the school-age child: Issues and procedures. New York: Grune & Stratton.

Senf, G. M. (1979). Can neuropsychology really change the face of special education? *The Journal of Special Education, 13*(1).

Spiers, P. (1981). Have they come to praise Luria or to bury him? The Luria–Nebraska controversy. *Journal of Consulting and Clinical Psychology, 49,* 331–341.

Telzrow, C. F., & Hartlage, L. C. (1984). A neuropsychological model for vocational planning for learning disabled students. In W. Cruickshank & J. Kleibhan (Eds.), *Early adolescence to early adulthood* (pp. 143–156). Syracuse, NY: Syracuse University Press.

Teuber, H. L., & Rudel, R. G. (1962). Behavior after cerebral lesions in children and adults. *Developmental Medicine and Child Neurology, 4,* 3–20.

Tuma, J. M. (1986). Clinical child psychology training: Report of the Hilton Head conference. *Journal of Clinical Child Psychology, 15*(1), 88–96.

VandenBos, G. R., Stapp, J., & Kilburg, R. R. (1981). Health service providers in psychology: Results of the 1978 APA human resources survey. *American Psychologist, 36,* 1395–1418.

Appendix

The Clinical Neuropsychologist
1987, Vol. 1, No. 1, **pp.** 29–34   @ Swets & Zeitlinger

Reports of the INS–Division 40 Task Force on Education, Accreditation, and Credentialing

GUIDELINES FOR DOCTORAL TRAINING PROGRAMS IN CLINICAL NEUROPSYCHOLOGY

Doctoral training in Clinical Neuropsychology should ordinarily result in the awarding of a Ph.D.-degree from a regionally accredited university. It may be accomplished through a Ph.D. programme in Clinical Neuropsychology offered by a Psychology Department or Medical Faculty or through the completion of a Ph.D. programme in a related specialty area (e.g., Clinical Psychology) which offers sufficient specialization in Clinical Neuropsychology.

Training programmes in Clinical Neuropsychology prepare students for health service delivery, basic clinical research, teaching, and consultation. As such they must contain (a) a generic psychology core, (b) a generic clinical core, (c) specialized training in the neurosciences and basic human and animal neuropsychology, (d) specific training in clinical neuropsychology. This should include an 1800-hour internship which should be preceded by appropriate practicum experience.

(A) Generic Psychology Core
1. Statistics and Methodology
2. Learning, Cognition, and Perception
3. Social Psychology and Personality
4. Physiological Psychology
5. Life-Span Developmental
6. History

(B) Generic Clinical Core
1. Psychopathology
2. Psychometric Theory
3. Interview and Assessment Techniques
    i. Interviewing
    ii. Intelligence Assessment
    iii. Personality Assessment
4. Intervention Techniques
    i. Counseling and Psychotherapy
    ii. Behavior Therapy/Modification
    iii. Consultation
5. Professional Ethics

(C) Neurosciences and Basic Human and Animal Neuropsychology
    i. Basic Neurosciences
    ii. Advanced Physiological Psychology and Pharmacology
    iii. Neuropsychology of Perceptual, Cognitive, and Executive Processes
    iv. Research Design and Research Practicum in Neuropsychology

(D) Specific Clinical Neuropsychological Training
    i. Clinical Neurology and Neuropathology
    ii. Specialized neuropsychological assessment techniques
    iii. Specialized neuropsychological intervention techniques
    iv. Assessment practicum (children and/or adults) in University-supervised assessment facility
    v. Intervention practicum in University supervised intervention facility
    vi. Clinical Neuropsychological Internship of 1800 hours preferably in noncaptive facility. (As per INS–Div. 40 Task Force guidelines). Ordinarily this internship will be completed in a single year, but in exceptional circumstance may be completed in a 2-year period.

(E) Doctoral Dissertation
It is recognized that the completion of a Ph.D. in Clinical Neuropsychology prepares the person to begin work as a clinical neuropsychologist. In most jurisdictions, an additional year of supervised clinical practice will be required in order to qualify for

licensure. Furthermore, training at the postdoctoral level to increase both general and subspecialty competencies is viewed as desirable.

GUIDELINES FOR NEUROPSYCHOLOGY INTERNSHIPS IN CLINICAL NEUROPSYCHOLOGY

The following report summarizes the recommendations of the subcommittee on internships of the INS/Division 40 Task Force. The report was prepared by Linus Bieliauskas and Thomas Boll.

At the outset, it is recognized that the Internship Program is designed primarily for students with degrees in clinical psychology. Such internship programs are those accredited by the American Psychological Association and or those listed in the Directory of the Association of Psychology Internship Centers.

Entry into a psychology internship program is a minimum qualification in a Neuropsychology Internship. Such entry must be based on completion of at least 2 years in a recognized Psychology Ph.D. Graduate Training Program in an area of Health Services Delivery (e.g., Clinical, Clinical Neuropsychology, Counseling, or School Psychology). Alternately, entry into a psychology internship program must be based on completion of a "retreading" Program designed to meet equivalent criteria as a Health Services Delivery Program per se. Within the training programs described above, the student must also have completed a designated track, specialization, or concentration in neuropsychology.

There are generally two models for psychology internship training: (1) Generic Clinical Psychology, and (2) specialty in Clinical Neuropsychology. The former does not concern us here since such training is not geared toward producing specialized experience or qualification. The latter type of internship program, when designed to provide specialized training in Neuropsychology, is what constitutes a Clinical Neuropsychology Internship.

A Clinical Neuropsychology Internship must devote at least 50% of a 1-year full-time training experience to neuropsychology. In addition, at least 20% of the training experience must be devoted to General Clinical Training to assure a competent background in Clinical Psychology. Such an internship should be associated with a hospital setting which has Neurological and/or Neurosurgical services to offer to the training background. Such an internship should not be associated only with a strictly psychiatric setting.

Experiences to Be Provided
The experiences to be provided to the intern in clinical neuropsychology should conform to the descriptions of professional activities in the Report of the Task Force on Education, Accreditation, and Credentialing of the International Neuropsychological Society and the American Psychological Association (1981). Necessary training should be provided in both a didactic and experiential format. Supervisors in such an internship should be board-certified clinical neuropsychologists.

Didactic Training
A. Training in neurological diagnosis.
B. Training in consultation to neurological and neurosurgical services.
C. Training in direct consultation to psychiatric, pediatric, or general medical services.
D. Exposure to methods and practices of neurological and neurosurgical consultation (grand rounds, bed rounds, seminars, etc.).
E. Training in neuropsychological techniques, examination, interpretation of tests results, report writing.
F. Training in consultation to patients and referral sources.
G. Training in methods of intervention specific to clinical neuropsychology.

Experiential Training
A. Neuropsychological examination and evaluation of patients with actual and suspected neurological diseases and disorders.
B. Neuropsychological examination and evaluation of patients with psychiatric disorders and/or pediatric or general medical patients with neurobehavioral disorders.
C. Participation in clinical activities with neurologists and neurosurgeons (bed rounds, grand rounds, etc.).
D. Direct consultation to patients involving neuropsychological issues.
E. Consultation to referral and treating professions.

Exit Criteria
At the end of the internship year, the intern in clinical neuropsychology should be able to undertake consultation to patients and professionals on an independent basis and meet minimal qualifications for competent practice of clinical neuropsychology as defined in Section B, Neuropsychological

roles and functions of the Report of the Task Force (1981).

GUIDELINES FOR POSTDOCTORAL TRAINING IN CLINICAL NEUROPSYCHOLOGY

Postdoctoral training, as described herein, is designed to provide clinical training to produce an advanced level of competence in the specialty of clinical neuropsychology. It is recognized that clinical neuropsychology is a scientifically based and evolving discipline and that such training should also provide a significant research component. Thus, this report is concerned with postdoctoral training in clinical neuropsychology which is specifically geared toward producing independent practitioner level competence which includes both necessary clinical and research skills. This report does not address training in neuropsychology which is focused solely on research.

Entry Criteria
Entry into a clinical neuropsychology postdoctoral training program ordinarily should be based on completion of a regionally accredited Ph.D. graduate training program in one of the health service delivery areas of psychology or a Ph.D. in psychology with additional completion of a "respecialization" program designed to meet equivalent criteria as a health services delivery program in psychology. In all cases, candidacy for postdoctoral training in clinical neuropsychology must be based on demonstration of training and research methodology designed to meet equivalent criteria as a health services delivery professional in the scientist-practitioner model. Ordinarily, a clinical internship, listed by the Association of Psychology Internship Centers, must also have been completed.

General Considerations
A postdoctoral training program in clinical neuropsychology should be directed by a board-certified clinical neuropsychologist. In most cases, the program should extend over at least a 2-year period. The only exception would be for individuals who have completed a specific clinical neuropsychology specialization in their graduate programs and/or a clinical neuropsychology internship (Subcommittee Report of the Task Force, 1984) provided the exit criteria are met (see below). As a general guideline, the postdoctoral training program should provide at least 50% time in clinical service and at least 25% time in clinical research. Variance within these guidelines should be tailored to the needs of the individual. Specific training in neuropsychology must be provided, including any areas where the individual is deemed to be deficient (testing, consultation, intervention, neurosciences, neurology, etc.).

Specific Considerations
Such a postdoctoral training program should be associated with hospital settings which have neurological and/or neurosurgical services to offer to the training background. Necessary training should be provided in both a didactic and experiential format and should include the following:

Didactic Training
A. Training in neurological and psychiatric diagnosis.
B. Training in consultation to neurological and neurosurgical services.
C. Training in direct consultation to psychiatric, pediatric, or general medical services.
D. Exposure to methods and practices of neurological and neurosurgical consultation (Grand Rounds, Bed Rounds, Seminars, etc.).
E. Observation of neurosurgical procedures and biomedical tests (Revascularization procedures, cerebral blood flow, Wada testing, etc.).
F. Participation in seminars offered to neurology and neurosurgery residents (Neuropharmacology, EEG, brain cutting, etc.).
G. Training in neuropsychological techniques, examination, interpretation of test results, report writing.
H. Training in consultation to patients and referral sources.
I. Training in methods of intervention specific to clinical neuropsychology.
J. Seminars, readings, etc., in neuropsychology (case conferences, journal discussion, topic-specific seminars).
K. Didactic training in neuroanatomy, neuropathology, and related neurosciences.

Experiential Training
A. Neuropsychological examination and evaluation of patients with actual and suspected neurological diseases and disorders.
B. Neuropsychological examination and evaluation of patients with psychiatric disorders and/or pediatric or general medical patients with neurobehavioral disorders.
C. Participation in clinical activities with neurologists and neurosurgeons (bed rounds, grand rounds, etc.).

D. Experience at a specialty clinic, such as a dementia clinic or epilepsy clinic, which emphasizes multidisciplinary approaches to diagnosis and treatment.

E. Direct consultation to patients involving neuropsychological assessment.

F. Direct intervention with patients, specific to neuropsychological issues, and to include psychotherapy and/or family therapy where indicated.

G. Research in neuropsychology, i.e., collaboration on a research project or other scholarly academic activity, initiation of an independent research project or other scholarly academic activity, and presentation or publication of research data where appropriate.

Exit Criteria

At the conclusion of the postdoctoral training program, the individual should be able to undertake consultation to patients and professionals on an independent basis. Accomplishment in research should also be demonstrated. The program is designed to produce a competent practitioner in the areas designated in Section B of the Task Force Report (1981) and to provide eligibility for external credentialing and licensure as designated in Section D of the Task Force Report (1981). The latter also includes training eligibility for certification in Clinical Neuropsychology by the American Board of Professional Psychology.

References

Meyer, M. J. (1981). Report of the Task Force on Education, Accreditation, and Credentialing of the International Neuropsychological Society. *The INS Bulletin,* September, pp. 5–10.

Report of the Task Force on Education, Accreditation, and Credentialing. *The INS Bulletin,* 1981, pp. 5–10. *Newsletter 40,* 1984, 2, 3–8.

Report of the Subcommittee on Psychology Internships. *Newsletter 40,* 1984, 2, 7. *The INS Bulletin,* 1984, p. 33. *APIC Newsletter,* 1983, 9, 27–28.

2

Development of the Child's Brain and Behavior

BRYAN KOLB AND BRYAN FANTIE

Introduction

Perhaps the central issue in neuropsychology over the past 100 years has been the question of how psychological functions are represented in the brain. At the turn of the century, the debate was largely whether or not functions were actually localized in the cortex. Although today this is no longer a subject of major discussion, the general problem of determining *what* is localized in the cortex remains. One way to examine this issue is to look at the way function and structure emerge in the developing child.

As we look historically at the consideration of structure–function relationships in development we are struck by the reluctance of researchers to engage in such analyses. Indeed, although Freud and Piaget were trained in biology, both carefully avoided inclusion of brain development in their theories of psychological development. It is likely that one major impediment to such theorists was an absence of biological data about developmental neuroscience (Segalowitz & Rose-Krasnor, 1992).

The development of structure–function relationships can be examined in three basic ways. First, we can look at the structural development of the nervous system and correlate it with the emergence of specific behaviors. Initially this approach seems ideal, as the development of both the nervous system and behavior is orderly and consistent across individuals. Unfortunately, it is not as simple as it appears.

The nervous system matures in a relatively unremitting way, unfolding to the dictates of time. Behavioral change, on the other hand, is often more highly dependent on environmental factors. Thus, the degree of damage caused by sensory deprivation is largely determined by *when* it occurs during an animal's life (Hubel & Wiesel, 1970). In contrast, whether or not someone can ice-skate will be more easily predicted when one knows if the person was raised in Canada or Brazil. In addition, age-related neural changes are seldom immediately observable *in vivo* so it is extraordinarily difficult to directly correlate structural and functional variables. Further, hypotheses regarding brain development are hard to verify, especially because the human nervous system cannot be manipulated during development. Nevertheless, despite these impediments, this approach is still possible.

The second way to examine morphological and psychological development is to scrutinize behavior and then make inferences about neural maturation. For example, we might carefully study the emergence of distinct cognitive stages, as Piaget (1952) and his followers have done, and then predict what alterations must have occurred in the nervous system to account for the behavioral change. This approach has not been widely used, largely because psychologists most interested in human development have not been very interested in brain function and many behaviors considered important to child development may not be related directly to neural growth. Nevertheless, this approach is promising and has been pursued actively by Gibson (1977).

BRYAN KOLB • Department of Psychology, University of Lethbridge, Lethbridge, Alberta T1K 3M4, Canada.   BRYAN FANTIE • Department of Psychology, American University, Washington, DC 20016-8062.

There is a tendency to emphasize school-related skills as the most important for study in child neuropsychology. This is reasonable because many types of childhood learning disorders are likely related to abnormalities in neural development. It must be remembered, however, that the human brain did not evolve in a schoolroom. Thus, the basic functions that are related to neural development may not be found easily by studying scholastic behaviors such as reading. Rather, the neural mechanisms underlying reading ability may best be understood by examining fundamental visuospatial or visuomotor skills.

The third way to study structure–function relationships is to relate brain malfunction to behavioral disorders. This method, which is prevalent in research dealing with adults, is difficult to apply to the developing brain. The major problem is that the function of a specific neural area may change over time. For instance, Goldman (1974) found that although juvenile rhesus monkeys that had sustained frontal cortex lesions in infancy could solve tasks sensitive to frontal-lobe damage in adults, they subsequently lost this ability as they matured. This result can be interpreted as showing that some other structure, probably the striatum, initially controlled the behaviors necessary for the successful performance of the tasks. Through the natural course of development, this function is eventually transferred to the frontal cortex as the original structure takes some other role in the production of behavior. Because, in this case, the frontal cortex was damaged, it was unable to assume the function when required and the task could not be fulfilled. Therefore, because the association of functions and brain sites that are applicable at one age may be inappropriate at other ages, there is not just one form of the immature brain.

The plasticity of the immature brain poses another problem to inferring structure–function relations from malfunction in the developing nervous system. Brain damage occurring in infants may produce very different behavioral effects than in adults because early injury has also altered fundamental brain organization. For example, Rasmussen and Milner (1977) showed that if neonatal speech zones, usually found in the left cerebral hemisphere, are damaged, language may develop in the right cerebral hemisphere. Similar damage at 5 years of age may cause the speech zones to move within the left hemisphere. In both cases, language would then occupy space normally serving other functions. The chronic behavioral loss would manifest itself in some other cognitive function, such as spatial orientation, even though the damage can be shown to have been in the cortical site that normally subserves language functions. Identical lesions could result in very different deficits depending on the age at which the damage occurred. Such effects do not occur in the adult.

We point out the pitfalls in developmental neuropsychology not to discourage the study of the child's brain, but to caution that what follows in this chapter must be considered in the light of these problems. We shall summarize research on neocortical development using each of the three approaches outlined above. We begin by considering the anatomical development of the cerebral cortex. We then consider functional development and try to draw correlations between the emergence of particular behaviors and neural development. Finally, we examine factors affecting brain development.

Anatomical Development of the Child's Brain

The process of brain growth can be understood by considering the composition of the nervous system. The cortex is a laminated structure of approximately six layers made up of neurons and glial cells. Some glial cells in the brain, called oligodendrocytes, insulate certain portions of many neurons by wrapping around them. Other glial cells, mainly astrocytes and microcytes, are believed to perform basic maintenance and support functions for neighboring neurons. Neurons receive input from other neurons across tiny spaces known as synaptic gaps through processes called dendrites while sending output to other neurons via processes called axons. Cortical neurons exchange information with other cortical neurons as well as with neurons located in subcortical structures. Additionally, the many projections each neuron usually receives from other neurons often use different chemical substances to transmit information. Basically, these chemicals excite or inhibit the activity of the target cell and it is the net total of these influences that determines whether or not the neuron fires. The successful development of the brain into a properly functioning, integrated organ requires that each component first be formed and then be correctly interrelated with the others.

The development of the different components of the nervous system can be categorized into distinct phases, illustrated in Figure 1. These include: (1) the birth of neurons (neurogenesis), (2) the migration of neurons to their correct location, (3) the differentiation of neurons into different types and their subsequent maturation of connections, and (4) the pruning back of connections and cells themselves. Each of these stages is dependent on the production of specific molecules that act to facilitate the respective process. These molecules include various growth factors, hormones, and specific proteins that act as a sort of traffic signal for cells or their processes to follow. We will consider the development processes in turn.

Neural Generation

The human brain follows a general pattern of development, beginning as a neural tube and gradually acquiring the features of the adult brain (illustrated in Figure 2), that is typical of all mammals. The basic neural tube surrounds a single ventricle where cells are generated along the ventricular wall and then migrate out to their proper location. In humans, approximately 10^9 cells are required to eventually form the mature neocortex of a single cerebral hemisphere (Rakic, 1975). During development, the cortex is composed of four embryonic regions: the ventricular, marginal, intermediate, and subventrical zones (as illustrated in Figure 3). These zones are transient features uniquely related to early development for each either disappears or becomes transformed so that they are no longer identifiable in the adult nervous system.

Sidman and Rakic (1973) combined the extensive studies of Poliakov (1949, 1961, 1965) with their own observations to produce a summary of the timing and phases of cortical development in humans (Figure 3). There is some disagreement over how

long cells destined for the cortex divide and migrate in the human, but cortical cell proliferation appears to be complete by the middle of gestation; although, at this stage, the cortex by no means appears like that of an adult. Cell migration may still proceed for some months after this time, possibly continuing postnatally, and the cortical lamination continues to develop and differentiate until after birth.

One curious feature of cortical development is that it progresses in an "inside-out" progression. Neurons destined to form layer VI form first, followed in sequence by layers V to II. Marin-Padilla (1970, 1988) studied the sequential lamination of the human motor cortex in ontogenesis and found that by the fifth embryonic month, cortical layers V and VI are visible, although not yet completely mature. Over the ensuing months the remaining layers develop (as summarized in Table 1). Thus, we see that successive waves of neurons pass earlier-arriving neurons to assume progressively more superficial positions. A second curious feature of brain development is that the cortex overproduces neurons, which are later lost through normal cell death. Layer IV in the motor cortex is a particularly clear example of this because cells that are visible there in the seventh month and at birth later degenerate, leaving an agranular layer.

As might be predicted, the precise timing of the development and migration of cells to different cytoarchitectonic regions varies with the particular area in question. For example, Rakic (1976) showed that while the ventricular zone is producing layer IV cells for area 17, the neighboring ventricular zone is generating layer III cells that will migrate to area 18. Thus, at any given moment during cortical ontogenesis, cells migrating from the ventricular zone are destined for different regions and layers of the cortex. One implication of this phenomenon is that events that might affect the fetus during cortical development, like the presence of a toxic agent such as alcohol, will affect different cytoarchitectonic zones differently. Furthermore, because specific populations of cells are migrating at different times to any given cortical laminae, it implies that toxic agents, or other environmental events, could perturb the development of a specific population of cells to a particular cytoarchitectonic area.

Cell Migration

Because cortical cells are born distal to the cortical plate and must migrate there, one can ask how this occurs, particularly as cells traveling to the

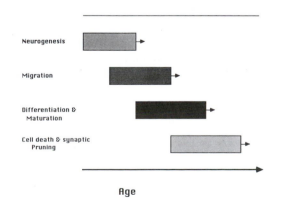

FIGURE 1. Stages of brain development.

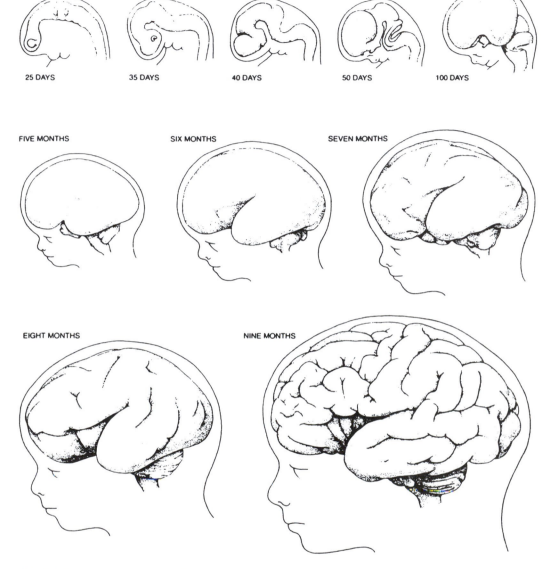

25 DAYS   35 DAYS   40 DAYS   50 DAYS   100 DAYS

FIVE MONTHS   SIX MONTHS   SEVEN MONTHS

EIGHT MONTHS   NINE MONTHS

FIGURE 2. Prenatal development of the human brain showing a series of embryonic and fetal stages (adapted from Cowan, 1979).

outer layers must traverse the cells and fibers of the inner layers. In a series of elegant studies, Rakic (1972, 1975, 1981, 1984) showed that neurons migrate to the appropriate laminae within the cortex along specialized filaments, known as radial glial fibers, which span the fetal cerebral wall at early ages. These radial glial cells originate in the ventricular zone and extend outward to the cortical plate. As the cortex develops, thickens, and sulci be-

gin to appear, the radial glial fibers stretch and curve, guiding the migrating neurons to their correct location (see Figure 4).

Axonal Development

As cells migrate along the radial glial fibers, they begin to develop axons that run to subcortical areas, other cortical areas, or across the midline as

CEREBRAL ISOCORTEX

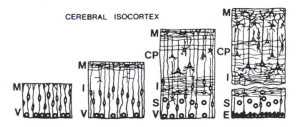

CEREBELLUM

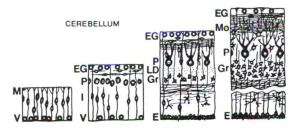

FIGURE 3. Schematic illustration of events occurring sequentially during development of the cerebral cortex and cerebellar cortex (from Jacobsen, 1978). Progressively later stages of development are shown from left to right. CP, cortical plate; E, ependymal layer; EG, external granule layer; Gr, granule layer; I, intermediate zone; LD, lamina dissecans; M, marginal zone; Mo, molecular layer; P, Purkinje cell layer; S, subventricular zone (also called subependymal zone); V, ventricular zone.

commissural fibers. The rate of axon development is extremely rapid, apparently on the order of 1 mm/day. In addition to axons of cortical cells growing out, axons from the thalamus enter the cortex after the principal cortical target cells complete their migrations and assume the appropriate positions within the developing cortical plate (Rakic, 1976).

Dendritic Development

Two processes occur during development of the dendrite: dendritic arborization and spine growth. The dendrites begin as individual processes protruding from the cell body. Later, they develop increasingly complex extensions, looking much like the branches of trees in winter. Spines are little appendages, resembling thorns on a rose stem, that begin to appear in the seventh intrauterine month (Poliakov, 1961). Before birth, they are observed only on the biggest neurons (mainly those found in layer V). After birth, they can also be found on other neurons where they spread and densely cover the dendritic surface. Although dendritic development begins prenatally in the human, it continues for a long time postnatally. In laboratory animals, the development of both dendritic branches and spines has been shown to be influenced dramatically by

TABLE 1. Sequential Lamination of the Human Motor Cortex in Ontogenesis[a,b]

Case	Cortical layers						
			III				
	I	II	Upper	Lower	IV	V	VI
5-month fetus	++	0	0	0	0	+	+
7-month fetus	++ − +++	+	+	+ − ++	+	++	++
7½-month fetus	+++ − ++++	++	++	++ − +++	++	+++	+++
Newborn infant	++++	+++	+++	++++	++++	++++	++++
2½-month-old infant	++++	+++	++++	++++	Very Thin	++++	++++
8-month-old infant	++++	+++	++++	++++	Agranular	++++	++++

[a]From Marin-Padilla (1970).
[b]Key: 0, unrecognizable; +, immature; ++, developing; +++, established; ++++, fully developed.

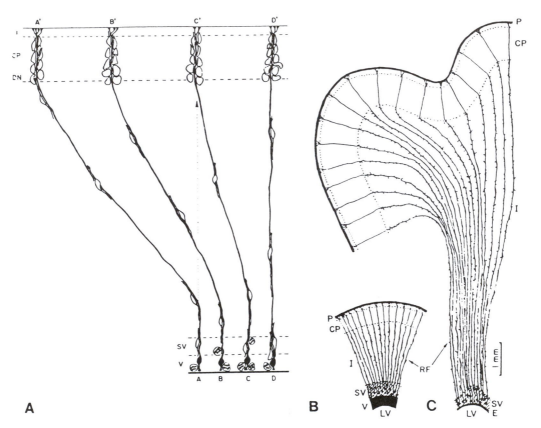

FIGURE 4. Schematic representations of the pattern of neural migration along the radial glial cells (from Rakic, 1981). (A) Migrating neurons leave the ventricular (V) and subventricular (SV) zones and travel to more superficial layers of the cortical plate (CP). En route they pass through the deeper neurons (DN), which are already in place. (B) Portion of the fetal cortex showing the radial glial fibers. (C) Section of the corresponding region in an older fetal cortex showing the changes in the radial glial fibers that allow the formation of gyri.

environmental stimulation (Greenough, 1976), a phenomenon that is probably very important in relation to the human child's development. In addition, it is now clear that dendritic development is also affected by gonadal hormones, leading to the development of a male or female cerebral structure (Juraska, 1990). The influence of gonadal hormones is not limited to birth but continues into adulthood and may play an important role in the processes related to aging (Stewart & Kolb, 1994).

In contrast to the development of axons, dendritic growth usually commences after the cell reaches its final position in the cortex and proceeds at a relatively slow rate, on the order of micrometers per day. The disparate developmental rates of axons and dendrite are important because the faster-growing axon can contact its target cell before the dendritic processes of that cell are elaborated, suggesting that the axon may play a role in dendritic

differentiation (Berry, 1982). The morphological changes associated with dendritic growth in the frontal cortex are illustrated in Figure 5.

Synaptic Development

The mechanism that controls synapse formation is one of the major mysteries of developmental neurobiology, largely because synapses are perceptible only by electron microscopy, which does not allow direct observation of their sequence of development in living tissue. The onset of synaptogenesis is abrupt and the appearance of synapses in any particular area is remarkably rapid although neurons may be juxtaposed for days before they actually make synaptic connections. Synapses usually form between the axon of one neuron and the dendrites, cell body, axons, or established synapses of other cells. Because synaptogenesis begins before

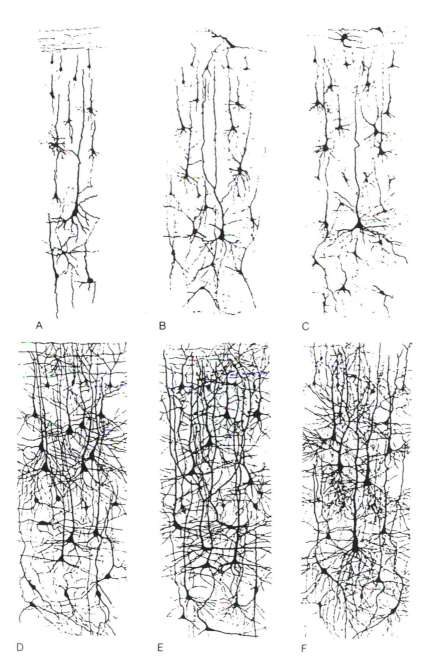

FIGURE 5. Postnatal development of human cerebral cortex around Broca's area as taken from camera lucida drawings of Golgi–Cox preparations (from Conel, 1939–1967). (A) Newborn; (B) 1 month; (C) 3 months; (D) 6 months; (E) 15 months; (F) 24 months.

neurogenesis is complete, neurons migrating to the superficial layers of the cortex must bypass cortical neurons on which synapses have already formed or are in the process of forming.

Little is known of the details of synapse formation in humans. Simple synaptic contacts have been observed during the fifth gestational month, and by the seventh fetal month there is extensive synaptic development on the deepest cortical pyramidal neurons. After birth, spine development spreads rapidly, which is reflected in a rapid increase in synapses. In the visual cortex, synaptic density almost doubles between the second and fourth months and then continues to increase until 1 year. After 1 year, synaptic density begins to decline to adult values, which occurs around age 11 (Huttenlocher, 1990). In the frontal cortex, synaptic density also reaches maximum levels at about 1 year, but this density is far higher than in visual cortex and does not begin to decline until about 5–7 years of age (Figure 6). It then takes until about 16 years of age to decline to adult levels (Huttenlocher, 1984). During the peak of maximum synaptic loss in humans, it has been estimated by Pasko Rakic that as many as 100,000 synapses may be lost per second! It is little wonder that children seem to change moods and behaviors so quickly.

It is interesting that the synaptic density of infants appears to exceed that of adults, for it has generally been assumed that a larger number, or a greater density, of synapses implies a higher functional capacity. Evidence of decreasing synaptic

density coincident with increasing cognitive skill is thus intriguing, especially because high numbers of synapses have been found in certain cases of mental retardation (Cragg, 1975). It is not surprising that intellectual ability cannot be predicted merely by its relation to the quantity of some anatomical feature, such as synapses, and, perhaps, the process involved in reducing synaptic density represents some sort of qualitative refinement.

Glial Development

The differentiation and growth of neurons, which are generally produced before their associated glia, appear to play some role in stimulating the growth and proliferation of glial cells, but the mechanisms are unknown (Jacobsen, 1978). In contrast to neurons, glial cells continue to proliferate after birth and may continue to do so throughout life.

Myelin Development

Myelination is the process by which the glial cells of the nervous system begin to surround axons and provide them with insulation. Although nerves can become functional before they are myelinated, it was assumed in the 1920s and 1930s that they only reach adult functional levels after myelination is complete (Flechsig, 1920). This notion now appears to be an oversimplification but is, nonetheless, useful as a rough index of cerebral maturation.

In contrast to other aspects of cortical development, myelin appears late, at a time when cellular proliferation and migration are virtually complete. The primary sensory and motor areas begin to myelinate just before term whereas the frontal and parietal association areas, the last to myelinate, begin postnatally and continue until about age 15 years or, sometimes, even later. Because different regions of the cortex myelinate at different times, and myelination begins in the lower layers of each cortical area and gradually spreads upward, the upper layers of the motor and primary sensory areas are myelinating at the same time that the lower areas of some association areas are just beginning to myelinate.

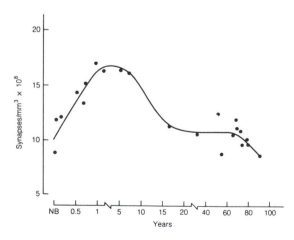

FIGURE 6. Synapse counts in layer 3 of the middle frontal gyrus of the human brain as a function of age. The number of synapses increases until 1 year of age and decreases, reaching asymptote at about age 16. There is further decline in old age, after about age 70. (After Huttenlocher, 1979.)

Neurochemical Development

Chemical neurotransmitters serve as the primary means of interneuronal communication, yet virtually nothing is known about the neurochemical development of the human cortex. Although there are numerous studies of neurotransmitter development in the rat, knowledge about the relationships among transmitters in the adult neocortex is still limited and the most completely described neurochemical systems make only a modest contribution to the overall synaptic activity of the neocortex (see Table 2). There are, however, some developmental studies using nonhuman primates that are worth reviewing as the human brain is likely to be similar (see also Parnavelas, Papadopoulos, & Cavanagh, 1988).

Goldman-Rakic and Brown (1981, 1982) investigated the regional distribution of catecholamines in rhesus monkeys ranging in age from newborns to young adults. Their overall findings were that, although monoaminergic systems are present in the cortex at birth, these networks continue to develop for years. Catecholamine development varies greatly between different cortical regions and the most striking postnatal increases in content were observed in the frontal and parietal association areas. Perhaps most interesting was their observation that catecholamine development (especially that of the monoamines) parallels functional development in the prefrontal cortex over the first 2–3 years of life. These data support the suggestion that catecholamines may play an important role in the development of functional activity in the frontal cortex and likely affect the morphological development of various neuronal processes such as dendritic fields.

Postnatal Brain Development

After birth, the brain does not grow uniformly but rather tends to increase its mass during irregular periods commonly called growth spurts. In his analysis of brain/body weight ratios, Epstein (1978, 1979) found consistent spurts in brain growth at 3–10 months, accounting for an increase of 30% in brain weight by the age of $1\frac{1}{2}$ years, as well as between ages 2 and 4, 6 and 8, 10 and 12, and 14 and 16+ years. The increments in brain weight were about 5–10% over each 2-year period. This expansion takes place without a concurrent increase in neuronal proliferation and is unlikely to be accounted for by increases in the number of glial cells. Rather, it most likely results from the growth of dendritic processes and myelination. Such an increase in cortical complexity would be expected to correlate with increased complexity in behavioral functions, and it could be predicted that there would be significant, and perhaps qualitative, changes in cognitive function during each growth spurt. It may be significant that the first four brain growth stages coincide with the classically given ages of onset of the four main stages of intelligence development described by Piaget. We return to this later.

Cell Death

One of the most intriguing stages in brain development is cell death. Consider the following analogy. If one wanted to make a statue, it would be possible to do so either by starting with grains of sand and glueing them together to form the desired shape or by starting with a block of stone and chiseling the unwanted pieces away. The brain uses the latter procedure. The "chisel" in the brain could be of several forms including genetic signal, environmental stimulation, gonadal hormones, stress, and so on. Similarly, the same processes are likely to affect the development of dendrites, axons, and synapses. Cell death does not end in infancy but rather may continue well into adolescence. The possibility that environmental events may alter the brain by influencing cell death is intriguing because it implies a permanence to at least some effects of early experience.

One example of the effect of environmental stimulation on brain development comes from the work of Werker and Tees (1992). They studied the

---

TABLE 2. Neocortical Neurotransmitters[a]

Transmitter type	Cell location
Afferents	
Norepinephrine	Locus coeruleus
Dopamine	Substantia nigra A10
Serotonin	Raphe
Acetylcholine	Globus pallidus magnocellular
Intrinsic	
GABA	Aspinous stellate (all layers)
Neuropeptides (somatostatin, neuropeptide Y, vasoactive intestinal polypeptide, cholecystokinin)	Aspinous bipolar stellates
Efferents	
Glutamate	Pyramidal cells (layer V corticostriatal)

[a]After Coyle (1982).

ability of infants to discriminate phonemes taken from widely disparate languages such as English, Hindi, and Salish. Their results showed that infants can discriminate speech sounds of different languages without previous experience, but there is a decline in this ability, over the first year of life, as a function of specific language experience. One might speculate that neurons in the auditory system that are not stimulated early in life may be selected against and die, although there are other explanations.

Not only is there cell death during development but there is also a process of pruning synapses as mentioned earlier. Recall that there is synapse elimination in the frontal lobe until adolescence (Figure 6). Thus, it seems likely that just as the nervous system uses the block-and-chisel method for choosing neurons, a similar process is used for selecting neuronal connections. The difference, however, is that it seems reasonable to expect that the brain could replace pruned connections later in life whereas the replacement of lost neurons is unlikely.

Cortical Function at Birth

The extreme paucity of behavioral skill in the newborn leads to the notion that, shortly after birth, the cortex has not yet begun to function. Thus, the cortically injured infant was once believed to be indistinguishable from the normal child at birth (Peiper, 1963). Several lines of evidence suggest that the cortex is indeed functioning, if only at a rudimentary level. It is now known that cortically hemiplegic infants can be distinguished from normal babies on the basis of muscle tone (Gibson, 1977) and cortically damaged infants may also have abnormal sleep–waking cycles and abnormal cries (Robinson, 1966). There are also several measures of electrical activity that imply cortical activity is present at birth. EEG activity can be recorded from the fetal brain (Bergstrom, 1969) and epileptic seizures of cortical origin can occur in the neonate (Caveness, 1969). Perhaps the most compelling evidence of early cortical activity comes from the extensive work of Purpura (Purpura, 1976, 1982). In his study of cortical activity in premature human infants, Purpura took advantage of the fact that, between 26 and 34 weeks of gestation, cortical pyramidal cells in primary visual cortex undergo significant growth and branching. These changes are associated with corresponding maturational changes in the electrophysiological characteristics

of the visual evoked potentials (VEPs) in preterm infants. Although, even at birth, the VEPs are not identical to those of adults, they are present and indicate that at least primary visual cortex is functioning in some capacity.

Chugani and Phelps (1986) studied glucose utilization in the brain of infants using positron emission tomography. Their results showed that, in infants 5 weeks of age or younger, glucose utilization, which can be taken as a crude measure of neural activity, was highest in the sensorimotor cortex, a result that is in accordance with anatomical evidence that this is the most mature cortical region at birth. By 3 months of age, glucose metabolism had increased in most other cortical regions with subsequent increases in frontal and posterior association cortex occurring by 8 months. Thus, by about 8–9 months there is evidence of activity throughout the cerebral cortex, although it probably changes in the years to come.

Abnormal Development of the Child's Brain

We have seen that the anatomical development of the child's brain consists of the proliferation and migration of cells, the growth of axons and dendrites, synapse formation and loss, myelin growth, and so on. These processes begin early in embryonic development and continue until late adolescence. In view of the complexity of the cortex and its prolonged development, it is reasonable to expect that normal cortical development could be disrupted by any number of events. These include abnormalities in the normal genetic program of neural growth, the influences of exogenous factors such as toxic substances or brain trauma, and nutritional or other environmental circumstances. We do not propose to discuss all of these possibilities, but will confine our discussion to those events that are most likely to be important to the neuropsychologist, namely, abnormal neural differentiation and early brain damage.

Abnormal Neural Structure

In the event that either neurogenesis or neural migration is abnormal, one would expect gross abnormalities in cortical development. Clinically, a variety of conditions are recognized (Table 3), but little is known about the details of cell differentiation in these disorders. The major experimental study of disturbed migration in the cerebral cortex involves the reeler mouse mutant. Caveness (Caviness, 1982; Caviness & Rakic, 1978; Caviness &

TABLE 3. Types of Abnormal Development

Type	Symptom
Anencephaly	Absence of cerebral hemispheres, diencephalon, and midbrain
Holoprosencephaly	Cortex forms as a single undifferentiated hemisphere
Lissencephaly	The brain fails to form sulci and gyri and corresponds to a 12-week embryo
Micropolygyria	Gyri are more numerous, smaller, and more poorly developed than normal
Macrogyria	Gyri are broader and less numerous than normal
Microencephaly	Development of the brain is rudimentary and the person has low-grade intelligence
Porencephaly	Symmetrical cavities in the cortex, where cortex and white matter should be
Heterotopia	Displaced islands of gray matter appear in the ventricular walls or white matter, caused by aborted cell migration
Agenesis of the corpus callosum	Complete or partial absence of the corpus callosum
Cerebellar agenesis	Portions of the cerebellum, basal ganglia, or spinal cord are absent or malformed

Sidman, 1973) showed that, in this animal, the cortex is inverted relative to that of a normal mouse; the cells generated first lie nearest the cortical surface and those generated last lie deepest. In addition, many of the pyramidal cells are abnormally oriented, in some cases with their major dendrites (the apical dendrites) oriented downward rather than upward as in the normal mouse. Despite their aberrant position, the cells develop connections as they would have had they been normally situated. Caviness and his colleagues studied the cortex of humans with various similar abnormalities, finding some of the same aberrant features (Caviness & Williams, 1979). Thus, in lissencephalic cortex, Williams, Ferrante, and Caviness (1975) found that cells failed to migrate into the appropriate layers and some cells were abnormally oriented, much as in the reeler mouse. The cause of these anomalies remains unknown.

Injury and Brain Development

If the brain is damaged during development, it is reasonable to suppose that its development might be fundamentally altered. There are few studies of human brains with early lesions but there is a considerable literature from work with laboratory animals. In an extensive examination of monkeys with prenatal or perinatal frontal cortex injuries, Goldman-Rakic has shown a variety of changes in cortical development including abnormal gyral formation and abnormal corticostriatal connections (Goldman & Galkin, 1978; Goldman-Rakic, Isseroff, Schwartz, & Bugbee, 1983). Similarly, Kolb and his colleagues have found abnormal corticostriatal and subcorticocortical connections, abnormal myelination, altered cortical catecholamine distribution, thalamic shrinkage, reduced gliosis relative to animals with similar injuries in adulthood, and markedly thinner cortex following early frontal lesions in rats (for a review, see Kolb, 1995). The thin cortex appears to result both from a loss in the number of cortical cells as well as from a loss in dendritic arborization. In sum, there is good reason to presume that early damage to the human brain produces significant changes in cortical morphology that extend far beyond the boundaries of the tissue directly traumatized.

One of the clearest abnormalities in the developing human brain can be seen in studies comparing the brains of normal and profoundly retarded subjects. Golgi studies have shown abnormally long, thin spines on dendrites of cortical neurons in retarded children with no known genetic abnormality (Figure 7). The degree of abnormality is related to the severity of retardation. The dendritic abnormalities in retarded children are strikingly similar to those seen in rats with cortical injuries around the time of birth and may reflect similar etiologies.

One of the difficulties in applying the results of studies of laboratory animals to humans is the difficulty in equating the developmental age of the brain in different species. For example, when rats are born their brain is very immature relative to the human brain, which is reflected in the fact that their eyes and ears are not open, and not functional. Cats are somewhat older developmentally than rats but still are much less mature than humans. In contrast, at birth rhesus monkeys are more mature than humans. Thus, as we try to compare developmental ages we must not be overly impressed by the "birth day" but rather we need to focus on the developmental age of the brain. In comparing rats and humans, it therefore appears that newborn humans are roughly equivalent to 10-day-old rats; newborn rats are probably

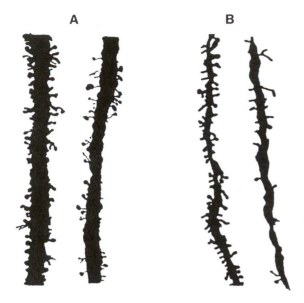

FIGURE 7. Camera lucida representations of Golgi preparations showing typical dendritic segments of medium-sized pyramidal neurons. (A) Left: Example of apical segment from a normal 7-year-old child (accident case). Right: Example of apical segment from a 12-year-old profoundly retarded child. (B) Left: Example of apical segment from a normal rat. Right: Example of apical segment from a rat with a frontal lesion on the day of birth. (After Kolb & Gibb, 1993; Purpura, 1974.)

roughly equivalent to 8-month-old fetuses (Kolb, 1995).

Behavioral Correlates of Brain Development

Two types of behavior have been extensively studied and correlated with anatomical development, namely, motor behavior and language. We shall consider each separately, and then consider the development of their asymmetrical representation in the cortex. Finally, we will discuss the behavior of children on standardized tests typically used by clinical neuropsychologists. We shall not attempt to be exhaustive in our coverage of each, but rather try to give a flavor of the findings to date.

Motor Systems

The development of locomotion in human infants is quite familiar to most of us. Infants are, at first, unable to move about independently, but eventually they learn to crawl and then to walk. The way

in which other motor patterns develop is less obvious but one has been described in an elegant study by Twitchell (1965) who documented the stages an infant passes through while acquiring the ability to reach out with one limb and bring objects toward itself. Before birth the fetus's movements are essentially of the whole body. Shortly after birth the infant can flex all of the joints of an arm in such a way that it could scoop something toward its body, but it is not clear that this movement is executed independent of other body movements. Between 1 and 3 months it orients its hand toward, and gropes for, objects that have contacted it. Between 8 and 11 months it develops the "pincer grasp," using the index finger and thumb in opposition to each other. The development of the pincer grasp is extremely significant, because it allows the infant to make a very precise grasping movement that enables the manipulation of small objects. In summary, there is a sequential development of the grasping reaction: first scooping, then reaching and grasping with all fingers, then independent finger movements.

The fact that motor cortex lesions in adults abolish the grasp reaction with independent finger movements implies that there could be anatomical changes within the motor strip that correlate with the original development of the behavior. Although there are probably multiple changes occurring, especially in the development of dendritic arborizations, a correlation has been noted between myelin formation and the ability to grasp. In particular, the small motor fibers become myelinated at about the same time that reaching and grasping with the whole hand develop while the giant Betz cells of the motor cortex become myelinated at about the time the pincer grasp develops. These different motor fibers are thought to control arm and finger movements, respectively (Kolb and Whishaw, 1996).

The correlation between myelin development and motor behaviors can also be found in many other activities. Table 4 summarizes the development of a variety of behavioral patterns and myelin formation. It is of course difficult to be certain which correlations are meaningful and, as we have noted, there are obviously many other anatomical changes occurring concurrently. Careful study of these data, however, does show some intriguing associations that warrant more detailed study.

Language Development

The onset of speech consists of a gradual appearance of generally well-circumscribed events that

TABLE 4. Summary of Postnatal Human Development[a]

Age	Visual and motor function	Average brain weight (g)[a]	Degree of myelination[b]
Birth	Reflex sucking, rooting, swallowing, and Moro reflexes; infantile grasping; blinks to light	350	Motor roots $+++$; sensory roots $++$; medial lemniscus $++$; superior cerebellar peduncle $++$; optic tract $++$; optic radiation $\pm$
6 weeks	Extends and turns neck when prone; regards mother's face, follows objects	410	Optic tract $++$; optic radiation $+$; middle cerebral peduncle $\pm$; pyramidal tract $+$
3 months	Infantile grasp and suck modified by volition; keeps head above horizontal for long periods; turns to objects presented in visual field; may respond to sound	515	Sensory roots $+++$; optic tract and radiation $+++$; pyramidal tract $++$; cingulum $+$; frontopontine tract $+$; middle cerebellar peduncle $+$; corpus callosum $\pm$; reticular formation $\pm$
6 months	Grasp objects with both hands, will place weight on forearms or hands when prone; rolls supine to prone; supports almost all weight on legs for very brief periods; sits briefly	660	Medial lemniscus $+++$; superior cerebellar peduncle $+++$; middle cerebellar peduncle $++$; pyramidal tract $++$; corpus callosum $+$; reticular formation $+$; associational areas $\pm$; acoustic radiation $+$
9 months	Sits well and pulls self to sitting position; thumb–forefinger grasp; crawls	750	Cingulum $+++$; fornix $++$; others as previously given
12 months	Able to release objects; cruises and walks with one hand held; plantar reflex flexor in 50% of children	925	Medial lemniscus $+++$; pyramidal tracts $+++$; frontopontine tract $+++$; fornix $+++$; corpus callosum $+$; intracortical neuropil $\pm$; associational areas $\pm$; acoustic radiation $++$
24 months	Walks up and down stairs (two feet a step); bends over and picks up objects without falling; turns knob; can partially dress self; plantar reflex flexor in 100%	1065	Acoustic radiation $+++$; corpus callosum $++$; associational areas $+$; nonspecific thalamic radiation $++$
36 months	Goes up stairs (one foot a step); pedals tricycle; dresses fully except for shoelaces, belt, and buttons; visual acuity 20/20 OU	1140	Middle cerebellar peduncle $+++$
5 years	Skips; ties shoelaces; copies triangle; gives age correctly	1240	Nonspecific thalamic radiation $+++$; reticular formation $++$; corpus callosum $+++$; intracortical neuropil and associational areas $++$
Adult	—	1400	Intracortical neuropil and associational areas $++$ to $+++$

[a]Source: Spreen, Tupper, Risser, Tuokko, & Edgell (1984).
[b]From Yakovlev and Lecours (1967). Estimates are made from their graphic data ($\pm$, minimal amounts; $+$, mild; $++$, moderate; $+++$, heavy).

take place during the first 3 years of life (Tables 4 and 5). Language development is dependent not only on the development of appropriate perceptual abilities, such as the identification and categorization of speech sounds, but also on the development of motor capacities, especially those that control the lips and tongue. It therefore comes as little surprise that the precise movements of the lips and tongue needed for speech are fully developed well before the acquisition of finger and hand control.

The perceptual and motor processes necessary for language development are dependent on the maturation of the temporal and frontal lobes which may be highly variable in developmental rate in some children. Thus, some children have a markedly delayed speech acquisition but later turn out to have normal intelligence and normal skeletal and gross motor development. For example, such children may not begin to speak in phrases until after age 4, in spite of an apparently normal environment and the absence of any obvious neurological signs that might suggest brain damage.

Experiential factors clearly influence speech development (e.g., Werker & Tees, 1992) so it could

TABLE 5. Summary of Postnatal Development of Basic Social and Language Functions[a]

Approximate age	Basic social and language functions
Birth	Comforted by sound of human voice; reflexive smile. Most common sounds are discomfort and hunger cries and vegetative sounds; by end of 1st month the cries become differentiated; noncrying speechlike sounds usually during feeding
6 weeks	Makes eye contact with mother; spontaneous smile. Responds to human voice and being held by quieting; smiles when played with; makes cooing and pleasure noises; cries to gain assistance
2 months	Begins to distinguish different speech sounds; cooing becomes more guttural or "throaty"; seeing people causes excitement; unselective social smile
3 months	Discriminates between some individuals; recognizes mother; selective social smile; orients head to voices; makes a vocal response to others' speech; "babbling"—a phase characterized by the "spontaneous" production of sounds. Usually begins in month 2 or 3 and continues to month 12–15 or later although typically decreasing as echolalia increases
4 months	Selective attention to faces; prefers to look at happy rather than angry expressions; localizes to sounds; can discriminate individual faces; smiles at other babies; varies pitch of vocalizations; imitates tones
6 months	Laughs aloud; conveys pleasure and displeasure in prosody; smiles at self in mirror; "echolalia," the imitation of sounds made by others, usually beginning at month 4–7. Imitation of prosody occurs long before that of articulated speech segments; forms the dominant linguistic activity through the 2nd year with decreasing importance, except during the acquisition of new words, until at least month 30–36
9 months	Waves bye-bye; plays patty-cake; makes distinct intonational patterns; social gestures
12 months	May kiss on request. Sentences, the long and progressive process of learning the symbolic significance of speech sounds enabling the capacity to understand and generate meaningful words and sentences; in most individuals maximum capacity is probably not achieved until the middle of the second decade or later; a 12-month-old may have a vocabulary of 5–10 words that will double in the following 6 months
24 months	"Vocabulary" can be approximately 200–300 words by the 2nd year; names most common everyday objects; "morphological–syntactical"—most of child's utterances will be unitary, i.e., single, nonassociated linguistic units up to 18–24 months and occasionally later; next 5–6 years, at least, will be devoted to the acquisition of the complex, multistaged process of developing a mastery of a morphological–syntactical system
36 months	Has vocabulary of 900–1000 words; 3- to 4-word simple construction sentences (subject–verb); can follow two-step commands; curses
4 years	Has a vocabulary of more than 1500 words; asks numerous questions; sentences become more complex
5 years	The typical 5-year-old may have a vocabulary of approximately 1500–2200 words; discusses feelings; the average 5- to 7-year-old will be expected to have acquired a slow but fluent ability to read; handwriting will also likely be slow; graphism, however, should be well differentiated and regular; competent "phonetic" writing; the mastery of the orthographic system can be expected to extend for several more years
6 years	Expressive vocabulary of about 2600 words; receptive vocabulary of 20,000–24,000 words; uses all parts of speech
Adult	Has vocabulary of 50,000+ words by age 12

[a]Adapted from Lecours (1975) and Owens (1984).

be argued that language development is not so much dependent on the maturation of some neural structure as it is on some form of environmental stimulation. Although this is possible, it is unlikely that speech development is constrained exclusively by some environmental event. Indeed, it is a common observation by parents that children may have markedly different histories of language acquisition. Thus, the emergence of speech and language habits is most easily accounted for by assuming that there are maturational changes within the brain. The difficulty is in specifying what these changes might be. Indeed, in view of the complexity of the neural control of language, it is futile to look for any specific growth process that might explain language acquisition. Nonetheless, it is likely to be instructive to know in what ways the cortex is different before the onset of language (age 2) and after the majority of language acquisition is completed (about age 12).

It will be recalled from our discussion of neural maturation that by 2 years of age there is no longer any cell division and most cells have migrated to their final location in the cortical laminae. The major changes that occur between the ages of 2 and 12 years are in the interconnection of neurons, largely through a decrease in the number of synapses as well as increase in the complexity of their dendritic arborizations. If one assumes that language acquisition requires the development of *functional* connections between neurons, much as hypothesized by Hebb (1949) in his concept of cell assemblies, then these changes in synaptic density and dendritic detail may be logical candidates as constraints of speech development. The postnatal changes in dendritic complexity within the speech areas are among the most impressive in the brain. As illustrated in Figure 5, the dendrites are simple at birth and develop slowly until about 15 months when the major dendrites are present. Between 15 and 24 months there is a dramatic increase in the density of the neuropil. A similar observation can be made from examination of the cortex of the posterior speech zone. Given the correlation between language development and maturation of the language areas, we can infer that language development may be constrained, at least in part, by the maturation of these areas and that individual differences in language acquisition may be accounted for by differences in this neural development. Furthermore, given the known effect of environmental stimulation on dendritic development, we might also predict that those differences in language acquisition that have some environ-

mental influence may do so by changing the maturational rate of the dendritic fields within these areas.

Cerebral Asymmetry

Just as the asymmetrical function of the adult's brain has been a focal point for neurological study, the development of asymmetry has been a focal point of developmental studies. As asymmetry is the subject of another chapter in this volume (see Kinsbourne, this volume), we shall consider this topic only briefly.

Most of the research with children that has been designed to demonstrate lateralization of function has emphasized the age at which asymmetry first appears. Table 6 gives examples of a number of representative functions and the side and earliest age of demonstrated asymmetry. A central theoretical issue is whether or not functions are disproportionately represented in the two hemispheres because they depend on certain anatomical asymmetries that develop independent of environmental stimulation. The fact that anatomical asymmetries can be observed in the cortex prenatally (Chi, Dooling, & Gilles, 1977; Wada, Clarke, & Hamm, 1975) and, therefore, exist before the expression of the behaviors, implies that asymmetry is relatively innate. Nevertheless, several major problems arise when we try to correlate functional and anatomical asymmetry. First, the functions that are most lateralized in adults are not easily assessed in children. For example, it is extremely difficult, if not impossible, to determine handedness for writing in infants, unless, of course, one is willing to assume that some other indirect measure, such as hand strength, in this case, will serve as a reliable predictor. Second, correlations between function and anatomical asymmetry in adults are far from perfect. Although the left planum temporale is thought to be the posterior substrate of language functions, it is larger in only about 70% of right-handed people, whereas speech is lateralized to the left hemisphere in about 99% of right-handers. What then does a similar anatomical asymmetry in the fetal brain imply?

Development of Problem-Solving Ability

As each cortical layer within an area develops, it interacts with and modifies the function of the existing structure. Gibson (1977), therefore, suggested

TABLE 6. Studies Showing Age of Asymmetry for Different Behaviors

System	Age	Dominance	Reference
Auditory			
Speech syllables	Preterm	Right ear	Molfese & Molfese (1980)
Music	22–140 days	Left ear	Entus (1977)
Phonemes	22–140 days	Right ear	Entus (1977)
Words	4 years	Right ear	Kimura (1963)
Environmental sounds	5–8 years	Left ear	Knox & Kimura (1970)
Visual			
Rhythmic visual stimuli	Newborn	Right	Crowell, Jones, Kapuniai, & Nakagawa (1973)
Face recognition	7–9 years	Left field	Marcel & Rajan (1975)
	6–13 years	Left field	Witelson (1977)
	9–10 years	None	Diamond & Carey (1977)
Somatosensory			
Dichhaptic recognition	All ages	Left	Witelson (1977)
Motor			
Stepping	<3 months	Right	Peters & Petrie (1979)
Head turning	Neonates	Right	Turkewitz (1977)
Grasp duration	1–4 months	Right	Caplan & Kinsbourne (1976)
Finger tapping	3–5 years	Right	Ingram (1975)
Strength	3–5 years	Right	Ingram (1975)
Gesturing	3–5 years	Right	Ingram (1975)
Head orientation	Neonates	Right	Michel (1981)

that behavior patterns would be expected to emerge exactly in the manner described by Piaget (1952):

> Behavior patterns characteristic of different stages do not succeed each other in a linear way (those of a given stage disappearing at the time when those of the following one take form) but in the manner of the layers of a pyramid (upright and upside down), the new behavior patterns simply being added to the old ones to complete, correct or combine with them. (p. 329)

Thus, for example, because the deepest layers of the cortex myelinate first, and these are the efferent or output layers, one would expect to observe motor responses preceding the development of perceptual capacity. Indeed, according to Piaget, motor actions must come first, as motor actions provide data from which to build perceptions. The question to consider is just how well the stage of cognitive development coincides with changes in neural maturation. This is a difficult question that has not been extensively studied. Nevertheless, there is at least suggestive evidence that there may be a significant relationship between cortical development and the classical Piagetian stages. [We note that the Piagetian stages of cognitive development are a source of some debate and there are several other conceptual schemes to describe the development of cognition

in children (Carey, 1984). We will restrict our discussion to Piaget, however, because we wish merely to demonstrate the type of study that can be done and because we are unaware of any attempt to correlate other schemes of cognitive development to cortical maturation.]

Piaget was a biologist by training and considered the acquisition of knowledge and thought to be closely related to brain function. He believed that cognitive development was a continual process and that the child's strategies for exploring the world were constantly changing. These changes were not simply a result of the acquisition of specific pieces of knowledge but rather, at some specifiable points in development, were fundamental changes in the organization of the child's strategies for learning about the world. Piaget identified four major stages of cognitive development: stage I, Sensorimotor, birth to 18 months; stage II, Preoperational or Symbolic, 18 months to 7 years; stage III, Concrete Operational, 7 to 11 years; and stage IV, Formal Operational, 11+ years). In stage I the infant learns to differentiate itself from the external world, learns that objects exist when not visible, and gains some appreciation of cause and effect. In stage II, the child begins to represent things with something else, such as drawing. Stage III is characterized by the child's ability to mentally manipulate concrete ideas such as dimensions of objects and the like. Finally, in stage IV, the child is able to reason in the abstract. Having identified the stages, the challenge for the neuropsychologist is to identify those changes in neural structure that might underlie these apparent qualitative changes in cognitive activity.

The first four brain growth stages described earlier coincide with the usual given ages of onset of the four main Piagetian stages (Epstein, 1979). A fifth stage of development, which would correlate with the fifth brain growth stage, was not described by Piaget but has been proposed by Arlin (1975). The concordance of brain growth and Piagetian stage is intriguing but, to date, remains too superficial. We need to know what neural events are contributing to brain growth, and just where they are occurring. Little is known of this in children after 6 years of age but the question remains important to the neuropsychologist seeking to understand the maturation of cortical operations. A detailed hypothetical analysis of stage I has been attempted by Gibson (1977).

Development of Neuropsychological Test Performance

Neuropsychologists have developed an amazing array of tests since World War II with which to assess the behavior of patients with cortical injuries (e.g., Lezak, 1995). In principle, it is logical to suppose that if a test is sensitive to restricted cortical lesions in adults, and if a normal child performs poorly on such a test, it could then be inferred that the requisite cortical tissue is not yet functioning normally. This logic is seductive but is not without difficulties. First, the method assumes that tests will be sensitive to focal lesions: Few tests are. Second, a child may perform poorly on a test for many reasons. For example, a child may have difficulty with a verbal test because the speech areas are slow to develop or because he or she has an impoverished environment and has acquired only a limited vocabulary. Furthermore, just because a child does well on a test does not mean that the child's brain is solving the problem in the same manner as the adult brain. Indeed, there are examples of tests in which children do well, only to do more poorly the following year, followed later by improvement again. Thus, in their studies of facial recognition in children, Carey, Diamond, and Woods (1980) found that children improved in performance between ages 6 and 10, declined until age 14, and then attained adult levels

by age 16. This result can be taken to imply that the younger children were solving the problem in a different manner than the older children and adults while, presumably, using different cortical tissue. In sum, although there are clear limitations to the inferences that can be made about the development of specific brain regions, we feel that much can be learned using this type of approach. We will illustrate this by focusing on our own studies using tasks that test frontal lobe function and the perception of faces and facial expression.

Frontal Lobe Tests

Segalowitz and Rose-Krasnor (1992) edited a special issue of *Brain and Cognition* that was devoted to the general premise that an understanding of cognitive development in children is dependent on understanding the role of the frontal lobe in development. Their argument is based on the idea that the frontal lobe plays a central role in generating cognitive strategies (as opposed to habits) as well as in the evaluation of those strategies, the monitoring of their own behaviors, and the effects of one's behavior on other people. If their argument is correct, then an understanding of correlations between frontal lobe development and behavioral maturation is critical in developmental neuropsychology.

The idea that the frontal lobes play a special role in cognitive development is not new. Hebb (1949) speculated from his analyses of children with perinatal cerebral injuries that the frontal lobes were critical to cognitive development. In fact, Hebb believed that the frontal lobes played a more important role during development than in adulthood. More recently, Case (1992) has argued that between the ages of 1½ and 5 years, and again between the ages of 5 and 10 years, a sequence of changes takes place in children's behavior that indicates a fundamental reorganization of their attentional and executive processes. Case correlates these functional changes with physiological changes in the frontal lobe of children (Stuss, 1992; Thatcher, 1992).

One way to investigate correlations between frontal lobe maturation and cognitive maturation is to study the behavior of children on tests performed poorly by people with acquired frontal lesions in adulthood. Two tests are especially sensitive to frontal lobe injury, namely, the Wisconsin Card Sorting Test and the Chicago Word Fluency Test (Milner, 1964). In the first test the subject is presented with four stimulus cards, bearing designs that differ in color, form, and number of elements. The subject's task is to sort the remaining cards into piles in front of one or another of the stimulus cards. The only help the subject is given is being told whether the choice is correct or incorrect. The test works on this principle: the correct solution is first to sort by color; once the subject has figured this out, the correct solution then becomes, without warning, to sort by form. Thus, the subject must now inhibit grouping the cards on the basis of color and shift to form. Once the subject has succeeded at sorting by form, the relevant feature again changes unexpectedly, this time to number of elements. This cycle of color, form, and number is repeated. The subject's score is the number of target categories completed after sorting 128 cards, and the task is terminated when all of the cards have been used or six categories have been completed, whichever comes first. Shifting strategies is particularly difficult for patients with left frontal lobe lesions. In the second test the subjects must write as many words as they can beginning with the letter "S" in 5 minutes. Following this, they must write as many four-letter words beginning with "C" as possible in 4 minutes and the final score is the total number of words generated. Frontal lobe patients do very poorly on this test. This deficit is not simply a problem of verbal ability, however, as frontal lobe patients perform at normal levels when asked to write the names of as many objects or animals as they can think of within a fixed time. We note that frontal lobe patients perform normally on many other tests as well. For example, on tests of visual recognition, which are performed poorly by patients with right posterior lesions, frontal lobe patients achieve normal levels of performance.

Kolb and Fantie (1989) tested children on the card sorting and verbal fluency tests and predicted that if the frontal lobes were slow to mature relative to other cortical areas, then children should reach adult levels very late, probably in adolescence on tests of frontal lobe function. In contrast, children should perform at adult levels much sooner on the tests performed normally by patients with frontal lobe lesions. This is indeed the case. Children perform poorly on all frontal lobe-sensitive tests when very young but improve as they develop. As predicted, performance on tests performed normally by adults with frontal lobe injuries improves more quickly, however, than performance on tests sensitive to frontal lobe injuries.

Frontal lobe patients are also notorious for their difficulties in social situations, although it is more difficult to quantify their behavior (Kolb & Whishaw, 1996). Kolb and Taylor (1981, 1990) showed that one way to analyze the unique frontal contributions to social interaction is to focus on the ability of frontal lobe patients to produce and to recognize facial expressions. Kolb, Wilson, and Taylor (1992) gave children a series of tests of facial perception ranging from simple tests of facial recognition and closure to more complex tests in which facial expression had to be understood from the context of a cartoon. Children aged 5–6 years performed as well as normal adults on the tests of facial recognition but did not approach adult levels on the context-dependent facial perceptual tests until about age 14 years. Furthermore, in a small sample of adults with frontal lobe injuries in early childhood we have shown abysmal performance on the context-related tests. This result is consistent with a series of case histories showing that children with frontal lobe injuries at the time of birth do not develop anything approaching normal strategies for coping with social situations (e.g., Ackerly, 1964; Eslinger & Damasio, 1985; Grattan & Eslinger, 1992).

Abnormal Brain Development and Behavior

Earlier we described abnormalities in neural migration that are probably found throughout the brain but it is reasonable to predict that there will be conditions in which such abnormalities might be restricted to relatively small zones of cortex. In fact, there is now reason to suppose that at least some forms of developmental dyslexia result from abnormal structural development. Drake (1968) examined the brain of a 12-year-old learning-disabled boy who died of cerebral hemorrhage. Autopsy showed that there were atypical gyral patterns in the parietal lobes, an atrophied corpus callosum, and neurons underlying the white matter that should have migrated to the cortex. More recently, Galaburda and his colleagues have reported analogous results from several dyslexic brains (Galaburda & Eidelberg, 1982; Galaburda & Kemper, 1979; Geschwind & Galaburda, 1985). Thus, in the brain of a 20-year-old male who previously had a reading disability despite average intelligence, they found an abnormal pattern of cytoarchitecture, especially in the posterior speech region of the temporal–parietal cortex. Although other details varied in these cases, the left posterior region was always abnormal. These abnormalities were believed to be the result of disordered neuronal migration and/or assembly. The right hemisphere was either completely or largely normal in all of these cases. Finally, Geschwind and Galaburda (1985) claimed to have evidence of similar anomalies in living dyslexic patients, with arteriovenous malformations in the left temporal region.

The finding of left temporal–parietal abnormality in dyslexics leads to the question of how these people, even as children, might perform on tests sensitive to focal cortical lesions. Few studies have directly compared dyslexic children to adults with left posterior lesions, but studies of dyslexic children have found behavioral deficits on tests that are particularly disrupted by left posterior lesions including tests of short-term verbal memory, left/right differentiation, and verbal fluency (Sutherland, Kolb, Schoel, Whishaw, & Davies, 1982; Whishaw & Kolb, 1984). We must point out that it is likely that not all children with learning disabilities have left posterior abnormalities. It would be interesting, however, to determine the correlation between neuropsychological test performance in learning-disabled children and the presence of left posterior abnormalities.

Early Brain Injury and Behavior

There is little doubt that humans and other animals sustaining brain damage in infancy can show more rapid and more complete recovery of a particular function than when comparable damage is sustained later in life (Kennard, 1936, 1940). At the same time, there is also little doubt that this apparent sparing of function is not without some cost (Fletcher, Levin, & Landry, 1984; Milner, 1974; Taylor, 1984; Teuber, 1975; Woods, 1980). Thus, although recuperation may appear total for many specific verbal and academic skills, more global assessments of cognitive status suggest that the recovery is often accompanied by new deficits that affect other functions and may be overlooked (St. James-Roberts, 1981; Taylor, 1984). Furthermore, there is some evidence that brain damage during the first year of life, a time during which there are tremendous changes in brain morphology, may actually have more severe consequences than similar damage later. Consider the following examples.

Effect of Brain Damage on Language

It is common to find that language deficits resulting from cerebral injury in childhood are usually short-lived, and that recovery of conversa-

tional speech is nearly complete (e.g., Hécaen, 1976). Cognitive function is by no means normal, however. Studies of children with unilateral brain damage in infancy by Woods and Teuber (Woods, 1980; Woods & Teuber, 1973) and Rasmussen and Milner (1975, 1977) lead to several conclusions in this respect. (1) Language survives early left-side injury. (2) If lesions are incurred prior to age 5 and include both language areas in the left hemisphere, language functions shift to the right hemisphere. (3) If lesions are restricted to the anterior or posterior speech zones, only the affected language area is likely to shift, leading to bilateral representation of speech. (4) When language shifts to the right hemisphere, it is not without a price for visuospatial functions are impaired. These functions would not be impaired if the damage were incurred later in life. (5) Childhood injuries to the left hemisphere, occurring after age 5, seldom change speech representation. The observed recovery of language function is assumed to be mediated by some sort of intrahemispheric reorganization. (6) Children with lesions incurred before their first birthday had verbal and performance IQ scores below the mean of the normal population. In contrast, the effects of lesions after the first birthday depend on the side of the lesion. The left-hemisphere lesions lowered both verbal and performance IQ scores whereas later right-hemisphere lesions adversely affected only the performance IQ scores.

Emergence of Deficits

One of the difficulties in assessing the effects of early brain injury in children is the problem of knowing when to investigate the behavior. After all, it is pointless to try to investigate the extent of language loss in a 1-year-old infant. In an interesting and important study, Banich, Cohen-Levine, Kim, and Huttenlocher (1990) studied the development of performance on two subtests of the Wechsler Intelligence Scale for Children, namely, vocabulary and block design, in children with congenital cerebral injuries. The authors found that at 6 years of age there were no differences in performance but as the children aged, significant deficits emerged in the brain-damaged children relative to matched normal controls (Figure 8). It thus appears that as the children's brains matured, they "grew into their deficits." This observation illustrates the difficulty in making predictions regarding the prognosis for children with cerebral injuries.

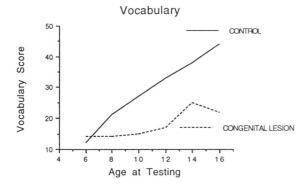

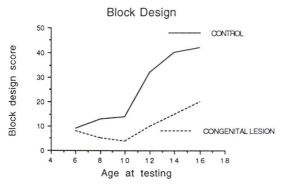

FIGURE 8. Summary of the developmental changes in performance on two subtests of the Wechsler Intelligence Scale for Children, Revised. Note that children with congenital lesions are equivalent to normal children at age 6, but they fail to improve and thus fall progressively behind as they age. (After Banich, Cohen-Levine, Kim, & Huttenlocher, 1990.)

Further evidence for the emergence of deficits during development comes from the work of Goldman-Rakic and her colleagues. In her early studies she was impressed with apparent recovery of functions after frontal lobe injuries in infant monkeys (e.g., Goldman, 1974). As she continued her investigations, it became clear that she and others had overestimated the extent of recovery because the animals were tested when still young. She found that as animals with prefrontal lesions developed, they became progressively more impaired at cognitive tasks such as delayed alternation (Goldman-Rakic *et al.*, 1983). Parallel results have also been found in studies on hamsters by Kolb and Whishaw (1985).

Frontal Lobe Damage

We have already discussed the functional development of the frontal cortex as inferred from the performance of children on neuropsychological tests

sensitive to frontal lobe function. We also noted that Hebb (1949) believed that the integrity of the frontal lobe was so important to normal cognitive development that he predicted that injuries to the developing frontal lobe might actually have more severe consequences than similar injury later in life. There is accumulating evidence that this might indeed be the case. Although there are likely differences in etiology and extent of injuries in the children in different studies, the overriding conclusion that intelligence is severely compromised by early frontal injuries is inescapable (e.g., Kolb & Fantie, 1989; Vargha-Khadem, Watters, & O'Gorman, 1985). Furthermore, even in other cognitive functions thought to be dependent on the frontal lobe in adulthood, there is no evidence of recovery after early frontal lobe injury, with the exception of language. For example, Milner (1974) found that in those patients with childhood damage to the left frontal lobe, there was a shift in language to the right hemisphere, but there was still a marked impairment of the performance of other tests of frontal lobe function such as the Wisconsin Card Sorting Test. We have seen similar results in a small sample of patients with unilateral frontal lobe injuries in childhood (largely head trauma and birth injury) (Kolb & Fantie, 1989).

The failure to see dramatic recovery from early frontal lesions finds support from the literature on laboratory animals: both Kolb and his colleagues (e.g., Kolb, 1995) and Goldman-Rakic and her colleagues (e.g., Goldman-Rakic *et al.*, 1983) have found less than complete recovery following early lesions in rodents and primates, respectively. Indeed, Kolb (1987) found that frontal lesions acquired just as cortical neuronal proliferation is completed (i.e., on the day of birth for rats) have greater behavioral and morphological effects than similar lesions even a couple of days later. In particular, although the lesion size appears the same at surgery, the early frontal lesion apparently also interrupts cell migration to the remaining sensorimotor cortex, resulting in a larger effective lesion in these rats. It is possible that a similar result might hold for the child's brain as well, particularly in those cases of prenatal injury.

To summarize, disruption of the normal growth and differentiation of the human brain is associated with a variety of pathological states, the nature of the behavioral changes depending on the developmental state of the brain at the time of injury. Although it was once believed that there was nearly complete recovery following cortical injuries during development, the bulk of the evidence does not support this view. Rather, it appears that events that produce abnormal development of the brain will also produce abnormal behavior, although certain behavioral functions such as speech appear to survive differentially relative to other functions, especially visuospatial functions. For the clinical neuropsychologist the assessment of children with brain injuries and the subsequent prediction of outcome is especially difficult regarding damage to the frontal and posterior associational cortices because one must wait until at least 10–12 years of age, the time at which these areas assume adultlike function, to determine how well the child will fare. It seems certain, however, that when such children are given a broad assessment battery, there will be significant neuropsychological deficits.

Effects of Hemidecortication

During the course of treatment for severe and often life-threatening neurological disorders, it has sometimes proven necessary to remove an entire hemisphere (hemispherectomy) or all of the cortex of one hemisphere (hemidecortication). The behavior of people with such surgery is especially interesting for there is remarkable behavioral recovery, especially in children. Perhaps the most striking result is that regardless of age, after complete removal of the left hemisphere most people are capable of some language and do not experience the dense global aphasia seen in patients with large left-hemisphere strokes. There are, however, significant behavioral sequelae of hemidecortication (e.g., Vargha-Khadem & Polkey, 1992). Full-scale IQ is usually at least one standard deviation below normal, but it is surprisingly high in view of the extent of the removal. There is also rather dramatic variability in the outcome, as several patients have been reported to have IQs that are above average (e.g., Smith, 1984). The outcome of hemidecortication varies with the etiology. Children with early seizure onset (before year 1) have a very poor outcome (IQ less than 70) relative to those with later disease onset. Left hemisphere "recovery" is more complete than right hemisphere "recovery." Indeed, although most left hemisphere patients show surprisingly good language functions, visuospatial and constructional capacities are compromised in most patients with removal of either hemisphere. In contrast to most patients with restricted lesions, there is much higher variation in the extent of behavioral dysfunction after hemidecortication. This may be related to the severity of residual seizure or other neurological disorders. Finally, functional recovery is very slow and may continue for many years. Overall,

it seems likely that recovery from hemidecortication is the slowest of all injuries in humans, but this may not be surprising in view of the severity of the brain damage.

Conclusion

The process of brain maturation is long, lasting at least into early adolescence. We have approached the problem of assessing the nature of functional localization in the cortex by examining the way in which structure and behavior emerge in the developing child. Neurons, the elementary components of the brain, are born, migrate, and, as their processes elaborate, establish connectional relationships with other neurons. Behavioral and cognitive capacities follow a similar sequence of development from the rudimentary to the complex. Structure–function relationships can be inferred by matching the developmental timetables of brain anatomy and physiology with those of behavior. In addition, we have demonstrated that neuropsychological tests that are sensitive to focal cortical damage in adults can be used to assess whether certain areas have reached functional maturity in normal, developing children. Further, by studying the abnormal development of the brain and behavior we may make inferences regarding the importance of particular developmental events on behavior.

The study of anatomical and behavioral development of the brain of the child is admittedly far from complete. However, we believe that the data obtained to date are beginning to answer the questions about the nature of the brain of the child. The continued study of developmental neuropsychology promises to change our understanding of the biological bases of the development of human behavior.

References

Ackerly, S. S. (1964). A case of prenatal bilateral frontal lobe defect observed for thirty years. In J. M. Warren & K. Ackert (Eds.), *Frontal granular cortex and behavior* (pp. 192–218). New York: McGraw–Hill.

Arlin, P. K. (1975). Cognitive development in adulthood: A fifth stage? *Developmental Psychology, 11*(5), 602–606.

Banich, M. T., Cohen-Levine, S., Kim, H., & Huttenlocher, P. (1990). The effects of developmental factors on I.Q. in hemiplegic children. *Neuropsychologia, 28*, 35–47.

Bergstrom, R. M. (1969). Electrical parameters of the brain during ontogeny. In R. J. Robinson (Ed.), *Brain and early behavior* (pp. 15–37). New York: Academic Press.

Berry, M. (1982). Cellular differentiation: Development of dendritic arborizations under normal and experimentally altered conditions. *Neurosciences Research Program Bulletin, 20*(4), 451–461.

Caplan, P. J., & Kinsbourne, M. (1976). Baby drops the rattle: Asymmetry of duration of grasp by infants. *Child Development, 47*, 532–534.

Carey, S. (1984). Cognitive development: The descriptive problem. In M. S. Gazzaniga (Ed.), *Handbook of cognitive neuroscience* (pp. 37–66). New York: Plenum Press.

Carey, S., Diamond, R., & Woods, B. (1980). Development of face recognition—A maturational component? *Developmental Psychology, 16*(6), 257–269.

Case, R. (1992). The role of the frontal lobes in the regulation of cognitive development. *Brain and Cognition, 20*, 51–73.

Caveness, W. F. (1969). Ontogeny of focal seizures. In H. H. Jasper, A. A. Ward, Jr., & A. Pope (Eds.), *Basic mechanisms of the epilepsies* (pp. 517–534). Boston: Little, Brown.

Caviness, V. S., Jr. (1982). Development of neocortical afferent systems: Studies in the reeler mouse. *Neurosciences Research Program Bulletin, 20*(4), 560–569.

Caviness, V. S., & Rakic, P. (1978). Mechanisms of cortical development: A view from mutations in mice. *Annual Review of Neuroscience, 1*, 297–326.

Caviness, V. S., Jr., & Sidman, R. L. (1973). Time of origin of corresponding cell classes in the cerebral cortex of normal and reeler mutant mice: An autoradiographic analysis. *Journal of Comparative Neurology, 148*, 141–152.

Caviness, V. S., & Williams, R. S. (1979). Cellular pathology of developing human cortex. *Research Publications of the Association for Research in Nervous and Mental Diseases, 57*, 69–98.

Chi, J. G., Dooling, E. C., & Gilles, F. H. (1977). Left–right asymmetries of the temporal speech areas of the human fetus. *Archives of Neurology, 34*, 346–348.

Chugani, H. T., & Phelps, M. E. (1986). Maturational changes in cerebral function in infants determined by [18]FDG positron emission tomography. *Science, 231*, 840–843.

Conel, J. L. (1939–1967). *The postnatal development of the human cerebral cortex* (Vols. I–VIII). Cambridge, MA: Harvard University Press.

Cowan, W. M. (1979). The development of the brain. *Scientific American, 241*, 112–133.

Coyle, J. T. (1982). Development of neurotransmitters in the neocortex. *Neurosciences Research Program Bulletin, 20*(4), 479–491.

Cragg, B. G. (1975). The density of synapses and neurons in normal, mentally defective and ageing human brains. *Brain, 98*, 81–90.

Crowell, D. H., Jones, R. H., Kapuniai, L. E., & Nakagawa, J. K. (1973). Unilateral cortical activity in newborn humans: An early index of cerebral dominance? *Science, 180*, 205–208.

Diamond, R., & Carey, S. (1977). Developmental changes in the representation of faces. *Journal of Experimental Child Psychology, 23*, 1–22.

Drake, W. (1968). Clinical and pathological findings in a child with a developmental learning disability. *Journal of Learning Disabilities, 1*, 468–475.

Entus, A. K. (1977). Hemispheric asymmetry in processing of dichotically presented speech and nonspeech stimuli by infants. In S. J. Segalowitz & F. A. Gruber (Eds.), *Language development and neurological theory* (pp. 63–73). New York: Academic Press.

Epstein, H. T. (1978). Growth spurts during brain development: Implications for educational policy and practice. In J. S. Chall & A. F. Mirsky (Eds.), *Education and the brain* (pp. 343–370). Chicago: University of Chicago Press.

Epstein, H. T. (1979). Correlated brain and intelligence development in humans. In M. E. Hahn, C. Jensen, & B. C. Dudek (Eds.), *Development and evolution of brain size: Behavioral implications* (pp. 111–131). New York: Academic Press.

Eslinger, P. J. & Damasio, A. R. (1985). Severe disturbance of higher cognition after bilateral frontal lobe ablation: Patient EVR. *Neurology, 35*, 1731–1741.

Flechsig, P. (1920). *Anatomie des menschlichen Gehirns und Ruckenmarks*. Leipzig: Thieme.

Fletcher, J. M., Levin, H. S., & Landry, S. H. (1984). Behavioral consequences of cerebral insult in infancy. In C. R. Almli & S. Finger (Eds.), *Early brain damage* (Vol. 1, pp. 189–213). New York: Academic Press.

Galaburda, A. M., & Eidelberg, D. (1982). Symmetry and asymmetry in the human posterior thalamus. II. Thalamic lesions in a case of development dyslexia. *Archives of Neurology, 39*, 333–336.

Galaburda, A. M., & Kemper, T. L. (1979). Cytoarchitectonic abnormalities in developmental dyslexia: A case study. *Annals of Neurology, 6*, 94–100.

Geschwind, N., & Galaburda, A. M. (1985). Cerebral lateralization: Biological mechanisms, associations, and pathology. 1. A hypothesis and a program for research. *Archives of Neurology, 42*, 428–459.

Gibson, K. R. (1977). Brain structure and intelligence in macaques and human infants from a Piagetian perspective. In S. Chevalier-Skolnikoff & F. E. Poirer (Eds.), *Primate biosocial development: Biological, social, and ecological determinants* (pp. 113–157). New York: Garland.

Goldman, P. S. (1974). An alternative to developmental plasticity: Heterology of CNS structures in infants and adults. In D. G. Stein, J. J. Rosen, & N. Butters (Eds.), *Plasticity and recovery of function in the central nervous system* (pp. 149–174). New York: Academic Press.

Goldman, P. S., & Galkin, T. W. (1978). Prenatal removal of frontal association cortex in the fetal rhesus monkey: Anatomical and functional consequences in postnatal life. *Brain Research, 152*, 451–485.

Goldman-Rakic, P. S., & Brown, R. M. (1981). Regional changes of monoamines in cerebral cortex and subcortical structures of aging rhesus monkeys. *Neuroscience, 6*, 177–187.

Goldman-Rakic, P. S., & Brown, R. M. (1982). Postnatal development of monoamine content and synthesis in the cerebral cortex of rhesus monkeys. *Developmental Brain Research, 4*, 339–349.

Goldman-Rakic, P. S., Isseroff, A., Schwartz, M. L., & Bugbee, N. M. (1983). The neurobiology of cognitive development. In P. Mussen (Ed.), *Handbook of child* psychology: Biology and infancy development (pp. 281–344). New York: Wiley.

Grattan, L. M., & Eslinger, P. J. (1992). Long-term psychological consequences of childhood frontal lobe lesion in patient DT. Brain and Cognition, 20, 185–195.

Greenough, W. T. (1976). Enduring brain effects of differential experience and training. In M. R. Rosenzweig & E. L. Bennett (Eds.), Neural mechanisms of learning and memory (pp. 255–278). Cambridge, MA: MIT Press.

Hebb, D. O. (1949). Organization of behavior. New York: Wiley.

Hécaen, H. (1976). Acquired aphasia in children and the ontogenesis of hemispheric functional specialization. Brain and Language, 3, 114–134.

Hubel, D. H., & Wiesel, T. N. (1970). The period of susceptibility to the physiological effects of unilateral eye closure in kittens. Journal of Physiology (London), 206, 419–436.

Huttenlocher, P. R. (1979). Synaptic density in human frontal cortex—Developmental changes and effects of aging. Brain Research, 163, 195–205.

Huttenlocher, P. R. (1984). Synapse elimination and plasticity in developing human cerebral cortex. American Journal of Mental Deficiency, 88, 488–496.

Huttenlocher, P. R. (1990). Morphometric study of human cerebral cortex development. Neuropsychologia, 28, 517–527.

Ingram, D. (1975). Motor asymmetries in young children. Neuropsychologia, 13, 95–102.

Jacobsen, M. (1978). Developmental neurobiology (2nd ed.). New York: Plenum Press.

Juraska, J. (1990). The structure of the rat cerebral cortex: Effects of gender and environment. In B. Kolb & R. Tees (Eds.), Cerebral cortex of the rat (pp. 483–506). Cambridge, MA: MIT Press.

Kennard, M. A. (1936). Age and other factors in motor recovery from precentral lesions in monkeys. American Journal of Physiology, 115, 138–146.

Kennard, M. A. (1940). Relation of age to motor impairment in man and in subhuman primates. Archives of Neurology and Psychiatry, 44, 377–397.

Kimura, D. (1963). Speech lateralization in young children as determined by an auditory test. Journal of Comparative and Physiological Psychology, 56, 899–902.

Knox, C., & Kimura, D. (1970). Cerebral processing of nonverbal sounds in boys and girls. Neuropsychologia, 8, 227–237.

Kolb, B. (1987). Factors affecting recovery from early cortical damage in rats. 1. Differential behavioral and anatomical effects of frontal lesions at different ages of neural maturation. Behavioral Brain Research, 25, 205–220.

Kolb, B. (1995). Brain plasticity and behavior. Hillsdale, NJ: Lawrence Erlbaum.

Kolb, B., & Fantie, B. (1989). Development of the child's brain and behavior. In C. R. Reynolds & E. Fletcher-Janzen (Eds.), Handbook of clinical child neuropsychology (pp. 17–39). New York: Plenum Press.

Kolb, B., & Gibb, R. (1993). Possible anatomical basis of recovery of function after neonatal frontal lesions in rats. Behavioral Neuroscience, 107, 799–811.

Kolb, B., & Taylor, L. (1981). Affective behavior in patients with localized cortical excisions: Role of lesion site and side. Science, 214, 89–91.

Kolb, B., & Taylor, L. (1990). Neocortical substrates of emotional behavior. In N. L. Stein, B. Levethal, & T. Trabasso (Eds.), Psychological and biological approaches to emotion (pp. 115–144). Hillsdale, NJ: Erlbaum.

Kolb, B., & Whishaw, I. Q. (1985). Neonatal frontal lesions in hamsters impair species-typical behaviors and reduce brain weight and neocortical thickness. Behavioral Neuroscience, 99, 691–706.

Kolb, B., & Whishaw, I. Q. (1996). Fundamentals of human neuropsychology (4th ed.). New York: Freeman.

Kolb, B., Wilson, B., & Taylor, L. (1992). Developmental changes in the recognition and comprehension of facial expression: Implications for frontal lobe function. Brain and Cognition, 20, 74–84.

Lecours, A. R. (1975). Myelogenetic correlates of the development of speech and language. In E. H. Lenneberg & E. Lenneberg (Eds.), Foundations of language development: A multidisciplinary approach (Vol. 1, pp. 121–135). New York: Academic Press.

Lenneberg, E. H. (1967). Biological foundations of language. New York: Wiley.

Lezak, M. D. (1995). Neuropsychological assessment (3rd ed.). New York: Academic Press.

Marcel, T., & Rajan, P. (1975). Lateral specialization for recognition of words and faces in good and poor readers. Neuropsychologia, 13, 489–497.

Marin-Padilla, M. (1970). Prenatal and early postnatal ontogenesis of the motor cortex: A Golgi study. 1. The sequential development of cortical layers. Brain Research, 23, 167–183.

Marin-Padilla, M. (1988). Early ontogenesis of the human cerebral cortex. In A. Peters & E. G. Jones (Eds.), Cerebral cortex (Vol. 7, pp. 1–34). New York: Plenum Press.

Michel, G. F. (1981). Right handedness: A consequence of infant supine head-orientation preference? Science, 212, 685–687.

Milner, B. (1964). Some effects of frontal lobectomy in man. In J. M. Warren & K. Akert (Eds.), The frontal granular cortex and behavior (pp. 313–334). New York: McGraw-Hill.

Milner, B. (1974). Sparing of language function after early unilateral brain damage. Neurosciences Research Program Bulletin, 12, 213–217.

Molfese, D. L., & Molfese, V. J. (1980). Cortical responses of preterm infants to phonetic and nonphonetic speech stimuli. Developmental Psychology, 16(6), 574–581.

Owens, R. E., Jr. (1984). Language development: An introduction. Columbus, OH: Charles E. Merrill Publishing.

Parnavelas, J. G., Papadopoulos, G. C., & Cavanagh, M. E. (1988). Changes in neurotransmitters during development. In A. Peters & E. G. Jones (Eds.), Cerebral cortex (Vol. 7, pp. 177–209). New York: Plenum Press.

Peiper, A. (1963). Cerebral function in infancy and childhood. New York: Consultants Bureau.

Peters, M., & Petrie, B. J. F. (1979). Functional asymmetries in the stepping reflex of human neonates. Canadian Journal of Psychology, 33, 198–200.

Piaget, J. (1952). *The origins of intelligence in children.* New York: Norton.

Poliakov, G. I. (1949). Structural organization of the human cerebral cortex during ontogenetic development. In S. A. Sarkisov, I. N. Filimonov, & N. S. Preobrazenskaya (Eds.), *Cytoarchitectonics of the cerebral cortex in man* (pp. 33–92). Moscow: Medgiz (In Russian).

Poliakov, G. I. (1961). Some results of research into the development of the neuronal structure of the cortical ends of the analyzers in man. *Journal of Comparative Neurology, 117,* 197–212.

Poliakov, G. I. (1965). Development of the cerebral neocortex during first half of intrauterine life. In S. A. Sarkosov (Ed.), *Development of the child's brain* (pp. 22–52). Leningrad: Medicina. (In Russian)

Purpura, D. P. (1974). Dendritic spine "dysgenesis" and mental retardation. *Science, 186,* 1126–1127.

Purpura, D. P. (1976). Structure–dysfunction relations in the visual cortex of preterm infants. In M. A. B. Braxier & F. Coceani (Eds.), *Brain dysfunction in infantile febrile convulsions* (pp. 223–240). New York: Raven Press.

Purpura, D. P. (1982). Normal and abnormal development of cerebral cortex in man. *Neurosciences Research Program Bulletin, 20*(4), 569–577.

Rakic, P. (1972). Mode of cell migration to the superficial layers of fetal monkey neocortex. *Journal of Comparative Neurology, 145,* 61–84.

Rakic, P. (1975). Timing of major ontogenetic events in the visual cortex of the rhesus monkey. In N. A. Buchwald & M. Brazier (Eds.), *Brain mechanisms in mental retardation* (pp. 3–40). New York: Academic Press.

Rakic, P. (1976). Prenatal genesis of connections subserving ocular dominance in the rhesus monkey. *Nature, 261,* 467–471.

Rakic, P. (1981). Developmental events leading to laminar and areal organization of the neocortex. In F. O. Schmitt, F. G. Worden, G. Adelman, & S. G. Dennis (Eds.), *The organization of the cerebral cortex* (pp. 7–8). Cambridge, MA: MIT Press.

Rakic, P. (1984). Defective cell-to-cell interactions as causes of brain malformations. In E. S. Gollin (Ed.), *Malformations of development—Biological and psychological sources and consequences* (pp. 239–285). New York: Academic Press.

Rasmussen, T., & Milner, B. (1975). Clinical and surgical studies of the cerebral speech areas in man. In K. J. Zulch, O. Creutzfeldt, & G. C. Galbraith (Eds.), *Cerebral localization* (pp. 238–257). Berlin: Springer-Verlag.

Rasmussen, T., & Milner, B. (1977). The role of early left-brain injury in determining lateralization of cerebral speech functions. *Annals of the New York Academy of Sciences, 299,* 355–369.

Robinson, R. J. (1966). Cerebral function in the newborn child. *Developmental Medicine and Child Neurology, 8,* 561–567.

St. James-Roberts, I. (1981). A reinterpretation of hemispherectomy data without functional plasticity of the brain. 1. Intellectual function. *Brain and Language, 13,* 31–53.

Segalowitz, S. J., & Rose-Krasnor, L. (1992). The construct of brain maturation in theories of child development. *Brain and Cognition, 20,* 1–7.

Sidman, R. L., & Rakic, P. (1973). Neuronal migration, with special reference to developing human brain: A review. *Brain Research, 62,* 1–35.

Smith, A. (1984). Early and long-term recovery from brain damage in children and adults: Evolution of concepts of localization, plasticity, and recovery. In C. R. Almli & S. Finger (Eds.), *Early brain damage: Research orientations and clinical observations* (pp. 299–324). New York: Academic Press.

Spreen, O., Tupper, D., Risser, A., Tuokko, H., & Edgell, D. (1984). *Human developmental neuropsychology.* London: Oxford University Press.

Stewart, J., & Kolb, B. (1994). Dendritic branching in cortical pyramidal cells in response to ovariectomy in adult female rats: Suppression by neonatal exposure to testosterone. *Brain Research, 654,* 149–154.

Stuss, D. T. (1992). Biological and psychological development of executive functions. *Brain and Cognition, 20,* 8–23.

Sutherland, R. J., Kolb, B., Schoel, M., Whishaw, I. Q., & Davies, D. (1982). Neuropsychological assessment of children and adults with Tourette syndrome: A comparison with learning disabilities and schizophrenia. In A. J. Freidhoff & T. N. Chase (Eds.), *Gilles de la Tourette syndrome* (pp. 311–322). New York: Raven Press.

Taylor, H. G. (1984). Early brain injury and cognitive development. In C. R. Almli & S. Finger (Eds.), *Early brain damage: Research orientations and clinical observations* (pp. 325–345). New York: Academic Press.

Teuber, H.-L. (1975). Recovery of function after brain injury in man. *Ciba Foundation Symposium, 34,* 159–186.

Thatcher, R. W. (1992). Cyclic cortical reorganization during early childhood. *Brain and Cognition, 20,* 24–50.

Turkewitz, G. (1977). The development of lateral differentiation in the human infant. *Annals of the New York Academy of Sciences, 299,* 213–221.

Twitchell, T. E. (1965). The automatic grasping responses of infants. *Neuropsychologia, 3,* 247–259.

Vargha-Khadem, F., & Polkey, C. E. (1992). A review of cognitive outcome after hemidecortication in humans. In F. D. Rose & D. A. Johnson (Eds.), *Recovery from brain damage* (pp. 137–168). New York: Plenum Press.

Vargha-Khadem, F., Watters, G., & O'Gorman, A. M. (1985). Development of speech and language following bilateral frontal lesions. *Brain and Language, 37,* 167–183.

Wada, J. A., Clarke, R., & Hamm, A. (1975). Cerebral hemispheric asymmetry in humans: Cortical speech zones in 100 adult and 100 infant brains. *Archives of Neurology 32,* 239–246.

Werker, J. F., & Tees, R. C. (1992). The organization and reorganization of human speech perception. *Annual Review of Neuroscience, 15,* 377–402.

Whishaw, I. Q., & Kolb, B. (1984). Neuropsychological assessment of children and adults with developmental dyslexia. In R. N. Malatesha & H. A. Whitaker (Eds.), *Dyslexia: A global issue* (pp. 375–404). The Hague: Nijhoff.

Williams, R. S., Ferrante, R. J., & Caviness, V. S., Jr. (1975). Neocortical organization in human cerebral malformation: A Golgi study. *Neuroscience Abstracts, 1,* 776.

Witelson, S. F. (1977). Early hemisphere specialization and interhemisphere plasticity: An empirical and theoretical review. In S. J. Segalowitz & F. A. Gruber (Eds.), *Language development and neurological theory* (pp. 213–287). New York: Academic Press.

Woods, B. T. (1980). The restricted effects of right-hemisphere lesions after age one; Wechsler test data. *Neuropsychologia, 18,* 65–70.

Woods, B. T., & Teuber, H.-L. (1973). Early onset of complementary specialization of cerebral hemispheres in man. *Transactions of the American Neurological Association, 98,* 113–117.

Yakovlev, P. E., & Lecours, A.-R. (1967). The myelogenetic cycles of regional maturation of the brain. In A. Minkowski (Ed.), *Regional development of the brain in early life.* Oxford: Blackwell.

3

Neurodevelopmental Anomalies and Malformations

GEORGE W. HYND, ALLISON E. MORGAN, AND MELANIE VAUGHN

Neuropsychologists frequently work with patients who have specified brain lesions that produce well-documented cognitive or behavioral effects. However, for those clinicians working with children or adolescents who suffer developmental disorders, the pathogenesis of cognitive and behavioral deficits may be poorly understood. This chapter reviews the anomalies of neurological development that not infrequently are seen in children and adolescents with developmental disorders. Most typically the neuropsychological manifestations of these anomalies impact on widely distributed functional systems, thus producing generalized and severe impairment. However, there are exceptions, especially with regard to anomalies of neuronal migration. Some basic understanding of these effects should aid neuropsychologists in a better conceptualization of how disorders of neurological development produce different effects than do discrete lesions of the central nervous system.

There is wide variability in neuroanatomical development and, unfortunately, there is still incomplete understanding of neurodevelopmental anomalies. Our ability to define these anomalies by pathogenesis or prognosis is greater than our ability to relate them to functional or behavioral deficits. Essentially three categories of anomalies can be specified: (1) those incompatible with life, (2) those not necessarily incompatible with life but

that severely impair functioning, and (3) those of variable consequences such that they can be asymptomatic or associated with subtle cognitive and behavioral deficits.

In this chapter, five general types of neurodevelopmental anomalies, as defined by pathogenesis, will be addressed: (1) bulk brain growth abnormalities, (2) cerebral hemisphere dysplasias, (3) cerebral cortex malformations, (4) congenital hydrocephalus and associated anomalies, and (5) neural tube abnormalities and fusion deficits.

Abnormalities in the Bulk Growth of the Brain

The usual brain-to-body weight ratio is 1:30, but there is great variability in brain bulk that can be caused by a wide range of factors. In the middle portions of the distribution, brain size is not typically correlated with functional differences. At the extreme ends of the distribution, as in the cases of micrencephaly and megalencephaly, there are associations between brain size and behavior (Hynd & Willis, 1988).

Micrencephaly

Micrencephaly is the term for small brain size with a brain-to-body weight ratio sometimes as little as 1:100. It is diagnosed when the head circumference is less than two or three standard deviations below the mean for age and gender. The term is of-

GEORGE W. HYND, ALLISON E. MORGAN, AND MELANIE VAUGHN • Center for Clinical and Developmental Neuropsychology, University of Georgia, Athens, Georgia 30602.

ten used interchangeably with microcephaly, which refers to a small head vault (Aicardi, 1992; Friede, 1989). Micrencephaly, however, is the preferred term because it specifies that the cause of the small head is an abnormally small brain or cerebral hemisphere (Friede, 1989).

Individuals with micrencephaly may have a small cranial vault in contrast to a near-normal face size, thickened scalp and cranial bones, and/or folded scalp. Frequently in cases of micrencephaly, the convolutional pattern of the brain is simplified with normal, or near-normal, sized gyri that are somewhat coarsened. The basal ganglia are usually of normal size and the cerebellum may appear disproportionately large (Friede, 1989). The brain tissue often has cytoarchitectonic anomalies. Males and females seem equally affected.

Micrencephaly is sometimes associated with epilepsy and moderate to severe retardation with delayed speech and motor function (Friede, 1989). Surprisingly, however, there are patients with normal intelligence (Hecht & Kelly, 1979). The deficits in autosomal recessive transmitted cases have been reported to be more severe than those in autosomal dominant transmitted cases (Haslam & Smith, 1979). The expected life span for individuals with micrencephaly varies, with some individuals surviving into adulthood but many others dying young because of intercurrent disease (Friede, 1975).

A variety of causal factors have been linked with micrencephaly. It can be produced experimentally by interfering with cell replication with the greatest damage seen when the interference occurs during the period of most active replication (Friede, 1989). Micrencephaly has been associated with radiation exposure. For example, Yamazaki and Schull (1990) reported that of 205 children who were exposed *in utero* to the Hiroshima bombing, 7 had microcephaly with mental retardation. Whereas mothers of only 4 nonmicrocephalic children were within 1200 m of the blast's center, the mothers of all 7 of these children were within this distance.

Winick and Rosso (1969) proposed a link between malnutrition and micrencephaly. In a study of individuals who died of malnutrition in their first year, the authors found that in comparison with normally nourished children, the fatalities had severe deficits in brain weight, protein, RNA, and DNA. The authors speculated that malnutrition disrupts cell division and migration and thus leads to small brains. However, other research, as reviewed by Hynd and Willis (1988), indicates that most cases of micrencephaly are probably not the result of mal-

nutrition because (1) moderate malnutrition seems to affect the maturation of myelinated cells rather than brain size, (2) the cerebellum may be most negatively impacted by malnutrition, and (3) rat studies have indicated that malnourishment does not slow the development of the brain to a significant extent. Friede (1989) suggests that it is difficult to test the malnutrition hypothesis because of the variability in normal human brain weights at autopsy.

Other proposed etiological factors include infection by rubella, toxoplasmosis, cytomegalic disease, and herpes simplex (Baron, Youngblood, Siewers, & Medeatis, 1969; South, Tompkins, Morris, & Rawls, 1969); prenatal exposure to toxins; and metabolic disorders such as phenylketonuria (McLone, 1982; Stevenson & Huntley, 1967). There is also evidence of a genetic basis for micrencephaly, perhaps related to an autosomal recessive gene, chromosomal deletions, trisomies (Hynd & Willis, 1988), or an autosomal dominant gene (Haslam & Smith, 1979).

In diagnosing micrencephaly it is important to distinguish between acquired and genetic micrencephaly. Neuroimaging is useful for finding evidence of brain damage leading to acquired micrencephaly, but the absence of this evidence does not necessarily indicate that the micrencephaly was not acquired. Prenatally, micrencephaly is difficult to diagnose unless there are associated malformations, and it is necessary to make multiple examinations of the entire skull shape (Aicardi, 1992).

Megalencephaly

Megalencephaly was first used to describe hyperplasia of the brain involving the overdevelopment of neural tissue (Fletcher, 1900). This consists of excessive neuronal and glial elements (Menkes, 1985). There is conflicting evidence as to whether or not cell size is abnormally large. The excess tissue may result from overproduction of neurons or from reduced neuronal death (Friede, 1989). In some cases, the brains weigh twice as much as expected for age and gender (Aicardi, 1992). Friede (1989) suggests that an adult brain weighing over 1600 g, with cerebrospinal fluid (CSF) drained and increases from edema and lesions excluded, is megalencephalic. More conservatively, Escourolle and Poirier (1973) reserve that diagnosis for brain weights over 1800 g.

Megalencephaly is sometimes used to refer to abnormally large brains that result from a variety of factors including astrocytomas, tuberous sclerosis, metabolic errors, or hydrocephalus. This is an inaccurate use of the term as the large brains in these instances are symptoms of another problem rather than the result of the overproduction of cerebral parenchyma (Hynd & Willis, 1988).

In infancy, megalencephaly may be apparent when a head of originally normal size grows more rapidly than ordinary, particularly in the first 4 months (DeMyer, 1972; Lorber & Priestley, 1981). Usually there is no specific disfigurement (Friede, 1989). In most cases, all sections of the brain are proportionately enlarged, whereas in others, all are abnormally large, but certain areas are enlarged disproportionately (Friede, 1989). Sectioning of a megalencephalic brain reveals normally sized ventricles and a corpus callosum that may or may not be enlarged. The cerebral cortex is often thicker and the underlying white matter is of greater volume than in normal brains. It is these differences that cause megalencephalic brains to be so large. Cytoarchitectonic structure is usually normal (Friede, 1989; Hynd & Willis, 1988).

There have been some unilateral cases of megalencephaly reported (e.g., Laurence, 1964) but most cases are bilateral. Some have suggested that unilateral megalencephaly may represent hemihypertrophy because some of the unilateral cases were found in association with a unilaterally large face, unilateral scalp hair excess, and unilaterally large extremities (Ward & Lerner, 1947).

Clinical implications of megalencephaly vary. It can be associated with mental retardation, seizures, and other neurological abnormalities (Aicardi, 1992; DeMyer, 1972; Hynd & Willis, 1988; Lorber & Priestley, 1981). In a study by Lorber and Priestley (1981), 13% of the megalencephalic children were mentally retarded or neurologically abnormal. In contrast, megalencephaly has also been associated with normal intelligence and even giftedness. In a study by Jakob (1927) of megalencephalic individuals with brain weights ranging from 1600 to 2850 g, 50 were gifted and 39 were mentally impaired. Clearly there is great variability in the effect megalencephaly has on cognitive abilities. Behavioral deficits associated with megalencephaly are typically related to deficient cognitive abilities (Hynd & Willis, 1988).

In characterizing true megalencephaly, it is important to rule out other possible causal factors for a large head size because some, like hydrocephalus, require medical attention. Lorber and Priestley (1981) examined 510 children with a head circumference greater than the 98th percentile and found that only 109 had primary megalencephaly with

normal pressure. DeMyer (1972) suggests that in making the differential diagnosis, the most important factor to consider is intracranial pressure.

There is some evidence for familial transmission of megalencephaly by both autosomal dominant and autosomal recessive mechanisms (DeMyer, 1972; Friede, 1989; Lorber & Priestley, 1981). The true incidence of megalencephaly is unknown, largely because asymptomatic cases are not reported (Hynd & Willis, 1988). There is a 4:1 male-to-female ratio (DeMyer, 1972; Lorber & Priestley, 1981). Table 1 summarizes the abnormalities of the bulk growth of the brain and other anomalies discussed in this chapter.

Dysplasias of the Cerebral Hemispheres

Holoprosencephaly

Holoprosencephaly results from a failure of the prosencephalon to cleave completely into two telencephalic hemispheres (Malamud & Hirano, 1974). This leaves a small forebrain containing a single ventricle (Evans, 1987). In the worst cases, the brain may weigh less than 100 g (Friede, 1989). The most severe form, alobar holoprosencephaly, is characterized by a completely undivided forebrain, little neocortex, fused thalami on the midline, and a well-developed brain stem and cerebellum (Aicardi, 1992). Holoprosencephaly is associated with abnormal facial features that in the most extreme cases can include cyclopia in which one or two eyeballs are contained in a partially fused orbit. Other orbitofacial anomalies include cebocephaly (nose is represented by a flattened bridge between the eyes with one or two nostrils), hypotelorism (close orbits), microphthalmia (narrowed eyelids), ethomocephaly (nose is replaced by proboscis with one or two nostrils), and cleft lip or palate (Birnholz, 1989; Evans, 1987; Friede, 1989; Hynd & Willis, 1988). There are also visceral deformities associated with holoprosencephaly including polydactyly and cardiac anomalies (Aicardi, 1992; Friede, 1975). To an extent, the severity of facial deformities is related to the extent of cerebral deformities, although the relationship is not perfect (Friede, 1989). Cases of semilobar holoprosencephaly, in which the brain is divided into hemispheres posteriorly, are associated with less severe or nonexistent facial abnormalities (Aicardi, 1992).

TABLE 1. Neurodevelopmental Malformations[a]

Malformation	Description	Clinical manifestations
Abnormalities of bulk growth		
Micrencephaly	Subnormal brain size associated with abnormally small head (<2 SD below mean for age and gender)	Size of face near normal; folded scalp, possibly epilepsy, and most typically intellectual retardation
Megalencephaly	Abnormally large brain from overproduction of cerebral parenchyma. Males > females	Associated with mental subnormality, normality, or hypothetically giftedness. Epilepsy may occur
Dysplasias of cerebral hemispheres		
Holoprosencephaly	Two hemispheres fail to develop. A large fluid-filled cavity results. No interhemispheric fissure present. 1:13,000 live births	Faciocerebral dysplasias, cebocephaly, apnea spells, severe mental retardation, hypotelorism, and other systemic deformities. Usually incompatible with life
Agenesis of the corpus callosum	Complete or partial failure of the corpus callosum to develop. Males > females	Occasionally asymptomatic or found in association with spina bifida, facial and ocular deformities, micrencephaly, and hydrocephalus. Epilepsy and mental retardation may occur
Malformations of the cerebral cortex		
Agyria/pachygyria	Smooth lissencephalic surface of brain. Few coarse gyri may be present	Commonly found in association with agenesis of corpus callosum, micrencephaly, epilepsy, severe mental retardation, and early death
Polymicrogyria	Development of many small gyri. Microscopically they may form an overlapping folded cortex	Found in association with learning disabilities (dyslexia), severe mental retardation, and epilepsy. Also appear asymptomatically
Focal dysplasia	Focal abnormalities in the cortical architecture usually consisting of disordered cells and layering of cortex	Reported in cases of epilepsy and learning disabilities (dyslexia)
Malformations associated with congenital hydrocephalus		
Dandy–Walker malformation	Malformation of the cerebellum associated with a dilation of the fourth ventricle. Males > females	Hydrocephalus, agenesis of the corpus callosum, Klippel–Feil and DeLange syndromes, and severe psychomotor retardation
Arnold–Chiari malformation	Congenital deformation of the brain stem and cerebellum	Congenital hydrocephalus, spina bifida, and severe psychomotor retardation
Stenosis of the aqueduct of Sylvius	Obstruction of the aqueduct and CSF circulation	Often insidious onset of symptoms associated with hydrocephalus. Shunted children may suffer learning/behavioral problems. Nonverbal IQ < Verbal IQ
Abnormalities of the neural tube and fusion defects		
Spina bifida occulta	Usually asymptomatic lesion discovered incidentally	Can be associated with lipoma, dermal sinuses, and dimples
Spina bifida cystica	Spinal defect that includes a cystic-like sac which may or may not contain the spinal cord	Hydrocephalus a frequent complication. Cognitive deficits related to extent of hydrocephalus. Arnold–Chiari malformation not uncommon
Cranium bifidum and encephalocele	Fusion defects of skull referred to as cranium bifidum; myelomeningoceles or meningoceles on the skull are referred to as encephaloceles. Males < females	Many associated difficulties with hydrocephalus including ataxia, cerebral palsy, epilepsy, and mental retardation
Anencephaly	Vault of skull absent and brain represented by vascular mass. Face is grossly normal. 1 male:4 female	Condition incompatible with life
Hydranencephaly	Cerebral hemispheres replaced by cystic sacs containing CSF	Difficult initially to distinguish from hydrocephalus. Hypnoatremia, eye movement disturbances, and death
Porencephaly	Large cystic lesion develops on the brain. May occur bilaterally or unilaterally	Occasionally asymptomatic but typically associated with mental retardation, epilepsy, and other neurodevelopmental malformations

[a]Modified and updated from Hynd and Willis (1988).

Holoprosencephaly has previously been called arhinencephaly under the terminology proposed by Kundrat (1882) who noted the frequent presence of aplasia of the olfactory bulbs and tracts. Since holoprosencephaly can occur with the presence of the olfactory bulb (Gilles, Leviton, & Dooling, 1983), the term arhinencephaly is now typically reserved for defects involving a primary olfactory bulb malformation (Friede, 1989). It is also possible to have olfactory aplasia in nonholoprosencephalic brains (Kobori, Herrick, & Urich, 1987).

The most severe cases of holoprosencephaly typically do not survive the neonatal period, and infants who do survive often develop seizures. The extent of neurological impairment varies, but mental retardation, usually severe, is always present (Aicardi, 1992). A semilobar patient described by Kobori et al. (1987) who lived until the age of $2\frac{1}{2}$ years had intact vision, hearing, and reflexes but failed to thrive and did not reach any developmental milestones. Rarely, however, some individuals survive into adulthood (Aicardi, 1992).

This abnormality develops within the fourth to sixth week of gestation during the period of embryogenesis when the hemispheres normally differentiate. There is some evidence from animal research that holoprosencephaly may result from exposure to neurotoxins (Hynd & Willis, 1988). Maternal diabetes may also be a risk factor (Barr et al., 1983; Kobori et al., 1987). There have been familial cases of holoprosencephaly reported in the literature suggesting the possibility of autosomal recessive inheritance (DeMyer, Zeman, & Palmer, 1963; Hintz, Menking, & Sotos, 1968). In cases of holoprosencephaly involving multiple extracephalic malformations, it is often associated with 13–15 trisomy. It is possible, however, to diagnose trisomy 13 in cases of holoprosencephaly not accompanied by extracephalic abnormalities (Verloes et al., 1991). Additionally, holoprosencephaly can occur in the absence of chromosomal irregularities (Friede, 1989; Verloes et al., 1991).

Verloes et al. (1991) reported on five unrelated children with holoprosencephaly, all of whom had a normal karyotype. The children had secondary facial abnormalities, visceral abnormalities, and polydactyly. They proposed that holoprosencephaly and the associated abnormalities in these cases and in other syndromes involving holoprosencephaly may result from an initial genetically determined disturbance altering brain development that leads to secondary developmental field defects. They proposed, based on this hypothesis and the fact that the true pathophysiology of these syndromes are uncertain, that holoprosencephaly "could be specific enough to justify the delineation of a provisionally 'new' syndrome" (p. 302). As of yet there is no validation of this notion.

Diagnosis of holoprosencephaly is fairly simple when accompanied by facial abnormalities. It can be diagnosed prenatally by ultrasonography from the 16th week of pregnancy. For antenatal diagnosis, orbital hypotelorism is the most reliable feature (Aicardi, 1992). In severe cases, Birnholz (1989) suggests that it can be diagnosed prenatally around the 9th week of gestation when the bony orbital margins are visible. In these cases, abnormal intracranial appearance and orbitofacial deformities provide evidence for diagnosis. Holoprosencephaly is estimated to occur in 1 of 13,000 births (Frutiger, 1969). The abnormality does not show gender preference (Friede, 1989; Hynd & Willis, 1988).

Agenesis of the Corpus Callosum

Agenesis of the corpus callosum is characterized by the complete or partial absence of the corpus callosum. In partial agenesis, typically the rostrum and genu are intact and the splenium and corpus are absent because of the anteroposterior direction in which the corpus callosum develops (Aicardi, 1992; Hynd & Willis, 1988). Usually the absent corpus callosum is replaced by two longitudinal bundles, called the longitudinal corpora callosa or Probst bundles (Aicardi, 1992). Usually the interhemispheric cortex is irregular in that the cingular gyrus may be missing and the gyral patterns are abnormal (Friede, 1989).

Agenesis of the corpus callosum may occur asymptomatically, and there is some evidence that a hypertrophied anterior commissure is involved in functional compensation (Fischer, Ryan, & Dobyns, 1992). It may also be found in association with other neurodevelopmental anomalies such as spina bifida, facial and ocular abnormalities, micrencephaly, megalencephaly, heterotopias, and hydrocephalus (Friede, 1989; Hynd & Willis, 1988; Jeret, Serur, Wisniewski, & Fisch, 1987). In some cases, it may be difficult to differentiate from holoprosencephaly (Aicardi, 1992). Epilepsy may be present, and mental retardation is frequently associated with callosal agenesis (Jeret et al., 1987).

In cases that appear asymptomatic, however, there are usually cognitive deficits. Selnes (1974) demonstrated that the corpus callosum is necessary for semantic–linguistic dominance to develop in the left hemisphere. Related to this finding, Dennis (1981) reported that acallosal individuals have difficulty on tasks involving syntactic–pragmatic ability and do poorly on semantic–linguistic information-processing tasks on suppressing ipsilateral input. These deficits are common in children with learning disabilities (e.g., Hynd & Obrzut, 1981; Hynd, Obrzut, Weed, & Hynd, 1979). Koeda and Takeshita (1993) described a 15-year-old acallosal, mentally retarded female who could write dictated sentences accurately but not read them, suggesting alexia. Sanders (1989) described a 6-year-old acallosal female who had deficits in syntactic comprehension because of a difficulty in assigning appropriate semantic roles to some sentence forms. Drake (1968) reported a thinned corpus callosum in the first reported autopsy of a learning-disabled individual. These findings lend support to speculation about the role of the corpus callosum in learning disabilities.

Most recently, Hynd et al. (1995) reported that the genu of the corpus callosum was significantly smaller in dyslexics and that area measurements of various regions correlated significantly with reading ability. These findings support the view that morphological variation in the corpus callosum may be related to cognitive deficits.

Other neuropsychological deficits have also been reported. One study reported that acallosal subjects were shown to respond more slowly, although they could perform the tasks successfully, than IQ-matched normal controls on tasks requiring inter- and intrahemispheric comparisons of visual and tactile stimuli (Lassonde, Sauerwein, McCabe, Laurencelle, & Geoffroy, 1988). Koeda and Takeshita (1993) reported on disconnection deficits in two patients with complete agenesis, mental retardation, and daily epileptic seizures. Specifically, they exhibited tactile naming disorder of the left hand. Importantly, the diagnostic process indicated the absence of amorphognosia and astereognosia which are gross sensory deficits rather than disconnection deficits. Although disconnection syndromes have not been commonly reported in cases of agenesis, the authors speculated that because of the severe impairments of the children, brain capacity and neural plasticity were insufficient to compensate for the absent corpus callosum.

In Chiarello's (1980) report on acallosal individuals, the 27 cases described had a mean verbal IQ of 89 (SD = 12.45). For the 25 cases for which both verbal and performance IQs were reported, the mean verbal IQ was 88.52 (SD = 12.58) and the mean performance IQ, 88.76 (SD = 15.75). These differences are not statistically significant. Hynd and Willis (1988) concluded from these studies that in cases where agenesis is incidentally discovered, general cognitive ability is approximately on standard deviation below normal. In addition, they noted that verbal scale IQ scores do not reflect the subtle neurolinguistic deficits present in these patients.

The prognosis of individuals with agenesis of the corpus callosum varies according to whether it is asymptomatic or whether it is associated with other deformities. Blum, André, Broullé, Husson, and Leheup (1990) found that of 12 infants diagnosed prenatally, 6 developed normally from age 2 to 8 years. Jeret et al. (1987) reported evidence suggesting that the life expectancy of acallosal males is greater than that of acallosal females.

Agenesis of the corpus callosum is diagnosed by neuroimaging. Angiography reveals the wandering appearance of the anterior cerebral artery which turns back on itself at the genu. "Batwing" or "butterfly" ventricles are evident in pneumoencephalograms. The disconnection of the cerebral hemispheres is also evident on CT and MRI scans (Hynd & Willis, 1988). Prenatal diagnosis is possible beginning at week 20 of gestation (Aicardi, 1992).

The disruption in embryogenesis is thought to occur between weeks 12 and 22 of gestation (Hynd & Willis, 1988). There is evidence for familial transmission of agenesis of the corpus callosum and autosomal recessive inheritance has been postulated (Dogan, Dogan, & Lovrencic, 1967; Menkes, Philippart, & Clark, 1964; Shapira & Cohen, 1973). There have also been suggestions of autosomal dominant inheritance (Aicardi, 1992) and X-linked transmission (Aicardi, 1992; Jeret et al., 1987; Vles et al., 1990). Further, agenesis has been associated with metabolic disorders of fetal (Bamforth, Bamforth, Poskitt, Applegarth, & Hall, 1988) and maternal origin (Aicardi, 1992) including fetal alcohol syndrome (Jeret et al., 1987; Wisniewski, Dambska, Sher, & Qazi, 1983). Figure 1 shows a brain with callosal agenesis.

Since agenesis of the corpus callosum is sometimes asymptomatic, the exact incidence is unknown. Although the incidence has been suggested to be 0.7%, Hynd and Willis (1988) note that the percentage of individuals with agenesis of the corpus callosum may be lower because the estimate was derived from a probably nonrepresentative population. Jeret, Serur, Wisniewski, and Fisch (1985–1986) reported an incidence of 2.3% among

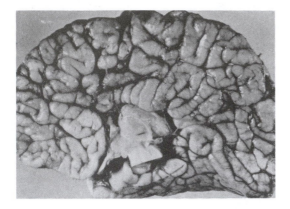

FIGURE 1. Agenesis of the corpus callosum. This sectioned brain shows the absence of the corpus callosum. Note the lack of a cingular gyrus.

a developmentally disabled population. There is evidence that it is more common among males (Jeret *et al.*, 1987).

Malformations of the Cerebral Cortex

Dysplasia, abnormal tissue growth, can occur in any region of the brain. Although it is likely that most instances of dysplasia are asymptomatic, dysplasias have been associated with behavioral and learning difficulties (Hynd & Semrud-Clikeman, 1989; Hynd & Willis, 1988). Dysplasias result from a disruption in neuronal migration. In the cases of agyria, pachygyria, and heterotopia, it has been speculated that they are variations of the same process that differ in severity (Friede, 1989). The review of radiologic and neuropathologic findings by Palmini *et al.* (1991) supported this theory. Similarly, a comparison of a child with generalized pachygyria, one with subcortical laminar heterotopias (or double cortex), and one with periventricular band heterotopia suggested to Palmini *et al.* (1993) that the pathogenesis for each of these disorders involves a disruption during the migration process, specifically neuron–glia interactions. They suggested that this disturbed interaction could lead to the halt of centrifugal neuronal movement as well as to failure of the neuron to detach from the glial guide when reaching the cortical plate. They hypothesized that the interaction of three factors—the period of migration during which injury occurred, degree of radial glial fiber involvement, and location of damage on

the glial fibers—determined the severity and site of the diffuse heterotopia.

Agyria (Lissencephaly) and Pachygyria

Agyria and lissencephaly are terms that have been used interchangeably. Owen (1868) originally used the term lissencephaly as a descriptor of brains in lower species that are smooth, flat, and unfolded. The term was later used to characterize brains that were malformed and lacked gyri. Agyria, however, is the preferable term because it refers specifically to the lack of gyri (Hynd & Willis, 1988).

Pachygyria, also called macrogyria, is used to describe brains with few gyri that are usually coarse and wide. Although agyria and pachygyria are sometimes used equivalently, it is better to distinguish between the two because they represent different levels of severity (Crome, 1956; Daube & Chou, 1966; McLone, 1982).

Children with agyria typically present with microencephaly, thickened skull (Hynd & Willis, 1988), bitemporal hollowing, and small jaw (Pavone, Gullotta, Incorpora, Grasso, & Dobyns, 1990). There are different pathological types with distinct clinical features as delineated by Aicardi (1992) and Pavone *et al.* (1990). Unilateral agyria has been reported (Hager *et al.*, 1991).

In classical agyria, the cerebral cortex is thick and the white matter is reduced. Kuchelmeister, Bergmann, and Gullotta (1993) reported a 4:1 gray-to-white matter ratio. The cortex typically consists of the following four layers (from top down): (1) cell-sparse, molecular layer; (2) superficial cellular layer containing a variety of cells, including large pyramidal cells usually found in layer five; (3) thin layer of white matter with no or few cells; and (4) thick bands of ectopic neurons (Aicardi, 1992; Friede, 1989).

In pachygyria, the extent of malformation is less severe and in layers two and four the expected small neurons are present (Aicardi, 1992). Both agyria and pachygyria often are accompanied by agenesis of the corpus callosum, suggesting that these anomalies occur during the first trimester of gestation (Friede, 1975). Jellinger and Rett (1976) suggest that agyria develops during weeks 11–13 of gestation and pachygyria, around week 13. Agyria is associated with postnatal microcephaly (Pavone, Rizzo, & Dobyns, 1993). A relationship between pachygyria and tuberous sclerosis has been reported (Sener, 1993).

Severe neurological problems are associated with agyria including severe mental retardation, motor retardation, diplegia, hypotonia, decere-brate posture, reduced spontaneous activity, and seizures (especially infantile spasms) (Aicardi, 1992; Friede, 1989; Hynd & Willis, 1988; Pavone *et al.*, 1990, 1993; Tachibana, 1990). Poor growth and feeding problems are also common (Pavone *et al.*, 1993). Interestingly, Barkovich, Koch, and Carrol (1991) reported, based on a study of ten patients, that the clinical manifestations did not appear to correlate with the severity of agyria. The cognitive and behavioral manifestations in pachygyria are less severe, although severe mental retardation and seizures are still common (Hynd & Willis, 1988).

Most infants with agyria die before the age of 2 (Friede, 1989; Hynd & Willis, 1988; Palmini *et al.*, 1991). These children often die of intercurrent disease. Respiratory infections, including pneumonia, are common (Pavone *et al.*, 1993). Münchoff and Noetzel (1965), however, described a child who lived until age 6 and Kuchelmeister *et al.* (1993) reported on a patient who reached age 20. The expectancies for individuals with pachygyria are better. Palmini *et al.* (1993) described a 7-year-old female who, while developmentally delayed and epileptic, was able to attend, with difficulties, a special first grade class. Aicardi (1992) reports that he has had patients with pachygyric brains who survived into adulthood, could walk, and had limited language abilities.

Diagnoses of agyria and pachygyria are made through neuroimaging techniques (i.e., CT, MRI). Agyria can be recognized in neonates and young infants through ultrasonography, but the diagnosis of pachygyria is more difficult and usually requires CT or MRI. In addition, EEG abnormalities associated with agyria and pachygyria can contribute to diagnostic decisions (Aicardi, 1992).

As noted previously, agyria and pachygyria are the result of arrested or disrupted neuronal migration. In the schema developed by Palmini *et al.* (1993), diffuse pachygyria results from an early injury (before most neurons have arrived at the cortex and thus providing insufficient material to form gyral patterns) and severe and distal radial glial fiber damage. In agyria, the disruption occurs earlier. Palmini *et al.* (1991), following a model proposed by Richman and colleagues, propose that in cases of agyria, most neurons are heterotopic which does not allow the availability of the amount of neurons necessary for gyration.

A variety of factors have been suggested to cause the disrupted migration. Aicardi (1992) sug-gests that most cases of agyria are sporadic but that there have been some cases indicating dominant inheritance. Pavone *et al.* (1990) found evidence of autosomal recessive inheritance and the possibility of X-linked recessive inheritance. When agyria is part of the Miller–Dieker syndrome, it is thought to result from a chromosomal microdeletion. Postconceptional factors perhaps responsible for the development of agyria or pachygyria are ischemia or viral infection (Pavone *et al.*, 1990) including congenital cytomegalovirus (Hayward, Titelbaum, Clancy, & Zimmerman, 1991). The incidence and gender ratios for agyria and pachygyria are unknown (Hynd & Willis, 1988).

Focal Dysplasia/Heterotopia

Heterotopia is the term used to describe the presence of ectopic gray matter in the cerebral hemispheres. It is thought to be on the other end of the continuum from agyria (Palmini *et al.*, 1993). In laminar heterotopias, the gray matter appears as symmetrical ribbons in the centrum semiovale (Friede, 1989). In pure cases of laminar heterotopia, called generalized band or "double" cortex heterotopia, the gray matter is continuous under the cortical surface and appears like a double cortex. The gray matter is most noticeable in the frontocentroparietal regions, but is typically found throughout the neocortex (Palmini *et al.*, 1991). Although there may be slightly fewer gyri than normal, the cortex is usually not malformed. Nodular heterotopias are characterized by clustered masses of gray matter in irregularly formed nodules that are separated by thin myelinated fibers. They are usually located near the lateral ventricles (Friede, 1989; Hynd & Willis, 1988).

Laminar heterotopia is usually associated with few, if any, deficits (Hynd & Willis, 1988), but it has occasionally been associated with epilepsy and mental retardation (Miura *et al.*, 1993; Palmini *et al.*, 1991, 1993; Ricci, Cusmai, Fariello, Fusco, & Vigevano, 1992). One 6-year-old female with double cortex syndrome was described as slightly developmentally delayed, clumsy, easily upset, and as having poor impulse control. It was unclear whether or not she was epileptic. Her daily living appeared to be affected only slightly by her cortical anomalies (Hashimoto, Seki, Takuma, & Suzuki, 1993). Palmini *et al.* (1993) note that while there may be a relationship between the extent of the migration deficit and clinical manifestations, the severity of epilepsy and retardation among patients may depend on the type of epileptic syndrome that develops. The severity of mental retardation is also thought to be related to the extent the cortex over the heterotopia is disorganized (Palmini *et al.*, 1991).

Nodular heterotopias, in small numbers, are usually asymptomatic (Aicardi, 1992; Hynd & Willis, 1988). They may be associated, however, with malformations such as agenesis of the corpus callosum and micrencephaly (Friede, 1989). Focal dysplasias have also been found in the brains of dyslexic individuals (Galaburda, Sherman, Rosen, Aboitiz, & Geschwind, 1985). Hynd and Willis (1988) speculate that the distribution and severity of focal dysplasias may dictate whether cortical arousal, learning, or attention is negatively impacted. Life expectancy depends on associated clinical features and can be normal (Palmini *et al.*, 1991).

Diagnosis of heterotopias is made through neuroimaging. In making the diagnosis, it is important to differentiate them from the tubers of tuberous sclerosis which they may resemble and with which they may be associated (Aicardi, 1992).

As with agyria and pachygyria, focal heterotopias are thought to develop from disrupted neuronal migration. It has been suggested that the disruption does not completely terminate neuronal migration at a certain point. Instead, only some waves of migration are unsuccessful. In the double cortex syndrome, the superficial layers receive close to the normal number of neurons so that gyration is possible (Palmini *et al.*, 1991). Palmini *et al.* (1993) propose that in heterotopia the migration is arrested late in the process and that radial glial fiber damage is mild and distal.

The etiology for the disrupted migration is uncertain. There are reports, however, of familial cases of double cortex syndrome, suggesting a possible genetic basis (Palmini *et al.*, 1991). In the examination of ten patients with "double cortex" described by Palmini *et al.* (1991), it was found that maternal drug ingestion occurred in two mothers and X-ray exposure occurred in a third, leading to the conclusion that these teratogens may have been related to disrupted neuronal migration. Fever, lasting one or more days before weeks 4 and 14 of gestation, has also been implicated (Pleet, Graham, & Smith, 1981). The incidence of focal dysplasias is unknown. There is some limited evidence, however, that they may occur more frequently in males than in females (Hynd & Willis, 1988).

Polymicrogyria

Polymicrogyria is characterized by crowded, small gyri, in an atypical convolutional pattern (Aicardi, 1992; Friede, 1989; Hynd & Willis, 1988). However, at gross inspection, there does not always appear to be an excessive number of gyri. Instead it may appear to be pachygyria (Byrd, Osborn, & Radkowski, 1991) because the gyri are not separated as a result of the fusion of molecular layers (Aicardi, 1992; Friede, 1989). The extent of polymicrogyria may not be evident until sectioning (Hynd & Willis, 1988). Polymicrogyria can cover the entire cortex unilaterally or bilaterally. They are more commonly localized, however, around arterial territories, and porencephalic or hydranencephalic areas (Aicardi, 1992; Friede, 1989). Brain weight may be reduced (Friede, 1989). Polymicrogyria may co-occur with other abnormalities including cellular heterotopias, agenesis of the corpus callosum, signs of fetal infection, and cortical and vascular anomalies (Aicardi, 1992; Friede, 1989).

The clinical manifestations of polymicrogyria vary. It has been found incidentally in the autopsies of individuals without neurological impairment, and small areas are usually asymptomatic (Aicardi, 1992; Hynd & Willis, 1988). It has also been found in association with severe mental retardation (Crome, 1960; Malamud, 1964), learning disabilities (Galaburda & Kemper, 1979; Galaburda *et al.*, 1985), seizures, and bilateral or unilateral neurological signs (Aicardi, 1992). Cohen, Campbell, and Yaghmai (1989) reported on a 7-year-old girl with developmental dysplasia who died of mononucleosis. Figure 2 shows a microgyria from her brain that was found in the language-related cortex. Life expectancies vary according to associated anomalies, but the evidence does not suggest that polymicrogyria is incompatible with a normal life span.

Diagnosing polymicrogyria is extremely difficult, if possible, even with the use of neuroimaging (Aicardi, 1992). Byrd *et al.* (1991) reported that 25% of the children they examined with polymicrogyria had MRI findings resembling pachygyria and that the polymicrogyria was revealed through histological studies.

The evidence suggests that rather than resulting from a disruption in neuronal migration, polymicrogyria develops postmigration and is the product of a disturbance of cortical gyration around the fifth and sixth months of gestation (Aicardi, 1992; Friede, 1989). The precipitating events may include severe trauma, carbon monoxide intoxica-

A

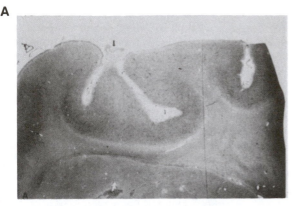

B

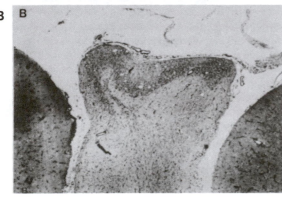

FIGURE 2. Microgyrus. (A) Section of the left insular cortex showing dysplastic microgyrus (arrow) adjacent to normal gyri. (B) Detail of the dysplastic gyrus. (From Cohen, Campbell, & Yaghmai, with permission.)

tion, maternal asphyxia, perfusion failure, and intrauterine infections (Aicardi, 1992; Hynd & Willis, 1988). There is also evidence of genetic transmission (Andermann, Palmini, Andermann, Tampieri, & Leonard, 1992). The incidence and gender ratios for polymicrogyria are unknown (Hynd & Willis, 1988).

Hydrocephalus and Associated Malformations

Hydrocephalus

Hydrocephalus results from excess CSF in the ventricles. It can develop through intra- or extraventricular obstruction of flow, excessive CSF production, or loss of brain tissue (Chervenak, 1989).

Hydrocephalus can have a variety of damaging effects on the cortex and underlying white matter of the developing brain, including (1) stretching and disruption of neural tracts, particularly long fiber tracts; (2) shifting of the internal capsule, which may contribute to motor difficulties; (3) atrophy of white matter; (4) stretched or extremely thin cortex; and (5) disruption of corpus callosum myelination. Congenital malformations are causally associated with hydrocephalus, particularly the Dandy–Walker malformation, the Arnold–Chiari malformation, and stenosis of the aqueduct of Sylvius (Dyken & Miller, 1980). In one study, approximately 37% of the hydrocephalic infants had congenital deficits not related to hydrocephalus among which trachosophageal fistula and genitourinary, cardiac, and multiple anomalies were most common (Wiswell, Tuttle, Northam, & Simonds, 1990). Ocular abnormalities, motor deficits, and seizures are also often associated with hydrocephalus (Dennis *et al.*, 1981).

Prior to the development of shunting, which transports CSF from the ventricular system or subarachnoid space to another area where it can be absorbed, the prognosis for hydrocephalus was very poor. Reporting on 182 unoperated cases of fetal hydrocephalus, Laurence and Coates (1962) computed survival estimates into adult life as falling between 20 and 23%. In a study by Raimondi and Soare (1974) of 200 shunted infants, only 9 died, with a mean age at death of 38 months.

In the Raimondi and Soare (1974) study, the mean IQ for 29 white infants with hydrocephalus was 84.5, SD = 25.8. This is approximately one standard deviation below average intelligence but within the normal range. For the total group of 50 hydrocephalic children (white and black), the mean IQ was 71.7, SD = 30.3. This IQ score approaches the range of mental retardation. The hydrocephalic children with associated problems, specifically porencephaly or Dandy–Walker cyst, had much lower IQs. McCullough and Balzer-Martin (1982) reported that the mean IQ of 37 shunted children was 96, SD = 22. Approximately two-thirds of the children in their study had normal or borderline IQs. Similarly, the average intelligence of children with uncomplicated hydrocephalus was reported to be 108 in another study (Shurtleff, Foltz, & Loeser, 1973). The average IQ of 78 hydrocephalic children in a study by Dennis *et al.* (1981) was 90.80, SD = 13.34. Some cases of superior intelligence in shunted children have been reported (Lorber, 1968). These studies indicate that in uncomplicated

cases of hydrocephalus treated with shunting, mental impairment is not necessarily an associated clinical feature.

Dennis *et al.* (1981) reported verbal intelligence as being superior to nonverbal intelligence in hydrocephalic individuals. They suggest that nonverbal intelligence is impaired, even with the benefits of shunting, for several reasons. First, the biomechanical effects of hydrocephalus damage some regions of the brain more than others. In children with intraventricular hydrocephalus, there is an asymmetric cortex thinning in the anteroposterior direction leading to greater thinning in the vertex and occipital regions. This has a negative impact on the development of nonverbal intelligence. Additionally, they proposed that associated deficits such as disturbed visual function, motor deficits, and seizures may further impair the development of nonverbal intelligence.

Of interest, Fernell, Gillberg, and von Wendt (1991) reported that when hydrocephalus was not associated with mental retardation, hydrocephalic children did not exhibit significantly more behavior problems than control children. Hydrocephalic children with mental retardation, however, had significantly more behavior problems, particularly inattentiveness and hyperactivity, than hydrocephalic children without mental retardation and controls.

Hydrocephalus can be diagnosed prenatally through the use of sonography. Chervenak (1989) notes that the ability to measure the ventricles is particularly helpful because the ventricles often dilate before the cranium enlarges. In children below the age of 2, hydrocephalus can usually be diagnosed easily. The skull volume develops rapidly and the child may be developmentally delayed. Ocular symptoms are also associated with hydrocephalus (Aicardi, 1992).

A variety of etiological factors may lead to hydrocephalus including meningitis and arachnoid fibrosis, subdural hematoma, cysts, vascular anomalies, tumors, and major cerebral dysplasias (Milhorat, 1982). Hydrocephalus is often associated with other abnormalities, such as spina bifida, and its exact incidence is thus unknown. As a congenital disorder, its incidence has been estimated to range from 0.9 to 1.5 per 1000 births (Milhorat, 1982). In a study of 763,364 live and stillborn infants born in U. S. Army hospitals from 1971 through 1987, 370 had hydrocephalus (0.48 per 1000 births). The population characteristics of the sample were similar to the United States as a whole. There were no significant racial differences found

or seasonal or yearly trends in incidence. There were significantly more males diagnosed than females and hydrocephalus was significantly more common among births in the Pacific region (South Korea and Hawaii) than in the other four regions examined (Europe, East Coast, Midwest, and West Coast) (Wiswell *et al.,* 1990).

Dandy–Walker Malformation

Three characteristics are typical of the Dandy–Walker malformation: (1) distension of the fourth ventricle; (2) complete or partial agenesis of the vermis; and (3) enlarged posterior fossa with vertical displacement of lateral sinuses, tentorium, and torcular. The cortex may be nonfoliated. The lateral ventricles, as they converge with the sagittal sinus, form an inverted Y shape (Friede, 1989). At one time, the Dandy–Walker syndrome was thought to be the same as atresia of the cerebellum which refers to the absence or closure of the cerebellum. It became evident, however, that atresia of the cerebellum is not an essential component of the Dandy–Walker malformation (Hynd & Willis, 1988). Benda (1954) suggested the term Dandy–Walker malformation to distinguish it as a separate entity.

The occipital region in children with the Dandy–Walker malformation is prominent which helps to distinguish them from children with hydranencephaly, aqueductal stenosis, or meningomyelocele which is associated with the Arnold–Chiari malformation (Hynd & Willis, 1988). Congenital anomalies that sometimes co-occur with the malformation include aqueductal stenosis, agenesis of the corpus callosum, craniofacial deformities, Klippel–Feil syndrome, Cornelia DeLange syndrome, polydactyly, syndactyly, and cytoarchitectonic irregularities (Evans, 1987; Friede, 1989; Hart, Malamud, & Ellis, 1972; Hynd & Willis, 1988). More than 80% of individuals with the Dandy–Walker malformation have early signs of hydrocephalus (Friede, 1989) although it is not usually present at birth (Hirsch, Pierre-Kahn, Renier, Sainte-Rose, & Hoppe-Hirsch, 1984).

Associated neurological deficits include mental retardation, slow motor development, cranial nerve palsies, nystagmus, and truncal ataxia. Mental retardation is usually pronounced (Hynd & Willis, 1988). In a study by Raimondi and Soare (1974), the mean IQ for hydrocephalic children with the Dandy–Walker malformation was 48.3. Most individuals survive past the first year without shunting and some survive into adulthood (Friede,

1989). Among 144 cases reviewed by Hirsch *et al.* (1984), the mortality rate was 27%. Approximately half of the survivors, however, had a normal IQ.

Diagnosis is usually not difficult if the child presents with the three classic symptoms (Friede, 1989). In approximately 80% of cases it is not diagnosed, however, until after the first birthday when hydrocephalus is evident (Aicardi, 1992).

Some have suggested that the Dandy–Walker malformation results from a developmental arrest in the hindbrain occurring sometime before the third month of gestation with persistence of the fourth ventricle's anterior membranous area. The malformation has been found among siblings (Friede, 1989) suggesting some familial–congenital mechanisms of transmission. Incidence is unknown (Hynd & Willis, 1988). Gender ratios may be equal (Friede, 1989) but some evidence suggests that males may outnumber females (Hynd & Willis, 1988).

Arnold–Chiari Malformation

The Arnold–Chiari malformation is characterized by brain stem and cerebellar deformities that crowd the hindbrain. Cleland (1883) first described this syndrome and illustrated the herniation of the vermis, the malformed medulla, and other brain stem abnormalities. Chiari (1891, 1896) further described the malformation and distinguished between three types: I, a syndrome involving herniation of the cerebellar tonsils; II, a syndrome now called the Arnold–Chiari malformation; and III, a syndrome involving cervical spina bifida with cerebellar encephalocele. Arnold (1894) reported on an infant with a ribbonlike cerebellar herniation. Thus, the term Arnold–Chiari malformation was introduced by Schwalbe and Gredig (1907) in an attempt to address the brain stem abnormalities described by Chiari and the cerebellar herniation described by Arnold.

Cranial bone and cervical spine anomalies are a component of the syndrome. The brain stem and cerebellum are downwardly displaced and are tightly crowded. Cranial projection and elongation of the cranial nerves occurs because of the brain stem's caudal displacement. Cerebellar tissue herniates into the cervical spinal cord. The brain stem is deformed as the dorsal part of the medulla oblongata, the fourth ventricle, and the choroid plexus are shifted dorsally. The caudal end of the fourth ventricle and its choroid plexus are shifted into the spinal canal where they frequently form a pouch in which herniated cerebellar tissue may enter. Cases vary as to whether malformations of the vermis and medulla are equally prominent or if one type of deformity is more pronounced. There are additional malformations of posterior fossa structures (Friede, 1989).

The most consistent symptoms are increased intracranial pressure and hydrocephalus (Friede, 1989). Ford (1926) reported that of 100 cases of infantile hydrocephalus, 16 were caused by the Arnold–Chiari malformation. It is also associated with lumbrosacral spina bifida and myelomeningocele (Hynd & Willis, 1988). The Arnold–Chiari malformation can occur, however, in the absence of spina bifida, and hydrocephalus in spina bifida can be produced by other causes (Friede, 1989). Children with the Arnold–Chiari malformation frequently have severe psychomotor retardation (Hynd & Willis, 1988). It is not, however, necessarily incompatible with normal intelligence. McCullough and Balzer-Martin (1982) reported the mean IQ of four children with Arnold–Chiari myelodysplasia to be 110.

Four classes of hypotheses exist to explain the pathogenesis of the syndrome: (1) downward traction (from the myelomeningocele anchoring the bottom portion of the spinal cord); (2) pressure from above (as the result of congenital hydrocephalus); (3) a primary dysgenesis of the brain stem; and (4) a primary malformation of the basicranium (Friede, 1989). Friede (1989) suggests that the fourth class of hypotheses is most tenable. Incidence and gender ratios are unknown (Hynd & Willis, 1988).

Stenosis of the Aqueduct of Sylvius

Stenosis of the aqueduct of Sylvius refers to the obstruction of the aqueduct and CSF circulation. The aqueduct is the most commonly blocked CSF pathway because it is the longest and most narrow (Friede, 1989). The blockage can occur through the following four mechanisms: (1) narrowing caused by congenital factors; (2) a thin membrane lying on the aqueduct; (3) narrowing resulting from pressure by an adjacent tumor; and (4) a herniation of the cerebellum and shifting of the fourth ventricle as found in the Arnold–Chiari malformation (Hynd & Willis, 1988).

Stenosis of the aqueduct of Sylvius is a common cause of hydrocephalus. For example, Elvidge (1966) found that of 44 hydrocephalic children, 13 had aqueductal stenosis. In 100 cases of infantile hydrocephalus, Ford (1926) found that 14 had aqueduct stenosis alone.

The symptoms of stenosis are those of hydro-cephalus. A study by Dennis *et al.* (1981) revealed that the mean Full Scale IQ of children with aque-ductal stenosis was 86.73, SD = 14.99, which is slightly less than one standard deviation below average intelligence. However, these children had significantly better verbal than performance skills as indicated by a 20-point discrepancy between scale scores.

There are reports of several familial forms of aqueductal stenosis (Bickers & Adams, 1949; Drachman & Richardson, 1961; Edwards, Norman, & Roberts, 1961; Shannon & Nadler, 1968; Warren, Lu, & Ziering, 1963). Incidence and gender ratios are unknown (Hynd & Willis, 1988).

Abnormalities of the Neural Tube and Fusion Deficits

Spina Bifida

Spina bifida has long been recognized and it is thought that Hippocrates and medieval Arab physi-cians noted the defect (Reigel, 1982). It is a defect that occurs because of the failure of the caudal por-tion of the developing neural tube to fuse properly (Hynd & Willis, 1988). The lesions involve malfor-mations of both the vertebral column and the spinal cord (Friede, 1989). Since dermal development is related to neural tube development, there may be as-sociated malformations of the skin, vertebrae, and soft tissues (Evans, 1987).

The degree of severity of spina bifida varies with some cases being found incidentally and others being associated with so many other anom-alies that it leads to early death (Hynd & Willis, 1988). The most severe form is cranioarchischisis totalis in which the nervous system is completely open (Evans, 1987). Associated anomalies include skeletal, gastrointestinal, pulmonary, craniofacial, cardiovascular, and genitourinary anomalies (Hynd & Willis, 1988). Wiswell *et al.* (1990) reported that of 526 cases of spina bifida, 22% had additional congenital anomalies, of which gastrointestinal, genitourinary, and cardiac malformations were most common.

In spina bifida occulta, the neural structures do not herniate and are covered by skin (Aicardi, 1992). The tissue over the lesion is often normal and the defect is frequently discovered only incidentally via X ray (Hynd & Willis, 1988). There may be one

or more lesions and the defect may be associated with lipoma, dimples, and congenital dermis si-nuses (Anderson, 1975; James & Lassman, 1981). It is often asymptomatic, but it may be accompanied by pain, foot deformities, abnormal gait, abnormal reflexes, shortening of one leg, and incontinence (James & Lassman, 1972). In this case, hydro-cephalus is not an associated problem (Aicardi, 1992). Individuals with uncomplicated lesions have a slightly increased incidence of occult intraspinal lesions (Reigel, 1982).

Spina bifida cystica involves a vertebral de-fect and a visible cystic lesion on the back. In myelomeningocele, part of the spinal cord is in-volved in the cyst (Friede, 1989; Hynd & Willis, 1988). Eighty to ninety percent of the lesions oc-cur in the lumbosacral region. The lesion may not correspond with the bone malformation (Friede, 1989). Aicardi (1992) distinguishes between myelomeningocele and myeloschisis in that in the former the lesion is bulging while in the latter the lesion is flat.

Myelomeningoceles are associated with a variety of neurological deficits particularly when located in the lumbosacral region. Deficits may in-clude unresponsiveness to pain and temperature, incontinence, flaccid paralysis, and weakness of the lower extremities. Foot deformities may also co-occur (Friede, 1989). The severity and location of the lesion determine the pattern of deficits (Evans, 1987). Approximately 70% of children with myelomeningoceles have the Arnold–Chiari malformation (Aicardi, 1992). Complications in-clude meningitis, hydrocephalus, and pneumonia (Friede, 1989).

Laurence and Tew (1971) reported that with-out modern surgical treatment, life expectancy to age 11 was 12.8%. With the improvements in the in-terventions for hydrocephalus as discussed previ-ously and surgical interventions specific to spina bifida, however, the prognosis has improved. In the past 80 years, mortality has been reduced from about 50% to 10% (Hynd & Willis, 1988).

There are cognitive deficits associated with co-morbid hydrocephalus. Cull and Wyke (1984) re-ported that the mean IQ of ten children with surgically treated spina bifida and hydrocephalus was 76. Compared with IQ-matched controls, they were significantly less skilled in recalling lists of unrelated words. Interestingly, however, they were not significantly different from children with nor-mal intelligence or matched controls in their recall of meaningful verbal material in the form of a short story. This pattern of performance suggested to the authors that these children may be impaired at using appropriate semantic strategies when encoding. The three groups were equal in their performance on a pictorial memory test. This is inconsistent with the finding of Dennis *et al.* (1981) that hydrocephalic children had better-developed verbal abilities than nonverbal abilities. Hynd and Willis (1988) suggest that the discrepancy between the results is likely related to the confounding effect of general ability.

A variety of etiological factors pertaining to maternal health have been suggested. These include fevers, viruses, hormonal and ovulatory changes, folic acid and zinc deficiencies, and maternal diabetes (Friede, 1989; Hynd & Willis, 1988). Suspected teratogens include alcohol, hypervitaminosis A, and valproic acid (an anticonvulsant) (Friede, 1989; Hynd & Willis, 1988). There is also evidence that chromosomal anomalies and genetic susceptibility sometimes play an etiological role (Friede, 1989).

Screening for spina bifida can take place prenatally through analysis of α-fetoprotein (AFP) levels—preferably during weeks 16 to 18 of gestation. At this time, the levels in open spina bifida pregnancies are usually four times greater than in nonaffected pregnancies. Closed lesions cannot be detected biochemically. Ultrasound can be used to identify the spina bifida lesion (Wald & Cuckle, 1992).

The incidence of spina bifida varies by the type of lesion. Since spina bifida occulta is asymptomatic, it is difficult to ascertain its incidence. Reigel (1982) has estimated that it may occur in 20 to 30% of the population but a true incidence this high seems unlikely. In one study, 1172 routine radiological examinations of autopsied individuals revealed that 5% had spina bifida occulta (James & Lassman, 1972). This latter estimate of incidence seems more likely.

Alter (1962) reported the incidence of spina bifida cystica to be 0.7 per 1000 live births. Wiswell *et al.* (1990), in their 17-year epidemiological study of U. S. Army hospital births, reported an incidence of 0.68 per 1000 when cases of spina bifida occulta and meningoceles were excluded. They noted a significant decline in the incidence of spina bifida among female infants from 1971 through 1987.

There are significant geographic variations in the incidence of spina bifida with the British Isles having the highest incidence. India, China, and parts of the Middle East are also high-risk areas. In contrast, Japan, Hong Kong, and countries in north and sub-Saharan Africa have low rates (Little & Elwood, 1992a). However, in the Wiswell *et al.* (1990)

study, no geographic variation for spina bifida was found. Several studies have provided evidence that spina bifida is less common in blacks than in whites (Little & Elwood, 1992b). For example, Wiswell *et al.* (1990) reported that white infants and infants of other races were more likely to have spina bifida than black infants. It is also more common among children born of low-socioeconomic-status mothers and those at the extreme ages for childbearing (Chervenak & Isaccson, 1989). There are also sex differences in spina bifida with it being slightly more common in females. Approximately 56% of individuals with spina bifida in Canada and the United States are females (Elwood & Little, 1992).

Cranium Bifidum and Encephalocele

Cranium bifidum is a fusion defect of the skull that typically affects the midline sutures. Lesions not containing tissue are called cranial meningoceles and are rare (Aicardi, 1992; Friede, 1989). Lesions that contain cerebral tissue are referred to as encephaloceles (Friede, 1989). Approximately 10% of myelomeningoceles fit this description (Eckstein, 1983). They are most frequently found in the occipital region and are less commonly found in the frontal region. Frontal encephaloceles typically involve some frontal lobe tissues as well as olfactory tissue (Friede, 1989). Lesions in the frontal and nasopharyngeal regions are often associated with holoprosencephaly, agenesis of the corpus callosum, and ocular hypertelorism (Hynd & Willis, 1988). Encephaloceles are rare at other midline locations (Friede, 1989).

The extent of herniation is not necessarily correlated with the size of swelling (Hynd & Willis, 1988). Encephaloceles are not usually associated with a primary skin deficit although ulcerated skin may develop. Tissue within the encephalocele connects with usually just one cerebral hemisphere through glial tissue. Encephaloceles affect the shape of the brain with the attached hemisphere usually being smaller and the contralateral hemisphere extending past the midline. This sometimes distorts cranial nerves, cerebral arteries, and the hypothalamus. Gyri radiate from the site of the encephalocele and the lateral ventricles are deformed (Friede, 1989).

Encephaloceles are sometimes associated with agenesis of the corpus callosum (Friede, 1989). Wiswell *et al.* (1990) reported that 40% of newborns with encephaloceles had additional congenital anomalies. Among their sample, they most frequently found multiple anomalies, cleft lip and palate, and limb defects.

Hydrocephalus sometimes develops. Clinical manifestations related to hydrocephalus include mental retardation, ataxia, cerebral palsy, epilepsy, and visual–perceptual problems (Hynd & Willis, 1988), Of 45 patients with encephaloceles and hydrocephalus described by Lorber (1967), only 4 had IQs in the normal range and only 20 survived. Surgery to remove occipital encephaloceles somewhat improves the prognosis. In one study that followed patients approximately 9 years after the operation, 25 of 40 patients were still living and had normal or near-normal intelligence (Mealey, Dzenitis, & Hockey, 1970). Wilkins, Radtke, and Burger (1993) described the case of a 36-year-old woman with an anteroinferior temporal encephalocele. She had a 23-year history of simple and complex partial seizures which were controlled after surgical treatment for the encephalocele.

Encephaloceles are considerably more rare than spina bifida. Friede (1989) cites the incidence as 0.1 to 0.3 per 1000 live births. In the Wiswell *et al.* (1990) study, the incidence for live- and stillbirths was 0.14 per 1000. They reported a significant reduction in incidence among white females during the 17-year period covered by the study. They also found that among white infants, encephaloceles were more common among females. This is consistent with reports that the sex distribution of encephaloceles is similar to that of spina bifida cystica and anencephaly (Friede, 1989).

Anencephaly

Anencephaly is a defect in which the vault of the skull is typically missing and the midbrain and forebrain consist of highly vascularized tissue containing mainly glial and scattered neurons (Friede, 1989; Hynd & Willis, 1988). The face is grossly normal, although the eyelids bulge and the nose is enlarged. Cranial nerves can be identified from the trigeminal down. Maxillofacial bones show some deformity. The extent of the involvement of the spine varies. Often there is abnormal vertebral segmentation. The body is disproportional in that the neck is very short while the upper extremities are large and long in comparison with the lower extremities. The term rachischisis is used to describe those severe cases in which many spinal segments are involved in an open defect at the back. This is essentially the same as spina bi-fida but rachischisis is the conventional term of choice (Friede, 1989).

Anencephaly is incompatible with life and is estimated to account for 29.5% of all abnormal stillbirths (Coffey & Jessop, 1957). Most infants die minutes to hours (Hynd & Willis, 1988) or weeks (Aicardi, 1992) after birth. McAbee, Sherman, Canas, and Boxer (1993), however, have described two infants with anencephaly who survived for 7 and 10 months without prolonged mechanical ventilation.

In a case reported by Dyken, an anencephalic male had spinal and brain stem reflexes, hypertrophied muscles, rigid limbs, hypothermia, and suckling and swallowing reflexes. He had no associated systemic abnormalities. He died after 6 days and structures above the diencephalon were not identified during the autopsy (Dyken & Miller, 1980). In the study by Wiswell *et al.* (1990), 20% of anencephalic infants had additional anomalies. The most frequent included multiple anomalies, cleft lip and palate, and other neural tube defects.

Anencephaly can be diagnosed antemortem through elevated maternal AFP levels. It results from failure of the neural tube to form at approximately the fourth week of gestation (Friede, 1989). The cause of anencephaly is not certain but several factors have been suggested. Proposed etiological factors include maternal diabetes (Gilles *et al.,* 1983), trauma, radiation (Rugh & Grupp, 1959), and hypervitaminosis A (Brett, 1983).

The incidence of anencephaly is estimated to be between 0.5 and 2.0 per 1000 births in the United States and most of Europe. The incidence is higher in Britain and lower in Africa, Asia, and South America (Friede, 1989). In the Wiswell *et al.* (1990) study, the incidence was 0.36 per 1000 live- and stillbirths. They also reported that it was more common among females. This is consistent with other research that has revealed a 3:1 to 4:1 female-to-male ratio. With longer gestation periods, however, the proportion of females decreases (Friede, 1989).

Hydranencephaly

Hydranencephaly is a deficit in which cystic sacs containing CSF replace the cerebral hemispheres as a result of massive necrosis. A thin, translucent membrane containing attenuated blood vessels makes up the walls of the sac. The membrane lies adjacent to the dura mater. There is usually some preservation of the thalamus, brain stem, and basal ganglia. In some cases, portions of the temporal and occipital lobes are present (Friede, 1989). See Figure 3.

Early in life it may be difficult to distinguish hydranencephaly from hydrocephalus. The size of the head is usually not enlarged at birth but it begins to grow at an abnormal rate during the first weeks of life (Friede, 1989). Deficits include feeding difficulties, atypical eye movements, hypnoatremia, seizures, dystonic posturing, persistence of primitive reflexes, and disturbed thermoregulation (Friede, 1989; Hynd & Willis, 1988).

Aylward, Lazzara, and Meyer (1978) described the case of a hydranencephalic male infant. As a newborn he was described as well developed, irritable, and as having a high-pitched persistent cry, primitive reflexes, and intact cranial nerves. The only abnormal physical signs were a slightly enlarged head and aberrant ocular movements. He was assessed at 41, 42, and 48 weeks. The infant was able to habituate to noise and light and was sometimes able to track a high-contrast schematic face. The infant was hyperirritable and had difficulty attending to social stimuli. However, he displayed some socially appropriate automatisms in addition to reflex automatisms. His motor activity displayed a high number of spontaneous activities at a medium speed and at a high level of intensity. He was hypertonic and had poor head control. At 7 months, he was still alive.

In making the differential diagnosis between hydrocephalus and hydranencephaly, translumination of the head is an important clinical feature

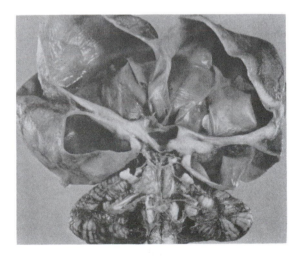

FIGURE 3. Hydranencephaly. Note large cystic sacs that are filled with CSF.

although it is not always present. EEGs may also be helpful since in most cases of hydranencephaly electrical activity is absent. Neuroimaging also contributes to the diagnostic process (Sutton, Bruce, & Schut, 1980).

The necrosis of the hemispheres has been speculated to result from infarction related to vascular occlusion. This may occur through mechanical problems such as umbilical cord strangulation or through the secondary effects of other etiological agents such as toxoplasmosis or gas intoxication (Friede, 1989; Hynd & Willis, 1988). There have been some reports of blunt trauma to the abdomen during pregnancy (Friede, 1989). In addition, some familial cases have been reported (Aicardi, 1992). Incidence and gender ratios are unknown (Hynd & Willis, 1988).

Porencephaly

Porencephaly is a deformity in which there is a circumscribed, large cystic lesion resulting from necrosis. Here we will address those of neurodevelopmental nature that occurred before the appearance of adult hemispheric characteristics. Thus, we exclude lesions occurring postnatally or during the terminal stages of pregnancy (Friede, 1989; Hynd & Willis, 1988). This usage of porencephaly is synonymous with schizencephaly, a term offered by Yakovlev and Wadsworth (1946a,b).

The term porencephaly was first used by Heschl (1859, 1868) who reported the case of a 26-year-old beggar who had symptoms similar to cerebral palsy. Autopsy revealed that he had an asymmetric skull which was thicker on the left. He also had a large perisylvian cyst which was in communication with the brain surface and the lateral ventricles.

The defect may occur unilaterally but is most often found bilaterally, typically in the insula region. The neurodevelopmental nature of the deficit is apparent because of minimal scar tissue and the anomalies in adjoining cortex. The lesion is not space occupying so it does not increase pressure. Often the septum pellucidum is absent which allows better communication between bilateral defects. Usually the thalamus is small because of atrophy of thalamic projection nuclei, but focal lesions are typically not found in the basal ganglia, cerebellum, or brain stem (Aicardi, 1992; Friede, 1989).

Friede (1989) distinguishes between two types. In the first type, polymicrogyria is associated with the lesion. In the second type, polymicrogyria is not present but the gyral patterns are atypical, often radiating toward the defect. Often the laminar architecture is disrupted.

Behavioral manifestations vary according to factors such as the size of the lesion, location of the lesion, amount of disturbance in surrounding cortex, the extent that the cyst infiltrates the ventricular system, and whether or not the lesions are bilateral (Aicardi, 1992; Hynd & Willis, 1988). Clinical features may include mental retardation, epilepsy, cerebral diplegia, quadriplegia, macrocephaly, facial apraxia, and speech disorders (Aicardi, 1992; Hynd & Willis, 1988). Some cases may be discovered incidentally and are largely asymptomatic. Life expectancy varies according to associated complications.

The diagnosis of porencephaly is usually made through neuroimaging but it may also be detected by sonography. The diagnosis is usually easy to make but in cases involving large cysts it may be difficult to distinguish from holoprosencephaly (Aicardi, 1992).

It has been suggested that porencephaly results from an ischemic event, leading to necrosis, during the fifth fetal month. Aicardi (1992) suggests that in porencephaly, the mantle is damaged early and is inadequately repaired. In association with the damage, neuronal migration is also disrupted. It is not certain if the etiologies or time of injury for the two types of porencephaly are different (Friede, 1989). There have been a few reported cases of familial porencephaly with dominant inheritance (Aicardi, 1992). The incidence and gender ratios for this disorder are unknown (Hynd & Willis, 1988).

Conclusions

In this chapter we have reviewed in some detail the spectrum of neurodevelopmental abnormalities including those that impact on the bulk growth of the brain, dysplasias of the cerebral hemisphere, malformations of the cerebral cortex, malformations associated with congenital hydrocephalus, and abnormalities of the neural tube and fusion defects. As Crome (1960) noted, however, over three decades ago, "it seems likely that future refinements in techniques will rise to the surface other, still submerged anomalies" (p. 903). Advances in microimaging, staining, and in understanding the architecture of the neurotransmitter systems will undoubtedly improve our con-

ceptualization of normality and its neurological deviations.

Clearly, the seminal work of Galaburda and his colleagues in articulating the neurodevelopmental pathology associated with developmental dyslexia deserves our attention (Galaburda et al., 1985; Humphreys, Kaufman, & Galaburda, 1990; Rosen, Sherman, Richman, Stone, & Galaburda, 1992). Their research demonstrates not only that cytoarchitectonic anomalies are associated with a syndrome long thought to have a neurological etiology (Hynd & Cohen, 1983), but also the vast complexity of factors that may produce some of the more subtle neurodevelopmental anomalies found in disorders of cognition.

Although this research and that of others is profoundly exciting, caution against overinterpretation must always be kept in mind. There is no one-to-one relationship between the behavioral and cognitive symptoms we may see in patients with developmental disorders and the manifestation of neuropathology seen at postmortem. In disorders such as severe or profound mental retardation there is almost always associated neuropathology (Crome, 1960; Freytag & Lindenberg, 1967); however, it is not unlikely that in cases of dyslexia or congenital dysphasia the anomalies occur only in the micro-structure, if at all. It should be kept in mind, for example, that the IQs of the patients studied at postmortem by Galaburda et al. (1985) ranged from 88–117. Thus, if one were to generalize, it might be said that the more severe the neurodevelopmental pathology, the more serious the impact on widely distributed functional systems (such as porencephaly), but the more focal the pathology, the more likely the effects will be negligible or more specific to the functional system disrupted.

Science is rarely without an agenda. Thus, it would serve us well to recall that it was less than 100 years ago that neuroanatomists attempted to quantify the relationship between intelligence and the estimated number of neurons in the brain (Gould, 1981). Unfortunately, some of these scholars were guided by racial preconceptions and an agenda that precluded objective inquiry. If anything is evident from our more refined understanding of how the brain grows and develops, it is that alterations occurring at specific stages of CNS development are likely to produce well-documented abnormalities. What is less clear is what causes the deviations to occur, but it seems evident that the etiology of many, if not most, of these disorders is multifactorial (e.g., genetic, environmental, vascular). Continued neurobiological research will serve to disentangle these complex relationships, and it can be presumed that neuropsychological research will equally contribute to a better conceptualization of the cognitive and behavioral effects of these neurodevelopmental anomalies.

ACKNOWLEDGMENT

Supported in part by a grant (ROI-HD26890-02) awarded to G.W.H. from the National Institute of Child Health and Human Development, National Institutes of Health.

References

Aicardi, J. (1992). *Diseases of the nervous system in childhood.* New York: MacKeith Press.

Alter, M. (1962). Anencephalus, hydrocephalus, and spina bifida. Epidemiology with special reference to a survey in Charleston. *Archives of Neurology, 7,* 411–422,

Andermann, E., Palmini, A., Andermann, D., Tampieri, D., & Leonard, G. (1992). Familial bilateral congenital perisylvian syndrome: Genetic determination of a localized neuronal disorder. *Neurology, 42* (Suppl. 3), 354.

Anderson, F. M. (1975). Occult spinal dysraphism: A series of 73 cases. *Pediatrics, 55,* 826–835.

Arnold, J. (1894). Myelocyste, transposition von gewebskeimen und sympodie. *Beitraege zur Pathologischen Anatomie, 16,* 1–28.

Aylward, G. P., Lazzara, A., & Meyer, J. (1978). Behavioral and neurological characteristics of an hydranencephalic infant. *Developmental Medicine and Child Neurology, 20,* 211–217.

Bamforth, F., Bamforth, S., Poskitt, K., Applegarth, D., & Hall, J. (1988). Abnormalities of corpus callosum in patients with inherited metabolic diseases. *The Lancet, 2,* 451.

Barkovich, A. J., Koch, T. K., & Carrol, C. L. (1991). The spectrum of lissencephaly: Report of ten patients analyzed by magnetic resonance imaging. *Annals of Neurology, 30,* 139–146.

Baron, J., Youngblood, L., Siewers, C. M. F., & Medeatis, D., Jr. (1969). Incidence of cytomegalovirus, herpes simplex, rubella, and toxoplasma antibodies in microcephalic, mentally retarded, and normocephalic children. *Pediatrics, 44,* 932.

Barr, M., Hanson, J. W., Currey, K., Sharp, S., Toriello, H., Schmickel, R., & Wilson, G. N. (1983). Holoprosencephaly in infants of diabetic mothers. *Journal of Pediatrics, 102,* 565–568.

Benda, C. E. (1954). The Dandy–Walker syndrome or the so-called atresia of the foramen Magendie. *Journal of Neuropathology and Experimental Neurology, 13,* 14–29.

Bickers, D. S., & Adams, R. D. (1949). Hereditary stenosis of the aqueduct of Sylvius as a cause of congenital hydrocephalus. *Brain, 72,* 246–262.

Birnholz, J. C. (1989). Ultrasonic fetal neuro-ophthalmology. In A. Hilland & J. J. Volpe (Eds.), *Fetal neurology* (pp. 41–56). New York: Raven Press.

Blum, A., André, M., Broullé, P., Husson, S., & Leheup, B. (1990). Prenatal echographic diagnosis of corpus callosum agenesis: The Nancy experience 1982–1989. *Genetic Counseling, 38,* 115–126.

Brett, E. M. (1983). Hydrocephalus and congenital anomalies of the nervous system other than myelomeningocele. In E. M. Brett (Ed.), *Paediatric neurology* (pp. 396–423). Edinburgh: Churchill Livingstone.

Byrd, S. E., Osborn, R. E., & Radkowski, M. A. (1991). The MR evaluation of pachygyria and associated syndromes. *European Journal of Radiology, 12,* 53–59.

Chervenak, F. A. (1989). Current perspectives on the diagnosis, prognosis, and management of fetal hydrocephalus. In A. Hill & J. J. Volpe (Eds.), *Fetal neurology* (pp. 231–251). New York: Raven Press.

Chervenak, F. A., & Isaccson, G. (1989). Current perspectives on the diagnosis, prognosis, and management of fetal spina bifida. In A. Hill & J. J. Volpe (Eds.), *Fetal neurology* (pp. 257–264). New York: Raven Press.

Chiarello, C. (1980). A house divided? Cognitive functioning with callosal agenesis. *Brain and Language, 11,* 128–158.

Chiari, H. (1891). Ueber veranderungen des kleinhirns infolge von hydrocephalie des grosshirns. *Deutsche Medizinische Wochenschrift, 17,* 1172–1175.

Chiari, H. (1896). Ueber veranderungen des kleinhirns, des pons, und der medulla oblongata in folge von congenitaler hydrocephalie des grosshirns. *Denkschriften Akademie der Wissenschaften Wein, 63,* 71–116.

Cleland, J. (1883). Contributions to the study of spina bifida, encephalocele, and anencephalus. *Journal of Anatomy and Physiology, 17,* 257–291.

Coffey, V. P., & Jessop, W. J. E. (1957). Study of 137 cases of anencephaly. *British Journal of Preventative and Social Medicine, 11,* 174–189.

Cohen, M., Campbell, R., & Yaghmai, F. (1989). Neuropathological abnormalities in developmental dyslexia. *Annals of Neurology, 25,* 567–570.

Crome, L. (1956). Pachygyria. *Journal of Pathology and Bacteriology, 71,* 335–352.

Crome, L. (1960). The brain in mental retardation. *British Medical Journal, 1,* 897–904.

Cull, C., & Wyke, M. A. (1984). Memory function of children with spina bifida and shunted hydrocephalus. *Developmental Medicine and Child Neurology, 26,* 177–183.

Daube, J., & Chou, S. M. (1966). Lissencephaly: Two cases. *Neurology, 16,* 179–191.

DeMyer, W. (1972). Megalencephaly in children. *Neurology, 22,* 634–643.

DeMyer, W., Zeman, W., & Palmer, C. G. (1963). Familial alobar holoprosencephaly (arhinencephaly) with median cleft lip and palate: Report of patient with 46 chromosomes. *Neurology, 13,* 913–918.

Dennis, M. (1981). Language in a congenitally acallosal brain. *Brain and Language, 12,* 33–53.

Dennis, M., Fitz, C. R., Netley, C. T., Sugar, J., Harwood-Nash, D. C. F., Hendrick, E. B., Hoffman, H. J., & Humphreys, R. P. (1981). The intelligence of hydrocephalic children. *Archives of Neurology, 38,* 607–615.

Dogan, K., Dogan, S., & Lovrencic, M. (1967). Agenesis of the corpus callosum in two brothers. *Lijecnicki Vjesnik, 89,* 377–386.

Drachman, D. A., & Richardson, E. P., Jr. (1961). Aqueductal narrowing, congenital and acquired. *Archives of Neurology, 5,* 552–559.

Drake, W. E. (1968). Clinical and pathological findings in a child with a developmental learning disability. *Journal of Learning Disabilities, 1,* 486–502.

Dyken, P. R., & Miller, M. D. (1980). *Facial features of neurologic syndromes.* St. Louis: Mosby.

Eckstein, H. B. (1983). Myelomeningocele. In E. M. Brett (Ed.), *Paediatric neurology* (pp. 385–396). Edinburgh: Churchill Livingstone.

Edwards, J. H., Norman, R. M., & Roberts, J. M. (1961). Sex-linked hydrocephalus: A report of a family with 15 affected members. *Archives of Diseases of Children, 36,* 481–485.

Elvidge, A. R. (1966). Treatment of obstructive lesions of the aqueduct of Sylvius and the fourth ventricle by interventriculostomy. *Journal of Neurosurgery, 27,* 11–23.

Elwood, M., & Little, J. (1992). Distribution by sex. In J. M. Elwood, J. Little, & J. H. Elwood (Eds.), *Epidemiology and control of neural tube defects* (pp. 306–323). London: Oxford University Press.

Escourolle, R., & Poirier, J. (1973). *Manual of basic neuropathology.* Philadelphia: Saunders.

Evans, O. B. (1987). *Manual of child neurology.* Edinburgh: Churchill Livingstone.

Farmer, T. W. (1975). *Pediatric neurology* (2nd ed.). New York: Harper & Row.

Fernell, E., Gillberg, C., & von Wendt, L. (1991). Behavioral problems in children with infantile hydrocephalus. *Developmental Medicine and Child Neurology, 33,* 388–395.

Fischer, M., Ryan, S. B., & Dobyns, W. B. (1992). Mechanisms of interhemispheric transfer and patterns of cognitive function in acallosal patients of normal intelligence. *Archives of Neurology, 49,* 271–277.

Fletcher, H. M. (1900). A case of megalencephaly. *Pathological Society of London, 51,* 230–232.

Ford, F. R. (1926). Cerebral birth injuries and their results. *Medicine, 5,* 121–194.

Freytag, E., & Lindenberg, R. (1967). Neuropathologic findings in patients of a hospital for the mentally deficient. A survey of 359 cases. *Johns Hopkins Medical Journal, 121,* 379–392.

Friede, R. L. (1975). *Developmental neuropathology.* Berlin: Springer-Verlag.

Friede, R. L. (1989). *Developmental neuropathology* (2nd ed.). Berlin: Verlag.

Frutiger, P. (1969). Zur Frage der Arhinencephalie. *Acta Anatomica, 73,* 410–430.

Galaburda, A. M., & Kemper, T. C. (1979). Cytoarchitectonic abnormalities in developmental dyslexia: A case study. *Annals of Neurology, 6,* 94–100.

Galaburda, A. M., Sherman, G. F., Rosen, G. D., Aboitiz, F., & Geschwind, N. (1985). Developmental dyslexia: Four consecutive patients with cortical anomalies. *Annals of Neurology, 18,* 222–233.

Gilles, F. H., Leviton, A., & Dooling, E. C. (1983). *The developing human brain: Growth and epidemiologic neuropathology.* Boston: John Wright.

Gould, S. J. (1981). *The mismeasure of man.* New York: Norton.

Hager, B. C., Dyme, I. Z., Guertin, S. R., Tyler, R. J., Tryciecky, E. W., & Fratkin, J. D. (1991). Linear nevus sebaceou syndrome: Megalencephaly and heterotopic gray matter. *Pediatric Neurology, 7,* 45–49.

Hart, M. N., Malamud, N., & Ellis, W. G. (1972). The Dandy–Walker syndrome. *Neurology, 22,* 771–780.

Hashimoto, R., Seki, T., Takuma, Y., & Suzuki, N. (1993). The 'double cortex' syndrome on MRI. *Brain Development, 15,* 57–59; discussion, 83–84.

Haslam, R. H. A., & Smith, D. W. (1979). Autosomal dominant microcephaly. *Journal of Pediatrics, 95,* 701–705.

Hayward, J. C., Titelbaum, D. S., Clancy, R. R., & Zimmerman, R. A. (1991). Lissencephaly–pachygyria associated with congenital cytomegalovirus infection. *Journal of Child Neurology, 6,* 109–114.

Hecht, F., & Kelly, J. V. (1979). Little heads: Inheritance and early detection. *Journal of Pediatrics, 95,* 731–732.

Heschl, R. (1859). Gehirndefekt und hydrocephalus. *Vierteljahrsschrift fuer Praktikale Heilkunde, 61,* 59.

Heschl, R. (1868). Neue fälle von porencephalie. *Vierteljahrsschrift feur Praktikale Heilkunde, 100,* 40.

Hintz, R. L., Menking, M., & Sotos, J. F. (1968). Familial holoprosencephaly with endocrine dysgenesis. *Journal of Pediatrics, 59,* 726–733.

Hirsch, J. F., Pierre-Kahn, A., Renier, D., Sainte-Rose, C., & Hoppe-Hirsch, E. (1984). The Dandy–Walker malformation. *Journal of Neurosurgery, 61,* 515–522.

Humphreys, P., Kaufman, W. E., & Galaburda, A. (1990). Developmental dyslexia in women: Neuropathological findings in three patients. *Annals of Neurology, 28,* 727–738.

Hynd, G. W., & Cohen, M. (1983). *Dyslexia: Neuropsychological research, theory and clinical differentiation.* New York: Grune & Stratton.

Hynd, G. W., Hall, J., Novey, E. S., Eliopulos, D., Black, K., Gonzalez, J. J., Edmonds, J. E., Riccio, C., & Cohen, M. (1995). Dyslexia and corpus callosum morphology. *Archives of Neurology, 52,* 32–38.

Hynd, G. W., & Obrzut, J. E. (1981). Reconceptualizing cerebral dominance: Implications for reading and learning disabled children. *Journal of Special Education, 15,* 447–457.

Hynd, G. W., Obrzut, J. E., Weed, W., & Hynd, C. R. (1979). Development of cerebral dominance: Dichotic listening asymmetry in normal and learning disabled children. *Journal of Experimental Child Psychology, 28,* 445–454.

Hynd, G. W., & Semrud-Clikeman, M. (1989). Dyslexia and brain morphology. *Psychological Bulletin, 106,* 447–482.

Hynd, G. W., & Willis, W. G. (1988). *Pediatric neuropsychology.* Boston: Allyn & Bacon.

Jakob, A. (1927). *Normale und pathologische anatomie und histologie des grosshirns.* Leipzig: Deuticke.

James, C. C. M., & Lassman, L. P. (1972). *Spinal dysraphism. Spina bifida occulta.* London: Butterworth.

James, C. C. M., & Lassman, L. P. (1981). *Spina bifida occulta. Orthopaedic, radiological, and neurosurgical aspects.* New York: Academic Press.

Jellinger, K., & Rett, A. (1976). Agyria-pachygyria (lissencephaly syndrome). *Neuropädiatrie, 7,* 66–91.

Jeret, J. S,, Serur, D., Wisnlewski, K., & Fisch, C. (1987). Frequency of agenesis of the corpus callosum in the developmentally disabled population as determined by computerized tomography. *Pediatric Neuroscience, 12,* 101–103.

Kobori, J. A., Herrick, M. K., & Urich, H. (1987). Arhinencephaly: The spectrum of associated malformations. *Brain, 110,* 237–260.

Koeda, T., & Takeshita, K. (1993). Tactile naming disorder of the left hand in two cases with corpus callosum agenesis. *Developmental Medicine and Child Neurology, 35,* 65–69.

Kuchelmeister, K., Bergmann, M., & Gullotta, F. (1993). Neuropathology of lissencephalies. *Childs Nervous System, 9,* 394–399.

Kundrat H. (1882). *Arhinencephalie als typische art von missbildung.* Graz: Leuschner & Lubensky.

Lassonde, M., Sauerwein, H., McCabe, N., Laurencelle, L., & Geoffroy, G. (1988). Extent and limits of cerebral adjustment to early section or congenital absence of the corpus callosum. *Behavioural Brain Research, 30,* 165–181.

Laurence, K. M. (1964). A case of unilateral megalencephaly. *Developmental Medicine and Child Neurology, 6,* 585–590.

Laurence, K. M., & Coates, S. (1962). The natural history of hydrocephalus. *Archives of Disease in Childhood, 37,* 345–362.

Laurence, K. M., & Tew, B. J. (1971). Natural history of spina bifida cystica and cranium bifidum cysticum. Major central nervous system malformations in South Wales, Part IV. *Archives of Disease in Childhood, 46,* 127–138.

Little, J., & Elwood, M. (1992a). Geographical variation. In J. M. Elwood, J. Little, & J. H. Elwood (Eds.), *Epidemiology and control of neural tube defects* (pp. 96–145). London: Oxford University Press.

Little, J., & Elwood, M. (1992b). Ethnic origin and migration. In J. M. Elwood, J. Little, & J. H. Elwood (Eds.), *Epidemiology and control of neural tube defects* (pp. 146–167). London: Oxford University Press.

Lorber, J. (1967). The prognosis of occipital encephalocele. *Developmental Medicine and Child Neurology, 13* (Suppl.), 75–87.

Lorber, J. (1968). The results of early treatment of extreme hydrocephalus. *Developmental Medicine and Child Neurology, 16* (Suppl.), 21–29.

Lorber, J., & Priestley, B. L. (1981). Children with large heads: A practical approach to diagnosis in 557 children, with special reference to 109 children with megalencephaly. *Developmental Medicine and Child Neurology, 23,* 494–504.

McAbee, G., Sherman, J., Canas, J. A., & Boxer, H. (1993). Prolonged survival of two anencephalic infants. *American Journal of Perinatology, 10,* 175–177.

McCullough, D. C., & Balzer-Martin, L. A. (1982). Current prognosis in overt neonatal hydrocephalus. *Journal of Neurosurgery, 57,* 378–383.

McLone, D. G. (1982). Congenital malformations of the brain. In R. L. McLaurin (Ed.), *Pediatric neurosurgery: Surgery of the developing nervous system* (pp. 95–110). New York: Grune & Stratton.

Malamud, N. (1964). Neuropathology. In H. A. Stevens & R. Heber (Eds.), *Mental retardation* (pp. 429–452). Chicago: University of Chicago Press.

Malamud, N., & Hirano, A. (1974). *Atlas of neuropathology.* Berkeley: University of California Press.

Mealey, J., Jr., Dzenitis, A. J., & Hockey, A. A. (1970). The prognosis of encephaloceles. *Journal of Neurosurgery, 32,* 209–218.

Menkes, J. H. (1985). *Textbook of child neurology* (3rd ed.). Philadelphia: Lea & Febiger.

Menkes, J. H., Philippart, M., & Clark, D. B. (1964). Hereditary partial agenesis of corpus callosum. *Archives of Neurology, 11,* 198–208.

Milhorat, T. H. (1982). Hydrocephalus: Historical notes, etiology, and clinical diagnosis. In R. C. McLaurin (Ed.), *Pediatric neurosurgery: Surgery of the developing nervous system* (pp. 197–210). New York: Grune & Stratton.

Miura, K., Watanabe, K., Maeda, N., Matsumoto, A., Kumagi, T., Ito, K., & Kato, T. (1993). Magnetic resonance imaging and positron emission tomography of band heterotopia. *Brain Development, 15,* 288–290.

Münchoff, C., & Noetzel, H. (1965). Uber eine nahezu totale agyrie bei einem 6 jahre alt gewordenen knaben. *Acta Neuropathologica, 4,* 469–475.

Owen, R. (1868). *On the anatomy of vertebrates* (Vol. 3). London: Longmans, Green.

Palmini, A., Andermann, F., Aicardi, J., Dulac, O., Chaves, F., Ponsot, G., Pinard, J. M., Goutières, F., Livingston, J., Tampieri, D., Andermann, E., & Robitaille, Y. (1991). Diffuse cortical dysplasia, or the 'double cortex' syndrome: The clinical and epileptic spectrum in 10 patients. *Neurology, 41,* 1656–1662.

Palmini, A., Andermann, F., de Grissac, H., Tampieri, D., Robitaille, Y., Langevin, P., Desbiens, R., & Andermann, E. (1993). Stages and patterns of centrifugal arrest of diffuse neuronal migration disorders. *Developmental Medicine and Child Neurology, 35,* 331–339.

Pavone, L., Gullotta, F., Incorpora, G., Grasso, S., & Dobyns, W. B. (1990). Isolated lissencephaly: Report of four patients from two unrelated families. *Journal of Child Neurology, 5,* 52–59.

Pavone, L., Rizzo, R., & Dobyns, W. B. (1993). Clinical manifestations and evaluation of isolated lissencephaly. *Childs Nervous System, 9,* 387–390.

Pleet, H., Graham, J. M., Jr., & Smith, D. W. (1981). Central nervous system and facial defects associated with maternal hyperthermia at four to 14 weeks' gestation. *Pediatrics, 67*, 785–789.

Raimondi, A. J., & Soare, P. (1974). Intellectual development in shunted hydrocephalic children. *American Journal of Diseases of Childhood, 127*, 665–671.

Reigel, D. H. (1982). Spina bifida. In R. L. McLaurin (Ed.), *Pediatric neurosurgery: Surgery of the developing nervous system* (pp. 23–47). New York: Grune & Stratton.

Ricci, S., Cusmai, R., Fariello, G., Fusco, L., & Vigevano, F. (1992). Double cortex. A neuronal migration anomaly as a possible cause of Lennox–Gastaut syndrome. *Archives of Neurology, 49*, 61–64.

Rosen, G. D., Sherman, G. F., Richman, J. M., Stone, L. V., & Galaburda, A. M. (1992). Induction of molecular layer ectopias by puncture wounds in newborn rats and mice. *Developmental Brain Research, 67*, 285–291.

Rugh, R., & Grupp, E. (1959). Exencephalia following X-irradiation of the preimplantation mammalian embryo. *Journal of Neuropathology and Experimental Neurology, 18*, 468–481.

Sanders, R. (1989). Sentence comprehension following agenesis of the corpus callosum. *Brain and Language, 37*, 59–72.

Schwalbe, E., & Gredig, M. (1907). Uber entwicklungsstorunger des kleinhirns, hirnstamus und halsmarks bei spina bifida (Arnold'sche und Chiari'sche Missbildung). *Beitraege zur Pathologischen Anatomie und Allgemeinen Pathologie, 40*, 132–194.

Selnes, O. A. (1974). The corpus callosum: Some anatomical and functional considerations with special reference to language. *Brain and Language, 1*, 111–140.

Sener, R. N. (1993). Tuberous sclerosis associated with pachygyria. CT findings, *Pediatric Radiology, 23*, 489–490.

Shannon, M. W., & Nadler, H. L. (1968). X-linked hydrocephalus. *Journal of Genetics, 5*, 326–328.

Shapira, Y., & Cohen, T. (1973). Agenesis of the corpus callosum in two sisters. *Journal of Medical Genetics, 10*, 266–269.

Shurtleff, D. B., Foltz, E. L., & Loeser, J. D. (1973). Hydrocephalus: A definition of its progression and relationship to intellectual function, diagnosis, and complications. *American Journal of Diseases of Childhood, 125*, 688–693.

South, M. A., Tompkins, W. A. F., Morris, C. R., & Rawls, W. E. (1969). Congenital malformation of the central nervous system associated with genital type (type 2) herpesvirus. *Journal of Pediatrics, 75*, 13–18.

Stevenson, R. E., & Huntley, C. C. (1967). Congenital malformations in offspring of phenylketonuria mothers. *Pediatrics, 44*, 33.

Sutton, L. N., Bruce, D. A., & Schut, L. (1980). Hydranencephaly versus maximal hydrocephalus: An important clinical distinction. *Neurosurgery, 6*, 35–38.

Tachibana, Y. (1990). Special etiologies in the classification of epilepsy—with special reference to brain malformations. *Japanese Journal of Psychiatry and Neurology, 44*, 335–339.

Verloes, A., Aymé, S., Gambarelli, D., Gonzales, M., Le Merrer, M., Mulliez, N., Philip, N., & Roume, J. (1991). Holoprosencephaly–polydactyly ('pseudotrisomy 13') syndrome: A syndrome with features of hydrolethalus and Smith–Lemli–Opitz syndromes. A collaborative multicentre study. *Journal of Medical Genetics, 28*, 297–303.

Vles, J. S., Fryns, J. P., Folmer, K., Boon, P., Buttiens, M., Grubben, C., & Janeveski, B. (1990). Corpus callosum agenesis, spastic quadriparesis and irregular lining of the lateral ventricles on CT-scan. A distinct X-linked mental retardation syndrome? *Genetic Counseling, 1*, 97–102.

Wald, N., & Cuckle, H. (1992). Antenatal screening and diagnosis. In J. M. Elwood, J. Little, & J. H. Elwood (Eds.), *Epidemiology and control of neural tube defects* (pp. 711–726). London: Oxford University Press.

Ward, J., & Lerner, H. H. (1947). A review of subject of congenital hemihypertrophy and complete case report. *Journal of Pediatrics, 31*, 403–414.

Warren, M., Lu, A. T., & Ziering, W. H. (1963). Sex-linked hydrocephalus with aqueductal stenosis. *Journal of Pediatrics, 63*, 1104–1110.

Wilkins, R. H., Radtke, R. A., & Burger, P. C. (1993). Spontaneous temporal encephalocele. Case report. *Journal of Neurosurgery, 78*, 492–498.

Winick, M., & Rosso, P. (1969). The effect of severe early malnutrition on cellular growth of human brain. *Pediatric Research, 3*, 181–184.

Wisniewski, K., Dambska, M., Sher, J., & Qazi, Q. (1983). A clinical neuropathological study of the fetal alcohol syndrome. *Neuropediatrics, 14*, 197–201.

Wiswell, T. E., Tuttle, D. J., Northam, R. S., & Simonds, G. R. (1990). Major congenital neurologic malformations. A 17-year survey. *American Journal of Diseases of Childhood, 144*, 61–67.

Yakovlev, P. I., & Wadsworth, R. C. (1946a). Schizencephalies. A study of the congenital clefts in the cerebral mantle. I. Clefts with fused lips. *Journal of Neuropathology and Experimental Neurology, 5*, 116–130.

Yakovlev, P. I., & Wadsworth, R. C. (1946b). Schizencephalies. A study of the congenital clefts in the cerebral mantle. II. Clefts with hydrocephalus and lips separated. *Journal of Neuropathology and Experimental Neurology, 5*, 169–206.

Yamazaki, J. N., & Schull, W. J. (1990). Perinatal loss and neurological abnormalities among children of the atomic bomb: Nagasaki and Hiroshima revisited, 1949 to 1989. *Journal of the American Medical Association, 264*, 605–609.

4

Development of Higher Brain Functions in Children

Neural, Cognitive, and Behavioral Perspectives

LAWRENCE V. MAJOVSKI

Introduction

Higher cortical functions in children proceed through defined stages of development. Significant limitations in our knowledge exist as to the processes involved in the normal developing human brain with respect to neurophysiological, neurochemical, neuroanatomical, metabolic, and other related neuroscience disciplines. Attempts have been made to correlate anatomical and behavioral data in a direct manner, leading to a surfeit of postulations in the literature against a shortage of supporting data for known brain–behavior relationships in children (Taylor, Fletcher, & Satz, 1984). Much emphasis tends to be placed on proposed neural mechanisms and theories accounting for changes regarding development of the human central nervous system (CNS) versus description of changes taking place with respect to normal development of the human brain. Major difficulties exist in drawing fixed conclusions because each human brain is unique with respect to its molecular blueprint, cellular differentiation pattern, acculturation factors, and neural growth patterns (Cooke, 1980; McConnell, 1991).

Luria (1969a; personal communication, 1977) stressed that what was lacking in the area of clinical child neuropsychology was an integrative scheme outlining a conceptual blueprint of normal brain development with concomitant motor, sensory, perceptual, and cognitive processes involved in children's higher cortical functions. During the past 10 years, however, neuroimaging and brain metabolism (^{1}H magnetic resonance spectroscopy and functional imaging) technologies are producing quantitative means of mapping human brain function onto brain structure (Kreis, Ernst, & Ross, 1993; Raichle, 1987; Raichle et al., 1994; Reynolds, McCormick, Roth, Edwards, & Wyatt, 1991; Stehling, Turner, & Mansfield, 1991; Tzika, Vigneron, Bull, Dunn, & Kirks, 1993).

The main goal of this chapter is to address highly significant facts and concepts related to the normal developing brain from the perspective of human conception through childhood. Major emphasis will be placed on the normal developmental perspective with selected pathological consequences that can result from abnormal influences for the clinical practitioner's interest. Recent advances in neuroimaging measurement and *in vivo* techniques of cerebral and cognitive developmental processes will be addressed in the final section of the chapter.

Development of the Human CNS

Throughout its development, one of the brain's many functions is to act in generating behavior. The question of how the brain effects

LAWRENCE V. MAJOVSKI • Department of Psychiatry and Behavioral Sciences, University of Washington School of Medicine, Harbor View Medical Center, Seattle, Washington 98104-2499.

control over behavior is central to the study of human developmental neuroscience. The brain can be viewed in one sense as a decision-making organ system for information processing (Hillyard, 1987). Understanding the development of the human CNS poses a basic problem of how inhibition brings about the regulation and integration of higher cortical processes involved in the brain's development. Two major themes of importance throughout the course of neuroembryological development are the integrative action of the component parts of the nervous system, and cellular differentiation, i.e., how the component parts are derived (cellular differentiation) (Humphrey, 1978; McConnell, 1991; Nilsson, 1978).

A major problem in understanding the brain's development stems from the lack of a blueprint as to nature's original design. Completion of the human brain took place some 50,000 years ago. To date, knowledge is incomplete as to the original model. In studying the brain's development, neuroanatomists have discovered that the brain develops much more rapidly than other organs. Why this is so is not known. The influence of external signals in the environment, e.g., acculturation, on the brain is incalculable and is changing its structure more rapidly today than ever before (McConnell, 1991).

The human nervous system contains an estimated 10^9 neurons in the CNS, another 30×10^9 in the cerebellum itself, plus some 10^{11} granular cells within the cerebellum's macromolecular layers. There are an estimated 10^{12} glial cells crucial to the function and support of neurons. It is the association of these cells and their neurochemical communication links that makes humans human.

The human nervous system can be divided into three major aspects: central, peripheral, and autonomic. All three act in concert to control behavioral activities (e.g., motor, sensory, acoustic, optic). It is commonly held that the brain is the organ system that controls human behavior (Gottlieb, 1976a,b). A key element in attempting to understand how the brain works is the problem of inhibition and its role in human behavior. Exactly how the brain accomplishes control (inhibition) is not fully understood but part of the answer lies in the unfolding of the brain's morphology through the process of cellular differentiation.

Morphology

The CNS is usually defined as the brain (encephalon) and spinal cord (medulla spinalis) which develops from the *medullary plate* of the ectoderm. The brain lies in the cranial cavity surrounded by a bony capsule. The spinal cord is situated in the vertebral canal surrounded by vertebrae. Both are covered by cranial or spinal meninges that enclose a space filled with cerebrospinal fluid (CSF). The peripheral nervous system (PNS) is composed of cranial and spinal nerves (31 pairs) with associated ganglia consisting of motor fibers and sensory fibers. There are two types of motor fibers: (1) somatic motor fibers, which terminate in skeletal muscles, and (2) autonomic fibers, which furnish innervation to cardiac muscle, smooth muscles, and glands. Sensory fibers receive stimuli from receptive organs of various types. Nerves of the PNS supply the head, trunk, and limbs. The CNS and PNS together serve conscious perception, voluntary movement, and the processing of sensory-based messages and integration (Arey, 1974; Kahle, Leonhardt, & Platzer, 1978; Moore & Persand, 1993a; Nilsson, 1978).

In the autonomic nervous system (ANS), there are two antagonistic components, the *sympathetic* and the *parasympathetic* systems. They are responsible for preserving a constant internal environment (homeostasis). All viscera, blood vessels, and glands are innervated by the ANS. The human nervous system, the organism, and the environment are functionally interrelated.

The human organism not only responds to its surroundings, it acts spontaneously on them as well through functional circuits. The action that is instigated by the CNS (transmitted via efferent nerves) is registered by the sense organs and information is then returned to the CNS via the efferent nerves. An integrative process follows until regulation occurs involving both *exteroceptive* and *proprioceptive* sensations (Afifi & Bergman, 1980; B. M. Carlson, 1994).

The importance of the above phenomena is seen in the control and regulation of the muscular responses achieved via sensory cells in the muscles that provide a feedback circuit through sensory nerves to the CNS (Crelin, 1973; Kahle *et al.*, 1978). Luria (1973a) and others have pointed out the functional interrelations between the nervous system, the organism, and the environment from which emerge higher cortical processes. These three components, together, serve conscious perception, voluntary movement, and the processing of messages through *polysensory integration*. To better appreciate the interplay between structure and function, it is useful to first understand the development of the brain, starting with the formation of the embryonic disc, the nervous system's point of origin (Humphrey, 1978; Moore & Persand, 1993a,b).

Neuroembryonic Structure Formation

The nervous system starts developing approximately 18–22 days after fertilization. The egg is composed of ectoderm and endoderm with mesoderm developing between the two. The nervous system is derived from the *ectodermal layer.* During embryological development, the neural plate, the neural tube, and the neural crest form. The neural crest becomes elevated to form the neural folds which, in turn, approximate each other in the midline and then fuse to form the neural tube. Cells at margins of the folds are not included in the wall of the neural tube. The partial fusion of the neural folds occurs approximately 23 to 24 days postfertilization (Crelin, 1974; Hamilton & Mossman, 1974; Kahle *et al.,* 1978; Le Douarin, 1980; Lowrey, 1978; Moore & Persand, 1993a,b). In its formative stages, the neural tube appears as a straight structure. During its organogenesis, cervical somites deviate from the shape of the simple neural tube. This portion, destined to become the brain, forms various bulges and cavities, each of which has significance in the embryological plan of development (Jones & Cowan, 1978; Moore & Persand, 1993a).

Three primary bulges appear in the brain region of the neural tube: the forebrain (prosencephalon), midbrain (mesencephalon), and hindbrain (rhombencephalon). When the development of the caudal end of the tube is completed, the *optic vesicles* appear and protrude from each side of the forebrain. Otic invagination also occurs at day 28 postfertilization. In terms of the ventricles of the future brain, a *cephalic flexure* and a *cervical flexure* become visible with cavities at sites of the prosocele of the forebrain, mesocele of the midbrain, and rhombocele of the hindbrain.

Each optic vesicle will differentiate to form a characteristic pattern: first, the optic cup; then stalk; and, later on, optic nerves that becomes part of the eyeball. The original connection of each optic vesicle becomes located in the diencephalon, a subdivision of the forebrain.

By day 36, the forebrain divides into two parts. The caudal subdivision becomes the *diencephalon,* and the anterior component further differentiates to form the *telencephalic vesicles* which eventually become the cerebral hemispheres (B. M. Carlson, 1994; Hamilton & Mossman, 1974; Jones &

Cowan, 1978; Moore 1977). Simultaneous with the subdivision of the forebrain, the original cavity (the prosocele) undergoes subdivisions. Two telencephalic vesicles (teloceles) are formed and become the *lateral ventricles.* The median telocele, which lies between these two teloceles, together with the diocele, becomes the *third ventricle.* The mesocele develops into the *cerebral aqueduct.* As the forebrain divides into the telencephalon and diencephalon, the hindbrain is forming into two structures: the *anterior metencephalon,* which becomes the *pons* and the *cerebellum;* and the posterior *myelencephalon,* which becomes the *medulla oblongata.* The fourth ventricle forms from the cavity of the metencephalon *(metacele),* together with the cavity of the myelencephalon *(myelocele).*

By day 34, the cerebellar plate, cervical and mesencephalic flexures, lens invagination, otic vesicles, and olfactory placodes are visible. By day 45, olfactory evagination will have occurred as well as formation of the cerebral hemispheres. Lens fiber migration of retinal cells will begin in earnest at this point.

Growth and development by 3 months postfertilization take place in terms of the two smooth-walled telencephalic vesicles. These are easily identified as *cerebral hemispheres.* Each emerging hemisphere of the telencephalon will have divided by this time into three parts, each of which has different functions. The first component is the *rhinencephalon;* the second is the thick basal *(striatal)* region, which develops into the *basal ganglia;* and the third is a *suprastriatal region,* which forms the *cerebral cortex* and related underlying white matter (Arey, 1974; Crelin, 1974; Kahle *et al.,* 1978; Moore & Persand, 1993a).

The rhinencephalon begins as an outgrowth from the telencephalon, e.g., the olfactory lobes. Each olfactory lobe forms part of the wall of the cerebral hemispheres. The second major portion of the rhinencephalon forms part of the wall of the cerebral hemispheres, e.g., the *hippocampus,* a bulging mass that appears on the medial wall of the lateral ventricles, bilaterally. In humans, the rhinencephalon includes, in addition to the bilaterally placed olfactory bulbs and hippocampi, such structures as the bilateral *pyriform lobes,* midline *septum pellucidum,* and midline *fornix.* The rhinencephalon differentiates into structures referred to as the *limbic lobe,* which contains interconnections with structures such as thalami, epithalamus, and hypothalamus. This constitutes the *limbic system.*

The functional significance of the limbic system lies in its association with emotional responses and the integration of olfactory information subserving both visceral and somatic information. The limbic system is involved in "emotional expression," whereas the hypothalamus is involved in the regulation "control" of emotions through hormonal substances. The thalamus serves as the "portal" to the cerebral cortex, which is inextricably bound together in the processing of sensory information leading to human conscious activity. Other bilaterally placed structures of the rhinencephalon include the *stria terminalis; septum; amygdaloid bodies; medial* and *lateral olfactory gyria; parahippocampal gyri;* and *cingulate gyri* (Carpenter, 1978; Crelin, 1974; Hamilton & Mossman, 1974; Kahle *et al.,* 1978; Moore, 1977).

Basal Ganglia

The second part of the telencephalon that is formed is the *basal ganglia* (or *basal nuclei*). They are formed in the thickened portion of the striatal region of the telencephalic area, composed of several groups of neuronal cell bodies. One of the major groups of these *ganglia* (i.e., nerve cell bodies outside the brain and spinal cord) is the *corpus striatum,* which becomes related to the thalamus of the diencephalon. Up to the third month, the corpus striatum and thalamus are separated by a deep fissure. The corpus striatum bulges into the lateral ventricle while the thalamus protrudes into each side of the third ventricle. Beginning about the fourth month, the groove between these two structures will disappear and fuse into a common mass. When fully matured, the basal ganglia comprise the following main structures: *caudate nucleus, claustrum, amygdaloid body,* and *corpus striatum.* These structures will become involved with motor control (N. R. Carlson, 1994; Carpenter, 1978; Kahle *et al.,* 1978; Nauta, 1986a,b).

In the suprastriatal region, the third component of the telencephalon forms all of the externally visible cerebral hemispheres. The hemispheres increase in size and completely envelop the mesencephalon and the upper portion of the cerebellum, and the originally smooth surfaces begin to show convolutions at around 7 weeks. The formation of the surface convolutions, known as *sulci,* and the deeper depressions, termed *fissures,* allows the outer layer of neurons (the six cell layers in the cerebral cortex) to increase greatly in depth without a major change in the overall size of the brain in relation to its final volume. By the completion of its development, the cerebral cortex will range in thickness from approximately 1.5 to 4.0 mm with a surface area of 2.3 to 2.5×10^3 cm^2 (Crelin, 1973, 1974).

The first major fissure to appear on the lateral aspect of each cerebral hemisphere is the *lateral Sylvian sulcus* (or *fissure*) which becomes evident by the third month. The slowly growing floor of the sulcus, which is lateral to the corpus striatum of the basal ganglia, is the *insula*. It eventually becomes completely covered by adjacent areas of the hemisphere. Beneath the convolutions of the cerebral cortex lies the substrate of the highest centers of the cortical integration in the human nervous system. Cortical layers I–VI subserve *higher cortical functions* involving conscious activity, memory processing of information, decision-making, planning, voluntary action, and ultimately reflection (Luria, 1966, 1969b, 1970, 1973a,b; Posner & Rothbart, 1992).

Ventricle Formation and CSF

Important changes are also occurring in various parts of the brain after the third month, particularly ventricle formation. The lateral ventricles each develop three horns that protrude into the various lobes of the cerebral hemispheres: the *anterior* horn projects into the frontal lobe, the *inferior* horn into the temporal lobe, and the *posterior* horn into the occipital lobe. Each lateral ventricle occupies a more lateral position relative to the third ventricle and the formerly broad *interventricular foramen* (*foramen of Monro*) becomes a narrow canal. The third ventricle connects with the lateral ventricles of each hemisphere by the foramen of Monro and continues caudally into the *cerebral aqueduct of Sylvius,* expanding beneath the cerebellum to form the fourth ventricle (Humphrey, 1978; Moore & Persand, 1993a).

Simultaneously, the egg-shaped thalami bulge into a third ventricle. Eventually the two thalami, with normal development, bridge this ventricle, come in contact with each other, fuse, and produce an interthalamic bridge. The *cerebral aqueduct of Sylvius* becomes a long, slender tube connecting the third and fourth ventricles. Two major foramina become prominent: the left lateral opening (*foramen of Luschka*) and the median opening (*foramen of Magendie*), both comprising the fourth ventricle (Kahle *et al.,* 1978; Moore & Persand, 1993a,b).

A region of invagination, the *choroid plexus,* will occur along the choroid fissure of the lateral ventricle. Functionally, the choroid plexus serves as a source of CSF, the three main functions of which are to support the weight of the brain in the skull, to protect the brain from physical trauma during injury to the skull, and to provide a stable chemical environment for the CNS, despite plasma's chemical composition changes (Afifi & Bergman, 1980; N. R. Carlson, 1994).

Ependymal cells lining the brain's ventricles form the medial surfaces of each lateral ventricle, the roofs of the third and fourth ventricles, and portions of the plexus. As these cells grow and invaginate, they are accompanied by blood vessels known as *choroidal vessels*. CSF escapes through the median (foramen of Magendie) and lateral (foramen of Luschka) openings of the fourth ventricle into the *subarachnoid* space surrounding the brain and spinal medulla. The lining of the choroid plexus also forms a physiological barrier known as the *blood–brain barrier system* between the CSF and the blood supply to the brain.

The brain barrier system is more permeable in newborns than in adults, becoming less permeable as the brain matures. Bilirubin, for example, in high concentration in infants can cause brain damage because it passes through the brain barrier system. Conversely, high levels of bilirubin do not affect the adult brain (B. M. Carlson, 1994; Moore, 1977; Moore & Persand, 1993b).

Spinal Cord Formation, Alar and Basal Plates

During neuroembryological development, the neural tube is divided into longitudinal zones; the ventral half of the lateral wall differentiates early into the *basal plate*. It is thought to be the site of origin of the motor nerve cells. The dorsal portion of the lateral wall differentiates later and is termed the *alar plate*. It is the site of origin of sensory nerve cells. Between the alar and the basal plates lies an area from which autonomic nerve cells are thought to arise. Viewing the structural plan of the spinal cord and brain stem in this fashion aids in understanding how various parts of the brain are organized. Because it is held that the basal plate does not participate in the formation of the brain areas beyond the midbrain (metencephalon), the diencephalic and telencephalic vesicles are thought to arise from the alar plate (Kahle *et al.,* 1978). Alar plate cell bodies are composed of *sensory* and *coordinating* (internuncial) neurons. These are located in the layer of gray matter (*mantle layer*). Gray matter is the region of the brain and cord that contains aggregates of nerve cell bodies, as distinct from *ganglia,* which are nerve cell bodies that lie outside

the brain and spinal cord. Differentiation of the diencephalon from the alar plate results in division into dorsal and ventral portions. The dorsal portion becomes the thalamus and consists of cell bodies of sensory and coordinating neurons. These *nuclei* are nerve cell groups within the brain. The ventral portion of the alar plate develops into the hypothalamus, which is composed of motor control neurons. The dorsal (alar) plate thus becomes the site of sensory and coordinating neuronal cell bodies. The ventral basal plate becomes the site of motor control neuronal cell bodies (Crelin, 1973, 1974; Moore, 1977; Moore & Persand, 1993b).

The thalamus exerts control through its *projectional* (internuncial) neurons, which synapse with parts of the brain other than the cerebral hemispheres, and in particular, with the hypothalamus. Thalamocortical interaction exists in what is known as the *thalamocortical projection system.* Two major structures of importance in terms of cortical–cortical and cortical–subcortical interneuronal connections are the major fiber tracts that arise in the *internal capsule* and the *median forebrain bundle* (MFB). The last projectional pathway from thalami to cerebral cortex takes place through the *nuclealis reticularis thalami.* It is thought that through this projection pathway, there is ongoing monitoring and modulation of information from lower levels of nervous activity to the upper cortical regions of the CNS. The thalami also serve a role in pacemaking activities seen in the electroencephalogram (EEG). Another important function is *selective awareness* involved in conscious activity (Bear, 1986; Bloom, 1979; Crelin, 1973; Hamilton & Mossman, 1974; Scheibel & Scheibel, 1961, 1963). A significant portion of the human thalami is composed of a group of nuclei that receive proprioceptive and general cutaneous, visceral, visual, and acoustic impulses, which are relayed to the cerebral cortex via other projectional (internuncial) neurons. The structural and functional relationships of the component parts of thalamic nuclei are inextricably comingled (Riss, 1972; Scheibel & Scheibel, 1966, 1972).

The hypothalamus, derived from the alar plate of the diencephalon, is part of the limbic system and is considered to be the headquarters for central motor control of the ANS. It regulates emotional responses and certain visceral functions, such as appetite, thirst, digestion, sleep, sexual drive, heart rate, body temperature, general smooth muscle action of internal organs, and control of the anterior lobe of the hypophysis. The hypothalamus is involved in the releasing of neuroregulatory factors.

By the seventh week, the *infundibulum* (posterior lobe of the hypophysis) appears and develops as an extension of the hypothalamus. The *parathyroid* structure appears in association with the *thyroid* gland. During the eighth to tenth weeks, thyroid follicles emerge as well as production of adrenaline and noradrenaline (Crelin, 1974; Hamilton & Mossman, 1974; Lemire, Loeser, Alvord, & Leech, 1975).

The basal portion of each cerebral hemisphere, situated anterior and lateral to the hypothalamus, is derived from the ventral portion of the *alar plate.* This basal area contains the *basal ganglia.* Other important anatomical structures that emerge from the telencephalon include the cerebral cortex and the septal–hippocampal–amygdaloid nuclei complex.

Fiber tract systems are also developing with nerve fibers of the brain and spinal cord that have a common origin and destination. This anatomical feature should be kept in mind when thinking about the development and differentiation of white matter versus fiber tract systems. It is the cell bodies of neurons (the functional and anatomical unit of the human nervous system) that are involved in human thought, memory, and voluntary and regulatory motor control over the entire nervous system. These neurons are localized in the cerebral cortex and are responsible for executing higher cortical functions (Afifi & Bergman, 1980; Kahle *et al.,* 1978; McConnell, 1988; Szentagothai, 1975, 1978).

Hippocampi

The hippocampi have been described in recent as well as past studies going back to Santiago Ramón y Cajal (Anderson, 1975; Ramón y Cajal, 1911; O'Keefe & Nadel, 1978; Storm-Mathisen, 1979). The hippocampi play a significant role in the generation and retrieval of memory processes. They also serve a key role in the generation of conscious activity in humans. Studies on active memory capabilities of infants have shown that this feature of cognition occurs as early as 6 months after birth (Kagan, 1985; Kagan & Moss, 1983). The hippocampal commissure (fornix) is the second set of major connections to appear in the *lamina terminalis,* a major component of the early telencephalon (the first set to appear is the *anterior commissure* and the third commissure will be the *corpus callosum*). These connections begin to cross from one cerebral hemisphere to the other toward the end of the first trimester of fetal life (B. M. Carlson, 1994; Altman, Brunner, & Bayer, 1973).

Findings from magnetic resonance imaging (MRI) of human cortical development in autistic 8-year-olds to 53-year-olds, support the observation that brain abnormalities responsible for autism likely occur in the first 6 months of gestation (Courchesne *et al.,* 1994; Saitoh *et al.,* 1995; Piven, 1990). Brain stem auditory evoked responses (BAER) of young children with autism suggest brain stem dysfunction affecting the processing of sensory input through the auditory pathway. Viewed from this perspective, an anomalous development of brain stem or posterior fossa may be only part of a generalized process of neurodevelopmental dysfunction that might account for deviant language, cognitive, and social development in the spectrum of autistic disorder (Wong & Wong, 1991). The hippocampal commissure could be a key maturational component of compromise, along with other structures (telencephalic) involved in the cognitive informational processing pathways forming during the sixth month of fetal brain development.

Cellular Differentiation of the Nervous System

Structural and functional organization of the nervous system is based on cellular organization in which the neuron is the basic building block of the nervous system. In terms of the nervous system's network, neurons are interconnected in a specialized array of systems via synaptic connections (Crelin, 1973, 1974; Hebb, 1949; Kuffler & Nicholls, 1977; Lund, 1978; McConnell, 1988; Szentagothai, 1978). Inhibitory synapses are as important as excitatory ones. Inhibitory synapses limit and select continual impulse inflow. Selected signals are transmitted for further information processing and unimportant signals are suppressed.

Spinal Medulla. As the neural tube forms, three cell layers develop and differentiate from its walls: the ependymal layer, the mantle layer, and the marginal layer. These layers form distinct zones: the ependymal zone, the mantle zone (gray matter), and the marginal zone (white matter). The outermost layer becomes the *pia mater* derived from pial cells. The organizational patterns formed from these zones are best seen from the viewpoints of the spinal medulla (cord), the cerebellar hemispheres, and the cerebral hemispheres (Arey, 1974; Crelin, 1974; Kahle *et al.,* 1978; Moore & Persand, 1993a,b).

The basic three-zone pattern of the spinal medulla structure will be retained into maturity as follows: The ependymal zone remains as columnar cells lining the lumen of the central canal; the cells of the mantle zone form the gray matter; and the marginal zone becomes the white matter. The gray matter of the spinal medulla assumes the anatomical appearance of an H-shaped mass surrounded by white matter. The *association* and *commissural (internuncial)* neurons of the gray matter of the spinal medulla are formed by other mantle zone neurons. The white matter lacks neurons. Instead, there are bundles of axons arising from those nerve cells located throughout all levels of the spinal medulla and brain to form various fiber tract systems. White matter, in contrast to gray matter's large number of cell bodies (neurons), contains only scattered bodies of cells, which are chiefly supportive in nature, e.g., *glial* cells, which outnumber neurons in the nervous system by a ratio of 10:1. With increased specialization of the brain, more complex arrangements of the axonal tracts occur constituting brain white matter.

Cerebellum. Research in the past decade indicates that an enormous amount of integration occurs within the cerebellum, specifically with the bursting of Purkinje fibers and the quenching of Purkinje cells (Ito, 1984; Thach, Goodkin, & Keating, 1992). The organizational pattern in the cerebellum shows pronounced deviation, neurohistologically, from the basic structural pattern of the mesencephalon, metencephalon, and medulla oblongata, which develop from neuroblasts of the dorsal portion of the mantle layer. Cells of the cerebellum are involved in motor control and have interconnections via the basal ganglia that may serve a role in monitoring and coordinating muscle activity in relation to all forms of sensory input (Carpenter, 1978; Kahle *et al.,* 1978; Thach *et al.,* 1992).

The cerebellum serves many functions. It repeats activities in a regulated, precise manner; smooths out all motor activities; plays a role in sensory activity; and may even be involved in affective responses. It is the center for the smooth coordination of muscular responses, especially those involved with subconscious maintenance of normal posture. Because of its primitive three-layer system, i.e., molecular, Purkinje, and granular cells, it is also involved in feedback and dampening circuits that operate as a "servomechanistic system" to control complicated integrative movements such as talking and writing. Many cerebellar cells serve an inhibitory

role, e.g., "turn off" cells such as Mugwump and Golgi II cells. The cerebellum may even be viewed as similar to a computer in that it may be able to generate programs on its own (Scheibel, 1978).

Thalamocortical Fiber System. The thalami receive all types of sensory input relayed by projectional neurons either to various nuclei of the brain stem or to the cerebral cortex. Nearly all of the axons conveying sensory input to each thalamus cross from the opposite side of the spinal medulla or brain stem. Those fibers that have not crossed include half of optic nerve fibers entering the thalami from the same side. From each thalamus, projectional neurons relay sensory impulses to the cerebral cortex for which there is a corresponding area in each thalamus. Activation of a minute portion of the thalamus will stimulate the corresponding (and much larger) portion of cerebral cortex via the axons from the *thalamocortical projectional neurons.* The cerebral cortex contains cell bodies of *associational neurons,* which send their axons through the white matter of the hemisphere and in another part of the cortex of the same side. The cortex also contains cell bodies of *commissural neurons,* which send their axons via the hemisphere's white matter ending on the opposite cerebral hemisphere. It is via the commissures (originating from the *lamina terminalis*) that a bridge is formed to allow the *functional integration* between the two sides of the brain (Arey, 1974; B. M. Carlson, 1994; Carpenter, 1978; Crelin, 1973; Kahle *et al.,* 1978).

During development, the first commissure to appear is the anterior commissure. It interconnects the olfactory amygdaloid nuclei and cortical portions of the cerebral hemispheres. Second to appear is the hippocampal commissure (region of the fornix), which will unite the two hippocampal olfactory portions of the hemispheres. Then, posteriorly, in the region of the pineal body, the *habenular* and *posterior commissures* interconnect with the diencephalon. The last of the commissures to form (and the largest of all) is the *corpus callosum.* It is known that myelination begins in the brain at about embryonic week 16 and typical layers in the cerebral cortex are observed around week 24. At birth, there will be continuing organization of axonal networks, cerebral corticospinal tract development, motor coordination, and myelination pattern formation (B. M. Carlson, 1994; Moore, 1977).

Glial Cells. White matter and gray matter are made up almost entirely of cell constituents: White matter consists chiefly of bundles of axons, glial cells, and blood vessels; and gray matter is composed primarily of neuronal cell bodies, dendrites, axons, glial cells, and blood vessels (Afifi & Bergman, 1980; N. R. Carlson, 1994). Glial cells are the supporting structures of the CNS. There are three types of glial cells in the human CNS: *astrocytes, oligodendrocytes,* and *microglia* cells. Glial cells outnumber neurons by 10:1. Type II astrocytes are thought to derive from oligodendrocytes. The latter are derived from either precursor cells in the neural tube or neural crest precursor cells. Microglia cells primarily arise from mesodermal embryonic connective tissue from which *all* layers of blood vessels of the brain and spinal medulla arise. They serve a phagocytic function after damage to the brain and are not found in the developing brain until blood vessels are present (N. R. Carlson, 1994).

Astrocytes are composed principally of two different functional forms. The first are the fibrous *astrocytes,* which are abundant in white matter, providing both support and binding for the tracts of nerve fibers. The second, *type II astrocytes (radial glial cells),* are present in large numbers in the gray matter and serve many different purposes. They establish close contacts with neuronal cell bodies, blood capillaries, and pia mater. In conjunction with endothelial cells of capillaries, they form a highly selective blood–brain barrier (Crelin, 1973, 1974; Hamilton & Mossman, 1974; Moore & Persand, 1993a,b).

Cerebral Hemispheres. Beginning at approximately the third fetal month, migrating neuroblasts from the mantle zone pass into the marginal zone, giving rise to the cerebral cortex. Stratification within the cortex proceeds at an ever-increasing rate. At approximately 6 months, the six layers of cell bodies and their associated interconnections that characterize the cerebral cortex become identifiable. Final differentiation of the outer layers continues through the second decade of life (and perhaps even longer). The outer layers (I–III) become more highly developed in humans than in any other mammalian species (Arey, 1974; Crelin, 1973, 1974; Moore, 1977; Moore & Persand, 1993a,b).

The pattern of neuronal development in the cerebral cortex during infancy is integral to the complex functions of the cortex, which ultimately consists of a vast information storage and processing ensemble, e.g., cognitive reasoning abilities, memory, communication, reflective thinking, and individual mental performance skills. From infancy through the first 3 to 5 years of life, the subcortical–cortical

connections serve prominent roles in the storage of the myriad patterns of motor responses that can be elicited at will in order to control motor functions of the developing human body. It is the neocortex that gives humans voluntary control over how they will react to sensory–perceptual stimuli, integrate information, and decide whether or not to act on it in a deliberate manner (Scheibel & Scheibel, 1973).

In humans, voluntary control of muscles is almost exclusively regulated through the descending projectional tract systems arising from neurons in the cerebral motor cortex, e.g., the *pyramidal motor system.* One major system is the *corticospinal* tract that begins to form during embryonic week 9, reaching its outer limits by week 29. Fibers from the projectional neurons located in the cerebral cortex form fiber tracts and pass from the cerebral cortex to the other parts of the CNS (Bear, 1986; Carpenter, 1978; Kahle *et al.,* 1978; Majovski & Jacques, 1982; Nauta, 1986a,b).

Axons of the pyramidal neurons pass from each cerebral hemisphere to form the corticospinal tract portion of each *internal capsule* situated in the *basal ganglia.* These two corticospinal tracts pass through the mesencephalon as part of the cerebral peduncles through the lower portion of the medulla oblongata. It is at the level of the medulla oblongata that most of the fibers of the tracts will *decussate* across the midline to pass down to the opposite side of the spinal medulla and become the *lateral corticospinal tract.* The uncrossed fibers, which remain ipsilateral, make up the *ventral corticospinal* tract and eventually cross to the opposite side at the lower levels of the spinal medulla. It is estimated that approximately 30% of the corticospinal tract fibers remain uncrossed, and that 70% are involved in decussation. Axons of the pyramidal motor control neurons of the cerebral cortex synapse with ventral gray column motor neurons (Arey, 1974; Carpenter, 1978). Functionally, the cerebral hemisphere on one side, from the decussation pattern manifested, exerts voluntary motor control over the opposite side of the body and also receives sensory inputs from the opposite side of the body via fibers that are crossed to enter each thalamus (Crelin, 1974; Lund, 1978).

Axons, whether myelinated or unmyelinated, become surrounded by glial cells (oligodendrocytes). Within the CNS, commissural, projectional, somatic, associational, and autonomic motor neurons become encapsulated by parts of other cells. The only exceptions are the *boutons* at synapses and nodes of Ranvier. From the PNS, the neurons become completely encapsulated parts of other cells, except at the terminal endings and at the nodes of Ranvier (Kahle *et al.,* 1978).

Unmyelinated axons are those that are surrounded (sheathed) by parts of either oligodendrocytes (those within the CNS) or neurilemmal cells (those peripheral to the CNS). In contrast, myelinated axons are those that are sheathed by numerous layers of the cell membranes of either oligodendrocytes or neurilemmal (Schwann) cells. Major differences, neurohistologically, exist between the myelin sheath formed by each type. Oligodendrocytes and neurilemmal cells form myelin sheaths by similar processes but at different times.

Myelin Sheath Formation. Sheath cells become wrapped around the axon many times, with the sheath cell, the axon, or both, causing the spiraling motion. Fiber tracts begin to function maturely at the time they are covered with myelin. The process of myelination in the human brain begins 3 months postfertilization in peripheral site nerve fibers produced by adjacent Schwann cells. Myelination of nerve fibers in the CNS starts later and is produced by oligodendrocytes (Dietrich & Hoffman, 1992; Dietrich *et al.,* 1988; Yakovlev & Lecours, 1967). However, at birth, only a few areas of the brain and tract systems are completely myelinated, e.g., brain stem centers serving subcortical functions such as certain primitive reflexes. Generally, tracts become myelinated at the same time they become functional.

As the wrapping process occurs around the axon, the cytoplasm of the sheath cell retracts such that it is extruded so that the two layers of plasma membrane of the sheath cell fuse together. Myelin is actually formed by numerous fused layers of lipoprotein membrane composed of 70–80% lipid and 20–30% protein (Valk & Van der Knapp, 1989). Tracts of white, myelinated axons make up the majority of white matter of the nervous system. The majority of *preganglionic sympathetic* axons are myelinated and responsible for the appearance of the white *ramus communicans.* In contrast, the majority of *postganglionic sympathetic* axons are unmyelinated.

Myelination is a process closely associated with the development of the functional capacity of neurons. One of its chief characteristics is the promotion of impulse conduction, which enhances the functional efficiency of the neurons. Unmyelinated neurons tend to have a low conduction velocity and show fatigue earlier, whereas myelinated neurons

fire rapidly and have long periods of activity before fatiguing occurs. Neurons that are capable of rapid transmission of impulses become fully functional at about the time their axons are completely insulated with myelin (B. M. Carlson, 1994; N. R. Carlson, 1994; Crelin, 1974; Lemire *et al.,* 1975; Valk & Van der Knapp, 1989).

Formation of myelin in the spinal medulla begins during the middle of fetal life but is not completed until puberty. The last spinal tracts to be myelinated are the descending motor tracts, such as the corticospinal (pyramidal) and the tectospinal tracts. These become myelinated during the first 2 years of life. At birth, only a few of the 15 dissectable descending tracts are completely myelinated (Crelin, 1974; Kahle *et al.,* 1978; Yakovlev & Lecours, 1967). In the human brain, myelination continues into the fourth decade of life and even beyond (Dietrich & Hoffman, 1992; Valk & Van der Knapp, 1989; Yakovlev, 1962; Yakovlev & Lecours, 1967). The increased staining of myelin during the first and second decades occurs in the subicular region. During the fourth through sixth decades, it progressively shows lateralization along the surface of the presubiculum (including cingulum bundle projections). Data point to the importance of both early and late postnatal increases of myelination which occur in a key cortical limbic relay area of the human brain. This holds importance when applying a neurodevelopmental perspective to the study of normal versus psychopathological processes during early childhood and even adulthood (Bennes, Turtle, Khan, & Farol, 1994).

Motor neurons of the cranial nerves show myelination patterns before their sensory counterparts. Optic nerve fibers begin to show early myelination at birth and will be completed by the end of the third month including optic tracts, lateral geniculate body, optic radiations, and calcarine cortex.

Axons of the cerebral hemispheres are among the last to become myelinated, beginning around birth. At first, only the axons of cortical neurons of the olfactory, optic, and acoustic areas are myelinated, followed by those arising from cell bodies in the somesthetic and motor cortices. Fibers that become myelinated after birth are those of the projectional, commissural, and associational axons of the cerebral hemispheres. By 4 to 6 months of life, the splenium of the corpus callosum becomes myelinated. The infant will now begin to develop binocular vision and visual accommodation in order to identify objects. These skills, however, require interhemispheric connections and myelination of the fiber tracts between the visual cortex and associational areas of the brain. Myelination of axons of the associational cortices of the cerebral cortex will continue into adulthood (Carpenter, 1978; Crelin, 1973, 1974; Yakovlev & Lecours, 1967).

Neurotransmitters and Neurohormones. Neurons secrete specific neurotransmitters, neuropeptides, or neurohormone substances at the axonal terminal endings (boutons). Boutons are the sites where information is transferred from one neuron to the next and where electrochemical changes in the release properties of the presynaptic terminals take place. This might be thought of as a "chemical language" system within the brain. Neurohormones attach to the membrane of the cell on which the axon terminates and induce internal changes in that cell. Neurotransmitter substances serve as neurotransmitters, i.e., to either stimulate or inhibit the secretory process in concert with other neuromodulators. Once the secretory process is stimulated, physiochemical changes occur within the cell that are intimately related to the changes in the permeability of the cell's membrane (Cooper & Bloom, 1991; Lehninger, 1968, 1993; Zucker & Lando, 1986).

Neurohistologically, many neurons that become highly specialized evolved from glandular cells. Certain cells of the body are structurally and functionally intermediate to typical endocrine cells and neurons. These cells possess axon terminations in the posterior lobe of the hypophysis (pituitary gland), rich in both cytoplasmic material and hormones. Hormones are produced by the neurons and pass along the axons to the hypophysis, where they are stored for release as required (Halasz, 1994). After being released, these posterior lobe hormones pass to the responsive tissues of the body through the vascular system. Other similar hypothalamic cells secrete hypophysiotropic substances that pass on to the endocrine cells of the anterior lobe of the hypophysis through the blood vessels and regulate endocrine hormone secretion. The sympathetic and parasympathetic components of the ANS are under the regulation of the neuroendocrine system via the pituitary gland (Daughaday, 1981; Imura, 1994; Kaplan, Grumbach, & Aubert, 1976; Kuffler & Nicholls, 1977; Snyder, 1980).

In the region of the *substantia nigra,* the dopaminergic (DA) nigrostriatal system affects motor balance and affectual response. This site also is implicated in the etiology of schizophrenia and parkinsonism (Majovski, Jacques, Hartz, & Fogwell, 1981). Different ascending arousal activating systems are located in the basal forebrain, upper brain stem, and hypothalamus releasing various neurotransmitters, as follows.

Serotonin (5-hydroxytryptamine) molecules are found in the raphe nuclei of the brain stem. The pathways that originate from them are distributed in a manner similar to those for adrenergic neurons. Serotonin (5-HT) can produce both inhibition and excitation of neuronal activity as well as depression of behavioral activity in the mature brain (Jacobs, 1994; Smith & Sweet, 1978a,b).

γ-Aminobutyric acid (GABA) is a transmitter substance released by inhibitory interneurons, as well as by cerebellar Purkinje cells. High concentrations of GABA are present in the striatonigral pathway within the substantia nigra, reticular thalamic nuclei, thalamocortical nuclei, and cortical pyramidal cells. The reticular nucleus is an important GABA-containing neuronal structure in that it is thought to influence the flow of information between the thalamus and cerebral cortex. GABA release in the ascending activating system, putatively, is implicated as having a role in helping to achieve and maintain the waking state.

Acetylcholine (ACh) is released at both excitatory terminals in the sensorimotor cortex, as well as visual cortex, and inhibitory terminals such as the olivocochlear bundle. In addition, it has been found in the *nucleus basalis of Meynert* (Dunn, 1980; Steriade, McCormick, & Sejnowski, 1993). ACh is involved in the dreaming state and plays a major role in influencing the cortex, thalamus, and forebrain structures (Cooper & Bloom, 1991; Steriade *et al.,* 1993).

Monoamine transmitter substances can produce excitation or inhibition of neuronal activity. When this effect is exerted on inhibitory neurons, the net result is often facilitation via noradrenaline. Such a mechanism may account for the behavioral arousal produced by the catecholamines (i.e., noradrenaline and DA), which are believed to be involved in the facilitation of inhibition (Bloom, 1973, 1979, 1994; Cooper & Bloom, 1991; Majovski *et al.,* 1981; Smith & Sweet, 1978b).

It has been theorized that DA and other peptides may play a role in the mechanisms of memory. A large body of evidence implicates pituitary hormones, particularly adrenocorticotropic hormone (ACTH), melanocyte-stimulating hormone (MSH), and vasopressin, in learning. The action of ACTH, MSH, and vasopressin may improve memory processes by modifying motivational and attentional factors. ACTH may act to stimulate the metabolism of DA and/or norepinephrine (NE). It is also thought by some that vasopressin may act to affect catecholamine metabolism in a rather complex manner. In this regard, arousal is thought to be associated with the activation of central NE systems and the release of hormones such as ACTH, vasopressin, and glucocorticoids. In the neonate's brain, modulators (neuropeptides) may play a role in terms of the mode of information storage and not necessarily have a direct effect on information stored. Even though not completely understood, it is currently thought that catecholaminergic as well as neurohormonal factors may play some type of role in the storage of memory (Bloom, 1994).

Some have suggested that opiate receptors may even play a role in the filtering of sensory stimuli at the cortical level involved with emotion-induced selective attention. This suggestion offers the possibility that neural mechanisms may exist whereby the limbic-mediated emotional states, essential for individual and species survival, may influence which sensory stimuli are selected for attention (Bear, 1986; Dunn, 1976; Kety, 1970). By implication, endogenous opiates may exert progressively greater influences at higher levels of sensory information processing in the cortex. Whether this holds true in the neonate's brain over the course of the earliest years of development is unknown. However, sensory stimuli at the cortical level may play a role in selective attention, which can have a significant bearing on the processes of cognition and learning mechanisms since they involve ACh, GABA, 5-HT, NE, glutamate, glycine, and aspartate, all of which can stimulate neurons. These substances, collectively, act to innervate the entire regions of the cerebral cortex and have a major influence on forebrain functioning (Steriade *et al.*, 1993).

Neuroanatomical specific sites with neurotransmitter systems regulate attentional networks that have connections with subcortical areas. The latter structures and their diversity affect the developing brain by influencing orientation to sensory input, maintaining wakefulness, or carrying out various cognitive operations. Also involved in this modulatory neurotransmitter–neurohormone system is the fine tuning aspect of the state and level of excitability of the different parts of the nervous system so that analysis of sensory, cognitive processing and memory storage can lead to performance and behavioral responses once learned (Bloom,

1994; Posner & Petersen, 1990; Posner & Rothbart, 1992; Zola-Morgan & Squire, 1993).

Summary

Phylogenetically, the brain can be thought of as a blueprint of nature's original design in which we currently lack the original complete set of plans. To understand the brain's architectural plan today is like looking in a house in which additions have been made but without having access to the original plans to guide us. Clues that have been left behind concerning the functional aspects of the additions to the phylogenetic blueprint of the brain appear as follows. At the midbrain level, for example, children born with anencephaly will be able to live for only a few days or weeks, but they can nonetheless exhibit laughing and crying responses.

Another clue to understanding the functional neuroanatomy of the developing brain is in terms of its serving as a communication system where there is biological (neurochemical) information transfer. The principal components involved in this communication network are axonal conduction, synaptic transmission, and local cell processes. Another clue is the phenomenon of *supersegmental control* over lower processes of the human nervous system which also occurs at the midbrain level. The spinal cord as a mode of neural organization is yet another clue. Its chief characteristics are seen in *segmental* and *suprasegmental reflexes.*

The functional anatomy of sensation is another important clue in understanding the human CNS and its development. Distinguishing aspects are as follows: receptors and transduction processes; pain systems; discriminative sensory systems; and systems for automatic adjustment. Other important aspects are the descending motor control systems such as commissural, associational, and projectional fiber systems; basal ganglia; extrapyramidal mechanisms; and brain stem control centers of behaviors essential in development. The cerebellum is another system crucial in the functional understanding of the developing brain's neuroanatomy. It is involved in the modulation of motor and sensory mechanisms and may even have a role in decision-making responses as well, including perhaps emotional expression.

Other major clues are the brain stem and internal states. Both play a prominent role in the regulation and maintenance of sleep, wakefulness, emotional affect, pain, pleasure, and suppression of pain. In addition, there are various support systems and the internal milieu, e.g., the autonomic and endocrinological mechanisms that influence neuronal activity and ultimately human behavior.

The developing brain's higher cortical functions are the ultimate expression of human information processing consisting of an array of psychological processes (Luria, 1973a,b, 1980; Posner, 1993; Posner & Petersen, 1990; Zola-Morgan & Squire, 1993).

Factors Affecting Normal Brain Development and Higher Cortical Functions

There are six major events of significance that occur in normal human brain development: (1) dorsal induction, (2) ventral induction, (3) neuronal proliferation, (4) neuronal migration, (5) neural cell assembly organization, and (6) myelination. Any disruption in these processes will result in maturational dysfunction in the brain's early pattern of organization. The significance of this fact for developmental/pediatric/child clinical neuropsychology as a discipline is that the incidence of all major CNS anomalies diagnosed at or after birth is approximately 33%. It has only been in the last 10 years that myelogenesis and dysmyelination patterns could be studied and quantitatively measured *in vivo* or sequentially in the same child (Cohen & Roesmann, 1994; Dietrich, 1990; Dietrich *et al.,* 1988; Dietrich & Hoffman, 1992; Valk and Van der Knapp, 1989; Zimmerman, Bilaniuk, & Grossman, 1983; Zimmerman, Bilaniuk, & Gusnard, 1992).

The development of higher cortical pathways used to the best advantage of the neonate, rests on the above six maturational processes that affect conscious and unconscious programs of behavior. The formation of higher (cortical) mental processes involved in concept acquisition during early development is limited by unmaturated neural organizational and myelination patterns that are affected by several variables: timing, nutrition, environment, teratogenicity, and genetics, among others. Knowledge about these factors with regard to normal infant development of mental abilities and cognitive development is an essential aspect in the clinical exercise of diagnosis and establishment of remediation/intervention programs for neuropsychological deficits in young children (Gaddes, 1980; Rourke, Bakker, Fisk, & Strang,

1983; Spreen, Tupper, Risser, Tuokko, & Edgell, 1984).

General Factors Involved in Human Brain Growth

At the time of adult maturation, the human brain accounts for approximately 2–3% of the body's weight, but utilizes about 20% of cardiac output (oxygen consumption), and 70% of the body's glucose, which it is almost exclusively dependent on in the *oxidative phosphorylation* process (Davison & Dobbing, 1968; Humphrey, 1978; Lemire *et al.,* 1975; Nilsson, 1978). Even though the body may be starving, the brain receives a disproportionate share of nutrients, thriving almost exclusively on oxygen and glucose. Because of these metabolic requirements and dependence on the above two principal constituents, and the fact that the human neocortex is poorly vascularized, states of anoxia, hypoxia, and hypoglycemia can seriously damage the brain's normal functions during early infancy. A child may suffer from extreme malnutrition and weigh only half of his or her normal weight and yet the brain may only be 15% underweight.

Ninety percent of neurons are located in the brain. It is an electrochemical network of some 10 to 15×10^9 nerve cells, all present at birth, that regulate sensory–perceptual, motor, language, and other functions, as well as the higher psychological processes that we define as human behavior. Brain work occurs whether we are awake or not. For example, breathing alone requires the complex coordination of some 90 muscles that must be regulated precisely in order to execute one breath.

Processing over approximately 10^2 bits of information per second, simultaneously, the human brain distinguishes between aspects of reality, memory (declarative and procedural), and fantasy as it matures. As the brain develops in its inhibitory capacity to effect control over behavior, it regulates the various human drives and emotions that it spawns throughout its development course. In some brain regions, 10^7 cell bodies can fit into a cubic inch; each one of them can be connected by their arborization pattern to as many as perhaps 6×10^4 neurons and none of them are exactly alike (Scheibel & Scheibel, 1973; Szentagothai, 1975, 1978; Szentagothai & Arbib, 1974). The neuroelectrochemical pulses reaching the inner ear, for example, pass through at least four increasingly elaborate stages of analysis and refinement before any sound reaches conscious awareness for perceptual discrimination.

Insults to the brain early in gestation may arrest development with resulting gross malformations, such as anencephaly (failure to develop a prosencephalic outpouching), holoprosencephaly (failure of the forebrain to separate and develop normal commissures), and lissencephaly (failure of fissures to occur, resulting in a smooth surface of the brain) (Dietrich & Hoffman, 1992; Langman, 1975; Smith, 1976; Zimmerman et al., 1992). There are very few recorded cases in which the timing of a damaging stimulus to the fetus can be determined accurately. In a recent report (Cohen & Roesmann, 1994), brain damage caused by fetal injury showed a dual pattern involving the globus pallidus (basal ganglia) during the second trimester and thalamic nuclei during the third. This pattern of prenatal insult to the brain in various gestational periods is essential in relation to timing of sensitive regions for normal versus anomalous brain growth patterns.

Nutritional requirements, as well as effects of malnutrition (especially protein deficiency, which can affect brain weight and result in cognitive deficiencies later in life), are critical during postnatal months 6 to 18. Throughout childhood (and well into adult life), brain function increases tremendously, despite a brain weight gain during this time that remains relatively low, i.e., 350 to 400 g (Dodge, Prensky, & Feigin, 1975; Hamilton & Mossman, 1974).

Mass Growth of the Brain

Brain weight has been used as a quantitative index of brain growth, as well as a traditional indicator of quantitative aspects of CNS development. The brain of the newborn weighs approximately 300 to 350 g. By 12 months, the weight has more than doubled since birth and is approximately two-thirds that of the adult. The average weight of the adult brain is 1300 to 1500 g and is related to body size. Larger people usually have heavier brains although there is no proven correlation between brain weight and intelligence. Growth of the CNS during early fetal life reflects an increase in volume in the first trimester from 4% to 16%, compared to 42% at birth. The brain's weight is 21% that of the body at the sixth fetal month, 15% at birth, and approximately 3% at adulthood (Dodge et al., 1975; Hamilton & Mossman, 1974; Yakovlev, 1962; Yakovlev & Lecours, 1967).

The increase in volume of the cerebral hemispheres is slow and steady between fetal months 2 and 6 but rapidly accelerates thereafter. The postnatal growth of the cerebral hemispheres results mainly from an increase in myelination. Myelination has begun in most areas by 8 months of age reaching its greatest deposit in the first 2 years of life. After this period, the process will continue at a slower rate into adulthood. The brain stem grows most rapidly between fetal months 2 and 6 and less rapidly thereafter. The cerebellum grows slowly between fetal months 2 and 5, followed by an exceptionally rapid increase in volume commencing at fetal month 6 and continuing until postnatal month 6. The weight of the brain more than doubles during the first 9 months postnatally, and reaches 90% of its adult weight by age 6.

The hemispheric surface of the brain more than doubles during the postnatal growth to reach an adult value of approximately 1600 m^2. This growth is accompanied by an increase in the size and number of gyri so that the intrasulcal portion of the adult cortex is about the same as that in the newborn. The adult cortical surface area is reached by the second year of life. The entire hemispheric surface is gyrated by approximately fetal week 32, despite the fact that these gyri are less numerous than in the adult brain.

Normal thickness of brain tissue between the ventricles and the cortical surface is approximately 4.5 mm. There are many reports in the literature that people of normal or above-average intelligence, on CT scans, have only a thin layer of mantle between ventricles and cortical surfaces measuring 1 mm versus the normal 4.5 mm. Several such cases have been documented in the medical literature (Lorber, 1980).

White Matter Development

Hemispheric white matter develops slower than cortical gray matter during gestation. Postnatally, white matter will continue to develop long after gray matter has reached a specified volume. The growth of the cortex subsides by the second year of life while hemispheric white matter continues even through the second decade as a result of accumulation of myelinated fibers with their increased diameters. Myelination is closely associated with development of the functional capacity of neurons; they fire more rapidly and have a longer refractory period. Different fiber tracts show myelination patterns at different developmental periods. The component populations of a given tract system may differ as to the timing of myelination (Davison & Peter, 1970; Dobbing, 1975; Dobbing & Sands, 1973; Valk & Van der Knapp, 1989; Zimmerman *et al.,* 1983).

Myelination of tracts typically follows in a caudorostral direction, the cortical association fibers being the last to myelinate. The schedule for myelination was first elaborated by Flechsig (1883). Around fetal month 4, myelinated fibers appear in the ventral and dorsal spinal roots. Last to receive this investment are the associational fibers of higher cortical centers, e.g., the cerebral cortex's thalami. Some tracts are not fully myelinated until several years after birth (Crelin, 1973, 1974; Dobbing & Sands, 1970; Dobbing & Smart, 1974; Yakovlev & Lecours, 1967).

Sensorimotor Functions and the Appearance of Neurological Reflexes

Motor control behavior of the newborn is largely under the control of the spinal cord and medulla, whereas motor control in adults occurs at different levels of the nervous system. At birth, several neurological responses are present. The appearance and disappearance of neurological (primitive reflex) signs are essentially transient mechanisms either subserving life-sustaining functions or forming preliminary patterns of future voluntary activity, e.g., the stepping reaction that precedes voluntary step-walking. The most important responses that appear and disappear in early postnatal life are reflexes of position and movement, e.g., the Moro reflex; asymmetric tonic neck reflex (TNR); neck righting reflex; Landau response; palmar grasp reflex; abductor spread of knee jerk; plantar grasp reflex; Babinski response; and parachute reaction. The Landau response and the neck righting reflex are the first to appear around the time of birth and the last to disappear (at 1–2 years) (Siqueland & Lipsitt, 1966). Reflexes to sound that appear at the time of birth include the blinking response and the turning response. The reflexes of vision include blinking to threat; horizontal following; vertical following; opticokinetic nystagmus; postrotational nystagmus; lid closure to light; and macular light reflex (Barnet, 1966; Franz, 1963). The feeding reflexes include rooting response-awake, rooting response-asleep, and sucking response, all of which appear at the time of birth; the last to disappear is the sucking response at approximately 12 months.

The level of neural functioning during the neonatal period can be determined only with great approximation. Some of these reflexes will drop out of an infant's behavioral repertoire at around postnatal month 3 or 4. This is presumably the result of increasing cortical inhibition of lower centers in the brain. Reflex arcs exist below the cortical level, and before integration occurs between subcortical and cortical structures, stimulation of the infant elicits an involuntary, subcortically mediated reflex response. As the maturing cortical centers become integrated with subcortical areas, primitive reflex behavior then becomes inhibited. The fact that most of the activity of a normal newborn can be observed in an anencephalic infant possessing only a brain stem and certain components of the basal ganglia indicates that cerebral cortex participates very little, if at all, in the function of the CNS during this stage of life. Children with these morphogenetic anomalies do not survive usually more than 2 months, but while alive, they do show reflex development similar to the patterns of normal infants of the same age (Davison & Dobbing, 1968; Dodgson, 1962; Humphrey, 1964; Moore, 1977; Smith, 1976).

Concerning development of the cerebral cortex, upper, central, and hindmost regions tend to mature early, such as those concerned with bodily sensations involved in the control of movements, hearing, and vision. Frontal and lower sides (frontal lobe area) in the region of the temporal lobe mature at a slower rate. In the motor strip area, for example, parts that control trunk and arm movements appear in advance of parts that will control leg and finger movements.

Prematurity and Low Birth Weight

The fact that babies who are born prematurely but go on to develop without complications suggests that only when the brain is ready, and not before, will it start to develop in earnest. Infants who are 4 weeks preterm, generally speaking, will tend to "catch up" after 12 months. Judging by the immature state of the cerebral cortex, it can be speculated that the latter phenomenon plays a minor role in the life of the child at the time of birth. Support for this notion comes from recent studies showing correlation of myelin deposition with measurements of local glucose metabolism from [18]FDG-PETT research which is an indication of functional activity (Chugani & Phelps, 1986). The infant may be completely dependent on the inner regions of the brain, especially subcortical structures, since not until postnatal month 3 does the roof of the brain begin to intervene in a dominant manner, e.g., control of arm movements involved with the first signs of coordination of hand and eye movements (Davies & Stewart, 1975; Lemire *et al.,* 1975; Levene & Dubowitz, 1982).

Studies in the past 10 years have shown that babies of very low birth weights (LBW $<$ 1500 g) are at high risk for cognitive development problems. Premature infants (weighing $<$2500 g or $5\frac{1}{2}$ lb) are at a far higher risk for birth-related defects and infant mortality than full-term infants. Developmental abnormalities of the brain account for 30–40% of deaths during the first 12 months of life. Survivors tend to develop intellectual impairment (Hack *et al.,* 1994; Weisberg, Strub, & Garcia, 1989). White matter abnormalities such as perinatal leukoencephalopathies (PLE) are significantly higher in preterm infants. Cerebral palsy is 30 times greater in infants weighing less than 1.5 kg (53 oz) at birth. LBW infants can develop bronchopulmonary dysplasia that can lead to neurological and cognitive impairment as well (Leviton & Paneth, 1990; Vohr *et al.,* 1991).

Hack *et al.,* (1994) recently tracked 68 children born 5 to 9 years ago weighing under 750 g (0.5% of 4×10^6 births in the United States each year). This group makes up just under 7% of the 292,000 premature infants (under 2500 g, or $5\frac{1}{2}$ lb) born every year in the United States. Results from this study show these children to have higher incidences of cerebral palsy, intellectual retardation, distractability/inattention, delayed speech/language problems, and learning difficulties (mathematics skills, in particular). While the researchers showed about one-third living normal lives, the majority of these children face major problems, both physical and mental, which affect their scholastic and social development.

Frontal Lobe Maturation

The slowly maturing frontal lobes play a significant role required for a young child to respond correctly to verbal instructions. Luria pointed out that in young children, the immaturity of brain structures may be such that it is physically impossible for a child not to say or do what he or she is told not to do (Luria, 1960, 1961). This situation bears close resemblance to that of adults with damage to the frontal lobes. Not until the frontal regions of the brain are well developed can a child become capable of consistently obeying certain verbal commands. It is usually not until $3\frac{1}{2}$ to 4 years of age that children are capable of learning to carry out a com-

plex program of actions deliberately, in accordance with unrepeated verbal instructions. The timing of myelination of the frontal lobes, starting at approximately 12 months, correlates with the development of fear response (anxiety) in infancy (Kagan, 1985; Kagan & Moss, 1983).

Stratification within the cortex proceeds according to a definite plan in terms of neuronal organization. Neurons with connections in certain parts of the brain differ from others with respect to the cerebral hemispheres. For example, in the posterior portion of the cerebral cortex, the development of the layers proceeds according to a clear-cut, typically six-layer plan with a distinct layer (IV) as the main site of termination of afferent impulses from the subcortical divisions of perceptual analyzer regions. There is a difference that exists between the structural differentiation of the anterior versus posterior divisions of the cortex in early ontogenesis. This may account for slowly developing cortical–cortical connections, essential to the later differentiation and organization of the outer three layers in middle and later childhood (Luria, 1969b; Stuss & Benson, 1986; Warren & Akert, 1964; Zimmerman *et al.,* 1992).

Nutrition and Malnutrition

Human fetal nutrition depends largely on the size and functional capacity of the trophoblasts in the placenta and the villous surface area through which the exchange of nutrients takes place. In the placenta, three phases of growth occur by about 34 to 36 weeks of gestation. Cell division ceases while weight and protein increase nearly until full term. Placentas from infants who had experienced intrauterine growth failure tend to show fewer numbers of cells and an increased RNA/DNA ratio relative to control placentas. Studies of placentas from malnourished populations in different parts of the world have confirmed that fewer cells are present relative to normal placentas. Maternal malnutrition, vascular insufficiency, and abnormal influences with regard to intrauterine growth contingent on the placenta will adversely affect cell division in the placenta. During intrauterine life, all fetal organs are in a hyperplastic phase of growth and probably at no other time is the human organism more susceptible to nutritional stresses. Fetal malnutrition can result from any number of causes, e.g., reduced nutrients within the maternal circulation, faulty placental transport of specific nutrients, and abnormal maternal circulation. Deficiencies in specific nutrients are not known to affect fetal brain development. Reduction in either total calorie or total protein intake by the fetus can lead to retarded growth (Cravioto & Arrieta, 1979, 1983; DeLong, 1993).

Studies of the effects of malnutrition on human brain cell development have been limited. Infants who died as a result of failure to thrive (marasmus) during the first year of life had correlations of reduced protein, total RNA, total cholesterol, total phospholipid, and total DNA content. The rate of DNA synthesis was also found to be reduced. Cell division showed limitations, too. These factors collectively suggest that if malnutrition persists beyond 8 months postnatally, not only the cell number but also the size becomes reduced, disproportionately. Malnutrition in humans tends to reduce the rate of cell division in all brain areas. Early malnutrition affects cell division, myelination, and vulnerability as to neural tissues' optimal rate of synthesis of DNA. Nutritional deprivation up to an age of 18 months causes permanent intellectual impairment (Dobbing, 1990).

Cerebral Oxygen Consumption and Blood Flow

In the developing brain of the newborn, oxygen consumption is relatively low but gradually increases with maturation. That the neonatal brain is able to tolerate states of anoxia is suggested by the low cerebral oxygen consumption at birth. This ability to tolerate anoxic conditions may also be related to the brain's dependence (prior to birth) on anaerobic glycolysis as an energy source. The level of enzymes needed for aerobic glycolysis just prior to birth shows an increase as the brain's metabolism begins to change from anaerobic to aerobic.

Cerebral blood flow (CBF) is relatively low in the newborn but increases with age to a maximum of 105 ml/100 g per min starting at approximately 3 or 4 years of age. Disruption of CBF and oxygen consumption will affect oxidative phosphorylation as the brain develops. The average CBF for an adult is between 45 and 55 ml/100 g per min. In adults, a value below 20 ml/100 g per min will begin a process of metabolic degradation within neuronal mitochondria, leading to failure in synaptic transmission and EEG changes. Abnormalities that arise as a result of this degradation process are as follows: perinatal asphyxia; hypoxic–ischemic birth-related episodes; and extended decrease of CBF that is interrupted in terms of cardiac output (Finkelstein et al., 1980; Ingvar, Sjölund, & Ardö, 1976; Mazziotta & Phelps, 1985; Mazziotta,

Phelps, & Miller, 1981; Phelps, Mazziotta, & Schelbert, 1986; Roberts, 1986).

Changes in cerebral function result in demonstrable changes in metabolism and blood flow. EEG frequency correlates with the metabolic rate of the brain. Total CBF correlates with oxygen consumption. Activation of specific areas of the brain associated with sensory, motor, and mental functions has been widely shown to cause increases in regional cerebral blood flow (rCBF) and metabolism. It has been proposed that neural activity results in the release of vasoactive substances, e.g., adenosine triphosphate (ATP), which has been implicated as a possible mediator responsible for the local coupling of blood flow and metabolism (Bruns et al., 1987).

The response to hypoxia appears to depend on the level of neural tissue oxygenation rather than arterial pressure. The role of oxygen can be viewed in terms of *mitochondrial oxygen metabolism* which accounts for 80–90% of total cellular oxygen consumption (Lehninger, 1993). The provision of energy for the nerve cell via oxidative phosphorylation (the process in which cellular oxygen consumed produces usable energy) is the main function of oxygen. Most of the energy used by a cell comes from ATP and the electron transport chain, which yields free energy changes that occur in a series of bioenergetic steps. Inadequate delivery of oxygen to brain tissues may result from hypoxemia (inadequate arterial oxygen amount), ischemia (inadequate blood flow), or a combination of these two. Several mechanisms exist in order to protect tissue oxygenation, including local cerebral blood flow.

Mechanisms underlying brain damage in newborns are poorly understood (Cross, Gadian, Connelly, & Leonard, 1993). The first human neonatal applications of magnetic resonance spectroscopy (^{31}P-MRS) to measure relative metabolite concentrations in newborn brain tissues *in vivo* were described 10 years ago (Cady et al., 1983; Hope et al., 1984). Since then, the value of ^{31}P-MRS, as a research tool and investigation technique, has been widely confirmed as a useful prognostic tool in asphyxiated infants; hypoxic–ischemic states; cerebral oxidative metabolism and hemodynamics involved in perinatal brain injury; and early normal brain development (Hope & Moorecraft, 1991; Reynolds et al., 1991).

CBF has been studied using PETT investigation to address the suggestion that newborn human brains may be more resistant to ischemic injury than are adult brains. Altman et al. (1988) studied preterm and term newborns and found the range of mean CBF in preterm infants to be 4.9 to 23 ml/100 g per min whereas the range of CBF in term infants was 9.0 to 73 ml/100 g per min. This study shows that the CBF requirement for brain tissue viability in newborns is lower than in adults in contrast to normal findings on neurological examinations and Bayley Scales of 80 or greater.

Recently, ^{1}H-MRS investigation was used to examine (within the first month of life) the brains of 11 infants born at term (10 showing signs of hypoxic–ischemic encephalopathy, 1 neurologically intact). All infants had peak resonances on their spectra that could be correlated with N-acetyl-aspartate (NAA), choline compounds (Cho), and creatine/phosphocreatine (Cr and PCr). Neurodevelopmental outcome was correlated with initial spectroscopy findings as to reflecting clinical outcome (Peden et al., 1993). This study provides the latest information about five major chemical changes occurring in the brains of infants with hypoxic–ischemic encephalopathy. It demonstrates quantitatively useful in vivo MRS-based biochemical information in newborns' brains in a noninvasive manner, as to normal and abnormal metabolic brain development. This same type of study using ^{1}H-MRS has demonstrated that NAA and Cr are determined by gestational age whereas the concentration in terms of milliliters correlates best with postnatal age (Kreis et al., 1993). The central key lies in obtaining ^{1}H-MRS quantitative information regarding these chemicals, i.e., in the confirmed ability to diagnose and monitor living functional tissue as a "metabolic window" into biochemical events in normal and pathological developmental processes, since metabolic ratios are often misleading (Goplerud & Delivoria-Papadopoulos, 1993; Kreis et al., 1993; Tzika et al., 1993).

The functional activation of the human brain can be visualized with MR imaging as a method of mapping brain structure to function (Connelly et al., 1993). Neuronal activity changes through in utero and neonatal brain development causing local changes in CBF, blood oxygenation, blood volume, and oxidative phosphorylation (bioenergetic changes in the mitochondria) by using intrinsic blood-tissue contrast via functional MR imaging (FI). This technology opens a spatial–temporal window into individual brain physiology (Connelly et al., 1993; Kwong et al., 1992; Stehling et al., 1991). Because of FI and ^{1}H-MRS investigating methods, it is possible to extend metabolic and developmental brain physiology in vivo beyond immediate cellular response, e.g., asphyxia, to chronic

adaptation in the newborn. Clinically applied, this now enables researchers and clinicians to quantitatively identify brain injury that is reversible, in some cases, to have sufficient time to diagnose and intervene. The prospect for future prevention and potential therapies is a clinical revolution not achieved until now (Goplerud & Delivoria-Papadopoulos, 1993; Kwong et al., 1992; Martin, Grutter, & Boesch, 1990; Peden et al., 1993; Tzika et al., 1993).

EEG Development

Human fetal EEG activity has been recorded as early as day 43 (Bernstine, Borkowski, & Price, 1955). Fetal EEG activity evolves in a rapid and specific manner. In a 5-month-old fetus, cerebral activity lacks organization, rhythmicity, and regularity. At 6 months, organization emerges; rhythmic theta activity (4–6 Hz) appears in flurries lasting about 2 s. In the seventh month, activity tends to become continuous at about 1 Hz with voltages ranging from approximately 100 to 200 µV. This slower activity is interspersed with faster frequencies around the seventh and eighth months. Differences between active and quiet sleeping states become more pronounced (Ellingson, 1964; Lindsley, 1939).

Bursts in the electrical activity pattern at 6 to 7 months are associated with an increase in enzymatic activity in the brain. The major difference between the immature and maturing infant's brain is the definite change in EEG between periods of wakefulness and sleep. As a generalization, the amount of quiet sleep increases with maturation. In the eighth month, during active sleep, fast waves of approximately 2–3 Hz appear with no localization and often imposed on low-voltage faster waves, and become dominant. Frequency measurements of photically evoked responses recorded from the occipital area show a progressive shortening with maturation. Responses to auditory stimuli also show clear differences in waveform, amplitude, and latency of wave components with maturation (Ellingson, 1964; Hagne, 1972).

Rate of maturation of brain electrical activity decreases with age. After birth, maturity of changes occurs within the first 3 years. Fewer alterations are noted between 3 and 8 years of age. Five stages have been shown to be synchronous across regions during the first $10\frac{1}{2}$ years of life. Thereafter, the four maturation times show independence from one another based on maturational trajectories for quantitative EEG frequencies in brain regions. This suggests a strong relationship between neuroanatomical and neurolinguistic development (Semrud-Clikeman, Hynd, Novey, & Elipulos, 1991). Because of the continually changing aspects of the EEG during childhood, problems of interpretation are more numerous than for adult recordings.

Newborns have only brief periods of wakefulness with eyes open. They sleep 16 h a day, and half of that is REM sleep. Fetuses spend most of their sleeping time in REM sleep. Two well-defined types of sleep patterns are noted in 32- to 39-week premature and in full-term neonates: active sleep and quiet sleep. Early in the newborn's life, 2- to 4-Hz waves are present, which will be replaced by those of 4 to 7 Hz at approximately 5 years of age. Faster activity in the occipital regions of the brain (8 to 12 Hz) begins to dominate, and *alpha* rhythm of the mature brain starts to emerge. Occipital alpha rhythm changes rapidly in the first year from a 3- to 4-Hz rhythm to twice that frequency by the end of the first year. Changes in frequency have been postulated to be correlated with neurohormone growth factors, brain growth, and myelination.

Changes in the EEG's alpha frequency with age have important behavioral consequences. Periods of rapid change in EEG activity can help to identify critical periods for behavioral change. One of these periods occurs at the end of the third month of life when the alpha rhythm first appears. Another important period extends from the end of the first to the completion of the second year of life when the alpha rhythm attains adult values. Alpha frequency can be construed as one key variable in brain maturation signaling critical behavioral changes.

Lindsley (1939; Lindsley & Wicke, 1974) proposed that the onset of organized rhythmic occipital activity reflects a significant change in cortical organization and may mark a point at which the infant progresses from a subcortical to a cortical level of functioning. It is suspected that visual behavior in early infancy is processed by subcortical mechanisms with the cortex usually taking over in earnest at about the time rhythmic occipital EEG patterns begin to emerge.

Recent studies using quantitative complex statistical analyses of EEGs in an effort to map the physical maturational stages of the developing brain in humans from ages 1 to 21 have demonstrated five distinct stages of maturation (Hudspeth & Pribram, 1992). Immediate and abrupt changes were observed in specific brain regions throughout maturation in 500 *Ss* studies as follows: parieto-occipital (PO), temporotemporal (TT), centrocentral (CC), and frontotemporal (FT). In the first stage, all regions of the brain, including those governing somatic, visuospatial, and visuoauditory, show signs of synchronous development up to approximately age 6. Sensory and motor systems (PO, TT, and CC) mature in concert until about $7\frac{1}{2}$. At this age, the FT region begins development in earnest. The third stage involves visuospatial functions (PO) and some visuoauditory (TT) regions. The fourth stage shows maturation of the visuoauditory, visuospatial, and somatic systems (CC) occurring from ages 13 to 17. The fifth stage, ages 17–21, in the FT region, governs frontal functions and shows significant maturation. The five physical brain development stages in the quantitative EEG analyses show a high degree of correlation to stages of psychological development in children, especially in light of Jean Piaget's theories (Hudspeth & Pribram, 1992).

Magnetic source imaging (MSI) is a technological advance that makes use of the physical principle that every electric signal creates a magnetic field around it. MSI tracks tiny electrical signals that are generated as the brain and muscle tissue go about their routine functions. The instrument uses superconducting quantum interference devices (SQUIDs) that enable researchers to image the function of brain tissues as well as structure. SQUIDs measure magnetic fields, which do not become distorted as they pass through the body, unlike the EEG, which cannot determine the exact location because the signals are distorted as they pass through bone and tissue (Gallen *et al.,* 1993; Huk & Vieth, 1993; Orrison, Davis, Sullivan, Mettler, & Flynn, 1990).

Currently, researchers are using MSI to map the brain before surgery. MSI has the capability to be able to tell immediately whether brain tissue is working or not. This technique has applications for better understanding of normal versus abnormal brain activity, e.g., epilepsy, Parkinson's disease, and behavioral neurology (Gallen *et al.,* 1993). A broader goal is to combine SQUID technology with data from MRI studies in order to create a dynamic, functional image of higher mental processes occurring in the brain (Wang, Kaufman, & Williamson, 1993).

Speech and Oral Communication Development

Speech (oral communication) is a basic tool in interpersonal relationships and serves as a key indicator of brain development in the early years of life.

Interference with speech development or subsequent distortion of speech may have a profound effect on social competency and cognitive and interpersonal development in the child (Goodglass & Kaplan, 1972; Luria, 1969c; Neville, 1984). An understanding of the neuropsychological development of the speech process is needed prior to any professional advice or instruction with regard to the causes and treatment of speech-related disorders. Such diverse elements as neurological maturation, acquisition of fine muscle control, and development of symbolic formulation abilities crucial to development of cognitive processing of information can all be related to speech development. It is these neuroanatomical, neuropsychological, and neurophysiological aspects that provide the content and control from which speech is created. In later stages, especially in acquisition of words and sentences, contributions of learned behavior emerge (Darley & Fay, 1980; DeVilliers & DeVilliers, 1979; Lenneberg, 1964, 1967; Milner, 1976; Siegel, 1979).

In the early stage, any division of speech development into discrete stages can be misleading. Generally, all basic behaviors that appear at different ages function throughout childhood and into adulthood. After the prespeech stage (from birth to 3 months), speech starts with the *reflex stage*. The birth cry can be considered the beginning of speech, but any true expression is doubtful. Shortly after birth, reflex crying appears in response to discomfort or fear. Cries often vary and become differentiated from other noises, such as gurgling, sucking, cooing, and laughing. From 3 to 12 months babbling occurs. Basic changes in vocal expression are observed in the rapid increase in the number and varieties of sounds. As a child develops early awareness of vocalizations and moves into a period of vocal exploration, practice and repetition occurs in greater frequency. A child at this stage begins to modify imitations and is aware that he or she is "imitating" oneself. In many instances, early imitations of others' speech result from the repetition of sounds that the child has produced. Later, as the adult model initiates imitative responses with familiar new sounds, the basis for learning speech pattern emerges. In the earlier phase, various sounds are repeated. Sounds that approximate language are usually selected based on the most intense reinforcement derived by the child.

Another step in the development of speech emerges when the child integrates babblings and imitations into sequential patterns that sound more like true speech onset at about 12 months. Individual sounds tend to be reasonably accurate, vocal quality approaches that of voices heard, and sounds are grouped into nonsense forms and even phrases. Occasionally, what appear to be recognizable words are heard by adults, but may not represent meaningful speech at this stage.

True speech stages begin to emerge when characteristic features include motor control of breathing, phonation, and articulation. Ability to echo, complex mechanical patterning of speech, and other skills are practiced to assist in the leap to a distinctly different level of function. Complementary interlanguage is a prerequisite as recognition of familiar objects in the environment requires inner language. As the child develops into later years, this type of language would be similar to what adults sometimes use when talking to oneself (Molfese, Freeman, & Palermo, 1975; Segalowitz & Chapman, 1980). The child comes to develop an awareness that certain sounds spoken by the parents stand for objects (auditory receptive language). Inner language and auditory receptive language have been suggested to precede actual production of meaningful words (Luria, 1961, 1982; Luria & Yudovich, 1959).

The *word stage* emerges from approximately 11 to 24 months in which true first words are usually names of concrete objects. Sentences start to appear at approximately 18 to 36 months. With the advent of an increasing vocabulary containing a variety of representations for objects, people and actions in the child's environment provide the opportunity for the child to discover more complex meanings and verbal reinforcement. This is a variable period for the beginning of sentences and there may be periods of little progress after sentences are first used.

Complex speech development takes place from approximately 24 months up to 7 years of age. All parts of speech increase at a rapid rate. The word "no" will cover a vast number of situations, behaviorally, and provide a distinct measure of control over individuals in the child's environment. Extrapolations of grammatical structures cause difficulty with some irregular verbs, but the process of such abstracting indicates increasing degrees of complexity of symbolic thinking. Categories are learned, e.g., male versus female, dog versus cat. Children start to learn that matching reality to a symbol requires relative concepts as well as absolutes. This quality of assigning symbol to meaning is lacking, for example, in severely autistic children in their speech development (DeVilliers & DeVilliers, 1979; Luria, 1960; Piven *et al.,* 1990; Siegel, 1979; Wertsch, 1979). As the expansion of potential for expression continues to develop, not only does oral communication serve as an efficient tool for exploring and understanding the people and the world that surround the child, it also becomes a means for controlling and manipulating the environment. It serves to provide an extension in a variety of emotional expressions that goes beyond methods such as tensing muscles, throwing a tantrum, crying, and engaging in uncontrolled movements (Darley & Fay, 1980).

During the child's first 12 to 20 months, a transition occurs from visual representation to a verbalization mode in which the child's ability to participate in sequences of interpersonal exchanges via speech emerges (Mills, Coffey, & Neville, 1993). Children use language as a medium to communicate messages that become more syntactically refined over age. It is the process of assigning a memory code to a symbolic form that raises the questions of "how does a child retain what is learned?" and "how are coding errors corrected or adaptations to a changing environment effected?" (Grossberg, 1980; Vygotsky, 1980). Partial answers to these questions are seen from recent memory and auditory brain stem studies (Roncagliolo, Benitez, & Perez, 1994; Semrud-Clikeman *et al.,* 1991; Squire & Zola-Morgan, 1991; Zola-Morgan & Squire, 1993).

It would be myopic to view speech development as an isolated process. It is integrally linked with physical, psychological, and sociological maturational processes. Disruptions or distortions in any of these areas can have serious repercussions. It is particularly important that speech be developed uninterrupted during early childhood, since there is compelling evidence suggesting that lack of developmental opportunity or severe inhibitory factors have serious and permanent effects on linguistic–symbolic–intellectual development (Jernigan, Hesselink, Sowell, & Tallal, 1991; Kulynych, Vladar, Jones, & Weinberger, 1994; Roncagliolo *et al.,* 1994; Semrud-Clikeman *et al.,* 1991; Wong & Wong, 1991). The child may never become a completely functional human being in the developmental sense if speech is arrested or not developed by 7 years of age (Curtiss, 1979). Professionals and parents involved in a child's development have a significant responsibility to detect aberrant patterns during develop-

ment as early as possible (Goodglass & Kaplan, 1972).

Symptoms of possible difficulty may be noted in several ways during the first year of life. In the prespeech period, the most critical characteristic is the lack of progressive change in the nature of babbling or, conversely, deterioration of vocalization to that representing earlier stages of development. At ages when response to and imitation of sounds of others may be expected, any unusual delay may suggest difficulty in learning to talk. Failure to engage in jargon conversation is likewise an important indicator of problems. It is when more advanced behaviors have failed to materialize that one becomes concerned in terms of delay. Continuation of earlier forms of vocalizations during later months of the prespeech period is not evidence that progress is delayed. As long as speech is inclusive enough for useful communication and can be reasonably well understood by strangers by 4 years of age, concern over development of a serious problem lessens. In addition to articulation aspects, there is the possibility, during this period of development, of difficulties in fluency. For example, all children have numerous dysfluencies in speech. At certain times and under certain circumstances, these are more frequent and noticeable. The distinction between normal dysfluencies and stuttering is not always easy to make, particularly as there is variability from individual to individual. In general, however, major concern is not necessary unless there are signs of struggling behavior, tensions, anxiety, or reactions to specific dysfluencies in the child. Persistent rudimentary sentences may indicate a broader developmental delay but it must be emphasized that the total environmental background must be considered before assuming that a child has basic inadequacies.

Recognition of a speech problem versus undue concern over what are essentially individual differences in oral communication patterns can affect a child's cognitive, social, and emotional development. In this sense, appropriate evaluation can be reached by the integration of several factors: sequence and nature of speech skills; relationship of these to the child's experience and development; and the acculturation process in which others in the child's environment can influence these developments.

Acculturation Processes

Brain growth and the acculturation process are inextricably bound in human development. Neural networks are being set and affected by specific experiences related to environmental events (Szentagothai, 1978; Witelson, 1985). Acquisition of cognitive operations, which in part is influenced by a particular culture, has an effect on elaboration of neural circuitry. Neural circuits are formed during a period of acquisition and development of cognitive neural codes. Brain morphogenesis during a prolonged period of exposure to significant novel experiences can be expected to be modeled in accordance with ongoing experience (Goldman, 1975; Gottlieb, 1976a,b; McConnell, 1991; Mills et al., 1993; Plante, Swisher, Vance, & Rapcsak, 1991; Semrud-Clikeman et al., 1991; Taylor, 1969).

Data collected from studies of heredity and environment suggest that morphogenetic development of the brain's intellectual nature is attributable to both genetic and social environmental influences, the former having slightly greater effect than the latter (Oates, 1979; Plomin & Rowe, 1979; Posner, 1993). What this suggests is that several different cortical–cortical and cortical–subcortical systems are operative during the process of learning and information storage. What the infant senses, then, may be in part the result of what is neurally "set" to sense or competent to sense via a selective attending process (Dietrich, 1990; DiGuilio, Seidenberg, O'Leary, & Raz, 1994; Hudspeth & Pribram, 1992; Posner & Petersen, 1990; Pribram, 1976; Siegel, 1979).

Postnatal Perceptual, Cognitive, and Motor Development

Perception can be considered a multichannel process of visuomotor, auditory, sensorimotor, and other skills in which motor components of perceptual acts may be seen as a control process over sensory input mechanisms. Sensory input data contribute significantly to the following: perceptual processing of information; decision-making; readiness-to-act; and motor control commands, all the way from motor reflexes to the highest neocortical levels involving planning, organizational abstract thought. The significance of these processes as to the phenomenon of control lies in the success (or failure) of the infant's development and behavioral repertoire (Petersen et al., 1994; Raichle et al., 1994).

During the earlier stage in development (the first 2 years of life), an infant changes from having little awareness of the environment, to a child who is aware of the environment via its developing sensoriperceptual systems and neurological growth

processes. If development proceeds normally, the child is capable of discriminating among the various environmental stimuli. During the second stage (2 to 5 years), preconceptual representation as described by developmental psychologists such as Piaget and Bruner takes place in which the child develops pictorial (ideograph) images as symbols. The child also begins to advance in language competency. During the third stage (5 to 7 years), symbolic representation occurs in which the child becomes aware that he or she is not alone in the universe and begins to interact with several environmental forces that impinge on the child's development. The fourth stage (7 to 12 years) is characterized by operational thinking in which the child begins to recognize certain relationships between objects and appreciate their relative values, e.g., the concept of mass, size, distance, length, and time (Bower, 1977; Mistretta & Bradley, 1978; Siegel, 1979; Tulving, 1985).

Several attempts have been made to match developmental stages in cognition with defined structural changes in the brain (Epstein, 1978; Milner, 1976; Ploog, 1979; Vygotsky, 1974). Until recently, such efforts have met with very limited success except for recent studies (Hudspeth and Pribram, 1992; Kwong et al., 1992). Major obstacles in trying to correlate behavioral, motor, and sensorimotor development in finite stages include neural and metabolic processes involved in cellular differentiation, synaptic process formation, dendritic arborization, and myelination development discussed previously. Actual alterations or modifications can arise as a result of metabolic factors that affect function, e.g., decreased CBF; oxygen use by cerebral tissues; glucose use by cerebral tissues; cerebral vascular alterations leading to ischemic, hypoxic, or anoxic episodes; and periventricular leukomalacia (PVL). As glucose and oxygen are the primary constituents providing the metabolic energy requirements of neurons, rates at which these substrates are used can provide a quantitative assessment of the level of neuronal function in the brain (Martin et al., 1990).

Maturational changes in cerebral function in human infants have been studied by quantitative methods using 2-deoxy-2-fluoro-D-glucose (2-DFG) and positron emission tomographic technique (PETT) (Chugani & Phelps, 1986). Studies of infants at various times during development reveal significant changes in a progressive manner in local cerebral glucose metabolism. Chugani and Phelps (1986) studied 5-week-old, 3-month-old, and older infants and found glucose metabolic activity increasing in anatomical regions in agreement with behavioral, anatomical, and neurophysiological alterations that are known to occur in the first 12 months according to established patterns of infant CNS development. More recent studies have extended this growing body of information on human infants by using PETT and functional imaging (fMRI) (Chugani, 1992, 1993, 1994; Chugani & Jacobs, 1994; Kreis *et al.*, 1993).

Although it is not yet possible to specify which brain mechanisms are specifically involved in perceptual processing, it is believed that many of the events are distributed throughout the brain. Perception represents functions drawing from systems at diverse anatomical sites, both in upper and in lower regions of the brain (Bower, 1977; Livingston, 1978; Majovski & Jacques, 1982; Posner, 1993).

Connections conceivably involved with central information processing of context-dependent and context-free events in the environment may involve cortex-to-basal ganglia and frontolimbic pathways. Sensorimotor readiness, in part, is dependent on cognitive–spatial mapping properties thought to be carried out in the hippocampal formation and neocortical structures (Izquierdo, 1975; Liben, Patterson, & Newcombe, 1981; Nauta, 1986a,b; O'Keefe, 1994; Squire & Zola-Morgan, 1991).

Memory underlies the highest functions of the brain, from multiplying two numbers to developing a sense of oneself. All memories come from the world outside of the mind. Whereas visual images leave shadows on the retina for less than a second, sounds taper off into echoes lasting no more than 4 s. A major question arises: How does a coded memory process, specific to certain environmental events, differ from those that organize and lay down a long-term memory code? Partial answers have issued from a recent developmental study by DiGuilio *et al.* (1994) of procedural versus declarative memory. Structures implicated as crucial for forming new and enduring memories include the hippocampi, frontal lobes, and medial–temporal structures (Squire & Zola-Morgan, 1991). It is at this level that human thought, planning, decision-making, and organization of information involved in higher cortical functions are taking place, and where sensory impressions leave their "traces" in neurons. How this process works is not fully understood because only selected features are allowed to pass on to the cortex.

A child's functional memory capacity develops across years from early infancy onward. Recall performance increases reaching a plateau in adolescence (Kail & Hagen, 1977; Meudell, 1983). Procedural and declarative memory have been studied extensively in adults but research on the development of memory in childhood has been focused mainly on declarative memory from a developmental perspective. The dissociation between procedural and declarative memory systems in amnestic patients may serve as a model for a better understanding of the type of memory tasks children are capable of learning early in their cognitive development and subsequently improve with aging.

Developmental differences seen at different ages on measures of declarative memory may correspond to anatomical changes occurring in such structures as the hippocampi, diencephalon, and medial temporal lobes (Nadel & Zola-Morgan, 1984; Squire & Zola-Morgan, 1991; Zola-Morgan & Squire, 1993). Procedural memory is thought to reach maturation by middle childhood although no consensus has been reached concerning the neural mechanisms responsible. Tulving (1985) suggested that procedural memory is analogous to that of lower animals which is subserved by subcortical structures. Evidence from several animal and human studies has shown a role of the striate system, independent from corticolimbic circuit responsible for recognition and recall, involved in mediating procedural memory (Heindel, Salmon, Shults, Walicke, & Butters, 1989; Mishkin & Petri, 1984; Saint-Cyr, Taylor, & Lang, 1987).

DiGuilio *et al.* (1994) have demonstrated in children that the level of procedural memory performance stabilizes during a period of development when declarative memory continues to improve. A plausible explanation may come from myelination and neuronal dendritic proliferation processes that continue in the diencephalon; ongoing maturation in hippocampal formation; and associated connections involving the temporal lobe regions. The absence of age differences found in procedural memory may suggest that these brain regions are functionally and neuroanatomically mature by middle childhood.

How other information is inhibited is a mystery. How neurons are "tuned in" to the ongoing events of the environment, such that they can abruptly change in firing patterns on sensing the smell of food, the perception of fear or threat, the sight of something stimulating, is unresolved at present. Functional imaging (MR), MRS, and MSI are quantitative methods that are providing a major gain in examining the *in vivo* process of how cognition takes place.

The question of "how does a cognitive code become established?" involves understanding how neurons record symbolization of the representational objects from the environment. How representations, symbolically, achieve distinctiveness as to properties of global consistency and stability (once encoded) in the brain remains one of the major challenges for researchers of infant cognitive development (Grossberg, 1980).

Representation of environmental events receives continuous updating, in part, via the thalamocortical processing of spatiotemporal events, such as formation of a spatiotemporal "envelope" of reality leading to consciousness. The thalami are the major structures and gateways for the flow of information toward the cortex and are the first point at which information can be blocked by synaptic inhibition during sleep. Lashley, Chow, and Semmes (1951) asserted that the core function of the CNS lies in the spatial and temporal integration of perception and motor activity in order to provide refined adaptation of behavior. Since then, major progress has been made in investigating the role of the thalamocortical mechanism involved in arousal and sleep (Steriade *et al.,* 1993).

Some important clues related to how brain mechanisms operate in terms of sensory processing and an infant's behavioral output come from a consideration of noncorrespondence with past experiences. The infant discovers through action that stored codes are connected after his or her behavior achieves success. Perhaps it is at that particular moment that perception itself is projected in symbolic form in a predictive manner for the desired behaviors to follow. Behavior, in this sense, is essential to the shaping process of stored sensory information and not simply its goal. Memory storage might be deposited in the neural substrates of various brain centers that are accessed according to a given contextlike paging system such as is found in a library cataloging system. Delays in matching stored percepts to sensory input would then be experienced when the context is suddenly altered (Majovski & Jacques, 1982; Petersen *et al.,* 1994; Saint-Cyr *et al.,* 1987; Sergent, Ohta, & MacDonald, 1992; Zola-Morgan & Squire, 1993).

Some crucial steps considered operational in this process include rapid matching stage; hypothesis formation; internal sorting from possibilities; and testing the selections made via behavioral acts. Siqueland and Lipsitt (1966) demonstrated that infants can exhibit learning during the first day of postnatal life. Head turning is a regular response in which hypothesis testing conceivably is occurring. Memory storage is taking place together with suppression of interhemispheric transfer of memory codes. The suppression phenomenon introduced here has the potential effect of expanding the capacity of the neocortex for memory storage in its early stages. The anterior commissure of the corpus callosum, which interconnects the two temporal lobes, is believed to participate in memory storage bilaterally in a yet unspecified process.

Studies that have examined the relationship between abilities of infants and subsequent cognitive functioning indicate a strong relationship between infant behaviors and cognitive and linguistic abilities in early childhood, despite rather low correlations of test scores and measurements from infant intelligence tests. It has been suggested that later cognitive development correlates more highly with early problem-solving skills, whereas language development tends to correlate more highly with a child's understanding of both object–concept and means–end relationships (Siegel, 1979). Current research on dyslexia has addressed the issue of the extent reading deficits of dyslexic children are related to processing deficits at the levels of sensory–visual, cognitive–linguistic, or both. Using evoked potential brain mapping at the P110 and N400 microstates has shown critical factors for successful identification of specific processing deficits in brain mapping studies (Brandeis *et al.,* 1994).

Studies have also shown that cerebral functions are not necessarily localized as was previously believed based on older theories regarding left and right brain functions because children, as well as adults, involve both hemispheres. Perhaps in early development, both hemispheres serve linguistic functions, prior to left-hemisphere lateralization in the majority of right-handed individuals for language capacity (Benson & Zaidel, 1985; DeVos *et al.,* 1995; Mills *et al.,* 1993; Semrud-Clikeman *et al.,* 1991). This would suggest the possibility that greater cortical plasticity is most likely present in the earlier stages of infant language development (Molfese, 1977; Witelson, 1985). Despite the appearance of a high degree of hemispheric specialization during child maturation, the human brain can be viewed as a "single-channel system" in the earlier stages of infant development and later, shifts as a result of changes in its subsequent cognitive and linguistic development (Bennes *et al.,* 1994; Kinsbourne, 1976; Taylor, 1969; Witelson, 1977).

Some of the rather striking consistent correlations between maturation of the brain and development of behavioral processes are emerging from recent MRI, functional imaging (MR), and MRS investigations in infants (Chugani, 1992; Kreis *et al.,* 1993; Kwong *et al.,* 1992). The visual processing area in the brain has been studied and shows development early in the first year. Limbic areas develop later in the first year. Sensorimotor areas develop in earnest in the second year whereas auditory areas continue to develop well into the fourth year (Bronson, 1982; Bushnell, 1982; Levine, 1982; Selnes & Whitaker, 1976). The brain's highest areas (those involved in thinking, abstraction, reasoning, and problem-solving) continue to mature into the teens and perhaps into the third decade. Development of social competency can be viewed as a mixture of maturing of perceptual, sensorimotor, motor, and linguistic mechanisms in the brain, in conjunction with the social conditions of the acculturation process (Oates, 1979; Siegel, 1979).

CNS Maturation in Early Cognitive Development

Maturation of cognitive abilities in relation to brain development, previously discussed, also can influence emotional and personality development in an as yet unspecified manner (Emde, Gaensbauer, & Harmon, 1976). Kagan (1985) proposed a maturational sequence of cognitive abilities as follows. First, the infant demonstrates the capacity of memory for past experiences; second, active memory formation occurs; third, there is a symbolic framework that takes shape; fourth, the infant is able to infer causality; and finally, the child is able to exhibit self-awareness. Kagan and co-workers assert that these five steps occur in sequence by 24 months in normal brain development (Kagan, 1981; Kagan, Kearsley, & Zelazo, 1978; Kagan & Moss, 1983).

Kagan's research has demonstrated that a normal developing child by 8 months has the ability to retrieve hidden objects, whereas earlier, if "out of sight," it was "out of mind." Beginning approximately at 8–9 months, incoming information is related to knowledge for the first time, giving rise to the emergence of active memory processing. At 8 to 10 months, cardiac acceleration occurs in relation to exposure to the visual cliff experiment. This does not occur prior to 8 months, indicating that the sympathetic nervous system is having greater influence

and affects what has been commonly termed the separation anxiety phenomenon. Infants all over the world have been shown to manifest separation anxiety features between 8 and 12 months (Kagan, 1985). This may reflect the fact that myelination occurs in the frontal regions by about 12 months reaching greatest deposition of myelin by age 2 (Dietrich & Hoffman, 1992). As growth of the CNS continues, new capabilities emerge. At 17 to 24 months, several important behaviors emerge: appreciation of right versus wrong; appreciation that physical aggression is wrong; appearance of anxiety in relation to failure; the ability to experience empathy; and acknowledging anxiety in relation to unsolved problems.

At 1 to 3 years of age, children begin to recognize themselves with a sense of self-appreciation. It is thought that the maturing brain's anatomical structures and neurochemical pathways permit the concept of self-awareness to emerge, implicating structures such as the hippocampi, thalamocortical nuclei systems, corpus callosum development, and frontal lobe maturation (Aboitiz, Scheibel, Fisher, & Zaidel, 1992; Bekkers, 1993; Cowell, Allen, Kertesz, Zalatimo, & Demenberg, 1994; Mills *et al.,* 1993; Posner & Rothbart, 1992). Kagan's (1981) studies show that in a child of approximately 2–3 years, fear is prevalent. The more a child is capable of inhibiting an unfamiliar experience, the better stabilized the child becomes. Separation anxiety is a cognitive mediated event and the environmental context dictates the value placed on the notion of a child's "inhibitedness" (Smith & DeVito, 1984). The latter consideration may be causally related to aspects of temperament that can be influenced with experience throughout child development. The parasympathetic system quells sympathetic arousal to unfamiliar and unregistered events in the child's repertoire of behavioral experiences. The development of temperament heavily influences a child's behavioral choices in later years in many subtle ways, e.g., children with ADD/H or behavioral adjustment difficulties show adverse effects concerning decision-making strategy.

Cerebral Asymmetry and Cerebral Lateralization

To date, there is no firm conclusion as to the nature and cause of cerebral hemisphere asymmetry. However, the structure and function of each hemisphere are indeed different (Connelly *et al.*, 1993; Mazziotta & Phelps, 1985; Sperry, Gazzaniga, & Bogen, 1969). An explanation of the functional differences solely in terms of a dichotomy of verbal or nonverbal nature of information processing also has not been adequately substantiated. Many researchers have proposed theories and models of the development of cerebral asymmetry and its function, including Buffery (1976), Corballis (1980), Kimura (1967), Kinsbourne (1974), Kinsbourne and Hiscock (1977), Krashen (1973), Lenneberg (1967), Moscovitch (1977), and Witelson (1977).

Some investigators have suggested that within the left and right cerebral hemispheres, at all ages and in both sexes, different functions are served (Benson & Zaidel, 1985; Bradshaw & Nettleson, 1983; Bryden, 1979; Corballis, 1982; Kinsbourne, 1976; Morgan, 1977; Taylor, 1969; Witelson & Pallie, 1973). It is believed that bilateral integration of information is mainly subserved by the corpus callosum. Problems arise when growth is delayed or when dysmyelination or other neural pathway dysfunctions occur in the between-hemisphere interplay during cognitive information processing (Aboitiz *et al.*, 1992; Cowell *et al.*, 1994; Dietrich, 1990; Dietrich & Hoffman, 1992; Witelson, 1985). A majority of studies and theories that deal with the body of scientific evidence on cerebral asymmetry have focused on the lateralized aspects of cognitive functioning in children.

Other investigators have reported studies that have pointed away from the content-dictated, verbal–spatial dichotomies of the encoding process to a process-determined, "analytical/sequential" versus "gestalt/holistic" information processing style (Bogen, 1969; Levy, 1972; Levy-Agresti & Sperry, 1968; Luria & Simernitskaya, 1977; Sperry, 1974; Sperry *et al.*, 1969). Kinsbourne and Hiscock (1977, 1978) have presented compelling arguments leading away from the concept of progressive lateralization with age. Kinsbourne (1982) discussed in depth the importance of the collaborative efforts of the two hemispheres of the brain. Arguing from the viewpoint of cerebral lateralization theory, Kinsbourne stated that mental activities that relate to action in the real world impose demands for integral and coordinated action of both sides of the brain.

Luria (1966, 1973a) places emphasis on each hemisphere contributing a different strategy of cognitive information-processing and does not isolate each process within a specific hemisphere of the brain. He views the human brain as hierarchically organized in order to integrate messages from its lower centers as well as across hemispheres. Luria asserts that dichotomy of functioning does not do justice to the complexity of the human brain's hemispheres. Rather, it is the manner in which the hemispheres organize or represent information versus the type of information organized that is the important distinguishing feature (Luria, 1970, 1973a,b).

Witelson's (1977) earlier review of selected developmental studies on different sensory modalities pertaining to cerebral asymmetries, handedness, sensorimotor, perceptual, and even genetic studies shows that development of cognitive functions follows a definite order. Several changes occur, some of which can be genetically determined (but influenced by the environment). Hemispheric shifts in which side of the brain handles what type of information, related to alterations in the structural development of the brain, also occur (Annett, 1978; Bakan, 1971; Satz, Strauss, Hunter, & Wada, 1994). Cerebral dominance is related not only to linguistic processes but also to underlying morphogenetic factors that are influenced by several factors including gender differences in the normal developing infant as well as pathological conditions affecting early brain development (Satz, 1993; Satz, Orsini, Saslow, & Henry, 1985; Satz *et al.*, 1994).

The *planum temporale* (PT) has been a major focus of brain laterality research that has looked at asymmetry relative to other brain regions and neuropsychological evidence linking this structure to language development. Kulynych *et al.* (1994) have perhaps made this the first *in vivo* study reported to show evidence of gender differences in the asymmetry of PT. Left plana were significantly larger than right plana among normal males. No significant differences between left and right areas were present among females. The lack of a significant main effect of gender was interpreted to mean no difference in overall (left and right) planum size was observed, although left plana alone were significantly larger in men and women.

This finding corresponds remarkably close to Witelson and Kigar's (1992) findings concerning asymmetries of the horizontal portion of the Sylvian fissure, the posterior extent of which reflects PT length. These results also show a consistent correlation with earlier neuropsychological reports of gender differences in patterns of functional asymmetry (Kimura & Harshman, 1984). The divergence in patterns of PT laterality suggests that sex differences in the lateralization of language need major consideration in any discussion of the relationship between human psychopathology and developmental abnormal cerebral asymmetries.

Intermodal hemispheric processing of information can show differential effects when the child approaches age 8 and older, a result of the late structural maturation of the corpus callosum (Aboitiz *et al.,* 1992; Cowell *et al.,* 1994). This can lead to various forms of difficulties, for example, dominance problems, dyslexia, and learning difficulties (Satz *et al.,* 1985; Schonhaut & Satz, 1983; Sips, Catsman-Berrevoets, Van Dongen, Van der Werff, & Brooke, 1994). Currently there are conflicting theories and hypotheses related not only to cerebral dominance and hemispheric specialization but also to the onset, development, sexual orientation, and maturation of the brain's lateralization (Geschwind & Galaburda, 1984; McCormick & Witelson, 1994; Satz *et al.,* 1985; Witelson, 1985).

Conclusion

Inadequate encoding of early experience, brain insult, nutritional deficiency, anoxia at birth, perinatal asphyxia, teratogenicity factors, and certain congenital hereditary/metabolic defects can impose severe restrictions on the developmental capacities essential for sensory processing of motor, visual, acoustic, and haptic information. Until normal brain development and the mechanisms involved in higher mental processes are more precisely measured and adequately described by newer technologies and improved experimental designs, educational, diagnostic, remedial, and therapeutic efforts will only be partially effective.

An essential first step in making scientific progress regarding normal brain maturation is to describe the events and conditions defining psychological functions before proceeding to hypotheses and constructs of brain–behavior relationships. Experimental studies of brain mechanisms and developmental issues, coupled with neurophysiological, neuropsychological, neuroimaging, and neurobiological data will yield broader generalizations and more precise knowledge leading to better understanding of the child's developing brain structures, functions, and cognitive processes involved in extracting meaning from the external environment. The next section discusses the most recent advances in brain imaging techniques and methods for mapping brain function onto structure *in vivo.*

Research Techniques for Studying Normal Brain Development and Its Functions

New Brain Imaging Techniques for Studying Normal Brain Development and Its Functions

The major new brain imaging tools in the past decade have led to advances in imaging of brain anatomy, CNS development, metabolic measurement of hemodynamics, and electrochemical physiological properties of nervous tissue that reflect a wide array of neuronal activities. With regard to cognitive human neuroscience, the major consequence of these newer technologies lies in their ability to identify, localize, and more precisely study higher cognitive processes. Methods based on noninvasive magnetic resonance imaging (MRI), magnetic resonance spectroscopy (MRS), functional MRI imaging (FI or EPI), magnetic source imaging (MSI or MEG), and positron emission tomographic technique (PETT) have each demonstrated their impact on the dynamic changes occurring in the human brain. This extends beyond sensory neural systems to higher mental processes, e.g., thinking, reading, problem-solving, and how the brain attends (selects) to certain stimuli versus inhibits ("brain work" in the words of David Ingvar, M.D.).

It is now possible to apply these newer techniques to the study of normal and abnormal brain development and certain mental functions. These new tools and their clinical impact will be briefly reviewed. Emphasis will be placed on their respective capabilities, applications in clinical and neuroscientific investigation, and potential to go beyond the two major tools used, i.e., MRI and PETT.

MRI

MRI (nuclear magnetic resonance) is based on proton (hydrogen) nuclei in which resonating hydrogen atoms give off radio waves (radio frequency) that reveal tissue structure, noninvasively, and can detect physical abnormalities. (For a complete discussion, see Stark & Bradley, 1992.) MRI has been applied to study human brain development as to neuroanatomical patterns of myelination and dysmyelination (Dietrich, 1990; Dietrich & Hoffman, 1992; Dietrich *et al.*, 1988; Hittmair *et al.*, 1994; Zimmerman *et al.*, 1992).

EPI

Recent advances in neuroimaging technology have led to the adaptation of MRI to look not just at structure but also at function. Echo-planar imaging (EPI) was invented by Sir Peter Mansfield and colleagues (Stehling *et al.*, 1990, 1991). It makes use of high-speed computers and mathematical algorithms to generate images of high rate frequency so that second-to-second changes in one's brain activity can be recorded. EPI lends itself to functional imaging (FI) of the CNS, depiction of blood and CSF flow dynamics, and movie imaging of the mobile fetus *in utero* (Stehling *et al.*, 1990). Basic changes are viewed in the blood supply of the brain. Strong magnetic fields in an MRI scanner induce a magnetic field in hemoglobin, the basic molecule in blood that transports oxygen via heme–heme interaction. This magnetic field then distorts the signal given off by proton atoms (hydrogen) and shows up in the skin. Active areas of the brain require more blood since they thrive on glucose but they do not use more oxygen. When blood flow to an active area of the brain increases, the concentration of oxygen-poor hemoglobin leaving the area decreases noticeably. The principle works with respect to cognitive activity in that it is possible using EPI to see where thought patterns are forming since it is that region of the brain that suddenly starts to utilize more blood. Some of these areas can be quite small, but using EPI, changes are revealed in the blood supply to components of the brain as small as 1 mm in diameter. Neuronal activity causes local brain changes in the cerebral blood flow, blood volume, and blood oxygenation; by using intrinsic blood–tissue contrast, functional MRI (EPI technology) thus opens a spatiotemporal window onto individual brain physiology (Jackson *et al.*, 1994; Kwong *et al.*, 1992).

EPI's accuracy lies in its ability to demonstrate the differences between two brains and establish that the sites under observation do not shift over time, which is a significant advance made over the general maps of similar areas showing where specific stimuli exert their effects using PETT technology. This method of relating brain structure to function uses equipment that has become widely available in the past few years and has considerable implications for investigations of many neurologic diseases, and for understanding brain functions and dysfunctions (Connelly *et al.*, 1993). Researchers have been us-

ing this technique in human studies of frontal cortex activation during word generation, language, and memory functioning (McCarthy, Blamire, Rothman, Gruetter, & Shulman, 1993; Shulman, Blamire, Rothman, & McCarthy, 1993). PETT studies have shown that an area of the left frontal lobe plays a role in language. However, EPI studies reveal that a part of the right-hand frontal lobe lights up as well (McCarthy *et al.*, 1993; Shulman *et al.*, 1993). These studies also reveal short-term memory associated with the frontal lobes. EPI as a tool assists surgeons as it has been shown that critical structures to be preserved versus excised may show slight variation from patient to patient. It is an accurate method of locating and displaying the structures while surgery is in progress. The value of functional MRI studies versus PETT is that it allows examination of brain activity in an individual in relation to his or her own brain structure in order that differences in one's brain anatomy can be studied in direct relation to mental operations (McCarthy *et al.*, 1993). These anatomical applications allow progress to be made in considering what structures are involved in such higher cortical functions as awareness, voluntary control of information storage, motor responses under cerebral regulation, organization, and higher thought planning (decision-making).

PETT

PETT averages, among individuals, cerebral blood flow (CBF). Only one such study can be implemented at a time. Because of safety regulations, women of childbearing age cannot be scanned. CBF requirement for brain viability in newborns has been demonstrated and correlated to be lower than in adults (Altman *et al.*, 1988). The fundamental links between blood flow and neuronal activity have remained obscure up to the recent advent of EPI. CBF measurement enables one to determine where neurons are more or less active relative to a control situation. However, increase in neuronal activity has its drawbacks. For example, it can signal either inhibitory or excitatory synaptic events. By its use in research, the task undertaken requires measurement that must be related to the efficiency of the task's performance because blood flow lags behind in neural activity and real time (Raichle, 1987; Raichle *et al.*, 1994).

The major advantages of the EPI technique are that it is fast, safe, yields maximum data in the least amount of time, resolution is of the highest degree, and the technique is readily available without the constraints of a cyclotron needed to make isotopes for PETT. With respect to infants, especially in terms of perfusion imaging, this is the major advance for early infant detection of hemorrhages and ischemic conditions based on the utility of the navigation technique for EPI and rapid imaging in millisecond-to-millisecond recordings (Stehling *et al.*, 1990, 1991). The PETT method requires averaging among subjects within a normalized brain situation as opposed to functional MRI (EPI) studies, which allow examination of brain activity of *an individual* in relation to *his or her own* brain structure.

MRS

Phosphorus nuclear magnetic resonance spectroscopy (^{31}P-MRS) is a noninvasive investigation technique that measures intracellular metabolism in the brain of humans including infants. The acronym "NMR" has been replaced by "MRS" (Ross & Michaels, 1994). MRS can be used to measure relative metabolite concentrations in human tissues and organs *in vivo*; study energy metabolites and intracellular pH; and as a research tool and an investigative technique in cases of infant asphyxia. MRS is unique in that it provides quantitative information about a wide range of intracellular metabolites. The first neonatal applications were described in 1983 (Cady *et al.*, 1983). The technique allows important metabolic consequences of cellular hypoxia to be detected rapidly and is being used in medical centers to investigate normal and abnormal conditions in neurodevelopment (Hope & Moorecraft, 1991). *In vivo* MRS provides biochemical information on living organisms in a noninvasive manner. Clinical correlations have been made regarding intractable seizures of both children and adults with long-term neurologic sequelae associated with decreased phosphocreatine; neuronal loss or damage (e.g., increased rates of Cr and Cho reflecting astrocytosis); metabolic ratios (orthophosphate); and information on morphologic and metabolic brain development (Gadian *et al.*, 1994; Martin *et al.*, 1990).

Recent studies have shown, preliminarily, that MRS can contribute to the evaluation of CNS abnormalities of infants and children, namely, neurodegenerative disorders that show low levels of *N*-acetylaspartate. This particular metabolite has been shown to be significantly lower in infants with a tendency to increase in teens. MRS investigations have provided new information about metabolic

changes in early childhood in terms of elevation peaks on metabolites that have been attributable to myelination; in addition, membrane synthesis differences, useful for the determination of brain maturation and diagnosis of pathology as well as retardation, have been recorded by this technique (Gadian *et al.*, 1994; Graham *et al.*, 1994; Kreis *et al.*, 1993; Tzika *et al.*, 1993).

MRS imaging has permitted sequential *in vivo* analysis of CNS maturation in the perinatal period that is superior in anatomical resolution, and especially in the characterization of myelination, to either cranial ultrasound or radiographic CT. As a result, accurate detection and recognition of brain lesions associated with hypoxic–ischemic encephalopathy is possible, including conditions of periventricular leukoencephalopathy. This has advanced our understanding of the associated risk factors for abnormal neurodevelopment outcome with specific lesions. In this regard, MRS provides a metabolic "window" into the biochemical events during and following asphyxia. The potential application of this noninvasive technology may lie in its ability to identify brain injury that is reversible in sufficient time to intervene based on imaging studies. The importance of combining MRI with MRS is that MRI could improve spectroscopy interpretation by identifying the observed tissue whereas MRS may help to better clarify diagnosis of anatomic lesions detected by MRI in newborns (Goplerud *et al.*, 1993; Peden *et al.*, 1993; Reynolds *et al.*, 1991).

MSI

MSI is an investigative technique that tracks electrical signals generated as the brain and muscle tissue carry out their routine activities. MSI scans can identify the precise functions of different parts of the brain. For example, sensors placed around the skull detect increased electrical activity where movement originates. The system's computer can then generate an image that pinpoints the brain regions that control motion. The principle on which MSI operates is based on the fact that every electrical signal creates a magnetic field around it. In the body, the difficulty is that such magnetic fields are extremely small, i.e., a billionth of the earth's gravitational pull in the case of the brain. Surface (depth) recording of electrical or magnetic potentials via this technology allows precise measurement (milliseconds) of changes between experimental and controlled conditions. This is particularly advantageous in tracing the circuitry of a specific mental activity. Research in this field has identified specific generators of electrical signals and has led to developments relating to measurements of what the brain does when neuronal systems are involved in a given task, and how this takes place in terms of mapping function onto structure (Gallen *et al.*, 1993; Huk & Vieth, 1993; Orrison *et al.*, 1990).

Studies have investigated neuroanatomical localization of cerebral function by magnetoencephalography (MEG) combined with MRI and CT (Orrison *et al.*, 1990). Unlike traditional EEG, these studies cannot determine the exact location because electrical signals are destroyed as they pass through bone and tissue. Because MSI monitors electrical activity, it will be possible to tell immediately whether or not the brain tissue is responding. This holds great promise for diagnostic studies involving head injuries, strokes, and psychiatric conditions. This technology, in comparison with EPI as discussed above, which measures the rate at which blood flows in the brain and is only a means to an end, lends itself to more precise measurement of the electrical activity that is the physical manifestation of thought. The latter is too rapid and subtle for EPI to address at present.

SQUIDs

MEG is based on the principle of magnetic field detection of the tiniest electrical currents that flow along nerve cells. These fields are so sensitive that they can only be detected with SQUIDs (superconducting quantum interference devices).

Research in this area has been conducted by investigators who have been able to demonstrate imaging of regional changes in the spontaneous activity of the brain (Wang *et al.*, 1993). Investigators in New Mexico (Orrison *et al.*, 1990) are using a system with 37 SQUIDs in order to link to a supercomputer that can determine where the brain's electrical activity is occurring. By combining MEG and EPI, one can achieve precision in studies currently in progress regarding seizure activity, neurogenerative disorders, and certain psychiatric conditions. It is not yet applicable to the neurodevelopment of infants, but as technology develops, refinements may enable viewing the signals that scintillate over the landscape of cerebral conditions in early abnormal processes (Gallen *et al.*, 1993). Researchers will seek to create a dynamic, functional image of how

mental processes such as perception, memory, attention, problem-solving, and decision-making proceed in the brain. SQUIDs may pave the road toward a new level of analysis regarding both baseline information for normal brain processes, as well as dysfunctional states. It is well known that disruptions caused by brain damage correlate highly with abnormal patterns of magnetic fields which can be traced by using MEG recordings and SQUIDs.

US

Cranial ultrasonography (US) has proven to be of value in predicting neurodevelopmental outcome in preterm infants in conjunction with MRI in early human development (Leviton & Paneth, 1990; Van de Bor, Den-Ouden, & Guit, 1992).

In summary, the new brain imaging techniques and methodologies for studying normal brain development and its functions and abnormal processes have the potential of better defining and more precisely describing brain–behavior functions, *in vivo* and in real-time dynamic processes at different stages in development. Combining these technologies for diagnostic purposes, understanding human cognitive processes involved in higher mental functions, and assessing clinical conditions for infants at high risk suggests a vital and necessary role for clinical neuropsychology as this science and practice advances.

Research Designs and Methodologies

The choice of experimental designs and research methodologies available for investigation of scientific and clinical questions in the field of developmental neuropsychology poses significant problems, e.g., replication, proper statistical means of analyzing sample data, group differences, and power as to the conclusions that can be drawn from research studies. Spreen *et al.* (1984) addressed some of the methodological concerns regarding developmental neuropsychology research and made the following point regarding the importance of replication in competent research.

> The goals of the replication study are to answer the following questions. Can the original investigator or an independent investigator following the information provided by the original investigator replicate the results of the original study? Have social, cultural, economic, medical, etc., changes in the population made previous findings obsolete or misleading? Are the findings generalizable to a new set of sub-

jects, test items, test settings, etc.? In sum, replication is a powerful tester for determining the relevance of an investigation and for weeding out findings that may show significance by pure chance or may have become obsolete. (pp. 88–89)

The future of clinical research in developmental neuropsychology will radically change in the next few decades, reflecting the fact that available instruments are being technologically refined for pragmatic use with different age levels of populations starting with fetal life. The key to making a systematic investigation of mapping brain function onto structure during development in order to correlate cortical processes in the functional organization of the brain lies in the combination of imaging techniques (MRI, PETT, ^{1}H-MRS) together with functional source localization (Hillyard, 1987) and neuropsychological measurement (Magnun, Hillyard, & Luck, 1993; Posner & Rothbart, 1992; Taylor et al., 1984).

The horizons that lie ahead for developmental neuropsychological research will be shaped chiefly through these emerging technological innovations. These include imaging of in vivo brain chemistry, metabolism, and physiology by quantifying individual ($N = 1$) maturational changes in cerebral functioning via mapping brain function onto structure. A radically new data base from which to make generalizations about normal brain–behavior relationships in the developing infant will come about through more refined observations and accurate measurement regarding structure, function, and metabolic requirements of the brain during development.

A current review of the literature of developmental psychology and developmental neuropsychology reveals a lack of replication in many studies. There exists considerable controversy in the area of human lateralization studies, cerebral asymmetry theories, and implications for brain development. These controversies will abound until research on normal brain–behavior relationships in infants and young children begins to fill in the gaps in our knowledge.

Despite the impressive existing array of technological capabilities for measurement, a major aspect is missing. Measurement of the brain's sensory, motor, and cognitive processes provides only indirect assessment of task performance. Even noninvasive techniques, such as EEG or event related potential (ERP), are indirect in that they only measure electrophysiological phenomena arising from electrochemical brain activity, not actual cognitive activity (Gevins et al., 1981). Details of cognitive activities must be inferred from knowledge of the underlying physiology and the task being performed by the subject (Fender, 1985). What is needed to overcome these limitations is a systematic, comprehensive investigation correlating patterns of brain activity with selected behaviors; and mapping of function onto brain structure. This will allow researchers to acquire information about the functional organization of the working brain (Gallen et al., 1993; Huk & Vieth, 1993; Orrison et al., 1990; Posner, 1993).

It is now possible to map brain function onto structure by bringing together neuropsychological assessment data about structural changes and correlating structural damage with change in cerebral function and altered cortical processes. Various determinants, which can be quantitatively measured and correlated, will allow more accurate description of the maturational changes in cerebral function with reasonable behavioral correlates. Cognitive tasks administered during physiological neuroimaging measurements allow for clinical and experimental investigation of specific variables affecting regional brain activity involved in cognitive information processing (Chugani & Phelps, 1986; Gur & Reivich, 1980; Posner & Petersen, 1990; Risberg & Ingvar, 1973; Roland, Eriksson, Widen, & Stone-Elander, 1989; Sergent et al., 1992). These studies have demonstrated specific behavioral effects of cognitive tasks on regional CNS activation.

Conclusion

Relatively little is known about the normal developing brain with respect to higher cortical function development, especially during early infancy. Recent studies and neurotechnologies discussed have begun to make an impact on this situation. Significant information on the development of normal brain–behavior functions is emerging from combined efforts using imaging methods (MRI and EPI) (which reveal structure); neuropsychological assessment techniques (which determine consequences of neurological function); neural source localization techniques (which can identify the site of those neural populations that subserve specific brain functions); and metabolic and spectral measurements (PETT and MRS) of human physiology (metabolic tissue competency) (Gallen et al., 1993; Kwong et al., 1992; McCarthy et al., 1993; Phelps et al., 1986; Shulman et al., 1993; Taylor et al., 1984).

Standardized quantitative *in vivo* correlations of structure, function, metabolism, brain electrical activity, and neuropsychological factors are leading toward a different and more accurate data and knowledge base, enabling developmental scientists and clinicians to approach this area with a greater depth in their understanding of the development of higher cortical functions from a normal developmental perspective. The possibility now exists of linking knowledge regarding brain structure, function, and cerebral physiology with quantitative measurement techniques in a standardized fashion for gathering data so as to produce the needed correlation lacking in previous research studies concerning developing brain structures, function, and normal versus aberrant higher cortical processes in infants and children. The implications for future treatment and clinical prevention strategies are obvious. The role for the profession of clinical pediatric/child neuropsychology is very bright and filled with great promise of advancing the science, practice, and more importantly, the health and welfare of children.

References

Aboitiz, F., Scheibel, A. B., Fisher, R. S., & Zaidel, E. (1992). Fiber composition of the human corpus callosum. *Brain Research, 598,* 143–153.

Afifi, A. K., & Bergman, R. A. (1980). *Basic neuroscience.* Munich: Urban & Schwarzenberg.

Altman, D. I., Powers, W. J., Perlman, J. M., Herscovitch, P., Volpe, S. L., & Volpe, J. J. (1988). Cerebral blood flow requirements for brain viability in newborn infants is lower than adults. *Annals of Neurology, 24,* 218–226.

Altman, J., Brunner, R. L., & Bayer, S. A. (1973). The hippocampus and behavioral maturation. *Behavioral Biology, 8,* 557.

Anderson, P. (1975). Organization of hippocampal neurons and their interconnections. In R. L. Isaacson & K. H. Pribam (Eds.), *The hippocampus* (Vol. I). New York: Plenum Press.

Annett, M. (1978). Genetic and nongenetic influences on handedness. *Behavior, 8,* 227–249.

Arey, L. B. (1974). *Developmental anatomy* (7th ed.). Philadelphia: Saunders.

Bakan, P. (1971). Handedness and birth order. *Nature, 229,* 195.

Barnet, A. B. (1966). Visual responses in infancy and their relation to early visual experience. *Clinical Proceedings Children's Hospital National Medical Center, 22,* 273.

Bear, D. M. (1986). Hemispheric asymmetries in emotional functioning. In B. K. Doane & K. E. Livingston (Eds.), *The limbic system: Functional organization and clinical disorders.* New York: Raven Press.

Bekkers, J. M. (1993). Enhancement by histamine of NMDA-mediated synaptic transmission in the hippocampus. *Science, 261,* 104–106.

Bennes, F. M., Turtle, M., Khan, Y., & Farol, P. (1994). Myelination of a key relay zone in the hippocampal formation occurs in the human brain during childhood, adolescence and adulthood. *Archives of General Psychiatry, 51,* 477–484.

Benson, D. F., & Zaidel, E. (Eds.). (1985). *The dual brain: Hemispheric specialization in humans.* New York: Guilford Press.

Bernstine, R. L., Borkowski, W. J., & Price, A. H. (1955). Prenatal fetal electroencephalography. *American Journal of Obstetrics and Gynecology, 70,* 623.

Bloom, F. E. (1973). Dynamic synaptic communication: Finding the vocabulary. *Brain Research, 62,* 229–305.

Bloom, F. E. (1979). *Neurobiological research and selective attention.* H. G. Birch Memorial Lecture, 1979 International Neuropsychological Society, San Francisco.

Bloom, F. E. (Ed.). (1994). Neuroscience: From the molecular to the cognitive. *Progress in Brain Research, 100.* New York: Elsevier.

Bogen, J. E. (1969). The other side of the brain: Parts I, II, III. *Bulletin of the Los Angeles Neurological Society, 34,* 73–105, 135–162, 191–203.

Bower, T. G. R. (1977). *The perceptual world of the child.* Cambridge, MA: Harvard University Press.

Bradshaw, J. L., & Nettleson, N. C. (1983). *Human cerebral asymmetry.* Englewood Cliffs, NJ: Prentice–Hall.

Brandeis, D., Vitacco, D., & Steinhausen, H. C. (1994). Mapping brain electric microstates in dyslexic children during reading. *Acta-Paedopsychiatrica, 56,* 239–247.

Bronson, G. W. (1982). *The scanning patterns of human infants: Implications for visual learning.* Norwood, NJ: Ablex.

Bruns, F. J., Fraley, D. S., Haigh, J., Marquez, J. M., Martin, D. J., Matuschak, G. M., & Snyder, J. V. (1987). Control of blood flow in organs. In J. V. Snyder & M. R. Pinsky (Eds.), *Oxygen transport in the critically ill* (pp. 87–125). Chicago: Year Book Medical.

Bryden, M. (1979). Evidence for sex differences in cerebral organization. In M. Wittig & A. Peterson (Eds.), *Determinants of sex-related differences in cognitive functioning.* New York: Academic Press.

Buffery, A. W. H. (1976). Sex differences in the neuropsychological development of verbal and spatial skills. In R. M. Knights & D. J. Bakker (Eds.), *The neuropsychology of learning disorders.* Baltimore: University Park Press.

Bushnell, E. W. (1982). Visual–tactual knowledge in 8-, $9\frac{1}{2}$-, and 11-month-old infants. *Infant Behavior and Development, 5,* 63–75.

Cady, E. B., Costello, A. M., Dawson, M. J., Delpy, D. T., Hope, P. L., Reynolds, E. O., Tofts, P. S., & Wilkie, D. R. (1983). Non-invasive investigation of cerebral metabolism in newborn infants by phosphorus nuclear magnetic resonance spectroscopy. *Lancet, 8333,* 1059–1062.

Carlson, B. M. (1994). *Human embryology and developmental biology* (pp. 204–251). St. Louis: Mosby.

Carlson, N. R. (1994). *Physiology of behavior* (5th ed.). Boston: Allyn & Bacon.

Carpenter, M. B. (1978). *Core text of neuroanatomy* (2nd ed.). Baltimore: Williams & Wilkins.

Chugani, H. T. (1992). Functional brain imaging in pediatrics. *Pediatric Clinics of North America, 39,* 777–799.

Chugani, H. T. (1993). Positron emission tomographic scanning: Applications in newborns. *Clinic in Perinatology, 20,* 395–409.

Chugani, H. T. (1994). The role of PET in childhood epilepsy. *Journal of Child Neurology, 9* (Suppl.), 582–588.

Chugani, H. T., & Jacobs, B. (1994). Metabolic recovery in caudate nucleus following cerebral hemispherectomy. *Annals of Neurology 36,* 794–797.

Chugani, H. T., & Phelps, M. E. (1986). Maturational changes in cerebral function in infants determined by ^{18}FDG positron emission tomography. *Science, 231,* 840–843.

Cohen, L. B. (1979). Our developing knowledge of infant perception and cognition. *American Psychologist, 34,* 894–899.

Cohen, L. B., DeLoache, J. S., & Strauss, M. S. (1979). Infant perceptual development. In J. D. Osofsky (Ed.), *Handbook of infant development.* New York: Wiley.

Cohen, M., & Roesmann, U. (1994). *In utero* brain damage: Relationship of gestational age to pathological consequences. *Developmental Medicine and Child Neurology, 36,* 263–268.

Connelly, A., Jackson, G. D., Frackowiak, R. S., Belliveau, J. W., Vargha-Khadem, F., & Gadian, G. D. (1993). Functional mapping of activated human primary cortex with a clinical MR imaging system. *Radiology, 188,* 125–130.

Cooke, J. (1980). Early organization of the central nervous system: Form and pattern. In R. K. Hunt (Ed.), *Neural development.* New York: Academic Press.

Cooper, J. R. & Bloom, F. E. (1991). *The biochemical basis of neuropharmacology* (6th ed.). London: Oxford University Press.

Corballis, M. C. (1980). Is left-handedness genetically determined? In J. Herron (Ed.), *Neuropsychology of left handedness.* New York: Academic Press.

Corballis, M. C. (1982). Asymmetries in spatial representation: Anatomical or perceptual? In R. N. Malatesha & L. C. Hartlage (Eds.), *Neuropsychology and cognition* (Vol. 1). The Hague: Nijhoff.

Courchesne, E., Townsend, J., & Saitoh, O. (1994). The brain in infantile autism: Posterior fossa structures are abnormal: *Neurology, 44,* 214–223.

Cowell, P. E., Allen, L. S., Kertesz, A., Zalatimo, N. S., & Demenberg, V. H. (1994). Human corpus callosum: A stable mathematical model of regional neuroanatomy. *Brain and Cognition, 25,* 52–66.

Cravioto, J., & Arrieta, R. (1979). Stimulation and mental development of malnourished infants. *Lancet, 2,* 899.

Cravioto, J., & Arrieta, R. (1983). Malnutrition in childhood. In M. D. Rutter (Ed.), *Developmental neuropsychiatry.* New York: Guilford Press.

Crelin, E. S. (1973). *Functional anatomy of the newborn.* New Haven, CT: Yale University Press.

Crelin, E. S. (1974). Development of the nervous system: A logical approach to neuroanatomy. *Ciba Clinical Symposia, 26,* 1–32.

Cross, J. H., Gadian, D. G., Connelly, A., & Leonard, J. V. (1993). Proton magnetic resonance spectroscopy studies in lactic acidosis and mitochondrial disorders. *Journal of Inherited Metabolic Disorders, 16,* 800–811.

Curtiss, S. (1979). Genie: Language and cognition. *UCLA Working Papers in Cognitive Linguistics, 1,* 15–62.

Damasio, H. (1989). Anatomical and neuroimaging contribution to the study of aphasia. In H. Goodglass (Ed.), *Handbook of neuropsychology* (Vol. II). Amsterdam: Elsevier.

Darley, F. L., & Fay, W. H. (1980). Speech mechanism. In F. M. Laasman, R. O. Fisch, D. K. Vetter, & E. S. Benz (Eds.), *Early correlates of speech, language, and hearing.* Littleton, MA: PSG Publishing.

Daughaday, W. H. (1981). The adenohypophysis. In R. H. Williams (Ed.), *Textbook of endocrinology.* Philadelphia: Saunders.

Davies, P., & Stewart, A. L. (1975). Low birthweight infants: Neurological sequelae and later intelligence. *British Medical Bulletin, 31,* 85.

Davison, A. N., & Dobbing, J. (1968). The developing brain. In A. N. Davison & J. Dobbing (Eds.), *Applied neurochemistry.* Oxford: Blackwell.

Davison, A. N., & Peter, A. (1970). *Myelination.* Springfield, IL: Thomas.

DeLong, G. R. (1993). Effects of nutrition on brain development in humans. *American Journal of Clinical Nutrition, 57,* (Suppl. 2), 2868–2905.

DeVilliers, P. A., & DeVilliers, J. G. (1979). *Early language.* Cambridge, MA: Harvard University Press.

DeVos, K. J., Wyllie, E., Geckler, C., Kotagal, P., & Comair, Y. (1995). Language dominance in patients with early childhood tumors near left hemisphere language areas. *Neurology, 45,* 349–356.

Dietrich, R. B. (1990). Myelin disorders of childhood: Correlation of MR findings and severity of neurological impairment. *Journal of Computer Assisted Tomography, 14,* 693.

Dietrich, R. B., Bradley, W. G., Zaragoza, E. J., Otto, R. J., Taira, R. K., Wilson, G. H., & Kangarbo, H. (1988). MR evaluation of early myelination patterns in normal and developmentally delayed infants. *American Journal of Roentgenology, 150,* 889–896.

Dietrich, R. B., & Hoffman, C. H. (1992). Myelination and dysmyelination. In D. D. Stark & W. G. Bradley (Eds.), *Magnetic resonance imaging.* St. Louis: Mosby–Year Book.

DiGuilio, D. V., Seidenberg, M., O'Leary, D. S., & Raz, N. (1994). Procedural and declarative memory: A developmental study. *Brain and Cognition, 25,* 79–91.

Dobbing, J. (1975). Prenatal nutritional and neurological development. In N. A. Buchwald & M. A. B. Brazier (Eds.), *Brain mechanism in mental retardation.* New York: Academic Press.

Dobbing, J. (1990). Early nutrition and later achievement. Boyd Memorial Lecture. *Proceedings of the Nutrition Society, 49,* 103–118.

Dobbing, J., & Sands, J. (1970). Timing of neuroblast multiplication in developing human brain. *Nature, 226,* 639.

Dobbing, J., & Sands, J. (1973). Quantitative growth and development of human brain. *Archives of Disabled Children, 48,* 757.

Dobbing, J., & Smart, J. L. (1974). Vulnerability of developing brain and behavior. *British Medical Bulletin, 30,* 164.

Dodge, P., Prensky, A., & Feigin, R. (1975). *Nutrition and the developing nervous system.* St. Louis: Mosby.

Dodgson, M. C. H. (1962). *The growing brain: An essay in developmental neurology.* Bristol, England: Wright Press.

Dunn, A. J. (1976). The chemistry of learning and the formation of memory. In W. H. Gispen (Ed.), *Molecular and functional neurobiology.* Amsterdam: Elsevier.

Dunn, A. J. (1980). Neurochemistry of learning and memory: An evaluation of recent data. *Annual Review of Psychology, 31,* 343–390.

Ellingson, R. J. (1964). Studies of the electrical activity of the developing human brain. *Progress in Brain Research, 9,* 26–53.

Emde, R. N., Gaensbauer, T. J., & Harmon, R. J. (1976). *Emotional expression of infancy: A behavioral study* (Vol. 10). New York: International University Press.

Epstein, H. T. (1978). Growth spurts during brain development: Implications for educational policy and practice. In J. S. Chall & A. F. Mirsky (Eds.), *Education and the brain: The 77th yearbook of the National Society for the Study of Education* (Part II). Chicago: University of Chicago Press.

Fender, D. H. (1985). Source localization of brain electrical activity. In A. Gevins & A. Remond (Eds.), *Handbook of electroencephalography and clinical neurophysiology* (Vol. 3A). Amsterdam: Elsevier.

Finkelstein, S., Alpert, N. M., Ackerman, R. H., Buonano, F. S., Correia, J. A., Chang, J., Kulas, S., Brownell, G. L., & Taveras, J. M. (1980). Positron imaging of the normal brain—Regional patterns of cerebral blood flow and metabolism. *Transactions of the American Neurological Association, 105,* 8–10.

Flechsig, P. (1883). *Plan des menschlichen Gehirns.* Leipzig: Veit.

Franz, R. L. (1963). Pattern vision in newborn infants. *Science, 140,* 296.

Gaddes, W. H. (1980). *Learning disabilities and brain function: A neuropsychological approach.* Berlin: Springer-Verlag.

Gadian, D. G., Connelly, A., Duncan, J. S., Cross, J. H., Kirkhan, F. J., Johnson, C. L., Vargha-Khadem, F., Nevile, B. G., & Jackson, G. D. (1994). 1H magnetic resonance spectroscopy in the investigation of intractable epilepsy. *Acta Neurological Scandinavica, 152,* 116–121.

Gallen, C. C., Sobel, D. F., Schwartz, B., Copeland, B., Waltz, T., & Aung, M. (1993, August 28). Magnetic source imaging: Present and future. *Investigative Radiology, 3,* (Suppl.), 5153–5157.

Geschwind, N., & Galaburda, A. M. (Eds.). (1984). *Cerebral dominance.* Cambridge, MA: Harvard University Press.

Gevins, A. S., Doyle, J. C., Cutillo, B. A., Schaffer, R. E., Tannehill, R. S., Ghannam, J. H., Gilcrease, V. A., & Yeager, C. L. (1981). Electrical potentials in human brain during cognition—New method reveals dynamic patterns of correlation. *Science, 213,* 918–921.

Goldman, P. S. (1975). Age, sex and experience as related to the neural basis of development. In N. A. Buchwald & M. A. B. Brazier (Eds.), *Brain mechanisms in mental retardation.* New York: Academic Press.

Goodglass, H., & Kaplan, E. (1972). *The assessment of aphasia and related disorders.* Philadelphia: Lea & Febiger.

Goplerud, J. M., & Delivoria-Papadopoulos, M. (1993). Nuclear magnetic resonance imaging and spectroscopy following asphyxia. *Clinical Perinatology, 20,* 345–367.

Gottlieb, G. (1976a). Conceptions of prenatal development: Behavioral embryology. *Psychological Review, 83,* 215–234.

Gottlieb, G. (1976b). The roles of experience in the development of behavior and the nervous system. In G. Gottlieb (Ed.), *Neural and behavioral specificity.* New York: Academic Press.

Graham, S. H., Myerhoff, D. J., Bayne, L., Sharp, F. R., & Weiner, M. W. (1994). Magnetic resonance spectroscopy of N-acetylaspartate in hypoxic-ischemic encephalopathy. *Annals of Neurology, 35,* 490–494.

Grossberg, S. (1980). How does a brain build a cognitive code? *Psychological Review, 87,* 1–51.

Gur, R. C., & Reivich, M. (1980). Cognitive task effects on hemispheric blood flow in humans; evidence for individual differences in hemispheric activation. *Brain and Language, 9,* 78–92.

Hack, M., Taylor, H. G., Klein, N., Eiben, R., Schatschneider, C., & Mercuri-Minich, N. (1994). School-age outcomes in children with birth weights under 750 g. *New England Journal of Medicine, 331,* 753–759.

Hagne, I. (1972). Development of the EEG in the normal infants during the first year of life. *Acta Paediatrica Scandinavica, 232* (Suppl. 1), 5.

Halasz, B. (1994). Hypothalamo-anterior pituitary system and pituitary portal vessels. In H. Imura (Ed.), *The pituitary gland* (2nd ed., pp. 1–28). New York: Raven Press.

Hamilton, W. J., & Mossman, H. W. (1974). *Human embryology: Prenatal development of form and function* (4th ed.). London: Heffer.

Hebb, D. O. (1949). *The organization of behavior.* New York: Wiley.

Heindel, W. C., Salmon, D. P., Shults, C. W., Walicke, P. A., & Butters, N. A. (1989). Neuropsychological evidence for multiple implicit memory strategies: A comparison of Alzheimers, Huntington, and Parkinson disease patients. *Journal of Neuroscience, 9,* 282–287.

Hillyard, S. J. (1987). Electrophysiology of cognition. In V. Mountcastle, F. Plum, & S. Geiger (Eds.), *Handbook of physiology: Sec. I. The Nervous System: Vol. V.* (pp. 519–584). Bethesda: American Physiological Society.

Hittmair, K., Wimberger, D., Rand T., Prayer, L., Bernert, G., Kramer, J., & Imhof, H. (1994). MR assessment of brain maturation: Comparison of consequences. *American Journal of Neuroradiology, 15,* 425–433.

Hope, P. L., Costelo, A. M., Cady, E. B., Delpy, D. T., Tofts, P. S., Chu, A., Hamilton, P. A., Reynolds, E. O., & Wilkie, D. R. (1984). Cerebral energy metabolism studied with phosphorus NMR spectroscopy in normal and birth-asphyxiated infants. *Lancet, 2,* 366–370.

Hope, P. L., & Moorecraft, J. (1991). Magnetic resonance spectroscopy. *Clinical Perinatology, 18,* 535–548.

Hudspeth, W. J., & Pribram, K. H. (1992). Psychophysiological indices of cerebral maturation. *International Journal of Psychophysiology, 12,* 19–29.

Huk, W. J., & Vieth, J. (1993). Functional imaging of the brain. *Radiologe, 33,* 633–638.

Humphrey, T. (1964). Some correlation between the appearance of human fetal reflexes and the development of the nervous system. In D. P. Purpura & J. P. Schade (Eds.), *Progress in brain research: Growth and maturation of the brain* (vol. 4). Amsterdam: Elsevier.

Humphrey, T. (1978). Function of the nervous system during prenatal life. In U. Stave & A. A. Weech (Eds.), *Perinatal physiology.* New York: Plenum Medical.

Imura, H. (1994). *The pituitary gland* (2nd ed.). New York: Raven Press.

Ingvar, D. H., Sjölund, B., & Ardö, A. (1976). Correlation between dominant EEG frequency, cerebral oxygen uptake and blood flow. *Encephalography and Clinical Neurophysiology, 41,* 268–276.

Ito, M. (1984). *The cerebellum and neural control.* New York: Raven Press.

Izquierdo, I. (1975). The hippocampus and learning. *Progress in Neurobiology, 5,* 37–75.

Jackson, G. D., Connelly, A., Cross, J. H., Gordon, I., & Gaidan, D. E. (1994). Functional magnetic resonance imaging of focal seizures. *Neurology, 44,* 850–856.

Jacobs, B. L. (1994). Serotonin, motor activity, and depression-related disorders. *American Scientist, 82,* 456–463.

Jernigan, T. L., Hesselink, J. R., Sowell, E., & Tallal, P. A. (1991). Cerebral structure on magnetic resonance imaging in language and learning-impaired children. *Archives of Neurology, 48,* 539–545.

Jones, E. G., & Cowan, W. M. (1978). Nervous tissue: Development of nervous tissue. In E. Weiss (Ed.), *Textbook of histology.* New York: McGraw-Hill.

Kagan, J. (1981). *The second year.* Cambridge, MA: Harvard University Press.

Kagan, J. (1985). The human infant. In A. M. Rogers & C. J. Scheirer (Eds.), *The G. Stanley Hall lecture series* (Vol. 5). Washington, DC: American Psychological Association.

Kagan, J., Kearsley, R. B., & Zelazo, P. R. (1978). *Infancy: Its place in human development.* Cambridge, MA: Harvard University Press.

Kagan, J., & Moss, H. A. (1983). *Birth to maturity.* New Haven, CT: Yale University Press.

Kahle, W., Leonhardt, H., & Platzer, W. (1978). *Color atlas and textbook of human anatomy* (Vol. 3). Chicago: Year Book Medical.

Kail, R. V., Jr., & Hagen, J. W. (1977). *Perspectives on the development of memory and cognition.* Hillsdale, NJ: Erlbaum.

Kaplan, S. L., Grumbach, M. M., & Aubert, M. L. (1976). The ontogenesis of pituitary hormone and hypothalamic factors in the human fetus: Maturation of the central nervous system regulation of anterior pituitary function. *Recent Progress in Hormone Research, 32,* 161.

Kety, S. S. (1970). The biogenic amines in the central nervous system: Their possible roles in arousal, emotion and learning. In F. O. Schmitt (Ed.), *The neurosciences: Second study program.* New York: Rockefeller University Press.

Kimura, D. (1967). Functional asymmetry of the brain in dichotic listening. *Cortex, 3,* 163–178.

Kimura, D., & Harshman, R. (1984). Sex differences in brain organization for verbal and nonverbal functions. In G. De Vries, J. De Bruin, H. Vylings, & M. Conner (Eds.), *Progress in brain research.* Amsterdam: Elsevier.

Kinsbourne, M. (1974). Mechanisms of hemisphere interaction in man. In M. Kinsbourne & W. L. Smith (Eds.), *Hemisphere disconnection and cerebral function.* Springfield, IL: Thomas.

Kinsbourne, M. (1976). The ontogeny of cerebral dominance. In R. Reiber (Ed.), *The neuropsychology of language.* New York: Plenum Press.

Kinsbourne, M. (1982). Hemispheric specialization and the growth of human understanding. *American Psychologist, 37,* 411–420.

Kinsbourne, M., & Hiscock, M. (1977). Does cerebral dominance develop? In S. J. Segalowitz & F. A. Gruber (Eds.), *Language development and neurological theory.* New York: Academic Press.

Kinsbourne, M., & Hiscock, M. (1978). Cerebral lateralization and cognitive development. In J. S. Chall & A. F. Mirsky (Eds.), *Education and the brain: The 77th yearbook of the National Society for the Study of Education* (Part II). Chicago: University of Chicago Press.

Krashen, S. (1973). Lateralization, language, learning, and the critical period: Some new evidence. *Language and Learning, 23,* 63–74.

Kreis, R., Ernst, T., & Ross, B. D. (1993). Development of the human brain: *In vivo* quantification of metabolite and water content with proton magnetic resonance spectroscopy (1H-MRS). *Magnetic Resonance Medicine, 30,* 424–437.

Kuffler, S. W., & Nicholls, J. G. (1977). *From neuron to brain: A cellular approach to the function of the nervous system.* Sunderland, MA: Sinauer Associates.

Kulynych, J., Vladar, K., Jones, D., & Weinberger, D. (1994). Gender differences in the normal lateralization of the supratemporal cortex: MRI surface-rendering morphometry of Heschel's gyrus and planum temporale. *Cerebral Cortex, 4* (2), 107–118.

Kwong, K. K., Belliveau, J. W., Chesler, D. A., Goldberg, I. E., Weisskoff, R. M., Poncelet, B. P., Kennedy, D. N., Hoppel, B. E., Cohen, M. S., & Turner, R. (1992). Dynamic magnetic resonance imaging of human brain activity during primary sensory stimulation. *Proceedings of the National Academy of Sciences, USA, 89,* 5675–5679.

Langman, J. (1975). *Medical embryology: Human development—normal and abnormal* (3rd ed.). Baltimore: Williams & Wilkins.

Lashley, K. S., Chow, K. L., and Semmes, J. (1951). An examination of the electrical field theory of cerebral integration. *Psychology Review, 58,* 123–136.

Le Douarin, N. (1980). Migration and differentiation of neural crest cells. In R. K. Hunt (Ed.), *Neural development.* New York: Academic Press.

Lehninger, A. L. (1968). The neuronal membrane. *Proceedings of the National Academy of Sciences, USA, 60,* 1069–1080.

Lehninger, A. L. (1993). *Principles of biochemistry.* New York: Worth.

Lemire, R. J., Loeser, J. D., Alvord, E. C., & Leech, R. W. (1975). *Normal and abnormal development of the human nervous system.* New York: Harper & Row.

Lenneberg, E. H. (1964). The natural history of language. In F. Smith & G. A. Miller (Eds.), *The genesis of language: A psycholinguistic approach.* Cambridge, MA: MIT Press.

Lenneberg, E. H. (1967). *Biological foundation of language.* New York: Wiley.

Levene, M. I., & Dubowitz, L. M. S. (1982). Low-birth weight babies long-term follow-up. *British Journal of Hospital Medicine, 24,* 487.

Levine, S. (1982). Comparative and psychobiological perspectives on development. In A. Collins (Ed.), *Minnesota symposium* (Vol. 15). Hillsdale, NJ: Erlbaum.

Leviton, A., & Paneth, N. (1990). White matter damage in preterm newborns: An epidemiologic perspective. *Early Human Development, 24* (1), 1–22.

Levy, J. (1972). Lateral specialization of the human brain: Behavioral manifestation and possible evolutionary basis. In J. A. Kiger (Ed.), *Biology of behavior.* Corvaillis: Oregon State University Press.

Levy-Agresti, J., & Sperry, R. W. (1968). Differential perceptual capacities in major and minor hemispheres. *Proceedings of the National Academy of Sciences, USA, 61,* 1151.

Liben, L. S., Patterson, A. H., & Newcombe, N. (1981). *Spatial representation and behavior across the life span: Theory and application.* New York: Academic Press.

Lindsley, D. B. (1939). A longitudinal study of the occipital alpha rhythm in normal children: Frequency and amplitude standards. *Journal of Genetic Psychology, 55,* 197–213.

Lindsley, D. B., & Wicke, J. D. (1974). The electroencephalogram: Autonomous electrical activity in man and animals. In R. F. Thompson & M. M. Patterson (Eds.), *Bioelectric recording techniques. Part B. Electroencephalography and human brain potentials.* New York: Academic Press.

Livingston, R. B. (1978). *Sensory processing, perception, and behavior.* New York: Raven Press.

Lorber, J. (1980). Is your brain really necessary? *Science, 210,* 1232–1234.

Lowrey, G. H. (1978). *Growth and development of children* (7th ed.). Chicago: Year Book Medical.

Lund, R. D. (1978). *Development and plasticity of the brain: An introduction.* London: Oxford University Press.

Luria, A. R. (1960). Verbal regulation of behavior. In M. Brazier (Ed.), *The CNS and behavior.* New York: Josiah Macy Jr. Foundation.

Luria, A. R. (1961). *The role of speech in the regulation of normal and abnormal behavior.* Elmsford, NY: Pergamon Press.

Luria, A. R. (1966). *The human brain and psychological processes.* New York: Harper & Row.

Luria, A. R. (1969a). Origin and brain organization of conscious activity. *Evening lecture to the 19th International Congress of Psychology.* London: Dorset Press.

Luria, A. R. (1969b). Frontal lobe syndromes. In P. J. Vinken & G. W. Bruyn (Eds.), *Handbook of clinical neurology* (Vol. 2). Amsterdam: North-Holland.

Luria, A. R. (1969c). Speech development and the formation of mental processes. In J. Cole & I. Maltzman (Eds.), *A handbook of contemporary Soviet psychology.* New York: Basic Books.

Luria, A. R. (1970). The functional organization of the brain. *Scientific American, 222,* 66–78.

Luria, A. R. (1973a). *The working brain.* New York: Basic Books.

Luria, A. R. (1973b). The frontal lobes and the regulation of behavior. In A. R. Luria & K. H. Pribram (Eds.), *The behavioral psychophysiology of the frontal lobes.* New York: Academic Press.

Luria, A. R. (1980). *Higher cortical functions in man* (2nd ed.). New York: Basic Books.

Luria, A. R. (1982). *Language and cognition.* New York: Wiley–Interscience.

Luria, A. R., & Simernitskaya, E. G. (1977). Interhemispheric relations and the functioning of the minor hemisphere. *Neuropsychologia, 15,* 175–178.

Luria, A. R., & Yudovich, F. I. (1959). *Speech in the development of mental processes in the child.* London: Staples.

McCarthy, G., Blamire, A. M., Rothman, D. L., Gruetter, R., & Shulman, R. G. (1993). Echo-planar magnetic resonance imaging studies of frontal cortex activation during word generation in humans. *Proceedings of the National Academy of Sciences, USA, 90,* 4952–4956.

McConnell, S. K. (1988). Development of decision-making in the mammalian cerebral cortex. *Brain Research Review, 13,* 1–23.

McConnell, S. K. (1991). The generation of neuronal diversity in the central nervous system. *Annual Review of Neuroscience, 14,* 269–300.

McCormick, C. M., & Witelson, S. F. (1994). Functional cerebral asymmetry and sexual orientation in men and women. *Behavioral Neuroscience, 108,* 525–531.

Magnun, G. R., Hillyard, S. A., & Luck, S. J. (1993). *Attention and performance XIV* (pp. 219–244). Cambridge, MA: MIT Press.

Majovski, L. V., & Jacques, D. B. (1982). Cognitive information processing and learning mechanisms of the brain. *Neurosurgery, 10,* 663–677.

Majovski, L. V., Jacques, D. B., Hartz, G., & Fogwell, L. A. (1981). Dopaminergic (DA) systems: Their role in pathological neurobehavioral symptoms. *Neurosurgery, 9,* 751–757.

Martin, E., Grutter, R., & Boesch, O. (1990). *In vivo* NMR spectroscopy: Investigation of brain metabolism in neonates and infants. *Pediatre, 45,* 877–882.

Mazziotta, J. C., & Phelps, M. E. (1985). Metabolic evidence of lateralized cerebral function demonstrated by positron emission tomography in patients with neuropsychiatric disorders and normal individuals. In D. F. Benson & E. Zaidel (Eds.), *The dual brain.* New York: Guilford Press.

Mazziotta, J. C., Phelps, M. E., & Miller, J. (1981). Tomographic mapping of human cerebral metabolism. Normal unstimulated state. *Neurology, 31,* 503–516.

Metcof, J. (1974). Biochemical markers of intrauterine malnutrition. In M. Winick (Ed.), *Current concepts in nutrition* (Vol. 2). New York: Wiley.

Meudell, P. R. (1983). The development and dissolution of memory. In A. Mayes (Ed.), *Memory in animals and humans.* Princeton, NJ: Van Nostrand–Reinhold.

Mills, D. L., Coffey, C. S., & Neville, H. J. (1993). Language acquisition and cerebral specialization in 20-month-old infants. *Journal of Cognitive Neuroscience, 5,* 317–334.

Milner, E. (1976). CNS maturation and language acquisition. In H. Whitaker & H. A. Whitaker (Eds.), *Studies in neurolinguistics* (Vol. I). New York: Academic Press.

Mishkin, M., & Petri, H. L. (1984). Memories and habits: Some implications for the analysis of learning and retention. In L. R. Squire & N. Butlers (Eds.), *Neuropsychology of memory.* New York: Guilford Press.

Mistretta, C. M., & Bradley, R. M. (1978). Effect of early sensory experience on brain and behavioral development. In G. Gottlieb (Ed.), *Studies on the development of behavior and the nervous system* (Vol. 4). New York: Academic Press.

Molfese, D. L. (1977). Infant cerebral asymmetry. In S. J. Segalowitz & F. A. Gruber (Eds.), *Language development and neurological theory.* New York: Academic Press.

Molfese, D., Freeman, R., & Palermo, D. (1975). The ontogeny of brain lateralization for speech and nonspeech stimuli. *Brain Language, 2,* 356–368.

Moore, K. L., & Persand, T. V. N. (1993a). *Before we were born: Essentials of embryology and birth defects* (4th ed., pp. 45–59). Philadelphia: Saunders.

Moore, K. L., & Persand, T. V. N. (1993b). *The developing human. Clinically oriented embryology* (5th ed.). Philadelphia: Saunders.

Moore, R. Y. (1977). The developmental organization of the fetal brain. In L. Gluck (Ed.), *Intrauterine asphyxia and the developing fetal brain.* Chicago: Year Book Medical.

Morgan, M. (1977). Embryology and inheritance of asymmetry. In S. Harnad, R. Doty, L. Goldstein, J. Jaynes, & G. Lruthamer (Eds.), *Lateralization in the nervous system.* New York: Academic Press.

Moscovitch, M. (1977). The development of lateralization of language functions and its relation to cognitive and linguistic development: A review and some theoretical speculations. In S. J. Segalowitz & F. A. Gruber (Eds.), *Language development and neurological theory.* New York: Academic Press.

Nadel, L., & Zola-Morgan, S. (1984). Infantile amnesia: A neurobiological perspective. In M. Moscovitch (Ed.), *Infant memory.* New York: Plenum Press.

Nauta, W. H. (1986a). Circuitous connections linking cerebral cortex, limbic system and corpus striatum. In B. K. Doane & K. E. Livingston (Eds.), *The limbic system: Functional organization and clinical disorders.* New York: Raven Press.

Nauta, W. H. (1986b). A simplified perspective on the basal ganglia and their relation to the limbic system. In B. K. Doane & K. E. Livingston (Eds.), *The limbic system: Functional organization and clinical disorders.* New York: Raven Press.

Negergaard, M. (1994). Direct signaling from astrocytes to neurons in cultures of mammalian brain cells. *Science, 263,* 1768–1774.

Neville, H. (1984). Effects of early sensory and language experience on the development of the human brain. In J. Mehler & R. Fox (Eds.), *Neonate cognition: Beyond the blooming buzzing confusion.* Hillsdale, NJ: Erlbaum.

Nilsson, L. (1978). *A child is born.* New York: Delacorte Press.

Oates, J. (Ed.). (1979). *Early cognitive development.* New York: Wiley.

O'Keefe, J. (1994). Developmental psychology. Cognitive maps in infants. *Nature, 370,* 57–59.

O'Keefe, J., & Nadel, L. (1978). *The hippocampus as a cognitive map.* Oxford: Clarendon Press.

Orrison, W. W., Davis, L. E., Sullivan, G. W., Mettler, F. A., & Flynn, L. R. (1990). Anatomic localization of cerebral cortical function by magnetoencephalography combined with MR imaging and CT. *American Journal of Neuro-Radiology, 11,* 713–716.

Peden, C. J., Rutherford, M. A., Sargentorri, J., Cox, I. J., Bryant, D. J., & Dubowitz, L. M. (1993). Proton spectroscopy of the neonatal brain following hypoxic-ischemic injury. *Developmental Medicine and Child Neurology, 35,* 502–510.

Petersen, S. E., Fox, P. T., Posner, M. I., Mintun, M., & Raichle, M. E. (1989). Positron emission tomographic studies of the processing of single words. *Journal of Cognitive Neuroscience, 1,* 153–170.

Petersen, S. E., Gorbetta, M., Miezin, F. M., & Shulman, G. L. (1994). PET studies of parietal involvement in spatial attention: Comparison of different task types. *Canadian Journal of Experimental Psychology, 48,* 319–338.

Phelps, M. E., Mazziotta, J., & Schelbert, H. R. (1986). *Positron emission tomography and autoradiography: Principles and applications for the brain and heart.* New York: Raven Press.

Piven, J., Berthier, M. L., Storkstein, S. E., & Nehme, E. (1990). Magnetic resonance imaging evidence for a defect of cerebral cortical development in autism. *American Journal of Psychiatry, 147,* 734–739.

Plante, E., Swisher, L., Vance, R., & Rapcsak, S. (1991). MRI findings in boys with specific language impairment. *Brain and Language, 41,* 52–66.

Plomin, R. A., & Rowe, D. C. (1979). Genetic and environmental etiology of social behavior in infancy. *Developmental Psychology, 15,* 62–72.

Ploog, D. (1979). Phonation, emotion, cognition with reference to the brain mechanisms involved. *Ciba Foundation Symposia, 69,* 79–98.

Posner, M. I. (1993). Seeing the mind. *Science, 262,* 673–674.

Posner, M. I., & Petersen, S. E. (1990). The attentional system of the human brain. *Annual Review of Neuroscience, 13,* 25–42.

Posner, M. I., & Rothbart, M. K. (1992). Attentional mechanisms and conscious experience. In A. D. Milner & M. D. Rugg (Eds.), *The neuropsychology of consciousness* (pp. 91–112). Orlando: Academic Press.

Pribam, K. H. (1976). Modes of central information processing in human learning and remembering. In T. J. Tyler (Ed.), *Brain and learning*. Baltimore: Graylock Press.

Raichle, M. E. (1987). Circulatory and metabolic correlations of brain function in normal humans. In V. Mountcastle, F. R. Plum, & S. Geiger (Eds.), *Handbook of physiology: Sec. 1. The nervous system: Vol. V. (1,2)* (pp. 643–674). Bethesda: American Physiological Society.

Raichle, M. E., Fiez, J. A., Videen, T. O., MacLeod, A. M., Pardo, J. V., Fox, P. T., & Petersen, S. E. (1994). Practice-related changes in human brain functional anatomy during nonmotor learning. *Cerebral Cortex, 4,* 8–26.

Ramón y Cajal, S. (1911). *Histologie du Systeme Nerveaux de l'Homme et des Vertebres.* Paris: Maloine (Republished 1955, *Histologie du Systeme Nerveux.* Translated by L. Azoulay. Madrid: Inst. Ramón y Cajal).

Reichlin, S. (1974). Neuroendocrinology. In R. H. Williams (Ed.), *Textbook of endocrinology.* Philadelphia: Saunders.

Reynolds, E. O., McCormick, D. C., Roth, S. C., Edwards, A. O., & Wyatt, J. S. (1991). New non-invasive methods for the investigation of cerebral oxidative metabolism and hemodynamics in newborn infants. *Annals of Medicine, 23,* 681–686.

Risberg, J., & Ingvar, D. H. (1973). Patterns of activation in the gray matter of the dominant hemisphere. *Brain, 96,* 737–756.

Riss, W. (1972). Nonspecific thalamic projection system: Introduction. *Brain, Behavior, and Evolution, 6,* 329–331.

Roberts, E. (1986). Metabolism and nervous system disease: A challenge for our times (Part I). *Metabolic Brain Disease, 1,* 1–25.

Roland, P. E., Eriksson, L., Widen, L., & Stone-Elander, S. (1989). Changes in regional cerebral oxidative metabolism induced by tactile learning and recognition in man. *European Journal of Neuroscience, 1,* 3–18.

Roncagliolo, M., Benitez, J., & Perez, M. (1994). Auditory brainstem responses of children with developmental language disorders. *Developmental Medicine and Child Neurology, 36,* 26–33.

Ross, B., & Michaels, T. (1994). Clinical applications of magnetic resonance spectroscopy. *Magnetic Resonance Quarterly, 10,* 191–247.

Rourke, B. P., Bakker, D. J., Fisk, J. L., & Strang, J. D. (1983). *Child neuropsychology: An introduction to theory, research, and clinical practice.* New York: Guilford Press.

Saint-Cyr, J. A., Taylor, A. E., & Lang, A. E. (1987). Procedural learning impairment in basal ganglia disease. *Journal of Clinical and Experimental Neuropsychology, 9,* 280.

Saitoh, D., Courchesne, F., Egaas, B., Lincoln, A. J., & Schreibrion, L. (1995). Cross-sectional axia of posterior hippocampus in autistic patients with cerebral and corpus collosum abnormalities. *Neurology, 45,* 317–324.

Satz, P. (1993). Brain reserve capacity on symptom onset after brain injury: A formulation and review of evidence of threshold theory. *Neuropsychology, 7,* 293–295.

Satz, P., Orsini, D. L., Saslow, E., & Henry, R. (1985). The pathological left-handedness syndrome. *Brain and Cognition, 4,* 27–46.

Satz, P., Strauss, E., Hunter, M., & Wada, J. (1994). Reexamination of the crowding hypothesis: Effects of age of onset. *Neuropsychology, 8,* 255–262.

Scheibel, A. B. (1978). Clinical neuroanatomy lecture. *Anatomy and Physiology 103: Winter–Spring Quarter 1978,* UCLA School of Medicine, Los Angeles.

Scheibel, M., & Scheibel, A. (1961). On circuit patterns of brain stem reticular core. *Annals of the New York Academy of Sciences, 89,* 857–865.

Scheibel, M., & Scheibel, A. (1963). Some neural substrates of postnatal development. In E. Hoffman (Ed.), *First annual review of child development.* New York: Russell Sage Foundation.

Scheibel, M. E., & Scheibel, A. G. (1966). Patterns of organization in specific and nonspecific thalamic fields. In D. Purpura & M. D. Yahr (Eds.), *The thalamus.* New York: Columbia University Press.

Scheibel, M. E., & Scheibel, A. B. (1972). Input–output relations of the thalamic nonspecific system. *Brain, Behavior, and Evolution, 6,* 332–358.

Scheibel, M. E., & Scheibel, A. B. (1973). Dendrite bundles as sites for central program: An hypothesis. *International Journal of Neuroscience, 6,* 195–202.

Schonhaut, S., & Satz, P. (1983). Prognosis for children with learning disabilities: A review of follow-up studies. In M. Rutter (Ed.), *Developmental neuropsychiatry.* New York: Guilford Press.

Schulte, F. J. (1974). The neurological development of the neonate. In J. A. Davis & J. Dobbing (Eds.), *Scientific foundation of pediatrics.* Philadelphia: Saunders.

Segalowitz, S., & Chapman, J. (1980). Cerebral asymmetry for speech in neonates: A behavioral measure. *Brain Language, 9,* 281–288.

Selnes, D. A., & Whitaker, H. A. (1976). Morphological and functional development of the auditory system. In R. W. Rieber (Ed.), *The neuropsychology of language.* New York: Plenum Press.

Semrud-Clikeman, M., Hynd, G. W., Novey, E. S., & Elipulos, D. (1991). Dyslexia and brain morphology: Relationship between neuroanatomical variation and neurolinguistic tasks. *Learning and Individual Differences, 3,* 225–242.

Sergent, J., Ohta, S., & MacDonald, B. (1992). Functional neuroanatomy of face and object processing: A positron emission tomography study. *Brain, 115,* 15–36.

Shulman, R. G., Blamire, A. M., Rothman, D. L., & McCarthy, G. (1993). Nuclear magnetic resonance imaging and spectroscopy of human brain function. *Proceedings of the National Academy of Sciences, USA, 90,* 3127–3133.

Siegel, L. S. (1979). Infant perceptual, cognitive, and motor behavior as predictors of subsequent cognitive and language development. *Canadian Journal of Psychological Reviews, 33,* 382–395.

Sips, H. J. W. A., Catsman-Berrevoets, C. E., Van Dongen, H. R., Van der Werff, P. J. J., & Brooke, L. J. (1994). Measuring right-hemisphere dysfunction in children: Validity of two new computer tests. *Developmental Medicine and Child Neurology, 36,* 57–63.

Siqueland, E. R., & Lipsitt, L. P. (1966). Conditioned head turning in newborns. *Journal of Experimental Child Psychology, 3,* 356–376.

Smith, B. H., & Sweet, W. H. (1978a). Monoaminergic regulation of central nervous system function. I. Noradrenergic systems. *Neurosurgery, 3,* 109–119.

Smith, B. H., & Sweet, W. H. (1978b). Monoaminergic regulation of central nervous system function. II. Serotonergic systems. *Neurosurgery, 3,* 257–272.

Smith, D. W. (1976). *Recognizable patterns of human malformation: Genetic, embryologic and clinical aspects* (2nd ed.). Philadelphia: Saunders.

Smith, O. A., & DeVito, J. L. (1984). Central neural integration for the control of autonomic responses associated with emotion. *Annual Review of Neuroscience, 7,* 43–65.

Snyder, S. (1980). Brain peptides as neurotransmitters. *Science, 209,* 976–983.

Sperry, R. W. (1974). Lateral specialization in the surgically separated hemispheres. In F. O. Schmitt & F. G. Worden (Eds.), *Neurosciences: Third study program* (pp. 5–19). Cambridge, MA: MIT Press.

Sperry, R. W., Gazzaniga, M. S., & Bogen, J. E. (1969). Interhemispheric relationships: The neocortical commissures; syndromes of hemisphere disconnection. In P. J. Vinken & G. W. Bruyn (Eds.), *Handbook of clinical neurology* (Vol. 4, pp. 273–290). Amsterdam: Elsevier.

Spreen, O., Tupper, D., Risser, A., Tuokko, H., & Edgell, D. (1984). *Human developmental neuropsychology.* London: Oxford University Press.

Squire, L. R., & Zola-Morgan, S. (1991). The medial-temporal lobe memory system. *Science, 253,* 1380–1386.

Stark, D. D., & Bradley, W. G. (Eds.). (1992). *Magnetic resonance imaging* (2nd ed., Vols. 1,2). St. Louis: Mosby–Year Book.

Stehling, M. K., Mansfield, P., Ordidge, R. J., Coxon, R., Chapman, B., Blamire, A., Gibbs, P., Johnson, I. R., Symonds, E. M., Worthington, B. S., *et al.* (1990). Echo-planar imaging of the human fetus *in utero. Magnetic Resonance in Medicine, 13,* 314–318.

Stehling, M. K., Turner, R., & Mansfield, P. (1991). Echo-planar imaging in a fraction of a second. *Science, 254,* 43–50.

Steriade, M., McCormick, D. A., & Sejnowski, T. J. (1993). Thalamocortical oscillations in the sleeping and aroused brain. *Science, 262,* 679–685.

Storm-Mathisen, J. (1979). Localization of transmitter candidates in the brain: The hippocampal formation as a model. *Progress in Neurobiology, 8,* 381–388.

Stuss, D. T., & Benson, D. F. (1986). *The frontal lobes.* New York: Raven Press.

Szentagothai, J. (1975). The "module concept" in the cerebral cortex architecture. *Brain Research, 95,* 475–496.

Szentagothai, J. (1978). The Ferrier Lecture. The neuron network of the cerebral cortex: A functional interpretation. *Proceedings of the Royal Society of London, 201,* 219–248.

Szentagothai, J., & Arbib, M. A. (1974). Conceptual models of neural organization. *Neurosciences Research Program Bulletin, 12,* 307–501.

Taylor, D. (1969). Differential rates of cerebral maturation between sexes and between hemispheres. *Lancet, 2,* 140–142.

Taylor, H. G., Fletcher, J. M., & Satz, P. (1984). Neuropsychological assessment of children. In L. Halpern & G. Goldstein (Eds.), *Handbook of psychological assessment.* Elmsford, NY: Pergamon Press.

Thach, W. T., Goodkin, H. P., & Keating, J. G. (1992). The cerebellum and the adaptive coordination of movement. *Annual Review of Neuroscience, 15,* 403–442.

Tulving, E. (1985). On the classification problem in learning and memory. In L. Nilsson & T. Archer (Eds.), *Perspectives on learning and memory.* Hillsdale, NJ: Erlbaum.

Tzika, A. A., Vigneron, D. B., Ball, W. S., Dunn, R. S., & Kirks, D. R. (1993). Localized proton MR spectroscopy of the brain in children. *Journal of Magnetic Resonance Imaging, 3,* 719–729.

Valk, J., & Van der Knapp, M. S. (1989). White matter and myelin. In J. Valk & M. S. Van der Knapp (Eds.), *Magnetic resonance of myelin, myelination, and myelin disorders* (pp. 9–21). Berlin: Springer-Verlag.

Van de Bor, M., Den-Ouden, L., & Guit, G. L. (1992). Value of cranial ultrasound and magnetic resonance imaging in predicting neurodevelopmental outcome in preterm infants. *Pediatrics, 90,* 196–199.

Vohr, B. R., Coll, C. E., Lobato, D., Yunis, K. A., O'Dea, C., & Oh, W. (1991). Neurodevelopmental and medical status of low birth weight survivors of broncho-pulmonary dysphasia at 10–12 years of age. *Developmental Medicine and Child Neurology, 33,* 690–697.

Vygotsky, L. S. (1974). The problem of age-periodization of child development (translated by A. Zender & B. F. Zender). *Human Development, 17,* 24–40.

Vygotsky, L. S. (1980). *Mind in society: The development of higher psychological process* (edited by M. Coles, V. John-Steiner, S. Scribner, & E. Souberman). Cambridge, MA: Harvard University Press.

Wang, J. Z., Kaufman, L., & Williamson, S. J. (1993). Imaging regional changes in the spontaneous activity of the brain: An extension of the minimum-norm least-squares estimate. *Encephalography and Clinical Neurophysiology, 86,* 36–50.

Warren, J. M., & Akert, K. (Eds.) (1964). *The frontal granular cortex and behavior.* New York: McGraw-Hill.

Weisberg, L. A., Strub, R. L., & Garcia, C. A. (1989). Neurological disorders of childhood. In L. A. Weisberg, R. L. Strub, & C. A. Garcia (Eds.), *Essentials of clinical neurology* (2nd ed.). Rockville, MD: Aspen.

Wertsch, J. V. (1979). The regulation of human action and the given new organization of private speech. In G. Zivin (Ed.), *The development of self-regulation through private speech.* New York: Wiley.

Witelson, S. (1977). Early hemispheric specialization and interhemispheric plasticity: An empirical and theoretical review. In S. J. Segalowitz & F. A. Gruber (Eds.), *Language development and neurological theory.* New York: Academic Press.

Witelson, S. F. (1985). On hemispheric specialization and cerebral plasticity from birth: Mark II. In C. Best (Ed.), *Hemi-*

spheric function and collaboration in the child (pp. 33–85). New York: Academic Press.

Witelson, S., & Kigar, D. (1992). Sylvian fissure morphology and asymmetry in men and women: Bilateral differences in relation to handedness in men. *Journal of Comparative Neurology, 323,* 326–340.

Witelson, S., & Pallie, W. (1973). Left hemisphere specialization for language in the newborn. *Brain, 96,* 641–646.

Wong, V., & Wong, S. N. (1991). Brainstem auditory evoked potential study in children with autistic disorder. *Journal of Autism and Developmental Disorders, 21,* 329–340.

Yakovlev, P. I. (1962). Morphological criteria of growth and maturation of the nervous system in man. *Research Publications, Association for Research in Nervous and Mental Diseases, 39,* 3.

Yakovlev, P. I., & Lecours, A. R. (1967). The myelogenetic cycles of regional maturation of the brain. In A. Minkowski (Ed.), *Regional development of the brain.* Oxford: Blackwell.

Zimmerman, R. A., Bilaniuk, L. T., & Grossman, R. I. (1983). Computed tomography in migratory disorders of human brain development. *Neuroradiology, 25,* 257–269.

Zimmerman, R. A., Bilaniuk, L. T., & Gusnard, D. A. (1992). Pediatric cerebral anomalies. In D. D. Stark & W. G. Bradley (Eds.), *Magnetic resonance imaging* (2nd ed.). St. Louis: Mosby-Year Book.

Zola-Morgan, S., & Squire, L. R. (1993). Neuroanatomy of memory. *Annual Review of Neuroscience, 16,* 547–564.

Zucker, R. S., & Lando, L. (1986). Mechanism of transmitter release: Voltage hypothesis and calcium hypothesis. *Science, 231,* 574–579.

5

Mechanisms and Development of Cerebral Lateralization in Children

MARCEL KINSBOURNE

The Normative Endpoint of Hemisphere Specialization in the Adult

The sequences of cognitive development to be considered in this discussion culminate in an endpoint of lateralization in the mature human nervous system that in its broad definition is no longer in dispute. In the right-handed majority, language-related processes are left lateralized in almost every case. The right hemisphere does contribute toward certain aspects of verbal behavior, however (Hécaen, 1978; Searleman, 1977, 1983), notably comprehension of logical relationships, inference, metaphor, and humor (Beeman, 1993; Gardner, Ling, Flamm, & Silverman, 1975), and at the output stage, intonation, particularly when it reflects the emotional tone of the utterance (Ross & Mesulam, 1979). The left hemisphere is also specialized for rapid sequential recognition of familiar input, nonverbal as well as verbal, and also the recall and recognition of order information and the formulation of action plans, both motor and conceptual. Right hemisphere dominance is best documented for certain spatial-relational processes, particularly in the visual modality, and for the processing of emotional information (Kinsbourne, 1982). Non-right-handers deviate from the dextral norm in the following manner: in addition to left-sided representation of language, which is as prevalent in non-right-handers as in right-handers, language is also represented on the right in up to 70% of the cases (Gloning, Gloning, Haub, &

Quatember, 1959). In non-right-handers, spatial-relational functions are right lateralized as in right-handers, but involve the left hemisphere also in more than half of all instances (Bryden Hécaen, & DeAgostini, 1983). Within each hemisphere the territory involved in cognitive function is more extensive in the left- than the right-hander (Kinsbourne, unpublished analysis of data from Bryden *et al.,* 1983). Gender-related differences in lateralization are more contentious (Lewis & Harris, 1990), and the claim that language and visuospatial functions are more bilateralized in females than males, and even that left intrahemispheric organization differs between the sexes, are not yet well substantiated. With respect to development, existing knowledge is virtually restricted to language functions on the one hand and spatial-relational functions on the other. This discussion will therefore be confined to considering how peripheral laterality, notably hand preference, is established in the developing child, and how the differential hemispheric representation of language and spatial-relational functions develops, first in the normal case, and then in certain types of developmental disability.

At birth the human infant's cerebrum has not yet assumed its ultimate functions. The functions that will emerge over time can be subdivided into those for which hemispheric specialization has been ascertained, and those for which no lateralization has (as yet) been established. Although a good deal is now known about the changes in number, configuration, and connectivity of neurons in the two developing hemispheres, it is not yet clear how they relate to emerging higher mental functions. One can only time the origin of the various lateralized men-

MARCEL KINSBOURNE • New School for Social Research, New York, New York 10011.

tal skills by observing their appearance at the behavioral level. The developmental sequences involved in the emergence of language and spatial-relational skills have been reasonably well specified. Once each begins to emerge, and subsequently to become more refined, it becomes possible to ask, what is the basis of this developing skill?

A distinction has to be drawn between hemispheric specialization and lateralization of function to a hemisphere. It cannot be taken for granted that the developing skill in its earliest stages is based on the same cerebral hemisphere as it is ultimately. The hypothesis that the lateralization to one hemisphere is constant is termed "invariant lateralization" (Kinsbourne, 1975). An alternative view is that in the earlier stages mental functions in general (and language in particular) are based on the activity of both cerebral hemispheres and that lateralization of verbal functions to the left and spatial–relational to the right occurs over time during childhood. This is the "progressive lateralization" hypothesis (Lenneberg, 1967). Virtually all that is known about the emergence of hemispheric specialization in the child can be formulated in terms of these two hypotheses.

Insofar as lateralization and its development are subject to biological variation, one can ask whether a particular topography of hemispheric representation of function is more conducive to efficient mental function than other topographies [as has been assumed for more than a century (reviewed by Harrington, 1987)], and whether anomalous topographies characterize certain developmental disabilities and even account for some or all of the behavioral deficits involved. These questions can be addressed most directly in the case of the fully mature nervous system, but lags in achieving that endpoint can also be considered.

Asymmetries in the Evolutionary Context

Asymmetric cerebral and somatic functioning are chiefly of interest in clinical child neuropsychology for any implications they might have for adaptive performance and behavior. An appropriate point of departure for considering these issues is therefore an inquiry into the evolutionary origin of these asymmetries. Why did they evolve and what might have been their adaptive relevance to natural selection? If we could discover a role that asymmetry of function plays in adaptive behavior, then we

could better predict the ways in which lack or distortion of such asymmetries might affect the functioning of the human infant, child, and adult.

The Origin of Bisymmetry

Somatic bisymmetry is an adaptation to the needs of motile organisms. In addition to the obvious advantage of the streamlining that results, the bisymmetric organism is well adapted for the basic decision continually made by organisms as they move from point to point: to turn right or to turn left (Loeb, 1918). Given that whatever benefits and hazards the environment might present occur with equal probability to either side, the organism needs to be able to deploy its sensorimotor capabilities to either side with comparable speed and efficiency (Gardner, 1967). To meet this need, the receptor equipment and the musculature are both bilaterally arranged, and the corresponding control centers in the nervous system (contralaterally in the chordate phylum, ipsilaterally in the other phyla; Hyman, 1940) are reciprocally inhibitory opponent processors. Sessile organisms are not bisymmetric, and organisms that regress from a motile to a sessile state concurrently lose their bisymmetric organization. Organisms whose life cycle divides into a motile larval and a sessile mature phase exhibit the relationship most strikingly. The motile larva is bisymmetric, the sessile adult is not. Fishes, which also freely swim up and down, usually exhibit dorsal–ventral somatic symmetry as well (Braitenberg, 1977).

Asymmetry (Somatic)

Minor asymmetries abound and have been documented in all species studied in sufficient detail (Ludwig, 1932). An instructive example relates to the pelvic and pectoral fins of fishes. These, though bilateral, are asymmetric, it being the general rule that the right-sided fins are more bony and muscular than the left (Hubbs & Hubbs, 1944). This is the case even though the fishes' musculature itself is bisymmetric. This appears to be because their asymmetry poses no problem for the function of fins as rudders to direct efficient swimming movements. This is an example of an asymmetry that does not appear to have evolved to meet a specific adaptive need, but rather exists because the engineering of exact bisymmetry was not needed to meet the adaptive pressures in the context of which the species evolved.

Asymmetry (Neural)

In behaviorally simple organisms the functions of the nervous system distribute across two domains: the regulation of the internal environment and the control of behavior that is oriented in space. The former does not call for bisymmetric control, and certain striking brain asymmetries in behaviorally limited species may relate to vegetative function (Braitenberg & Kemali, 1970). In the more behaviorally sophisticated vertebrates, including mammals and birds, the repertoire includes a third domain: higher mental function as involved in communication, memory, and problem solving. Not being targeted toward specific locations in the physical environment, these processes can serve their purpose without being bilaterally represented. Whereas central representation of sensorimotor processes is topographic, representation of higher mental functions is abstract (Young, 1962). If an abstract representation deviates, even substantially, from bisymmetry, this need not be because the asymmetric topography confers specific adaptive advantage. A diminished adaptive advantage of bisymmetrical organization may sufficiently account for deviation from bisymmetry (Kinsbourne, 1974). Ringo *et al.* (1994) suggest that lateralization is adaptive to limitations in the efficiency of the corpus callosum in integrating bihemispheric neuronal computations in mammals with large brains. However, lateralization characterizes brains as small as those of rats, whereas left-handed humans are cognitively unimpaired by substantial bisymmetry.

Dramatic functional asymmetry exists in certain male songbirds whose song is largely controlled from the left brain (Nottebohm, 1971). The relevant brain area, the Higher Vocal Control Center, is paralleled by a comparable area on the right side of the brain, though in the intact organism its functions are unknown. If the left-sided control area for song is destroyed or disconnected from its effector, the right side assumes control over bird song, but only if the lesion is made early, before singing has fully developed. Bird song is communicative, and is targeted at no particular point in space but simply at ambient space. Bilateral control of such a function would not seem to be necessary and in fact unilateral control prevails. Nevertheless, the mirror image area does develop and is available as a reserve. This is not to suggest that it is there in order to be in reserve in case of left-sided brain damage. Rather, nature is conservative in the manner in which it refines neural control mechanisms, and there was perhaps no provision (or environmental adaptive trigger) to preclude the unutilized right-sided area from evolving in parallel with the left. This issue is of interest because there are human specializations that can be similarly interpreted, notably the left-sided control of speech. If the left speech area is totally destroyed, the right side does seem to be able to control speech output (Searleman, 1977, 1983). Should we suppose that in the intact state the unilateral facility that controls behavior maintains its control by actively suppressing (inhibiting) its potential rival on the other side (Kinsbourne, 1974)? If so, it can also do so in the reverse direction in some species, and in yet others control of bird song is bilateral (Hauser, 1996). The latter species are analogous to left-handed humans who are bilateralized for language, without apparent detriment to their control of vocalizations. Thus, both in songbirds and in humans, lateralization of control of rapidly sequential utterances is prevalent, but evidently not a condition for its efficient performance.

The analogy with the neural basis of bird song captures one attribute of human brain organization, the usual (but not mandatory) restriction of the control of a skill not targeted to a specific external location to one side of the brain. It fails to capture another attribute: the complementarity of human hemispheric specialization (Kinsbourne, 1982). A much simpler animal model illustrates complementary specialization. The paired claws of the lobster differentiate into a stout crusher driven by slow muscle fibers, and a slender cutter, largely driven by faster muscle fibers (Govind & Pearce, 1986). The asymmetry develops under central neuron control, and is mediated by lateral differences in the degree of reflex activity. In humans, the cerebral hemispheres contribute differentiated but complementary components to skilled behavior, to the point that many real-life activities simply cannot be effectively controlled by one hemisphere alone. Bresson, Maury, Pierant-LeBonniec, and deSchonen (1977) found that human infants prefer the right hand for some activities, the left for others. Whether to press the analogy with the lobster one step further is conjectural. Govind and Pearce found that exercising one claw facilitated its development into the crusher. In humans, we have no comparable observations. But experimentally controlled studies of this kind are hardly practicable. A child's first words are accompanied by pointing to the named object

(Kinsbourne & Lempert, 1979; Lempert & Kinsbourne, 1985). Whether manipulating the side on which attention-attracting stimuli appear, or the limb used to point, would qualify the genetically preprogrammed left brain speech laterality is doubtful. But if, as Annett (1973) suggested, sinistrals lack an overriding "right shift factor," it is quite possible that in them lateralization could be influenced by such environmental factors.

When one applies these considerations to the human brain, one learns that lateralization of higher mental functions cannot be assumed to be adaptively necessary simply because it happens to be the general rule (but see Ringo & Doty, 1991). Whether deviating from the norm of lateralization exacts a penalty in terms of behavioral control is an empirical issue not to be prejudged. It follows that we have to consider separately the following two questions: under what circumstances do humans deviate from the usual laterality patterns and when they do, what if any are the consequences for adaptive behavior?

Morphological Asymmetries in the Human

The internal organs of the human exhibit well-known major asymmetries. Deviation from the usual pattern has also been well documented, such as in the form of a complete lateral reversal (situs inversus), reversal of a single organ (e.g., dextrocardia), and absence of asymmetry, as in horseshoe kidney in which a single bilaterally symmetric kidney straddles the midline. Abnormal position of the internal organs may compress adjacent structures, but the functioning of the organs themselves does not seem to depend on their location. In the human brain and musculature, a number of less radical asymmetries exist. None of them has been convincingly tied to function.

The right-hander's body is subtly asymmetric. Most bones and muscles on the right are reported to be somewhat more massive than on the left (Latimer & Lowrance, 1965) and this is not secondary to differential use, as it already obtains in the infant (Pande & Singh, 1971). Asymmetries in fingerprints, hair whorls, and other ectodermal structures have been documented. More relevant to the brain, the skull, the shape of which is determined by the growth of the brain, is more protuberant anteriorly on the right and posteriorly on the left (LeMay, 1976; LeMay & Culebras, 1972). The parietal operculum is longer on the left. The right frontal lobe and the left occipital lobe are somewhat bulkier than the corresponding lobes on the opposite side.

Function could be inferred from these morphological findings (Galaburda, 1984) if the mass of a given area were to correlate with the efficiency with which the individual performs the activities it is specialized to control. Also, individuals who lack the asymmetry in question should have a correspondingly different profile of functional capabilities. The evidence is far from conclusive along either of these two lines. In particular, by far the greatest variability with respect to relative size of parts of right and left brain (and the body in general; Hicks & Kinsbourne, 1978) is to be found in the non-right-handed population (Hochberg & LeMay, 1975; LeMay, 1992; McRae, Branch, & Milner, 1968). No one has been able to attribute any functional differences between right-handers and non-right-handers (or among non-right-handers) to these morphological variations among the latter.

Galaburda and his colleagues have studied the neurogenesis of cerebral asymmetry in detail (Rosen et al., 1989). They found more collateral interconnections between symmetrical than asymmetrical cerebral areas. This would be consistent with the localization of lateralized functions in asymmetrical cortex. That the mere bulk of the brain may not be a good index of functional efficiency is not unexpected, since the amount of normal variance in intelligence accounted for by overall brain size, though significant, is quite slight. Also, the greater average bulk of the male than the female brain is not accompanied by an overall greater intellectual capability. A more refined measure of brain size would perhaps take account of local differences in the amount of infolding of cortex, the gray matter being layered around the folds. There is a dissociation between the size of Broca's area, which is greater on the right, and its infolding, which is greater on the left (Falzi, Perrone, & Vignolo, 1982). However, other areas are known to have more bulk on the left side in right-handers, notably the planum temporale (Geschwind & Levitsky, 1968; Witelson & Kigar, 1988). In any case, bulk of a brain area may not only reflect the number of its neurons. An area that is demarcated by gyral boundaries is not necessarily demarcated architectonically, or unitary in its function. There may be variation in how tightly packed neurons are, in the richness of their connections or the excellence of their organization and normality of their morphology. In the four cases of dyslexia documented by Galaburda, Sherman, Rosen, Aboitiz, and Geschwind (1985) in whom dysgenesis of neurons in various left cerebral areas was found at autopsy, brain bulk as observed on CT scan did not deviate from the norm. But a special case exists, a structure the cross-sectional area of which does reflect the number of nerve fibers it transmits: the corpus callosum. Its area in cross-section did correlate positively with performance in certain tests of laterality and attention in multiple sclerosis (Reinvang, Bakke, Hugdahl, Karlsen, & Sundet, 1994), and in normals (Yazgan, Wexler, Kinsbourne, Peterson, & Leckman, 1995).

A further impediment to linking brain asymmetry with differential skill in higher mental functions derives from comparative data. Yeni-Komshian and Benson (1976) found that the planum temporale is larger on the left than on the right in chimpanzees, a species not noted for its verbal ability. In summary, although it is intriguing that morphological asymmetries are "invariant" across development, they have not been validated as indices of function, and correspondingly their existence in the newborn cannot be used as evidence that language precursors are lateralized.

Precursors of Lateralization of Function

Peripheral Laterality

The infant cannot do the things that are used to classify more mature individuals into those who are right-handed and those who are not. However, certain motor biases may predict hand preference. The newborn infant is not capable of behavior so differentiated as to involve the use of one hand and arm only. But within his or her repertoire is a lateral orienting synergism, the asymmetric tonic neck response, which includes turning of head and eyes to one side, extension of the ipsilateral arm and leg, and flexion of the contralateral arm and leg. This can be seen as a precursor of locomotion toward one side, though the infant is lying supine. The outstretched arm may be a precursor for reaching and pointing. Be that as it may, Gesell and Ames (1947) first observed that spontaneous head turning in infants is more often to the right than to the left, and in a follow-up study with a small sample they found a relationship between the direction of the most frequent head turning in the infant and subsequent hand preference. Notably, all four of the infants who showed predominantly leftward head turning subsequently became left-handers. There is now good circumstantial evidence for a developmental sequence of peripheral laterality arising from the asymmetric tonic neck response that is first evident after the intrauterine age of 32 weeks (Turkewitz, 1977). Nevertheless,

Liederman and Kinsbourne (1980a) were able to show that head turning asymmetry represents a motor, and not a sensory, bias, and it is indicative that an overall rightward turning bias was found in children of right-handed parents but not in a group of children with one non-right-handed parent (Liederman & Kinsbourne, 1980b). It is possible that asymmetric head turning takes place even *in utero*. The most frequent presentation of the fetal head at birth is left occipito-anterior (LOA). This indicates that the infant's head is most often turned to the right as it descends (headfirst and backward relative to the mother) through the birth canal. Churchill, Igna, and Senf (1962) reported that more LOA than ROA babies turn out to be right-handed at age 2 years. They attributed this to hypothesized hemisphere injury by pressure against the pelvic floor—right hemisphere in LOA, left hemisphere in ROA. This does presuppose a staggering amount of birth-related cerebral damage. If the child who is predisposed to become dextral (and with a more prominent left than right occipital region; LeMay, 1992) has a more vigorous rightward turning tendency, even *in utero,* and vice versa, and this is one determinant of the presentation of the fetal head, the findings can be accounted for without invoking uncorroborated pathology.

Subsequent work has shown that 2- and 3-month-old infants grasp an object longer with the right than with the left hand (Caplan & Kinsbourne, 1976; Hawn & Harris, 1983) and at 5 months infants reach more frequently to the right (Cohen, 1966; Hawn & Harris, 1983; Seth, 1973). After pointing has emerged toward the end of the first year, it more frequently is accomplished with the right hand (Bates, O'Connell, Vaid, Sledge, & Oakes, 1986). The situation is complicated by evidence that the hand preferred for activities at the appropriate developmental level fluctuates, perhaps systematically, within a subject during the first year of life (Halverson, 1937; Liederman, 1983; Ramsey, 1984). It could be that this reflects epochs in which one or the other hemisphere is in a phase of relatively more active development. A mechanism that might relate actively developing brain to the frequency of corresponding hand use was provided by Kinsbourne (1970) who proposed an activational model by which activities in a given hemisphere overflow to hemispheric facilities not primarily involved in the activity in question. Contrary to the assumption that handedness emerges from diffuse movement patterns in infancy, its antecedents are already differentiated at birth. In summary, a motor bias that in most individuals is targeted rightward clearly exists as early as at birth or even before, and is a major determinant of the side of the sub-sequently preferred hand.

Infant Central Laterality

The asymmetry in size of planum temporale has been documented in neonatal brains, and in the fetus as early as 29 weeks of gestation (Chi, Dooling, & Gilles, 1977; Wada, Clark, & Hamm, 1975; Witelson & Pallie, 1973). With respect to function, several studies of infants have documented differential response to speech and nonspeech input depending on its side of origin. Entus (1977) used the paradigm of high-amplitude nonnutritive sucking to indicate orienting to a change in stimulus state. At $2\frac{1}{2}$ months, infants demonstrated their habituation to a constant sound by discontinuing the sucking. If that sound changed discriminably, the sucking was dishabituated. Entus presented tape-recorded speech and music. Given changing speech sounds the interruption of sucking happened earlier if the change occurred in the sound presented to the right ear, and given music the same was true for the left. These outcomes could not be replicated (Vargha-Khadem & Corballis, 1979). But Best, Hoffman, and Glanville (1982) presented similar findings using a heart rate dishabituation paradigm, as did Molfese, Freeman, and Palmero (1975) using amplitude of evoked potential. Amplitudes were higher over the left brain for speech, over the right brain for music, in newborns. MacKain, Studdert-Kennedy, Spieker, and Stern (1983) found infants better able to coordinate seen (lip) and heard aspects of an observed speech act when turning right toward the speaker than when turning left. Young and Gagnon (1990) reported that newborns turn more to the right than left when they hear speech. Segalowitz and Chapman (1980), studying premature infants, found that a verbal input caused a quieting of movements of the right arm and leg and musical input a quieting on the left.

These findings are fragmentary and qualitative and not always confirmed (Shucard, Shucard, Cummins, & Campos, 1981). Nevertheless, precursors of aspects of verbal behavior are observably present and lateralized as predicted by the invariant lateralization hypothesis as early as at or even before birth. Given the immature and not yet functional state of the infant cerebrum the asymmetry must be at a brain stem level. Evidence for an involvement of left thalamic nuclei in verbal behavior and of right thalamus in visual behavior (Ojemann, 1977) fits well with the notion that subcortical mechanisms

are involved, if not in the actual mental processing of which the infant is not yet capable, then in facilitating its prospective occurrence, perhaps by implementing lateralized ascending activation of cortex. If there are lateralized selector mechanisms at a brain stem level, implementing a categorical (hemispheric) mental set (Kinsbourne, 1980), this could help to explain difficulties with particular categories of thinking exhibited by children with learning disability, to be discussed subsequently.

An isolated but intriguing finding relates to lateralization of emotion, which is right-sided in adults (Schwartz, Davidson, & Maer, 1975). In infants less than 1 year old, Davidson and Fox (1982) monitored power spectrum EEG changes while they discriminated faces. They offered evidence that even at this early age the right hemisphere is more involved than the left in the discrimination of facial affect. Subsequent research on right–left interactions of EEG activation and emotional state in infants are reviewed by Segalowitz and Berge (1995).

Lateralization of Function

Emergence of Hand Preference in Children

When the child has become capable of reaching, grasping, and pointing, movements analogous to the activities based on which hand preference is determined, the choice of hand used is under control of factors that will cease to operate as maturation proceeds. Notable is the tendency of infants not to cross the midline when they reach for things (Provine & Westerman, 1979). If the target is slightly to one side of center, the child will reach with the ipsilateral limb regardless of hand preference. It is not that there is any motor constraint on reaching across the midline. If the child is already holding a desired object in the ipsilateral hand, he or she does cross the midline in picking up the target with the free hand (Hawn & Harris, 1983). Otherwise, the infant's "prewired" tendency to orient to the side of stimulation (use the hand ipsilateral to the target) overrides motor preference. This could account for observations such as those of Goodwin (cited in Liederman, 1983) who found that right-hand preference on a reaching task at 19 weeks strongly predicted hand preference at 3 years, but left-hand reaching preference did not. Unimanual preference for reaching at 7 weeks predicts the dominant hand for bimanual manipulation at 13 weeks (Ramsey, 1980). The tendency not to cross the midline seems to be a consequence of brain organization. As such it has to be taken into consideration when failure to establish hand preference occurs in developmentally delayed individuals. Subject to developmental lag, they may remain under the control of the type of limiting factor that constrains the normal infant but not the normal older child. Even when it becomes possible to observe the child's choice of hand in a number of standard unimanual activities, the young child differs from the older individual in sometimes being inconsistent in which hand performs which activity (a factor separate from the question of which hand is preferred for activities overall). Palmer (1964) observed this so-called ambiguous hand preference (Silva & Satz, 1984) in normal children and we will return to it when discussing children with mental retardation and autism.

Consistent hand preference tends to be established in the preschool years and to persist unless the individual is subjected to contrary cultural pressure. Until recently it was customary to encourage if not constrain a child who showed left-handed tendencies to use the right hand instead, generating shifted sinistrals who would use the right hand at least for those activities that are socially conspicuous like writing and holding tableware. Such people might still be more dexterous on the left and their left-hand preference may be revealed by giving them a novel activity to perform. Nowadays this type of pressure has been relaxed in the West (though it persists in the Orient; Teng, Lee, Yang, & Chang, 1976). Presumably for this reason, Western offspring have a higher probability of being non-right-handed than their parents. Levy (1976) reported that left-handers were 2.2% of the U.S. population in 1932, but more than 11% by 1972.

Frequently documented within the left-handed population is the position of pen in hand, a distinction being made between the inverted position in which the point of the pen is below the tip of the thumb and index finger and the noninverted in which the pen is held as right-handers do. The inverted handwriting posture is considerably more common in males and develops during the grade school period. It is of interest in view of evidence that it reflects certain biological differences in brain organization (Levy & Reid, 1976). With respect to motor behavior the noninverter exhibits a more bilateralized or right hemispheric type of control and the inverter seems to be more ambidextrous (Parlow & Kinsbourne, 1981).

The prevalence of inverted writing position among left-handed developmentally disabled individuals is not known. It might be of interest, however, because Searleman, Porac, and Coren (1982) found it to be more common after birth stress.

Development of Central Laterality in Childhood

Most of the evidence derives from two sources, lateralized brain lesion effects and laterality testing in normal children, and relates to the language function. Laterality paradigms reveal the effects of functional lateralization on the control of behavior. Which hemisphere is dominant for a particular mental operation is revealed by a bias in how efficiently the relevant task is performed when the pertinent input originates from the right versus the left side of extrapersonal space. Each hemisphere also controls the elements of contralateral turning: faster orienting contralaterally, with consequent faster information pickup; and faster response in that direction by limb or gaze. Thus, the task-specific activation of the specialized hemisphere introduces a slight but observable contralateral turning bias. Kinsbourne (1972) demonstrated that verbal thinking generates rightward orienting (gaze and head turning), whereas spatial thought occasions more left than right gaze shifts. Conversely, verbal learning during rightward head turning was greater than during left turning (Lempert & Kinsbourne, 1982). This method has as yet been little used in developmental studies. However, Barrera, Dalrymple, and Witelson (1978) did report more left gaze during visual processing of faces by infants, and MacKain et al. (1983) found infants better able to map visual on auditory components of speech signals when orienting rightward.

The most generally used laterality measures for input processing are dichotic listening and visual half-field viewing. In dichotic listening, speech sounds, syllables, or words are simultaneously presented to both ears and the subject either tries to report all stimuli ("whole report") or listens separately, to the right ear only and to the left ear only ("selective listening"). In the first case a laterality index is computed to represent the extent to which the subject is able correctly to report input through the right ear as compared with the left. In the second case the subject's ability to identify input from the specified ear is compared for the two ears, and so also is the incidence of responses that represent interference from the ear not to be attended. Normal right-handed adults as a group exhibit right-ear advantage, i.e., they are better able to identify material presented to the right ear than the left under both whole and selective reporting conditions. More intruding stimuli from the right ear are normally reported when selectively listening to the left than vice versa (Treisman & Geffen, 1968).

As early as age 3, a right-ear advantage has been repeatedly demonstrated (Ingram, 1975, Kinsbourne & Hiscock, 1977; Nagafuchi, 1970; Piazza, 1977). Thus, a greater engagement of the left hemisphere in verbal auditory processing can be accepted. The question remains: is the degree of this effect as great in children as in adults or is it that although lateralization has already occurred to some extent by age 3, it will subsequently further increase?

Whereas the direction of group mean ear advantage is an acceptable index of the side of the cortex that is dominant for the task in question, the degree of asymmetry is a dubious index for "degree of lateralization," which is itself a dubious concept. There are numerous factors that interact with differential hemispheric specialization to generate ear advantages that differ in degree, even within the same subject tested under different circumstances or with different dichotic test material. The test–retest reliability for dichotic listening ranges between about 0.5 and 0.8 (e.g., Bakker, Van der Vlugt, & Claushuis, 1978; Hiscock & Kinsbourne, 1980a), hardly commensurate with an index of a fixed structural characteristic. Direction of gaze and direction of movement in the visual environment can both influence the degree of right ear advantage (Hiscock, Hampson, Wong, & Kinsbourne, 1985). Perhaps still more important is task difficulty. The extent to which items from one ear have to be held in memory while those from another are reported (Inglis & Sykes, 1967) can be a major factor if there is a bias to report a particular ear first (Bryden & Allard, 1981). For all of these reasons it would not have been immediately clear how to interpret any interaction between age of child and degree of right-ear advantage for verbal material, had such been found. In fact, most competent studies failed to find such an interaction. Instead, the degree of ear advantage is roughly invariant, consistent with the invariant lateralization hypothesis. The proportion of interfering response from right versus left ear is also invariant across a wide age range in childhood (Geffen, 1978; Geffen & Wale, 1979; Hiscock & Kinsbourne, 1977, 1980a). Progressive lateralization gains little support from dichotic listening studies both in its original strong form, positing a gradient of lateralization

culminating at puberty (Lenneberg, 1967), and in its weak form, restricting that gradient to the first 5 years of life (Krashen, 1973). If lateralization develops at all, its development is completed by age 3 (Porter & Berlin, 1975), the youngest age at which it is feasible to perform dichotic testing in the conventional manner. However, Lokker and Morais (1985) tested children aged $1\frac{3}{4}$–3 years old dichotically, using selective reaching for an object rather than speech as the response. They too found a right-ear advantage for children of right-handed parents.

The visual method of verbal laterality testing is less generally applicable to preschoolers because it relies on the written word. When grade-schoolers were presented with words that they could easily read, then the usual right half-field advantage was found, regardless of age, by Lewandowski (1982) and Marcel and Rajan (1975). Studies that find progression in the development of the right field advantage (Carmon, Nachson, & Starinsky, 1976; Forgays, 1953; Miller & Turner, 1973; Reynolds & Jeeves, 1978; Tomlinson-Keasey, Kelly, & Burton, 1979) are so much in conflict with each other in detail that their diverse outcomes must reflect methodological differences. In any case, no other findings support progressive lateralization into adolescence (for a comprehensive review see Hahn, 1987).

The method used for determining lateralization of speech output control in the intact individual is that of verbal–manual interference (Kinsbourne & Cook, 1971; Kinsbourne & Hicks, 1978). Subjects perform a unimanual activity, such as speeded repetitive finger tapping, with one hand or the other, with or without concurrent speaking. If speech control is lateralized, speaking interferes disproportionately with the finger tapping when they are both controlled by the same hemisphere (i.e., left lateralized speech will interfere more with right than with left finger tapping). When this paradigm is used, there is already at age 3 differential interference with right-hand performance, indicating that speech is already lateralized to the left at that age, supporting invariance of lateralization for speech production (Hiscock & Kinsbourne, 1978, 1980b; White & Kinsbourne, 1980).

Less is known about the ontogeny of lateralization for those nonverbal activities that are regarded as being right lateralized. Piazza (1977) found a left-ear advantage for the dichotic presentation of environmental sounds in 3-, 4-, and 5-year-olds, and Saxby and Bryden (1984) confirmed this for 5-year-olds [although in an earlier study, Knox and Kimura (1970) found somewhat weaker left-ear effects in 5- and 6- than in 7- and 8-year-olds]. Sidtis, Sadler, and Nass (1987) found no interaction with age of left-ear advantage in the discrimination of complex tunes in children aged 7–12 years. For tachistoscopic face recognition, left visual field advantages are found in quite young children, unaffected in degree by age (Marcel, Katz, & Smith, 1974; Turkewitz & Ross-Kossak, 1984; Young & Bion, 1980; Young & Ellis, 1976). With respect to the ability to discriminate shapes by active touching (haptic perception; Witelson, 1974), the typical left-hand advantage has been found as early as 2–3 (Rose, 1984). Other studies revealed left-hand advantages for nonsense shapes in preschoolers (Etaugh & Levy, 1981) and grade-schoolers (Affleck & Joyce, 1979; Coiffi & Kandel, 1976; Flanery & Balling, 1979; Klein & Rosenfield, 1980; Witelson, 1974, 1976), but only Flanery and Balling found a developmental trend. Recognition of verbalizable shapes yields less consistent data, perhaps because of variability in the degree of left-hemisphere participation in the task (e.g., Coiffi & Kandel, 1976; Witelson, 1974). Invariance is generally supported for males, but younger females are more apt than males to use a verbal strategy in coding input (e.g., Caplan & Kinsbourne, 1981).

Briefly exposed faces are equally well identified on either side of the midline until about age 7, subsequent to which a left half-field advantage begins to emerge, earlier in boys than in girls (Carey & Diamond, 1977; Levine, 1985). This finding illustrates a fundamental issue in interpretation. Whereas the gradual emergence of an asymmetry could indeed imply progressive lateralization, it could as readily indicate the emergence of a processor that had not been functional in the less mature brain. If space perception calls for particular processing skills that normally only emerge toward the end of the first decade of life, then presenting a spatial-relational task to younger children will yield a lack of asymmetry by default, rather than indicate that at that age both hemispheres were processing the material in question to a comparable extent. Carey and colleagues believe that the manner in which children process face information changes qualitatively at the time that the left half-field advantage emerges. If this is so, then what is being indexed is the increasing specialization of the right hemisphere with increasing age, and not a changing neural basis for an already available skill. With further increase in age, the degree of left-field advantage will not increase. Indeed, it may temporarily diminish at around puberty in concert with a de-

crease in overall efficiency. This effect has been speculatively related to endocrine changes around puberty (Diamond, Carey, & Black, 1983).

Degree of Lateralization

The absence of interaction between degree of lateral asymmetry and age in most studies simplifies the task of explanation. In addition to supporting lateralization invariance, it sidesteps the dilemma of interpreting between-group differences in the degree of laterality bias in the same direction. The assumption that degree of lateral asymmetry indexes degree of lateralization of the critical task-related mental operation (Shankweiler & Studdert-Kennedy, 1967) has never been substantiated (Allen, 1983). Indeed, it is unclear what is meant by greater or lesser degree of lateralization. Does the distinction assume that both hemispheres participate in the task, though to a varying extent unequally? If so, are they redundant in their contribution, or complementary? If unilateral brain damage occurs, should the function in question be compromised by damage on both sides, in proportion to the degree of lateralization on each side? If so, no such intimation from lateral brain injury exists. Given the many factors that, for instance, modify asymmetry in a dichotic test—task difficulty, task aptitude and motivation, the extent of stimulus dominance, and perhaps whatever else the subject is thinking about and how (happy or sad) he or she is feeling—it is hardly surprising that the literature on degree of lateralization is inconsistent in the extreme. Two related areas to which the concept has been vigorously applied are gender differences and age at puberty difference in degree of lateralization. It is little wonder that the literature in both fields (McGlone, 1980, and peer commentary; Newcombe & Bandura, 1983, respectively) is a morass of inconsistencies. Operationally, laterality tests (and lateral brain damage effects) can only guide us in a choice between three alternatives: left lateralized, right lateralized, bilateralized.

Whereas functional lateralization is not conclusively associated with the degree of asymmetry on laterality measures, one already mentioned anatomical measure yields strikingly powerful correlations: the cross-sectional area of the corpus callosum (CA). Specifically, the smaller the CA is, the greater the asymmetry both on verbal and on spatial laterality measures (Yazgan *et al.,* 1995). It appears that size of a laterality effect is more likely to reflect the manner in which the task engages lateralized facilities, than the extent to which their neural substrate is lateralized.

Lateralization Probed by Lateral Cerebral Damage

If language lateralization is invariant, then left-brain damage should be equally likely, and right-brain damage equally unlikely, to cause aphasia or delayed language development in right-handed children as in adults (acutely—whether the probability or rate of compensation changes with increasing age is a separate issue). Contrary to earlier impressions (Basser, 1962), this is approximately the case. In Woods and Teuber's (1978) series, the incidence of aphasia in right-handed children aged 2–14 was about 70% versus 7% for left- and right-sided cerebral damage, respectively. The implication that the left hemisphere is specialized early for language is corroborated by series of children who suffered lateral cerebral damage before the emergence of language would be expected. The long-term language outcome is less favorable if the early damage was left-sided (Kershner & King, 1974; Kiessling, Denckla, & Carlton, 1983; Rankin, Aram, & Horwitz, 1981; Vargha-Khadem, O'Gorman, & Watters, 1985), at least in terms of syntactic proficiency (Aram, Ekelman, Rose, & Whitaker, 1985; Dennis & Kohn, 1975; Rankin et al., 1981). But the selective syntactic difficulties (themselves questionable on methodological grounds; Bishop, 1988) are overshadowed by the recurrent finding that early lateral damage on either side, even when strictly lateralized, moderately impairs performance across a wide range of tests (Aram et al., 1985). Injuries sustained before age 5 years result in less favorable intellectual outcome than later injuries (Aram & Eisele, 1994) although the children still score well within the normal range of IQ. It follows that brain organization is not strictly modular, but draws on distributed as well as focalized neural processing, at least during mental development.

Although lateralization of language remains invariant throughout its development, the locus of compensation after damage to the language area of the child's brain does not. Penfield and Roberts (1959) reported on the incidence of aphasia after left temporal lobectomy in epileptic adults. When lesion onset was prior to age 2 years, the probability of aphasia was much less than when the damage had occurred subsequently in childhood. It appears that territories in both hemispheres have the potential to compensate for injury to the language area. Right-sided territories are more likely to assume a compensatory role the earlier the lesion occurred, and perhaps the more extensive it is. Perhaps right-hemisphere territories that normally control other processes are preempted for purposes of the compensatory functioning ("crowding hypothesis" of Teuber and Rudel, 1962) to the detriment of their customary role. Even adult aphasics may program their residual or recovered speech from the uninjured right side of the brain (Gainotti, 1993; Kinsbourne, 1971, in press). When Huttenlocher, Raichelson, Rye, and Wainer (1986) hemispherectomized infant rats, an ipsilateral corticospinal tract developed in addition to the normally present contralateral tract. The investigators subsequently found that the spared cortical area that contained pyramidal tract cells had greatly expanded, in response to the excision of the contralateral hemisphere. This provides an animal model for contralateral compensation for early lateralized injury.

We conclude that language precursors rely on the same hemisphere that subserves language in its full maturity. The earliest manifestation is perhaps a selective activation of that hemisphere in a verbal context, well before its neural substrate has matured to the point that language processing is feasible. As language ability differentiates, language processing may involve, not a shrinking, but an expanding neural base within that same hemisphere (Satz, Strauss, & Whitaker, 1990).

Supportive evidence for early right-sided lateralization derives from studies of right-hemisphere lesion effects in childhood (Ferro, Martins, & Tavora, 1984; Kershner & King, 1974; Kohn & Dennis, 1974; Stiles-Davis, Sugarman, & Nass, 1985). They all found spatial deficits analogous to those observed in adults after right-hemisphere damage.

The fact that lateralization is invariant is not contradicted by the claim that lateralized findings emerge serially over time within each hemisphere (Satz, Strauss, & Whitaker, 1990). The latter phenomenon is better characterized as progressive intrahemispheric specialization than lateralization. Obviously different specialized central facilities become functional at different times throughout childhood. Whether their intrahemispheric base shrinks, expands, or remains the same during this process has not been determined.

The impressively consistent evidence in favor of invariant lateralization for the major functions of both hemispheres offers a conveniently simple standard of reference against which to evaluate the frequently offered suggestion that children with a variety of developmental disabilities are anomalously lateralized, and that this causes the behavioral deficit.

Lateralization in Developmental Deficit

Introduction

Perhaps because developmental deficits offer so few clues beyond their surface phenomenology for their pathogenesis, lateralization has often been invoked as a possible factor. Allegedly, the normal lateralization of hemispherically specialized cognitive functions failed to occur, the assumption being that when cognitive processing is based on both hemispheres it is relatively primitive and necessarily inefficient. This logic depends crucially on the notion that lateralization is normally progressive and that when this progression is impaired, the end result is a cognitive deficit. As we have seen, the evidence for progressive lateralization is lacking; if anomalies of lateralization are to be found in developmental disabilities, some other explanation has to be sought. There is, in fact, a greater incidence of unusual forms of lateralization in developmental deficits, but the causes and implications of these differences remain quite obscure. They may be coincidental and nonspecific. Furthermore, there is a coincidence between absence of the usual left lateralization of language in various disabilities and an increased prevalence of non-right-handedness in the same conditions (though the central and peripheral laterality anomalies by no means correlate perfectly). I first consider the data on hand preference.

Hand Preference in Developmental Disabilities

Non-right-handedness is not only more common among the mentally retarded, and language and learning delayed, but the non-right-handed subgroups of these populations tend to be more severely affected. For example, Hicks and Barton (1975) found severe and profoundly mentally retarded individuals to be even more often non-right-handed than mild and moderate, who in turn were more often non-right-handed than the general population. Bradshaw-McAnulty, Hicks, and Kinsbourne (1984) confirmed this finding, and related greater severity of the mental retardation to a

greater probability of non-right-handedness in one or other parent. In infantile autism, non-right-handedness is particularly prevalent (Colby & Parkinson, 1977; Tsai, 1982), and several investigators have found the lower-functioning autistic individuals to be more often non-right-handed (e.g., Fein, Humes, Kaplan, & Lucci-Waterhouse, 1984). Indeed, in mental retardation, and particularly in autism, the hand preferred even for a single activity, is apt to change from trial to trial (ambiguous handedness, according to Silva & Satz, 1984; see also Soper, Satz, Orsini, Van Gorp, & Gireer, 1987). Non-right-handedness is relatively common in stuttering and in language delay. In selective reading disability (dyslexia), non-right-handedness is relatively prevalent, again especially among the most severely affected children, who are to be found in clinical settings and in special schools for the learning disabled (Satz, 1976). An excess of non-right-handedness is generally not found among relatively poor readers as compared with good readers in the general school population.

Sharply contrasting explanations for this conjunction of findings have been offered. (1) Presuming that peripheral non-right-handedness implies a corresponding absence of central lateralization, the latter deficiency is incriminated as inducing a processing inefficiency (Orton, 1937). (2) Some left-handedness (Satz, 1972) or even all left-handedness (Bakan, 1971) is related to early left-hemisphere pathology (syndrome of pathological left-handedness of Satz, Orsini, Saslow, & Henry, 1985), and such early pathology is also likely to induce diverse developmental disabilities. (3) An adverse influence early in development is postulated that tends both to diminish language lateralization and to impair the evolving competence of the language hemisphere (Geschwind & Behan, 1982). (4) Becoming non-right-handed and suffering from a wide range of developmental disorders are consequences of an adverse influence on the fetal brain ("maternal immune attack") which is generated by mothers who are susceptible to diseases of the immune system (Crawford, Kaplan, & Kinsbourne, 1994).

The second and third of these models are only applicable to those developmental deficits that can plausibly be attributed to malfunctioning of the left (language) hemisphere, rather than of the cerebral cortex as a whole. Language and reading disabilities are a case in point, and autism used to be so regarded (Rutter, Bartak, & Newman, 1971) although the evidence against this is now very strong (Fein *et al.,* 1984). However, it then also has to be explained why the right hemisphere does not compensate for the hypothesized left-sided malfunction, given its well-known ability to compensate for the effects of gross early left-hemisphere damage. For mental retardation and perhaps autism, in which conditions a more general cerebral deficit seems likely, explanations (2) and (3), targeted on the left hemisphere, lose force. However, conceivably more than one of the above-postulated mechanisms might come into play in the same individual. For instance, there is circumstantial evidence that right- as well as left-handed members of relatively sinistral families are more at risk for developmental deficit, or for having more severe deficit should early damage occur (Kinsbourne, 1986). The damage to which such individuals are vulnerable could in turn, when it implicates the left hemisphere, not only impair cognition, but also shift the hand preference phenotype to sinistral, in a genotypic dextral (pathological left-handedness). This would increase the prevalence of non-right-handedness among the affected family members beyond the level that prevails within their already relatively sinistral family (Bradshaw-McAnulty *et al.,* 1984).

Central Laterality in Developmental Deficits

The measurement of central laterality requires a degree of cooperation from subjects, and perhaps for that reason, has most often been attempted in people whose developmental deficits are relatively mild, namely, the learning disabled. These consist of two main subgroups: children with attention deficit and children with central processing difficulties (Kinsbourne & Caplan, 1979). A sample of the former was found to be normally lateralized by a dichotic (Hiscock, Kinsbourne, Caplan, & Swanson, 1979) and a visual (Naylor, 1980) laterality test. Therefore, studies have concentrated on the latter, and especially on the reading-disabled subgroup ("dyslexics"), under the influence of the persisting notion that dyslexia is the result of failure of left language lateralization (Orton, 1937; Zurif & Carson, 1970). But enough studies have found normal verbal laterality in learning-disabled children (e.g., Bouma & Legein, 1977; Caplan & Kinsbourne, 1982; McKeever & Van Deventer, 1975; Marcel *et al.,* 1974; Marcel & Rajan, 1975) to indicate that failure of left-sided language lateralization is not a viable explanation for selective reading disability (reviewed by Hiscock & Kinsbourne, 1995).

The lack of evidence for abnormal laterality does not imply, however, that the left-sided language areas are normal in dyslexic children. Patchy microdysgenesis has been identified at autopsy (Galaburda *et al.,* 1985). Alternatively, the left hemisphere might be undersupplied by ascending activation, rendering it hard for the child to muster verbal skills in full force to solve what is for him or her a difficult verbal problem (Kinsbourne, 1980). Such an activational insufficiency might also generate a relatively nonverbal (right hemispheric) cognitive style in dyslexic children (Caplan & Kinsbourne, 1982). Obrzut, Hynd, Obrzut, and Pirozzola (1981) found learning-disabled children better able than normally reading controls to listen selectively to left-ear input. Obrzut, Hynd, and Zellner (1983) obtained comparable results in visual laterality. The voluntary attentional shift could override a diminished rightward attentional bias engendered by the presumably relatively weak left-brain activation of the dyslexics. Yet another possibility is that dyslexic children fail to distribute verbal and spatial computation to different hemispheres (Obrzut, Boliek, Bryden, & Nicholson, 1994). If so, their behavior is analogous to that of normal adult left-handers, using the preferred direction of reflective lateral gaze as the dependent variable (Kinsbourne, 1972).

An electrophysiological approach has attempted to distinguish subgroups of dyslexics that are deficient in right- and left-hemisphere functioning, respectively (Bakker, Licht, Kok, & Bouma, 1980). Evoked potential studies lend support to the view that dyslexic children may exhibit abnormal responses in one hemisphere when tested, but the stability of those patterns has not been proven (Fried, Tanguay, Boder, Doubleday, & Greensite, 1981; Mecacci, Sechi, & Levi, 1983). If stable, they could reflect lateralized activational deficiencies.

Absent and reversed anatomical cerebral asymmetries abound in dyslexics (reviewed by Hynd, Marshall, Hall, & Edmonds, 1995). As these authors point out, the significance of such findings is qualified by their presence also in many people in the general population. Either they are devoid of functional significance, or, conversely, they account not only for extreme individual differences (as in learning disability) but also for individual differences considered to be within the normal range. Advances in quantitative MRI have now made the latter possibility amenable to study in the normal population.

Stuttering is an early arising deficit (age 3 to 5 years) in which maladaptive rivalry between the cerebral hemispheres for control of speech has long been suspected (Travis, 1927). The concept was dramatically supported by case studies of four left-handed stutterers with lateralized cerebrovascular congenital anomalies (Jones, 1966). They were found to be bilateralized for speech by intracarotid Amytal testing before operation. After operation, repeat Amytal testing showed that speech control had become restricted to the normal (unoperated) hemisphere. Also, after operation, the patients ceased to stutter. This could be because the operation had titled rivalry in favor of a single hemisphere. However, comparable studies of three more right-handed stutterers without brain damage have not yielded comparable findings (Andrews, Quinn, & Sorby, 1972), and both behavioral and EEG laterality were normal in stutterers (Pinsky & McAdam, 1980). As in dyslexia, it is more likely that in most stutterers any cerebral abnormality is of a dynamic rather than a static nature, for instance, an abnormality of left-hemisphere activation for stuttered speech acts only. We await findings from event-related measures selectively time-locked to stuttered utterances (nonstuttered utterances serving as control). The regional cerebral blood flow study of Wood, Stump, McKeehan, Sheldon, and Proctor (1980), in which stutterers were judged to have inadequate left-hemisphere activation (normalized when the stuttering was relieved by haloperidol), is a step in this direction.

Both bilateral failure to lateralize and right-brain dominance have been proposed. But it seems more likely that heterogeneous patterns of cerebral specialization occur within the autistic population, and that no one pattern of lateralization constitutes a necessary condition for autistic symptomatology to appear (Kinsbourne, 1987). Among the heterogeneous mentally retarded population, Down syndrome individuals have been credited with anomalous perceptual laterality (Hartley, 1981; Pipe, 1983), indicating reversed cerebral dominance. But Tannock, Kershner, and Oliver (1984) found a right-ear advantage in Down syndrome, and Parlow, Kinsbourne, and Spencer (in press) found no laterality differences between Down and non-Down severely mentally retarded adults and an overall pattern for both laterality of verbal input and output control that was comparable to the norm.

In summary, anomalous lateralization is not infrequent in diverse developmentally delayed populations. But there is no evidence that failure to lateralize causes any of the developmental delays.

References

Affleck, G., & Joyce, P. (1979). Sex differences in the association of cerebral hemisphere specialization of spatial function with conservation task performance. *Journal of Genetic Psychology, 134,* 271–280.

Allen, M. (1983). Models of hemispheric specialization. *Psychological Bulletin, 93,* 73–104.

Andrews, G., Quinn, P. T., & Sorby, A. (1972). Stuttering: An investigation into cerebral dominance for speech. *Journal of Neurology, Neurosurgery and Psychiatry, 35,* 414–418.

Annett, M. (1973). Handedness in families. *Annals of Human Genetics, 37,* 93–105.

Aram, D. M., & Eisele, J. A. (1994). Intellectual stability in children with unilateral brain lesions. *Neuropsychologia, 32(1),* 85–95.

Aram, D. M., Ekelman, B. L., Rose, D. F., & Whitaker, H. A. (1985). Verbal and cognitive sequelae following unilateral lesions acquired in early childhood. *Journal of Clinical and Experimental Neuropsychology, 7,* 55–78.

Bakan, P. (1971). Handedness and birth order. *Nature, 229,* 195.

Bakker, D. J., Licht, R., Kok, A., & Bouma, A. (1980). Cortical responses to word reading by right- and left-eared normal and reading-disturbed children. *Neuropsychologia, 2,* 1–12.

Bakker, D. J., Van der Vlugt, H., & Claushuis, M. (1978). The reliability of dichotic ear asymmetry in normal children. *Neuropsychologia, 16,* 753–758.

Barrera, M. E., Dalrymple, A., & Witelson, S. F. (1978). *Behavioral evidence of right hemisphere asymmetry in early infancy.* Paper presented to the Canadian Psychological Association, Ottawa.

Basser, S. (1962). Hemiplegia of early onset and the faculty of speech with special reference to the effects of hemispherectomy. *Brain, 85,* 427–460.

Bates, E., O'Connell, B., Vaid, J., Sledge, P., & Oakes, L. (1986). Language and hand preference in early development. *Developmental Neuropsychology, 2,* 1–15.

Beeman, M. (1993). Semantic processing in the right hemisphere may contribute to drawing inferences from discourse. *Brain and Language, 44,* 80–120.

Best, C. T., Hoffman, H., & Glanville, B. B. (1982). Development of infant ear asymmetries for speech and music. *Perception and Psychophysics, 35,* 75–85.

Bishop, D. V. M. (1988). Can the right hemisphere mediate language as well as the left? A critical review of recent research. *Cognitive Neuropsychology, 3,* 353–367.

Bouma, H., & Legein, C. P. (1977). Foveal and parafoveal recognition of letters by dyslexics and average readers. *Neuropsychologia, 15,* 69–80.

Bradshaw-McAnulty, G., Hicks, R. E., & Kinsbourne, M. (1984). Pathological left-handedness and familial sinistrality in relation to degree of mental retardation. *Brain and Cognition, 3,* 349–356.

Braitenberg, V. (1977). The concept of symmetry in neuroanatomy. *Annals of the New York Academy of Sciences, 299*, 186–196.

Braitenberg, V., & Kemali, M. (1970). Exceptions to bilateral symmetry in the epithalamus of lower vertebrates. *Journal of Comparative Neurology, 138*, 137–146.

Bresson, F., Maury, L., Pierant-LeBonniec, G., & deSchonen, S. (1977). Organization and lateralization of reaching in infants: An instance of asymmetric functions in hand collaborations. *Neuropsychologia, 15*, 311–320.

Bryden, M. P., & Allard, F. A. (1979). Dichotic listening and the development of linguistic processes. In M. Kinsbourne (Ed.), *Asymmetrical function of the brain* (pp. 392–404). London: Cambridge University Press.

Bryden, M. P., & Allard, F. A. (1981). Do auditory perceptual asymmetries develop? *Cortex, 17*, 313–318.

Bryden, M. P., Hécaen, H., & DeAgostini, M. (1983). Patterns of cerebral organization. *Brain and Language, 20*, 249–262.

Caplan, P. J., & Kinsbourne, M. (1976). Baby drops the rattle: Asymmetry of duration grasp by infants. *Child Development, 47*, 532–534.

Caplan, P. J., & Kinsbourne, M. (1981). Cerebral lateralization, preferred cognitive mode, and reading ability in normal children. *Brain and Language, 14*, 349–370.

Caplan, B., & Kinsbourne, M. (1982). Cognitive style and dichotic asymmetries of disabled readers. *Cortex, 18*, 357–366.

Carey, S., & Diamond, R. (1977). From piecemeal to configurational representation of faces. *Science, 195*, 312–314.

Carmon, A., Nachson, I., & Starinsky, R. (1976). Developmental aspects of visual hemifield differences in perception of verbal material. *Brain and Language, 3*, 463–469.

Chi, J. G., Dooling, E. C., & Gilles, F. H. (1977). Left–right asymmetries of the temporal speech areas of the human fetus. *Archives of Neurology, 34*, 346–348.

Churchill, J. A., Igna, E., & Senf, R. (1962). The association of position at birth and handedness. *Pediatrics, 29*, 307–309.

Cohen, A. I. (1966). Hand preference and developmental status of infants. *Journal of Genetic Psychology, 108*, 337–345.

Coiffi, J., & Kandel, G. (1976). Laterality of stereognostic accuracy of children for words, shapes, and bigrams: Sex differences for bigrams. *Science, 204*, 1432–1434.

Colby, K. M., & Parkinson, C. (1977). Handedness in autistic children. *Journal of Autism and Childhood Schizophrenia, 7*, 3–9.

Crawford, S. G., Kaplan, B. J., & Kinsbourne, M. (1994). Are families of children with reading difficulties at risk for immune disorders and nonrighthandedness? *Cortex, 30*, 281–292.

Davidson, R. J., & Fox, N. (1982). Asymmetrical brain activity discriminates between positive versus negative affective stimuli in ten month old infants. *Science, 218*, 1235–1236.

Dennis, M., & Kohn, B. (1975). Comprehension of syntax in infantile hemiplegics after cerebral hemidecortication: Left hemisphere superiority. *Brain and Language, 2*, 475–486.

Diamond, R., Carey, S., & Black, K. J. (1983). Genetic influences on the development of spatial skills during early adolescence. *Cognition, 13*, 167–185.

Entus, A. K. (1977). Hemispheric asymmetry in processing of dichotically presented speech and nonspeech stimuli by infants. In S. J. Segalowitz & F. A. Gruber (Eds.), *Language development and neurological theory* (pp. 63–73). New York: Academic Press.

Etaugh, C., & Levy, R. B. (1981). Hemispheric specialization for tactile–spatial processing in preschool children. *Perceptual and Motor Skills, 53*, 621–622.

Falzi, G., Perrone, P., & Vignolo, L. A. (1982). Right–left asymmetry in anterior speech region. *Archives of Neurology, 39*, 239–240.

Fein, D., Humes, M., Kaplan, E., & Lucci-Waterhouse, L. (1984). The question of the left hemisphere dysfunction in infantile autism. *Psychological Bulletin, 95*, 258–281.

Ferro, J. M., Martins, I. P., & Tavora, L. (1984). Neglect in children. *Annals of Neurology, 15*, 281–284.

Flanery, R. C., & Balling, J. D. (1979). Developmental changes in hemispheric specialization for tactile spatial ability. *Developmental Psychology, 15*, 364–372.

Forgays, D. G. (1953). The development of differential word recognition. *Journal of Experimental Psychology, 45*, 165–168.

Fried, I., Tanguay, P. E., Boder, E., Doubleday, C., & Greensite, M. (1981). Developmental dyslexia: Electrophysiological evidence of clinical subgroup. *Brain and Language, 12*, 14–22.

Gainotti, G. (1993). The middle of the right hemisphere's contribution to the recovery of language. *Journal of Disorders of Communications, 28*, 227–246.

Galaburda, A. M. (1984). Anatomical asymmetries. In N. Geschwind & A. M. Galaburda (Eds.), *Cerebral dominance: The biological foundations* (pp. 11–25). Cambridge, MA: Harvard University Press.

Galaburda, A. M., Sherman, G. F., Rosen, G. D., Aboitiz, F., & Geschwind, N. (1985). Developmental dyslexia: Four consecutive patients with cortical anomalies. *Annals of Neurology, 18*(2), 222–233.

Gardner, H., Ling, P. K., Flamm, L., & Silverman, J. (1975). Comprehension and appreciation of humor in brain-damaged patients. *Brain, 98*, 399–412.

Gardner, M. (1967). *The ambidextrous universe*. Baltimore: Penguin.

Geffen, G. (1978). The development of the right ear advantage in dichotic listening with focused attention. *Cortex, 14*, 169–177.

Geffen, G., & Wale, J. (1979). Development of selective listening in hemispheric asymmetry. *Developmental Psychology, 15*, 138–146.

Geschwind, N., & Behan, P. (1982). Left–handedness: Association with immune disease, migraine, and developmental learning disorder. *Proceedings of the National Academy of Sciences USA, 79*, 5097–5100.

Geschwind, N., & Levitsky, W. (1968). Human brain: Left–right asymmetries in temporal speech region. *Science, 161*, 186–187.

Gesell, A., & Ames, L. (1947). The development of handedness. *Journal of General Psychology, 70*, 155–157.

Gloning, I., Gloning, K., Haub, G., & Quatember, R. (1959). Comparison of verbal behavior in right-handed and non-righthanded patients with anatomically verified lesion of one hemisphere. *Cortex, 5*, 43–52.

Govind, C. K., & Pearce, J. (1986). Differential reflex activity determines claw and clasper muscle asymmetry in developing lobsters. *Science, 33,* 354–356.

Hahn, W. K. (1987). Cerebral lateralization of function: From infancy through childhood. *Psychological Bulletin, 101,* 376–392.

Halverson, H. (1937). Studies of the grasping responses of early infancy. *Journal of Genetic Psychology, 51,* 371–392; 392–424.

Harrington, A. (1987). *Medicine, mind and the double brain.* Princeton, NJ: Princeton University Press.

Hartley, X. Y. (1981). Lateralization of speech stimuli in young Down's syndrome children. *Cortex, 17,* 241–248.

Hauser, M. D. (1996). *The evolution of communication.* Cambridge, MA: MIT Press.

Hawn, P. R., & Harris, L. J. (1983). Hand differences in grasp duration and reaching in two- and five-month-old infants. In G. Young, S. Segalowitz, C. M. Cotter, & S. E. Trehub (Eds.), *Manual specialization and the developing brain.* New York: Academic Press.

Hécaen, H. (1978). Right hemisphere contribution to language function. In P. A. Buser & A. Rougeul-Buser (Eds.), *Cerebral correlates of conscious experience.* Amsterdam: North-Holland.

Hicks, R. E., & Barton, A. (1975). A note on left-handedness and severity of mental retardation. *Journal of General Psychology, 127,* 323–324.

Hicks, R. E., & Kinsbourne, M. (1978). Lateralized concomitants of human handedness. *Journal of Motor Behavior, 10,* 83–94.

Hiscock, M., Hampson, E., Wong, S. C. P., & Kinsbourne, M. (1985). Effects of eye movements on the recognition and localization of dichotic stimuli. *Brain and Cognition, 4,* 140–155.

Hiscock, M., & Kinsbourne, M. (1977). Selective listening asymmetry in preschool children. *Developmental Psychology, 13,* 217–224.

Hiscock, M., & Kinsbourne, M. (1978). Ontogeny of cerebral dominance: Evidence from time-sharing asymmetry in children. *Developmental Psychology, 16,* 70–82.

Hiscock, M., & Kinsbourne, M. (1980a). Asymmetries of selective listening and attention switching in children. *Developmental Psychology, 16,* 70–82.

Hiscock, M., & Kinsbourne, M. (1980b). Asymmetry of verbal–manual time-sharing in children: A follow-up study. *Neuropsychologia, 18,* 151–162.

Hiscock, M., & Kinsbourne, M. (1995). Progress in the measurement of laterality and implications for dyslexia research. *Annals of Dyslexia, 45,* 249–268.

Hiscock, M., Kinsbourne, M., Caplan, B., & Swanson, J. M. (1979). Auditory attention in hyperactive children: Effects of stimulant medication on dichotic listening performance. *Journal of Abnormal Psychology, 88,* 27–32.

Hochberg, F. H., & LeMay, M. (1975). Arteriographic correlates of handedness. *Neurology, 25,* 218–222.

Hubbs, C. L., & Hubbs, L. C. (1944). Bilateral asymmetry and bilateral variation in fishes. *Paper to Michigan Academy of Arts, Sciences and Letters, 30,* 229–311.

Huttenlocher, P., Raichelson, R. M., Rye, D. B., & Wainer, B. H. (1986). Hemispherectomy in infancy enlarges the distribution of motor neurons in the remaining cerebral hemisphere. *Annals of Neurology, 20,* 418.

Hyman, L. H. (1940). *The invertebrates.* New York: Mc-Graw–Hill.

Hynd, G. W., Marshall, R., Hall, J., & Edmonds, J. E. (1995). Learning disabilities: Neuroanatomic asymmetries. In R. J. Davidson & K. Hugdahl (Eds.), *Brain asymmetry* (pp. 617–635). Cambridge, MA: MIT Press.

Inglis, J., & Sykes, D. H. (1967). Some sources of variation in dichotic listening performance in children. *Journal of Experimental Child Psychology, 5,* 480–488.

Ingram, D. (1975). Cerebral speech lateralization in young children. *Neuropsychologia, 13,* 103–105.

Jones, R. K. (1966). Observations on stammering after localized cerebral injury. *Journal of Neurology, Neurosurgery and Psychiatry, 29,* 192–195.

Kershner, J. R., & King, A. J. (1974). Laterality of cognitive functions in achieving hemiplegic children. *Perceptual and Motor Skills, 39,* 1238–1284.

Kiessling, L. S., Denckla, M. B., & Carlton, M. (1983). Evidence for differential hemisphere function in children with hemiplegic cerebral palsy. *Developmental Medicine and Child Neurology, 25,* 727–734.

Kinsbourne, M. (1970). The cerebral basis of lateral asymmetries in attention. *Acta Psychologica, 33,* 193–201.

Kinsbourne, M. (1971). The minor cerebral hemisphere as a source of aphasic speech. *Archives of Neurology, 25,* 302–306.

Kinsbourne, M. (1972). Eye and head turning indicate cerebral lateralization. *Science, 176,* 539–541.

Kinsbourne, M. (1974). Lateral interactions in the brain. In M. Kinsbourne & W. L. Smith (Eds.), *Hemisphere disconnection and cerebral functions* (pp. 239–259). Springfield, IL: Thomas.

Kinsbourne, M. (1975). The ontogeny of cerebral dominance. *Annals of the New York Academy of Sciences, 263,* 244–250.

Kinsbourne, M. (1980). A model for the ontogeny of cerebral organization in non-right-handers. In J. Herron (Ed.), *Neuropsychology of left handedness* (pp. 177–185). New York: Academic Press.

Kinsbourne, M. (1982). Hemispheric specialization and the growth of human understanding. *American Psychologist, 37,* 411–420.

Kinsbourne, M. (1986). Sinistrality and risk for immune diseases and learning disorders: A pleiotropic gene effect? *Annals of Neurology, 20,* 416 (abstract).

Kinsbourne, M. (1987). Cerebral–brainstem interactions in infantile autism. In E. Schopler & G. Mesibov (Eds.), *Neurobiological theories of arousal and autism.* New York: Plenum Press.

Kinsbourne, M. (in press).

Kinsbourne, M., & Caplan, P. J. (1979). *Children's learning and attention problems.* Boston: Little, Brown.

Kinsbourne, M., & Cook, J. (1971). Generalized and lateralized effects of concurrent verbalization on a unimanual skill. *Quarterly Journal of Experimental Psychology, 23,* 341–345.

Kinsbourne, M., & Hicks, R. E. (1978). Functional cerebral space: A model for overflow, transfer and interference effects in human performance: A tutorial review. In J. Requin (Ed.), *Attention and performance VII.* Hillsdale, NJ: Erlbaum.

Kinsbourne, M. & Hiscock, M. (1977). Does cerebral dominance develop? In S. J. Segalowitz & F. A. Gruber (Eds.), *Language development and neurological theory* (pp. 171–191). Academic Press.

Kinsbourne, M., & Lempert, H. (1979). Does left brain lateralization of speech arise from right-biased orienting to salient percepts? *Human Development, 22,* 270–276.

Klein, S. P., & Rosenfield, W. D. (1980). The hemispheric specialization for linguistic and nonlinguistic tactile stimuli in third grade children. *Cortex, 16,* 205–212.

Knox, C., & Kimura, D. (1970). Cerebral processing of nonverbal sounds in boys and girls. *Neuropsychologia, 8,* 227–237.

Kohn, B., & Dennis, M. (1974). Selective impairments of visuospatial abilities in infantile hemiplegics after right hemidecortication. *Neuropsychologia, 12,* 505–512.

Krashen, S. D. (1973). Lateralization, language learning, and the critical period: Some new evidence. *Language Learning, 23,* 63–74.

Latimer, H. B., & Lowrance, E. W. (1965). Bilateral asymmetry in weight and length of human bones. *Anatomical Record, 152,* 217–224.

LeMay, M. (1976). Morphological cerebral asymmetries of modern man, fossil man, and nonhuman primate. *Annals of the New York Academy of Sciences, 280,* 349–366.

LeMay, M. (1992). Left–right dissymmetry, handedness. *American Journal of Neuroradiology, 13,* 493–504.

LeMay, M., & Culebras, A. (1972). Human brain-pathological differences in the hemispheres demonstrable by cortical arteriography. *New England Journal of Medicine, 287,* 168–170.

Lempert, H., & Kinsbourne, M. (1982). Effect of laterality of orientation on verbal memory. *Neuropsychologia, 20,* 211–214.

Lempert, H., & Kinsbourne, M. (1985). Possible origin of speech in selective orienting. *Psychological Bulletin, 97,* 62–73.

Lenneberg, E. H. (1967). *Biological foundations of language.* New York: Wiley.

Levine, S. C. (1985). Developmental changes in right hemisphere involvement in face-recognition. In C. Best (Ed.), *Hemisphere function and collaboration in the child* (pp. 157–191). New York: Academic Press.

Levy, J. (1976). A review of evidence for a genetic component in the determination of handedness. *Behavor Genetics, 6,* 429–453.

Levy, J., & Reid, M. (1976). Variations in writing posture and cerebral organization. *Science, 194,* 337–339.

Lewandowski, L. L. (1982). Hemispheric asymmetry in children. *Perceptual and Motor Skills, 54,* 1011–1019.

Lewis, R. S., & Harris, L. J. (1990). Handedness, sex and spatial ability. In S. Coren (Ed.), *Left-handedness: Behavioral implications and anomalies.* Amsterdam: North-Holland.

Liederman, J. (1983). Mechanisms underlying instability in the development of the hand preference. In G. Young, S. Segalowitz, C. M. Carter, & S. E. Trehub (Eds.), *Manual*

specialization and the developing brain. New York: Academic Press.

Liederman, J., & Kinsbourne, M. (1980a). The mechanism of neonatal rightward turning bias: A sensory or motor asymmetry? *Infant Behavior and Development, 3,* 223–238.

Liederman, J., & Kinsbourne, M. (1980b). Rightward motor bias in newborns depends upon parental right-handedness. *Neuropsychologia, 18,* 579–584.

Loeb, J. (1918). *Forced movements, tropisms and animal conduct.* Philadelphia: Lippincott.

Lokker, R., & Morais, J. (1985). Ear differences in children at two years of age. *Neuropsychologia, 23,* 127–129.

Ludwig, W. (1932). *Das Rechts-Links-Problem in Tierreich und beim Menschen.* Berlin: Springer.

McGlone, J. (1980). Sex differences in human brain asymmetry: A critical survey. *Behavioral and Brain Sciences, 3,* 215–263.

MacKain, K., Studdert-Kennedy, M., Spieker, S., & Stern, D. (1983). Infant intermodal speech perception is a left hemisphere function. *Science, 214,* 1347–1349.

McKeever, W. F., & Van Deventer, A. D. (1975). Dyslexic adolescents: Evidence of impaired visual and auditory language processing associated with normal lateralization and visual responsivity. *Cortex, 11,* 361–378.

McRae, D., Branch, D., & Milner, B. (1968). The occipital horns and cerebral dominance. *Neurology, 18,* 95–98.

Marcel, T., Katz, L., & Smith, M. (1974). Laterality and reading proficiency. *Neuropsychologia, 12,* 131–139.

Marcel, T., & Rajan, P. (1975). Lateral specialization for recognition of words and faces in good and poor readers. *Neuropsychologia, 13,* 489–497.

Mecacci, L., Sechi, E., & Levi, G. (1983). Abnormalities of visual evoked potentials by checkerboards in children with specific reading disability. *Brain and Cognition, 2,* 135–143.

Miller, L. K., & Turner, S. (1973). Development of hemifield differences in word recognition. *Journal of Educational Psychology, 65,* 172–176.

Molfese, D. L., Freeman, R. B., & Palmero, D. S. (1975). The ontogeny of brain lateralization for speech and nonspeech stimuli. *Brain and Language, 2,* 356–368.

Nagafuchi, M. (1970). Development of dichotic and monaural hearing abilities in young children. *Acta Otolaryngologica, 69,* 409–414.

Naylor, H. (1980). Reading disability and lateral asymmetry: An information processing analysis. *Psychological Bulletin, 87,* 531–545.

Newcombe, N., & Bandura, M. M. (1983). Effect of age at puberty on spatial ability in girls: A question of mechanism. *Developmental Psychology, 19,* 215–224.

Nottebohm. F. (1971). Neural lateralization of vocal control in a passerine bird. I. Song. *Journal of Experimental Zoology, 177,* 229–262.

Obrzut, J. E., Boliek, C. A., Bryden, M. P., & Nicholson, J. A. (1994). Age and sex-related differences in left and right hemisphere processing by learning disabled children. *Neuropsychology, 8,* 75–82.

Obrzut, J. E., Hynd, G. W., Obrzut, A., & Pirozzolo, F. J. (1981). Effect of directed attention on cerebral asymmetries in normal and learning-disabled children. *Developmental Psychology, 17, 118–125.*

Obrzut, J. E., Hynd, G. W., & Zellner, R. D. (1983). Attentional deficit in learning disabled children: Evidence from visual half-field asymmetries. *Brain and Cognition, 2,* 89–101.

Ojemann, G. A. (1977). Asymmetric function of the thalamus. *Annals of the New York Academy of Sciences, 299,* 380–396.

Orton, S. T. (1937). *Reading, writing and speech problems in children.* London: Chapman & Hall.

Palmer, R. D. (1964). Development of a differentiated handedness. *Psychological Bulletin, 62,* 257–272.

Pande, B. S., & Singh, I. (1971). One-sided dominance in the upper limbs of human fetuses as evidenced by asymmetry in muscle and bone weight. *Journal of Anatomy, 109,* 457–459.

Parlow, S. E., & Kinsbourne, M. (1981). Handwriting posture and manual motor asymmetries in sinistrals. *Neuropsychologia, 19,* 687–696.

Parlow, S. E., Kinsbourne, M., & Spencer, J. (1996). Cerebral laterality in severely mentally retarded adults. *Developmental Neuropsychology,* 299–312.

Penfield, W., & Roberts, L. (1959). *Speech and brain mechanisms.* Princeton, NJ: Princeton University Press.

Piazza, D. M. (1977). Cerebral lateralization in young children as measured by dichotic listening and finger tapping tasks. *Neuropsychologia, 15,* 417–425.

Pinsky, S. D., & McAdam, D. W. (1980). Electroencephalographic and dichotic indices of cerebral laterality in stutterers. *Brain and Language, 11,* 374–397.

Pipe, M. E. (1983). Dichotic listening performance following auditory discrimination training in Down's syndrome and developmentally retarded children. *Cortex, 19,* 481–491.

Porter, R. J., Jr., & Berlin, C. I. (1975). On interpreting developmental changes in the dichotic right-ear advantage. *Brain and Language, 2,* 186–200.

Provine, R. R., & Westerman, J. A. (1979). Crossing the midline: Limits of early eye–hand behavior. *Child Development, 50,* 437–441.

Ramsey, D. S. (1980). Beginnings of bimanual handedness and speech in infants. *Infant Behavior and Development, 3,* 67–77.

Ramsey, D. S. (1984). Onset of unimanual handedness in infants. *Infant Behavior and Development, 3,* 377–385.

Rankin, J. M., Aram, D. M., & Horwitz, S. J. (1981). Language ability in right and left hemiplegic children. *Brain and Language, 14,* 292–306.

Reinvang, I., Bakke, S. J., Hugdahl, K., Karesen, N. R., & Sundet, K., (1994). Dichotic listening performance in relation to callosal area on the MRI scan. *Neuropsychology, 8,* 445–450.

Reynolds, D. M. Q., & Jeeves, M. A. (1978). A developmental study of hemisphere specialization for alphabetical stimuli. *Cortex, 14,* 259–267.

Ringo, J. L., Doty, R. W., Demeter, S., & Simard, P. Y. (1994). Time is of the essence: A conjecture that hemispheric specialization arises from intrahemispheric conduction delay. *Cerebral Cortex, 4,* 331–343.

Rose, S. (1984). Developmental changes in hemispheric specialization for tactual processing in very young children: Evidence from cross-modal transfer. *Developmental Psychology, 20,* 568–574.

Ross, E. D., & Mesulam, M. M. (1979). Dominant language functions of the right hemisphere? Prosody and emotional gesturing. *Archives of Neurology, 36,* 144–148.

Rosen, G. D., Sherman, G. F. & Galaburda, A. M. (1989). Interhemispheric connection differ between symmetrical and asymmetrical brain regions. *Neuroscience, 33,* 525–533.

Rutter, M., Bartak, L., & Newman, S. (1971). Autism: A central disorder of cognition and language? In M. Rutter (Ed.), *Infantile autism: Concepts, characteristics and treatment.* London: Churchill.

Satz, P. (1972). Pathological lefthandedness: An explanatory model. *Cortex, 8,* 121–135.

Satz, P. (1976). Cerebral dominance and reading disability: An old problem revisited. In R. M. Knights & D. J. Bakker (Eds.), *The neuropsychology of learning disorders.* Baltimore: University Park Press.

Satz, P., Orsini, D. L., Saslow, E., & Henry, R. (1985). The pathological left-handedness syndrome. *Brain and Cognition, 4,* 27–46.

Satz, P., Strauss, E., & Whitaker, H. (1990). The ontogeny of hemispheric specialization: Some old hypotheses revisited. *Brain and Language, 38,* 596–614.

Saxby, L., & Bryden, M. P. (1984). Left-ear superiority in children for processing of auditory emotional material. *Developmental Psychology, 20,* 72–80.

Schwartz, G. E., Davidson, R. J., & Maer, F. (1975). Right hemisphere lateralization for emotion in the human brain: Interactions with cognition. *Science, 190,* 286–288.

Searleman, A. (1977). A review of right hemisphere linguistic capabilities. *Psychological Bulletin, 84,* 503–508.

Searleman, A. (1983). Language capabilities of the right hemisphere. In A. W. Young (Ed.), *Functions of the right cerebral hemisphere.* New York: Academic Press.

Searleman, A., Porac, C., & Coren, S. (1982). The relationship between birth stress and writing hand posture. *Brain and Cognition, 1,* 158–164.

Segalowitz, S. J., & Berge, B. E. (1995). Functional asymmetries in infancy and early childhood: A review of electrophysiologic studies and their implication. In R. J. Davidson & K. Hugdahl (Eds.), *Brain asymmetry* (pp. 579–616). Cambridge, MA: MIT Press.

Segalowitz, S. J., & Chapman, J. S. (1980). Cerebral asymmetry for speech in neonate: A behavioral measure. *Brain and Language, 9,* 281–288.

Seth, G. (1973). Eye–hand coordination and "handedness": A development study of visuomotor behaviour in infants. *British Journal of Educational Psychology, 43,* 35–49.

Shankweiler, D. P., & Studdert-Kennedy, M. A. (1967). A continuum of lateralization for speech perception? *Brain and Language, 2,* 212–225.

Shucard, J. L., Shucard, D. W., Cummins, K. R., & Campos, J. J. (1981). Auditory evoked potentials and sex-related differences in brain development. *Brain and Language, 13,* 91–102.

Sidtis, J. J., Sadler, A. E., & Nass, R. D. (1987). Dichotic complex pitch and speech discrimination in 7 to 12 year old children. *Developmental Neuropsychology, 3,* 227–238.

Silva, D., & Satz, P. (1984). Pathological left-handedness and ambiguous handedness: A new explanatory model. *Neuropsychologia, 22,* 511–515.

Soper, H. V., Satz, P., Orsini, D. L., Van Gorp, W. G., & Gireer, M. F. (1987). Handedness distribution within severe to profound mental retardation. *American Journal of Mental Deficiency, 92,* 94–102.

Stiles-Davis, J., Sugarman, S., & Nass, R. (1985). The development of spatial and class relations in four young children with right hemisphere damage: Evidence for an early spatial constructive deficit. *Brain and Cognition, 4,* 388–412.

Tannock, R., Kershner, J. R., & Oliver, J. (1984). Do individuals with Down's syndrome possess right hemisphere language dominance? *Cortex, 20,* 221–223.

Teng, E. L., Lee, P., Yang, K., & Chang, P. C. (1976). Genetic, cultural and neuropathological factors in relation to laterality. In D. O. Walton, L. Rogers, & J. H. Finzi-Fried (Eds.), *Conference on human brain function: Brain information service.* Los Angeles: BRC Publication, University of California.

Teuber, H.-L., & Rudel, R. G. (1962). Behavior after cerebral lesions in children and adults. *Developmental Medicine and Child Neurology, 4,* 3–20.

Tomlinson-Keasey, C., Kelly, R., & Burton, J. (1979). Hemispheric changes in information processing during development. *Developmental Psychology, 14,* 214–223.

Travis. L. E. (1927). Studies in stuttering. *Archives of Neurology and Psychiatry, 18,* 671–690, 998–1014.

Treisman A. M., & Geffen, G. (1968). Selective attention and cerebral dominance in perceiving and responding to speech messages. *Quarterly Journal of Experimental Psychology, 20,* 139–150.

Tsai, L. Y. (1982). Handedness in autistic children and their families. *Journal of Autism and Developmental Disorders, 12,* 421–423.

Turkewitz, G. (1977). The development of lateral differentiation in the human infant. *Annals of the New York Academy of Sciences, 299,* 309–317.

Turkewitz, G., & Ross-Kossak, P. (1984). Multiple modes of right hemisphere information processing: Age and sex differences in facial recognition. *Developmental Psychology, 20,* 95–103.

Vargha-Khadem, F., & Corballis, M. C. (1979). Cerebral asymmetry in infants. *Brain and Language, 8,* 1–9.

Vargha-Khadem, F., O'Gorman, A. M., & Watters, G. V. (1985). Aphasia and handedness in relation to hemispheric side, age at injury and severity of cerebral lesion during childhood. *Brain, 8*(3), 677–696.

Wada, J. A., Clark, R., & Hamm, A. (1975). Cerebral hemispheric asymmetry in humans. *Archives of Neurology, 32,* 239–246.

White, N., & Kinsbourne, M. (1980). Does speech output control lateralization over time? Evidence from verbal–manual time sharing tasks. *Brain and Language, 10,* 215–233.

Witelson, S. F. (1974). Hemispheric specialization for linguistic and nonlinguistic tactual perception using a dichotomous stimulation technique. *Cortex, 10,* 3–17.

Witelson, S. F. (1976). Sex and the single hemisphere: Right hemisphere specialization for spatial processing. *Science, 193,* 425–427.

Witelson, S. F., & Kigar, D. L. (1988). Asymmetry in brain function follows asymmetry in anatomical form: Gross, microscopic, postmortem and imaging studies. In F. Boller & J. Grafman (Eds.), *Handbook of neuropsychology* (Vol. I, pp. 114–142). Amsterdam: Elsevier.

Witelson, S. F., & Pallie, W. (1973). Left hemisphere specialization for language in the newborn. *Brain, 96,* 641–646.

Wood, F., Stump, D., McKeehan, A., Sheldon, S., & Proctor, J. (1980). Patterns of regional cerebral blood flow during attempted reading aloud by stutterers both on and off haloperidol medication: Evidence for inadequate left frontal activation during stuttering. *Brain and Language, 9,* 141–144.

Woods, B. T., & Teuber, H. L. (1978). Changing patterns of childhood aphasia. *Annals of Neurology, 32,* 239–246.

Yazgan, M. Y., Wexler, B. E., Kinsbourne, M., Peterson, B., & Leckman, J. F. (1995). Functional significance of individual variations in callosal area. *Neuropsychologia, 33,* 769–779.

Yeni-Komshian, G. H., & Benson, D. A. (1976). Anatomical study of cerebral asymmetry in the temporal lobe of humans, chimpanzees and rhesus monkeys. *Science, 192,* 387–389.

Young, A. W., & Bion, P. J. (1980). Absence of any developmental trend in right hemisphere superiority for face recognition. *Cortex, 16,* 113–221.

Young, A. W., & Ellis, H. D. (1976). An experimental investigation of developmental differences in ability to recognize faces presented to the left and right cerebral hemispheres. *Neuropsychologia, 14,* 495–498.

Young, G., & Gagnon, M. (1990). Neonatal laterality, birth stress, familial sinistrality, and left-brain inhibition. *Developmental Neuropsychology, 6,* 127–150.

Young, J. Z. (1962). Why do we have two brains? In V. B. Mountcastle (Ed.), *Interhemispheric relations and cerebral dominance.* Baltimore: Johns-Hopkins Press.

Zurif, E. B., & Carson, G. (1970). Dyslexia in relation to cerebral dominance and temporal analysis. *Neuropsychologia, 8,* 351–361.

6

Neuropsychology of Child Psychopathology

MICHAEL G. TRAMONTANA AND STEPHEN R. HOOPER

Introduction

In our chapter in the earlier edition of the *Handbook* (Tramontana & Hooper, 1989), we began with a series of questions. We asked: What is the relationship between brain dysfunction and psychopathology in childhood? Does it depend on the extent or type of brain dysfunction? What about the age or other attributes of the child at the time of onset? How might environmental factors potentiate the child's risk? Are certain forms of psychopathology more likely to arise than others? Does the form of psychopathology change over time? There were other questions raised, namely: Is brain dysfunction more likely in certain psychiatric disorders or behavioral syndromes than others? Does its presence explain the form of psychopathology manifested? How important is it relative to other factors contributing to the child's disturbance?

These questions remain pertinent in underscoring the complexity of the topic. Clearly there are mental, emotional, and behavioral sequelae for the child who has sustained brain damage or who shows an anomalous course of brain development. In many instances, such problems may persist and significantly impede the child's overall adjustment.

What is not so clear is how often this occurs, and the precise factors that influence it.

Conversely, there is little disagreement that there are multiple etiologies for psychopathology in childhood and that, in some cases, brain dysfunction can play an important contributing role. How often this is the case, however, is far from clear. Estimates of prevalence have varied greatly according to the methods of analysis and samples selected for study.

Once again the foregoing should help to define the scope of this chapter. We will begin with an examination of key conceptual issues, including the role and prevalence of brain dysfunction in child psychopathology. An updated summary of findings pertaining to selected areas of child psychopathology will be discussed and critically evaluated. Definitive conclusions still are not possible, but exciting developments continue to unfold. Lastly, we will highlight what we consider to be some of the major theoretical and methodological issues that will relate to further research and practice advances in this area.

Conceptual Issues

Psychiatric Sequelae of Childhood Brain Dysfunction

The presence of brain dysfunction in childhood appears to be associated with a greater risk for the development of a psychiatric disorder, far more so than with other physical handicaps (Brown,

MICHAEL G. TRAMONTANA • Division of Child and Adolescent Psychiatry, Vanderbilt University, Nashville, Tennessee 37212-3133. STEPHEN R. HOOPER • Department of Psychiatry and the Clinical Center for the Study of Development and Learning, University of North Carolina, Chapel Hill, North Carolina 27599.

Chadwick, Shaffer, Rutter, & Traub, 1981; Rutter, Graham, & Yule, 1970; Seidel, Chadwick, & Rutter, 1975; Shaffer, 1978). Moreover, the effects appear to persist and impede the child's long-range adjustment in many important respects (Breslau & Marshall, 1985; Milman, 1979; Shaffer *et al.*, 1985).

One of the best investigations on this topic comes from the well-known Isle of Wight epidemiological studies of school-aged children by Rutter and his colleagues (Rutter *et al.*, 1970). Using multiple assessment procedures, and controlling for rater bias, Rutter *et al.* found that about 6 to 7% of the general population of children studied had a psychiatric disorder consisting of some persistent emotional, behavioral, or social disability. The rate was nearly twice that (11.5%) for children having chronic handicapping physical conditions not involving the brain. This group consisted of children with disorders such as asthma, diabetes, heart disease, or orthopedic deformities, as well as diseases of the spinal cord or peripheral nervous system. In contrast, the rate of psychiatric disorder was over five times higher (34.3%) in their neuroepileptic group consisting of all children ranging from 5 to 14 years of age with cerebral palsy, epilepsy, or some other frank neurological disorder above the brain stem. Even when eliminating all cases who had an IQ of 85 or less (as low IQ, itself, was found to be associated with an increased risk for psychiatric disorder), the rate of psychiatric disorder was still twice as high in the neuroepileptic group than in the "other physical handicap" group.

Among children in the neuroepileptic group, psychiatric disorders were more likely in cases with seizures, more severe or widespread brain impairment, lower IQ, and other functional handicaps (e.g., reading deficits). An exception was in the case of children with extremely incapacitating conditions. For them the rate of psychiatric disorder was actually *less*, suggesting that protective factors may be operating when dealing with a profound level of disability.

In a further study, Seidel *et al.* (1975) were better able to control for the possibility that overt stigmata, such as crippling, may have been associated with the higher rate of psychiatric disorder that Rutter *et al.* found in their neuroepileptic group (neither obvious crippling nor other overt stigma was common in their "other physical handicap" group). Here, they compared two groups of children with visibly crippling conditions who were alike in all respects except for the presence of brain damage. All children ranged from 5 to 15 years of age and had

an IQ of 70 or higher. The two groups were matched in terms of age, sex, psychosocial factors, as well as the degree of physical disability. Again, based on both teachers' questionnaire responses and psychiatric ratings, the rate of disorder was about twice as high for children with cerebral disorders (mostly cerebral palsy) than for the group with noncerebral or peripheral conditions (including muscular dystrophy, polio, or spina bifida).

Clearly, the studies by Rutter *et al.* (1970) and Seidel *et al.* (1975) provided a strong case that an increased risk for psychiatric disorder was associated with the presence of brain damage in childhood. Neither study, however, demonstrated a causal relationship. Although the neurological conditions of the brain-damaged groups typically had an early onset that probably preceded the appearance of any psychiatric disorder, one still could argue that the relationship was merely coincidental. That is, some common vulnerability (whether it be genetic, congenital, or environmental), which may have predisposed a child to cerebral damage, also may have led independently to psychiatric or behavioral disturbance. A more convincing case for the existence of a causal relationship would come from demonstrating that previously normal children with *acquired* brain injuries are more likely to develop subsequent psychiatric disorders.

Children suffering from accidental head injury represent an excellent choice for examining this question. It must be recognized, however, that they do not constitute a random sample of the general population. These children, especially those suffering from mild as opposed to severe injuries, often show *preexisting* problems with impulsivity, aggression, and attention-seeking behavior that make them more susceptible to accidental injury (Klonoff, 1971). The families of these children, as a group, also differ from the general population in that they show more parental illness and mental disorder, more social disadvantages, and less adequate supervision of the child's play activities. Thus, the absence of adequate controls in many studies reporting intellectual impairment and behavioral disturbance following head injury makes it impossible to determine whether the psychological sequelae stem directly from cerebral damage rather than preexisting difficulties (Rutter, Chadwick, & Shaffer, 1983).

One of the better-controlled examinations of this topic comes from the prospective studies of head-injured children by Rutter and his colleagues (Brown *et al.*, 1981; Chadwick, Rutter, Brown, Shaffer, & Traub, 1981; Chadwick, Rutter, Shaffer, &

Shrout, 1981; Rutter, Chadwick, Shaffer, & Brown, 1980). Children ranging from 5 to 14 years of age who had experienced closed head injuries of sufficient severity to result in a posttraumatic amnesia (PTA) of 7 days or more were compared with a group of children having less severe head injuries (i.e., those with a PTA of less than 7 days but at least 1 hour). In addition, these groups were compared with a matched control group of hospital-treated children also suffering severe accidents, but with orthopedic rather than cranial injuries. There were 28 children in each group. All children were studied prospectively at 4 months, 1 year, and $2\frac{1}{2}$ years after their injuries. An important feature of this study was the care taken to determine the children's behavior before their accidents. This was done in an unbiased fashion by interviewing parents immediately after their child's injury, but *before* the child's postinjury psychiatric condition could have been known.

The children with milder head injuries had a higher rate of preinjury behavior problems than the other groups. The rate did not change significantly postinjury (roughly 10 to 18%). By contrast, children with severe head injuries did not differ from controls in their preinjury behavior, but they showed more than double the rate of psychiatric disorder at 4 months and at each subsequent follow-up period. This was true even when children with psychiatric disorders prior to their accidents were eliminated from the study, thereby focusing specifically on the comparative rate of new psychiatric disorders arising over the course of the follow-up period. Head-injured children tended to show greater impairment on timed visual–spatial and visual–motor tests than on verbal tests, but, apart from this, no pattern of cognitive deficit specific to head injury was identified. Likewise, the types of psychiatric disorder among the head-injured children were very similar to those found in controls. The only exception to this was in the case of grossly disinhibited social behavior, which was present only in children with very severe head injuries, and may have been linked directly to frontal lobe dysfunction.

Children with head injuries showed an increased risk for psychiatric disorder regardless of the age, sex, or social class of the child—factors that ordinarily show a striking mediating effect in the general population. Clearly, the risk was greater among those children with histories of preaccident behavior disorders as well as those experiencing various psychosocial adversities within their homes, but the effects were additive rather than interactive. Thus, although psychiatric disorders in childhood have a multifactorial etiology, the evidence from this series of studies indicated that brain injury can play an independent role.

An especially interesting finding was that Brown *et al.* observed a weaker and less consistent dose–response relationship between severity of head injury and behavior changes than was found in the case of intellectual impairment arising subsequent to injury. Also, the relationship between intellectual impairment and behavior disorder was weak, and was limited mainly to the early postinjury period. This raised the possibility that modifying factors, such as secondary family reactions, may play a critical role in the development of persistent behavior problems.

In another well-controlled study, Fletcher, Ewing-Cobbs, Miner, Levin, and Eisenberg (1990) compared 45 children, ages 3 to 15, with mild, moderate, and severe head injuries on standardized measures of behavioral adjustment. Behavior ratings were obtained at the time of injury (based on preinjury features) and at 6 and 12 months postinjury. Cases with preexisting neurological disorder, developmental disabilities, or behavioral disturbance were excluded. Children with severe head injuries significantly declined and differed from the other two groups over the 12-month follow-up on ratings of their adaptive behavior. They also were rated as having more school problems and as engaging in fewer social activities. Children with mild and moderate injuries did not differ from each other nor from average normative levels. No distinctive type of behavior disorder was found to be associated with head injury. Also, as was observed in the Brown *et al.* study, behavioral and cognitive outcome measures were related more strongly to indices of initial injury severity than to one another—again suggesting some dissociation or independence in the mechanisms for behavioral and cognitive outcomes.

Each of the preceding studies dealt with children having known or documented brain damage. One may ask whether a similar relationship exists between psychiatric disorder and so-called "soft" neurological signs or minimal brain dysfunction (MBD) in childhood. This has been a subject of much debate, as some investigators have regarded sensory or motor phenomena such as mirror movements, dysdiadochokinesis, dysgraphesthesia, and choreic or athetoid movements to be of little diagnostic value when elicited from patients not having a discrete neurological disorder (e.g., Ingram, 1973). Others (e.g., Rutter *et al.,* 1970) have argued that it is important to differentiate among different types of signs that are labeled as "soft." Some are considered as soft because: (1) they run a developmental course in which the signs may subside as the child grows older; (2) they are rather prevalent among otherwise normal children (with estimates ranging from 8 to 14%); and (3) they have no clear locus of origin and their neuropathological significance is obscure (Shaffer, 1978). They are not necessarily unreliable, however, and may show consistency over time (Shapiro, Burkes, Petti, & Ranz, 1978). Other signs, such as minor reflex or tone asymmetries, would tend to be less reliable because they are more difficult to detect.

Overall, the research on neurological soft signs has shown that: (1) there is a relationship with age, IQ, and sex (with soft signs occurring more frequently among boys), (2) they are more prevalent among children with psychiatric disorders and learning disabilities, (3) they are related to indices of emotional immaturity and dependency in childhood, and (4) the relationship with hyperactivity, aggression, and antisocial conduct is less clear, although soft signs are commonly seen among children who are described as impulsive and distractible (Shaffer, 1978; Shaffer, O'Connor, Shafer, & Prupis, 1983).

In a well-controlled prospective study, Shaffer and his colleagues (Shaffer et al., 1985) examined the comparative outcomes in adolescence of children with early soft neurological signs. Children with ($n = 83$) and without ($n = 79$) documented soft signs at age 7 received a careful follow-up assessment at age 17. Compared with controls, adolescents with early soft signs had lower IQs and were more likely to have a psychiatric disorder with symptoms of anxiety, withdrawal, and depression. These findings mainly pertained to boys, but all of the girls in this study with an anxiety–withdrawal diagnosis in adolescence showed early soft signs. The relationship was independent of IQ and, when taken together with the presence of anxious–dependent behavior at age 7, the presence of early soft signs was strongly predictive of persistent problems with anxiety and withdrawal. However, no relationship was found with attention deficit disorder or conduct disorder.

This was somewhat different than the pattern that Rutter et al. (1970) found in the Isle of Wight study. Children with frank brain damage showed a heterogeneous range of psychiatric disorders without specific features. Hyperactivity and psychosis were more prevalent in their neuroepileptic group, but these appeared to be related more specifically to the presence of mental retardation. However, besides Shaffer et al. (1985), several other studies have found an association between brain dysfunction and the type of behavior problems manifested, although the exact findings have varied according to factors such as age and chronicity.

In a 5-year follow-up of children and adolescents with physical disabilities secondary to brain damage, Breslau and Marshall (1985) found that problems with social isolation rather than aggression were more likely to persist. Dorman (1982) found that the relationship between neuropsychological impairment and the type of behavior problems observed varied as a function of age in a group of boys with school problems and no known neurological disorder. Whereas poor neuropsychological performance was associated with externalizing behavior problems in younger (7 to 8) boys, it was associated with internalizing symptoms in the older (9 to 14) subjects. It may be that internalizing rather than externalizing symptoms are more distinctively tied to brain dysfunction as the child grows older and encounters repeated failure and loss in self-esteem. The relationship eventually may become blurred as other factors enter and play a more important determining role in perpetuating the youngster's poor adjustment. Moreover, this process may be accelerated in cases with early histories of more severe disorder. This was suggested in a study by Tramontana, Hooper, and Nardolillo (1988) in which the presence of neuropsychological deficits was found to be associated with more extensive behavior problems among psychiatrically hospitalized boys, regardless of factors such as IQ and SES. However, the relationship mainly applied to younger (8 to 11) as opposed to older (12 to 16) subjects, and specifically involved internalizing rather than externalizing behavior problems. We will discuss more fully the question of the relationship between brain dysfunction and the form of psychopathology manifested.

Taken together, the studies reviewed in this section provide strong evidence that brain dysfunction in childhood is associated with an increased vulnerability for psychiatric disorder. The relationship appears to hold both for children with frank brain damage as well as those with so-called soft neurological signs. The risk is greater for children with more severe neurological disorders (with the possible exception of those with extreme impairment), especially when accompanied by low IQ and other neuropsychological deficits. It also is compounded by factors such as psychosocial adversity and any preexisting tendencies toward behavioral or emotional disturbance. The relationship is not trivial, as the effects appear to persist and influence long-range outcomes (Breslau & Marshall, 1985; Milman, 1979; Shaffer *et al.,* 1985). This certainly underscores the importance of accurate detection of the functional deficits and behavioral liabilities in the brain-impaired child as a first step in limiting the risk for the later development or progression of a psychiatric disorder (Tramontana, 1983).

Prevalence of Brain Dysfunction among Children with Psychiatric Disorders

Although brain dysfunction can play a significant contributing role in the development of child psychopathology, it is unclear just how often this occurs. Estimates of prevalence have varied greatly both as a function of the methods and criteria used in identifying brain dysfunction, and in terms of differences in the subject samples selected for study. For example, the prevalence would appear to be rather low if one simply used the presence of positive findings on a routine neurological examination as the basis of establishing neurological involvement. However, such an approach would likely be associated with an underestimation of prevalence because normal neurological examinations are common even among children with documented histories of head injury, encephalitis, or epilepsy (Rutter, 1977).

The findings from the few studies that have incorporated noninvasive neurodiagnostic methods such as computed tomography (CT) have been mixed. Much of the research examined children with autism or other major developmental handicaps for whom enlarged ventricles and other structural deficits have been found in subgroups of the subjects examined (Campbell *et al.,* 1982; Caparulo *et al.,* 1981; Damasio, Maurer, Damasio, & Chui, 1980; Rosenbloom *et al.,* 1984). Reiss *et al.* (1983) likewise found ventricular enlargement in a controlled comparison of CT scans for a mixed group of child psychiatric patients. The results were of questionable generalizability, however, because their subjects also tended to be among the more impaired with respect to psychiatric and developmental status, with about half of the group having a confirmed neurological disorder and a third showing mild mental retardation.

In another study, CT scans were compared across four subgroups of subjects with childhood disorders (infantile autism, attention deficit disorder, Tourette's syndrome, and language disorder) and a control group of medical patients without documented neurological disorder (Harcherik *et al.,* 1985). No differences were found among the groups with respect to ventricular volume, right–left ventricular ratios, asymmetries, or brain density. The study was very well done from a technical standpoint, but the interpretation of its results is complicated by several factors. The groups were not matched in age, and the neurological status and level of functioning of subjects (including controls) were poorly specified. The interested reader should refer to a review by Kuperman, Gaffney, Hamdan-Allen, Preston, and Venkatesh (1990), which provides an overview of the findings obtained in various child psychiatric samples using other brain imaging techniques, including magnetic resonance imaging (MRI) and positron emission tomography (PET).

Prevalence rates using neuropsychological criteria have tended to be comparatively high. For example, Tramontana, Sherrets, and Golden (1980) found a high rate of neuropsychological abnormality in a mixed sample of child and adolescent psychiatric patients without known brain damage. The subjects consisted of 20 hospitalized cases ranging from 9 to 15 years of age who had neither a history of brain damage nor positive findings on a routine neurological examination. From a neuropsychological standpoint, these were "nonreferred" cases for whom brain dysfunction was not suspected. Nonetheless, about 60% of the subjects showed at least mild impairment (with 25% showing more definite impairment) according to the normative rules established by Selz and Reitan (1979) on the Halstead–Reitan Neuropsychological Battery (HRNB). Impaired performance on the HRNB was associated with lower IQ and was more prevalent among cases whose psychiatric disorders were of at least 2 years' duration and who had a lag of at least 2 years in academic achievement.

One may question the meaning of the neuropsychological abnormalities found in the Tramontana *et al.* study, especially as to whether they indeed reflected underlying brain anomalies that were missed in a routine neurological examination or review of history. This was explored in a subsequent study with a similar sample of subjects in which neuropsychological results were compared with various quantified indices of brain structure examined through CT (Tramontana & Sherrets, 1985). Psychiatric cases without suspected brain damage again were found to show a high rate of neuropsychological abnormality (at least 50%) when examined on either the HRNB or the Children's Revision of the Luria–Nebraska Neuropsychological Battery (LNNB-C; Golden, 1981). Impaired performance was more likely among boys, younger subjects, and those with more chronic psychiatric histories. Interestingly, impaired performance was not associated significantly with IQ. The overall results of the two test batteries correlated quite highly, but it was the LNNB-C that corresponded more closely with CT scan results. Specifically, impairment on the LNNB-C was associated with *smaller* ventricular size and *less* density variability, suggesting the possibility of anomalous brain maturation. It also was associated with lesser regional densities, especially within the right cerebral hemisphere.

The absence of control subjects in the foregoing study did not permit one to conclude that the CT results, although associated with neuropsychological abnormality, were themselves necessarily abnormal according to any established normative standards. Nonetheless, the findings were noteworthy in that the presence of neuropsychological deficits among the psychiatric cases did correspond to variations in brain structure, and were not merely the product of nonneurological factors. This was a remarkable finding, especially in view of the restricted range of the sample because of the exclusion of cases having documented neurological involvement.

Taken together, the studies reviewed in this section indicate that the question of prevalence is inextricably tied to the methods and criteria used in assessing brain dysfunction. Children with cerebral palsy, epilepsy, and other obvious neurological conditions (as evidenced on routine neurological examination) probably comprise less than 5% of the total population of children with psychiatric disorders (Rutter, 1977). The rate is uncertain, but obviously would be higher if one were to include children with clumsiness, language impairment, mental retardation, and learning disabilities (Gualtieri, Koriath, Van Bourgondieu, & Saleeby, 1983; Rutter *et al.,* 1970) for whom there is at least the *suspicion* of underlying brain damage. The rate is higher still if one further includes children for whom brain damage is not suspected, but who nonetheless may show various neuropsychological deficits when they are comprehensively assessed. Although these deficits may have a relationship with underlying structural factors (see Tramontana & Sherrets, 1985), they cannot be interpreted as reflecting brain damage *per se.* Rather, they should be viewed as functional impediments, some of which may be tied to abnormalities

in brain structure or maturation, which in any event may play a role in the development of child psychiatric disorders. As was noted before, the presence of neuropsychological deficits has been found to be associated with more extensive behavior problems among younger boys, regardless of factors such as IQ, SES, and whether the deficits can be linked specifically with a history of brain injury (see Tramontana *et al.,* 1988). Neuropsychological deficits are important in their own right, as they appear to comprise an important index of increased psychiatric risk.

Relationship to Manifest Psychopathology

A number of mechanisms have been suggested whereby brain dysfunction may lead to psychopathology, although evidence as to their relative contribution is uncertain (Rutter, 1977, 1983). These include: (1) behavioral disruption that arises directly from abnormal brain activity; (2) a heightened exposure to failure, frustration, and social stigma related to associated disabilities; (3) the possible effects of brain damage on subsequent temperament and personality development; (4) adverse family reactions ranging from overprotection to scapegoating; (5) the child's own reaction to being handicapped and its effects on his or her actual capacity to cope and compete; and (6) possible adverse effects from treatments themselves (e.g., recurrent hospitalization) that may restrict normal activities and socialization. Thus, the effects may be direct or indirect. They also may be conceptualized as transactional and dynamic.

Direct effects, for example, would be seen in the case of frontal lobe damage resulting in pronounced impulsivity and social disinhibition. Other examples include organically induced psychosis or episodic aggressiveness that may arise from certain temporal lobe disorders. In other cases, however, brain dysfunction may play more of an *indirect* etiological role, one that essentially sets the stage for other factors to come into play that, themselves, act to produce an emotional or behavioral disturbance and perhaps further aggravate existing functional difficulties (Tramontana, 1983).

For example, brain dysfunction may give rise to learning disabilities that, in turn, render the child more likely to encounter frustration and failure on entry into school. This may lead to disruptive behavior problems consisting of inattention, anger, and defiance as an eventual (albeit indirect) outcome. There also may be a compounded difficulty in those areas of performance that have become anxiety-laden and aversive. Parents and teachers may come to view the child as lazy, apathetic, or otherwise difficult, and thereby generate expectations that would only serve to perpetuate the existing problems. The latter represents a *transactional* effect, namely, the differential reinforcement elicited from significant others by the brain-impaired child and his or her particular deficits. Lastly, the effects of behavior are *dynamic* rather than static. Just as the primary symptoms of brain dysfunction may change over time, so too they may vary in terms of their developmental significance and the reactions that they elicit from others, including the child. The pattern of behavioral disturbance itself may vary so that, for example, instead of hypersensitivity, defiance, and misconduct, the child later may show apathy, withdrawal, and resignation.

Besides the issue of how brain dysfunction may lead to psychopathology in childhood, there also is the question of what form manifest symptoms may take. Earlier thinking (e.g., Bakwin & Bakwin, 1966; Wender, 1971) suggested that the behavioral manifestations of cerebral dysfunction, whatever the cause, were uniform and comprised a rather distinctive behavioral syndrome consisting of symptoms such as hyperactivity, inattention, and impulsivity. However, there is little evidence of such a behavioral stereotype for the brain-impaired child. Symptoms such as hyperactivity, inattention, and impulsivity do not distinguish children with either frank brain damage (Brown *et al.*, 1981; Rutter *et al.*, 1970) or soft neurological signs (Shaffer *et al.*, 1983, 1985). This is not to say that such symptoms are not common among brain-impaired children—they are, but they also are common features of psychiatric disorder in general, regardless of whether neurological abnormality is present (Rutter, 1977).

One may argue that the relationship between brain dysfunction and psychopathology in childhood is *nonspecific* (e.g., Boll & Barth, 1981). That is, the presence of brain dysfunction, regardless of its pattern or cause, may contribute nonspecifically to a lowered adaptive capacity and a greater likelihood of exposure to adverse experiences. In this view, brain dysfunction operates indirectly by creating the functional deficits that make successful adjustment more difficult for the child. Any of a variety of behavioral and emotional problems may result, with the distribution of specific symptoms being similar to what is seen generally among children with psychiatric disorders.

There is some support for this position. In the Isle of Wight study (Rutter *et al.*, 1970), children with brain damage showed a heterogeneous range of psychiatric disorders with no specific features. Except for cases falling at the extreme of incapacity, the risk was greater in children with more severe injuries, seizures, and lower IQ. Also, apart from the possible relationship between frontal lobe dysfunction and gross social disinhibition, Brown *et al.* (1981) found no psychiatric symptoms that were specific to children with closed head injuries. From a different perspective, Tramontana and Hooper (1987) found that groups of adolescents with either conduct disorder or major depression were virtually identical in their pattern of neuropsychological functioning. Thus, although these represented two very different types of psychopathology (each falling at opposite ends of a continuum of externalizing and internalizing symptoms, respectively), there were no distinctive neuropsychological features. Kusche, Cook, and Greenberg (1993) found executive function deficits to be related to child psychopathology, in general.

On the other hand, it was noted before that a history of soft neurological signs or the presence of neuropsychological impairment tended to be associated specifically with *internalizing* behavior problems consisting of symptoms such as anxiety, depression, and withdrawal (Shaffer *et al.*, 1985; Tramontana, Hooper, & Nardolillo, 1988). In addition to cognitive deficits, children with physical disabilities secondary to brain damage are likely to show persistent problems with social isolation, but problems with aggression are less likely to persist (see Breslau & Marshall, 1985). Also, results from a study of children with localized (penetrating) head injuries showed a significant association between the presence of depression and lesions specifically involving right frontal and left posterior cerebral regions; this was true regardless of the child's age, sex, and psychosocial factors (Rutter, 1983). No relationship was found between the site of injury and symptoms such as hyperactivity, inattention, aggression, or antisocial conduct. Thus, although we are not suggesting the existence of an alternative behavioral stereotype, it may be that internalizing rather than externalizing symptoms are more distinctively tied to brain dysfunction in childhood, perhaps especially in terms of longer-range outcomes. These may emerge as the child grows older, continues to struggle with chronic handicaps, and encounters repeated failure and loss of self-esteem.

A major stride in linking behavioral outcomes with a particular pattern of neurodevelopmental deficits has come from the work of Rourke and associates (Rourke, 1987, 1989; Rourke & Fuerst, 1991) on the syndrome of nonverbal learning disability (NLD). This is an empirically derived model that posits a relationship, not only between nonverbal deficits and certain academic learning difficulties (especially in mechanical arithmetic), but to limitations in a broader range of psychosocial and adaptive functioning. Because of difficulties processing nonverbal cues, children with NLD are seen as overrelying on rote verbal memory skills in their coping. The capacity to adapt to novel situations suffers, as does the ability to relate in a flexible and appropriate fashion. Significant deficits in social perception, judgment, and interactional skills are likely. These, in turn, may lead to a tendency toward social withdrawal or isolation—i.e., *internalizing* forms of psychopathology—as age increases. The NLD syndrome may arise from various causes, although a disruption of cerebral white matter is seen as necessarily involved. However, apart from its anatomical underpinnings, the model is significant for positing a relationship between a particular syndrome—defined neuropsychologically—and a *specific* pattern of child psychopathology.

Findings in Selected Categories of Child Psychopathology

This section provides a review of neurodiagnostic findings in major categories of child psychopathology. Included here are findings pertaining to autism, attention deficit/hyperactivity disorder, conduct disorders, depression, and anxiety disorders. With this we will return to the question of specificity, i.e., the extent to which different patterns of brain dysfunction are associated with specific types of psychopathology.

Autistic Disorder

Autism is a behavioral syndrome characterized by impairment in reciprocal social interactions, poor communication abilities, and a pronounced restriction of interests and activities. It is distinct from mental retardation, although the majority of children with autism carry a concurrent diagnosis of mental retardation (Folstein & Rutter, 1987). It is also distinct from a number of other childhood disorders, including schizophrenia (Green *et al.,* 1984) and developmental receptive language disorder (Lincoln, Courchesne, Kilman, Elmasian, & Allen, 1988).

A variety of etiological processes for autism have been proposed but none has gained widespread acceptance to date. However, regardless of the specific anomaly or etiology that is hypothesized, the general consensus is that some form of brain impairment is involved (Damasio & Maurer, 1978). Children with autism tend to have a significant prenatal or perinatal history and show a high rate of soft neurological signs (Jones & Prior, 1985). Garreau, Barthelemy, Sauvage, Leddet, and LeLord (1984) further noted that the presence of neurological impairment was associated with an earlier onset of autistic features. An increased incidence of seizure disorders has been found in this population, particularly with increasing age, with approximately 25 to 30% of children with autism developing seizures by adulthood (Deykin & MacMahon, 1979). However, this finding may be applicable mainly to cases with IQs below 70 (Bartak & Rutter, 1976).

A number of brain imaging studies have documented the presence of structural abnormalities in autism, although the precise findings have varied greatly. Some of these have identified left hemispheric and, in some cases, bilateral defects, particularly involving frontal and temporal regions (Gillberg & Svendsen, 1983; Maurer & Damasio, 1982). Findings suggestive of reversed asymmetry have been noted as well (e.g., Hier, LeMay, & Rosenberger, 1979). Other findings have included anomalies involving various subcortical structures, such as the basal ganglia (Jacobson, LeCouteur, Howlin, & Rutter, 1988), brain stem (Gaffney, Kuperman, Tsai, & Minchin, 1988), and cerebellar regions (Courchesne, Yeung-Courchesne, Press, Hesselink, & Jernigan, 1988; Gaffney, Tsai, Kuperman, & Minchin, 1987). There also have been studies in which structural abnormalities were identified but no specific localizable pattern emerged (e.g., Balottin *et al.,* 1989; Caparulo *et al.,* 1981). Some studies have found no structural abnormalities of any kind (e.g., Harcherik *et al.,* 1985; Prior, Tress, Hoffman, & Boldt, 1984).

Electroencephalographic (EEG) abnormalities also have been identified, with a prevalence of 40 to 50% found in one study of autistic children (Tsai, Tsai, & August, 1985). The abnormalities generally have been varied, although a pattern consisting of excessive slow-wave activity and decreased alpha bilaterally has been reported (Cantor, Thatcher, Hrybyk, & Kaye, 1986). Small (1975) suggested that, among autistic children, the presence of a normal EEG is associated with a higher IQ and a more favorable developmental course. Auditory and visual evoked potentials (EP) also have been observed to be impaired in autistics, with auditory processing capabilities evidently more impaired than visual processing (Courchesne, Lincoln, Kilman, & Galambos, 1985; DeMyer, Hingtgen, & Jackson, 1981). Moreover, Courchesne *et al.* (1985) have identified two endogenous components of EP, Nc and P3b, that appear to be associated with abnormal neural responses among autistics, responses involving attention and general cognition to important external information.

Other assorted neurobiological findings have been reported. Using positron emission tomography (PET), Rumsey, Rapoport, and Sceery (1985) found diffusely elevated glucose utilization but no clear focal abnormalities among autistic adults. Coleman, Romano, Lapham, and Simon (1985) found no consistent differences in a postmortem cell count of selected left hemispheric regions between an autistic adult and a control subject. However, Bauman and Kemper (1985) found anatomical differences involving the forebrain and cerebellum in a postmortem comparison of a 29-year-old autistic man and a normal 25-year-old. The investigators suggested that the cerebellar abnormalities were of unknown etiology but probably were acquired early in development, possibly at or before 30 weeks of gestation.

Numerous neuropsychological aspects of autism have been reported. These have included poor motor imitation abilities (Jones & Prior, 1985), disproportionate impairment in sequential processing abilities (Tanguay, 1984), poor recall of meaningless material (Ameli, Courchesne, Lincoln, Kaufman, & Grillon, 1988), and, as a group, IQ scores that are significantly lower than normals but comparatively higher than mentally retarded children (Kagan, 1981). The neurocognitive profiles of autistic children also can be rather varied when compared with children with mental retardation (Fein, Waterhouse, Lucci, & Snyder, 1985), although a pattern indicative of better visual–perceptual abilities than language abilities typically has been asserted (e.g., Lincoln *et al.,* 1988).

Many of the neuropsychological studies have been directed toward investigating the presence of lateralized deficits in autistic children. The findings have included a reversal of ear advantage for speech sounds (i.e., left ear rather than right) on dichotic listening tasks (Blackstock, 1978; James & Barry, 1983; Prior & Bradshaw, 1979); increased prevalence rates of left and mixed handedness of about 20 and 34%, respectively (Soper *et al.,* 1986); and performance profiles on neuropsychological test batteries suggestive of predominantly left hemispheric dysfunction (Applebaum, Egel, Koegel, & Imhoff, 1979; Dawson, 1983; Hoffman & Prior, 1982). In a study by Dawson, Finley, Phillips, and Galpert (1986), there was evidence of an atypical pattern of hemispheric specialization, with about 70% of the autistic children showing right hemispheric dominance for speech. However, the investigators noted that many of the autistic children exhibited bilateral rather than unilateral dysfunction, and they also speculated that their dysfunction might involve subcortical as well as cortical levels. This interpretation is consistent with the findings in some of the brain imaging studies reported above.

Regardless of the issue of lateralization, the presence of disturbed language abilities in autism is critical. Bartak, Rutter, and Cox (1975) postulated that a language disability constitutes a necessary condition for the development of this disorder. They observed that autistic children showed more deviant language development, a severe comprehension deficit, and deficits in the social usage of language. Moreover, the degree of language impairment appears to be strongly predictive of the child's prognosis (Wing, 1971). Although related to childhood language disorders, the communication deficits in autistic children are qualitatively different from those seen in developmental dysphasia or acquired aphasia (Arnold & Schwartz, 1983). Semantic, prosodic, and pragmatic aspects of language development (i.e., possible right hemispheric contributions) may be particularly deviant (Cohen, Caparulo, & Shaywitz, 1976; Ferrari, 1982; Prizant, 1982; Simon, 1975; Tager-Flusberg, 1981).

Overall, as we concluded in our earlier review (Tramontana & Hooper, 1989), the research on autism provides a variable picture with respect to neurobiological and neuropsychological features. With the exception of aberrations in language development and communication skills, there is little agreement as to the neurodevelopmental features that are necessarily characteristic of this disorder. Some children with autism show significant anomalies in brain structure, whereas others do not. The same is true with respect to their neurophysiological and neuropsychological presentation. Although some autistic children show evidence of lateralized dysfunction involving the left cerebral hemisphere, this by no means is a definitive characteristic of the syndrome (Fein, Humes, Kaplan, Lucci, & Waterhouse, 1984). However, although the precise mechanisms remain unclear, there probably is not another category of child psychopathology for which the evidence of a neurobiological foundation is more compelling than in the case of autism.

Attention Deficit/Hyperactivity Disorder (ADHD)

This is another syndrome in which an organic etiology is commonly assumed, although the precise mechanisms are far from clear. Earlier thinking linked ADHD and MBD because of the purported behavioral similarities between children with ADHD and those with documented brain damage (Strauss & Lehtinen, 1947). However, problems in documenting the presence of underlying brain dysfunction (e.g., Rutter, 1983; Taylor, 1983) led to a more descriptive approach in conceptualizing the disorder. Children with ADHD have been characterized as showing inattention, impulsivity, and overactivity (Douglas, 1980, 1983); a deficit in self-directed instruction (Kendall & Broswell, 1985); poor self-regulation of arousal, particularly in meeting environmental demands (Douglas, 1983); and deficiencies in rule-governed behavior (Barkley, 1981a,b).

There have been numerous debates over diagnostic criteria, issues of heterogeneity, and whether ADHD is truly distinguishable from other forms of disruptive behavior problems. Nonetheless, it has been one of the most commonly diagnosed child psychiatric disorders (Mattison et al., 1986). The current diagnostic criteria [Diagnostic and Statistical Manual of Mental Disorders (DSM-IV), American Psychiatric Association, 1994] recognize three subtypes of ADHD: Predominately Inattentive; Predominately Hyperactive-Impulsive; as well as a Combined subtype.

There have been a number of theories regarding the neurological basis of ADHD (Riccio, Hynd, Cohen, & Gonzalez, 1993). To date, the evidence is strongest with respect to implicating frontal lobe dysfunction in the increased distractibility and impulsive orienting reactions to irrelevant stimuli often seen in children with ADHD (Passler, Isaac, & Hynd, 1986; Stuss & Benson, 1984; Zambelli, Stamm, Maitinsky, & Loiselle, 1977). Various specific patterns of localization have been proposed, including frontal regions anterior and medial to the

precentral motor cortex (Mattes, 1980), as well as frontolimbic pathways (Lou, Henriksen, & Bruhn, 1984; Newlin & Tramontana, 1980).

There has been a clustering of findings specifically implicating right frontal dysfunction. Voeller and Heilman (1988) found ADHD children to be markedly deficient on a task of motor persistence, a deficit ordinarily associated with right frontal lobe impairment. In a subsequent study (Voeller, Alexander, Carter, & Heilman, 1989), the motor persistence of children with ADHD improved significantly with the administration of methylphenidate. Similarly, in a study of regional cerebral blood flow (Lou et al., 1984), children with ADHD exhibited lower perfusion rates in the region of the caudate, an anterior subcortical structure known to be involved in the motor regulatory system. Metabolic levels normalized with the administration of methylphenidate, and then declined as the medication wore off. A subsequent study by Lou, Henriksen, Bruhn, Borner, and Nielsen (1989) replicated the earlier findings, but pinpointed the right striatal region as specifically deficient in children with ADHD. As before, the administration of methylphenidate resulted in a normalization of metabolic activity. From a different perspective, Hynd, Semrud-Clikeman, Lorys, Novey, and Eliopulos (1990) found that ADHD children did not demonstrate the typical right frontal asymmetry on MRI found in normal controls. The finding lacked specificity, however, in that both ADHD and dyslexic cases had significantly smaller right frontal widths relative to normal control children.

Barkley, Grodzinsky, and Du Paul (1992) have reviewed a total of 22 neuropsychological studies of frontal lobe functioning in children with attention deficit disorder, with and without hyperactivity. Tests of response inhibition were found to discriminate hyperactive cases from normals, although many measures presumed to assess frontal lobe dysfunction were not reliably sensitive to deficits in either ADD group. Numerous inconsistencies were noted, many of which were seen to reflect methodological differences across studies.

Conduct Disorders

Research in this broad category of child psychopathology has been beset with a number of problems. First, as a diagnosis, it pertains to a very heterogeneous range of disturbances in which the manifestation of socially unacceptable behavior is the primary common feature. Second, the bulk of research has focused on adolescents, particularly the juvenile offender. If one excludes children with ADHD, little is known with respect to the neurological and neuropsychological features of conduct disorders manifested at early ages. Third, youngsters with conduct disorders have a higher risk for accidental head injury (Lewis, Pincus, & Glaser, 1979; Lewis & Shanok, 1977; Pincus & Tucker, 1978); thus, although neurological abnormalities may be seen on examination, they may be the product—not the cause—of the initial conduct disorder. This problem obviously is compounded by the emphasis on studying older as opposed to younger conduct-disordered subjects. With these limitations in mind, the findings for this general category of psychopathology are summarized below.

A number of studies have reported abnormal neurological findings in youngsters with conduct disorders (Elliott, 1982; Korhonen & Sillanpaa, 1976; Krynicki, 1978; Woods & Eby, 1982). Electrophysiological studies (Coble *et al.,* 1984; Elliott, 1982; Krynicki, 1978; Luchins, 1983) have found EEG sleep abnormalities, specifically in the expression of slow-wave (delta) activity (Coble *et al.,* 1984); seizure activity that may contribute to recurrent and unprovoked rage attacks (Elliott, 1982); and in some cases, frontal lobe paroxysmal activity, particularly in conduct-disordered adolescents with a significant history of assaultive behavior (Krynicki, 1978). The latter finding bears some relationship to the work of Woods and Eby (1982) and Pontius and Ruttiger (1976) who postulated a delay in the development of normal inhibitory mechanisms (i.e., frontal lobe functions) in repetitively aggressive youngsters.

Children with conduct disorders have been reported to show a higher incidence of episodes of disturbed consciousness and, as already noted, to suffer more head injuries than other children (see Lewis & Shanok, 1977; Lewis *et al.,* 1979; Pincus & Tucker, 1978). However, they have not been found to differ from normal controls in terms of perinatal problems, except for more frequently being small for gestational age (McGee, Silva, & Williams, 1984). These findings further serve to suggest that the neurological features in some of these children may postdate the initial onset of their conduct disorders.

Conduct-disordered youngsters have been found to have a high rate of learning disabilities (Cannon & Compton, 1980; Robbins, Beck, Pries, Jacobs, & Smith, 1983; Zinkus & Gottlieb, 1978), as well as more generalized problems with language performance (Funk & Ruppert, 1984; Stellern, Marlowe, Jacobs, & Cossairt, 1985; Wardell & Yeudall, 1980). This appears to apply to both nonincarcer-

ated (Robbins *et al.,* 1983) as well as incarcerated (Cannon & Compton, 1980) populations. These findings suggest that the presence of cognitive impairments, perhaps particularly of a verbal nature, places the youngster at risk for acting out impulsively when placed in frustrating or provocative social situations. The degree of impulsivity *per se* is unrelated to either the type or the number of crimes committed by delinquent youth (Oas, 1985). Rather, it may be that the presence of faulty capacities in verbal reasoning and judgment, along with impulsivity, is a necessary ingredient in the production of chronic antisocial conduct. Thus, although unrelated to the degree of impulsivity, the presence of at least a 15-point inferiority in Verbal IQ versus Performance IQ on the Wechsler Intelligence Scale for Children-Revised (WISC-R) has been found to be predictive of recidivism in adjudicated white delinquent boys (Haynes & Bensch, 1981).

Some studies have examined the relative effects of language and executive function deficits. Linz, Hooper, Hynd, Isaac, and Gibson (1990) selected 20 adolescents meeting DSM-III criteria for conduct disorder from a juvenile evaluation center and compared them with 20 normal adolescents on nine Lurian tasks measuring behaviors attributed to frontal lobe functioning. Differences were obtained on the verbal conflict and verbal retroactive inhibition tasks, although these disappeared when controlling for receptive vocabulary. Cole, Usher, and Cargo (1993) examined the relationship between cognitive factors and risk for disruptive behavior disorders in a sample of 82 preschoolers. Verbal, visuospatial, and executive function abilities were examined in terms of their relationship with labeling emotions and behavioral control. Difficulties in both verbal and visuospatial processes were associated with a higher risk for behavioral difficulties. Additionally, whereas verbal abilities contributed to the prediction of emotion labeling accuracy, executive functions were predictive of behavioral control. The latter was noteworthy also for the examination of behavioral risk in a younger-aged sample.

Further investigations into the pattern of neuropsychological deficits in conduct disorders have produced mixed results. Berman and Siegal (1976) found that delinquents performed more poorly than normal controls on virtually every task of the HRNB. Whereas prominent deficits were observed in tasks requiring verbal mediation, concept formation, and perceptual organization, only minimal difficulties were found in memory and gross motor coordination. Brickman, McManus, Grapentine, and Alessi (1984) found that more violent youth tended to show more impairment on the LNNB than their nonviolent counterparts, with Expressive Speech and Memory being the distinguishing summary scales. This was true with respect to both male and female offenders. These findings were similar to the results of earlier studies by Lewis, Shanok, and Pincus (1982) and Voorhees (1981). However, in controlling for the presence of psychosis and a history of neurological disorder, Tarter, Hegedus, Alterman, and Katz-Garris (1983) failed to find differences in neuropsychological, intellectual, and psychoeducational performance across groups of adolescent offenders differing with respect to their type of offense (i.e., violent, nonviolent, sexual).

The previously noted problems limit the generalizations that one can make with respect to this category of child psychopathology. It is probably fair to say that, as a group, youngsters with conduct disorders tend to have more limited verbal abilities and a heightened rate of neurological signs (these, however, may arise secondarily as consequences of their behavior disorders). With the possible exception of cases with prominent histories of repetitive, assaultive behavior, the specific role of neurological factors in conduct disorders remains unclear.

Depression

MacAuslan (1975) reported that depressed children have an increased frequency of neurological soft signs relative to normal controls. Conversely, as was noted earlier, adolescents with early soft signs were more likely to have a psychiatric disorder characterized by symptoms such as anxiety, withdrawal, and depression (Shaffer et al., 1985); social isolation rather than aggression is more likely to be a persistent problem in children with physical disabilities secondary to brain damage (see Breslau & Marshall, 1985); and internalizing rather than externalizing symptoms have been found to be more clearly tied to neuropsychological impairment in psychiatrically hospitalized boys (Tramontana et al., 1988). Also, apart from gross social disinhibition, it will be recalled that depression was the only psychiatric symptom that bore a specific relationship to lesion localization in the series of studies on head injury by Rutter and his colleagues (Rutter, 1983). Thus, depression appears to be an important feature of the brain-impaired child, perhaps especially in terms of long-range outcomes.

Much of the neuropsychological investigation into childhood depression has focused specifically on the question of lateralization of dysfunction. Research demonstrating the specialized role of the right cerebral hemisphere in the processing of human emotion and affective cues, along with reports of right hemispheric dysfunction in adults suffering from depression (Tucker, 1980), prompted inquiries into the existence of such relationships in children. A number of studies have reported impaired nonverbal abilities relative to verbal abilities in children with depression. For example, Kaslow, Rehm, and Siegel (1984) found that higher scores on the Children's Depression Inventory (CDI) were associated with poor performance on the WISC-R subtests of Block Design, Coding, and Digit Span in a mixed group of childhood depressives. No significant relationships were found for WISC-R Vocabulary or the Trail Making Test of the HRNB. Blumberg and Izard (1985) found a similar pattern of results using the Peabody Picture Vocabulary Test and WISC-R Block Design, with the CDI again serving as the index of depression. In both studies, girls were found to perform more poorly than boys on Block Design. Children of bipolar probands likewise have been found to show a disproportionate inferiority in Performance IQ relative to Verbal IQ when compared with normal controls (Decina et al., 1983). However, the fact that left-handedness was overrepresented in their sample of children at risk for affective disorder would tend to argue against an inference of right hemispheric dysfunction. More generally, the findings in the preceding studies constitute very weak evidence of lateralized right hemispheric dysfunction. The obtained pattern of results simply may reflect the differential sensitivity of performance measures to the effects of depressed concentration and motor speed.

Several studies have reported improvements on neuropsychological measures suggestive of both right hemispheric and frontal lobe dysfunction subsequent to treatment with antidepressant medication (Brumback, Staton, & Wilson, 1980; Staton, Wilson, & Brumback, 1981; Wilson & Staton, 1984). Specifically, Staton et al. found that remission of melancholic symptoms was associated with improved performance on WISC-R Similarities, Comprehension, Block Design, and Coding, as well as on the Matching Familiar Figures Test, the Category Test of the HRNB, and the Visual Reception Subtest of the Illinois Test of Psycholinguistic Abilities. Although the localizing significance of this pattern of results is uncertain, two children in the study reportedly had a mild left-sided motor deficit which also seemed to improve subsequent to antidepressant treatment. The latter finding, if replicated, would constitute more convincing evidence of improvement in lateralized dysfunction.

A number of electrophysiological studies have been reported as well. Rochford, Weinapple, and Goldstein (1981) found greater EEG variance in the right hemisphere than in the left in a heterogeneous group of depressed adolescents. This pattern was distinct from that of normal controls, who demonstrated about equal hemispheric variance, and from adolescents with paranoid symptomatology, who exhibited greater variance in the left hemisphere. However, Knott, Waters, Lapierre, and Gray (1985) found no evidence of specific hemispheric abnormalities in a comparison of EEG patterns and auditory-evoked potentials in matched pairs of siblings discordant for affective disorder. They did find that the bipolar group spent less time in EEG alpha, suggesting a hyperarousal of the nervous system in this form of affective disorder. EEG abnormalities in REM sleep latencies also have been described in depressed adolescents, although this finding has not been documented in prepubescent children (Mendlewicz, Hoffman, Kerkhofs, & Linkowski, 1984).

Sackeim, Decina, and Malitz (1982) reviewed much of the earlier literature pertaining to functional brain asymmetry and affective disorders. They concluded that affective disorders, particularly unipolar depression, tend to be associated with right hemispheric cognitive dysfunction and/or electrophysiological overactivation. In contrast, bipolar patients may evidence right- or left-sided hemispheric hyperactivation depending on whether the individual is experiencing a depressive (right hemisphere) or manic (left hemisphere) episode. These assertions will require further validation with child and adolescent subjects.

Another perspective comes from the model of nonverbal learning disability of Rourke and associates noted earlier, and its relationship to internalizing forms of psychopathology, including depression. Rather than lateralized dysfunction *per se*, NLD is seen as more directly related to the extent of white matter disruption present. Lateralized findings may be explained, however, by the higher ratio of white matter to gray matter in the right versus left hemisphere (Rourke, 1987).

Anxiety Disorders

The relationship between anxiety and neuropsychological factors is complex. Much of the discussion of anxiety within the context of neuropsychological functioning has dealt with the disruptive effects it may exert on formal test performance. Thus, anxiety may be viewed as a source of interference contributing to false-positive diagnosis or invalid inferences of neuropsychological deficit, especially in situations with high base rates of psychiatric disorder (Tramontana, 1983).

Alternatively, anxiety may arise as a secondary reaction in situations in which a child's deficits are challenged or brought to the fore (Tramontana & Hooper, 1989). For example, a language-impaired child may react with avoidance or withdrawal in situations requiring spoken communication. In this case, the anxiety is symptomatic of a breakdown in the child's ability to cope effectively with his or her deficits. The child's actual performance may suffer from disruptive or distracting emotional reactions. Worse yet, the underlying deficits may become compounded in time if the child's anxiety leads to a chronic avoidance of appropriate learning and stimulation experiences.

Another perspective has to do with more of a direct relationship between neuropsychological processes and particular forms of anxiety disorder. For example, right parahippocampal abnormality has been posited in the case of panic disorder (George & Ballenger, 1992). A disturbance in a network of structures involving the basal ganglia, thalamus, as well as orbitofrontal and anterior cingulate cortex has been hypothesized as a pathogenic mechanism in obsessive–compulsive disorder (Modell, Mountz, Curtis, & Gredens, 1989). However, these findings are based on adults and their applicability to children is unclear. Studies of obsessive–compulsive disorder in adolescents have noted frontal and basal ganglia dysfunction (Cox, Fedio, & Rapoport, 1989; Behar *et al.,* 1984). There were also findings suggestive of possible right hemispheric dysfunction (visual–spatial deficits; left hemibody signs) together with larger ventricular–brain ratios on CT and a greater frequency of age-inappropriate synkinesias relative to matched controls.

Posttraumatic stress disorder (PTSD) is an especially noteworthy area of emerging interest. As in other areas, much of the neuropsychological investigation to date has been specifically with adults. One study, for example, compared the attention and memory performance of military personnel with and without PTSD (Vasterling, Roost, Brailey, Uddo, & Sutker, 1994). Those with PTSD were impaired on tasks of attention and mental control, especially where a visual component was involved. Poor organization on a constructional task and a greater susceptibility to proactive interference in verbal learning were also noted. The findings were seen as consistent with neurobiological models of PTSD emphasizing the role of hyperarousal and frontal–subcortical systems. Other findings have specifically related extreme stress with damage to the hippocampus and with associated deficits in memory function. Bremner *et al.* (1995) found that Vietnam combat veterans had a statistically significant 8% smaller right hippocampal volume on MRI relative to a matched comparison group. Deficits in short-term verbal memory were also noted.

Taken together, the implication is that some of the memory disturbances seen in PTSD result from experientially induced structural changes and are not merely the product of defensive processes. This is an exciting line of inquiry that hopefully will be extended to victims of child abuse and trauma as well.

Implications for Research and Practice

Many of the conclusions that we put forth in the previous edition of the *Handbook* still apply. As before, there continues to be little evidence of specificity in the type or pattern of brain dysfunction associated with different categories of child psychopathology. For example, we saw evidence suggestive of left hemispheric dysfunction in disorders as dissimilar as autism and conduct disorder; frontal lobe dysfunction was reported in one study or another for almost all of the categories of disturbance considered. With the neurodiagnostic findings overlapping to such an extent, these hardly could be used to provide a satisfactory explanation for the different forms of psychopathology manifested.

Methodological factors obviously had a limiting effect here. To some extent, the picture was blurred by differences in subject samples and the methods used in identifying brain dysfunction across studies. Inconsistencies in the use of diagnostic terminology and criteria obviously would confuse the picture when considering a particular disorder. We should not expect the neurodiagnostic findings to be any more cohesive than the particular behavioral syndrome or category of disturbance to which they refer.

Confusion also seems to have resulted from the faulty application of neuropsychological inference in a number of studies. It is one thing to use neuropsychological test data in making inferences regarding lesion localization for cases with documented brain damage; however, even here issues such as individual differences in compensatory development can obscure specific brain–behavior relationships (e.g., Bigler & Naugle, 1985; Rourke, Bakker, Fisk, & Strang, 1983). In any event, one is certainly on rather weak ground in making such inferences on cases for whom there is no corroborating evidence as to the presence or localization of injury. A relatively low Verbal IQ is not necessarily associated with left hemispheric impairment, nor is impulsivity necessarily a sign of frontal lobe dysfunction. Although such results may have localizing significance, they easily can be attributed to nonneurological factors as well.

At the same time, there have been some major strides in identifying more specific brain–behavior relationships. Promising leads have emerged, as in some of the newer studies on anxiety disorders. To no small degree, these discoveries have been made possible through the incorporation of more precise brain imaging techniques, such as MRI. As emphasized earlier (Tramontana, 1983), the use of such tools within a multimethod approach will be essential for knowledge in this field to grow.

Also highly welcome have been the theoretical advances that have begun to appear. This was exemplified clearly in the work of Rourke and colleagues on the syndrome of nonverbal learning disability—especially in terms of its hypothesized relationships with particular aspects of psychosocial functioning. Another example deserving particular mention comes from the work of Mirsky and associates and their empirically derived model of attention (Mirsky, Anthony, Duncan, Ahearn, & Kellam, 1991). Based on factor-analytic studies of tests considered to assess some aspect of attention, Mirsky *et al.* have conceptualized attention in terms of four components or elements: (1) focus-execute, (2) sustain, (3) encode, and (4) shift. Each of these is seen as supported by distinct brain regions that, if damaged, will result in specific deficits in the particular attentional processes involved. Because so many brain regions come into play, it explains why attentional disturbances of one form or another are commonly seen in different types of brain injury or disease. This is a heuristically powerful model that permits a far more refined conceptualization of brain–behavior relationships in a functional domain that holds such a key role in childhood behavior disorders and psychopathology.

The existing research has documented a heightened risk for psychopathology in the child with brain dysfunction. Emphasis should be given to gaining a better understanding of what factors might curtail that risk, and thereby maximize outcomes. At present, the natural history of behavioral disturbances secondary to brain dysfunction is poorly understood. There is some indication that the relationship may weaken or grow more indirect over time, as other factors perhaps come to assume a more important role in maintaining problem behaviors (Dorman, 1982; Tramontana *et al.,* 1988). The nature of behavioral disturbances also may show some convergence over time, with symptoms such as withdrawal and depression being among the more common outcomes associated with a history of chronic handicap (Breslau & Marshall, 1985; Shaffer *et al.,* 1985). It is important to know more precisely how this process unfolds so that it might be redirected more positively, if not prevented. The implications for clinical practice are similar. Accurate detection of the functional deficits and behavioral liabilities in the brain-impaired child is the first step in limiting the risk for the later development or exacerbation of psychopathology. The essence of the strategy is to identify, treat early, and thereby minimize the development of secondary disturbances.

Issues surrounding valid neuropsychological diagnosis with this population have been discussed elsewhere (Tramontana, 1983), and thus will not be elaborated here. Briefly, the major interpretive problem involves distinguishing the effects of *deficit versus disturbance versus delay* in the neuropsychological results of psychiatrically disordered children. The standard application of neuropsychological methods is associated with a greater likelihood of false-positive errors in diagnosis with this population. This is because a psychiatric disturbance in childhood or adolescence, in the absence of brain damage, may itself produce significant impairment on many neuropsychological tests. Impaired performance could result from the disruptive effects of psychogenically based problems with anxiety, depression, or frustration tolerance. Such conditions may not only disrupt present performance, but also could have impeded the past attainment of various skills that are prerequisite to age-appropriate performance in many of the areas that are assessed. It is just as undesirable to overdiagnose brain dysfunction as it is to overlook it when it does exist. This had led some authors (e.g., Tramontana, 1983) to argue for the use of more conservative detection criteria when applying neuropsychological methods in a child psychiatric population. Neuropsychological inferences regarding the presence of brain dysfunction should never be based solely on defective levels of performance,

but also should be supported by other features in the neuropsychological results.

Some outcomes in this population appear to be predicted especially well by neuropsychological assessment. This was seen clearly in a study that examined the determinants of academic achievement within a sample of hospitalized child psychiatric cases, all of whom had been referred for neuropsychological assessment because of suspected learning impediments or other deficits (Tramontana, Hooper, Curley, & Nardolillo, 1990). Achievement test scores were examined as a function of six variables: IQ, socioeconomic status, age, sex, neuropsychological status, and severity of behavioral disturbance. Neuropsychological status proved to be the best predictor overall. It even surpassed IQ, whether examined alone or in combination with demographic and behavioral variables. This differed from what is ordinarily the case with normal school-aged children, for whom IQ and socioeconomic status are generally the most important determinants of academic performance and educational outcomes. The findings underscored the relevance of neuropsychological factors in understanding the academic deficits of children with significant mental or emotional disturbance.

Overall, the neuropsychology of child psychopathology continues to represent an important and challenging aspect of the broader field of child neuropsychology. It is a complex area of investigation for the researcher and clinician alike, as there are many confounding factors that can obscure the study of brain–behavior relationships in child psychopathology. Our discussion of a number of these hopefully has given the reader an appreciation for both the importance and complexity of the topic. Judging from the progress over the past few years, this promises to be an exciting line of inquiry offering fresh insights into the neuropsychological underpinnings of child psychopathology.

References

Ameli, R., Courchesne, E., Lincoln, A., Kaufman, A., & Grillon, C. (1988). Visual memory processes in high-functioning individuals with autism. *Journal of Autism and Developmental Disorders, 18,* 601–615.

American Psychiatric Association. (1994). *Diagnostic and statistical manual of mental disorders* (4th ed.). Washington, DC: Author.

Applebaum, E., Egel, A. L., Koegel, R. L., & Imhoff, B. (1979). Measuring musical abilities of autistic children. *Journal of Autism and Developmental Disorders, 9,* 279–285.

Arnold, G., & Schwartz, S. (1983). Hemispheric lateralization of language in autistic and aphasic children. *Journal of Autism and Developmental Disorders, 13,* 129–139.

Bakwin, H., & Bakwin, R. M. M. (1966). *Clinical management of behavior disorders in children* (3rd ed.). Philadelphia: Saunders.

Balottin, U., Bejor, M., Cecchini, A., Martelli, A., Palazzi, S., & Lanzi, G. (1989). Infantile autism and computerized tomography brain-scan findings: Specific versus nonspecific abnormalities. *Journal of Autism and Developmental Disorders, 19,* 109–117.

Barkley, R. (1981a). Hyperactivity. In E. G. Mash & L. G. Terdal (Eds.), *Behavioral assessment of childhood disorders* (pp. 127–184). New York: Guilford Press.

Barkley, R. (1981b). *Hyperactive children: A handbook for diagnosis and treatment.* New York: Guilford Press.

Barkley, R. A., Grodzinsky, G., & Du Paul, G. J. (1992). Frontal lobe functions in attention deficit disorder with and without hyperactivity: A review and research report. *Journal of Abnormal Child Psychology, 20,* 163–188.

Bartak, L., & Rutter, M. (1976). Differences between mentally retarded and normally intelligent autistic children. *Journal of Autism and Childhood Schizophrenia, 6,* 109–122.

Bartak, L., Rutter, M., & Cox, A. (1975). A comparative study of infantile autism and specific developmental receptive language disorder. 1. The children. *British Journal of Psychiatry, 126,* 127–145.

Bauman, M., & Kemper, T. (1985). Histoanatomic observations of the brain in early infantile autism. *Neurology, 35,* 866–874.

Behar, D., Rapoport, J. L., Berg, C. J., Denekla, M. B., Mann, L., Cox, C., Fedio, P., Zahn, T., & Wolfman, M. G. (1984). Computerized tomography and neurological test measures in adolescents with obsessive–compulsive disorder. *American Journal of Psychiatry, 14,* 363–369.

Berman, A., & Siegal, A. (1976). Adaptive and learning skills in juvenile delinquents: A neuropsychological analysis. *Journal of Learning Disabilities, 9,* 583–590.

Bigler, E. D., & Naugle, R. I. (1985). Case studies in cerebral plasticity. *International Journal of Clinical Neuropsychology, 7,* 12–23.

Blackstock, E. (1978). Cerebral asymmetry and the development of early infantile autism. *Journal of Autism and Childhood Schizophrenia, 8,* 339–353.

Blumberg, S., & Izard, C. (1985). Affective and cognitive characteristics of depression in 10 and 11 year old children. *Journal of Personality and School Psychology, 49,* 194–202. (Abstract)

Boll, T., & Barth, J. (1981). Neuropsychology of brain damage in children. In S. B. Filskov & T. J. Boll (Eds.), *Handbook of clinical neuropsychology* (pp. 418–452). New York: Wiley.

Bremner, J. D., Randall, P., Scott, T. M., Bronen, R. A., Seibyl, J. P., Southwick, S. M., Delaney, R. C., McCarthy, G., Charney, D. S., & Innis, R. B. (1995). MRI-based measurement of hippocampal volume in patients with combat-related posttraumatic stress disorder. *American Journal of Psychiatry, 152,* 973–981.

Breslau, N., & Marshall, I. A. (1985). Psychological disturbance in children with physical disabilities: Continuity and change in a 5-year follow-up. *Journal of Abnormal Child Psychology, 13,* 199–216.

Brickman, A., McManus, M., Grapentine, W., & Alessi, N. (1984). Neuropsychological assessment of seriously delinquent adolescents. *Journal of the American Academy of Child Psychiatry, 23,* 453–457.

Brown, G., Chadwick, O., Shaffer, D., Rutter, M., & Traub, M. (1981). A prospective study of children with head injuries. III. Psychiatric sequelae. *Psychological Medicine, 11,* 63–78.

Brumback, R. A., Staton, R. D., & Wilson, H. (1980). Neuropsychological study of children during and after remission of endogenous depressive episodes. *Perceptual and Motor Skills, 50,* 1163–1167.

Campbell, M., Rosenbloom, S., Peery, R., George, A. E., Kricheff, I. I., Anderson, L., Small, A. M., & Jennings, S. J. (1982). Computerized axial tomography in young children. *American Journal of Psychiatry, 4,* 510–512.

Cannon, I., & Compton, C. (1980). School dysfunction in the adolescent. *Pediatric Clinics of North America, 27,* 79–96.

Cantor, D., Thatcher, R., Hrybyk, M., & Kaye, H. (1986). Computerized EEG analyses of autistic children. *Journal of Autism and Developmental Disorders, 16,* 169–187.

Caparulo, B. K., Cohen, D. J., Rothman, S. L., Young, G., Katz, J., Shaywitz, S., & Shaywitz, B. (1981). Computed tomographic brain scanning in children with developmental neuropsychiatric disorders. *Journal of the American Academy of Child Psychiatry, 20,* 338–357.

Chadwick, O., Rutter, M., Brown, G., Shaffer, D., & Traub, M. (1981). A prospective study of children with head injuries. II. Cognitive sequelae. *Psychological Medicine, 11,* 49–61.

Chadwick, O., Rutter, M., Shaffer, D., & Shrout, P. (1981). A prospective study of children with head injuries. IV. Specific cognitive deficits. *Journal of Clinical Neuropsychology, 3,* 101–120.

Coble, P., Taska, L., Kupfer, D., Kazdin, A., Unis, A., & French, N. (1984). EEG sleep "abnormalities" in preadolescent boys with a diagnosis of conduct disorder. *Journal of the American Academy of Child Psychiatry, 23,* 438–447.

Cohen, D. J., Caparulo, B., & Shaywitz, B. (1976). Primary childhood aphasia and childhood autism: Clinical, biological, and conceptual observations. *Journal of the American Academy of Child Psychiatry, 15,* 604–645.

Cole, P. M., Usher, B. A., & Cargo, A. P. (1993). Cognitive risk and its association with risk for disruptive behavior disorder in preschoolers. *Journal of Clinical Child Psychology, 22,* 154–164.

Coleman, P., Romano, J., Lapham, L., & Simon, W. (1985). Cell counts in cerebral cortex of an autistic patient. *Journal of Autism and Developmental Disorders, 15,* 245–255.

Courchesne, E., Lincoln, A., Kilman, B., & Galambos, R. (1985). Event-related brain potential correlates of the processing of novel visual and auditory information in autism.

Journal of Autism and Developmental Disorders, 15, 55–76.

Courchesne, E., Yeung-Courchesne, R., Press, G. A., Hesselink, J. R., & Jernigan, T. L. (1988). Hypoplasia of cerebellar vernal lobules VI and VII in autism. *New England Journal of Medicine, 318,* 1349–1354.

Cox, C. S., Fedio, P., & Rapoport, J. L. (1989). Neuropsychological testing of obsessive–compulsive adolescents. In J. L. Rapoport (Ed.), *Obsessive–compulsive disorder in children and adolescents* (pp. 73–86). Washington, DC: American Psychiatric Association Press.

Damasio, A. R., & Maurer, R. G. (1978). A neurological model for childhood autism. *Archives of Neurology, 35,* 777–786.

Damasio, H., Maurer, R. G., Damasio, A. R., & Chui, H. C. (1980). Computerized tomographic scan findings in patients with autistic behavior. *Archives of Neurology, 37,* 504–510.

Dawson, G. (1983). Lateralized brain dysfunction in autism: Evidence from the Halstead–Reitan Neuropsychological Battery. *Journal of Autism and Developmental Disorders, 13,* 269–286.

Dawson, G., Finley, C., Phillips, S., & Galpert, L. (1986). Hemispheric specialization and the language abilities of autistic children. *Child Development, 57,* 1440–1453.

Decina, P., Kestenbaum, C., Farber, S., Kron, L., Gargan, M., Sackeim, H., & Fieve, R. (1983). Clinical and psychological assessment of children of bipolar probands. *American Journal of Psychiatry, 140,* 548–553.

DeMyer, M., Hingtgen, J., & Jackson, R. (1981). Infantile autism reviewed: A decade of research. *Schizophrenia Bulletin, 7,* 388–451.

Deykin, E., & MacMahon, B. (1979). The incidence of seizures among children with autistic symptoms. *American Journal of Psychiatry, 136,* 1310–1312.

Dorman, C. (1982). Personality and psychiatric correlates of the Halstead–Reitan tests in boys with school problems. *Clinical Neuropsychology, 4,* 110–114.

Douglas, V. (1980). Higher mental processes in hyperactive children: Implications for training. In R. Knights & D. Bakker (Eds.), *Treatment of hyperactive and learning disordered children* (pp. 65–92). Baltimore: University Park Press.

Douglas, V. (1983). Attention and cognitive problems. In M. Rutter (Ed.), *Developmental neuropsychiatry* (pp. 280–329). New York: Guilford Press.

Elliott, F. A. (1982). Neurological findings in adult minimal brain dysfunction and the dyscontrol syndrome. *Journal of Nervous and Mental Disease, 170,* 680–687.

Fein, D., Humes, M., Kaplan, E., Lucci, D., & Waterhouse, L. (1984). The question of left hemisphere dysfunction in infantile autism. *Psychological Bulletin, 95,* 258–281.

Fein, D., Waterhouse, L., Lucci, D., & Snyder, D. (1985). Cognitive subtypes in developmentally disabled children: A pilot study. *Journal of Autism and Developmental Disorders, 15,* 77–95.

Ferrari, M. (1982). Childhood autism: Deficits of communication and symbolic development: I. Distinctions from language disorders. *Journal of Communication Disorders, 15,* 191–208.

Fletcher, J. M., Ewing-Cobbs, L., Miner, M. E., Levin, H. S., & Eisenberg, H. M. (1990). Behavioral changes after closed head injury in children. *Journal of Consulting and Clinical Psychology, 58,* 93–98.

Folstein, S. E., & Rutter, M. (1987). Autism: Familial aggregation and genetic implications. In E. Schopler & G. Mesibov (Eds.), *Neurological issue in autism* (pp. 83–105). New York: Plenum Press.

Funk, J. B., & Ruppert, E. (1984). Language disorders and behavioral problems in preschool children. *Journal of Developmental and Behavioral Pediatrics, 5,* 357–360.

Gaffney, G. R., Kuperman, S., Tsai, L. Y., & Minchin, S. (1988). Morphological evidence for brainstem involvement in infantile autism. *Biological Psychiatry, 24,* 578–586.

Gaffney, G. R., Tsai, L. Y., Kuperman, S., & Minchin, S. (1987). Cerebellar structure in autism. *American Journal of Diseases of Childhood, 141,* 1330–1332.

Garreau, B., Barthelemy, C., Sauvage, D., Leddet, I., & LeLord, G. (1984). A comparison of autistic syndromes with and without associated neurological problems. *Journal of Autism and Developmental Disorders, 14,* 105–111.

George, M. S., & Ballenger, J. C. (1992). The neuroanatomy of panic disorder: The emerging role of right parahippocampal region. *Journal of Anxiety Disorders, 6,* 181–188.

Gillberg, C., & Svendsen, P. (1983). Childhood psychosis and computed tomographic brain scan findings. *Journal of Autism and Developmental Disorders, 13,* 19–32.

Golden, C. J. (1981). The Luria–Nebraska Children's Battery: Theory and formulation. In G. W. Hynd & J. E. Obrut (Eds.), *Neuropsychological assessment and the school-age child* (pp. 277–302). New York: Grune & Stratton.

Green, W., Campbell, M., Hardesty, A., Grega, D., Gadron-Gayol, M., Shell, J., & Erlenmeyer-Kimling, L. (1984). A comparison of schizophrenic and autistic children. *Journal of the American Academy of Child Psychiatry, 23,* 399–409.

Gualtieri, C. T., Koriath, U., Van Bourgondieu, M., & Saleeby, N. (1983). Language disorders in children referred for psychiatric services. *Journal of the American Academy of Child Psychiatry, 22,* 165–171.

Harcherik, D. F., Cohen, D. J., Ort, S., Paul, R., Shaywitz, B. A., Volkmar, F. R., Rothman, S. L. G., & Leckman, J. F. (1985). Computed tomographic brain scanning in four neuropsychiatric disorders of childhood. *American Journal of Psychiatry, 142,* 731–734.

Haynes, J., & Bensch, M. (1981). The P>V sign on the WISC-R and recidivism in delinquents. *Journal of Consulting and Clinical Psychology, 49,* 480–481.

Hier, D. B., LeMay, M., & Rosenberger, P. B. (1979). Autism and unfavorable left–right asymmetries of the brain. *Journal of Autism and Developmental Disorders, 9,* 153–159.

Hoffman, W. L., & Prior, M. R. (1982). Neuropsychological dimensions of autism in children: A test of the hemispheric dysfunction hypothesis. *Journal of Clinical Neuropsychology, 41,* 27–41.

Hynd, G. W., Semrud-Clikeman, M., Lorys, A., Novey, E. S., & Eliopulos, D. (1990). Brain morphology in developmental dyslexia and attention deficit and disorder/hyperactivity. *Archives of Neurology, 47,* 919–926.

Ingram, T. T. S. (1973). Soft signs. *Developmental Medicine and Child Neurology, 15,* 527–530.

Jacobson, R., LeCouteur, A., Howlin, P., & Rutter, M. (1988). Selective subcortical abnormalities in autism. *Psychological Medicine, 18,* 39–48.

James, A. L., & Barry, R. J. (1983). Developmental effects in the cerebral lateralization of autistic, retarded and normal children. *Journal of Autism and Developmental Disorders, 13,* 43–56.

Jones, V., & Prior, M. (1985). Motor imitation abilities and neurological signs in autistic children. *Journal of Autism and Developmental Disorders, 15,* 37–46.

Kagan, V. E. (1981). Nonprocess autism in children: A comparative etiopathogenic study. *Soviet Neurology and Psychiatry, 14,* 25–30.

Kaslow, N., Rehm, L., & Siegel, A. (1984). Social-cognitive and cognitive correlates of depression in children. *Journal of Abnormal Child Psychology, 12,* 605–620.

Kendall, P., & Broswell, L. (1985). *Cognitive–behavioral therapy for impulsive children.* New York: Guilford Press.

Klonoff, H. (1971). Head injuries in children: Predisposing factors, accident conditions, and sequelae. *American Journal of Public Health, 61,* 2405–2417.

Knott, V., Waters, B., Lapierre, Y., & Gray, R. (1985). Neurophysiological correlates of sibling pairs discordant for bipolar affective disorder. *American Journal of Psychiatry, 142,* 248–250.

Korhonen, T., & Sillanpaa, M. (1976). MBD-like behavior and neuropsychological performances. *Acta Paedopsychiatrica, 42,* 75–87.

Krynicki, V. E. (1978). Cerebral dysfunction in repetitively assaultive adolescents. *Journal of Nervous and Mental Disease, 166,* 59–67.

Kuperman, S., Gaffney, G. R., Hamdan-Allen, G., Preston, D. F., & Venkatesh, L. (1990). Neuroimaging in child and adolescent psychiatry. *Journal of the American Academy of Child and Adolescent Psychiatry, 29,* 159–172.

Kusche, C. A., Cook, E. T., & Greenberg, M. T. (1993). Neuropsychological and cognitive functioning in children with anxiety, externalizing, and comorbid psychopathology. *Journal of Clinical Child Psychology, 22,* 172–195.

Lewis, D., Pincus, J., & Glaser, G. (1979). Violent juvenile delinquents: Psychiatric, neurological, psychological, and abuse factors. *Journal of the American Academy of Child Psychiatry, 18,* 307–319.

Lewis, D., & Shanok, S. (1977). Medical histories of delinquent and nondelinquent children: An epidemiological study. *American Journal of Psychiatry, 134,* 1020–1025.

Lewis, D., Shanok, S., & Pincus, J. (1982). A comparison of the neuropsychiatric status of female and male incarcerated delinquents: Some evidence of sex and race bias. *Journal of the American Academy of Child Psychiatry, 21,* 190–196.

Lincoln, A. J., Courchesne, E., Kilman, B. A., Elmasian, R., & Allen, M. (1988). A study of intellectual abilities in high-functioning people with autism. *Journal of Autism and Developmental Disorders, 18,* 505–524.

Linz, T. D., Hooper, S. R., Hynd, G. W., Isaac, W., & Gibson, R. (1990). Frontal lobe functioning in conduct disordered juveniles: Preliminary findings. *Archives of Clinical Neuropsychology, 5,* 411–416.

Lou, H. C., Henriksen, L., & Bruhn, P. (1984). Focal cerebral hypoperfusion in children with dysphasia and/or attention deficit disorder. *Archives of Neurology, 41,* 825–829.

Lou, H. C., Henriksen, L., Bruhn, P., Borner, H., & Nielsen, J. (1989). Striatal dysfunction in attention deficit and hyperkinetic disorder. *Archives of Neurology, 46,* 48–52.

Luchins, D. (1983). Carbamazepine for the violent psychiatric patient. *Lancet, 1,* 766.

MacAuslan, A. (1975). Physical signs in association with depressive illness in childhood. *Child-Care-Health-Development, 1,* 225–232.

McGee, R., Silva, P. A., & Williams, S. M. (1984). Perinatal, neurological, environmental and developmental characteristics of seven-year-old children with stable behavioral problems. *Journal of Child Psychology and Psychiatry and Allied Disciplines, 25,* 573–586.

Mattes, J. A. (1980). The role of frontal lobe dysfunction in childhood hyperkinesis. *Comprehensive Psychiatry, 21,* 358–369.

Mattison, R., Humphrey, F., Kales, S., Handford, H., Finkenbinder, R., & Hernit, R. (1986). Psychiatric background and diganoses of children evaluated for special class placement. *Journal of the American Academy of Child Psychiatry, 25,* 514–520.

Maurer, R. G., & Damasio, A. R. (1982). Childhood autism from the point of view of behavioral neurology. *Journal of Autism and Developmental Disorders, 12,* 195–205.

Mendlewicz, J., Hoffman, G., Kerkhofs, M., & Linkowski, P. (1984). EEG and neuroendocrine parameters in pubertal and adolescent depressed children: A case report study. *Journal of Affective Disorders, 6,* 265–272.

Milman, D. H. (1979). Minimal brain dysfunction in childhood: Outcome in late adolescence and early adult years. *Journal of Clinical Psychiatry, 40,* 371–380.

Mirsky, A., Anthony, B., Duncan, C., Ahearn, M., & Kellam, S. (1991). Analysis of the elements of attention: A neuropsychological approach. *Neuropsychology Review, 2,* 109–145.

Modell, J. G., Mountz, J. M., Curtis, G. C., & Gredens, J. G. (1989). Neurophysiological dysfunction in basal ganglia/limbic striatal and thalamocortical circuits as a pathogenic mechanism of obsessive–compulsive disorder. *Journal of Neuropsychiatry and Clinical Neuroscience, 1,* 27–36.

Newlin, D. B., & Tramontana, M. G. (1980). Neuropsychological findings in a hyperactive adolescent with subcortical brain pathology. *Clinical Neuropsychology, 2,* 178–183.

Oas, P. (1985). Impulsivity and delinquent behavior among incarcerated adolescents. *Journal of Clinical Psychology, 41,* 422–424.

Passler, M., Isaac, W., & Hynd, G. W. (1986). Neuropsychological development of behavior attributed to frontal lobe functioning in children. *Developmental Neuropsychology, 1,* 349–370.

Pincus, J., & Tucker, G. (1978). Violence in children and adults. *Journal of the American Academy of Child Psychiatry, 17,* 277–288.

Pontius, A., & Ruttiger, K. (1976). Frontal lobe system maturational lag in juvenile delinquents shown in narrative test. *Adolescence, 11,* 509–518.

Prior, M., & Bradshaw, J. (1979). Hemisphere functioning in autistic children. *Cortex, 15,* 73–81.

Prior, M. R., Tress, B., Hoffman, W. L., & Boldt, D. (1984). Computed tomographic study of children with classic autism. *Archives of Neurology, 41,* 482–484.

Prizant, B. M. (1982). Gestalt language and gestalt processing in autism. *Topics in Language Disorders, 3,* 16–23.

Rapoport, J., Buchshaum, M., Weingartner, H., Zahn, T., Ludlow, C., & Mikkelsen, E. (1980). Dextroamphetamine: Its cognitive and behavioral effects in hyperactive boys and normal men. *Archives of General Psychiatry, 37,* 933–943.

Rapoport, J., Elkins, R., & Langer, D. (1981). Childhood obsessive–compulsive disorder. *American Journal of Psychiatry, 138,* 1545–1554.

Reiss, D., Feinstein, C., Weinberger, D. R., King, R., Wyatt, R. J., & Brallier, D. (1983). Ventricular enlargement in child psychiatric patients: A controlled study with planimetric measurements. *American Journal of Psychiatry, 4,* 453–456.

Reitan, R. M. (1974). Methodological problems in clinical neuropsychology. In R. M. Reitan & L. A. Davison (Eds.), *Clinical neuropsychology: Current status and applications* (pp. 19–46). New York: Wiley.

Riccio, C. A., Hynd, G. W., Cohen, M. J., & Gonzalez, J. J. (1993). Neurological basis of attention deficit hyperactivity disorder. *Exceptional Children, 60,* 118–124.

Robbins, D. M., Beck, J. C., Pries, R., Jacobs, D., & Smith, C. (1983). Learning disability and neuropsychological impairment in adjudicated, unincarcerated male delinquents. *Journal of the American Academy of Child Psychiatry, 22,* 40–46.

Rochford, J., Weinapple, M., & Goldstein, L. (1981). The quantitative hemispheric EEG in adolescent psychiatric patients with depressive or paranoid symptomatology. *Biological Psychiatry, 16,* 47–54.

Rosenbloom, S., Campbell, M., George, A. E., Kricheff, I. I., Taleporos, E., Anderson, L., Reuben, R. N., & Korein, J. (1984). High resolution CT scanning in infantile autism. *Journal of the American Academy of Child Psychiatry, 23,* 72–77.

Rourke, B. P. (1987). Syndrome of nonverbal learning disabilities: The final common pathway of white-matter disease/dysfunction? *The Clinical Neuropsychologist, 1,* 209–234.

Rourke, B. P. (1989). *Nonverbal learning disabilities: The syndrome and the model.* New York: Guilford Press.

Rourke, B. P., Bakker, D. J., Fisk, J. L., & Strang, J. D. (1983). *Child neuropsychology: An introduction to theory, research, and clinical practice.* New York: Guilford Press.

Rourke, B. P., & Fuerst, D. R. (1991). *Learning disabilities and psychosocial functioning: A neuropsychological perspective.* New York: Guilford Press.

Rumsey, J. M. Rapoport, J. L., & Sceery, W. R. (1985). Autistic children as adults: Psychiatric, social and behavioral outcomes. *Journal of the American Academy of Child Psychiatry, 24,* 465–473.

Rutter, M. (1977). Brain damage syndromes in childhood: Concepts and findings. *Journal of Child Psychology and Psychiatry, 18,* 1–21.

Rutter, M. (1983). Issues of prospects in developmental neuropsychiatry. In M. Rutter (Ed.), *Developmental neuropsychiatry* (pp. 577–598). New York: Guilford Press.

Rutter, M., Chadwick, O., & Shaffer, D. (1983). Head injury. In M. Rutter (Ed.), *Developmental neuropsychiatry* (pp. 83–111). New York: Guilford Press.

Rutter, M., Chadwick, O., Shaffer, D., & Brown, G. (1980). A prospective study of children with head injuries. I. Design and methods. *Psychological Medicine, 10,* 633–645.

Rutter, M., Graham, P., & Yule, W. (1970). *A neuropsychiatric study in childhood* (Clinics in Developmental Medicine Nos. 35–36). London: Spastics International Medical Publications/Heinemann Medical Books.

Sackeim, H. A., Decina, P., & Malitz, S. (1982). Functional brain asymmetry and affective disorders. *Adolescent Psychiatry, 10,* 320–335.

Seidel, U. P., Chadwick, O., & Rutter, M. (1975). Psychological disorders in crippled children: A comparative study of children with and without brain damage. *Developmental Medicine and Child Neurology, 17,* 563–573.

Selz, M., & Reitan, R. M. (1979). Rules of neuropsychological diagnosis. *Journal of Consulting and Clinical Psychology, 47,* 258–264.

Shaffer, D. (1978). "Soft" neurological signs and later psychiatric disorder—A review. *Journal of Child Psychology and Psychiatry, 19,* 63–65.

Shaffer, D., O'Connor, P. A., Shafer, S. Q., & Prupis, S. (1983). Neurological "soft signs": Their origins and significance for behavior. In M. Rutter (Ed.), *Developmental neuropsychiatry* (pp. 144–163). New York: Guilford Press.

Shaffer, D., Schonfeld, I., O'Connor, P. A., Stokman, C., Trautman, P., Shafer, S., & Ng, S. (1985). Neurological soft signs. *Archives of General Psychiatry, 42,* 342–351.

Shapiro, T., Burkes, L., Petti, T. A., & Ranz, J. (1978). Consistency of "nonfocal" neurological signs. *Journal of the American Academy of Child Psychiatry, 17,* 70–78.

Simon, N. (1975). Echolalic speech in childhood autism: Consideration of possible underlying loci of brain damage. *Archives of General Psychiatry, 32,* 1439–1446.

Small, J. (1975). EEG and neurophysiological studies of early infantile autism. *Biological Psychiatry, 10,* 385–397.

Soper, H., Satz, P., Orsini, D., Henry, R., Mvi, J., & Schulman, M. (1986). Handedness patterns of autism suggest subtypes. *Journal of Autism and Developmental Disorders, 16,* 155–167.

Staton, R. D., Wilson, H., & Brumback, R. A. (1981). Cognitive improvement associated with tricyclic antidepressant treatment of childhood major depressive illness. *Perceptual and Motor Skills, 53,* 219–234.

Stellern, J., Marlowe, M., Jacobs, J., & Cossairt, A. (1985). Neuropsychological significance of right hemisphere cognitive mode in behavior disorders. *Behavior Disorders, 10,* 113–124.

Strauss, A., & Lehtinen, L. (1947). *Psychopathology and education of the brain-injured child.* New York: Grune & Stratton.

Stuss, D., & Benson, D. (1984). Neuropsychological studies of the frontal lobes. *Psychological Bulletin, 95,* 3–28.

Tager-Flusberg, H. (1981). On the nature of linguistic functioning in early infantile autism. *Journal of Autism and Development Disorders, 11,* 45–56.

Tanguay, P. (1984). Toward a new classification of serious psychopathology in children. *Journal of the American Academy of Child Psychiatry, 23,* 373–384.

Tarter, R. E., Hegedus, A. M., Alterman, A. I., & Katz-Garris, L. (1983). Cognitive capacities of juvenile violent, nonviolent, and sexual offenders. *Journal of Nervous and Mental Disease, 171,* 564–567.

Taylor, H. (1983). MBD: Meanings and misconceptions. *Journal of Clinical Neuropsychology, 5,* 271–287.

Tramontana, M. G. (1983). Neuropsychological evaluation of children and adolescents with psychopathological disorders. In C. J. Golden & P. J. Vincente (Eds.), *Foundations of clinical neuropsychology* (pp. 309–340). New York: Plenum Press.

Tramontana, M. G., & Hooper, S. R. (1987). Discriminating the presence and pattern of neuropsychological impairment in child psychiatric disorders. *International Journal of Clinical Neuropsychology, 9,* 111–119.

Tramontana, M. G., & Hooper, S. R. (1989). Neuropsychology of child psychopathology. In C. R. Reynolds & E. Fletcher-Janzen (Eds.), *Handbook of clinical child neuropsychology* (pp. 87–106). New York: Plenum Press.

Tramontana, M. G., Hooper, S. R., Curley, A. D., & Nardolillo, E. M. (1990). Determinants of academic achievement in children with psychiatric disorder. *Journal of the American Academy of Child and Adolescent Psychiatry, 29,* 265–268.

Tramontana, M. G., Hooper, S. R., & Nardolillo, E. M. (1988). Behavioral manifestations of neuropsychological impairment in children with psychiatric disorders. *Archives of Clinical Neuropsychology, 3,* 369–374.

Tramontana, M. G., & Sherrets, S. D. (1985). Brain impairment in child psychiatric disorders: Correspondences between neuropsychological and CT scan results. *Journal of the American Academy of Child Psychiatry, 24,* 590–596.

Tramontana, M. G., Sherrets, S. D., & Golden, C. J. (1980). Brain dysfunction in youngsters with psychiatric disorders: Application of Selz–Reitan rules for neuropsychological diagnosis. *Clinical Neuropsychology, 2,* 118–123.

Tsai, L., Tsai, M., & August, G. (1985). Brief report: Implications of EEG diagnosis in the subclassification of infantile autism. *Journal of Autism and Developmental Disorders, 15,* 339–344.

Tucker, D. M. (1980). Lateral brain function, emotion, and conceptualization. *Psychological Bulletin, 89,* 19–46.

Vasterling, J. J., Roost, L., Brailey, K., Uddo, M., & Sutker, P. B. (1994). *Attention and memory performances in posttraumatic stress disorder.* Paper presented at the 22nd Annual Meeting of the International Neuropsychological Society, Cincinnati, OH.

Voeller, K. K. S., Alexander, A. W., Carter, R. L., & Heilman, K. (1989). Motor impersistence in children with attention deficit hyperactivity disorder decreases in response to treatment with methylphenidate. *Neurology, 39,* 276.

Voeller, K. K. S., & Heilman, K. (1988). Attention deficit disorder in children: A neglect syndrome? *Neurology, 38,* 806–808.

Voorhees, J. (1981). Neuropsychological differences between juvenile delinquents and functional adolescents. *Adolescence, 16,* 57–66.

Wardell, D., & Yeudall, L. (1980). A multidimensional approach to criminal disorders. The assessment of impulsivity and its relation to crime. *Advances in Behavioral Research and Therapy, 2,* 159–177.

Wender, P. (1971). *Minimal brain dysfunction in children.* New York: Wiley.

Wilson, H., & Staton, R. D. (1984). Neuropsychological changes in children associated with tricyclic antidepressant therapy. *International Journal of Neuroscience, 24,* 307–312.

Wing, L. (1971). Perceptual and language development in autistic children: A comparative study. In M. Rutter (Ed.), *Infantile autism: Concepts, characteristics, and treatment.* London: Churchill Livingstone.

Woods, B. T., & Eby, M. D. (1982). Excessive mirror movements and aggression. *Biological Psychiatry, 17,* 23–32.

Zambelli, A. J., Stamm, J. S., Maitinsky, S., & Loiselle, D. L. (1977). Auditory evoked potentials and selective attention in formerly hyperactive adolescent boys. *American Journal of Psychiatry, 134,* 742–747.

Zinkus, P. W., & Gottlieb, M. I. (1978). Learning disabilities and juvenile delinquency. *Clinical Pediatrics, 17,* 775–780.

7

Pediatric Brain Injury

Mechanisms and Amelioration

THOMAS J. BOLL AND LISA D. STANFORD

The purpose of this chapter is not to provide a comprehensive review of the literature in the area of pediatric brain injury in neuropsychology. This has been accomplished multiple times, most recently by Ryan, LaMarche, Barth, and Boll (1995). Reviews of specific neurobehavioral recovery issues cited individually in this chapter are also available in reasonably recent form (Levin, Grafman & Eisenberg, 1987). The purpose of this chapter is to engage in a series of discussions about the issues that influence the outcome of pediatric brain injury, including those issues or mechanisms that predate the injury itself. Such mechanisms include the premorbid psychological characteristics of the patient (not just the injury the brain sustains, but the brain that sustains the injury) as well as the epidemiologic mechanisms that contribute to the nature of the injury and the specific characteristics of the individuals who sustain that injury. Amelioration of the injury, which has in many reviews been focused largely on rehabilitative techniques of a formal nature, are discussed in the broader context of psychological interventions, educational interventions, and family-based activities. One of the purposes of this chapter will be to enhance understanding of the importance of the individual who has the accident, and the context in which that individual lives, and will continue to live. The chapter begins with a discussion of the physiological, epidemiological, and psychological mechanisms that characterize a brain injury, and/or

characterize the patient who suffers the brain injury. Discussion then proceeds to multifactorial influences on outcome, including those that make outcome in certain instances so perplexing when to initial glance, "dose and response" seems hopelessly out of proportion. The emphasis of the final portion on school and family once again suggests the unique role in children's lives of those institutions, and the individuals who come into contact with children who have had a head injury, as well as the children who come into contact with the children who have had a head injury. Because considerable data have already been amassed on specific tests, treatment technologies, complicating factors such as bleeding and seizures, and developmental influences, this chapter can enjoy the luxury of going somewhat further afield in discussing those day-to-day and somewhat more mundane issues that cross the clinician's desk, and confront the treating doctor, be it psychologist, psychiatrist, neurologist, or other health professional.

The mechanisms of pediatric traumatic brain injury can be divided into three categories. The first is the physical and physiological mechanisms involved when brain injury occurs, and which provides a description of varying degrees of severity of brain injury. Gennarelli's classification into four major levels of severity provides the greatest amount of information. In this context, anterograde, event, and retrograde amnesia can be employed as markers of severity, albeit indirect, and in children, unfortunately possibly unreliable. Although these markers are still worth obtaining as part of the overall examination, there is need for correlation with the nature of the injury that is presented in the medical records. Appro-

THOMAS J. BOLL • Department of Psychology, University of Alabama at Birmingham, Birmingham, Alabama 35294.
LISA D. STANFORD • Department of Psychiatry and Psychology, Cleveland Clinic Foundation, Cleveland, Ohio 44195.

priate diagnosis requires understanding by caregivers of the actual condition of the child, and recognition that children's self-reports across a broad range of activities are subject to the full range of unreliability that characterizes children's mental state in general, and the impaired mental state of a child following brain injury in particular.

Physical and Physiological Mechanisms

The physical and physiological mechanisms of head injury and their neurosurgical and medical risks and requirements have been reviewed widely and frequently, and will not be dealt with in great detail here (Corkin, Hurt, Twitchell, Franklin, & Yen, 1987; Fletcher, Miner, & Ewing-Cobbs, 1987; Gennarelli, 1982; Grafman & Salazar, 1987; Papanicolaou, 1987). The mechanisms have not significantly changed since previous reviews have been published, and those reviews are, by themselves, quite sufficient. Nevertheless, a review of those portions of mechanism and categorizations most relevant to general day-to-day practice of assessment and treatment of children with pediatric head injury, be that practice medical, neuropsychological, psychiatric, educational, or other, will be considered.

Classification of injury into degrees of severity always carries with it a measure of arbitrariness. Nevertheless, agreed-on definitional statements can add much to the understanding of individual patients, their requirements for care, and eventual prognosis. Such definitions also add significantly to scientific communicability. Careful studies, like those of Dikmen and her colleagues on neuropsychological outcome, depend heavily on preestablished criteria that are well spelled out and can be replicated later, and are clearly understood in advance (Dikmen, Machamer, Winn, & Temkin, 1995). The largely normal outcomes described for patients who have sustained head injury in the "mild" category as documented by Dikmen, McLean, and Temkin (1986) and Dikmen, McLean, Temkin, and Wyler (1986) have been enormously reassuring to patients who have sustained these injuries. The significance of knowing that one is going to have a satisfactory outcome can have much to do with producing an even increasingly positive result. In like manner, the false implication that all head injuries produce irreversible damage can lead to misattributions, false convictions, and undue concern that may not only produce its own symptoms, but

lead to misunderstanding of existing related and unrelated symptoms. Such misunderstanding leads to failures of appropriate care, and applications of inappropriate care including polypharmacy. These misunderstandings and subsequent agglomeration of multifactorially based complaints also lead to incorrect imputations of disability which can be more disabling than the injury itself.

Penetrating Head Injury

Penetrating brain wounds are an entirely different neuropathological occurrence than closed head injury. Direct penetration of the skull, dura, and in many instances, actual brain tissue, produces on the one hand more specific and focal deficits, and on the other hand does not produce the level of general neurologic and subsequent neurocognitive disruption that is commonly found in closed head injuries of equal general severity classification. In fact, in very young children, as well as adults, such events as a skull fracture may be a positive rather than a negative prognostic sign (Klove & Cleeland, 1972), for reasons that have to do with dissipation of energy directly into the bone, and the relatively lesser effect on other brain structures, even while specific parts of the brain are being rather more badly injured.

The force of a penetrating head injury is determined by the nature of the object causing the penetration and other characteristics of that object. Such penetration may be produced by a small, very sharp object moving very rapidly, such as a bullet. A penetration may also be produced by a large, dull, slow-moving object, such as a baseball bat. Each of these can be seen to have rather different outcomes, structurally, medically, and very probably neurocognitively. The effects on the brain are influenced by: (1) damage to the tissue directly touched; (2) damage to surrounding tissue caused by the force of the object; (3) damage to the brain related to secondary bleeding; (4) damage to the brain resulting from swelling, anoxia, and increased intracranial pressure; and (5) damage to the brain caused by the entry, through the penetration site, of infectious agents. Although penetrating head injuries are less common in children than adults, trauma, in general, continues to be the leading cause of death in children aged 1 to 14, and the largest disabler of persons through age 44. Estimates of evidence of cerebral injury from trauma vary from 25 to 67% of emergency room trauma visits. For every 9 individuals who die secondary to head injury, 40 are hospitalized, and 1300 visit emergency departments.

Closed Head Injury

Gennarelli (1982) recognized four classifications of brain injury severity as follows: (1) mild concussion, (2) classical cerebral concussion, (3) diffuse injury, and (4) diffuse white matter shearing (shearing injury). For the purposes of the current discussion, we will adopt Gennarelli's general classification and also his subdivision of the first category into three subcategories, thereby leading to a total of six overall severity ratings. This is worthwhile, because different discussions of mild head injury have used various terms that are more equivalent to one or another of the separate definitions of degrees of severity within the category of mild. It is important to recognize that each of these descriptions continues to exist within the category of mild, and that it takes substantially greater damage than that to rise to the level at which such phenomena as diffuse brain injury and cortical and subcortical shearing occur. As this is a commonly made mistake, it is important to subdivide degrees of severity in such a way as to make it quite clear when these conditions do and do not pertain.

Category 1: Mild Concussion

According to Gennarelli, Category 1a, within the overall category of mild, results from an injury that produces confusion and disorientation that is only momentarily present, unaccompanied by amnesia, and without loss of consciousness. This syndrome is completely reversible and without any accompanying sequelae.

Category 1b involves confusion with amnesia, and is descriptive of that kind of difficulty that occurs when athletes are injured with what is commonly referred to as a "ding." Retrograde amnesia typically develops after 5 or 10 minutes, even following a period of time when the player can describe the event in question. Subsequent to the development of retrograde amnesia, however, the event itself is lost to memory. This degree of amnesia typically has a span of only a few minutes prior to the injury (retrograde amnesia) which may shrink as is common with all cases of retrograde amnesia, but always results in event amnesia of a permanent sort. Confusion, disorientation, or other aberrations in mental process completely resolve in a very short time, typically less than 1 minute.

Category 1c involves sufficient stress and strain to the brain that confusion and amnesia, including event amnesia, retrograde amnesia, and at least some limited amount of posttraumatic amnesia are always present. The confusional stage typically lasts several minutes, and in many instances more than that, with some permanent retrograde and posttraumatic amnesia, as well as persisting event amnesia. Obviously, with the presence of amnesia, the implication that memory mechanisms have been affected is direct. No other brain-related dysfunction appears to be at issue, and once again long-term sequelae are not a component of this condition. Rather, an existing and, on occasion, misunderstood and sometimes bothersome permanent retrograde and posttraumatic amnesia may be present. Although these have no necessary implications for day-to-day functioning, inappropriate explanation can create areas of concern.

Category 2: Classical Cerebral Concussion

Classical cerebral concussion is "that posttraumatic state which results in loss of consciousness. This state is always accompanied by some degree of retrograde and post-traumatic amnesia, and, in fact, the length of post-traumatic amnesia is a good measure of severity of cerebral concussion" (Gennarelli, 1982). Although the disturbance in consciousness is transient and reversible, full consciousness may not return for up to 24 hours. As described by Gennarelli, neuropathological examinations of experimental cerebral concussion have found some microscopic neuronal abnormalities (Adams, Graham, & Gennarelli, 1981; Groat, Windle, & Magoun, 1945). According to Gennarelli (1982),

> In patients with classical cerebral concussion, there is unconsciousness or coma from the moment of head impact. Although systemic changes, such as bradycardia, hypertension and apnea, or neurological signs, such as decerebrate posturing, pupillary dilatation, or flaccidity may occur, they do so only fleetingly and disappear within several seconds. The patient awakens and is temporarily confused before regaining full alertness and orientation. As in the mild concussion syndrome, classical cerebral concussion is always associated with both retrograde and post-traumatic amnesia. Although these states vary in length, they tend to be longer in cerebral concussion than in mild concussion syndromes. (pp. 86–87)

As pointed out by Gennarelli (1982),

Certainly some sequelae, such as headache or tinnitus, may reflect injuries to the scalp, inner ear, or other non-cerebral structures. However, subtle changes in personality and in psychological or memory functioning have been documented, and must be of cerebral cortical origin. Thus, although the great majority of patients with classical cerebral concussion have no sequelae other than amnesia for the events of impact, some patients may have more long-lasting, though subtle, neurological deficiencies. (p. 87)

Category 3: Diffuse Injury

According to Gennarelli (1982), this classification is

> more severe than classical cerebral concussion, it must be distinguished from shearing injury. Diffuse injury is evidenced by loss of consciousness from the time of injury, and which continues beyond 24 hours. It is common for patients with diffuse injury to be unconscious for days or weeks before recovery begins. Diffuse injury is distinguished from shearing injury in that there are few signs of decerebrate posturing, and no signs of increased sympathetic injury activity (hypertension, hyperhidrosis, hyperpyrexia). Permanent deficits of intellectual, cognitive, memory, and personality functions may be mild to severe. (pp. 87; 88)

These patients present with Glascow coma scores of 4–8, and thus fall into the group of severe head injuries.

Category 4: Shearing

> Patients with shearing injuries are immediately, deeply unconscious and remain so for a prolonged period of time. They are differentiated from patients with diffuse injury by the presence and persistence of abnormal brain stem signs, such as decorticate or decerebrate posturing. However, recovery rarely is good, and rather severe intellectual or bilateral sensory motor deficits occur. (Gennarelli, 1982, pp. 88, 89)

These patients remain in a vegetative state (36%), and although their eyes are open, they have no cognitive connection or response to their environment. The most common pattern with the shearing injury is death (55%).

Prognostically then, patients in Categories 3 and 4 very commonly have significant persisting deficits, and in some instances their lifelong functioning is significantly limited. Patients in Category 2 appear to experience the full range of possible difficulties from very mild and almost nonexistent deficits to measurable and disruptive neurocognitive difficulties. Categories 1a–c are generally characterized by few, if any, neuropsychological consequences, and these are typically transient and of importance only for their appropriate initial management. Appropriate initial management usually renders successful the overall reintegration of patients to work and school, while mismanagement, as mentioned above, can produce its own negative consequences. Mismanagement can occur not simply from ignoring these injuries and allowing patients to experience unusual, troubling, and unexplained difficulties resulting in short-term failure and long-term losses of confidence, but can also occur from mismanagement of an inappropriate diagnosis in which overeager examiners pronounce on the relationship between any pattern of neurocognitive variability and brain injury in such a way as to generate self-fulfilling expectations, misattributions, and unnecessary anxiety. Dikmen *et al.* (1993) point out, as many others are beginning to do, that other factors than those directly attributable to the effect of the injury on brain structure and function must be carefully evaluated in determining the reasons why some individuals, including children, appear to experience considerable difficulties after an injury for which the normal prediction would be a good outcome. Often, these difficulties are misattributed to brain-related activities, impairments, and dysfunctions, when, in fact, other causes are apparent or identifiable. These other causes (considered in the next sections of this chapter), all of which are subject, some more than others, to various forms of intervention, are important to identify. Without such identification, not only is the wrong treatment commonly provided, but the patient is thereby deprived of the right treatment.

Epidemiological Mechanisms

The second mechanism is epidemiological. Understanding of head injury is incomplete, unless one understands when, where, why, and how head injury occurs. This is not simply an issue of statistics or physical data gathering. This is also an issue that relies on these data to provide a broader understanding of head injury, its occurrence, and its consequences. By understanding the epidemiology of head injury, one understands not just when, where, why, and how head injury occurs, but also to whom it occurs. It is well recognized that head injury in general, and pediatric head injury in particular, is not random disease. The use of the term *accident* widely decried in the injury and epidemiology literature lends the unfortunate implication that these events are both random and uncontrollable. Neither is entirely true. Head injury occurs to an increasingly identifiable cross-section of the general population. This population is described in part as predominantly male, most frequently lower socioeconomic status, and very commonly characterized by high life stress, tumult, with a variety of behavioral propensities that lead to risk taking, and high action levels. These are frequently associated with other difficulties with social boundaries that may, in turn, lead to untoward events. As a simple example of that, while the majority of head injuries occur in children under the watchful eye of a caretaker, the most severe head injuries occur outside of such observation. Caretakers who are negligent, children who have no caretaker, or children who tend to absent themselves from caretaking observation hardly represent random cross-sections of the population with regard to risk for a wide variety of unfortunate occurrences. Such individuals are not randomly distributed as well with regard to difficulties academically, economically, occupationally, and socially in other regards.

The best epidemiological data continue to indicate that males outnumber females more than two to one, with an increasing frequency of males aged 15 to 29. Children between 3 and 8 tend to show an elevated incidence of head injury, followed by a relatively steady incidence of injury, until approximately 15 or 16 years of age when incidence goes up, very probably coinciding with the obtaining of a driver's license, and continues high until approximately age 29.

Spring and summer are the most common time of year for individuals to sustain head injuries. The weekend, and particularly Friday and Saturday, are the most common days of the week, the late afternoon and early evening the most common times of the day. Falls are the predominant injury for younger children, and motor vehicle accidents the most frequent injury-producing event for children over the age of 16. Motor vehicle accidents play a significant role for younger children as well, but here, children are very frequently victims as pedestrians of motor vehicle traffic rather than as participants in a motor vehicle accident. Simple preventative measures continue to be highly effective. For example, 18% of children who were injured in motor vehicles were injured in motor vehicles not involved in accidents. Rather, these children were thrown about and injured as the driver was swerving or braking so as to avoid an accident. The fact that the accident was avoided did not preclude injury from occurring. The force of the human body hurling against a hard object inside a car can be quite destructive, even when the driver avoids injury to the car (Annegers, Grabow, Purland, & Laws, 1980).

Risk factors over and above those related to time and day are well reviewed by Waaland, Burns, and Cockrell (1993). They point out, and other literature supports, the fact that patient characteristics, such as hyperactivity, emotional disturbance, delinquency, and family background, have a significant impact on the patient's risk and prognosis. Children at greatest risk are under 5, have prior adjustmental difficulties, have parents with psychiatric/marital difficulties, come from the lower socioeconomic strata of society, and frequently are experiencing difficulties academically. These children suffer more serious injuries than do children from more favorable circumstances (Ewing-Cobbs, Miner, Fletcher, & Levin, 1989).

Head injury tends to occur at a rate of 150 to 200 per 100,000 prior to age 5, increasing to more than 400 per 100,000 by age 15. The incidence for females is lower, with approximately 100 to 170 per 100,000 reported for girls under 5, and over 300 per 100,000 by age 15. Children have a better survival rate than do adults following closed head trauma (Bruce, Schut, Bruno, Wood, & Sutton, 1978). Although motor vehicle accidents account for over one-half of all closed head injuries in adults, they account for less than one-third among children, with falls comprising over 50% of the injuries. Children are less likely to have penetrating head injuries than are adults, all of which most probably leads to better survivability (Boll & Barth, 1981; Levin, Eisenberg, Wigg, & Kobayashi, 1982; Spreen, Tupper, Risser, Tuokko, & Edgell, 1984).

Psychological Competence

The third mechanism that needs to be understood when discussing pediatric head injury is the mechanism of psychological competence. Within the mechanism of psychological competence is included pre- and post-brain-injury social integration, family tolerance, school performance, and neurocognitive function and dysfunction, which contribute to and directly interact with other variables that are generally described as contributing to outcome. Describing mechanism in a manner that merges the purely mechanical, the environmental, and the inter- and intrapersonal makes it clear that the understanding of head injury must be taken as a continuum, as well as a continuous work in progress.

The finding that head injury is not random is now widely accepted, and Rutter (1981) was very probably the first to carefully spell out the implications of premorbid characteristics and behavior to post-head-injury problems. Parents burdened with the trauma of a severely injured child are understandably reluctant to grapple with their and the child's contribution to this injury, especially when this contribution appears terribly indirect. Nevertheless, Rutter found a strong relationship between children's preinjury behavior and psychiatric and other difficulties 1 year and further post-head injury. It is therefore important, not simply in the sense of assessing blame or making predictions, that all understand that children with preinjury behavioral difficulties are at greater risk. It is important because understanding the nature of those pre-head-injury risks gives substantial prognostic information and information of importance in designing a treatment program, and in attending to the appropriate variables that may not be apparent immediately subsequent to a brain injury. It is important to intergrade family functioning issues, and to understand that families of head-injured children may bring with them greater numbers of difficulties in coordinating this type of integrated effort. These factors must be dealt with by the care team. Assuming that a family is fully able to manage and cope with the changes following a closed head injury begins with an assumption that the family was able to cope with the child adequately prior to the injury. If that is false, then certainly the more important assumption of post-head-injury coping capacity is even more problematic. Understanding this suggests that a substantial amount of resources must be directed toward discovering, dealing with, and anticipating problems, even in the very early going, so that when a child is sufficiently recovered to return home, there is an environment that has been sufficiently prepared to facilitate rather than impede recovery. Waiting until difficulties occur, and assuming that all of those difficulties are, in fact, related to the head injury rather than preexisting, are two perfectly good ways of reducing the effectiveness of any post-brain-injury intervention program. Helping parents to come to the understanding that their behavior contributes to difficulties rather than

being merely a result of those difficulties, although probably unpleasant and prone to be met with substantial resistance, is, nevertheless, crucial if important behavior changes are to be made in areas where behavior is most important, namely, the family itself. The worsening of premorbid tendencies, especially those already having been found to produce difficulties, either academically, behaviorally, psychiatrically, or otherwise, is easy to predict, but all too seldom the focus of early intervention activities. Neuropsychological referrals, even less common in children than adults (Boll, 1983), should, in fact, be more frequent and be part of the overall secondary and eventually tertiary preventative efforts of any head injury treatment program (Boll, 1983). On the other hand, intervention is important, even for those individuals who have not been identified as having pre-head-injury behavioral difficulties. Patients with head injury have been found recently to have increased long-term risk for aberrant post-head-injury behavior. Rosenbaum et al. (1994) found that even among patients with no pre-head-injury behavioral difficulties, individuals who had sustained a head injury in childhood were at substantially greater risk for becoming partner-abusive men in adulthood. These authors found that—over and above the usual irritability, decreased impulse control, and increase in generalized aggressiveness that often temporarily characterize individuals with brain injury—specific behaviors such as partner abuse also characterized their sample. Lewis, Pincus, Feldman, Jackson, and Bard (1986) found a positive history of head injury in a disproportionate number of violent criminals. What Rosenbaum et al. found tends to continue the "piling on" of risk factors. Just as more abusers are low-socioeconomic-status individuals, so too when these risk factors become accumulated in any single individual, outcomes such as psychiatric disturbance and criminal behavior become substantially more commonplace. The fact that head injury, even occurring many years prior to marriage, plays a role in marital aggression, is one more point that must be weighed in any post-brain-injury long-term treatment and management plan. Many patients with head injury are substantially more sensitive to the effects of alcohol than they were prior to their head injury. Alcohol use is substantially associated with additional head injuries, noninjuring accidents, and aggression of all sorts, not limited to the marital relationship. Therefore, individuals who have sustained a head injury are not only more at risk for other difficulties, but also more susceptible to future risk factors, such as alcohol use. Furthermore, individuals with head injuries who have sustained cognitive compromise may be more inclined to experience occupational and educational difficulties, rendering them permanently in lower socioeconomic strata, further exacerbating difficulties, frustrations, and coping complications in an already compromised organism. Such an individual, then, significantly brain injured at an early age, carries with her or him substantial and continuing risk factors that must be contended with in a variety of ways. This can only be accomplished through appropriate treatment approaches that sustain contact with this individual and her or his support system, and provides sufficient types of support to attend to these issues as they occur on a developmental basis throughout the life span.

To assume that someone has received maximum treatment benefit, and has had all appropriate interventions applied because he or she has become able to walk, talk, and return to school, and is now obtaining appropriate special educational intervention, is to miss the fact that as these individuals grow, they become drivers, drinkers, and marriage partners. Although individuals with head injuries certainly deserve all of the freedom provided to any other person, their condition can best be understood as that of any other chronic disorder, which requires continuing attention, even though its manifestations may not be constantly apparent, continuously problematic, or evenly distributed across time. Much like asthma, which may be differentially important, depending on one's activities, weather conditions, and general state of health, so too a head injury may have differential influences under different circumstances. These variations may depend on the nature of the various provocations such as fatigue, emotional tension, alcohol use, and even subsequent head injuries. A mechanism for continuing attention to these identifiable risk factors is no less important and appropriate than are treatments utilized to provide care for individuals with cardiovascular and pulmonary difficulties on a lifelong, albeit occasional, nature.

Behavioral and personality changes after brain injury are among the family's most serious concerns (Ball & Zinner, 1994; Bond, 1983; Lezak, 1986; McKinlay & Hickox, 1988), and produce the greatest amount of stress on the family (Brooks & McKinlay, 1983). Family members struggle with responding to the new behaviors of their brain-injured child while experiencing a strong sense of loss for the child they once knew. It is as if a new person has been added to the family, and their grief often resembles the bereavement associated with the actual death of a child (Ball & Zinner, 1994). Poor fit can be as devastating as poor capacity. A child with limited abilities in an environment with limited expectations may be quite well integrated, and a child with substantially better but yet imperfect abilities may well be seen as having sustained an intolerable loss in environments where significantly more stringent demands for particular types of performance pervade. The ability of an environment to adjust to change in a child is multifactorial, and yet far more crucial to the satisfactory nature of outcome than any identifiable single intervention strategy *per se*. Therefore, intervention strategies aimed at increasing the malleability of the environment are far more functionally oriented than intervention strategies aimed at improving the actual capacity of the child.

Although family-oriented research dealing specifically with adjustment to a brain-injured child is limited, several studies based on families of adults with traumatic brain injury, as well as families with other chronic illness and disabilities, suggest that families go through several stages of adaptation (Blacher, 1984; Drotar, Baskiewicz, Irvin, Kennell, & Klaus, 1975; Lezak, 1986; Waaland & Kreutzer, 1988). After the initial period of shock and disbelief, the family is thankful for the patient's survival and anticipates recovery within the first year. Confusion and anxiety begin to set in as the recovery slows, and lack of motivation and uncooperativeness in the patient are viewed as impediments to recovery. As expectations for recovery diminish, feelings of depression surface, and a mourning process begins. In the final stages, the family comes to accept the permanence of the disability. It is at this time that family can benefit the most from strategies and planning for the patient's future adjustment. The availability of appropriate supportive and therapeutic resources at this time is critical to family adjustment outcome.

Each of these challenges, and the demands to understand the multifaceted etiology of difficulties secondary to traumatic brain injury, argue convincingly for the role of psychological treatment for the family, including siblings, and occasionally even more extended family members, as well as for the patient. The patient may not be in an adequate position to receive benefit from direct treatment because of cognitive and emotional impairments on a neurological basis. Even when the patient is perfectly capable of carrying on full involvement in psychological treatment, however, his or her symptom picture does not affect the patient alone. Rather, it has substantial influence on his or her entire environment. Treatment for the family has many foci. One focus, of course, is to help in the overall treatment programming, and provision of aid for the traumatic brain injury survivor. To understand the nature of the condition, to anticipate difficulties that will occur, to make preparations, and to make alterations within the family to cope with these changes are critical responsibilities that are very difficult to meet without professional help. A second focus is the stress that these demands place on family members. Stresses in marital relationships, stresses in sibling relationships, unevenness in care demands, drains on financial and temporal resources, and changes in life pattern and style often produce significant emotional reactions in family members, even when the necessity for them is clear and the cause well understood. Being deprived of a previously well-established lifestyle, devoting resources to medical treatments rather than family vacations, turning part of the home into a rehabilitation environment instead of a recreation room, and having a sibling who is no longer fully presentable under a variety of social circumstances is something that certainly can challenge the coping capacity and reservoir of goodwill of even the most well-adjusted child and adolescent sibling, not to mention the parents. The way in which a family copes with these difficulties can, in some instances, determine the overall outcome and satisfactory adjustment, not only of the survivor, but of the entire family.

Several studies examining preinjury familial differences relative to the general population have found increased psychopathology, fewer social advantages, lower SES, and greater marital instability (Klonoff, 1971; Rutter, Chadwick, Shaffer, & Brown, 1980). Psychosocial outcomes of pediatric traumatic brain injury are mediated by these same variables: family stability, parental mental health, and socioeconomic status (Brown, Chadwick, Shaffer, Rutter, & Traub, 1981). Thus, poor availability of social support, limited financial resources, and long-standing difficulty coping with family stressors may inhibit the opportunity for adjustment to a family member's brain injury.

In addition to being a direct consequence of traumatic brain injury, changes in social, emotional, and behavioral functioning may create problems over time in response to increased personal awareness of deficits. Children may engage in dangerous or risk-taking behaviors as a form of denying deficits (Barin, Hanchett, Jacob, & Scott, 1985) or in response to an inability to recognize cognitive, behavioral, and physical risks and limitations. Disinhibition, impulsivity, aggressiveness, and irritability may make maintaining previous social relationships difficult or prevent a child from establishing new relationships (Barin et al., 1985). Old friends may lose patience or interest in coping with the multifaceted changes that have occurred in their friend who has suffered traumatic brain injury. This creates a sense of isolation and alienation for the child who can no longer function in the manner that her or his friends had come to expect. For adolescents, there is often a sense of dependency on caretakers at the very developmental stage when issues such as identity and autonomy become most salient (Barin et al., 1985; Lehr, 1990).

Intervention programs should help the child recognize, understand, and learn to compensate for his or her deficits. A child with brain injury may need to experience the consequences of his or her behavior several times before generalization and learning will occur (Barin et al., 1985). Modeling the appropriate behavior, maintaining consistent and explicit behavioral directives, using time-out, and reinforcing compliance behaviors combined with continuous feedback and cues are appropriate and effective techniques (Divack, Herrle, & Scott, 1985). Inclusion with other children with similar difficulties through participation in support groups for children with traumatic brain injury provides opportunities for learning new behavior while decreasing the child's sense of social isolation. Finally, and of most importance, education of school personnel, family, and friends will often provide an appreciation for the child's difficulties, and allow for more adaptive responses to inappropriate behavior and disruptive social skills. This is most important because the child's outcome is dependent on the environment's ability to provide the physical, social, emotional, and educational support required by all children which has become at once doubly important and challenging by virtue of the traumatic brain injury.

Multifactorial Influences

Why do various sorts of head injuries, with neurologically good prognosis, seem to produce more problems for some patients than for others?

Factor 1

It is indeed possible that the neurological damage was more severe than realized, and it is also possible that the head injury-related damages have been overlooked because of medical complications requiring emergency attention. These non-neurological complications may, in fact, produce a need for long-term convalescence and multiple surgeries and may incapacitate the patient in a way that causes that individual to be hospitalized over a lengthy period of time, and to have few, if any, demands made on her or him. The situation may mask any impairment of cognitive process related to neurological incapacity. If the head injury does not produce specific neurological symptoms that require neurosurgical intervention, little mention may be made of it in the medical record. Therefore, the impression may be created that the individual was in fact, not badly injured. It may well be that part of the patient's amnesia is related to multiple surgical procedures, anesthetic and sedating medications, and other treatment-related interventions. Other parts of the amnesia may, in fact, be neurological in origin. Sorting this out after the fact can be extremely difficult, and without adequate immediate documentation, the fact of the head injury may be lost. This, in turn, will make it difficult to understand why the patient, after some months or even weeks of hospitalization and return home, appears to be experiencing difficulties that cannot be easily associated with chest and limb injuries, but could be associated with head injuries if such had been documented in the first place.

It is important to say, however, that multiple bodily injuries can, by themselves, produce substantial trauma, psychological upset, and physical dysfunction. Therefore, individuals who have suffered multiple bodily injuries should not be assumed to have had a head injury just because they are experiencing some of the typical postconcussive symptoms, such as headaches, memory difficulties, fatigue, loss of energy, irritability, affective lability, and sleep problems. Such consequences are well known secondary to multiple types of trauma and even in illness, and none of these symptoms is specifically neurological.

Factor 2

The second factor leading some patients to behave more poorly than their neurological injury might predict is that their injury may interact with ongoing difficulties, such as preexisting psychiatric disorders, and preexisting disorders such as learning disability, severe diabetes or asthma, and low intellectual capacity on a lifelong basis. Such patients are often premorbidly compromised in a variety of functions, or may have been able to just barely manage. The addition of even a relatively minor insult may be sufficient to produce enough of an increase in difficulty and limitation to cause a disproportionate increment in disability. Individuals with already limited physical stamina may, by reason of a mild head injury, lose some capacity for intellectual tasks, thus rendering them doubly restricted. In similar fashion, individuals with lifelong limitations of a psychiatric or intellectual sort who now sustain some physical injury, may find themselves with few, if any, alternatives for meaningful occupational activities because of the combination of difficulties rather than any one single factor.

Factor 3

The third factor influencing outcome is the age of the patient. It may be difficult to determine whether a very young child has sustained serious injury because of the absence of any meaningful baseline. This is especially true for children who have sustained injuries prior to attending school. Children without siblings, and in the absence of adequate evaluation of parental intellectual capacity, may be misunderstood to have lost substantial intellectual functioning, when in fact, they may be, on a familial basis, predicted to be relatively limited. On the other hand, the opposite end of the spectrum may also produce misidentifications. Children from exceptionally bright and high functioning families who are now performing in the average range, may be incorrectly perceived to be fully recovered, when in fact they have lost a substantial amount from their premorbid yet undocumented brilliance.

Factor 4

Coexisting habit patterns, which may produce difficulties in life functioning, such as alcohol and substance abuse, or the existence of previous head injuries that may make patients, at least in some instances, more susceptible to negative outcome, also need to be appreciated. The outcome following previous head injuries, and the person's overall recovery path, need to be well understood, and actual changes from pre-head-injury performance need to be well documented in order for the specific incident at hand to be understood.

Factor 5

Some individuals, including children, find themselves in barely tolerable situations that are being managed only with the greatest of effort. Patients who come from significantly disrupted families, who have preexisting learning disorders and attention deficit disorders, who are forced by family circumstances to move frequently, or who, for a variety of nonpathological reasons, are simply a poor fit in their overall family circumstances (the unathletic son of two very athletic parents) may find in their injury either an excuse for limiting activities in which their skill level has actually declined little if at all, or may find the addition of even a minor change sufficiently additionally burdensome, to produce a collapse in coping capacity that was already sorely strained. Also, loss of cognitive and motor functioning in a child may produce sufficient strain in an already marginally coping family, to cause loss of support in a variety of ways sufficient to produce more negative consequences than the neurological event itself. In order to provide appropriate treatment for children, their families, and their important environments, including their extracurricular activities, their friendship networks, and their school performance, an understanding of who the child was prior to the accident, how the family was and is functioning, and what the demands have been and continue to be in various aspects of their environment will be important to obtain. To the extent that that information can be integrated with the neuropsychological examination, an appropriate level of intervention can be directed toward the aid of the child independent of the neurological or nonneurological medical or environmental base for the difficulties. The important distinction, however, is that the etiology may well, to some extent, drive the nature of the intervention. Therefore, a determination of whether or not individuals performed poorly on a particular test because they have always been limited or because they have become significantly emotionally stressed, or because they have neurological limitations does have substantial importance.

A discussion of the multiple sources of impediments to full recovery would not be complete without a discussion of the work of Michael Rutter (1977), who has postulated that brain damage produces a significant disadvantage to the patient and to the patient's family through five areas of negative influence. These influences on the patient and patient's family and their interaction can be seen to increase the likelihood of coping difficulties and decrease adjustmental adequacy because of the direct and indirect effects of any brain injury. These influences are: (1) abnormal brain activity which, when present, can disrupt all aspects of psychological functioning. This hardly needs elaboration at this point, but rather simply describes the fact that sufficiently severe brain damage does influence neurocognitive functions, in some instances selectively, and in other instances in a generalized manner. (2) Mental deficits produced by brain damage have consequences related to the attendant reduction in general coping capacity demonstrated by the patient in many aspects of life. This is most specifically noted for children in academic performance. These reductions are also found in a variety of recreational capacities that, when less well managed, make the child a less companionable individual, and one whose overall self-confidence and self-concept are inevitably lower. (3) The direct effects of brain injury on personality functioning, such as irritability and lowered frustration tolerance, further compromise the child's capacity to manage difficult and challenging situations such as school, make her or him a less companionable individual with whom to interact among peers, and places undue stresses on the home as parents are torn between their role as disciplinarian and provider of appropriate level of expectations for good behavior on the one hand, and caregivers and understanding supporters of a neurologically compromised child on the other. (4) Effects of treatments such as hospitalization, drugs, and in some instances, restriction on activities must be considered as a significant two-edged sword. On the one hand, hospitalization, medication, and restriction of activities are frequently necessary in order to keep the child from having more untoward effects. Refusing a child with a head injury the opportunity to engage in contact sports such as football may be very good judgment. It may also deprive the child of valued social contacts, peer support, and activities associated with positive self-worth. Causing the child to take medication may have the very positive effect of reducing or preventing seizures. It may also result in physical and behavioral side effects that are not welcome. Being in the hospital, either acutely for obviously needed care, or for re-habilitational activities on a more chronic basis, undoubtedly is indicated in instances of severe brain injury. Nevertheless, the abnormal environment of a hospital and the restriction from home, friends, and familiar surroundings certainly can be seen to pose their own stresses. (5) The responses of the environment itself, especially among family members, to symptoms that are not understood as having a "respectable" cause, can be very devastating to a child's self-concept, and to family cohesion. This is especially true for children who have had moderate or milder head injuries without significant physical bodily damage. Such children often look quite normal, walk adequately, and are even able to carry on a reasonably respectable conversation. Nevertheless, their behavior may have been substantially changed, their academic work declines, their interpersonal skills are notably different and usually in a negative way, and, in fact, they are not at all the same children their families have come to know. These changes can cause embarrassment for siblings who no longer want to have friends around to be exposed to their brother or sister's poor behavior patterns, and can create challenging situations for parents who have to adopt different expectation standards for the brain-injured child in many circumstances. This leads to charges of unfairness, favoritism, and devotion of disproportionate family energies, which in turn leads to resentment, confusion, and pressures that the brain-injured child feels, as do other family members, and for which there is no good or immediate solution that is satisfactory to all.

Cognitive effects are the most common, persistent, and difficult consequence of traumatic brain injury (TBI), and the most susceptible to individual variability (Gronwall & Wrightson, 1974; Jennett, 1972b; Levin, Benton, & Grossman, 1982). A study done by Dikmen, Reitan, and Temkin in 1983 supported the following conclusions regarding the cognitive sequelae of TBI. (1) Cortical or higher-level cognitive functions appear more vulnerable to disruption than lower or subcortical functions; (2) improvement can occur across complex as well as simple functions; (3) difficulties with reasoning, conceptualization, mental flexibility, problem-solving, mental processing speed, and adaptability to tasks are common early deficits; (4) those with milder impairments show less improvement and less residual deficit and those with more substantial deficits show a relatively greater amount of improvement; (5) cognitive recovery does not necessarily stop or slow down after the first year postinjury.

School-Related Issues

Children with TBI often show impairment in the ability to learn new information whereas over-learned and familiar tasks are preserved or recover more quickly. Problems with attention and concentration or increased distractibility and variability of cognitive responsiveness are also common consequences of TBI (Lezak, 1986). Memory deficits following TBI such as recovery of long-term memories first, shrinking of retrograde amnesia, and disruption of semantic versus episodic memory have been described (Ewing-Cobbs, Fletcher, & Levin, 1985; Goodglass & Kaplan, 1979; Levin, Benton, & Grossman, 1982; Levin, Eisenberg, et al., 1982; Lezak, 1986). Concrete thinking, slow visual–motor dexterity, perceptual distortions, and disturbances of expressive and receptive language may also be present (Chadwick, Rutter, Shaffer, & Shrout, 1981; Klonoff et al., 1977; Lezak, 1986). Impairment in academic achievement, specifically reading and mathematical calculation, can be affected by mild, moderate, and severe brain injury, and proficiency will often be inconsistent (Boll, 1982; Goldstein & Levin, 1985; Hécaen, 1976).

Pediatric TBI has profound and sometimes persisting effects on the developing brain that extend across physical, sensory, behavioral, cognitive, and psychosocial domains, which are all factors in school success or failure. Because of modern medical and technical advances, more children are surviving TBI and subsequently must be accommodated in the public school systems. According to Blosser and De-Pompei (1991), inadequate communication between rehabilitation professionals and school personnel's lack of preparation for working with this population are barriers that interfere with efficient and effective reentry into the school. With this influx of children with unique special educational needs into an already burdened system, children with TBI are often placed in classrooms designed and modified for children with other health impairment (OHI), learning disabilities, seriously emotionally disturbed (SED), or mental retardation (Bengali, 1992).

Certainly, brain-injured children as a group demonstrate learning difficulties similar to more traditional special education classifications, such as problems with attention, impulse control and social judgment, and learning new information (Cohen,

Joyce, Rhoades, & Welks, 1985). They often, however, demonstrate greater discrepancies between abilities, more uneven patterns of progress, and often require a different academic focus in comparison with children with learning disabilities. Children with TBI may initially score poorly on tests of intellectual functioning, but the transient nature and variability of their deficits separate them from children with lifelong mental retardation or learning disability. Children with TBI may have the potential to improve cognitive and intellectual abilities, if not reestablish their premorbid IQs (Boll, 1983). Children with TBI often display behaviors that are new or are exacerbations of premorbid behaviors. They also display original difficulties, such as impulsivity, disinhibition, and poor planning skills. They may show increased irritability, overactivity, or increased lethargy due to fatigue as a direct effect of the injury. These behaviors, however, are very different from the often explosive, maladaptive, and long-standing difficulties exhibited by children who are severely emotionally disturbed, and whose inability to learn cannot be explained by intellectual, sensory, or health factors (Federal Register, 1977, p. 42478). Children with health impairments other than TBI are often more physically limited than children with TBI, and the focus of instruction tends to emphasize adaptive skill modification. Thus, trying to meet the special needs of children with TBI by placing them in a modified classroom created for children with more circumscribed difficulties, be these physical, emotional, or intellectual, fails to recognize the need for adjusting classroom strategies to accommodate the unique, multifaceted, and often rapidly changing sequelae of deficits (Bengali, 1992). Appropriately providing education to the child with TBI requires the application of general knowledge relevant to TBI, and a specific understanding of that injury's impact on learning. Therefore, while a program may be appropriate for some TBI children with specific, demonstrable characteristics and needs that are very close to those of children in various formal special education categories, these services do not meet the varied and multifaceted needs of most children with TBI.

Popular strategies routinely recommended, such as practice and repetition, consideration of learning styles for adaptive instruction, task analysis, compensatory skill development, and minimization of distractions, are effective for children with TBI. It is the well-trained professional who recognizes the need for utilizing instructional techniques to increase the chance for functional improvement. The best effect approach includes enhancement of compensation strategies for physical, sensory, behavioral, emotional, and cognitive difficulties (Bengali, 1992). The environment must accommodate multiple needs that result from insult to physical, psychosocial, behavioral, and cognitive functioning. As stated earlier, intervention strategies should be aimed at increasing the malleability of the environment to accommodate the multifactorial needs of children with TBI, as well as the improvement of the functional capacity of the child.

Physical Sequelae

Pediatric brain injury may produce lasting or temporary physical effects that must be taken into consideration for educational and rehabilitational planning, particularly during the initial reintegration and adjustment period of returning to school following even brief but unplanned absence. As a result of TBI, many children experience problems related to endurance and fatigue, regulation of bodily functions, and motor deficits resulting from focal impairment of neurological status. A child may also experience decreased stamina and chronic fatigue as a result of prolonged inactivity, medication, or increased mental and physical effort required to complete tasks that were premorbidly routine (Lezak, 1986). Thus, it may be necessary to reduce a child's courseload or length of school day. This may be accomplished by gradually introducing the student to the school regimen on a half-day basis until a reasonable return of endurance allows for an increase in time (Rosen & Gerring, 1986), rescheduling the most difficult classes during the student's most productive time (Ball & Zinner, 1994), and building in regular rest periods at critical times throughout the day.

Hypersensitivity to noise and lower thresholds for stress as a result of TBI will make class transition and lunchtime particularly difficult periods (Boll, 1982). A "buddy system" for the child with TBI may help to reduce the stress associated with having to manage several activities at once (i.e., maneuvering through crowded halls while remembering what class is next, finding a place to sit, and deciding what to eat in a noisy cafeteria). Brain centers that control appetite regulation, body temperature, and hormone production may have also been damaged. Recognition of the overt symptoms associated with changes in body comfort regulation should be encouraged through physical consultation with family members and school personnel, and systems for either monitoring or teacher awareness of these changes should be established.

Motor deficits, such as hemiparesis, ataxia, apraxia, visual deficits, or speech disturbances, may result from TBI, depending on the site and extent of damage. Secondary difficulties related to motor impairment, such as maneuverability of a wheelchair, usage of augmentative devices, and transfer of handedness, are often impediments to the child's learning process that can add increased frustration and fatigue. Although more likely in severe and penetrating TBI, these children are also at increased risk for developing seizures (Golden, Moses, Coffman, Miller, & Strider, 1983a,b; Hauser, 1983; Jennett, 1972a,b). They may often be placed on anticonvulsant medication as a precaution against the occurrence of seizures. Medication side effects could include drowsiness, decreased attention, lethargy, dizziness, speech disturbance, slowed mental processing, and incoordination, all of which decrease the child's ability to maximally benefit from traditional academic instruction.

Thus, school personnel need to be prepared to implement follow-up recommendations provided on discharge from a rehabilitation agency. These objectives should be included in the student's individualized educational program (IEP). Close contact with rehabilitation personnel should be encouraged to maximize the child's response to appropriate therapies (i.e., occupational, physical, and speech), and to academic modifications.

Several studies have suggested that there are no distinct or unitary behavior disorders following TBI, and that behavioral recovery is strongly influenced by characteristics of the environment before and after injury (Brown et al., 1981; Fletcher, Ewing-Cobbs, & Miner, 1990; Fletcher & Levin, 1988; Levin, Benton, & Grossman, 1982). Thus, an additional burden is placed on the school to create and maintain an environment that maximizes the brain-injured child's response to and compliance with educational modifications. School personnel and family members must also learn to recognize premorbid characteristics of the environment and of the child that may contribute to or impede recovery and adjustment.

Because of the paucity of research on prescriptive academic techniques for children with TBI and the heterogeneity of this group of learners, sound teaching practices applied with an understanding of and a sensitivity to possible cognitive, psychosocial, and physical sequelae are a good instructional starting point. This can best be accomplished by early planning, education, and training of school personnel and family members. Classmates and teachers should be made aware of procedures that will facilitate adjustment in a way that is sensitive to all parties. In preparation for reentry of a child with TB injury, coordination of efforts between hospital or rehabilitation personnel and school personnel should begin while the child is still in the hospital or under home-based care. This would include participation in the school's multidisciplinary team placement meeting or tentative IEP. The school should remain open to possible ongoing modifications in the child's educational objectives as the reentry process begins and the child is observed in the classroom setting. Because recovery from pediatric TBI is an ongoing, adaptational, dynamic process, the policy of retesting special educational students every 3 years is too infrequent (Ball & Zinner, 1994). Instead, a child with brain injury should be formally assessed every 6 to 12 months by a neuropsychologist trained in the subtleties of brain functioning and recovery.

Because not all children with TBI qualify for special education placement, regular education teachers should be included in the training process to make them aware of modifications that could be implemented throughout traditional instruction. Emphasis should be placed on functional development using process-oriented instructions. Ongoing consultations among teachers, administrators, the school nurse, school mental health professionals, and parents can be helpful in addressing day-to-day frustrations associated with the difficulties of educating a child with special needs. This may also be an effective mechanism for sharing success and progress. For the child with brain injury, gradual introduction to less predictable and more demanding situations will be needed to develop accurate environmental cues. Individual psychotherapy will help the child address issues related to increased awareness of deficits, social isolation, and adjustment changes in family and social dynamics.

It is safe to conclude that all of these residual cognitive and social deficits of TBI will have a detrimental effect on school performance, especially if they remain undetected or change without alteration in the IEP, and thus remain unremediated. Computer-assisted learning, systematic practice, memory books, self-talk and instruction, compensatory training, academic tutoring, task structuring, and multimodality presentation are just a few of the interventions that can be utilized within the regular TBI classroom to treat and continuously monitor a child with TBI. Appropriate educational intervention requires modifications in traditional academic instruction and gives new meaning to individualized educational planning.

Immediate awareness of TBI on the part of the school is also important across the range from mild to severe. Following very mild head injuries a small adjustment such as delaying an algebra test for 1 week after a football game, or allowing for slightly shorter attendance or a delay in final examinations, or provision for a tutor for a matter of weeks may be required. These adjustments are not automatically attainable, however. Someone has to understand that such adjustments are necessary, know how to present the request for these adjustments, and interact with an environment that is not typically used to dealing with children who have these temporary types of changes in their mental and personal capacities.

With more severely injured children, the demands for individual educational programming, which change from time to time, and the demands of a child who does not fit neatly into categories such as learning disabled, attention deficit, or emotionally conflicted place the school under real fiscal and administrative pressures to which its teachers and administrators may respond well or badly. Even the most well-intended administrator and teacher may not understand these demands. They may seem to be driven by a higher priority for pedagogical order or fiscal limits than for consideration of an individual child's educational requirements. By the time a child has been identified and processed through a cumbersome or resistant system she or he may have fallen far, far behind. Because of this failure to promptly respond to the child's needs, much additional damage has been done. Resources required in this circumstance will be even more extensive in order to make up for the secondary harm done by inadequate immediate educational planning. It is not at all unheard of to see a child return to school months or even weeks after a moderate or severe head injury and be in a state of modest confusion while sitting at his or her desk. To say that the child has obtained nothing from this experience understates the matter. When the child has fully recovered, it must be recognized that a period of time has elapsed during which no learning has occurred whatsoever. This period of time may be measured in months. This period may be characterized by frustration for the child and

teacher. Therefore, even though the child may eventually become ready to progress adequately, the background of knowledge necessary to benefit from current lessons is missing. The circumstances of school life may also have become negative enough to further impede academic progress related to the anger, confusion, and uncertain expectations produced by the child's condition, and the school's failure to manage the situation in an informed and appropriate manner from a time even before the child returns to school. This may mean repeat of the year, summer school, or a whole variety of individual resource interventions. In order to make an adequate determination of what is necessary, deficits must be appropriately appreciated, examinations accomplished, and various sorts of meetings and planning sessions held in order to make individualized arrangements that actually fit what it is that the child needs to make adequate progress. It is never sufficient to simply leave the child at home or to place the child in a special class without appreciating what it is that the child's neurological state and other aspects of the consequences of the head injury have resulted in by way of educational changes. Even a high level of irritability and low frustration tolerance without decline in cognitive capacity can make sitting in a classroom for a grade school or junior high school student intolerable. Poor behavior is at least as unacceptable within the school as is poor academic performance. Blame, additional pressures, and exclusion from learning environments are hardly therapeutic, and yet the reaction of the teacher, particularly one who is not aware of or unprepared to deal with the child's condition, is not difficult to predict. Teachers, too, have rights, and these rights include the expectation that children will attempt to learn in their class, and be in a class appropriate for the tasks at hand. If neither is possible on the part of the child, then other arrangements must be made. Simply placing them under some pious term like "inclusion," which may mean little more than ignoring the problem, is seldom if ever satisfactory. Pretending that the child will be all right if enough time passes misses the point entirely. During this period, the child may miss so much by way of academic instruction that the requirement then becomes one of reconstruction of an entire academic year. This, too, is discouraging and frustrating for the child who then may be separated from age mates of long standing either because of the severity of the head injury or because of inadequate academic management. In either case, this is an additional academic and coping challenge, and one that makes recovery from head injury all the more difficult.

All children are not alike. All head injuries are not alike, and the outcome of all head injuries is not alike. Children who have had head injuries, therefore, are not all alike. Neither are they, in an overall sense, like children with other conditions. Some children with head injuries do have low IQs, some have deficits in attention, and others have difficulties with specific or general learning issues, be these academic or social. In addition, others have physical limitations, including but not limited to motor and sensory deficits. Each child comes from a family and exists in an environment. The purpose of this chapter was to indicate that each of those factors, including but most assuredly not limited to the head injury, and including, but not limited to, the child him- or herself, must be taken into consideration and understood, if a full range of appropriate ameliorative activities is to be provided. These ameliorative activities in children with head injury, unlike children with many other chronic conditions affecting school, home, and social behavior, require changes in strategies from time to time. Even the intervals across which changes must be made, change as recovery rates alter from initially very rapid to eventually much more gradual. Who the child is, the family from which he or she comes, the social circumstances including stability and demand level that pertain, the academic prowess the child had before, and the academic flexibility of the school after, the apparent versus inapparent nature of the changes to the child, and the available resources, all significantly influence a child's outcome. The purpose of this chapter has been to bring those issues together and to discuss them in one place to give the practicing clinician an overview of the issues in as practical a way as the authors could manage. When an integrated set of efforts is directed toward the multifactorial issues that influence the occurrence as well as the outcome of head injury, the best interests of the child are maximally served.

References

Adams, H. J., Graham, D. I., & Gennarelli, T. A. (1981). Acceleration induced head injury in the monkey. *Acta Neuropathologica, 7,* 26–28.

Annegers, J. F., Grabow, J. D., Purland, L. T., & Laws, E. R. (1980). The incidence, causes, and circular trends in head trauma in Olmstead County, Minnesota, 1935–1974. *Neurology, 30,* 912–919.

Ball, J. D., & Zinner, E. S., (1994). Pediatric brain injury: Psychoeducation for parents and teachers, *Advances in Medical Psychotherapy, 7,* 39–50.

Barin, J. J., Hanchett, J. M., Jacob, W. L., & Scott, M. B. (1985). Counseling the head injured patient. In M. Ylvisaker (Ed.), *Head injury rehabilitation: Children and adolescents,* (pp. 361–383). San Diego: College-Hill Press.

Bengali, V. (1992). *Head injury in children and adolescents* (2nd ed.). Brandon, VT: Clinical Psychology Publishing Co.

Blacher, J. (1984). *Severely handicapped young children and their families.* Orlando, FL: Academic Press.

Blosser, J., & DePompei, R. (1991). Preparing education professionals for meeting the needs of students with traumatic brain injury. *Journal of Head Trauma and Rehabilitation, 6,* 73–82.

Boll, T. J. (1982). Behavioral sequelae of head injury. In P. Cooper (Ed.), *Head injury* (pp. 363–377). Baltimore: Williams & Wilkins.

Boll, T. J. (1983). Minor head injury in children: Out of sight but not out of mind. *Journal of Clinical Child Psychology, 12,* 74–80.

Boll, T. J., & Barth, J. T. (1981). Neuropsychology of brain damage in children. In S. B. Filskov & T. J. Boll (Eds.), *Handbook of clinical neuropsychology* (pp. 418–452). New York: Wiley.

Boll, T. J., & Barth, J. B. (1983). Mild head injury. *Psychiatric Developments, 3,* 362–375.

Bond, M. (1983). Standardized methods of assessing and predicting outcome. In M. Rosenthal, E. R. Griffith, M. R. Bond, & J. D. Miller (Eds.), *Rehabilitation of the head injured adult* (pp. 97–117). Philadelphia: Davis.

Brooks, D. N., & McKinlay, W. (1983). Personality and behavioral change after severe blunt head injury: A relative's view. *Journal of Neurology, Neurosurgery, and Psychiatry, 46,* 333–334.

Brown, G., Chadwick, O. Shaffer, D., Rutter, M., & Traub, M. (1981). A perspective study of children with head injuries: III. Psychiatric sequelae. *Psychological Medicine, 11,* 63–78.

Bruce, D., Schut, L., Bruno, L. A., Wood, J. H., & Sutton, L. N. (1978). Outcome following severe head injury in children. *Journal of Neurosurgery, 48,* 679–688.

Chadwick, O., Rutter, M., Shaffer, D., & Shrout, P. E. (1981). A prospective study of children with head injuries: IV. Specific cognitive deficits. *Journal of Clinical Neuropsychology, 3,* 101–120.

Cohen, S., Joyce, C., Rhoades, K., & Welks, D. (1985). Educational programming for head injured students. In M. Ylvisaker (Ed.), *Head injury rehabilitation: Children and adolescents* (pp. 383–411). San Diego: College-Hill Press.

Corkin, S. H., Hurt, R. W., Twitchell, R. E., Franklin, L. C., & Yen, R. K. (1987). Consequences of non-penetrating and penetrating injury: Retrograde amnesia and post-traumatic amnesia, and lasting effects on cognition. In H. Levin, J. Grafman, & H. Eisenberg (Eds.), *Neurobehavioral recovery from head injury* (pp. 318–329). London: Oxford University Press.

Dikmen, S. S., Machamer, J. E., Winn, H. R., & Temkin, N. R. (1995). Neuropsychological outcome at one year post head injury. *Neuropsychology, 9,* 80–90.

Dikmen, S., Machamer, J., & Temkin, N. R., (1993). Psychosocial outcome in patients with moderate to severe head injury: Two-year follow-up. *Brain Injury, 7* (2), 113–124.

Dikmen, S. S., McLean, A., & Temkin, N. R. (1986). Neuropsychological and psychosocial consequences of minor head injury. *Journal of Neurology, Neurosurgery, and Psychiatry, 49,* 1227–1232.

Dikmen, S. S., McLean, A., Jr., Temkin, N., & Wyler, A. R. (1986). Neuropsychologic outcome at one-month post injury. *Archives of Physical Medicine and Rehabilitation, 67,* 507–513.

Dikmen, S., Reitan, R. M., & Temkin, N. R. (1983). Neuropsychological recovery in head injury. *Archives of Neurology, 40,* 333–338.

Divack, J. A., Herrle, J., & Scott, M. B. (1985). Behavioral management. In M. Ylvisaker (Ed.), *Head injury rehabilitation: Children and adolescents* (pp. 347–360). San Diego: College-Hill Press.

Drotar, D., Baskiewicz, A., Irvin, N., Kennell, J. H., & Klaus, M. H. (1975). The adaptation of parents in the birth of an infant with congenital malformation: A hypothetical model. *Pediatrics, 56,* 710–717.

Ewing-Cobbs, L., Fletcher, J. M., & Levin, H. (1985). Neuropsychological sequelae following pediatric head injury. In M. Ylvisaker (Ed.), *Head injury rehabilitation: Children and adolescents* (pp. 3–91). San Diego: College-Hill Press.

Ewing-Cobbs, L., Miner, M. E., Fletcher, J. M., & Levin, H. S. (1989). Intellectual, motor, and language sequelae following closed head injury in infants and pre-schoolers. *Journal of Pediatric Psychology, 14,* 531–548.

Federal Register. (1977). 42 (250), p. 42478.

Fletcher, J. M., Ewing-Cobbs, L., & Miner, M. E. (1990). Behavioral changes after closed head injury in children. *Journal of Consulting and Clinical Psychology, 58,* 93–98.

Fletcher, J. M., & Levin, H. S. (1988). Neurobehavioral effects of brain injury in children. In D. Routh (Ed.), *Handbook of pediatric psychology* (pp. 258–298). New York: Guilford Press.

Fletcher, J. M., Miner, M. E., & Ewing-Cobbs, L. (1987). Age and recovery from head injury in children: Developmental issues. In H. Levin, J. Grafman, & H. Eisenberg (Eds.), *Neurobehavioral recovery from head injury* (pp. 279–291). London: Oxford University Press.

Gennarelli, T. A. (1982). Cerebral concussion and diffuse brain injury. In P. R., Cooper (Ed.), *Head injury* (pp. 83–97). Baltimore: Williams & Wilkins.

Golden, C. J., Moses, J. A., Coffman, J., Miller, W. R., & Strider, F. D. (1983a). *Clinical neuropsychology.* New York: Grune & Stratton.

Golden, C. J., Moses, J. A., Coffman, J., Miller, W. R., & Strider, F. D. (1983). *Clinical neuropsychology.* New York: Grune & Stratton.

Hauser, W. A. (1983). Post-traumatic epilepsy in children, In K. Shapiro (Ed.), *Pediatric head trauma* (pp. 271–287). Mount Kisco, NY: Futura.

Goldstein, F. C., & Levin, H. S. (1985). Intellectual and academic outcome following closed head injury in children and adolescents: Research strategies and empirical findings. *Developmental Neuropsychology, 1,* 195–214.

Goodglass, H., & Kaplan, E. (1979). Assessment of cognitive deficit in the brain-injured patient. In M. S. Gazzaniga (Ed.), *Handbook of behavioral neuropsychology* (Vol. 2, pp. 1–22). New York: Plenum Press.

Groat, R. A., Windle, W. F., & Magoun, H. W. (1945). Functional and structural changes in the monkey's brain during and after concussion. *Journal of Neurosurgery, 2,* 26–35.

Gronwall, D., & Wrightson, P. (1974). Delayed recovery of intellectual function after minor head injury. *Lancet, 2,* 605–609.

Hauser, W. (1983). Post-traumatic epilepsy in children. In K. Shapiro (Ed.), *Pediatric head trauma* (pp. 271–287). Mount Kisco, NY: Futura.

Hecaen, H. (1976). Acquired aphasia in children and the ontogenesis of hemispheric functional specialization. *Brain and Language, 3,* 114–134.

Jennett, B. (1972a). Head injuries in childhood. *Developmental Medicine and Child Neurology, 14,* 137.

Jennett, B. (1972b). Late effects of head injuries. In M. Critchley, J. O'Leary, B. Jennette (Eds.), *Scientific foundations of neurology* (pp. 441–451). Philadelphia: F. A. Davis.

Klonoff, H. (1971). Head injuries in children: Predisposing factors, accident conditions, accident proneness, and sequelae. *American Journal of Public Health, 61,* 2405–2417.

Klonoff, H., Low, M. W., & Clark, C. (1977). Head injuries in children: A prospective five-year follow-up. *Journal of Neurology, Neurosurgery, and Psychiatry, 40,* 1211–1219.

Klove, H., & Cleeland, C. S. (1972). The relationship of neuropsychological impairment to other indices of severity of head injury. *Scandinavian Journal of Rehabilitation Medicine, 4,* 55–60.

Lehr, E. (1990). A developmental perspective. In E. Lehr (Ed.), *Psychological management of traumatic brain injuries in children and adolescents* (pp. 99–132). Rockville, MD: Aspen.

Levin, H. S., Benton, A. L., & Grossman, R. G. (1982). *Neurobehavioral consequences of closed head injury.* London: Oxford University Press.

Levin, H. S., Eisenberg, H. M., Wigg, N. R., & Kobayashi, K. (1982). Memory and intellectual ability after head injury in children and adolescents. *Neurosurgery, 11,* 668–673.

Levin, H. S., Grafman, J., & Eisenberg, H. M. (Eds.). (1987). *Neurobehavioral recovery from head injury.* New York: Oxford University Press.

Lewis, D. O., Pincus, J. H., Feldman, M., Jackson, L., & Bard, B. (1986). Psychiatric, neurological, and psychoeducational characteristics of 15 death row inmates in the United States. *American Journal of Psychiatry, 143*(7), 838–845.

Lezak, M. D. (1986). Psychological implications of traumatic brain damage for the patient's family. *Rehabilitation Psychology, 31,* 241–250.

Lezak, M. D. (1985). *Neuropsychological assessment* (3rd ed.). London: Oxford University Press.

McKinlay, W. W., & Hickox, A. (1988). How can families help in the rehabilitation of the head injured? *Journal of Head Trauma and Rehabilitation, 3,* 64–72.

Papanicolaou, A. C. (1987). Electrophysiological methods for the study of attentional deficits in head injury. In H. Levin, J. Grafman, & H. Eisenberg (Eds.), *Neurobehavioral recovery from head injury* (pp. 379–389). London: Oxford University Press.

Pren, O., Tupper, D., Risser, A., Tuokko, H. & Edgell, T. (1984). *Human developmental neuropsychology.* London: Oxford University Press.

Rimel, R., (1982). Mild head injury. In R. Grossman & P. Gildenberg (Eds.), *Fourth Chicago Head Injury Symposium.* New York: Raven Press.

Rosen, C. D., & Gerring, J. P. (1986). *Head trauma: Educational reintegration.* San Diego: College-Hill Press.

Rosenbaum, A., Hodge, S. K., Adelman, S. A., Warnken, W. J., Fletcher, K. E., & Kane, R. L. (1994). Head injury in partner abusive men. *Journal of Consulting in Clinical Psychology, 62,* 1187–1193.

Rutter, M. (1981). Psychological sequelae of brain damage in children. *American Journal of Psychiatry, 138,* 1533–1544.

Rutter, M. (1977). Brain damage syndromes in childhood: Conceptual finding. *Journal of Child Psychology and Psychiatry, 18,* 1–21.

Rutter, M., Chadwick, O., & Shaffer, D. (1983). Head injury. In M. Rutter (Ed.), *Developmental neuropsychiatry* (pp. 83–111). New York: Guilford Press.

Rutter, M., Chadwick, O., Shaffer, D., & Brown, G. (1980). A perspective study of children with head injuries: I. Design and methods. *Psychological Medicine, 10,* 633–645.

Ryan, T. V., LaMarche, J. A., Barth, J. T., & Boll, T. J. (1996). Neuropsychological consequences and treatment of pediatric head trauma. In E. S. Batchelor & R. S. Dean (Eds.), *Pediatric neuropsychology* (pp. 117–137). New York: Pergamon Press.

Shaffer, D., Bijur, P., Chadwick, O., & Rutter, M. (1980). Head injury and later reading disability. *Journal of the American Academy of Child Psychiatry, 19,* 592–610.

Shaffer, D., Chadwick, O., & Rutter, M. (1975). Psychiatric outcome of localized head injury in children. In N. Porter & R. Fitzsimmons (Eds.), *Outcome of severe damage to the central nervous system. Ciba Foundation Symposia, 34.*

Spreen, O., Tupper, D., Risser, A., Tuokko, H., & Edgell, P. (1984). *Human developmental neuropsychology.* New York: Oxford University Press.

Waaland, P. K., Burns, C., & Cockrell, J. (1993). Evaluation of needs of high and low income families following pediatric traumatic brain injury. *Brain Injury, 7* (2), 135–146.

Waaland, P. K., & Kreutzer, J. S. (1988). Family response to childhood traumatic brain injury. *Journal of Head Trauma and Rehabilitation, 3,* 51–63.

8

Neuropsychological Bases of Common Learning and Behavior Problems in Children

ELIZABETH MURDOCH JAMES AND MARION SELZ

Increased interest and research into the possible neuropsychological bases of learning and behavior problems seen in children has been sustained in the past decade by promising results from researchers in the fields of learning disabilities, neuropsychology, neurophysiology, and cognitive psychology. Advances have been made in the neuropsychological assessment of children, accuracy of identification of specific subtypes of learning problems, identification and measurement of possible underlying neural mechanisms of childhood learning and behavioral disorders, and in the understanding of how these factors may interact.

Common Learning Problems in Children

Learning disorders in children (in the absence of mental retardation and/or emotional disturbance) are commonly referred to under the umbrella label of "learning disabilities." Although there has been disagreement as to whether "learning disability" constitutes a homogeneous or heterogeneous diagnostic entity, it was postulated early on that at least two subtypes of learning disability exist, namely, verbal and nonverbal (Johnson & Myklebust,

1971). The continuing work of such researchers as George Hynd and Byron Rourke leaves little doubt that within the categories of verbal and nonverbal learning disabilities there are varied and distinct dysfunctions that present different diagnostic patterns and require separate remedial efforts.

Within the literature "learning disability" has often been used to describe dyslexia, various expressive and receptive language disorders, differences between performance and verbal IQs, processing deficits (visual, auditory, kinesthetic, tactile), and other difficulties that interfere with a child's ability to learn when mental retardation and emotional disturbance conditions have been ruled out. Learning disabilities are thought to be related to dysfunction in the way that an individual perceives, processes, organizes, integrates, stores, and/or retrieves information. Probably the most current and widely used classification system for learning disabilities (and for behavior disorders and emotional disturbances as well) is the American Psychiatric Association's fourth edition of the *Diagnostic and Statistical Manual of Mental Disorders* (DSM-IV) (APA, 1994). Within this system learning disabilities are presented as specific, but not exclusive, developmental disorders that are identifiable through the comparison of achievement test scores and IQs. A diagnosis of one of the learning disorders described in the DSM-IV can be made only after ruling out lack of educational opportunity, poor teaching, cultural factors, impaired vision or hearing, and mental retardation as primary causes for the child's learning difficulties.

ELIZABETH MURDOCH JAMES • Department of Educational Psychology, Texas A&M University, College Station, Texas 77843. **MARION SELZ** • Carondelet Rehabilitation Services of Arizona, Tucson, Arizona 85716-5528.

At present, the DSM-IV offers no further definition of what constitutes a learning disability; it merely divides them into one of five categories: reading, mathematics, written expression, motor skills, and communication disorders. Using neuropsychological techniques and instruments, researchers (e.g., Fletcher, 1985; Rourke, 1985) have obtained results that have allowed them successfully to subdivide these five broad categories of disability into functional subtypes, and enabled them to make appropriate recommendations for remediation of each subtype of disability.

To date, much of the neuropsychological research investigating learning deficiencies has been conducted with adult subjects. It is assumed that adults have had enough schooling and experience to have mastered basic skills, that acquired lesions are interfering with communication of information from one area of the cerebral cortex to another, and that those lesions are therefore responsible for the deficits in academic skills (McCarthy & Warrington, 1990). When studying learning problems in children it is necessary to remember that part of what may appear to be a deficit may in fact reflect lack of instruction or practice with that particular skill, or motivational and emotional difficulties (Strang & Rourke, 1985).

Utility of Neuropsychological Assessment of Learning Disabilities

One of the first studies designed to test the utility of neuropsychological assessment with children with learning disabilities was conducted by Doehring (1968). He compared 39 boys between the ages of 10 and 14 who were disabled in reading but otherwise normal, with a control group of 39 boys with intact reading skills. Doehring found that the normal readers were significantly superior to the disabled readers on 62 out of 103 measures, and that the pattern of deficit included visual and verbal impairment. The disabled readers were superior to the normal readers on several measures using somesthetic input. Two experienced neuropsychologists gave subjects blind ratings of "no cerebral dysfunction" or "definite cerebral dysfunction." The trend for the judges to rate the normal subjects as having no cerebral impairment and the disabled readers as having definite cerebral impairment was significant. Here was evidence for the usefulness of neuropsychological assessment, objective and subjective in nature, in differentiating learning-disabled from nondisabled children.

Reitan and Boll (1973) also used objective and subjective analysis to distinguish children of varying abilities when they evaluated the neuropsychological correlates of minimal brain dysfunction (MBD; an earlier term for what we now call learning disabilities) in children 5 to 8 years of age. Their study examined four groups of approximately 25 children each. The categories were (1) normal controls, (2) brain-damaged, (3) children with MBD whose primary referral was related to academic problems, and (4) children with MBD who were described as having mainly behavioral problems in the classroom. The test results were subjected to statistical and clinical analysis (i.e., a blind overall judgment of whether each child appeared to have normal, mildly impaired, or abnormal brain function). Results indicated that children in the control group generally earned the highest scores on the neuropsychological tasks, the children with documented brain damage earned the lowest scores, and the two groups of children with MBD usually scored somewhere in between. The brain-damaged groups consistently performed significantly more poorly that the other three groups, but the differences between the two MBD groups and the control subjects generally were not significant. The blind judgment analysis was also able to distinguish between the groups. Using only the test protocols, Reitan identified correctly 64% of the normal children, approximately 85% of the MBD subjects (averaging the two groups), and 96% of the brain-damaged children.

Selz (1977) designed a research project in which she addressed the neuropsychological differences between children who function normally, children diagnosed with learning disabilities, and children with documented brain damage. She found significant differences between the three groups. Using analysis of variance on 3 summary IQ scores and 10 neuropsychological measures, she found significant ($p < 0.01$ and $p < 0.015$) differences between the groups on 12 of 13 measures. T-test comparisons indicated that the children with learning disabilities performed in a relatively normal manner on measures with a strong motor component. Their performance resembled that of the children with brain damage on tests with strong cognitive or attentional demands. A discriminant analysis that used all 13 measures classified subjects according to group membership with 80% accuracy. The 20% classification errors tended to be in the direction of classifying subjects as less impaired than their group membership implied (Selz & Reitan, 1979).

Studies by Rourke (1975; Rourke & Finlayson, 1978) also indicated that neuropsychological instruments could be used to distinguish children with learning disabilities from those without, specifically in the area of reading. Results of a 4-year longitudinal study comparing performances of children with and without reading disabilities showed that differences between the groups in their auditory–verbal and language abilities were consistent during the entire period, while differences in reading achievement grew with time. Initial significant differences on tests of visual motor coordination (e.g., Grooved Pegboard Test) did not continue through the fourth year, whereas initial insignificant differences on the Halstead Category Test became significant with the passage of time.

Rourke reported that his results supported the hypothesis that reading disabilities were likely associated with other neuropsychological deficits. The finding that children with reading disabilities did not "catch up" with their peers over the 4-year period but, in fact, fell further behind in reading achievement was seen to support the neurological deficit theory of learning disabilities, rather than the theory that learning disabilities are caused by developmental lags. Although Rourke's laboratory would also come up with evidence of developmentally related features of reading disability in children (Fisk & Rourke, 1978), later support for the neurological deficit hypothesis would also come out of his laboratory (see Rourke, Young, & Leenaars, 1989) when it was shown that learning disabilities often persist into adolescence and adulthood despite efforts at remediation and sufficient developmental time for the "lags" to ameliorate. Recent evidence indicates that a combination of the two theories may be the most accurate.

Subtypes of Learning Disability

Once it became clear that neuropsychological assessment and analysis could be used to differentiate children with learning disabilities from those without learning disabilities, researchers began to show an interest in discovering whether neuropsychological measures could assist them in the further differentiation of subtypes of learning disability. More recent application of neuropsychological analysis centers on attempts to do just that—to delineate categories of learning disability into functional subtypes. Common methods of data analysis include clinical assessment of patterns of performance (e.g., visual inspection of protocols,

right–left differences, performance levels and patterns, and pathognomonic signs) and multivariate statistical analyses of research results (e.g., cluster and Q-analyses of assessment results). Both clinical and statistical analyses have strengths, shortcomings, and a place in this type of research, but it is through the use of the more objective statistical analyses that most reported conclusions from this research have been reached (Fletcher & Satz, 1985).

Earlier investigations into the performance of children with learning disabilities on the Wechsler Intelligence Scale for Children (WISC; Wechsler, 1949) found a pattern of performance called the ACID pattern, so named because of poor performance on the Arithmetic, Coding, Information, and Digit Span subtests (Ackerman, Dykman, & Peters, 1976). Although some researchers believed this pattern to be typical of all children with learning disabilities (e.g., Swartz, 1974), subsequent research has found that the ACID pattern is not "individually characteristic" in the majority of children with learning disabilities, and it is not indicative of similarities in processing deficits in the children who do display its pattern (Joschko & Rourke, 1985, p. 67). Joschko and Rourke (1985) found at least two subtypes *within* the groups of children who exhibited the ACID pattern, one with poor tactile–perceptual, visual–perceptual, and motor skills and the other with poor sequencing skills.

Testing the hypothesis that cerebral dominance and organization as reflected in handedness might be useful in identification of subtypes of learning disability, Del Dotto and Rourke (1985) analyzed performance of left-handed versus right-handed children on various neuropsychological measures and the WISC. Although seven identifiable subtypes emerged, handedness in and of itself was not an important factor on which subtypes of learning disability could be based. The authors concluded that left-handedness "should be viewed as a 'red herring' not worthy of the pathognomonic importance attributed to it" (p. 125).

Neuropsychological assessment was used successfully by other researchers in their attempts to learn more about the nature of learning disabilities (e.g., Fletcher, 1985; Doehring, Trites, Patel, & Fiedorowicz, 1981; Sweeney & Rourke, 1978). Lyon, Stewart, and Freeman (1982), Lyon and Watson (1981), Rourke (1978), and Satz and Morris (1981), among many others, divided learning disabilities into functional subtypes.

TABLE 1. Examples of Functional Learning Disability Subgroups

Author	Group	Characteristics
Rourke (1978, 1983)	1	"Auditory–linguistic dyslexia" PIQ > VIQ; good visual–spatial skills, nonverbal concept formation; average motor and tactile functioning; delay in speech onset; language and expressive speech deficits; poor reading, spelling, especially phonologically; good math
	2	VIQ > PIQ; normal oral language and auditory perception; poor visual–spatial, motor, and tactile abilities; poor nonverbal concept formation; good phonetic analysis/synthesis of unknown words; poor reading, spelling; good auditory memory; poor visual memory
	3	VIQ = PIQ; poor sequential processing; poor auditory memory and visual memory; poor reading and spelling; poor phonological skills
Satz & Morris (1981)	1	Language dysfunction; average nonverbal perception
	2	Poor verbal fluency
	3	Overall neuropsychological impairment
	4	"Visual–perceptual–motor" nonverbal deficits
	5	Normal neuropsychological profile
Lyon & Watson (1981)	1	Auditory + visual deficits
	2	Mixed deficits
	3	Receptive, expressive language deficits
	4	Visual perceptual deficits
	5	Poor auditory sequential memory
	6	Normal profile

One of the most comprehensive, methodologically sound, and best known series of studies using neuropsychological measures to subtype learning disabilities has been conducted by Rourke and associates from 1975 through the present. In these studies Rourke investigated reading, spelling, writing, and arithmetic disabilities. Initially, he sought to determine if any or all of these deficits were the result of brain dysfunction (Rourke, 1975). Results of this series of studies has led Rourke to more specific conclusions regarding learning disability subtypes. Distinctions between verbal and nonverbal learning disabilities include differences in their academic and social presentations, as well as their possible etiologies. Children with receptive and expressive verbal learning disabilities are likely to present with dysfunction in the areas of reading, spelling, and writing, all skills believed to be subsumed largely by the hemisphere that is dominant for language. In the majority of the population this is the left hemisphere. Nonverbal learning disabilities primarily involve dysfunctions of spatial orientation, arithmetic, and social perception and skill, all of which are believed to be under the control of the hemisphere that is nondominant for language—most often the right hemisphere. Neuropsychological, neuroanatomical, and electrophysiological findings differ between disability subtypes, academic areas, and age groups.

Verbal Learning Disabilities

Learning difficulties for which a psycholinguistic basis is hypothesized are sometimes referred to as "verbal learning disabilities" and/or "left hemisphere-mediated learning disabilities." Included therein are reading, spelling, and writing disabilities. Deficits in visual, auditory, and motor perception and processing, as well as any combination of the three, have all been implicated in such learning disabilities.

Reading Disability/Developmental Dyslexia

Dyslexia is a reading disorder in which specific language deficits are most prominent, including deficits involving phonological awareness, analysis, synthesis, and memory (Denckla, 1993). Children with this disorder have normal IQs, but may be slow readers or nonreaders. Although Denckla describes "pure" dyslexics as children who are able to attend to stimuli, use learning strategies to their advantage, and develop skills that can compensate for their reading difficulties, she also acknowledges that most reading disorders are *not* "pure," but reside in children who have other difficulties that contribute to their reading dysfunction (e.g., attention deficit disorder with or without hyperactivity).

Denckla (1993) makes specific the definition of a neurologically based reading disability, indicating that the current DSM-IV guidelines for such a diagnosis are inadequate and unacceptable. If one is to speak of reading disability in terms of neurological dysfunction, then a significantly depressed score on a reading achievement test relative to IQ is not enough. Socioemotional factors will have to be ruled out and brain dysfunction will have to be ruled in. Developmental dyslexia is a term often used in an effort to make the distinction between a neurologically based disability which can have an environmental or genetic basis (Pennington, 1991), and reading disability diagnosed from low reading scores on achievement tests and/or low reading achievement resulting from low IQ. Earlier definitions of dyslexia included dysfunctional reading most often accompanied by difficulties in the areas of speech and language, gross and fine motor skills, spatial perception, directionality, temporal orientation, color-naming, social perception, spelling, and cerebral dominance (Yule & Rutter, 1976).

The study of subtypes of reading disability has been ongoing since at least the 1960s when researchers found different patterns of reading dysfunction among children with visual and/or auditory processing deficits (Ingram, 1960; Johnson & Myklebust, 1967) with genetic or environmental causes (Bannatyne, 1966). The 1970s saw a wide variety of research into possible single causes of a homogeneous reading disability and included studies involving visual and auditory processes and association, phonological processes, language processes, memory, neurological functioning, developmental factors, and genetic factors (see Doehring *et al.*, 1981). Other research in the 1970s involved actual subtyping of dyslexics into such categories as dysphonetic, dyseidetic (Boder, 1973), articulation-graphomotor dyscoordination (Mattis, French, & Rapin, 1975), global-mixed language disorder, anomic-repetition disorder, correlational disorder, dysphonemic sequencing disorder (Denckla, 1979), inner-language dyslexia, auditory dyslexia, visual–verbal agnosia, intermodal/crossmodal dyslexia (Myklebust, 1978), auditory–linguistic disorder, visual–spatial disorder (Pirozzolo, 1979), intermodal association disorder, and sequential relations disorder (Doehring & Hoshko, 1977). One of the first researchers to study reading disabilities and their subtypes extensively was Donald Doehring.

Doehring has conducted research into the nature of reading disabilities since the 1960s. His study with Hoshko (1977) and with Trites, Patel, and Fiedorowicz (1981) revealed three subtypes of disabled readers. In the 1977 study using 88 subjects, subtype 1 (38%) was characterized by "readers who were particularly poor in the oral reading of letters, nonsense syllables, and words, relative to their silent reading skills" (Doehring, 1985, p. 134). Subtype 2 members (25%) read slowly and made many mistakes. Subtype 3 children (19%) were better able to read single letters than to read words or syllables during either silent or oral reading. The rest of the sample (18%) presented with "mild reading problems" and were left unclassified.

Doehring *et al.* (1981) then administered language and neuropsychological tests to these children. Results of the neuropsychological measures revealed not unexpected results. The entire sample performed deficiently on the Verbal subtests of the WISC, and on tasks measuring finger agnosia, finger-tapping speed, and grip strength. After several statistical analyses and blind clinical evaluations of subject profiles the authors hypothesized that some reading and nonreading/neuropsychological abilities were possibly associated with each other. Although these findings were not as clear as the investigators had hoped, some "provisional interpretation(s)" were presented (Doehring, 1985, p. 137). Children who had difficulty reading orally did not exhibit any clear signs of brain dysfunction, but could be subdivided into groups that exhibited naming deficits, auditory–verbal short-term memory deficits, and poor motor planning and coordination. Children who read slowly did have signs of underlying brain dysfunction. Those children who presented with letter sequencing difficulties in reading tasks did not exhibit sequencing deficits on nonreading tasks, but performed in a manner that indicated they may have had visual–perceptual difficulties that would be mediated by the posterior bilateral areas of the cortex (Doehring, 1985). Doehring explained that the choice of tasks and subjects may have contributed to the lack of definitive evidence of relationships between reading subtypes and specific neuropsychological findings in this study.

Based on results of neuropsychological testing, Petrauskas and Rourke (1979) identified three subtypes of reading disability in a sample of 133 seven- and eight-year-olds with reading disability.

Briefly, the subtypes exhibited (1) language difficulties with intact visual–motor skills; (2) sequencing, visual memory, and finger identification difficulties; and (3) language and concept formation difficulties and poor visual–motor skills. As a result of ongoing research examining these subtypes, Rourke and Strang (1983) were able to take subtyping a step further and postulated cortical areas implicated in these subtypes. They hypothesized that subtype 1 exhibited dysfunction that was likely mediated by the left temporal lobe, subtype 2 by the left angular gyral area, and subtype 3 by the left frontal lobe.

Interhemispheric Processing and Temporal Aspects of Dyslexia

Dysfunctional interhemispheric processing that leads to disrupted communication between cerebral hemispheres has been suggested as a possible underlying cause of dyslexia. Banich and Shenker (1994) note that if such dysfunction does exist, it could mean that the perception of the form of a letter by the right hemisphere would not be passed correctly to the left hemisphere where phonological processing occurs. They cite studies in which interhemispheric dysfunction in dyslexics has been found during bimanual motor tasks (e.g., Gladstone, Best, & Davidson, 1989) and offer the hypotheses that (1) interhemispheric dysfunction may be a marker for, rather than a cause of, dyslexia, (2) poor motor coordination may be one indicator of a more global deficit in temporal processing that has been found to affect dyslexics, and (3) bimanual motoric processing may be linked specifically to language processing through temporal control mechanisms. (See also Wolff, 1993.)

Poor motor coordination in the form of poor oculomotor control, erratic eye movements, and abnormal visual processes in dyslexics have been hypothesized and reported by many other researchers (e.g., Conners, 1990; Dodgen & Pavlidis, 1990; Fowler, Riddell, & Stein, 1990; Pavlidis, 1985, 1990). Research results have implicated the parietal lobe and tectopulvinar pathway in disorders of visual persistence/attention (Conners, 1990). Lennerstrand, Ygge, and Jacobsson (1993) also report relatively poorer visual acuity at high levels in dyslexics than in controls, which, the authors hypothesize, may indicate visual system differences in processing transient and sustained stimuli.

Other researchers have examined reading dysfunction from the related area of temporal sequen-

tial processing of visual information (see Tallal, Galaburda, Llinas, & von Euler, 1993, for comprehensive coverage). Basing their research on the observations that decoding deficits and poor sound-symbol awareness underlie dyslexic dysfunction, that language development precedes reading development, and that language disabilities and reading dysfunction often co-occur, these researchers have reported evidence of prefrontal and parietal lobe involvement in dyslexics. Temporal processing of rapid incoming transient information has been hypothesized to be slower in dyslexic children, hindering them in their efforts to process and integrate incoming phonological and linguistic information at a rate fast enough to allow them to read. This "dyschronia" (Llinas, 1993) involves the disruption of rapid central nervous system communication, and includes difficulties with elements of the visual system, subcortical structures, and neurochemical interactions at a most basic, even cellular (Galaburda & Livingstone, 1993) level.

Neuroanatomical Findings

Reading disability is generally regarded as a language-based disability, and as such is believed to be mediated (in most people) by the dominant left hemisphere. Dejerine (1892) is given credit for being the first to observe the onset of reading and writing dysfunction in an adult who had a lesion to the left angular gyrus. Many subsequent studies have found anomalies in the left hemisphere functioning of dyslexics, but others have found neuroanatomical anomalies implicating different areas of the brain. Galaburda, Sherman, Rosen, Aboitiz, and Geschwind (1985) argued that the anomalies found in brains of dyslexics occurred as a result of prenatal or neonatal injury. Another hypothesis as to the origin of these anomalies is neonatal exposure to testosterone, which slows down left hemisphere maturation, creating a setting predisposed to faulty neuronal migration and organization (Geschwind & Galaburda, 1985). Geschwind based his working hypothesis in part on the greater prevalence of males identified as reading disabled. The research design, methodology, and limited samples on which Geschwind based this and other conclusions have been criticized (see Hynd & Semrud-Clikeman, 1989a). Anomalies similar to those reported by Geschwind and Galaburda have been found in female brains at postmortem (Humphreys, Kaufman, & Galaburda, 1990), and other studies have called into question the effect of gender on neuropsychological functioning (see Damasio, Tranel, Spradling, & Alliger, 1989), so the underlying hypothesis of a testosterone catalyst may be in question also.

McCarthy and Warrington (1990) indicate that studies of adults with acquired dyslexia have implicated the posterior regions of the left hemisphere, specifically in the parietotemporal region, in various forms of dyslexia. Some patients also have involvement of the angular gyrus, parieto-occipital area, and subcortical structures.

Postmortem studies of individuals who were dyslexic have found dysplastic and ectopic anomalies in the left parietal lobe, both temporal lobes, and corpus callosum (Drake, 1968), left planum temporale (Galaburda & Kemper, 1979), and medial geniculate nucleus and lateral posterior thalamic nucleus (Galaburda & Eidelberg, 1982). Although differences in normal brain asymmetry (see section on Electrophysiological Findings below) in the area of the planum temporale and parieto-occipital cortex were found to occur more frequently in the brains of dyslexics than in the general population, there is also evidence that close to 20% of the population studied at postmortem who also exhibited this structural anomaly were not dyslexic (Hynd & Hooper, 1992), calling into question the relationship between abnormal brain asymmetry and dyslexia.

Galaburda *et al.* (1985) reported dysplasias and ectopias in the form of abnormally placed neurons and disorganized cortical layering in the left frontal, left temporal, and right frontal cortex, as well as in the medial geniculate nucleus and posterior thalamic nuclei in postmortems of five adult male dyslexics. The medial geniculate nucleus and posterior thalamic nuclei have connections with the auditory and parietal areas of the cortex, and have been postulated to be involved in the linguistic and auditory processing deficits (e.g., rapid naming tasks, dichotic listening) often seen in dyslexics (Hynd & Semrud-Clikeman, 1989a). Hynd and Semrud-Clikeman (1989a) point out the importance of the bilateral frontal findings in the Galaburda *et al.* (1985) study, noting that both frontal lobes function to regulate several behaviors that are crucial to functional language and reading ability: sustained attention, regulation of emotional tone, prosody, set shifting, and planning. The interhemispheric processing hypotheses discussed by Banich and Shenker (1994) point to the likelihood that both inter- and intrahemispheric communication are necessary for such behaviors to occur, and that neither hemisphere alone is likely to be able to handle the complicated processes that are involved in language and reading. An earlier study by Hynd, Hynd, Sullivan, and Kingsbury (1987) would appear to support such a contention. They measured regional cerebral blood flow in children who were reading narrative text and found that both right and left central and posterior cortical areas were activated during the task.

Electrophysiological Findings

Brain imaging and postmortem studies have shown that most normal brains have smaller left frontal than right frontal regions (Weinberger, Luchins, Morihisa, & Wyatt, 1982), larger left anterior speech regions and auditory cortices, larger left posterior thalami (Eidelberg & Galaburda, 1982), larger left posterior than right posterior regions (LeMay, 1981), and larger left plana temporale (superior posterior area of the temporal lobe) (Geschwind & Levitsky, 1968). [The left posterior areas and plana temporale are believed to be necessary for the processing of the visual–spatial and neurolinguistic aspects of reading (Hynd & Hynd, 1984).] Hynd and Hooper (1992) reviewed nine studies that used computerized tomography (CT) or magnetic resonance imaging (MRI) to test the hypotheses that predicted reversed asymmetry or lack of normal symmetry in brains of individuals with reading difficulties. Results of these studies revealed no gross malformations, but specific anomalies led their authors to conclude that dyslexic brains are less asymmetric than normal brains, and further suggested that reversed or lessened asymmetry in the posterior regions, specifically in the planum temporale, adversely affect language processing. However, results of most of these studies are questionable given the poor methodology used in many of them (Semrud-Clikeman, Hynd, Novey, & Eliopulos, 1991), as well as the small sample size (often a case study of one) on which conclusions are based. Although there are studies that offer proof of differences in the brain asymmetry of some dyslexics, the lack of corroboration and agreement among studies, as well as the methodological flaws in those studies lead to the conclusion that, at present, there is no definitive proof that the brains of dyslexics are more or less asymmetric than those of nondyslexics.

In an attempt to perform a study in the absence of the methodological flaws of many CT and MRI studies, Semrud-Clikeman *et al.* (1991) undertook a study in which children were carefully diagnosed and placed in one of three subgroups: dyslexic,

ADD/H, or normal. MRI findings showed that the dyslexic children had smaller anterior regions than the other groups, rather than the expected smaller posterior regions. Reversed asymmetry in the anterior region correlated with poor performance on word attack tasks, though passage comprehension was not affected. Reversed or symmetric plana temporale were related to poor verbal comprehension skills. The researchers concluded that reversed asymmetry alone may not account for dyslexia, but may interact with a smaller anterior region in general to result in reading disability.

Hynd and Semrud-Clikeman (1989a,b) reviewed the body of literature reporting electrophysiological studies of dyslexics and noted that, although findings are neither conclusive nor consistent, there is some evidence that there is a greater incidence of brain symmetry in the dyslexic population (particularly left-handed dyslexics), that electrical activity in the language areas of the brain of dyslexics is less focused and organized, and that there are more anomalies in the left frontal and perisylvian regions of dyslexics.

When measuring event-related potentials in children with reading disabilities, lower P3 and Pc amplitudes have been found in the area of the parieto-occipital area when the children were exposed to word stimuli (Holcomb, Ackerman, & Dykman, 1985). The authors note that these amplitudes measure late activity (> 500 ms) during information processing (e.g., after word perception has taken place), indicating that the reading-disabled children in their study "made inefficient use of attentional resources with regard to lexical processing" (p. 665). In related research, Fawcett et al. (1993) found that children with dyslexia experienced a "temporal processing speed deficit" (p. 344) in P3 latency on tasks requiring them to make a choice dependent on specific auditory input. The authors conclude that children with dyslexia have processing deficits when presented with nonlinguistic stimuli as well as when presented with reading tasks.

PET was used by Gross-Glenn et al. (1990) to compare cerebral metabolic activity in a group of male right-handed dyslexics with controls when performing a word-reading task. Their findings indicate that reading is an activity in which several brain areas are involved to a greater or lesser extent. For both groups the prestrite cortex (believed to be involved in visual discrimination processes) and the inferior frontal cortex (involvement with reading comprehension) were significantly more activated than other cortical areas. Dyslexics showed significantly less activity in the area between the frontal and temporal lobes (peri-insular cortex), which, the authors note, is a region that is believed to be involved in language functioning. Dyslexic subjects showed greater activation in the midtemporal and lingual gyri, areas that are necessary for visual discrimination. The authors speculate that the higher level of activation may be related to the greater difficulty dyslexics have with visual discrimination tasks, which requires them to exert greater effort during those tasks. Dyslexic readers showed less asymmetry of activity in the frontal cortex, which may be related to specific fields of oculomotor control.

In a study that would appear to support the contention that dyslexics have greater difficulty with certain tasks, but that they do not maintain a greater attentional focus on such activities, Mattson, Sheer, and Fletcher (1992) reported differences in electroencephalograms (EEG) for children with reading disability relative to controls and to a group of children with arithmetic disability. Children with reading disability had less left hemisphere EEG activity (40 Hz) during a verbal task, possibly indicating their "inability to efficiently activate left hemisphere processing systems" (p. 714). Attentional focus in children with dyslexia has been of some interest to researchers, and has led to studies in which the performances of children with primary dysfunction in both areas (i.e., attention and reading) have been compared.

Dyslexia and ADD/H

Though arguments that ADD/H and learning disabilities are distinct and separate conditions appear to have been made with some conviction (e.g., Barkley, 1981), researchers continue to be intrigued by the co-occurence of these disorders (e.g., Robins, 1992). While it is less often the case that children with a primary diagnosis of ADD/H have the additional diagnosis of dyslexia, it is commonplace to find studies in which children diagnosed as reading disabled also exhibit behaviors characteristic of ADD/H to a great extent (e.g., Halperin, Gittelman, Klein, & Rudel, 1984; Shaywitz & Shaywitz, 1988). Conversely, there are also a few studies in which a great majority of the children diagnosed with ADD/H were also given the diagnosis of learning disabled, suggesting comorbidity of the disorders (McGee & Share, 1988; McGee, Williams, Moffitt, & Anderson, 1989), and other studies where no relationship between the two conditions was found (Dalby, 1985). Pennington notes that it may be the case that the symptoms of ADD/H (e.g., inattention, distractibility, impulsivity) arise in dyslexics as a reaction to their academic difficulties in school rather than from a neurological base, and may be secondary to their reading disabilities.

Pennington and his associates (reported in Pennington, 1991) undertook a series of studies in which they sought to determine the neuropsychological characteristics of children with diagnoses of ADD/H, dyslexia, or both. They found that the ADD/H group had significantly more indicators of executive dysfunction, and the dyslexic group had significantly more indicators of phonological dysfunction, signifying the separateness of the two disorders. The children diagnosed with both conditions performed as did the dyslexic group, enabling the authors to conclude that when diagnosed in the same child, dyslexia will be the primary dysfunction and ADD/H will be a secondary condition.

Additional support for the separateness of ADD/H and dyslexia comes from electrophysiological (CT and MRI) studies showing that characteristic morphological signs are found in dyslexics (e.g., reversed or symmetrical plana temporale length, smaller insula, and symmetrical frontal regions) but not in children diagnosed as ADD/H or normal (Semrud-Clikeman et al., 1991). Event-related potentials between the two groups have also been found to be significantly different (Holcomb et al., 1985) indicating differential processing speed between them.

Methodological flaws associated with many of these and other similar studies reportedly include difficulty of obtaining samples without comorbid features of ADD/H, dyslexia, and attention deficit disorder without hyperactivity (ADD/WO), inaccuracies in identification of children as ADD/WO or ADD/H, co-occurrence of conduct disorder in ADD/WO and ADD/H samples, use of inappropriate assessment instruments, use of neuropsychological batteries of questionable construct validity, influence of IQ, and problems in diagnostic definition (Goodyear & Hynd, 1992; McGee et al., 1989). Given that such far-reaching flaws may be present in the aforementioned research, the question of the separateness of dyslexia, ADD/WO, and ADD/H would still appear to be open.

Spelling Disabilities

Disorders involving sequencing of sounds and/or letters were first reported by Gerstmann (1927). These disorders typically involve letter or-

der, additions, omissions, substitutions, and a pattern of misspelling specific to a particular part of a work (e.g., initial, medial, or ending), and are greatly affected by word length (Dubois, Hécaen, & Marcie, 1969; Hillis & Caramazza, 1989; Kinsbourne & Warrington, 1963). Spelling disorders may also become evident only in situations where a child is asked to spell using a specific modality (e.g., orally or in writing).

Spelling disabilities have been subtyped by examining the pattern of errors a child makes while attempting to encode words. Types of errors have been categorized as phonetically accurate, phonetically inaccurate, disorders of sequencing sounds and letters, and modality-specific impairments (McCarthy & Warrington, 1990). (oral vs written)

Several studies have attempted to analyze neuropsychological aspects of spelling errors from the point of view of their degree of phonetic accuracy. The impetus for this line of research emerged from clinical interactions with children diagnosed as having learning disabilities and research evidence derived from studies of adults with well-documented lesions (e.g., Kinsbourne & Warrington, 1963). Consistent evidence was found that indicated the tendency for neurologically intact individuals to misspell in a phonetically accurate manner, while those individuals with lesions in areas of the left cerebral hemisphere believed to mediate language tended to spell in a phonetically inaccurate manner. Studies conducted by Newcombe (1969) and Nelson and Warrington (1974) found a positive relationship between spelling disability characterized by phonetically inaccurate errors and a general impairment in language functioning. A study conducted by Boder (1973) demonstrated a positive relationship between spelling performances characterized by an excess of phonetic accuracy (indicative of auditory memory skill) and poor memory for how words looked (visual memory). In other words, subjects who were unable to revisualize words in order to spell them were able to reauditorize words and spelled them phonetically.

Rourke and colleagues investigated the nature of errors and possible underlying neuropsychological functioning in phonetically accurate and inaccurate spellers. The subjects for the first study conducted by Sweeney and Rourke (1978) were children at age levels corresponding to grades four (mean age ~ 9.5 years) and eight (mean age ~ 13 years). There were three groups: a control group consisting of normal spellers (N), a group of phonetically inaccurate (PI) spellers, and a group of phonetically accurate (PA) spellers.

Results from performances on neuropsychological, intelligence, and achievement tests indicated that the PIs were inferior to the PAs and the Ns on most measures of psycholinguistic ability at the older (grade eight) age level, and that the basic psycholinguistic skills of the older PAS were essentially equivalent to the Ns. More specifically, PAs performed at a level equivalent to Ns and superior to PIs on the Verbal Fluency Test and WISC Similarities and Arithmetic subtests. PAs performed at a level inferior to Ns but superior to PIs on the Peabody Picture Vocabulary Test (PPVT), and at a level inferior to Ns and equivalent to PIs on the Comprehension, Vocabulary, and Information subtests of the WISC.

The authors concluded that, for the older group, PIs were linguistically disabled at a very basic level when receptive operations were required, and that this likely had great effect on development of their language skills. They noted the similarity between the performance of the PIs in their study and the performance of the adult patients of Luria (1980) who had lesions in the secondary zones of their left temporal lobe.

It was concluded further that though they had significant difficulties in using visual memory to spell correctly, "in relating the verbal information provided with other information, and encoding relatively complex word strings in response to verbal information provided" (Sweeney & Rourke, 1985, p. 154), older PAs were less likely to sustain severe disturbances in their overall language development. The authors compared the PAs' dysfunction to that of others of Luria's adult patients (1980) who had sustained lesions in the tertiary zone (area of the angular gyrus) of the left hemisphere.

Results for the younger group (grade four) revealed no significant differences on tasks other than the arithmetic subtest of the Wide Range Achievement Test (WRAT). This subtest differentiated the three groups, with the PIs exhibiting the poorest performance. The authors posited that these results suggested that one important deficiency in the PIs at this age level might be their inability to benefit from formal instruction in the use of rules and logical grammatical reasoning. This possibility prompted further analysis of these same fourth-grade subjects (Sweeney, McCabe, & Rourke, 1978) in which their performance on the Logico-Grammatical Sentence Comprehension Test (Wiig & Semel, 1974) was compared. The results indicated that PIs were significantly inferior to Ns in their logical grammatical reasoning. Although PAs performed at a level superior to PIs and inferior to Ns, such differences were not significant. This led the researchers to conclude that younger PIs have significant difficulties in dealing with basic linguistic operations, and they therefore have more difficulty in benefiting from formal academic instruction which is largely language based (Sweeney & Rourke, 1985).

Coderre, Sweeney, and Rourke (1979) went on to test their conclusions about PIs, as well as their suspicions that PAs had difficulty answering questions or performing operations when they were required to generate information to do so. The authors used tests of phonetic segmentation, spelling recognition, visual memory, and a cloze procedure to further assess the functioning of a younger group of spellers (ages 9–11). Results supported earlier findings, and indicated that significantly different performances on the cloze procedure and spelling recognition tasks followed the pattern: PIs < PAs < Ns. The same pattern held for performance on the visual memory tasks, but the differences were not significant. The phonetic segmentation task wherein children were to break an intact spoken word into phonemic subunits resulted in an unexpected different pattern: PIs <Ns < PAs. Coderre et al. concluded that PAs may have outperformed Ns on this task as a result of adhering strictly to (over)learned phonetic rules.

Neuroanatomical Findings

McCarthy and Warrington (1990) note that spelling is widely believed to be subserved by the posterior areas of the left hemisphere. Specific types of spelling deficits have been linked to different areas of the cortex. Spelling by sound (i.e., phonetically accurate spelling) is believed to be subserved by the parietal lobe. Roeltgen and Heilman (1984) and Baxter-Versi (1987) reported that lesions of the area comprising the juncture of the angular gyrus and the parieto-occipital lobe, in adults, resulted in a deficit in phonetically accurate spelling. Spelling errors that result from phonetic inaccuracy (without impairment of sight word spelling) are also believed to be subserved by the parietal lobes, but in the areas near the supramarginal gyrus, at times extending into the temporal lobe (Baxter & Warrington, 1985; Kremin, 1987; Roeltgen & Heilman, 1984).

Spelling disorders that involve sequencing difficulties were postulated by Gerstmann (1927) to be mediated by the left parietal lobe as well. McCarthy and Warrington (1990) cite studies involving three patients that led them to hypothesize that misspellings that cluster at a particular site in a word (e.g., the beginning or left margin of a word) may be indicative of a neglect syndrome in which the contralateral hemisphere is lesioned.

Writing Disability

Although closely aligned with spelling and reading, disabilities in writing can be manifested uniquely. Berninger, Mizokawa, and Bragg (1991) describe writing as a process whose end product may be constrained by neuropsychological, linguistic, and cognitive factors. Neuropsychological factors that are basic to beginning writing skills include visual memory and retrieval of letters, maturity and integrity of the motor system, and visual–motor integration. Deficits in these areas may result in ideational agraphia and spatial agraphia. Linguistic factors (e.g., writing sentences and paragraphs) and cognitive factors (e.g., planning and revising) are believed to interfere with writing at a later stage of development (Berninger et al., 1991).

Ideational agraphia is said to be present in situations in which a writer is unable to call up from memory the correct way to form letters or words when asked to write from dictation, but is able to successfully copy written text (McCarthy & Warrington, 1990). Zangwill (1954) described an adult patient with a glioma in his left parietal lobe who, despite being able to spell and recite the alphabet orally, was unable to successfully write the alphabet. Substitutions and poorly formed letters occurred during writing, and the end product of writing to dictation was unreadable. Similar cases are reported involving severe disability in spontaneous writing, dictated writing, and writing of individual letters (Baxter & Warrington, 1986; Crary & Heilman, 1988). Some patients appear to have difficulty related to production of cursive versus printed letters, and uppercase versus lowercase letters (Patterson & Wing, 1989).

Results of studies analyzing the writing of children also have been reported. Using an unreferred (for special services) group of 45 kindergarten students at the end of their kindergarten year, DeBruyn, Smith, and Berninger (1985) found that the ability of these children to print the alphabet in sequence in lowercase letters correlated significantly with their spelling achievement. A reassessment of the same sample at the end of first grade produced the same results. Errors included omissions, case confusion, missequencing of letters, reversals, and substitutions (Berninger & Alsdorf, 1989). Aware of the shortcomings and criticisms that could be leveled at such a study (e.g., age, developmental, and curricular factors), Berninger et al. (1991) reported that many older children in grades two to nine referred for writing difficulties also were found to be unable to write the alphabet correctly in 1 minute or less. This sample also exhibited retracings of letters and an apparent need to vocalize while writing the alphabet. The authors concluded that these older children may not have fully internalized the motor pattern needed to write the letters of the alphabet, and also may have needed to vocalize to assist them in retrieving the imprint of the letters from their visual memory.

Integrity of the motor system has been linked to the presence of neurological soft signs revealed through analysis of finger movements. Although use of finger tasks to predict reading achievement has come under fire (Fletcher, Taylor, Morris, & Satz, 1982), such tasks are viewed by some researchers as having some value in uncovering neuropsychological deficits in children that may interfere with the motor component of writing. Neurological soft signs related to finger movement tend to be developmental in nature, and although often outgrown, their presence at an earlier age may limit the abilities of a young child, and have a subsequent impact on that child's future skills and achievement. Berninger et al. (1991) describe the inability to mirror finger and hand movements, difficulty with repetitive finger opposition, and deficits in finger localization and finger recognition tasks as possible indicators of neurological dysfunction that may interfere with a child's ability to perform the fine motor functions needed to write. Visual–motor integration, which is also implicated in writing disability, also was measured in this study. Difficulties with completion of the Beery Test of Visual-Motor Integration (Beery, 1982) were found to be correlated with spelling achievement at the end of kindergarten and first grade.

Spatial agraphia is present when children are unable to orient their writing properly. Errors indicative of neurological dysfunction may include poor spacing between words, crowding of words onto one side of the page, sloping lines of text, and malformation of letters (Hécaen & Marcie, 1974). Difficulties in spatial awareness and organization also have been linked to nonverbal learning disabilities.

Neuroanatomical Findings

McCarthy and Warrington (1990) note that there is a paucity of reported cases of neurological lesion wherein writing disability is the sole finding. Researchers who have reported cases with a posited neuroanatomical basis for ideational agraphia implicate the posterior parietal regions of the language (usually the left) hemisphere, specifically the parieto-occipital region (Baxter & Warrington, 1986; Crary & Heilman, 1988; Zangwill, 1954). Spatial agraphia in the form of crowding/left- or right-side neglect was found to be associated with lesions of the contralateral hemisphere (Hécaen & Marcie, 1974).

In reporting results of studies with kindergartners, Berninger *et al.* (1991) referred to Luria's theory of Stage 4 development, which he hypothesized occurs at 5–7 years of age, the age of most children in kindergarten. At this stage the tertiary areas of the parietal, occipital, and temporal lobes are believed to be capable of communicating information received from their secondary areas. Inability of the tertiary areas to relay and subsequently integrate the needed information from the secondary areas would result in dysfunction.

Emotional Consequences of Verbal Learning Disabilities

It has been widely believed that children with learning disabilities are at greater risk than their nondisabled peers for emotional difficulties such as depression related to frustration, low self-esteem, and feelings of inadequacy. They also may be at risk from the underlying organic difficulty that causes their learning disabilities which may serve as a diathesis for emotional difficulties. Spreen (1988) points out that although children with learning disabilities are certainly at greater risk for emotional dysfunction than their nondisabled peers, positing a cause–effect relationship between learning disabilities and emotional disorders is tenuous because of the large number of interactions from several sources (e.g., environmental factors, school experiences, and severity of lesion) that impinge on the child with disabilities.

Porter and Rourke (1985) dispute the idea that children with learning disabilities are *as a group* more likely to suffer emotional disturbance than

TABLE 2. Socioemotional Functioning of Children with Learning Disabilities: Porter and Rourke's (1985) Study

Subtype	% of sample	Characteristics
1	44%	Well adjusted; balanced functioning
2	26%	Most seriously disturbed; significantly elevated scores on measures of adjustment, depression, psychosis, and social skills; comparatively higher scores on measures of anxiety and withdrawal
3	13%	Significant elevation on measure of somatic concerns
4	17%	Significantly elevated scores on measures of delinquency, adjustment, hyperactivity; comparatively elevated on measures of family relations

nondisabled children. Results of a study they conducted revealed that, as with their nondisabled peers, children with learning disabilities are heterogeneous in their emotional functioning. Porter and Rourke identified four subtypes within their sample, the largest group comprising children who were well adjusted and not in emotional distress. Other studies have been conducted in attempts to understand the kinds of emotional dysfunction that children with certain types of learning disabilities are likely to encounter, and include research conducted by Brumback and Staton (1983), Glosser and Koppell (1987), and Nussbaum and Bigler (1986).

Brumback and Staton (1983) posited that children with disorders of the left hemisphere (i.e., language-based) are more likely to encounter temporary depression that will interfere with achievement on language-intensive tasks. In a study comparing children with performance that indicated either dysfunctional left, right/bilateral, or nonlateralized learning disabilities, Glosser and Koppell (1987) reported results that indicated children with performances indicative of left-hemisphere dysfunction did exhibit higher rates of dysphoric, anxious, and socially withdrawn behaviors, and exhibited lower rates of aggression and attentional disorders.

Nussbaum and Bigler (1986) cluster-analyzed results from a population of children with learning disabilities on measures of intelligence, neurops chological functioning, behavioral functioning, and academic achievement, and derived three sub-groups. Group 1 appeared to be generally cerebrally dysfunctional, showing poorest functioning on verbal, visual–spatial, visual–constructional, and perceptual tasks. Group 2 presented with moderate levels of impairment, appearing to fit the characteristics of children with a general language disorder, and left-hemisphere deficits. Group 3 presented with minimal deficits on all but the constructional praxis task, better verbal than arithmetic performance, and appeared to fit the pattern of children with right-hemisphere deficits.

Nussbaum and Bigler report that results of two tests of emotional functioning given to these children revealed little differences between the groups, but definite difficulties for the sample as a whole. These learning-disabled children showed symptoms of depression, social withdrawal, hyperactivity, internalizing and externalizing presentation, overall maladjustment, delinquency, anxiety, psychosis, and poor social skills.

Kusche, Cook, and Greenberg (1993) presented results showing that children with verbal deficits indicative of left hemisphere dysfunction were more likely to be female and to report symptoms of anxiety, somatization, and withdrawal. They tended not to be disruptive in school and therefore went unnoticed by their teachers, and were consequently not as likely to be referred for special services as often as they should have been, given their level of verbal disabilities. This population was also much more likely than controls to suffer from depression, though they were not as severely depressed as children with right-hemisphere disabilities.

Summary

Verbal learning disabilities comprise a heterogeneous group of largely language-based disorders involving the skills and abilities needed for achievement in reading, spelling, and writing. Subtypes of disability within each of these broader categories have been demonstrated. Concomitant disorders are common from within the verbal learning disabilities group (e.g., reading and spelling disabilities occurring in the same child) and from without (e.g., ADD/H and emotional disorders occurring with reading disability in the same child). Various psycholinguistic, neuropsychological, and neuroanatomical theories as to the "why" and "how" of these dysfunctions abound in the literature. Although

areas of the posterior left hemisphere are identified most often with these difficulties, there is a large body of evidence that suggests the involvement of the right hemisphere and subcortical structures.

Nonverbal Learning Disabilities

Nonverbal learning disabilities (NLD), sometimes referred to as right hemispheric learning disabilities, are those in which reading, spelling, and writing deficits are *not* of primary importance. Rourke *et al.* (1989) describe the neuropsychological characteristics of children with NLD as involving difficulties of tactile perception (especially on the left side of the body), psychomotor coordination (especially on the left side of the body), visual–spatial organization, nonverbal problem-solving, concept formation, hypothesis testing, ability to benefit from feedback, dealing with cause–effect relationships, age-appropriate understanding of humor, adapting to new and/or complex situations, arithmetic calculation (relative to reading and spelling), language content (disordered pragmatics—"cocktail party" speech), receptive and expressive speech prosody, social perception, social judgment, and social interaction. Children with NLD have a tendency to withdraw socially, becoming social isolates, and to develop depression as a result of their difficulties with peer interaction (Fletcher, 1989; Rourke *et al.*, 1989). They have good verbal memory skills, reading (word recognition) and spelling skills, and rote learning skills and may be verbose in a "repetitive, straightforward, rote" manner (p.169). The characteristics of NLD are usually evident, and the syndrome diagnosable, in children by age 8 or 9.

Johnson and Myklebust (1971) and Myklebust (1975) provided an early description of children with NLD, describing their difficulties as being mainly ones of misperception of their environment. Myklebust (1975) believed these misperceptions interacted to create other disabilities including math dysfunction, temporal difficulties (telling time), spatial difficulties (reading maps), poor adaptive behavior, impaired self- and social perception, and impaired relationships, and coined the term "nonverbal learning disability" (Hynd & Hooper, 1992). Some authors (e.g., Pennington, 1991) also include children who have difficulties in handwriting caused by poor spatial skills. After reviewing other studies, Pennington (1991) estimated the prevalence of NLDs to be 0.1%–1.0% of the LD population, which is approximately 10% of the total population, and the sex ratio as 1.2:1, male:female.

Arithmetic Disabilities

Disabilities involving arithmetic are sometimes referred to as dyscalculia or acalculia, a term coined by Henschen in the early 1900s subsequent to his investigation of calculation skills in over 400 individuals with documented brain lesions (McCarthy & Warrington, 1990). Arithmetic disability often coexists with more language-intensive (e.g., reading, spelling, and writing) disabilities, with spatial and attentional disabilities, and with psychomotor disabilities. In fact, it has often been the case that dyscalculia was thought of as a language-based disorder, or at the very least one involving a fair amount of verbal memory (Strang & Rourke, 1985). There are studies in evidence that call this idea into question and allow arithmetic disability to stand alone as a distinct disability apart from language disabilities (Warrington, 1982).

Three subtypes of arithmetic disability were conceived by Hécaen and associates: an aphasic arithmetic disability; a spatial disability; and anarithmetia, or computational disability (Benton, 1987). McCarthy and Warrington (1990) grouped disorders of computation into two broad categories: comprehension and retrieval of numbers (which includes spoken and written number comprehension, number retrieval, and number alexia, and is infrequently reported) and calculation (which includes spatial acalculia, memory and retrieval deficits for operations and math facts, speed of processing, and problem-solving).

In order to differentiate subtypes of arithmetically disabled children, Rourke and associates undertook a series of studies (Brandys & Rourke, 1991; Ozols & Rourke, 1988, 1991; Rourke & Finlayson, 1978; Rourke & Strang, 1978; Strang & Rourke, 1983). The impetus for these studies came from results of previous research efforts by Rourke and his associates in the 1970s wherein they attempted to "determine neuropsychological significance of patterns of academic achievement" (Rourke, 1993).

In the first three studies (Rourke & Finlayson, 1978; Rourke & Strang, 1978; Strang & Rourke, 1983) a group of 45 children aged 9–14 were divided into three groups. Rourke and Finlayson (1978) administered neuropsychological tasks to these groups and found that Groups 1 and 2 performed at higher levels than Group 3 on tasks involving visual–perceptual and visual–spatial

TABLE 3. Group Membership for Rourke *et al.* Studies

Group	Relative deficiencies on WRAT[a]	IQ profiles
1	Reading, Spelling, Arithmetic	VIQ < PIQ
2	Reading, Spelling only	VIQ < PIQ
3	Arithmetic only	VIQ > PIQ

[a]All groups were impaired on Arithmetic, but groups 2 and 3 were superior in Arithmetic to group 1, and did not differ from each other in their Arithmetic abilities.

abilities (left hemisphere mediated), and Group 3 outperformed Groups 1 and 2 on tasks requiring the use of verbal and auditory–perceptual abilities (left hemisphere mediated). Since achievement test scores between Groups 2 and 3 were not significantly different, and since Group 2 did significantly outperform Group 3 on measures of visual–perceptual and visual–spatial skills, it was postulated that the underlying neurological cause of the arithmetic disability in Groups 2 and 3 was likely different. Group 2 might be expected to do poorly on arithmetic tasks because of linguistically based deficits, and Group 3 would do poorly because of impaired visual–spatial abilities.

Further testing with the same groups was undertaken next by Rourke and Strang (1978). The groups were administered neuropsychological measures designed to assess motor (e.g., Finger Tapping Test and Strength of Grip Test; Reitan & Davison, 1974), psychomotor (Maze Test, Grooved Pegboard Test; Klove, 1963; Tactual Performance Test; Reitan & Davison, 1974), and tactile–perceptual skills (Finger Agnosia, Finger-Tip Number Writing, and Coin Recognition; Reitan & Davison, 1974). Significant differences between groups were evident on complex psychomotor measures (Maze and Grooved Pegboard), with Groups 1 and 2 outperforming Group 3. Groups 1 and 3 showed right-hand superiority on the Tactual Performance Test (TPT), and Group 2 showed left-hand superiority. Groups 1 and 2 were superior to Group 3 when both hands were used on the TPT. Generally, and as expected, Group 3 was found to be deficient relative to the other groups on tasks measuring psychomotor and tactile–perceptual skills which are assumed to be right hemisphere mediated.

In 1983, Strang and Rourke sought to measure the nonverbal abstract reasoning, hypothesis testing, and cognitive flexibility of children chosen for their similarity to children in Groups 2 and 3 in th

1978 studies. Performance on the Halstead Category Test (Reitan & Davison, 1974) showed that Group 3 children performed in a distinctly inferior and age-inappropriate manner, and Group 2 children performed essentially normally. Specifically, Group 3 children performed much worse than Group 2 on subtests 4, 5, and 6, which are the most likely to tap complex visual–spatial abilities and memory. Results confirmed the hypothesis that children with arithmetic disabilities and other indicators of NLD would perform more poorly on tests designed to assess nonverbal reasoning and memory, hypothesis testing, and ability to modify behavior when given feedback.

Ozols and Rourke (1988, 1991) conducted two studies comparing the performances of 7- to 8-year-olds who fit the profile of Groups 1, 2, and 3 on the same measures as had been used in the earlier studies with 9- to 14-year-olds. These younger children performed similarly to their older cohort on tasks measuring verbal, auditory–perceptual, and visual–spatial skills. Less definitive results were found in the motor, psychomotor, and tactile–perceptual skill areas.

Rourke has successfully delineated two subtypes of arithmetic disability. Group 2 and Group 3 children are distinct and separate in their neuropsychological abilities and disabilities. Even though both groups of children are disabled in arithmetic, the underlying reasons for their disabilities are likely dissimilar. Group 2-type children experience difficulties in math as a result of reading deficits and inexperience with the material. Group 3-type children have a much more serious and pervasive arithmetic dysfunction. They tend to make mistakes seen in much younger children, indicating they may not be learning from the feedback they have received. These mistakes include errors involving spatial organization, visual detail, procedure, perseveration, graphomotor skills, memory, and judgment/reasoning (Rourke, 1993). Group 3 children demonstrate poor judgment and lack of knowledge of their own abilities by often undertaking arithmetic problems that are too difficult for them. These same children do not appear to be able to judge the reasonableness of their answers. Other studies (Fletcher & Satz, 1985; Korhonen, 1991; van der Vlugt, 1991) have found results similar to Rourke's.

Fletcher (1985) conducted a related study in which he tested groups of children with disabilities in reading/spelling, reading/spelling/arithmetic, spelling/arithmetic, and arithmetic on tasks measuring memory for verbal and nonverbal stimuli in the presence of selective reminding. He found that children with arithmetic disabilities had significantly more difficulty with memory storage and retrieval on nonverbal tasks, and children with reading disabilities had significantly more difficulty on verbal tasks, indicating that children with different learning disabilities also have differences in their memory abilities.

Emotional Consequences of NLD

Building on the discussion of the socioemotional difficulties of arithmetic-disabled children in Strang and Rourke (1985), Bigler (1989) and Rourke et al. (1989) have postulated that children with NLDs are at greater risk than their language-disabled peers for certain types of emotional disturbance and suicide related to their difficulties with social perception, judgment, interaction, and ability to use feedback to modify their behavior. NLD children are more likely to experience peer rejection, loss of self-esteem, withdrawal, and social isolation. Internalized distress leading to anxiety, depression, and in the most extreme cases, suicide attempts may follow. In their discussion of childhood depression, Hynd and Hooper (1992) review several studies (e.g., Blumberg & Izard, 1985; Brumback & Staton, 1983; Sackheim, Decina, & Malitz, 1982) in which right-hemisphere dysfunction was associated with depression. [In his review of studies examining the link between LD and emotional disorders, Spreen (1988) notes that Rourke's assignment of a higher likelihood of emotional disorder to children with arithmetic disability appears to occur only "in individual LD children" (p. 126), and very rarely.]

From her examination of 15 children with right-hemisphere lesions or dysfunctions, Voeller (1986) found that the majority of them were shy, withdrawn, isolated, and considered "weird" by peers; got into fights often as a result of pushing and crowding their classmates; and had difficulty maintaining friendships. Parents of some of the children had a difficult time understanding and getting along with their children. Five of the subjects were receiving therapy or counseling with minimal results. (It should be noted that 14/15 children were also diagnosed as having ADD with/without hyperactivity. The interaction of ADD/H with the right-hemisphere deficits almost certainly had some effect on their behavior and affective states.)

Results of Glosser and Koppell's 1987 study measuring depression/anxiety, aggression, attentional disorders, and somatization indicated that children with learning disabilities believed to be caused by right-hemisphere/bilateral dysfunction reported lower levels of depression/anxiety and higher rates of somatization than children with left-hemisphere dysfunction or nonlateralized dysfunction. The authors hypothesize that the higher somatic complaints in the right-hemisphere/bilateral group may be related to their disability in perceiving and communicating their affective discomforts, so much so that they "concretize" their emotional discomfort into "specific bodily pain or physical symptom" (p. 367). Glosser and Koppell go on to note that somatic conversion reactions have been observed to occur more frequently on the left side of the body, indicating right-hemisphere interaction.

In their 1993 study, Kusche, Cook, and Greenberg found that children with disabilities indicative of right-hemisphere dysfunction were more likely to be males who were significantly impaired, relative to a control group, in the areas of depression, frustration tolerance, social skills, and self-control. They were more likely to be referred for special education services than children with predominantly left-hemisphere/verbal learning disabilities.

Neuroanatomical Features of Children with NLDs

Difficulties in reading and writing numbers have been linked to lesions in the left parietal lobe in the region of the angular gyrus (McCarthy & Warrington, 1990). The same area has been implicated in dyscalculia (Jackson and Warrington, 1986; Levin & Spiers, 1985). It is likely that different cortical areas are involved in different types of arithmetic disability. Luria (1980) posited right-hemisphere dysfunction in cases of spatially related arithmetic disability, and bilateral dysfunction in cases of acalculia. Benton (1987) reminded readers that lesions of the occipital lobe would almost certainly have detrimental effects on arithmetic ability. Spiers (1987) noted that children with right-hemisphere damage may have very different problems in math than children with left-hemisphere damage. Children with right-hemisphere involvement may be much like Rourke's NLDs, and will exhibit deficits related to spatial difficulties and number conservation, whereas the children with left-hemisphere involvement may have difficulties in sequencing and memory for number facts. However, a study by Grafman, Passafiume, Gaflioni, and

Boller (1982) indicated that in individuals with unilateral lesions, those with left posterior lesions performed more poorly overall on calculation tasks, and made more errors of a spatial nature than did those individuals with lesions of the right posterior hemisphere.

Building on Goldberg and Costa's (1981) model and drawing on reports of arithmetic performance of children with identifiable cerebral trauma brought on by disease, congenital anomaly, or exposure to toxins, Rourke has posited that not only right-hemisphere lesions, but specifically white matter lesions in the form of "disordered myelinization and/or myelin functioning" (1993, p. 223) may be implicated in the type of arithmetic disability seen in children with NLD syndrome. Fletcher and Copeland (1988) and Shapiro, Lipton, and Krivit (1992) also posit white matter dysfunction as a contributing factor to NLDs.

Subcortical structures have also been implicated in the kinds of dysfunctional emotional abilities present in children with NLD that interfere with their social interactions. Cohen, Riccio, and Flannery (1994) reported the case of an adolescent female who had suffered a stroke to the basal ganglia of her right hemisphere. Magnetic resonance imaging showed the damage to be to the right putamen and caudate nucleus with extension into the corona radiata, but not to the cortex itself. In tasks designed to measure her receptive and expressive emotional prosody, this patient demonstrated her ability to understand emotional content of stimuli, but was unable to demonstrate her competence on tasks of repetition and expression of emotion. The authors conclude that this case study supports previous research (e.g., Cohen, Prather, Town, & Hynd, 1990; Ross & Mesulam, 1979) showing that the right hemisphere and its subcortical structures are implicated in emotional prosody.

Electrophysiological Findings in Children with NLDs

Rourke (1993) cited studies (e.g., Mattson et al., 1992; Stelmack & Miles, 1990) in which groups of children with arithmetic disabilities together with reading and spelling disabilities were differentiated from children with only arithmetic disabilities on the basis of evoked potentials. Semrud-Clikeman and Hynd (1990) reviewed several studies in which right-hemisphere cortical and subcortical functioning as measured by evoked-potential and electrical stimulation have been implicated in arithmetic calculation abilities. Adolescents who exhibit depression have been found to have an increase in EEG variance in their right hemispheres (Goldberg & Costa, 1981). Ternes, Woody, and Livingston (1987) reported the case of a boy with the features of NLD (e.g., arithmetic deficits, social dysfunction) whose EEG revealed right temporal spikes.

Mattson *et al.* (1992) provided evidence that children with arithmetic disabilities have underactivated right hemispheres (EEG ~ 40 Hz) during nonverbal tasks when compared with control and reading-disabled children. They mentioned the results of Grunau and Low's 1987 study in which the authors concluded, based on EEG activity, that arithmetic ability is dependent not strictly on right-hemisphere activity, but on communication between both hemispheres.

Summary

Children with NLDs also display difficulties in the areas of arithmetic, social perception, understanding and interactions, spatial awareness, receptive and expressive language prosody, emotional functioning, and other related areas believed to be subserved by the right cerebral hemisphere. As with verbal learning disabilities, studies have indicated more than a simple hemispheric dysfunction, and have posited communication between both hemispheres and involvement of subcortical structures as contributors to NLDs. These disabilities are believed to be more serious to the overall development of a child than verbal learning disabilities, in that the emotional difficulties that emerge in childhood are not as easily ameliorated as the academic difficulties, and have the potential to result in internalized psychopathologies that persist into adolescence and adulthood.

A Brief Look at Conduct Disorder and Other Behavioral/Emotional Disorders in Children

Conduct disorder (CD) is recognized by the DSM-IV as diagnosable and separate from other behavioral disorders. Characteristics include aggression shown to people or animals, willfull destruction of property, habitual lying, theft, and violation of rules which impair the child's social, academic, or occupational functioning (APA, 1994, pp. 90–91). Differential diagnoses include opposi-

tional–defiant disorder and ADD/H. CD is distinguished from oppositional–defiant disorder by the frequency and seriousness of the child's or adolescent's offenses. Although children with ADD/H may meet some of the criteria for CD, their behavior does not typically "violate age-appropriate societal norms" (p. 89).

Neuropsychological findings regarding children and adolescents with CD indicate that they may present with expressive language deficits (Faigel, Doak, Howard, & Sigel, 1992), academic difficulties (Hinshaw, 1992), lower than average IQs (Hirschi & Hindelang, 1977), PIQs > VIQs (Moffitt, 1992), age-inappropriate cognitive and motor skills (Werry, Elkind, & Reeves, 1987), cerebral asymmetry (Nussbaum, Bigler, Koch, & Ingram, 1988), and ADD/H (Biederman, Faraone, Keenan, & Tsuang, 1991; Hinshaw, 1994). Adolescents with CD who show deficits in executive functions subserved by the frontal lobes likely were diagnosed as both CD and hyperactive as children (Moffitt & Henry, 1989).

Kusche *et al.* (1993) reported findings from their study of 305 children (ca. 7–9 years old), 62 (20%) of whom had externalizing symptoms of CD and/or ADD without symptoms anxiety (group E), and 47 of whom (15%) had externalizing symptoms of CD and/or ADD with anxiety (group AE). The remaining children in the study were divided into a control group (56%) and a group (A) with primarily internalized pathologies in the forms of anxiety, withdrawal, and somatization. The authors administered measures of neuropsychological, emotional/behavioral (teacher and self-ratings), and intellectual functioning to these children.

Children in group E had the lowest scores on frustration tolerance, and exhibited deficits in the areas of visual perception, nonverbal understanding, depression, emotional understanding, and executive functioning. Minor motor dysfunction also was noted, implicating the motor strip of the left hemisphere. The authors posit a right-hemisphere dysfunction associated with ADD and depression. [Right-hemisphere dysfunction also has been postulated as a neurological substrate of NLD with ADD or ADD/H. Brumback and Staton (1983) proposed such an association, and Voeller (1986) found that 14 out of 15 children in her sample of children with right-hemisphere dysfunction also presented with symptoms of ADD or ADD/H.]

Children in group AE had the most significant psychopathology of all children in the sample in all areas—cognitive, emotional/behavioral, and intellectual. On measures of neuropsychological functioning, group AE earned significantly discrepant (from the other groups) scores on 10 out of 14 tasks. Depression, emotional disturbance, and left-ear preference were noted, and right-hemisphere dominance for language, as well as right-hemisphere dysfunction, were presumed. Interpretations of Kusche, Cook, and Greenberg's results with regard to children with CD must be made with caution, as both groups E and AE were composed of children not only with conduct problems but with other disorders as well.

In attempting to differentiate children diagnosed as ADD/WO from children diagnosed as ADD/H, Goodyear and Hynd (1992) noted that CD is diagnosed more frequently in children with ADD/H, who are then served in programs designed for children with behavior disorders, and oppositional–defiant disorder is diagnosed more frequently in children with ADD/WO, who are then typically served in programs for children with learning disabilities. Although their behavioral dysfunction overshadows their academic difficulties, children with CD and ADD/H do perform poorly in academic subjects, particularly in reading and spelling. Their lower academic performance tends not to be significantly lower than their IQs, precluding them from a diagnosis of learning disability.

[For more complete coverage of the neuropsychological aspects of attention, ADD/WO, and ADD/H, the reader is directed to the chapter by Carol Boliek and Jack Obrzut. For a more comprehensive review of the neuropsychological nature of childhood psychopathology the reader is referred to the chapter by Michael Tramontana and Stephen Hooper. Other chapters (e.g., by Ronald Brown *et al.* and Arthur MacNeill Horton) also may prove helpful.]

Conclusions

Research into the neuropsychological bases for learning disabilities and behavioral disorders in children has been ongoing and has produced a large body of literature. Learning disabilities are no longer referred to as a unitary disturbance, but are divided into those with verbal or nonverbal bases. Further delineation within each of those broad categories is also possible, and functional subtypes within each category of academic disability (i.e., reading, spelling, writing, math) have been shown to be viable. Though some overlap does occur, these subtypes do differ with respect to presenting symptomatology, neuropsychological functioning, neuroanatomical features, and electrophysiological findings.

Neurophysiological studies have revealed patterns of brain functioning and morphology that correspond to specific disabilities. There is not always agreement about the form these patterns take, but the fact that neurologic functional differences of some kind do exist between nondisabled and disabled populations, and between subtypes within the disabled population, is generally accepted.

Investigators studying learning and behavior problems in children have been criticized for poor design and methodology in their research. Inconsistencies in population definition, sample composition, comorbidity, measurement practices, instrumentation, and analyses have led knowledgeable and observant reviewers to question the results of many investigations. Given the growth of this field of study and the interest it continues to generate, it is hoped that sound research methods and increased vigilance regarding research design will be incorporated into future studies.

References

Ackerman, P. T., Dykman, R. A., & Peters, J. E. (1976). Hierarchical factor patterns on the WISC as related to areas of learning deficit. *Perceptual and Motor Skills, 42,* 583–615.

American Psychiatric Association. (1994). *Diagnostic and statistical manual of mental disorders* (4th ed.) Washington, DC: Author.

Banich, M. T., & Shenker, J. I. (1994). Investigations of interhemispheric processing: Methodological considerations. *Neuropsychology, 8,* 263–277.

Bannatyne, A. (1966). The color phonics system. In J. J. Money & G. Schiffman (Eds.), *The disabled reader.* Baltimore: Johns Hopkins Press.

Barkley, R. (1981). *Hyperactive children: A handbook for diagnosis and treatment.* New York: Guilford Press.

Baxter, D. M., & Warrington, E. K. (1985). Category specific phonological dysgraphia. *Neuropsychologia, 23,* 653–656.

Baxter, D. M., & Warrington, E. K. (1986). Ideational agraphia: A single case study. *Journal of Neurology, Neurosurgery, and Psychiatry, 49,* 369–374.

Baxter-Versi, D. M. (1987). *Acquired spelling disorders.* Unpublished doctoral dissertation, London University, London.

Beery, K. E. (1982). *Revised administration, scoring, and teaching manual for the Developmental Test of Visual–Motor Integration.* Cleveland, OH: Modern Curriculum Press.

Benton, A. (1987). Mathematical disability and Gerstmann syndrome. In G. Deloche & X. Seron (Eds.), *Mathematical disabilities: A cognitive neuropsychological perspective* (pp. 111–120). Hillsdale, NJ: Erlbaum.

Berninger, V. W., & Alsdorf, B. (1989). Are there errors in error analysis? *Journal of Psychoeducational Assessment, 7*, 209–222.

Berninger, V. W., Mizokawa, D. T., & Bragg, R. (1991). Theory-based diagnosis and remediation of writing disabilities. *Journal of School Psychology, 29*, 57–79.

Biederman, J., Faraone, S. V., Keenan, K., & Tsuang, M. T. (1991). Evidence of familial association between attention deficit disorder and major affective disorders. *Archives of General Psychiatry, 48*, 633–642.

Bigler, E. D. (1989). On the neuropsychology of suicide. *Journal of Learning Disabilities, 22*, 180–185.

Blumberg, S., & Izard, C. (1985). Affective and cognitive characteristics of depression in 10 and 11 year old children. *Journal of Personality and Social Psychology, 49*, 194–202.

Boder, E. (1973). Developmental dyslexia: A diagnostic approach based on three atypical reading–spelling patterns. *Developmental Medicine and Child Neurology, 15*, 663–687.

Brandys, C. F., & Rourke, B. P. (1991). Differential memory capacities in reading- and arithmetic-disabled children. In B. P. Rourke (Ed.), *Neuropsychological validation of learning disability subtypes* (pp. 73–96). New York: Guilford Press.

Brumback, R. A., & Staton, R. D. (1983). Learning disability and childhood depression. *American Journal of Orthopsychiatry, 53*, 269–281.

Coderre, D. J., Sweeney, J. E., & Rourke, B. P (1979). *Spelling recognition, word analysis, and visual memory in children with qualitatively distinct types of spelling errors.* Unpublished study, University of Windsor and Windsor Western Hospital Centre.

Cohen, M. J., Prather, A., Town, P., & Hynd, G. W. (1990). Neurodevelopmental differences in emotional prosody in normal children and children with left and right temporal lobe epilepsy. *Brain and Language, 38*, 122–134.

Cohen, M., Riccio, C., & Flannery, A. (1994). Expressive aprosodia following stroke to the right basal ganglia: A case report. *Neuropsychology, 8*, 242–245.

Conners, C. K. (1990). Dyslexia and the neurophysiology of attention. In G. T. Pavlidis (Ed.), *Perspectives on dyslexia: Vol. 1. Neurology, neuropsychology, and genetics* (pp. 163–195). New York: Wiley.

Crary, M. A., & Heilman, K. M. (1988). Letter imagery deficits in a case of pure apraxic agraphia. *Brain and Language, 34*, 147–156.

Dalby, J. T. (1985). Taxonomic separation of attention deficit disorders and developmental reading disorders. *Contemporary Educational Psychology, 10*, 228–234.

Damasio, H., Tranel, D., Spradling, J., & Alliger, R. (1989). Aphasia in men and women. In A. M. Galaburda (Ed.), *From reading to neurons* (pp. 307–325). Cambridge, MA: MIT Press.

DeBruyn, I., Smith, R., & Berninger, V. W. (1985, April). *Visual and linguistic correlates of beginning skill.* Las Vegas, NV: National Association of School Psychologists.

Dejerine, J. (1892). Contribution a l'etude anatomoclinique et clinique des differentes varietes de cecite verbal. *Memoires de la Societe de Biologie, 4*, 61–90.

Del Dotto, J. E., & Rourke, B. P. (1985). Subtypes of left-handed learning-disabled children. In B. P. Rourke (Ed.), *Neuropsychology of learning disabilities* (pp. 89–130). New York: Guilford Press.

Denckla, M. B. (1979). Childhood learning disabilities. In K. Heilman & E. Valenstein (Eds.), *Clinical neuropsychology* (pp. 535–573). London: Oxford University Press.

Denckla, M. B. (1993). A neurologist's overview of developmental dyslexia. In P. Tallal, A. M. Galaburda, R. R. Llinas, & C. von Euler (Eds.), *Temporal information processing in the nervous system: Special reference to dyslexia and dysphasia* (pp. 23–26). New York: New York Academy of Sciences.

Dodgen, C. E., & Pavlidis, G. T. (1990). Sequential, timing, rhythmic and eye movement problems in dyslexics. In G. T. Pavlidis (Ed.), *Perspectives on dyslexia: Vol. 1, Neurology, neuropsychology, and genetics* (pp. 221–251). New York: Wiley.

Doehring, D. G. (1968). *Patterns of impairment in specific reading disability.* Bloomington: Indiana University Press.

Doehring, D. G. (1985). Reading disability subtypes: Interaction of reading and nonreading deficits. In B. P. Rourke (Ed.), *Neuropsychology of learning disabilities* (pp. 133–146). New York: Guilford Press.

Doehring, D. G., & Hoshko, I. (1977). Classification of reading problems by the Q-technique of factor analysis. *Cortex, 13*, 281–294.

Doehring, D. G., Trites, R. L., Patel, P. G., & Fiedorowicz, C. A. M. (1981). *Reading disabilities: The interaction of reading, language, and neuropsychological deficits.* New York: Academic Press.

Drake, W. E. (1968). Clinical and pathological findings in a child with a developmental learning disability. *Journal of Learning Disability, 1*, 9–25.

Dubois, J., Hécaen, H., & Marcie, P. (1969). Pure agraphia. *Neuropsychologia, 7*, 271–286.

Eidelberg, D., & Galaburda, A. M. (1982). Symmetry and asymmetry in the human posterior thalamus: I. Cytoarchitectonic analysis in normal persons. *Archives of Neurology, 39*, 325–332.

Faigel, H. C., Doak, E., Howard, S. D., & Sigel, M. L. (1992). Emotional disorders in learning disabled adolescents. *Child Psychiatry and Human Development, 23*, 31–40.

Fawcett, A. J., Chattopadhyay, A. K., Kandler, R. H., Jarratt, J. A., Nicolson, R. I., & Proctor, M. (1993). Event-related potentials and dyslexia. In P. Tallal, A. M. Galaburda, R. R. Llinas, & C. von Euler (Eds.), *Temporal information processing in the nervous system: Special reference to dyslexia and dysphasia* (pp. 342–345). New York: New York Academy of Sciences.

Fisk, J. L., & Rourke, B. P. (1978, February). *Mental retardation and learning disabilities: A neurodevelopmental perspective.* Paper presented at the meeting of the International Neuropsychology Society, Minneapolis.

Fletcher, J. M. (1985). Memory for verbal and nonverbal stimuli in learning disability subgroups: Analysis by selective reminding. *Journal of Experimental Child Psychology, 40*, 224–259.

Fletcher, J. M. (1989). Nonverbal learning disabilities and suicide: Classification leads to prevention. *Journal of Learning Disabilities, 22,* 176–179.

Fletcher, J. M., & Copeland, D. R. (1988). Neurobehavioral effects of central nervous system prophylactic treatment of cancer in children. *Journal of Clinical and Experimental Neuropsychology, 10,* 495–537.

Fletcher, J. M., & Satz, P. (1985). Cluster analysis and the search for learning disability subtypes. In B. P. Rourke (Ed.), *Neuropsychology of learning disabilities* (pp. 40–64). New York: Guilford Press.

Fletcher, J. M., Taylor, H. G., Morris, R., & Satz, P. (1982). Finger recognition skills and reading achievement: A developmental neuropsychological analysis. *Developmental Psychology, 18,* 124–132.

Fowler, M. S., Riddell, P. M., & Stein, J. F. (1990). Vergence eye movement control and spatial discrimination in normal and dyslexic children. In G. T. Pavlidis (Ed.), *Perspectives on dyslexia: Vol. 1. Neurology, neuropsychology, and genetics* (pp. 253–273). New York: Wiley.

Galaburda, A. M., & Eidelberg, D. (1982). Symmetry and asymmetry in the human posterior thalamus: II. Thalamic lesions in a case of developmental dyslexia. *Archives of Neurology, 39,* 333–336.

Galaburda, A. M., & Kemper, T. L. (1979). Cytoarchitectonic abnormalities in developmental dyslexia: A case study. *Annals of Neurology, 6,* 94–100.

Galaburda, A., & Livingstone, M. (1993). Evidence for a magnocellular defect in developmental dyslexia. In P. Tallal, A. M. Galaburda, R. R. Llinas, & C. von Euler (Eds.), *Temporal information processing in the nervous system: Special reference to dyslexia and dysphasia* (pp. 70–82). New York: New York Academy of Sciences.

Galaburda, A. M., Sherman, G. F., Rosen, G. D., Aboitiz, F., & Geschwind, N. (1985). Developmental dyslexia: Four consecutive patients with cortical anomalies. *Annals of Neurology, 18,* 222–223.

Gerstmann, J. (1927). Fingeragnosie und isolierte Agraphie: Ein neues Syndrom. *Zeitschrift fur Neurologie und Psychiatrie, 108,* 152–177.

Geschwind, N., & Galaburda, A. (1985). Cerebral lateralization. *Archives of Neurology, 42,* 428–459, 521–552, 634–654.

Geschwind, N., & Levitsky, W. (1968). Human brain: Left–right asymmetries in temporal speech region. *Science, 161,* 186–187.

Gladstone, M., Best, C. T., & Davidson, R. J. (1989). Anomalous bimanual coordination among dyslexic boys. *Developmental Psychology, 25,* 236–246.

Glosser, G., & Koppell, S. (1987). Emotional–behavioral patterns in children with learning disabilities: Lateralized hemispheric differences. *Journal of Learning Disabilities, 20,* 365–368.

Goldberg, E., & Costa, L. D. (1981). Hemisphere differences in the acquisition and use of descriptive systems. *Brain and Language, 14,* 144–173.

Goodyear, P., & Hynd, G. W. (1992). Attention deficit disorder with (ADD/H) and without (ADD/WO) hyperactivity: Behavioral and neuropsychological differentiation. *Journal of Clinical Child Psychology, 21,* 273–305.

Grafman, J., Passafiume, D., Gaflioni, P., & Boller, F. (1982). Calculation disturbances in adults with focal hemisphere damage. *Cortex, 18,* 37–50.

Gross-Glenn, K., Duara, R., Yoshii, F., Barker, W. W., Chang, J. Y., Apicella, A., Boothe, T., & Lubs, H. A. (1990). PET scan reading studies: Familial dyslexics. In G. T. Pavlidis (Ed.), *Perspectives on dyslexia: Vol. 1. Neurology, neuropsychology, and genetics* (pp. 109–118). New York: Wiley.

Grunau, R. V. E., & Low, M. D. (1987). Cognitive and task-related EEG correlates of arithmetic performance in adolescents. *Journal of Clinical and Experimental Neuropsychology, 9,* 563–574.

Halperin, J. M., Gittelman, R., Klein, D. F., & Rudel, R. G. (1984). Reading-disabled hyperactive children: A distinct subgroup of attention deficit disorder with hyperactivity? *Journal of Abnormal Child Psychology, 12,* 1–14.

Hécaen, H., & Marcie, H. (1974). Disorders of written language following right hemisphere lesions: Spatial dysgraphia. In J. Beaumont & S. Dimond (Eds.), *Hemisphere function in the human brain* (pp. 345–366). London: Elek.

Hillis, A. E., & Caramazza, A. (1989). The graphemic buffer and attentional mechanisms. *Brain and Language, 36,* 208–235.

Hinshaw, S. P. (1992). Externalizing behavior problems and academic underachievement in childhood and adolescence: Causal relationships and underlying mechanisms. *Psychological Bulletin, 111,* 127–155.

Hinshaw, S. P. (1994). *Attention deficits and hyperactivity in children.* Thousand Oaks, CA: Sage.

Hirschi, T., & Hindelang, M. J. (1977). Intelligence and delinquency: A revisionist review. *American Sociological Review, 42,* 571–587.

Holcomb, P. J., Ackerman, P. T., & Dykman, R. A. (1985). Cognitive event-related potentials in children with attention and reading deficits. *Psychophysiology, 22,* 656–666.

Humphreys, P., Kaufman, W. E., & Galaburda, A. M. (1990). Developmental dyslexia in women: Neuropathological findings in three patients. *Annals of Neurology, 28,* 727–738.

Hynd, G. W., & Hooper, S. R. (1992). *Neurological basis of childhood psychopathology.* London: Sage.

Hynd, G. W., & Hynd, C. R. (1984). Dyslexia: Neuroanatomical/neurolinguistic perspectives. *Reading Research Quarterly, 19,* 482–498.

Hynd, G. W., Hynd, C. R., Sullivan, H. G., & Kingsbury, T., Jr. (1987). Regional cerebral blood flow (rCBF) in developmental dyslexia: Activation during reading in a surface and deep dyslexic. *Journal of Learning Disabilities, 20,* 294–300.

Hynd, G. W., & Semrud-Clikeman, M. (1989a). Dyslexia and brain morphology. *Psychological Bulletin, 106,* 447–482.

Hynd, G. W., & Semrud-Clikeman, M. (1989b). Dyslexia and neurodevelopmental pathology: Relationships to cognition, intelligence, and reading skill acquisition. *Journal of Learning Disabilities, 22,* 204–220.

Ingram, T. T. S. (1960). Pediatric aspects of specific developmental dysphasia, dyslexia, and dysgraphia. *Cerebral Palsy Bulletin, 2,* 254–277.

Jackson, M., & Warrington, E. K. (1986). Arithmetic skills in patients with unilateral cerebral lesions. *Cortex, 22,* 610–620.

Johnson, D. J., & Myklebust, H. R. (1967). *Learning disabilities.* New York: Grune & Stratton.

Johnson, D. J., & Myklebust, H. R. (1971). *Learning disabilities.* New York: Grune & Stratton.

Joschko, M., & Rourke, B. P. (1985). Neuropsychological subtypes of learning-disabled children who exhibit the ACID pattern on the WISC. In B. P. Rourke (Ed.), *Neuropsychology of learning disabilities* (pp. 65–88). New York: Guilford Press.

Kinsbourne, M., & Warrington, E. K. (1963). The developmental Gerstmann syndrome. *Archives of Neurology, 8,* 490–501.

Klove, H. (1963). Clinical neuropsychology. In F. M. Forster (Ed.), *The medical clinics of North America* (pp. 1647–1658). Philadelphia: Saunders.

Korhonen, T. T. (1991). An empirical subgrouping of Finnish learning-disabled children. *Journal of Clinical and Experimental Neuropsychology, 13,* 259–277.

Kremin, H. (1987). Is there more than ah-oh-oh? Alternative strategies for writing and repeating lexically. In M. Coltheart, R. Sartori, & R. Job (Eds.), *The cognitive neuropsychology of language* (pp. 295–335). Hillsdale, NJ: Erlbaum.

Kusche, C. A., Cook, E. T., & Greenberg, M. T. (1993). Neuropsychological and cognitive functioning in children with anxiety, externalizing, and comorbid psychopathology. *Journal of Clinical Child Psychology, 22,* 172–195.

LeMay, M. (1981). Are there radiological changes in the brains of individuals with dyslexia? *Bulletin of the Orton Society, 31,* 135–141.

Lennerstrand, G., Ygge, J., & Jacobsson, C. (1993). Control of binocular eye movements in normals and dyslexics. In P. Tallal, A. M. Galaburda, R. R. Llinas, & C. von Euler (Eds.), *Temporal information processing in the nervous system: Special reference to dyslexia and dysphasia* (pp. 231–238). New York: New York Academy of Sciences.

Levin, H. S., & Spiers, P. A. (1985). Acalculia. In K. M. Heilman & E. Valenstein (Eds.), *Clinical neuropsychology* (2nd ed., pp. 97–114). London: Oxford University Press.

Llinas, R. R. (1993). Is dyslexia a dyschronia? In P. Tallal, A. M. Galaburda, R. R. Llinas, & C. von Euler (Eds.), *Temporal information processing in the nervous system: Special reference to dyslexia and dysphasia* (pp. 48–55). New York: New York Academy of Sciences.

Luria, A. R. (1980). *Higher cortical functions in man.* New York: Basic Books.

Lyon, R., Stewart, N., & Freeman, D. (1982). Neuropsychological characteristics of empirically derived subgroups of learning disabled readers. *Journal of Clinical Neuropsychology, 4,* 343–365.

Lyon, R., & Watson, B. (1981). Empirically derived subgroups of learning disabled readers: Diagnostic characteristics. *Journal of Learning Disabilities, 14,* 256–261.

McCarthy, R. A., & Warrington, E. K. (1990). *Cognitive neuropsychology: A clinical introduction.* New York: Academic Press.

McGee, R., & Share, D. L. (1988). Attention deficit disorder–hyperactivity and academic failure: Which comes first and what should be treated? *Journal of the American Academy of Child and Adolescent Psychiatry, 27,* 318–325.

McGee, R., Williams, S., Moffitt, T., & Anderson J. (1989). A comparison of 13-year-old boys with attention deficit and/or reading disorder on neuropsychological measures. *Journal of Abnormal Child Psychology, 17,* 37–53.

Mattis, S., French, J. H., & Rapin, I. (1975). Dyslexia in children and young adults: Three independent neuropsychological syndromes. *Developmental Medicine and Child Neurology, 17,* 150–163.

Mattson, A. J., Sheer, D. E., & Fletcher, J. M. (1992). Electrophysiological evidence of lateralized disturbances in children with learning disabilities. *Journal of Clinical and Experimental Neuropsychology, 14,* 707–716.

Moffitt, T. E. (1992, April). *The neuropsychology of conduct disorder.* Paper presented at the National Institute of Mental Health Workshop on Conduct Disorders, Washington, DC.

Moffitt, T. E., & Henry, B. (1989). Neuropsychological assessment of executive functions in self-reported delinquents. *Development and Psychopathology, 1,* 105–118.

Myklebust, H. R. (1975). Nonverbal learning disabilities: Assessment and intervention. In H. R. Myklebust (Ed.), *Progress in learning disabilities* (Vol. 3, pp. 85–121). New York: Grune & Stratton.

Myklebust, H. R. (1978). Toward a science of dyslexiology. In H. R. Myklebust (Ed.), *Progress in learning disabilities* (Vol. 4, pp. 1–39). New York: Grune & Stratton.

Nelson, H., & Warrington, E. K. (1974). Developmental spelling retardation and its relation to other cognitive abilities. *British Journal of Psychology, 65,* 265–274.

Newcombe, F. (1969). *Missile wounds to the brain.* London: Oxford University Press.

Nussbaum, N. L., & Bigler, E. D. (1986). Neuropsychological and behavioral profiles of empirically derived subgroups of learning disabled children. *International Journal of Clinical Neuropsychology, 8,* 82–89.

Nussbaum, N. L., Bigler, E. D., Koch, W. R., & Ingram, J. W. (1988). Personality/behavioral characteristics in children: Differential effects of putative anterior versus posterior cerebral asymmetry. *Archives of Clinical Neuropsychology, 3,* 127–135.

Ozols, E. J., & Rourke, B. P. (1988). Characteristics of young learning disabled children classified according to patterns of academic achievement: Auditory–perceptual and visual–perceptual disabilities. *Journal of Clinical Child Psychology, 17,* 44–52.

Ozols, E. J., & Rourke, B. P. (1991). Classification of young learning disabled children according to patterns of academic achievement: Validity studies. In B. P. Rourke (Ed.), *Neuropsychological validation of learning disability subtypes* (pp. 97–123). New York: Guilford Press.

Patterson, K. E., & Wing, A. M. (1989). Processes in handwriting: *Cognitive Neuropsychology, 6,* 1–23.

Pavlidis, G. T. (1985). Eye movements in dyslexia: Their diagnostic significance. *Journal of Learning Disabilities, 18,* 42–50.

Pavlidis, G. T. (1990). Detecting dyslexia through ophthalmo-kinesis: A promise for early diagnosis. In G. T. Pavlidis (Ed.), *Perspective on dyslexia: Vol. 1. Neurology, neuropsychology, and genetics* (pp. 199–220). New York: Wiley.

Pennington, B. F. (1991). *Diagnosing learning disorders: A neuropsychological framework.* New York: Guilford Press.

Petrauskas, R. J., & Rourke, B. P. (1979). Identification of subgroups of retarded reading: A neuropsychological multivariate approach. *Journal of Clinical Neuropsychology, 1,* 17–37.

Pirozzolo, F. J. (1979). *The neuropsychology of developmental reading disorders.* New York: Praeger.

Porter, J. E., & Rourke, B. P. (1985). Socioemotional functioning of learning-disabled children: A subtypal analysis of personality patterns. In B. P. Rourke (Ed.), *Neuropsychology of learning disabilities* (pp. 257–280). New York: Guilford Press.

Reitan, R. M., & Boll, T. J. (1973). Neuropsychological correlates of minimal brain dysfunction. *Annals of the New York Academy of Sciences, 205,* 65–88.

Reitan, R. M., & Davison, L. A. (Eds.). (1974). *Clinical neuropsychology: Current status and application.* Washington, DC: Winston.

Robins, P. M. (1992). A comparison of behavioral and attentional functioning in children diagnosed as hyperactive or learning-disabled. *Journal of Abnormal Child Psychology, 20,* 65–82.

Roeltgen, D. P., & Heilman, K. M. (1984). Lexical agraphia. Further support for the two strategy hypothesis of linguistic agraphia. *Brain, 107,* 811–827.

Ross, E. D., & Mesulam, M. (1979). Dominant language functions of the right hemisphere? Prosody or emotional gesturing. *Archives of Neurology, 46,* 437–443.

Rourke, B. P. (1975). Brain–behavior relationships in children with learning disabilities: A research program. *American Psychologist, 30,* 911–920.

Rourke, B. P. (1978). Reading, spelling, arithmetic disabilities: A neuropsychologic perspective. In H. Myklebust (Ed.), *Progress in learning disabilities* (Vol. 4, pp. 97–120). New York: Grune & Stratton.

Rourke, B. P. (1985). *Neuropsychology of learning disabilities: Essentials of subtype analysis.* New York: Guilford Press.

Rourke, B. P. (1993). Arithmetic disabilities, specific and otherwise: A neuropsychological perspective. *Journal of Learning Disabilities, 26,* 214–226.

Rourke, B. P., & Finlayson, M. A. J. (1978). Neuropsychological significance of variation in patterns of academic performance: Verbal and visuo-spatial abilities. *Journal of Abnormal Child Psychology, 6,* 121–133.

Rourke, B. P., & Strang, J. D. (1978). Neuropsychological significance of variations in patterns of academic performance: Motor, psychomotor, and tactile-perceptual abilities. *Journal of Pediatric Psychology, 3,* 62–66.

Rourke, B. P., & Strang, J. D. (1983). Subtypes of reading and arithmetic disabilities: A neuropsychological analysis. In M. Rutter (Ed.), *Developmental neuropsychiatry* (pp. 473–488). New York: Guilford Press.

Rourke, B. P., Young, G. C., & Leenaars, A. A. (1989). A childhood learning disability that predisposes those afflicted to adolescent and adult depression and suicide risk. *Journal of Learning Disabilities, 22,* 169–175.

Sackheim, H. A., Decina, P., & Malitz, S. (1982). Functional brain asymmetry and affective disorders. *Adolescent Psychiatry, 10,* 320–335.

Satz, P., & Morris, R. (1981). Learning disability subtypes: A review. In F. J. Pirozzolo & M. C. Wittrock (Eds.), *Neuropsychological and cognitive processes in reading* (pp. 109–141). New York: Academic Press.

Selz, M. (1977). *A neuropsychological model of learning disability: Classification of brain function in 9–14 year old children.* Unpublished doctoral dissertation, University of Washington.

Selz, M., & Reitan, R. M. (1979). Neuropsychological test performance of normal, learning-disabled, and brain-damaged older children. *Journal of Nervous and Mental Disease, 167,* 298–302.

Semrud-Clikeman, M., & Hynd, G. W. (1990). Right hemispheric dysfunction in nonverbal learning disabilities: Social, academic, and adaptive functioning in adults and children. *Psychological Bulletin, 107,* 196–209.

Semrud-Clikeman, M., Hynd, G. W., Novey, E. S., & Eliopulos, D. (1991). Dyslexia and brain morphology: Relationship between neuroanatomical variation and neurolinguistic tasks. *Learning and Individual Differences, 3,* 225–242.

Shapiro, E. G., Lipton, M. E., & Krivit, W. (1992). White matter dysfunction and its neuropsychological correlates: A longitudinal study of a case of metachromatic leukodystrophy treated with bone marrow transplant. *Journal of Clinical and Experimental Neuropsychology, 14,* 610–624.

Shaywitz, S. E., & Shaywitz, B. A. (1988). Attention deficit disorder: Current perspectives. In J. F. Kavanaugh & T. J. Truss (Eds.), *Learning disabilities: Proceedings of the national conference* (pp. 369–523). Parkton, MD: York Press.

Spiers, P. A. (1987). Acalculia revisited: Current issues. In G. Deloche & X. Seron (Eds.), *Mathematical disabilities: A cognitive neuropsychological perspective.* (pp. 1–25). Hillsdale, NJ: Erlbaum.

Spreen, O. (1988). The relationship between learning disabilities, emotional disorders, and neuropsychology: Some results and observations. *Journal of Clinical and Experimental Neuropsychology, 11,* 117–140.

Stelmack, R. M., & Miles, J. (1990). The effect of picture priming on event-related potential of normal and disabled readers during a word recognition memory task. *Journal of Clinical and Experimental Neuropsychology, 12,* 887–903.

Strang, J. D., & Rourke, B. P. (1983). Concept-formation/nonverbal reasoning abilities of children who exhibit specific academic problems with arithmetic. *Journal of Clinical Child Psychology, 12,* 33–39.

Strang, J. D., & Rourke, B. P. (1985). Arithmetic disability subtypes: The neuropsychological significance of specific arithmetical impairment in childhood. In B. P. Rourke (Ed.), *Neuropsychology of learning disabilities* (pp. 167–186). New York: Guilford Press.

Swartz, G. A. (1974). *The language-learning system.* New York: Simon & Schuster.

Sweeney, J. E., McCabe, A. E., & Rourke, B. P. (1978). *Logical-grammatical abilities of retarded spellers.* Unpublished study, Windsor Western Hospital Centre and University of Windsor.

Sweeney, J. E., & Rourke, B. P. (1978). Neuropsychological significance of phonetically accurate and phonetically inaccurate spelling errors in younger and older retarded readers. *Brain and Language, 6,* 212–225.

Sweeney, J. E., & Rourke, B. P. (1985). Spelling disability subtypes. In B. P. Rourke (Ed.), *Neuropsychology of learning disabilities* (pp. 147–166). New York: Guilford Press.

Tallal, P., Galaburda, A. M., Llinas, R. R., & von Euler, C. (1993). *Temporal information processing in the nervous system: Special reference to dyslexia and dysphasia.* New York: New York Academy of Sciences.

Ternes, J., Woody, R. & Livingston, R. (1987). A child with right hemisphere deficit syndrome responsive to carbamarepine treatments. *Journal of the American Academy of Child & Adolescent Psychology, 26,* 586–588.

van der Vlugt, H. (1991). Neuropsychological validation studies of learning disability subtypes: Verbal, visual-spatial, and psychomotor abilities. In B. P. Rourke (Ed.), *Neuropsychological validation of learning disability subtypes* (pp. 140–159). New York: Guilford Press.

Voeller, K. K. S. (1986). Right-hemisphere deficit syndrome in children. *American Journal of Psychiatry, 143,* 1004–1009.

Warrington, E. K. (1982). The fractionation of arithmetical skills: A single case study. *Quarterly Journal of Experimental Psychology, 34A,* 31–51.

Wechsler, D. (1949). *Wechsler intelligence scale for children.* San Antonio, TX: Psychological Corporation.

Weinberger, D. R., Luchins, D. J., Morihisa, J., & Wyatt, R. J. (1982). Asymmetrical volumes of the right and left frontal and occipital regions of the human brain. *Neurology, 11,* 97–100.

Werry, J. S., Elkind, G. S., & Reeves, J. C. (1987). Attention deficit, conduct, oppositional, and anxiety disorders in children: III. Laboratory differences. *Journal of Abnormal Child Psychology, 15,* 409–428.

Wiig, E. H., & Semel, E. M. (1974). Development of comprehension of logico-grammatical sentences by grade school children. *Perceptual and Motor Skills, 18,* 171–176.

Wolff, P. H. (1993). Impaired temporal resolution in developmental dyslexia. In P. Tallal, A. M. Galaburda, R. R. Llinas, & C. von Euler (Eds.), *Temporal information processing in the nervous system: Special reference to dyslexia and dysphasia* (pp. 87–103). New York: New York Academy of Sciences.

Yule, W., & Rutter, M. (1976). Epidemiology and social implications of specific reading retardation. In R. M. Knights & D. J. Bakker (Eds.), *The neuropsychology of learning disorders: Theoretical approaches* (pp. 25–39). Baltimore: University Park Press.

Zangwill, O. L. (1954). Agraphia due to a left parietal glioma in a left-handed man. *Brain, 77,* 510–520.

9

Measurement and Statistical Problems in Neuropsychological Assessment of Children

CECIL R. REYNOLDS

The field of neuropsychology as practiced clinically has been driven in large part by the development and application of standardized diagnostic procedures that are more sensitive than medical examinations to changes in behavior, in particular higher cognitive processes, as related to brain function. The techniques and methods so derived have led to major conceptual and theoretical advances in the understanding of normal and abnormal patterns of brain–behavior relationships. Despite the apparent utility of many of the neuropsychological tests discussed in this volume, their psychometric properties leave much to be desired. Much of their utility comes from the clinical acumen and experience of their users and developers, a situation that has, historically, made clinical neuropsychology more difficult to teach than should be the case. In fact, much of today's practice and yesterday's theoretical advances in clinical neuropsychology stem from intense and insightful observation of brain-damaged individuals by such astute observers as Ward Halstead, A. R. Luria, Hans Teuber, Karl Pribram, Roger Sperry, and others. These superstars of clinical neuropsychology were state-of-the-art researchers (though the state of the art was often crude) to be sure, but their greatest inspirations came from their constant monitoring and informal interactions with the behavior of persons suffering from a variety of neurological trauma and disease. Halstead roamed the halls of Otho S. S. Sprague making notes as he observed behavior among brain-damaged individuals; Luria gained great insights into brain function with his rather informal, sometimes impromptu, bedside examination and discussions with soldiers with head injury; Sperry and his students followed and observed a series of "split-brain" patients going about their daily activities, even to the point of observing some as they dressed themselves and others in leisure activities.

Major advances have occurred because of the sheer clinical acumen of these individuals. Many clinical neuropsychologists continue to evaluate patients quite profitably on the basis of observation and informal assessment. Others have devoted themselves to more purely actuarial approaches to clinical work and research (e.g., see the prolific works of Reitan, Rourke, and Satz). Most clinicians engage the complementary of the two approaches, a modus operandi that has made neuropsychologists more and more accepted and contributing members to medical staff in teaching hospitals and clinics. Clearly, clinical neuropsychology has been successful in earning its riches in medicine and in psychology largely as a result of empirical research and clinical acumen in the field. Neuropsychological techniques have infiltrated assessment in special and remedial education for some time now (e.g., Haak, 1989; Hynd, 1981).

At the same time, many of the practices in neuropsychology, clinical and research, have been criticized extensively from inside (e.g., Cicchetti,

CECIL R. REYNOLDS • Department of Educational Psychology, Texas A&M University, College Station, Texas 77843.

1994; Parsons & Prigatano, 1978; Reynolds, 1982a, 1986; Ris & Noll, 1994; Willson & Reynolds, 1982) and outside the discipline (e.g., Coles, 1978; Reschly & Gresham, 1989; Sandoval, 1981) for a lack of attention to certain principles of research design in the field and the failure to incorporate the many advances in psychometric methods of the past 25 years. To be sure, our research methods and statistical tools have improved greatly since Halstead's early work; yet our ability (or our inclination) to apply them uniformly or to our best advantage certainly has not kept pace with the growth in our clinical acumen and with theoretical advances in the field. Neuropsychologists have shown an increasing interest in the educational problems of children categorized as learning disabled as well, bringing neuropsychological methods to bear on the recurring questions of neuropsychological dysfunction within this population. Clinical neuropsychological assessment of educational disorders such as learning disability offers a prime opportunity to meld theory and clinical acumen with good psychometric practice, but has not, apparently, come fully about, although improvements are clearly evident since the first edition of this work in 1989.

The failure to reach this coalescence in clinical neuropsychology has serious implications for the credibility and, ultimately perhaps, the survival of the clinical application of neuropsychological principles in medical and educational settings. Perhaps it is the youth of the field or its placement primarily in the medical setting, where good research design and statistical methods are too rare, that has retarded coalescence.

Problems of statistical methods and design in test development in clinical neuropsychology have been noted with frequency (e.g., Reynolds, 1982a, 1986). In reviewing the Halstead–Reitan Neuropsychological Test Battery (HRNB), Dean (1985) remarked that the "manual for the HRNB lacks the basic psychometric documentation needed in interpretation. Moreover, interpretations are more dependent on the psychologist's knowledge and clinical acumen than reported psychometric properties for the battery" (p. 645). The other major battery in the discipline, the Luria–Nebraska Neuropsychological Battery (LNNB), fares no better; as Adams (1985) remarked, "the methodological errors committed in the construction of the test [the LNNB] are both numerous and substantive" (p. 879). Other scales in common use by clinicians are equally guilty. The normative data for the Benton Test of Facial Recognition, Mirsky's Continuous Performance Test, Purdue Pegboard Test, Rey Complex Figures, Stroop Color and Word Test, National Adult Reading Test, the Wide Range Achievement Test, and numerous other measures used in neuropsychological testing are far below contemporary standards. It is a monument to the clinical acumen and tenacity of clinical neuropsychologists, and perhaps also the insensitivity of many medical practitioners to behavioral changes, that the field has survived and in fact prospered over the last 50 years.

The issues to be delineated in the following pages deal primarily with pragmatic concerns that affect the clinical practice of neuropsychology in patient care certainly, but also the study of brain–behavior relationships generally. These issues principally revolve around measurement problems evident in the neuropsychological literature, the resolution of which could enhance progress in research and practice in the field. The solutions are neither novel nor unknown nor are the problems restricted to neuropsychology. A number of difficulties in present practice are apparently the result of either a lack of psychometric sophistication among those in the field, ignoring certain well-known measurement principles, or some combination of these two reasons. The following discussion will present several examples of what may be seen as a lack of sophistication or attention to measurement issues in neuropsychology and propose alternative procedures. Rather than employ a single battery or procedure as an example throughout, a variety were chosen to illustrate the widespread nature of the problem and not to appear to be "picking on" any specific application. A series of statistical issues related to diagnostic research problems is next presented along with recommendations for improving this line of research as well.

Lest this work appear too negative, it is worth noting that neuropsychology has emerged as a major field within psychology and that the procedures critiqued herein have been and remain useful in clinical and research domains. The clinical acumen, insight, and dedication of the practitioners who use these scales are considerable and are not being questioned. Indeed, they have moved the field substantially in many ways. Nevertheless, the fact remains that our methods and techniques could be better—by following some well-known, widely accepted methods.

Normative Data and Standardization Samples

The systematic development and presentation of *normative* data has received far too little attention in neuropsychology. Perhaps this reflects the rather tedious, mundane nature of such tasks, but nevertheless, the lack of good normative data in neuropsychology is a distinct handicap to the field. Certainly one encounters reports of "normative data" in the professional literature. However, these reports either are typically based on very small samples (some even as small as $N = 10$ at yearly age intervals) or do not employ normal individuals. Too much of our neuropsychological data are based on impaired individuals; we do not know enough about how normal individuals respond to most neuropsychological tests. The latter issue is more serious clinically than most clinicians realize because in addition to the other problems it creates, it results in a lack of items with sufficient difficulty for assessment of premorbidly high-functioning individuals with less than massive neurological trauma. Most of the children with premorbid IQs of 130 or more who suffer general cerebral trauma but lose only 20 to 25 IQ points or less can easily go undetected in neuropsychological testing, i.e., they can appear normal and go untreated or even lose existing services once these levels have been reached even in the case of initial massive trauma.

Without adequate normative data drawn from large-scale samplings of the population, the clinician and the researcher are also unable to assess the effects of demographic variables such as race or ethnicity, gender, and socioeconomic status on neuropsychological test performance. Demographic variables do have a significant influence on test performance on any number of tasks. Often, neuropsychologists ignore such factors during test interpretation or believe that because brain function is being evaluated, demographic variables may be irrelevant. Systematic effects of many demographic variables have been noted on numerous tasks as illustrated by even simple tasks like Coding and Digit Symbol (some of the most sensitive of all of the Wechsler tasks to neurological trauma) from the Wechsler Scales where females (both black and white) consistently outscore males. Whether using a level of performance or an ipsative profile analysis (e.g., Davis, 1959; Reynolds & Gutkin, 1980), ignorance of such robust findings could mislead the clinician. Very little research has considered the influence of demographic variables on more strictly neuropsychological test results and some of the primary books in the field do not discuss the issue or its relationship to diagnosis (e.g., Golden, 1981). For such tests as the Wechsler scales, the major studies of demographic influence on scores have occurred

as a function of research involving the standardization samples of these instruments (see Reynolds & Kaufman, 1986, for a review; see also Kaufman, McLean, & Reynolds, 1988, and Reynolds, Chastain, Kaufman, & McLean, 1987).

A great deal is known about potential cultural biases and other effects of demographic and other nominal variables on tests of intelligence and personality (e.g., Reynolds, 1995). However, there is a dearth of research on the effects of demographic factors in neuropsychological assessment. Helms (1992) has argued that neuropsychological tests may be biased by cultural factors for three major reasons: (1) a lack of equivalence of testing conditions, (2) functional inequivalence across groups, and (3) linguistic inequivalence. Reynolds (1982b, 1995; Reynolds & Kaiser, 1990) has suggested additional reasons including different latent structures of the tests across groups, differential affective responses to the examination and/or the examiner, and differences in the reliability of measurement, validity of the interpretations of performance, and in the content validity of the items and the item selection process. All of these factors may be evident to some degree for any ethnic minority or possibly even across gender for neuropsychological tests, despite the lack of such findings for intelligence tests. The use of neuropsychological tests with Hispanic populations has attracted the most attention thus far (e.g., Ardila, Roselli, & Puente, 1994; Arnold, Montgomery, Castaneda, & Langoria, 1994) although cultural bias with regard to blacks and women has been evaluated thoroughly for the Test of Memory and Learning (TOMAL; Reynolds & Bigler, 1994) both during test development (Reynolds & Bigler, 1994) and in postpublication research (e.g., Mayfield & Reynolds, 1995a,b) with no cultural effects being detected that would bias test interpretation. Nevertheless, all neuropsychological measures must be evaluated for effects related to culture, ethnicity, gender, and other nominal variables as findings in this area do not generalize well across tests or necessarily across nominal groupings.

The failure to provide good, stratified samples in the development and standardization of neuropsychological tests has been a major inhibiting factor in efforts to understand demographic influences on neuropsychological test performance. Other writers have reached similar conclusions. The manual for the HRNB contains no standardization or normative data, yet age and other demographic variables are correlated with the test results. This greatly complicates test interpretation for individuals (Dean, 1985).

By good normative data, reference is made to the application of stratified, random sampling techniques now common, and applied to such tests as the WISC-III, the McCarthy Scales, and the K-ABC. Indeed, the standardization of the K-ABC (Kaufman & Kaufman, 1983) is an excellent model of the development of normative data. Good standardization samples provide a reliable standard against which to judge the performance of others and have additional benefits including at least the following: (1) communications between researchers, (2) training of clinical neuropsychologists, and (3) the deflation and exposure of a variety of clinical myths. After a brief discussion of the first two of these benefits, I will turn to a more extensive presentation of the "myth deflation advantage."

Communication among researchers is a difficult and expensive task but a necessary one; indeed, it is in communication among us that the foundation of the "community of scholars" must lie. It would certainly enhance the clarity of research communications in the field if a good normative reference sample were available against which research samples could be contrasted (provided other appropriate demographic variables were adequately controlled). The development of scaled scores for neuropsychological tests based on such a sample would simplify matters as well. The issue of training also is ultimately one of communication. The presence of normative data makes learning easier. Although the accuracy of the statement is not known, it has often been said that when asked about how to become a good clinical neuropsychologist, Ralph Reitan replied, "Work in the field for 30 years." Although this would probably work, much of this time would be spent in developing a set of "clinical norms" in one's own mind about how normal and various groups of impaired individuals perform on such tests as the HRNB. This is necessary because of the lack of a standardization sample for such scales as the HRNB and the Boder Test of Reading–Spelling Patterns (a scale clearly intended to assess developmental phenomena), and the less than adequate sample for such popular scales as the LNNB. The transmission of the knowledge and the clinical skills of neuropsychology could be greatly enhanced by the presence of accurate, high-quality normative data.

Norms also have the advantage of allowing us to evaluate certain aspects of the "clinical mythology" of assessment. For some time, statistically significant Verbal–Performance IQ differences on the Wechsler Scales were believed (and, unfortunately, still are by many) to be indicative of brain damage, neurological dysfunction, or almost certainly a learning disability if a child were involved. From the standardization sample of the WISC-R, Kaufman (1976a) developed normative data for the frequency of occurrence of these differences. Prior to reporting these data, he took an informal poll of clinicians asking what they believed, on the basis of their clinical experience, the typical Verbal–Performance IQ difference would be for normal children. The response indicated a belief that other than small differences were considered unusual. A 3- or 4-point difference was the typical response. Differences of 15 points have long been thought to be clinically significant and have been used (e.g., Dean, 1978) to document the presence of a learning disability.

Actual analyses of the frequency of occurrence of Verbal–Performance differences by Kaufman (1976a) with the 2200 normally functioning children in the WISC-R standardization sample revealed a very different picture. The average difference was more than 9 points, with 12-point differences (the difference required for significance at $p = 0.05$) occurring with one of three children, and 15-point differences ($p = 0.01$) occurring with one of four children. This should not have been surprising as this is essentially the same distribution of difference scores that was reported 20 years earlier for the WISC, but that had gone largely ignored until Kaufman published his analyses of the WISC-R standardization sample. Note that the availability of a proper standardization sample made the investigation possible at all.

This again points to the need to develop good normative data on which to evaluate one's clinical insights. Next I discuss another index of neurological dysfunction that was not normed until recently, serving as an example of how one goes about developing and reporting such data.

Gutkin and Reynolds's (1980) Norming of the Selz and Reitan Index of Neurological Dysfunction

Over the last several decades, hundreds of attempts have been made to develop diagnostically useful patterns based on Wechsler subtest scores (Matarazzo, 1972). In general, these attempts have not been successful (e.g., Ivnik, Smith, Malec, Kokmen, & Tangelos, 1994; Kaufman, 1979; Sattler, 1974). A variety of scatter indexes have been developed and investigated as potentially useful diagnostic indicators for exceptionality. The Wechsler scales, and especially the Wechsler Intelligence Scale for Children-Revised (WISC-R) (Wechsler, 1974), have been extensively investigated with regard to utility of scatter indexes in diagnosis. Scatter indexes from the WISC-R that have been investigated include Verbal–Performance IQ discrepancies (Kaufman, 1976a; Piotrowski, 1978; Reynolds, 1979a; Reynolds, Hartlage, & Haak, 1980), the range of subtest scores, i.e., highest minus lowest subtest score (Kaufman, 1976b; Tabachnick, 1979), and the "number of deviant signs" or number of subtests deviating significantly from the mean of all subtests (Kaufman, 1976b). Range of subtest scores in particular has attracted substantial attention as a potential technique with which normals and different pathological groups could be distinguished. Although some prior research has found statistically significant differences between diagnostic groups on this scatter index, other studies, such as Thompson (1980), have not. Even in those studies where significant differences in Wechsler subtest scatter have been found across groups of normal, brain-damaged, emotionally disturbed, and other categories of child psychopathology, the small actual differences and resulting substantial overlap of distributions have made scatter indexes such as the range of little diagnostic utility. As such results become more widely known, the search for more sensitive, sophisticated indexes of scatter has broadened and statistics such as the profile variance technique (Plake, Reynolds, & Gutkin, 1981) have been developed. The provision of full normative data has allowed such scatter indexes to be evaluated for their potential contribution (e.g., Ivnik *et al.*, 1994). (Comparable data have not been made available for the WISC-III, despite its widespread replacement of the WISC-R in clinical practice.)

Selz and Reitan (1979) presented another Wechsler scatter index that seemed to facilitate the accurate diagnosis of neurological dysfunction when combined with other perceptual and neurological tests. Specifically, scatter was calculated by subtracting the lowest subtest score from the highest subtest score and dividing the result by the mean of all subtests (i.e., it is calculated as the range/mean). Selz and Reitan reported three levels of diagnostic criteria in their study. A scatter index calculated with this technique that equaled or exceeded 1.0 was taken as a mild indication of neurological dysfunction. A scatter index that equaled 1.4 was interpreted as being consistent with the existence of a "probable" neurological problem. A scatter index equaling or exceeding 1.76 (rounded to 1.8 for the Gutkin & Reynolds, 1980, study) was viewed as part of a symptom complex indicating definite neurological impairment.

One of the most common shortcomings in the Wechsler scatter pattern body of research has been the failure of investigators to validate the abnormality of various diagnostic incidents with a normal population. Often, seemingly abnormal levels of subtest scatter have been found to be quite common among normal individuals (Davis, 1959; Kaufman, 1976a,b, 1990; Reynolds, 1979a), prompting the Gutkin and Reynolds (1980) study, which is reviewed here as an example of how to develop and present such data.

The subjects for their investigation were the white ($N = 1868$) and black ($N = 305$) children from the WISC-R standardization sample of 2200 children. The characteristics of these children are described in great detail elsewhere (Wechsler, 1974). It is noteworthy, however, that these groups accurately reflect the 1980 United States census and are thus excellent, nationally representative samples of normal white and black children. The sample of 2200 was chosen to be a stratified random sample of children of the United States with sample stratification occurring by age (20 at each year between $6\frac{1}{2}$ and $16\frac{1}{2}$), race, sex, geographic region of residence in the United States, urban versus rural residence, and socioeconomic status (as determined by occupation of the head of household). The Wechsler series generally provides one of the best models of test standardization available, one to be emulated by developers of more distinctly neuropsychological measures.

As per the procedure separately described by Selz and Reitan (1979), a scatter index was calculated for each subject by subtracting his or her lowest subtest score from his or her highest subtest score and dividing the result by his or her mean subtest score. This calculation was performed for both the 10 regularly administered subtests and the 12 total subtests comprising the WISC-R. A series of one-way ANOVAs was calculated to determine if subtest scatter varied as a function of the demographic and intellectual characteristics of subjects, for the stratification variables are known to be differentially related to overall performance on the various IQ scales (Reynolds & Gutkin, 1979). Socioeconomic status is typically related to level of performance on cognitive tests, whereas race has its greatest impact on pattern of performance (Reynolds, 1981a). Specifically, subjects were grouped according to age (less than 10, 10–12, greater than 12), sex (male, female), race (white, black), place of residence (urban or rural), and Full-Scale IQ (FSIQ) (less than 85, 85–115, greater than 115). Because Kaufman (1976b) found significant differences in Verbal–Performance IQ scatter as a function of FSIQ, one-way ANOVAs yielding significant results were further examined with a covariance analysis with FSIQ serving as the covariate. Demographic variables that yielded significant results with covariance analysis were used to segregate the study's data.

Analysis of variance on the dimensions of place of residence, sex, FSIQ, occupation of the head of household, age, and race revealed significant differences for the latter four variables. This again points out the need for careful consideration of these variables in neuropsychological test interpretation. Using the FSIQ as a covariate resulted in nonsignificant differences for occupation of the head of household, but statistically significant differences remained for the dimensions of age and race. Because further examination revealed that the means at the different age levels never differed from each other by more than 0.04, subsequent data analyses were broken out only according to subject race and FSIQ. Means, standard deviations, and the percentage of subjects equaling or exceeding each Selz and Reitan (1979) diagnostic criterion as found by Gutkin and Reynolds (1980) are represented according to subject race and FSIQ category in Tables 1–5.

As indicated by the data analysis, the utility of the Selz and Reitan (1979) scatter index varies with the level of criteria employed and the characteristics

TABLE 1. Means and Standard Deviations for Scatter Index Using 10 Subtests

FSIQ	Whites	Blacks	Totals
< 85			
Mean	0.98	1.01	0.99
SD	0.36	0.38	0.37
85–115			
Mean	0.64	0.70	0.65
SD	0.23	0.23	0.23
> 115			
Mean	0.51	0.62	0.51
SD	0.16	0.20	0.16
Totals			
Mean	0.65	0.84	0.68
SD	0.27	0.35	0.29

TABLE 2. Means and Standard Deviations for Scatter Index Using 12 Subtests

FSIQ	Whites	Blacks	Total
<85			
Mean	1.07	1.10	1.09
SD	0.35	0.37	0.35
85–115			
Mean	0.71	0.78	0.72
SD	0.23	0.22	0.23
> 115			
Mean	0.58	0.70	0.58
SD	0.17	0.14	0.17
Totals			
Mean	0.72	0.93	0.76
SD	0.27	0.34	0.29

of the subjects examined. The most stringent criterion (i.e., scatter index equal to or greater than 1.8) appears to set a standard that is almost never reached in the normal population except for 2–5% of the subjects in the lowest IQ group.

Using the second most stringent criterion (i.e., scatter index equals or exceeds 1.4) also yields satisfactory results with all but the lowest IQ group. As with the highest criterion, normal subjects with IQs of 85 and above virtually never equal or exceed the Selz and Reitan index of 1.4. It is noteworthy, however, that both black and white subjects in the lowest IQ group do exceed the 1.4 criterion at a rate that calls into question the validity of this index for this particular group, unless one assumes a rather high incidence of neurological impairment in children with IQs below 85, even though most of these children were functioning normally.

The most lenient of the Selz and Reitan criteria (i.e., scatter index equals 1.0) appears completely to lack validity with the lowest IQ group. Depending on whether one uses 10 or 12 subtests and whether the subjects were white or black, between 49 and

TABLE 3. Percentage of Subjects Equaling or Exceeding Scatter Index of 1.0

FSIQ	10 subtests		12 subtests	
	Whites	Blacks	Whites	Blacks
< 85	49	55	62	64
85–115	9	15	14	21
> 115	0	0	2	0

TABLE 4. Percentage of Subjects Equaling or Exceeding Scatter Index of 1.4

FSIQ	10 subtests		12 subtest	
	Whites	Blacks	Whites	Blacks
< 85	12	18	21	23
85–115	1	1	1	0
> 115	0	0	0	0

64% of the sample exceeded the 1.0 cutoff. Clearly, the use of this standard with this group of normal children would lead to an unacceptable number of false positives. The middle IQ group also meets or exceeds the 1.0 criterion in numbers that call the validity of the index into serious question. Only with the highest IQ group was the 1.0 standard sufficiently infrequent.

Although the differences are not highly pronounced, statistically significant differences were evidenced on the Selz and Reitan index between blacks and whites, with the former group consistently showing higher index scores (see Tables 1 and 2) across the entire IQ range. Even smaller, but statistically significant, differences were found as a function of the children's age. No consistent pattern emerged with regard to this variable, although the youngest group most often evidenced the highest Selz and Reitan index scores.

However, the overall data from the Gutkin and Reynolds (1980) study indicate that the utility of the Selz and Reitan index varies substantially according to subject characteristics, especially FSIQ. The presentation of normative data in the detail presented here should be required for all neuropsychological measures.

Designing and conducting a normative study on such a large scale as to be useful is time-consuming and quite expensive. Few and far be-

TABLE 5. Percentage of Subjects Equaling or Exceeding Scatter Index of 1.8

FSIQ	10 subtests		12 subtests	
	Whites	Blacks	Whites	Blacks
< 85	4	3	2	5
85–115	0	0	0	0
> 115	0	0	0	0

tween are the times when money is available for the wholesale assessment of normally functioning individuals. Neuropsychologists must move actively to seek federal funding for normative studies, and test publishing houses must become convinced of the viability of neuropsychological test construction projects. Major publishing houses have been responsive to the needs of psychology in some instances resulting in large investments in test construction projects such as the Wechsler scales. Clinical neuropsychologists must demand that neuropsychological tests meet the same psychometric standards as many other scales and move toward the development and norming of such scales. Nowhere is this more needed generally than in neuropsychology and child neuropsychology in particular. We have not done so effectively, at least to this point. In 1995, I received an ad from a major publisher of tests in the United States promoting a reading test for adults of all ages with a normative sample of less than 200 across the entire adult age range. The estimation of the characteristics of the score distributions across age with such a sample and involving some 70 years is hardly more than speculation and should be rejected heartily by the profession.

Reliability of Neuropsychological Measures

Reliability may be the single most influential of latent psychometric concepts because of its relationship to all other psychometric characteristics. It is the foundation of validity, and classical psychometric theory is known as reliability theory. The problem of reliability, particularly of internal consistency reliability such as represented in Cronbach's alpha and the various Kuder–Richardson formulas, has not been well attended in clinical neuropsychology. Observed test score variance can be divided into two components, true score variance and error variance. Only true score variance is "real," systematic, and related to true differences among individuals. Only true score variance can be shared or related between two variables; thus, we see that the criterion-related validity of any test is restricted as a function of the square root of the product of the reliabilities of the two measures [i.e., $(r_{xx}r_{yy})^{1/2}$].

Variance Definitions of Reliability and Validity

Classical test theory's variance definitions of reliability and validity are useful for understanding these two constructs and the relation between them. Briefly, a person's score on a test is a product of two things: that person's true (but unknown) score, and error. Similarly, the variance in a set of scores is a function of true-score variance (V_t) and error variance (V_e):

$$V = V_t + V_e$$

This relation is displayed pictorially in Figure 1. Using this definition, reliability is simply the proportion of true-score variance (V_t) to total variance (V). If a test is error-laden, it is unreliable. Conversely, if scores on a test are primarily the result of the test takers' *true* scores, the test is relatively reliable.

The true-score variance, a reflection of the reliability of the test, may also be subdivided. Suppose we administer several measures of reading comprehension. One measure requires children to read a passage and point to a picture that describes the passage read; the second requires the child to fill in a blank with a missing word; and the third requires the child to act out a sentence or passage (e.g., "Stick out your tongue"). Each method measures reading comprehension, and may do so very reliably. But each method also measures something else in addition to reading comprehension. In the first case, the child has to comprehend the passage, but also has to be able to recognize and interpret a picture depicting that passage; in the third measure, we are also requiring the child to be able to translate the passage into action. In other words, each method measures reading comprehension, but each also measures something *specific* to that measure, although both components may be measured reliably.

Of course, the degree to which each test measures reading comprehension is the validity of that test. In Figure 1, we can further divide the V_t (reliability) into the variance each measure shares with the other (V_c, or common variance, in this example representing reading comprehension), and the variance that is specific to the test (V_s, representing pictorial understanding, etc.). As is the case with reliability, the validity of the test is simply the proportion of common variance to total variance (V_c/V). The relation of validity to reliability is clear using this definition: We may consider validity as simply a subset of reliability. This, then, is the reason for the rule learned (and often confused) by students of measurement: A test cannot be valid unless it is reliable (all valid tests are reliable; no unreliable tests may be valid; reliable tests may or may not be valid). A more extensive and informative review of these problems may be found in Cronbach (1990), Guilford (1954), and Feldt and Brennan (1989).

Calculating and Reporting Reliability

Reliability of neuropsychological measures has received attention in the literature as an area of special need (e.g., Parsons & Prigatano, 1978; Reynolds, 1982a). Reliability of neuropsychological measures is equally important to individual diagnosis and to research, as reliability will influence the likelihood that any experimental or treatment effects will be detected. In short, reliability is the foundation on which validity, the most important of measurement concepts, is built. Nonetheless, even in the research literature, reliability data are seldom presented and the most frequently used of the various batteries, the HRNB, does not even have a discussion of reliability in its manual. Reliability of the LNNB is reported but is based on highly heterogeneous groups, across a too wide age span, and is likely spuriously inflated. The Boder Test of Reading–Spelling Patterns, developed by a pediatric neurologist as a neuropsychological measure of educational deficits, provides a good example of how not to assess reliability of neuropsychological measure, although the authors must be acknowledged for at least attending to the issue.

In studying the reliability of the Boder Test, Boder and Jarrico (1982) reported on several aspects of reliability. *Test–retest* (represented as r_{12}) or stability of scores is reported for 2-month and 1-year intervals. The sample size for the 2-month study was 50 and for the long-term study, N was 14. Three aspects of the test (the Boder not actually

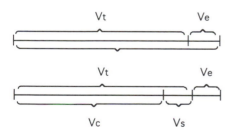

FIGURE 1. Variance definitions of reliability and validity. Variance in test scores may result from true-score variation (V_t) or error variance (V_e). True-score variation may be further divided into common variance (V_c) and specific variance (V_s), as in the bottom panel. Reliability is a function of V_t; validity is a function of V_c.

being divided into subtests) were evaluated, those yielding scores for Reading Level, Correctly Spelled Known Words, and the number of Good Phonetic Equivalents produced by the child. Both test–retest reports of reliability are based on wide age spans; for Reading Level an r_{12} of 0.98 is reported for ages 6–9, and 0.96 for ages 10–15. These rs are inflated to an unknown degree by the correlation of Reading Level with age. The use of a wide age range with rs based on raw scores or other age-related scores such as grade equivalents and age equivalents is a common method of exaggerating the observed reliability of test scores. When corrected for the confounding with age, which is certainly correlated to some substantial degree with Reading Level, these reliabilities are far less impressive. The original r_{12} for correctly spelled known words is but 0.64 for ages 6–9 and 0.84 for ages 10–15. For Good Phonetic Equivalents, the values are 0.89 and 0.85. After correction for spurious correlations with age, it would be surprising to find these reliabilities within any commonly accepted range for diagnosing individual cases. Also, the Ns are extremely small (ages 6–9, $N = 27$; ages 10–15, $N = 23$) for making any decision about the stability of scores on the Boder. The long-term rs were 0.81 for Reading Level, 0.62 for spelling, and 0.79 for Good Phonetic Equivalents, values that were clearly unacceptable for individual cases, but based only on $N = 14$, an unacceptable sample size in any case.

Internal consistency (corrected split-half) reliability estimates are reported for 46 cases randomly selected (by Boder and Jarrico's description) from Boder's private patient files. If truly random, the age range of these 46 children is 6 to 18 years. This tremendous age range greatly inflates internal consistency estimates and is unacceptable for assessing reliability. (This spurious increase in reliability estimates is the result of an artifactual, i.e., age-related, increase in item variances relative to total score variances on any test where item difficulties are correlated with age, i.e., on any test of a variable with a developmental nature). Though considerably inflated, the values were 0.97 for Reading Level, 0.82 for spelling (known words), and 0.92 for Good Phonetic Equivalents. The degree of spurious inflation is indeterminate.

The errors made in the estimation of the reliability of the Boder Test are serious but are all too common, not only in neuropsychology but in several areas of testing (e.g., see Reynolds, 1983). Lack of attention to standard psychometric methods

seems all too rampant in clinical neuropsychology and is retarding developments in the field. One other piece of relevant data is reported in the Boder Test manual's reliability section—the agreement on diagnosis of one of three reading disorders for the two testings with the test-retest reliability samples. Chi-square tests were used, appropriately, to evaluate changes in classification across testings, yet even these results are interpreted improperly. According to Boder and Jarrico (1982, p. 95), when the chi-square is evaluated, "a significant result shows high agreement between the classifications at the two testings." Rather, the significant chi-squares only show a statistically significant relationship between the two classifications; that is, the two sets of classifications were not independent. The actual number of children given the same classification on each testing was not reported and is necessary for a more proper interpretation of these results. The reliability of the Boder Test remains an open question specifically as does the reliability of the most popular of neuropsychological tests generally.

Because the validity of a test is restricted as a function of the square root of the product of the reliability coefficients of the test and the criterion [i.e., the theoretical limit placed on a test's validity coefficient is equal to $(r_{xx}r_{yy})^{1/2}$], one method of improving the validity of existing neuropsychological tests then obviously is to work toward enhancing the reliability of these scales. Too frequently, neuropsychologists rely on the "clinical" nature of certain tests and procedures to the extent that such important concepts as reliability are overlooked.

Reliability of our testing and assessment procedures is equally important to research in neuropsychology. The most direct implication of reliability for research is in the detection of experimental effects. As reliability decreases, so does the likelihood that a significant effect will be found in any experimental or clinical treatment. Marcel Kinsbourne has made reference to just this problem in consistently detecting hemispheric differences on certain tasks under a specified set of conditions (1981, personal communication). As anyone acquainted with the neuropsychology literature will be quick to recognize, the results of research employing dichotic listening procedures and tachistoscopic split-visual field presentation methods are not in great agreement. Dichotic listening and split-visual field methods are both very unreliable from a purely psychometric perspective. The reliabilities reported (albeit infrequently) in the literature are seldom better than 0.5 to 0.65. The reliability problems here possibly lie with the techniques themselves but a more likely problem seems to be the stimulus materials, i.e., the test that is presented through these methods. The proper application of traditional psychometric methods in the construction of tests to be presented through these methods would undoubtedly enhance the reliability of these techniques. Increases in the reliability of neuropsychological measures could increase the discriminability of the tests in studies of differential diagnosis as well. Error variance cannot contribute to the general problem of distinguishing among clinical groups, although, as reviewed later in this chapter, error variance can contribute spuriously in single studies without internal replication. Although increasing reliability will most certainly not alleviate all of the interpretive problems existing in this literature, it is better not to base arguments over the interpretation of data on what is essentially error variance and little else. Accuracy of scoring is crucial as well (Reynolds, 1979b).

Scaling Problems in Neuropsychological Testing

Children are in a constant state of development and change in many ways but perhaps most dramatically in their neurological and higher cortical development. Children are acquiring knowledge at the most rapid pace of their lifetime and their reasoning processes and insights into their learning grow in a dramatic manner. All are nevertheless moving at an uneven pace. Consequently, the scaling of any tests or measurement devices designed to aid the assessment of brain–behavior relations is crucial. This is true regardless of whether one takes a "key approach," looks simply at level of function, or assesses profiles of performance. The scaling of neuropsychological tests has been sporadic, with some scaled well, some poorly, and a significant number not at all. Even when scaling is handled well from a technical perspective, the quality of the standardization sample providing the estimates of population parameters from which standard scores are subsequently determined will influence the utility of the derived scores.

Raw scores, e.g., the number correct, the time to completion, or the number of errors, are problematic but common. The HRNB does not provide any transformed scores. Without standard score transformation, it is difficult to make any meaningful comparisons of scores. The dominant approaches to interpretation of the HRNB include assessing levels of performance and contrasting performance among the various tasks. Raw scores cannot be compared or assessed directly for a variety of reasons, the most potent being the lack of comparability of the raw score distributions among the tasks of the battery and for any one task across age. As Dean (1985) noted, in reviewing the HRNB, "without standard score transformation data, it is difficult to make any meaningful comparison between scores on individual tests" (p. 645). The use of raw scores is not necessarily wrong and is typically superior to the use of inaccurate score transformations. Appropriate use of raw scores does require extensive work and numerous calculations on the part of the person interpreting the test scores. The LNNB provides standardized or scaled scores in the form of the familiar T-score (mean = 50, standard deviation = 10) although the scaling is questionable because of the shape of the distributions obtained and the sample used in their standardization. Other attempts to scale neuropsychological measures have been made but use inappropriate scales, particularly age (AEs) or grade equivalents (GEs). Neuropsychological reports, even textbook examples, often contain performance reported in GEs. The Boder Test can again provide an illustration of some of the problems with scaling as practiced in clinical neuropsychology.

The Boder Test does not actually provide any type of standard score although the test's authors treat the various scores as though they are standardized or scaled scores. The Boder Test provides a Reading Level (RL) (analogous to a GE), a Reading Quotient (RQ), and a Reading Age (RA). Without adequate normative data, which the Boder does not possess, these scores are not very meaningful. Even if carefully normed, using state-of-the-art methods, these scores have serious limitations and should be used with extreme caution if at all and never as the featured scores for any contemporary scale, neuropsychological or otherwise.

RL and RA

The RL and RA of the Boder Test of Reading–Spelling Patterns (BTRSP) have similar problems. RL has the greatest difficulties even if calculated on the basis of good normative data, so the RL (the Boder Test's analogue of a GE) will be featured here. Given the interdependence of the RL and the RA as calculated on the Boder Test, their problems are almost identical.

The GE, i.e., RL, of the BTRSP is based in the grade level at which the words from the reading lists of the Boder are estimated to be introduced into the curriculum, and assumes that half of the children master these words for reading and spelling. True GEs are based on actual student knowledge of the curriculum content as reflected in mean scores on achievement tests. When content is introduced and when it is actually mastered by 50% of the pupils may not be closely related. Actual performance must be assessed.

GEs as a score on which to base decisions about individual pupils have serious deficiencies that have been presented in detail in a variety of sources (e.g., Angoff, 1971; Cronbach, 1990; Petersen, Kolen, & Hoover, 1989; Reynolds, 1981a,b, 1982a; Thorndike & Hagen, 1977). Though frequently treated as a standard score, GEs are not standard scores, and attempts to standardize them (Burns, 1982) have been largely unsuccessful (Reynolds & Willson, 1983); and indeed the true meaning of the GE is often distorted if understood at all. Most of the problems with GEs can be traced to one of two factors, or both: (1) GEs are calculated independent of the dispersion or distribution of scores about the mean and (2) the regression of the age, grade, and raw score is nonlinear, and varies across subject matter within grade as well as across grade within subject matter or content areas (AEs have analogous problems). Essentially, this tells us the GEs are on an ordinal scale of measurement and not an interval scale as so frequently interpreted. This makes many common uses of GEs entirely inappropriate.

Boder and Jarrico (1982, p. 5) defined significant reading retardation as performance 2 years below grade level for age according to the Boder Test RL. Other diagnoses are dependent on the RL and its discrepancy with expected level of performance as well. The "2 years" criterion for a reading disorder has been a common ground for diagnosis for some time and only recently abandoned (see also Reynolds, 1984). The use of GE scores at a constant discrepancy level irrespective of actual grade placement produces considerable irregularity for diagnosis, however. The distortions in interpreting discrepancies between GE scores and grade placement are readily apparent in Table 6, which was developed from data available in the norms or technical manuals of the Wide Range Achievement Test (WRAT), Peabody Individual Achievement Test (PIAT), Woodcock Reading Mastery Test (WRMT), and the Stanford Diagnostic Reading Test (SDRT). As is typical of GE scores, some occasional interpo-

lation was necessary to derive the exact values in Table 6. It is apparent, however, that a third-grader who reads "2 years below grade level for age" has a much more severe problem than say a seventh- or eighth-grader reading 2 years below grade level. In fact, a twelfth-grader with an IQ of 90 on a Wechsler scale and reading 2 years below grade level for age has no reading problem at all, but rather reads at a level slightly higher than what might be expected. Standard scores are by far a more accurate representation of an individual's achievement level than GEs because they are based not only on the mean at a given level but also on the distribution of scores about the mean. Thus, in the case of deviation standard scores, such as the Wechsler IQs, the relationship between standard scores is constant across age, and there are no excuses for the failure to provide such scores. Certainly the Boder Test provides no rationale for the lack of standard scores or even the preference for GEs. Nor do most clinical neuropsychologists have an adequate rationale for continued use of AEs and GEs in reports or in their application to profile analysis.

GEs are also inappropriate for use in any other sort of discrepancy analysis of an individual's test performance or key or profile analyses for the following reasons:

1. The growth curve between age and achievement in basic academic subjects flattens out at upper grade levels. This can be observed in Table 6 where it is seen that there is very little change in standard score values corresponding to 2 years below grade level for age after about grade 7 or 8. In fact, GEs have almost no meaning at this level, for reading instruction typically stops by high school and GEs are really only representing extrapolations from earlier grades. An excellent example of the difficulty in interpreting GEs beyond about grade 10 is apparent using an analogy with AEs. Height can be expressed in AEs just as reading can be expressed in GEs. However, although it might be helpful to describe a tall first-grader as having the height of an $8\frac{1}{2}$-year-old, how does one then characterize the 5'10" 14-year-old female, for at no age does the mean height of females equal 5'10"? Because the average reading level in the population changes very little after junior high school, GEs at these ages become virtually nonsensical, with large fluctuations in GEs sometimes resulting from a raw score difference of 2 or 3 points on a 100-item test.

2. GEs assume that the rate of learning is constant throughout the school year and that there is no gain or loss during summer vacation.

TABLE 6. Standard Scores Corresponding to Performance "Two Years below Grade Level for Age" on Four Major Reading Tests[a]

| Grade placement | Two years below placement | Standard scores[b] | | | |
		Wide Range Achievement Test	Peabody Individual Achievement Test[c]	Woodcock Reading Mastery Test[d]	Stanford Diagnostic Reading Test[c]
1.5	Pk.5	65	—	—	—
2.5	K.5	72	—	—	—
3.5	1.5	69	—	64	64
4.5	2.5	73	75	77	64
5.5	3.5	84	85	85	77
6.5	4.5	88	88	91	91
7.5	5.5	86	89	94	92
8.5	6.5	87	91	94	93
9.5	7.5	90	93	96	95
10.5	8.5	85	93	95	95
11.5	9.5	85	93	95	92
12.5	10.5	85	95	95	92

[a]Adapted from Reynolds (1981a).
[b]All standard scores have been converted for ease of comparison to a common scale having a mean of 100 and a standard deviation of 15.
[c]Reading Comprehension subtest only.
[d]Total test.

3. As partially noted above, GEs involve an excess of extrapolation, especially at the upper and lower ends of the scale. However, because tests are not administered during each month of the school year, scores between the testing intervals (often a full year) must be interpolated on the assumption of constant growth rates. Interpolation between extrapolated values on an assumption of constant growth rates is at best a highly perilous activity. The assumption underlying score derivations on the Boder Test that each word read correctly represents 2 months of academic achievement is even more perilous, and most likely cannot be substantiated. For the Boder Test, this adds to the error and the unfounded assumption already present in *properly derived* GEs, which the RL of the Boder Test is not. Popular achievement tests in neuropsychology have similar problems. The front of the protocol for the WRAT, for example, notes that standard scores only and not the so-called grade rating (the WRAT's GE) should be used for interpretive purposes.

4. Different academic subjects are acquired at different rates and the variations in performance differ from one content area to another. As a consequence, "2 years below grade level for age" may be a much more serious deficiency in mathematics than, say, in reading comprehension. The degree of academic deficit in Reading versus Spelling, as on

the Boder Test, denoted by the "2 years" marker, will differ as well.

5. GEs exaggerate small differences in performance between individuals and for a single individual across tests. Some test authors (e.g., Jastak & Jastak, 1978) even provide a caution on test record forms that standard scores only, and not GEs, should be used for comparison purposes.

RQ

The Boder Test also provides an RQ calculated in accordance with one of three formulas offered in the Boder Manual, with the choice of derivation given to the examiner. Giving a choice of three formulas to the examiners is problematic in itself. Though some general guidelines are provided concerning when to use each formula, the choice is left to the examiner, and it is entirely probable that, faced with a similar or even identical set of scores, different examiners will arrive at different RQs; the same examiner may well fall to the same plight over time, being inconsistent in the choice of formulas given a common set of circumstances. However, this is one of the more minor problems with the Boder Test RQ. The RQ is derived from a faulty score to begin with, the RA, as noted in the previous section. The RQ, as calculated to be

(RA/CA) × 100 (where CA is chronological age), will not have a constant standard deviation across age and is not a standard score as thought by many. It is conceptually the antiquated notion of a ratio IQ that was abandoned many years ago in favor of more refined standard score systems. The standard deviation of the first version of the RQ will almost certainly range from at least 10 to 29, leading to the confusing (and unaccounted for in the Boder Test's diagnostic system) state wherein, depending on age, RQs of 80 and 90 represent the same overall level of performance at different ages. The actual range of standard deviations could be larger or smaller; whichever it turns out to be is less important than the fact that the standard deviation will not be constant across age and that the standard deviation at any age is unknown.

Use of either of the two alternative formulas given below for calculating the RQ is even more problematic. These formulas

$$RQ = \frac{2RA}{MA + CA} \times 100 \qquad (1)$$

$$RQ = \frac{3RA}{MA + CA + grade\ age} \times 100 \quad (2)$$

are quite similar to expectancy formulas proposed by the U. S. Office of Education (1976) in their attempt to define severe discrepancies between aptitude and achievement. Commentary on such formulas has shown them to be grossly inadequate for use in any kind of normative reporting or discrepancy analysis and far more sophisticated approaches are needed (Reynolds, 1984). The standard deviation of the scores derived from these formulas will also vary and is unknown. The same number of children will not be identified at each IQ level *or each age level* using the BTRSP classification rules. There is no established validity for either formula; they are only intuitive in their appeal.

Given the problems of age- and grade-based equivalency scores and the amount of severe criticism they have received in the literature, it is difficult to imagine a justification for their use in place of standard scores. Certainly, standard scores should be provided at a minimum with AEs and GEs and related derived scores (e.g., RQ) provided as supplementary if at all. Because AEs and GEs are representing only ordinal scale data (and thus cannot be averaged or otherwise manipulated with any confidence except under special conditions), it is particu-

larly important that these scores not be used for comparative purposes. Standard scores could not be reported for the Boder Test because there are no normative data on which to base these calculations.

Ratios and Quotients

Probably the best known of all scores to the layperson is the ratio IQ, originated for use with the Binet scales early in the century. As every introductory psychology course student knows, IQ = (mental age/chronological age) × 100. This forms the ratio or quotient from which the designation IQ was derived. Such ratios or quotients have numerous psychometric problems and are no longer used by the major test publishers but do persist in certain areas of neuropsychology, even to the point of developing ratios of "hold" to "don't hold" subtests for estimating premorbid functioning. Such ratios are nonsensical for most interpretive purposes, however, and lead primarily to confusion. Although they may be used to rank individuals who take a common test, no comparisons beyond rank on the common measure are possible—including profile analysis or any comparisons across tests. The so-called ratio IQ is a ratio of numbers with radically different underlying distributions and mathematical properties. Chronological age is a ratio scale of measurement. Mental age is on an ordinal scale of measurement. Creating a ratio of two such disparate scales is a conceptual nightmare of some proportion. The standard deviation of the distribution of such ratios will also vary across age. The 1937 Stanford–Binet Intelligence Scale, which yielded such a ratio IQ, showed a standard deviation that ranged from about 9 to 32 depending on the age of the individual assessed. The familiar standard deviation of 16 used then, and now, by the Binet Scales, was the average standard deviation across ages 2 to about 16. Gross inaccuracies of interpretation are facilitated by such scales and they are not standard or scaled scores in any sense of contemporary uses of these terms. Various ratio scores and quotients such as the early IQ remain in use in neuropsychological assessment but do not possess the properties of standard scores that make the latter so useful in all areas of testing and assessment.

Standard or Scaled Scores

The primary advantage of standardized or scaled scores lies in the comparability of score interpretation across age. By standard scores is meant scores of the Wechsler Deviation IQ genre, referred to more properly as age-corrected deviation scaled scores. This designation is used because the mean and the standard deviation of the scaled score distribution are reset or rescaled periodically, typically every 2 to 4 months at preschool ages and every 4 to 6 months thereafter until the adult years when much larger age groupings may be used. Standard scores of the deviation IQ type have the same percentile rank across age, for they are based not only on the mean but the variability in scores about the mean at each age level. For example, a score that falls two-thirds of a grade level below the average grade level has a different percentile rank at every age.

Standard scores are more accurate and precise. When constructing tables for the conversion of raw scores into standard scores, interpolation of scores to arrive at an exact score point is typically not necessary, whereas the opposite is true of GEs. Extrapolation is also typically not necessary for scores within three standard deviations of the mean, which accounts for more than 99% of all scores encountered.

Standard scores are on an equal interval scale in many cases (see Gordon, 1984), making profile analysis possible across subtests of a common scale. Ipsative analysis of performance only makes mathematic sense with an interval or higher scale of measurement. Score comparisons among different batteries or subparts of different measuring devices are also possible provided the reliability of each measure is known, and, for some purposes, the correlation between the various pairs of scores must also be known. If the reliability coefficients are comparable, the score distributions are normal, and the percentile rank of scores is known, Table 7 can be used to place scores on a commonly expressed metric, i.e., a scale having the same mean and standard deviation. The choice of standard score scales is often arbitrary but is sometimes dictated by the standard deviation of the raw score distribution, such that the score points should not be artificially spread over too many standard score points nor should too many raw score points be collapsed into a single scaled score point. Such problems are usually avoided by the choice of an appropriate scale and finding a suitable scale is easy enough that it is seldom a serious problem in the application of scaled scores to most practical problems of assessment. There are few instances when other score systems are superior to scaled scores, and methods are now available for the use of scaled scores even at the most extreme points in the distributions of intelligence, achievement, and other special abilities (e.g., see Reynolds & Clark, 1985, 1986).

Differential Diagnosis: Determining Membership in Clinical Populations

One of the major problems for psychologists in professional practice has historically been that of differential diagnosis of mental disorders. In the area of clinical neuropsychology, differential diagnosis has been of particular importance. The major area of research in clinical neuropsychology has had as its purpose the development of clinical tests and procedures to differentiate reliably between brain-injured and neurologically intact individuals and to separate brain-injured groups into subsamples according to location, cause, time of onset, and, in some cases, prognosis. Many neuropsychologists still earn a considerable portion of their "keep" differentiating organic from nonorganic psychiatric referrals and evaluating the nature and extent of lesions for the neurology service. This does bring out another major area of methodological and statistical problems in clinical neuropsychology—one that, oddly enough, is nearly the opposite of the preceding discussions. In differential diagnosis, rather than being naive about the underlying psychometrics or scaling, the tendency has been to perform analyses that are too sophisticated for the data.

To their credit, researchers have, over the last two decades, brought to bear the most sophisticated statistical methodologies directly on the problem of diagnosis and classification of mental disorders in the form of various multivariate analytical techniques. In the quest to provide accurate diagnosis of neurological disturbances, a large set of behaviors is typically assessed. Rourke (1975), in discussing more than two decades of research on differential diagnosis, indicated that children referred to his laboratory are typically administered

> the WISC, the Peabody Picture Vocabulary Test, the Halstead Neuropsychological Test Battery for Children, the Reitan Indiana Neuropsychological Test Battery, the Wide Range Achievement Test, an examination for sensory–perceptual disturbances, the Klove–Mathews Motor Steadiness Battery, and a number of other tests for receptive and expressive language abilities. (p. 912)

This continues to be a common practice in the field. Multivariate classification techniques are very powerful in the determination of group membership.

TABLE 7. Conversion of Standard Scores Based on Several Scales to a Commonly Expressed Metric

$\bar{X} = 0$ SD = 1	$\bar{X} = 100$ SD = 15	$\bar{X} = 100$ SD = 16	$\bar{X} = 100$ SD = 20	$\bar{X} = 500$ SD = 100	$\bar{X} = 50$ SD = 10	$\bar{X} = 50$ SD = 15	$\bar{X} = 36$ SD = 6	$\bar{X} = 10$ SD = 3	Percentile rank
2.6	139	142	152	760	76	89	52	18	>99
2.4	136	138	148	740	74	86	51	17	99
2.2	133	135	144	720	72	83	49	17	99
2.0	130	132	140	700	70	80	48	16	98
1.8	127	129	136	680	68	77	47	15	96
1.6	124	126	132	660	66	74	46	15	95
1.4	121	122	128	640	64	71	44	14	92
1.2	118	119	124	620	62	68	43	14	88
1.0	115	116	120	600	60	65	42	13	84
0.8	112	113	116	580	58	62	41	12	79
0.6	109	110	112	560	56	59	40	12	73
0.4	106	106	108	540	54	56	38	11	66
0.2	103	103	104	520	52	53	37	11	58
0.0	100	100	100	500	50	50	36	10	50
−0.2	97	97	96	480	48	47	35	9	42
−0.4	94	94	92	460	46	44	34	9	34
−0.6	91	90	88	440	44	41	33	8	27
−0.8	88	87	84	420	42	38	31	8	21
−1.0	85	84	80	400	40	35	30	7	16
−1.2	82	81	76	380	38	32	29	6	12
−1.4	79	78	72	360	36	29	28	6	8
−1.6	76	74	68	340	34	26	26	5	5
−1.8	73	71	64	320	32	23	25	5	4
−2.0	70	68	60	300	30	20	24	4	2
−2.2	67	65	56	280	28	17	23	3	1
−2.4	64	62	52	260	26	14	21	3	1
−2.6	61	58	48	240	24	11	20	2	<1

Unfortunately, with such a large set of variables, small numbers of subjects can all be grouped and classified purely on the basis of random or chance variation that takes maximum advantage of correlated error variances. Thus, the need for large numbers of subjects in such research is a crucial one.

In the study of clinical disorders, however, one is frequently limited to relatively small samples of design. Although most researchers acknowledge this difficulty, few realize the devastating effect of subject/variable ratios approaching 1 on the generalizability of studies of differential diagnosis. This is not to say that excellent studies have not been done. Studies of discriminability by Satz and his colleagues (e.g., Satz, Taylor, Friel, & Fletcher, 1978) use large numbers of variables but have considerable subject populations. Large-N studies of clinical populations continue to be the exception rather than the rule. Willson and Reynolds (1982) evaluated the effects of small samples on the validity of research attempting to discriminate among clinical disorders on the basis of neuropsychological test performance and have reported on many of the statistical problems that seem to plague the area.

Some Statistical Considerations

In predicting group membership from a set of variables (e.g., neuropsychological test scores) there are several considerations. First, procedures that use *samples* of the target populations involve sampling error in the estimation of the relationships being examined. This means that results are expected to fluctuate from sample to sample as a result of the random differences inherent in the samples. The usual measure of prediction is the squared multiple correlation (R^2). In applying results of a particular sample to a second sample, R^2 is expected to decrease because correlation is a maximizing operation—R^2 was made as big as possible for the first sample capitalizing on correlated error variances whenever possible. It is unlikely the same fit of the data will occur in a second sample. Thus, rules for classification derived from a particular sample cannot necessarily be expected to generalize to any other sample without a cross-validation effort to demonstrate such an effect.

A second consideration in prediction occurs when the prediction used a strategy for selecting a small number of variables from a much larger initial set of variables (e.g., Purisch, Golden, & Hammeke, 1979). In the same, some correlations underestimate the population value and others overestimate it. In stepwise regression or discriminant procedures and related multivariate methods, the overestimates are always chosen. When a large number of predictors is available, stepwise procedures maximize the chance of selecting random or near-random predictors. These are variables that do not predict well in the population but by chance correlate highly with the outcome in the particular sample being used.

The degree of decrease in R^2 from sample to population can be estimated. The most commonly used estimate is from Wherry (1932; see also Lord & Novick, 1968, p. 286) and is

$$R_p^2 = 1 - (1 - R^2)(N - 1)/(N - K - 1) \quad (3)$$

N is the number of observations, K the number of predictors, R^2 the observed squared multiple correlation between outcome and predictors, and R_p^2 the population squared multiple correlation. This formula holds for either multiple regression or discriminant analysis.

Formula (3) has been widely cited. A review by Cattin (1980) suggested that for small N and K, another approximation should be used:

$$\hat{R}^2 = \frac{(N - K - 3)p^4 + p^2}{(N - 2K - 2)p^2 + K} \quad (4)$$

where

$$p^2 = 1 - \frac{N - 3}{N - K - 1}(1 - R^2)$$

$$\left[1 + \frac{2(1 - R^2)}{N - K - 1} + \frac{8(1 - R^2)^2}{(N - K + 1)(N - K + 3)}\right]$$

Although $\hat{R}^2$ is biased, the amount of bias is on the order of 0.01–0.02 for $N = 60$ and $K = 50$.

Of special interest is the case where there are more predictors than people. In equation (4), the shrunken $\hat{R}^2$ may become negative or greater than 1.0. What this really means is that mathematically

with more predictors than observations of the outcome, there is no unique solution to a best prediction. In discriminant analysis this may result in perfect classification entirely at random by the predictors. Mathematically, this results from having more parameters to estimate than data points. Either one is forced to make enough side conditions to constrain the solution or one accepts a solution that results from a particular order of entering predictors. As it is mathematically impossible to estimate all regression coefficients, there will be

$$\frac{K}{N} = \frac{K!}{N!(N - K)!}$$

different solutions that would provide perfect classification but would not generalize to any other samples. In particular, it may be quite likely to find a solution that maximizes R^2 based entirely on chance correlations if there are enough correlations from which to choose.

Even when there are fewer predictors than subjects, the shrunken R^2 estimate will rapidly approach zero as the number of predictors becomes a significant proportion of the number of subjects. When small samples of subjects are involved, as with many neuropsychological studies, the use of a large number of tests as predictors frequently fulfills this condition.

Multiple regression and discriminant analysis have been discussed interchangeably to this point, but some distinctions need to be made about them. Formally, they are identical in two-group prediction, e.g., brain-damaged versus non-brain-damaged. For more than two groups, discriminant analysis must be used. There have been a number of different classification rules proposed using discriminant analysis. These pertain to assumptions about prior probabilities for population composition and about homogeneity of within-group covariances. In any case the R of relationship between predictor and between group distance is computed. It is a canonical correlation (see Cooley & Lohnes, 1971, p. 249). Because there may be more than one discriminant function, there will be a canonical R for each. Their squares do not necessarily add together to get a total R^2, as there may be redundancy between functions (Cooley & Lohnes, 1971, p. 170), but their squared sum is the maximum possible R^2. This may be useful as a liberal estimate because if it can be shown that $\hat{R}_p^2$ is near zero, there is no need to estimate the study's R^2, because it will produce an even smaller estimate of $\hat{R}_p^2$.

For two groups, multiple regression and discriminant analysis yield the same results. For more than two groups, the canonical R^2 is still useful as an approximation to a multiple regression R^2. This interpretation can be a useful one but is rare in clinical neuropsychology, as multiple group discriminant analysis is so seldom applied by clinical researchers. The omission is significant in that although researchers in neuropsychology may not be familiar with or do not apply this technique for other reasons, it may be quite useful in discriminating among several populations.

The Willson and Reynolds Examples of Classification Problems

To illustrate the problems that can be created by these statistical considerations, Willson and Reynolds (1982) examined all articles in three journals (*Psychology in the Schools, Journal of Consulting and Clinical Psychology,* and *Clinical Neuropsychology*) for the years 1979–1981. They selected studies that used test batteries, socioeconomic or demographic variables, or a combination of these variables to predict clinical group membership and that could help illustrate the difficulties of such work. Nine studies were found. Such studies

are not unique to this era and the problems noted below continue (e.g., Bernard, Houston, & Natoli, 1993; Boone, Ghaffarian, Lesser, & Hill-Gutierrez, 1993; Miles & Stelmack, 1994; Thienemann & Koran, 1995) although well-accomplished works are becoming more frequent and continue to come from the laboratories of Rourke and of Satz as noted earlier as well as other research centers (e.g., Guilmette & Rasile, 1995; Ivnik *et al.*, 1994).

The studies are listed in Table 8 (from Willson & Reynolds, 1982). Also listed are sample sizes (N), total number of predictors used in stepwise procedures (K_T), and number of predictors used in the final or discriminant equation (K_F). In one case, R_F was determined indirectly through a 2×2 classification table that was reported in the studies. The tetrachoric correlation was computed and squared (see Glass, 1978, and Pedhazur & Schmelkin, 1991, for a discussion of estimating correlation effects).

Table 8 lists several other statistics that represent estimated values of R_F^2 and their significance via their associated F-statistic. The statistic $\hat{R}_T^2$ represents the estimated R shrunken by equation (3) to account for all predictors originally considered. Because in no study was the overall R_T^2 reported for

TABLE 8. Summaries of Prediction Studies from Three Special Population Journals

Study		Sample size	Total number of predictors	Number of predictors used	R_F^2 (reported)	$\hat{R}_T^2$	$\hat{R}_F^2$
Dean (1978)		120	14	4	0.25*	0.09	0.21*
Selz & Reitan (1979)[a]		75	37	37	0.57	0.57	0.57
Wallbrown, Vance, & Pritchard (1979)		200	8	3	0.19*	0.13	0.17*
Purisch, Golden, & Hammeke (1979)	(a)	100	282	40	1.00*	0[b]	0[b]
	(b)	100	14	14	0.88*	0.84*	0.84*
Taylor & Imivey (1980)	(a)	30	16	5	0.44*	0.00	0.26
	(b)	30	3	1	0.08	0.00	0.05
	(c)	30	16	5	0.30	0.00	0.10
	(d)	30	3	1	0.14*	0.02	0.12
	(e)	30	16	2	0.25*	0.00	0.22*
	(f)	30	2	1	0.11	0.03	0.09
Dunleavy, Hansen, & Baade (1981)		24	37	3	0.82*	0[b]	0.79*
Fuller & Goh (1981)		80	22	12	0.38*	0.05	0.19
Golden, Moses, Graber, & Berg (1981)	(a)	60	11	2	0.55*	0.37*	0.54*
	(b)	120	11	2	0.68*	0.62*	0.68*
Malloy & Webster (1981)[c]	(a)	36	14	14	0.57	0.57	0.57
	(b)	36	14	14	0.94*[d]	0.94*	0.94*

[a]Trinomial classification table was reported; it was converted to a binomial (normal versus brain-damaged or LD) and the tetrachoric correlation computed, which was squared to obtain $\hat{R}_F^2$. Because it was based on a prediction equation from another study, no shrinkage was expected.
[b]An R^2 of 0.00 is expected in an overdetermined system, in which there are more predictors than subjects. Perfect classification is always possible.
[c]Binomial classification was reported. The tetrachoric correlation was computed as in footnote a.
[d]The R^2 values were estimated from a misclassification rate of 20% with 36 subjects. Although the actual study was trinomial, the R^2 represents the equivalent for binomial classification for ease of computing.
*$p < 0.05$.

all predictors, it was necessary to use the R_F^2 based on the final regression. Thus, $\hat{R}_T^2$ underestimated the shrunken R_p^2 to some degree. Its upper bound is given by $\hat{R}_F^2$, the shrunken estimate based on the number of predictors actually used. This is an *overestimate* of the actual shrunken R_p^2.

A second set of statistics was calculated from the nine studies to estimate loss of classification power resulting from shrinkage and is presented in Table 9. For the reported R_F^2 and the $\hat{R}_T^2$ the *t*-statistic equivalent was computed according to

$$ t = \left[\frac{R^2/K}{(1 - R^2)/(N - K - 1)} \right]^{1/2} \tag{5} $$

Although most studies had only two groups, in Selz and Reitan (1979), the *t*-statistic was based on a reduction of three groups to two (normal versus abnormal). Then, an effect size was computed.

$$ \epsilon = t(1/n_1 + 1/n_2)^{1/2} \tag{6} $$

as defined by Glass (1978). This statistic is the number of standard deviations separating the two groups. Finally, the percentile point under the normal curve for *half* the effect is presented. This is the point that minimizes misclassification assuming equal cost for either false-positive or false-negative errors, and the equal population base rates.

Of the 17 R_F^2 obtainable from the studies, 12 were initially significant. After correcting the shrinkage, only 4 were significant as $\hat{R}_T^2$, and 8 as $\hat{R}_F^2$. Thus, half the results reported in these studies are attributable to chance large correlations. Under the most optimistic of circumstances, the upper limit of shrinkage R^2 estimate shows a mean R^2 of 0.37 versus a mean obtained R^2 value of 0.48 for all studies considered. The lower bound estimate of the shrunken R^2 yields even more pessimistic results, demonstrating a mean value of but 0.25. The chance variation that can appear on the surface to be reliable discrimination with powerful multivariate techniques is thus rather considerable. The importance of large subject/variable ratios and proper cross-validation becomes immediately obvious in considering the results summarized in Tables 8 and 9. Interested professionals must consider with special care the prediction rules generated from those studies when R dropped to nonsignificance.

In examining the misclassification rates (see Table 9), there is a change from about one-third expected in the original studies (35%) to almost half (44%) using the corrected values, the chance rates

under no knowledge, and very unimpressive when contrasted against base rates in referral populations. This is not surprising given the considerable decline in effect sizes shown in Table 9.

It must be reiterated that the shrinkage occurs in research in which correlation maximizing procedures have been used: stepwise multiple regression, stepwise discriminant analysis, and canonical correlation. The R^2 does not shrink in a fixed variable study in which all variables are included and in which order is unimportant (balanced ANOVA design) or in which order is predetermined (path analysis design, causal model design). Diagnosis seeks to find the best empirical discriminators, but it is most subject to chance.

The shrunken estimate of R^2 and the expected misclassification rate are part of the technique of cross-validation. Cross-validation requires two independent samples. Ideally both are drawn independently from the same population. Often a single sample is split into two halves. In either case the regression is computed on one sample and the weights applied to the scores of the second population to predict the outcome or group membership as appropriate. The R^2 is a one-sample estimate of the R^2 in the nonvalidation sample, but it is not nearly so convincing. First, it is a statistic itself that may vary; second, it uses information from one sample, not nearly as good as that available from two samples. In clinical samples the N is typically so small that splitting it is not a good idea. The regression weights and R^2 will become even more changeable as the subject/variable ratio is halved. This leaves two-sample cross-validation. Samples should be drawn from the same population initially. There may also be considerable value in determining the generalizability of the results to other populations in an effort to improve the clinical utility of the classification rules. These are separate problems; the sampling procedure in the first case is obvious and has been discussed. Sampling in the second case will be dictated by the specific design of the study.

Should prediction studies be cross-validated prior to publication? Is it the responsibility of the researcher to provide this evidence? If actuarial rules for diagnosis are used, the obvious answer is yes. Even in more purely clinical decision-making, the repeatability of one's results from a referral pool cannot be ignored. The Selz and Reitan (1979) research is an example where this procedure was followed, with quite credible results. The application of such a prediction rule to new populations requires new cross-validation, however. To those who

TABLE 9. Expected Misclassifications from Nine Studies

		t-equivalent for		Estimated effect[a] size for two populations for		Two-population % misclassification for	
		$\hat{R}_F^2$	$\hat{R}_T^2$	$\hat{R}_F^2$	$\hat{R}_T^2$	$\hat{R}_F^2$	$\hat{R}_T^2$
Dean (1978)		2.76	0.86	0.50	0.16	39%	47%
Purisch, Golden, & Hammeke (1979)	(a)	0	0	0	0	50%	50%
	(b)	6.27	6.27	1.25	1.25	27%	27%
Selz & Reitan (1979)[b]		1.15	1.15	0.27	0.27	45%	45%
Wallbrown, Vance, & Pritchard (1979)		3.12	1.89	0.44	0.27	41%	45%
Taylor & Imivey (1980)	(a)	1.69[c]	0.00	0.62	0.00	38%	50%
	(b)	1.21[c]	0.00	0.44	0.00	41%	50%
	(c)	0.73[c]	0.00	0.27	0.00	45%	50%
	(d)	1.95[c]	0.42	0.71	0.15	36%	47%
	(e)	2.84[c]	0.00	0.73	0.00	36%	50%
	(f)	1.76[c]	0.65	0.64	0.24	37%	45%
Dunleavy, Hansen, & Baade (1981)		5.01	0	2.05	0	16%	50%
Fuller & Goh (1981)		1.14	0.37	0.25	0.06	45%	49%
Golden, Moses, Graber, & Berg (1981)	(a)	5.78	1.61	1.49	0.42	23%	42%
	(b)	11.15	4.00	2.04	0.73	15%	36%
Malloy & Webster (1981)[b]	(a)	1.19	1.19	0.40	0.40	42%	42%
	(b)	5.04	5.04	1.68	1.68	20%	20%
Mean		3.11	1.38	0.81	0.33	35%	44%

[a]Effect = $t(1/n_1 + 1/n_2)^{\frac{1}{2}}$ (Glass, 1978)
[b]No shrinkage occurred.
[c]Single group statistics; effects were computed as if for two groups. Single group results are smaller than reported here.

argue it is difficult to obtain subjects in rare disorder categories, hold the results until a second population is sampled. There will be no real loss to the discipline. On the contrary, there will be a new gain, for only the cross-validated results will achieve publication. Given the sometimes harsh attacks on the application of clinical neuropsychological techniques (e.g., Coles, 1978; Reschly & Gresham, 1989; Sandoval, 1981) to the rehabilitation of learning and related problems, it certainly behooves researchers to be careful in deciding when research is ready to report. The external validity of one's "findings" must be clear.

Cross-validation, when it is presented as evidence for the consistency of results in one population, does not provide evidence for generalizability to other populations. This can be done by additional studies. There is no reason to believe that the regression weights that discriminate two groups will discriminate either from a third. This point is not restrictive to prediction studies but occurs in all behavioral research.

A related issue should be obvious and of great significance to the practicing clinician in neuropsy-chology and other subdisciplines involved in differential diagnosis. When actuarial rules for the diagnosis of psychological and neuropsychological disorders appear in refereed professional journals, those in applied settings, especially those keeping closest to current developments in the field, may feel very confident in applying such rules in diagnosis and in the development of treatment plans. Clearly, the Willson and Reynolds (1982) results show that in the absence of proper cross-validation, many diagnoses or classifications may be made on the basis of random relationships. This constitutes an unacceptable situation for all involved, but especially for the patient and her or his physician.

Profile Reliability

A related problem when multiple scores are being used in classification or individual diagnoses and decision-making is the reliability of the set of scores for each individual considered. Perhaps stability is a better conceptualization, as the question is whether (or how much) the profile of scores, taken as a whole, would change and whether this change would affect clinical decision-making. Stability of profiles over at least very short periods of time (largely depending on the clinical disorder under investigation) needs investigation and yet has gone largely ignored. The problems of such research, which may at first seem simple, are difficult ones, but can be solved.

The most difficult problem is that of differential practice effects among the various scales that go into making up the score profile. This introduces methodological artifacts that require statistical control through estimation of regression effects for each part of the battery prior to comparing the two profiles obtained—in such a case, only the second profile should be corrected. Following this set of corrections, profile stability or reliability can then be assessed. Profile reliability is essentially a multivariate problem and thus requires a multivariate solution. A variety of statistical approaches may be used and the specific purpose of the study may dictate different approaches. Roffe and Bryant (1979), in a study of profile reliability for the McCarthy Scales, used the Pearson correlation. This approach is problematic from several perspectives. If the Pearson correlation is employed, profiles must first be "standardized" as described by Nunnally (1978). However, even under these circumstances, the Pearson correlation is likely to be inaccurate, for it does not consider level, dispersion, shape, and accentuation of the various profiles. Several very powerful techniques have been developed that accurately determine the similarity of profiles, including D^2 (Cronbach & Gleser, 1953; Osgood & Suci, 1952) and the coefficient of pattern similarity, r_p (Cattell, 1966). These two approaches in particular are accurate, sophisticated measures of profile similarity and should be employed whenever possible (see also Nesselroade & Cattell, 1988).

Sensitivity, Specificity, and Diagnostic Accuracy

Neuropsychologists and other clinical researchers are, as I have noted, often interested in how well a disorder is detected or how well it is diagnosed. Too often, researchers fail to consider and report on the sensitivity, specificity, and diagnostic accuracy of their procedures, retarding the clinician's ability to understand the utility of a diagnostic procedure.

In any diagnostic question, there are four outcomes. The clinician can be: (1) right about the presence of a disorder (a true positive), (2) wrong about the presence of disorder (a false positive),

(3) right about the absence of a disorder (a true negative), or (4) wrong about the absence of a disorder (a false negative). These conditions are illustrated in Figure 2, and seldom are reported in research on diagnosis.

Sensitivity in diagnosis refers to the ability to detect a disorder when it is present. Sensitivity thus refers to the probability that a disorder will be diagnosed when a patient has the disorder. Of course, if we diagnose every child-patient we see as having a learning disability, we will "miss" none who do, making our diagnostic decision highly sensitive—but we would lack specificity.

Specificity refers to the ability to differentiate among conditions or, in essence, to detect the absence of a disorder. In the above example, we guard against false-negative diagnostic errors at the expense of creating a large number of false-positive errors.

Often we must seek a balance between specificity and sensitivity in diagnosis. It is a given in neuropsychology that we will not be 100% accurate in diagnosis. All four conditions in Figure 2 are likely to occur in any set of diagnostic decisions. Through our research, we seek to enhance both sensitivity and specificity through maximizing squares 1 and 4, thereby minimizing squares 2 and 3 (see Figure 2). Often, however, by increasing one we often decrease the other. Researchers should always report a table such as represented by Figure 2 (e.g., see Guilmette & Rasile, 1995, Tables 4–6) so that specificity, sensitivity, and diagnostic accuracy can be assessed and preferably using multiple cutoff scores of classification rules. Sensitivity is

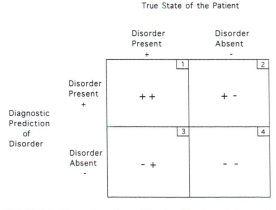

FIGURE 2. Illustration of possible classification of diagnostic decisions. Square 1 = true positives, square 2 = false positives, square 3 = false negatives, square 4 = true negatives.

represented by the ratio of square 1 to the sum of squares 1 and 3 while specificity is represented by the ratio of square 4 to the sum of squares 2 and 4. As this ratio approaches 1.00, sensitivity and specificity improve.

Diagnostic accuracy is a related concept that is determined to be the ratio of square 1 plus square 4 to the sum of all four squares. As this value approaches 1.00, diagnostic accuracy improves. These values are relatively easy to determine and will vary by diagnostic rule. Clinicians need to assess these concepts in deciding whether to apply a given diagnostic rule.

Is it better to make the error of a false-positive diagnosis or a false-negative diagnosis? This is a very complex question (see also Reynolds, 1984) that will vary in correct response as a function of the disorder and the consequences of each type of error. Errors will be made, however, and clinicians should be informed about the sensitivity, specificity, and diagnostic accuracy of their techniques so that a truly informed decision can be made about adopting a new test or a new interpretive rule.

Summary

It has become customary over the years to end reports of research with cautionary statements and call for further research. If diagnostic or classification studies with small samples and large numbers of variables employing powerful, sophisticated multivariate classification techniques are to continue to appear without concurrent cross-validation, and multivariate profiles are to be considered, much stronger cautions are needed to avoid the inadvertent leading of the diagnostician into potential malpractice. The most obvious, and the most sound solution is not to publish such small-*N* studies without concurrent replication, and not to rely on profiles with unknown stability in differential diagnosis research or clinical practice.

Many problems related to measurement and statistics in clinical neuropsychological research and in clinical diagnosis have been reviewed here. Many other problems exist but a substantial portion of these difficulties can be resolved by avoiding the problems noted in this chapter. By so doing, other, now fuzzy, issues, methodological, statistical, and clinical, should be brought into a sharper focus and new problems can be identified. The failure to resolve basic measurement issues in clinical neu-

ropsychological research can do nothing except restrain progress in the field at a time when sophisticated technology is experiencing explosive growth all around us. Specificity, sensitivity, and diagnostic accuracy are all information to be gathered and reported as new techniques (and old) are evaluated and reevaluated.

References

Adams, R. L. (1985). Review of the Luria–Nebraska Neuropsychological Battery. In J. V. Mitchell (Ed.), *The ninth mental measurements yearbook.* Lincoln: University of Nebraska Press.

Angoff, W. H. (1971). Scales, norms, and equivalent scores. In R. L. Thorndike (Ed.), *Educational measurement* (2nd ed.). Washington, DC: American Council on Education.

Ardila, A., Roselli, M., & Puente, T. (1994). *Neuropsychological evaluation of the Spanish speaker.* New York: Plenum Press.

Arnold, B. R., Montgomery, G. T., Castaneda, I., & Langoria, R. (1994). Acculturation and performance of Hispanics on selected Halstead–Reitan neuropsychological tests. *Assessment, 1,* 239–248.

Bernard, L. C., Houston, W., & Natoli, L. (1993). Malingering on neuropsychological memory tests: Potential objective indicators. *Journal of Clinical Psychology, 49,* 45–53.

Bersoff, D. N. (1982). The legal regulation of school psychology. In C. R. Reynolds & T. B. Gutkin (Eds.), *The handbook of school psychology.* New York: Wiley.

Boder, E., & Jarrico, S. (1982). *Boder Test of Reading–Spelling Patterns.* New York: Grune & Stratton.

Boone, K., Ghaffarian, S., Lesser, I., & Hill–Gutierrez, E. (1993). Wisconsin Card Sorting Test performance in healthy, older adults: Relationship to age, sex, education, and IQ. *Journal of Clinical Psychology, 49,* 54–60.

Burns, E. (1982). The use and interpretation of standard grade equivalents. *Journal of Learning Disabilities, 15,* 17–18.

Cattell, R. B. (1966). *Handbook of multivariate experimental psychology.* Chicago: Rand McNally.

Cattin, P. (1980). Note on the estimation of the squared cross-validated multiple correlation of a regression model. *Psychological Bulletin, 87,* 63–65.

Cicchetti, D. V. (1994). Multiple comparison methods: Establishing guidelines for their valid application in neuropsychological research. *Journal of Clinical and Experimental Neuropsychology, 16,* 155–161.

Coles, G. S. (1978). The learning disabilities test battery: Empirical and social issues. *Howard Educational Review, 4,* 313–340.

Cooley, W. W., & Lohnes, P. R. (1971). *Multivariate data analysis.* New York: Wiley.

Cronbach, L. J. (1990). *Essentials of psychological testing* (5th ed.). New York: Harper & Row.

Cronbach, L. J., & Gleser, G. C. (1953). Assessing similarity between profiles. *Psychological Bulletin, 50,* 456–473.

Davis, F. B. (1959). Interpretation of differences among average and individual test scores. *Journal of Educational Psychology, 50*, 162–170.

Dean, R. S. (1978). Distinguishing learning-disabled and emotionally disturbed children on the WISC-R. *Journal of Consulting and Clinical Psychology, 46*, 4381–4382.

Dean, R. S. (1985). Review of the Halstead–Reitan Neuropsychological Test Battery. In J. V. Mitchell (Ed.), *The ninth mental measurements yearbook*. Lincoln: University of Nebraska Press.

Dunleavy, R. A., Hansen, J. L., & Baade, L. E. (1981). Discriminating powers of Halstead Battery tests in assessment of 9 to 14 year old severely asthmatic children. *Clinical Neuropsychology, 3*, 99–12.

Feldt, L. S., & Brennan, R. L. (1989). Reliability. In R. Linn (Ed.), *Educational measurement* (3rd ed.). New York: Macmillan Co.

Fuller, G. B., & Goh, D. S. (1981). Intelligence, achievement, and visual-motor performance among learning disabled and emotionally impaired children. *Psychology in the Schools, 18*, 262–268.

Glass, G. V. (1978). Integrating findings: The meta-analysis of research. In L. Shulman (Ed.), *Review of Research in Education, 5*, 351–379.

Golden, C. J. (1981). *Diagnosis and rehabilitation in clinical neuropsychology* (2nd ed.). Springfield, IL: Thomas.

Golden, C. J., Moses, J. A., Jr., Graber, B., & Berg, T. (1981). Objective clinical rules for interpreting the Luria–Nebraska Neuropsychological Battery: Derivation, effectiveness, and validation. *Journal of Consulting and Clinical Psychology, 49*, 616–668.

Gordon, R. A. (1984). Digits backward and the Mercer–Kamin law: An empirical response to Mercer's treatment of internal validity of IQ tests. In C. R. Reynolds & R. T. Brown (Eds.), *Perspectives on bias in mental testing*. New York: Plenum Press.

Guilford, J. P. (1954). *Psychometric methods* (2nd ed.). New York: McGraw–Hill.

Guilmette, T. J., & Rasile, D. (1995). Sensitivity, specificity, and diagnostic accuracy of three verbal memory measures in the assessment of mild brain injury. *Neuropsychology, 9*, 338–344.

Gutkin, T. B., & Reynolds, C. R. (1980, September). *Normative data for interpreting Reitan's index of Wechsler subtest scatter*. Paper presented to the annual meeting of the American Psychological Association, Montreal.

Haak, R. (1989). Establishing neuropsychology in a school setting: Organization, problems, and benefits, In C. R. Reynolds & E. Fletcher–Janzen (Eds.), *Handbook of clinical child neuropsychology* (pp. 489–502). New York: Plenum Press.

Helms, J. E. (1992). Why is there no study of cultural equivalence in standardized cognitive ability testing? *American Psychology, 47*, 1083–1101.

Hynd, G. (Ed.). (1981). Neuropsychology in schools. *School Psychology Review, 10*(3).

Ivnik, R. J., Smith, G. E., Malec, J. F., Kokmen, E., & Tangelos, E. G. (1994). Mayo cognitive factor scales: Distinguishing normal and clinical samples by profile variability. *Neuropsychology, 8*, 203–209.

Jastak, J. F., & Jastak, S. (1978). *Wide Range Achievement Test*. Wilmington, DE: Jastak.

Kaufman, A. S. (1976a). A new approach to the interpretation of test scatter on the WISC-R. *Journal of Learning Disabilities, 9*, 160–167.

Kaufman, A. S. (1976b). Verbal–performance IQ discrepancies on the WISC-R. *Journal of Learning Disabilities, 9*, 739–744.

Kaufman, A. S. (1979). *Intelligence testing with the WISC-R*. New York: Wiley–Interscience.

Kaufman, A. S. (1990). *Assessing adolescent and adult intelligence*. Boston: Allyn & Bacon.

Kaufman, A. S., & Kaufman, N. L. (1983). *Kaufman Assessment Battery for Children: Interpretive manual*. Circle Pines, MN: American Guidance Service.

Kaufman, A. S., McLean, J. E., & Reynolds, C. R. (1988). Sex, race, residence, region, and education differences on the 11 WAIS-R subtests. *Journal of Clinical Psychology, 44*, 231–248.

Lord, F. M., & Novick, M. R. (1968). *Statistical theories of mental tests*. Reading, MA: Addison–Wesley.

Malloy, P. F., & Webster, J. S. (1981). Detecting mild brain impairment using the Luria–Nebraska Neuropsychological Battery. *Journal of Consulting and Clinical Psychology, 49*, 768–770.

Matarazzo, J. D. (1972). *Wechsler's measurement and appraisal of adult intelligence*. Baltimore: Williams & Wilkins.

Mayfield, J. W., & Reynolds, C. R. (1995a). *Factor structure of the Test of Memory and Learning for blacks and for whites*. Paper presented to the annual meeting of the National Association of School Psychologists, Chicago.

Mayfield, J. W., & Reynolds, C. R. (1995b). *Black–white differences in performance on measures of memory and learning*. Paper presented to the annual meeting of the National Academy of Neuropsychology, San Francisco.

Miles, J., & Stelmack, R. (1994). Learning disability subtypes and the effects of auditory and visual priming on visual event-related potentials to words. *Journal of Clinical and Experimental Neuropsychology, 16*, 43–64.

Nesselroade, J., & Cattell, R. B. (1988). *Handbook of multivariate experimental psychology* (2nd ed.). New York: Plenum Press.

Nunnally, J. C. (1978). *Psychometric theory* (2nd ed.). New York: McGraw–Hill.

Osgood, C. E., & Suci, G. J. (1952). A measurement of relation determined by both mean differences and profile interpretation. *Psychological Bulletin, 49*, 251–262.

Parsons, O. A., & Prigatano, G. P. (1978). Methodological considerations in clinical neuropsychological research. *Journal of Consulting and Clinical Psychology, 46*, 608–619.

Pedhazur, E. J., & Schmelkin, L. P. (1991). *Measurement, design, and analysis*. Hillsdale, NJ: Erlbaum.

Petersen, N. S., Kolen, M. J., & Hoover, H. D. (1989). Scaling, norming, and equating. In R. Linn (Ed.), *Educational measurement*, 3rd ed. (pp. 221–262). New York: MacMillan.

Piotrowski, R. J. (1978). Abnormality of subtest score differences on the WISC-R. *Journal of Consulting and Clinical Psychology, 46*, 569–570.

Plake, B. S., Reynolds, C. R., & Gutkin, T. B. (1981). A technique for the comparison of profile variability between independent groups. *Journal of Clinical Psychology, 37,* 142–146.

Purisch, A. D., Golden, C. J., & Hammeke, T. A. (1979). Discrimination of schizophrenic and brain injured patients by standardized version of Luria's neuropsychological tests. *Clinical Neuropsychology, 1,* 53–59.

Reschly, D., & Gresham, F. M. (1989). Current neuropsychological diagnosis of learning problems: A leap of faith. In C. R. Reynolds, & E. Fletcher-Janzen (Eds.), *Handbook of clinical child neuropsychology* (pp. 503–520). New York: Plenum Press.

Reynolds, C. R. (1979a). Interpreting the index of abnormality when the distribution of score differences is known: Comment on Piotrowski. *Journal of Consulting and Clinical Psychology, 47,* 401–402.

Reynolds, C. R. (1979b). Objectivity of scoring for the McCarthy Drawing Tests. *Psychology in the Schools, 16,* 367–368.

Reynolds, C. R. (1981a). The problem of bias in psychological assessment. In C. R. Reynolds & T. B. Gutkin (Eds.), *The handbook of school psychology.* New York: Wiley.

Reynolds, C. R. (1981b). Screening tests: Problems and promises. In N. Lamberts (Ed.), *Special Education Assessment Matrix.* Monterey, CA: CTB McGraw Hill.

Reynolds, C. R. (1982a). The importance of norms and other traditional psychometric concepts to assessment in clinical neuropsychology. In R. N. Malathesha & L. C. Hartlage (Eds.), *Neuropsychology and cognition* (Vol. II, pp. 55–76). The Hague: Nijhoff.

Reynolds, C. R. (1982b). The problem of bias in psychological assessment. In C. R. Reynolds & T. B. Gutkin (Eds.), *The handbook of school psychology* (pp. 178–208). New York: Wiley.

Reynolds, C. R. (1983). Some new and some unusual educational and psychological tests. *School Psychology Review, 12,* 481–488.

Reynolds, C. R. (1984). Critical measurement issues in learning disabilities. *Journal of Special Education, 18,* 451–476.

Reynolds, C. R. (1986). Clinical acumen but psychometric naivete in neuropsychological assessment of educational disorders. *Archives of Clinical Neuropsychology, 1,* 121–138.

Reynolds, C. R. (1995). Test bias and the assessment of personality and intelligence. In D. Saklofske & M. Zeidner (Eds.), *International handbook of personality and intelligence,* (pp. 545–573). New York: Plenum Press.

Reynolds, C. R., & Bigler, E. D. (1994). *Manual for the Test of Memory and Learning.* Austin, TX: PRO-ED.

Reynolds, C. R., Chastain, R., Kaufman, A. S., & McLean, J. (1987). Demographic influences on adult intelligence at ages 16 to 74 years. *Journal of School Psychology, 25,* 323–342.

Reynolds, C. R., & Clark, J. H. (1985). Profile analysis of standardized intelligence test performance of very low functioning individuals. *Journal of School Psychology, 23,* 227–283.

Reynolds, C. R., & Clark, J. H. (1986). Profile analysis of standardized intelligence test performance of very low functioning individuals. *Psychology in the Schools, 23,* 5–12.

Reynolds, C. R., & Gutkin, T. B. (1979). Predicting the premorbid intellectual status of children using demographic data. *Clinical Neuropsychology, 1,* 36–38.

Reynolds, C. R., & Gutkin, T. B. (1980). Statistics related to profile interpretation of the Peabody Individual Achievement Test. *Psychology in the Schools, 17,* 316–319.

Reynolds, C. R., Hartlage, L. C., & Haak, R. (1980, September). *Lateral preference as determined by neuropsychological performance and aptitude/achievement discrepancies.* Paper presented to the annual meeting of the American Psychological Association, Montreal.

Reynolds, C. R., & Kaiser, S. M. (1990). Test bias in psychological assessment. In T. B. Gutkin & C. R. Reynolds (Eds.), *The handbook of school psychology* (2nd ed., pp. 487–525). New York: Wiley.

Reynolds, C. R., & Kaufman, A. S. (1986). Clinical assessment of children's intelligence with the Wechsler Scales. In B. Wolman (Ed.), *Handbook of intelligence* (pp. 601–662), New York: Wiley.

Reynolds, C. R., & Willson, V. L. (1983, January). *Standardized grade equivalents: Really! No. Well, sort of, but they lead to the valley of the shadow of misinterpretation and confusion.* Paper presented to the annual meeting of the Southwestern Educational Research Association, Houston.

Ris, M. D., & Noll, R. B. (1994). Long-term neurobehavioral outcome in pediatric brain tumor patients: Review and methodological critique. *Journal of Clinical and Experimental Neuropsychology, 16,* 21.

Roffe, M. W., & Bryant, C. K. (1979). How reliable are MSCA profile interpretations? *Psychology in the Schools, 16,* 14–18.

Rourke, B. P. (1975). Brain–behavior relationships in children with learning disabilities: A research program. *American Psychologist, 30,* 911–920.

Sandoval, J. (1981, August). *Can neuropsychology contribute to rehabilitation in educational settings? No.* Paper presented to the annual meeting of the American Psychological Association, Los Angeles.

Sattler, J. M. (1974). *Assessment of children's intelligence.* Philadelphia: Saunders.

Satz, P., Taylor, H. G., Friel, J., & Fletcher, J. (1978). Some developmental and predictive precursors of reading disabilities: A six year follow-up. In A. L. Benton & D. Pearl (Eds.), *Dyslexia: An appraisal of current knowledge.* London: Oxford University Press.

Selz, M., & Reitan, R. M. (1979). Rules for neuropsychological diagnosis: Classification of brain function in older children. *Journal of Consulting and Clinical Psychology, 47,* 258–264.

Tabachnick, B. G. (1979). Test scatter on the WISC-R. *Journal of Learning Disabilities, 12,* 60–62.

Taylor, R. L., & Imivey, J. K. (1980). Diagnostic use of the WISC-R and McCarthy Scales: A regression analysis approach to learning disabilities. *Psychology in the Schools, 17,* 327–330.

Thienemann, M., & Koran, L. M. (1995). Do soft signs predict treatment outcome in obsessive–compulsive disorder? *Journal of Neuropsychiatry and Clinical Neurosciences, 7,* 218–222.

Thompson, R. J. (1980). The diagnostic utility of WISC-R measures with children referred to a developmental evaluation center. *Journal of Consulting and Clinical Psychology, 48,* 440–447.

Thorndike, R. L., & Hagen E. P. (1977). *Measurement and evaluation in psychology and education* (4th ed.). New York: Wiley.

U. S. Office of Education. (1976). Education of handicapped children: Assistance to state: Proposed rulemaking. *Federal Register, 41,* 52404–52407.

Wallbrown, F. H., Vance, H., & Pritchard, K. K. (1979). Discriminating between attitudes expressed by normal and disabled readers. *Psychology in the Schools, 4,* 472–477.

Wechsler, D. (1974). *Wechsler Intelligence Scale for Children-Revised.* New York: Psychological Corporation.

Wherry, R. J., Sr. (1932). A new formula for predicting the shrinkage of the coefficient for multiple correlation. *Annals of Mathematical Statistics, 2,* 404–457.

Willson, V. L., & Reynolds, C. R. (1982). Methodological and statistical problems in determining membership in clinical populations. *Clinical Neuropsychology, 4,* 134–138.

Wright, L., Schaefer, A. B., & Solomons, G. (1979). *Encyclopedia of pediatric psychology.* Baltimore: University Park Press.

10

Models of Inference in Evaluating Brain–Behavior Relationships in Children

EILEEN B. FENNELL AND RUSSELL M. BAUER

Introduction

Neuropsychologists generally measure behavior as a means for making inferences about brain function. Regardless of whether such measurement takes place in the clinic or the laboratory, the basic process is the same: Behavioral and cognitive performances that are readily observable "stand in," as it were, for the less observable "brain states" they are thought to reflect. Once measurement is completed, the quantitative and qualitative relationships among such performances are assembled according to certain rules in order to make probabilistic statements about brain function. The rules that are applied in the given case depend on the inferential model one uses in relating behavioral performance to brain function. This basic process characterizes all of neuropsychology, transcends theoretical persuasion or tests employed, and, in fact, is a fundamental aspect of the clinical-inferential method in general.

Making inferences about brain functioning from behavioral data is a fundamental aspect of the neuropsychological approach to assessment. However, because such inferences are so routinely made, it is important not only to articulate the various levels at which they play a part in our thinking but also to understand the specific theoretical assumptions on which they are based. The goal of this chapter is

to describe major inferential models that relate behavior to brain function in child neuropsychology. In working toward this goal, we will first describe basic issues in clinical inference as they relate to child neuropsychology. In doing so, we will outline a hypothesis testing approach to neuropsychological assessment that borrows from classical methods of inductive inference. We will articulate some of the basic models of inference of particular relevance to child neuropsychological assessment. Finally, we will briefly discuss several misconceptions in child neuropsychology that, if utilized by an examiner, may lead to faulty conclusions about the meaning of clinical test data.

Basic Issues of Clinical Inference

Clinical-Inferential Methods

Inference refers to the process of arriving at a conclusion by reasoning from evidence. Inferences generally take place according to organized systems of rules that stipulate (1) the kind of evidence on which conclusions can be drawn, (2) the kinds of conclusions that are possible given certain evidence, and (3) a set of logical connections between evidence and conclusions. In child neuropsychology, the performance of the child on cognitive or neuropsychological tests is the evidence on which inferences about brain functioning are based. It is assumed that the conclusions of interest are couched

EILEEN B. FENNELL AND RUSSELL M. BAUER • Department of Clinical and Health Psychology, University of Florida, Gainesville, Florida 32610.

in terms of some aspect of brain function that is not directly observable by the neuropsychologist. In general, we do not observe or measure functions; we see only the behavioral indicators of spared and impaired brain functions. Thus, for example, we make inferences about language *function* on the basis of performance on tests of language *ability,* or we may infer that there is some disturbance in brain-based attentional mechanisms when the child cannot stay on task, repeat digits, or shows inconsistent performance across a set of homogeneous test items. As Taylor and Schatschneider (1992) note, interpretations of child neuropsychological findings are based on two assumptions regarding the utility of the tests employed: (1) that these tests have neurological validity (i.e., reflect the state of the central nervous system) and (2) that these tests also have psychological validity (i.e., reflect meaningfully some aspect of childhood functioning).

In what follows, we presume that there are complex differences between children and adults in terms of how brain pathology leads to neuropsychological and behavioral deficits. Thus, the meaning or utility of a behavioral "sign" that has been well validated with adults may be different when that sign is applied to child neuropsychology cases (Fletcher & Taylor, 1984; Rourke, 1983). Similarly, the predictive value of knowing that a patient has had a specific brain insult may critically depend on the age at which the damage was incurred (Rasmussen & Milner, 1977; Woods & Teuber, 1973).

Despite the fact that the behavioral effects of the brain disease are complexly dependent on such factors as age and stage of development, we believe that one fruitful approach to understanding childhood neuropsychological data is the classical inferential method commonly used in adult neurology (Adams & Victor, 1977).This method involves the collection of clinical data in terms of signs (e.g., neuropsychological impairments) and symptons (clinical complaints). These findings are then correlated with similar signs and symptoms occurring in neurological disorders in which the underlying anatomy is known. By making analogy with these better-known disorders, and by reasoning from anatomic data, the findings in an individual case can be interpreted in terms of some pathophysiological mechanism. With children, however, the additional knowledge regarding normal developmental change must also be factored into the inferential process in order to take into account the changing nature of skills and abilities that occur with maturation.

The classical inferential method can be applied to the individual case or can form the framework for a general conceptualization of a childhood disorder that is as yet poorly understood. An excellent example is that of a neurobehavioral model of autism (Damasio & Maurer, 1978; Maurer & Damasio, 1982). These authors observed various abnormalities in a group of autistic children, including disturbances of motility (stereotyped movements, abnormal posturing and gait), attention (unpredictable response to sensory stimuli, gaze aversion), communication (mutism, use and comprehension of nonverbal signs), and social behavior (poor cooperative play, failure to initiate social interaction). They related each of these signs and symptoms to findings in specific acquired neurological diseases (e.g., basal ganglia disease, acquired mutism from mesial frontal lobe lesions) in which the pathogenesis and localization were more firmly established. On the basis of this analysis, they proposed a specific neuroanatomy for autism that included the mesolimbic cortex (mesial temporal and frontal lobes), the neostriatum, and the anterior and medial thalamic nuclei. For our purposes, the specific merits of this hypothesis, and its ability to explain core features of autism, are not at issue. What is important, however, is that the hypothesis was derived by starting with observable signs and symptoms and by inferring from them a possible functional anatomy.

Levels of Inference

Thus far, we have discussed clinical inference as if it were a simple process of reasoning from neuropsychological test performance to brain function. In fact, there are several types of inference involved here, each of which exists at a different level of analysis. For purposes of discussion, consider a 5-year-old male child who has received a closed head injury in a vehicular accident. He is given a battery of neuropsychological tests including assessment of intellectual ability, memory, language, visual and auditory perception, attentional ability, sensorimotor skill, and achievement. Results indicate low average intellectual ability, attentional and recent memory problems, and poor beginning reading skills. We are asked to relate the child's current status to the recent head injury and to assist in educational planning. There are three basic levels of analysis involved in utilizing our test data to answer such questions. At the first level, we are concerned with the degree to which the behavior elicited by the test battery is representative of the domain of behavior that would have been elicited given unlimited testing time (Cronbach, Rajaratnam, & Gleser, 1963). The basic issue here is whether our test findings are generalizable to other settings or conditions. At the second level of analysis, we are interested in the specific meaning of each of the test findings. Each test finding might have a formal statistical (see Wiggins, 1973) relationship with a specific form of brain impairment or may suggest a qualitative feature seen in other known brain disease (Adams & Victor, 1977). In either event, we are inferring what the outcome of each test means in terms of some nontest behavior or variable. This is a process that Holt (1968) termed primary inference. Thus, we make inferences regarding the status of verbal memory ability (and its constituent variables) by individually noting performance on tests to which this ability contributes. At the third level, we are concerned with integrating the diverse test findings to arrive at a general interpretation or conceptualization of their meaning. We are concerned here with the degree to which the pattern of spared and impaired abilities suggests a specific neuropsychological mechanism that can best account for the test findings and the clinical complaints. Holt (1968) indicated that this level

> demands a knowledge of the range of expectable syndromes, what their constituent variables are, and some means of measuring the strength of each variable. By drawing on this knowledge and on his [sic] knowledge of theory, the diagnostician puts together his primary inferences and in an act of secondary inference locates the subject with reference to diagnostic syndromes. (p. 15)

It is important to note that the specific inferences the clinician makes at each of these three levels will differ depending on the purpose of assessment and will at least in part be related to the assumptions the clinician makes about the relationship between test behavior and brain function. Such differences are most apparent at the second and third levels. For example, clinicians who favor an actuarial or statistical approach to test interpretation will be most concerned with the formal quantitative relationships between test findings and specific forms of neuropsychological impairment. Those who favor qualitative approaches might be more interested in demonstrating the presence of one or more "pathognomic signs" that are considered crucial indicators of functional impairment. In either case, an attempt is made to relate the pattern of test findings to previously available data on children

with head injuries. With quantitative data, the clinician might focus efforts on determining the degree to which this child is similar to other head-injured children in terms of specific neurobehavioral mechanisms that can best account for their neuropsychological deficit pattern. In actual practice, the responsible clinician frequently uses a mixture of actuarial and clinical methods in making inferences from test data (Lezak, 1995; Meehl, 1957). The final goal of the assessment, to assist in educational planning, assumes that the inferences about brain functioning are valid and can be utilized to provide specific recommendations to remediate behavioral difficulties resulting from the observed test deficits (Taylor & Fletcher, 1990).

Fundamentals of Hypothesis Formation: The Logic of Strong Inference

In the previous section we briefly considered three levels at which inferences about brain function may be made from test performances. The specific nature and content of such inferences will depend in large part on the assumption the clinician makes about the relationship between test behavior and brain function. That is, inferential processes in neuropsychological assessment are inextricably related to the theoretical or conceptual basis of one's assessment approach. Regardless of whether one adopts a quantitative or a qualitative approach, or some mixture of the two, an important concern is the manner in which clinical data contribute to hypotheses about the nature of the child's neuropsychological status.

In this section, we outline a general approach to forming and testing hypotheses derived from neuropsychological test data that seems equally well suited to both quantitative and qualitative models. This approach is based on our belief that there is no fundamental distinction between scientific and clinical hypotheses. That is, we believe that the same inferential processes one uses in the research laboratory for distinguishing between viable and invalid scientific hypotheses can be used in deriving and testing clinical hypotheses (see also Landy, 1986, who takes a hypothesis-testing approach to the process of test validation). Our approach is based on a model of inductive inference outlined by Platt (1964), a model that abounds in the physical sciences, particularly molecular biology and high-energy physics. Platt called his approach *strong inference* because its systematic application seems related to rapid scientific advance in the fields that utilize its strengths. It is based primarily on disconfirmatory logic (Popper, 1959) and consists mainly of the sequential evaluation of hypotheses that survive disconfirmation in experimental (clinical) test. Strong inference consists of the systematic application of the following steps:

1. Devising alternative hypotheses
2. Devising "crucial experiments' with alternative possible outcomes, each of which will exclude one of the alternative hypotheses
3. Carrying out the experiments "cleanly"
4. Recycling the procedure with surviving hypotheses

These four steps are recognizable to all neuropsychologists as the basic elements of inductive inference. The difference, however, is in the systematic, formal applications of all of these steps to every clinical problem.

We will illustrate the utility of this approach by describing a series of simple "experiments" designed to determine more precisely the nature of a specific neuropsychological deficit. As an example, assume we have a child who performs poorly on WISC-III Block Design and assume that we have reason to believe from the medical history that a significant neuropsychological factor is involved. Because Block Design measures more than one ability, a question of some relevance might be to determine more specifically the nature of the child's failure. On an *a priori* basis, the Block Design test can be thought of as tapping motor, visuoperceptual, visuomotor, constructional, and problem-solving abilities. A strong inference approach to isolating the reason(s) for a deficit in Block Design performance would proceed first by devising a series of tests that systematically eliminate one or more of these constituent abilities and then observing the resulting effects on the child's performance. Assuming relatively good control over difficulty level, performance on Block Design could be contrasted with performance on visuoperceptual tasks without motor demands (e.g., tests of form discrimination, visual synthesis). The relative role of visuomotor versus motor abilities could be assessed by contrasting performance on motor tests not requiring visual tracking (e.g., finger tapping, fine finger movements) with tasks with high visuomotor demands (e.g., drawing, visual reaching, grooved pegboard) and so on. Alternatively, the role of motor abilities could be excluded by requiring the child to perform on a match-to-sample task which empha-

sized the perceptual demands rather than motor components of the Block Design assembly task. By such a systematic approach to ruling out alternative hypotheses for the deficient Block Design performance, attention is gradually directed toward surviving hypotheses. For example, a pattern of good performance on visual, problem-solving, and motor tasks would tend to rule these abilities out as explanations, leaving the hypothesis that it was the visuomotor or constructional aspect of Block Design that specifically contributed to the child's difficulties on this task. It is our view that almost any complex test behavior can be broken down into its constituent features in this way in order to develop more precise hypotheses about performance deficits.

The strong inference approach, with its emphasis on disconfirmation, is quite different from the logic typically used in traditional approaches to neuropsychological testing. Traditional approaches typically utilize a pattern of test performance (e.g., lateralized motor or sensory findings, poor nonverbal memory performance) as confirmatory evidence for a particular hypothesis. This is the fundamental assumption underlying the so-called "sign" approach. Our view is that although this approach may result in correct inferences, it does so inefficiently and at the risk that alternative explanations for a test sign or performance have not been entirely ruled out. The qualitative approach also depends heavily on the ability of any given "sign" to discretely predict to a specific brain system or locus. A good example of the weakness of this sign approach is the so-called "Gerstmann syndrome." This combination of clinical signs (acalculia, agraphia, left–right confusion, and finger agnosia) frequently points to dominant parietal lesions in adults but is less reliably diagnostic among children with developmental disorders (Kinsbourne & Warrington, 1963; Spellacy & Peter, 1978).

Clinical Judgment in Neuropsychology

We have implied in the previous section that the theoretical model the clinician espouses will be an important factor governing the kinds of inferences made about neuropsychological test data. Although this makes the clinician an additional source of variation in test interpretation, which some (e.g., Rourke, Bakker, Fisk & Strang, 1983) find somewhat undesirable, we believe that the "cognitive activity of the clinician" is an integral and inevitable aspect of neuropsychological test interpretation. This issue has received little systematic attention within neuropsychology, though some guidance is available from the contemporary application of the Brunswick Lens Model (Brunswick, 1956) to the practice of psychodiagnosis (Hammond, Hursch, & Todd, 1964; Hursch, Hammond, & Hursch, 1964; Meehl, 1960; Wiggins, 1973).

The basic idea is that inference in neuropsychology is dependent not only on the specific relationship among test signs and brain function (so-called criterion-oriented validity), but also on the manner in which the neuropsychologist uses such test signs in arriving at interpretive statements. There are two basic issues involved here. First is the degree to which the clinician accurately uses the test results to arrive at a clinical diagnosis. This issue can be understood if one assumes that the separate test performances function as variables that, separately and in combination, predict to some criterion (e.g., brain function). The intercorrelations among test performances, and their individual relationships to the criterion, determine the relative importance (weighting) each performance has in predicting the criterion. In an ideal setting, the neuropsychologist utilizes the various test performances in a manner that accurately reflects the separate and combined relationship such performances actually have with the criterion. In this ideal world, the clinician's inferences directly reflect the empirical validities of the various test performances vis-à-vis the criterion; the test performances that bear stronger relationships with the criterion are given more weight than are those that correlate less highly. However, in actual clinical practice, the clinician may not have precise knowledge of the predictive relationship between test performance and criterion. What might result from this situation is a method of combining test performances that does not accurately reflect their predictive validity with respect to the criterion. In this case, it becomes important to distinguish empirical validity (the statistical relationship that exists between predictor variables and criterion) and cue utilization (the relationship between test performance and the inferences made by the clinician) (see Wiggins, 1973, p. 157).

A second issue is the manner in which test results are combined to arrive at a clinical conclusion. Do neuropsychologists combine test findings in the linear fashion implied by multiple regression accounts of empirical validity, or do they adopt a more complex, nonlinear method of combining data in which certain test scores are viewed as *a priori* more important than others? An example of a nonlinear approach to test score interpretation is the use of the "pathognomonic sign" approach in neuropsychology. Pathognomonic signs are performances that are seen rarely, if ever, in persons with normal brain function. When they do appear, therefore, they more than likely suggest some brain impairment. For example, the appearance of aphasia is regarded as a pathognomonic sign of left hemisphere impairment; significant discrepancies in right- and left-handed finger tapping speed are pathognomonic of lateralized motor system impairment. In terms of this discussion, pathognomonic signs could be weighted very heavily and could form the basis of the clinical judgment even in the absence of other supportive clinical evidence. In this situation, the clinician could elect, perhaps unwisely, to ignore the relationships among other test performances and the criteria if pathognomonic signs are present.

Summary

In discussing these basic issues, our purpose has not been to argue for one or another approach to interpretation, but rather to articulate the processes entering into the inferential process in child neuropsychology. Our view is that it is important to be explicitly aware of the crucial role such processes play in making sense out of neuropsychological test data. In large part, the concepts that are invoked to explain neuropsychological test performances (e.g., attention, memory capacity) are unobservable and must be inferred from overt behavior. Whether one elects to deal at the individual test level or at the level of pattern analysis, the same basic inferential processes are involved. In this section, we have purposely emphasized the context, rather than the content, of inductive inference in the clinical setting. As we have stated, this is important because the inferential method is such a fundamental aspect of the neuropsychological approach. We have outlined a strong inference model that, for us, is a useful way of conceptualizing the process of hypothesis formation and hypothesis testing in child neuropsychology. Finally, we have attempted to point out some of the general issues involved when a clinician attempts to derive meaningful interpretations of multiple test performances. With these broad issues as a background, the specific nature and content of the inferences made by the neuropsychologist will in large part depend on the level of data analysis and on the conceptual model that governs the assessment approach. We now turn to a discussion of the major inferential models of relevance to the child neuropsychologist.

Models of Inference in Child Neuropsychology

As Tarter and Edwards (1986) noted, clinical neuropsychological assessment is descriptive, correlational, and inferential rather than explanatory, causal, and direct. Neuropsychological procedures provide descriptive information regarding behavior in both normal and neurologically impaired children. This description of behavior on standardized and formal observations (tests) is then correlated with suspected or known pathological lesions derived from other tests (concurrent validity) in order to enable the neuropsychologist to: (1) infer the presence or absence of brain pathology from test signs (*primary* inference) or (2) classify the individual child according to test and historical variables into some classification group (e.g., brain injured, learning disabled, attention deficit disordered) by a process of *secondary* inference. Although the inferential *process* may be similar in adult and child neuropsychology, major differences exist in the *context* of that process.

The Inferential Context of Child Neuropsychology

Several recent texts devoted to child or developmental neuropsychology emphasize the critical differences in the neuropsychological organization and functioning of children relative to adults (Baron, Fennell, & Voeller, 1995; Hartlage & Telzrow, 1986; Rourke *et al.,* 1983; Spreen, Risser, & Edgell, 1995). Furthermore, as the analytic focus for the child neuropsychologist is on the developing brain, inferential processes regarding brain function must rest on models that account for differences in development at different ages (Dean, 1986; Fletcher & Taylor, 1984; Segalowitz & Gruber, 1977; Van der Vlugt, 1979) rather than rely on the models of adult brain functions and acquired pathologies (Heilman & Valenstein, 1993; Lezak, 1995). In addition, basic descriptions of the neuropsychological effects of developmental and acquired pathologies of childhood are still emerging (Baron *et al.,* 1995; Berg & Linton, 1989; Boll, 1983; Boll & Barth, 1981; Menkes, 1990; Netley & Rovet, 1983; Pirozzolo, Campanella, Christensen, & Lawson-Kerr, 1981; Rutter, 1983; Spreen *et al.,* 1995). Our understanding of the influence of individual differences in development and how these may affect the descriptive and inferential processes in child neuro-

psychology (Bakker, 1984; Bolter & Long, 1985; Clark, 1984; Dean, 1986; Rourke & Adams, 1984) is still incomplete. Finally, only recently has an emphasis been placed on the discriminative validity of various test signs and historical indicators of certain subgroups of childhood disorders such as learning disabilities (Lyon, 1994; Morris, Blashfield, & Satz, 1986; Rourke, Fisk, & Strang, 1986), developmental language disorders (van Santen, Black, Wilson, & Risucci, 1994), minimal brain dysfunctions (Chadwick & Rutter, 1983; Denckla, 1979; Ross & Ross, 1992; Satz & Fletcher, 1980), nonverbal learning disabilities (Rourke, 1995), or attention deficit disorder (Barkley, 1994). Specific information regarding the neuropsychological profiles of children with a variety of psychiatric disorders has recently emerged (Bornstein, King, & Carroll, 1983; Tramontana & Hooper, 1989). To the extent that the content of neuropsychological knowledge of the developing brain is still emerging, primary and secondary inference in child neuropsychology is affected by maturational and experiential variables to a more significant degree than is typically assumed in adult neuropsychology. At the same time, methods of assessing neuropsychological functioning in children were historically rooted in the work on adult assessment (Incagnoli, Goldstein, & Golden, 1986). It is not surprising, therefore, to find that there are many clinicians who have approached child neuropsychology with techniques of assessment that were modified from adult batteries or that use "scaled-down" versions of adult tests, the results of which form the data for their clinical inferences (Golden, 1989).

Assessment Methods in Child Neuropsychology

Broadly speaking, assessment approaches in child neuropsychology can be classified into three major types: a fixed battery approach, a flexible battery approach, and an individualized or patient-centered approach. In the fixed battery approach, the same set of tests, designed to tap a very broad spectrum of functions and abilities, is administered to each child regardless of the referral question. This approach may be either empirically or theoretically based. In the former instance, the test battery is selected according to its ability to separate groups and is typified by the work of Reitan and his associates. Theoretically based batteries, in contrast, are founded on a theory of development as it relates to rather broad or narrow dimensions of behavior and is typified by the Florida Longitudinal Project Battery (Satz & Morris, 1981). Fixed batteries may also include formal decision rules for clinical interpretation (Reynolds, 1989; Rourke *et al.,* 1986). The advantages of a fixed battery approach include the breadth and depth of functions assessed, the normative data bases frequently provided, and the ease with which a systematic data base for clinical interpretation of large numbers of clinical groups can be gathered (Hartlage & Telzrow, 1986; Tarter & Edwards, 1986). However, a fixed battery approach, particularly one that is empirically rather than theoretically based, may not be designed to describe age-related differences in problem-solving behaviors because the emphasis is often on quantitative discrimination between diagnostic groups. Frequently, educational and other experiential variables are not treated in the content of the battery itself. Often the battery may not be designed to address specific referral questions such as prescription of remediation programs for a developmental impairment. Finally, many fixed batteries suffer from dependence on the match between the validation and cross-validation samples and the base rate of clinical problems for the sample to which it is applied. Thus, for example, batteries developed at a hospital-based referral clinic may or may not be as capable of detecting cognitive disorders in a school-based or psychiatry inpatient setting (Tramontana & Hooper, 1987).

In the flexible battery approach, a core set of standardized tests are administered to which are added a selected set of additional tests designed to enhance examination for specific referral questions (Rourke *et al.,* 1986) or to examine problem behaviors that are detected on the core battery (Bauer, 1994; Hartlage & Telzrow, 1986). Like the fixed battery, such an approach may be empirically derived or theoretically based or some mixture of the two. For example, a screening battery, empirically derived, may be followed by a theoretically based complement of tests designed to test the best fit to a syndrome type. The advantage of such a flexible battery is that the neuropsychologist is able to employ both a nomothetic and an ideographic approach to child assessment. Thus, this approach permits the evaluation of broad classes of behaviors as well as subcomponents of a specific ability or symptom related to a particular referral question.

In the individualized or patient-centered approach to assessment (Goodglass, 1986), the set of test procedures employed is driven by two interacting factors: the referral question that includes the child's history and presenting symptoms and the child's test performance (successes and failures) (Christensen, 1975; Luria, 1973). More than any other approach, the patient-centered assessment requires that the clinician have substantial clinical knowledge of the specific as well as nonspecific effects of brain lesions on brain development and neuropsychological functioning. The patient-centered approach has, as a primary goal, the isolation of a specific neurobehavioral mechanism to account for the pattern of test findings. In this sense, the logic underlying this approach is most easily adapted for use in the strong inference model outlined earlier.

A number of lesion-related factors have been shown to have a differential impact on the developing brain, including age at time of insult (e.g., prenatal versus adolescence), type of lesion (e.g., vascular versus infectious), site of lesion (e.g., primary versus association cortex), and etiology (e.g., anoxia versus trauma). As yet, however, detailed descriptions of the neuropsychological functions and organization of behaviors in many children with development or acquired neuropathologies are not available (Baron *et al.,* 1995). As a result, the clinical-inferential approach of the patient-centered battery is less frequently seen in practice (Fennell, 1994).

Quantitative Inferences in Child Neuropsychology

There are four major inferential approaches that focus on quantitative aspects of performance in child neuropsychological assessment. These interpretive approaches derive primarily from the fixed battery methods in clinical assessment outlined by Reitan and others and focus on: (1) level of performance, (2) differential score patterns, (3) comparisons between sides of the body, and (4) comparisons of performance across time (Boll, 1983; Rourke *et al.,* 1986).

In the level of performance approach, the child's performance on a variety of measures is individually compared with normative data available for age-matched normal subjects or for selected clinical comparison subgroups (Satz & Morris, 1981; Spreen *et al.,* 1995). One risk of this approach is a high number of false-positive errors resulting from the large number of factors (e.g., psychiatric disturbance) besides brain dysfunction that can lead to poor performance.

The differential score or pattern approach evaluates an individual's set of performances on a battery of tests and may compare relative strengths or weaknesses in the total performance or may attempt to match a pattern or profile of scores to a clinical subtype. This is frequently done in the learning disabilities literature. This latter inferential approach is often difficult because of the fact that all measures do not equally allow for a comparison between the idealized referent group and the individual case (Morris, Blashfield, & Satz, 1986) or because of the absence of a well-defined ideal subtype to which the individual case is compared (Boll, 1983).

Comparisons between sides of the body may be made on the basis of speed of performance (e.g., finger tapping rate), skill of performance (e.g., manual dexterity), preferred performance (e.g., handedness), or accuracy of performance on sensory or motor tasks (e.g., tactile form discrimination). Transfer of learning from one side to the other may also be compared (e.g., dominant versus nondominant hand time to complete Tactual Performance Test; Reitan & Davison, 1974). In this analysis, differential performance between the sides of the body or in transfer of learning is the basis for inferring differential functional integrity at the level of the brain (Reitan & Davison, 1974).

The fourth approach, the longitudinal approach, compares performance on a battery of tests over time. In this approach, pretest versus posttest comparisons can be made of the effects of a known acquired lesion (e.g., surgical excision of an epileptic lesion), of the effects of recovery or restoration of function following an acquired lesion (e.g., recovery of memory functions subsequent to head trauma), or of the effects of a treatment intervention (e.g., pharmacological therapy for attention deficit disorder with hyperactivity).

In all of these quantitative approaches, the reliability and validity of the interpretation made rest on the data base available. Although normative data continue to be developed, there is still a paucity of data about the neuropsychological performance of various childhood neurologic disorders as well as a paucity of longitudinal studies of these clinical groups against which normal versus abnormal inferences can be derived.

Qualitative Inferences in Child Neuropsychology

Reflecting the emphasis of U.S. psychology on a psychometric approach, it is an unfortunate truth that only recently have developmental neurologists begun to collect data on the qualitative aspects of performance in both normal and abnormal development and attempted to relate these findings to neurologic models of brain development and to cognitive development (Fletcher & Taylor, 1984; Taylor & Schatschneider, 1992; Waber & Holmes, 1985). The focus of a qualitative approach is the emphasis on the qualitative features of performance (how a test is performed) rather than solely on the quantitative features of performance (what is achieved). By examining these qualitative features of performance, inferences are derived about the processes involved in executing a given behavioral task. These processes are then related to the differential functions of the right or left cerebral hemispheres or to other subcortical functional processes (Van der Vlugt, 1979). To some degree, this approach has also been applied to an analysis of errors in performance, for example, among different subgroups of learning-disabled children (Hynd, Obrzut, Hayes, & Becker, 1986) and to understanding the neurobehavioral deficits of autistic children (Damasio & Maurer, 1978). Similarly, this qualitative approach also underlies the pathognomonic sign approach in models of developmental delay versus deficit (Hartlage & Telzrow, 1986), in the analysis of "soft" versus "hard" neurologic signs among learning-disabled children (Denckla, 1979; Shafer, Shaffer, O'Connor, & Stokman, 1983; Shaffer, O'Connor, Shafer, & Prupis, 1983), and in the search for behavioral signs of "organicity" such as rotations in drawings (Boll, 1983). In this latter context, the neuropsychologist infers that the presence of the "sign" indicates the presence of brain damage or brain dysfunction. As Rourke *et al.* (1983) pointed out, however, the risk of relying on this approach is the likelihood of increasing false-negative errors, for the absence of sign is interpreted to reflect the absence of pathology. In fact, it is now recognized that behavioral signs of brain pathology are age related and may appear, disappear, and reappear at different stages of development reflecting the late versus early effects of a lesion as well as the capacity of the developing brain to adapt and to compensate for brain pathology (Boll, 1983; Spreen *et al.,* 1995; Stein, Rosen, & Butters, 1974). As noted with regard to quantitative inference, qualitative inference also depends on carefully documented empirical data relating qualitative aspects of performance to normal and abnormal development, which are still not widely available to clinical practitioners (Spreen *et al.,* 1995). Finally, both quantitative and qualitative approaches depend on the fundamental validity of the measures employed (Taylor & Schatschneider, 1992) as well as the accuracy with which quantitative techniques (e.g., multivariate clustering) or clinical techniques (e.g., clinical subtyping) are applied to the assessment data (Reynolds, 1989).

Inferential Fallacies in Child Neuropsychology

Fletcher and Taylor (1984) pointed out a number of inferential fallacies about the relationship between a child's test performance and the integrity of that child's brain. These fallacies include: (1) the differential-sensitivity fallacy, (2) the similar-skills fallacy, (3) the special-sign fallacy, and (4) the brain–behavior isomorphism fallacy.

In the differential-sensitivity fallacy, it is assumed that neuropsychological test findings associated with brain lesions in adults will be useful signs of brain disease in children. Instead, Fletcher and Taylor (1984) argued that one must document that a particular measure is a sensitive neurobehavioral measure in children whether or not it is helpful in the description of brain pathology in adults. Although it has been argued that the type and locus of childhood brain pathologies often do not lead to a picture of focal deficits (Boll, 1983; Boll & Barth, 1981), wherever possible, appropriate neurological and neurodiagnostic criteria must be utilized to assess the sensitivity of behavioral tests to brain pathology.

The similar-skills fallacy focuses on the belief that tests developed and normed on adult subjects measure the same abilities in children. Thus, for example, age norms that step down from adult age groups to younger children have been published for such widely used adult measures as the Wechsler Memory Scale (Ivinskis, Allen, & Shaw, 1971). In this example, it is assumed that children process these task demands in a fashion similar to adult subjects, despite clear evidence of age-based differences in the capacity and processes of verbal memory in children (Kail, 1984). Other major differences between children and adults are widely recognized in such important behavioral domains as language (Segalowitz, 1983); right-hemisphere functions (Witelson, 1977); and early versus later acquired reading skills and the role of the right versus the left hemisphere (Bakker, 1984).

The special sign fallacy occurs when neuropsychologists utilize specific test behaviors (e.g., rotations in drawings) as signs of brain pathology or infer from the presence of minor, accompanying or correlated signs that the major pathology from which these signs derive is present. A variant of this same fallacy occurs through the overreliance on analogies between signs of CNS pathology in adults and the assumption that such signs must also mean CNS pathology in children. As Boll (1983) and Fletcher and Taylor (1984) noted, there is very little evidence that similar behavioral pathologies seen in adults and children reflect similar etiologies. We do not want to imply that lessons learned from adult neurology should not be applied to children—only that they must be applied with caution. The major advantage of such application would be to generate new hypotheses capable of being put to subsequent disconfirmatory trials.

Finally, the brain–behavior isomorphism fallacy consists of mistaking dysfunction on behavioral tests as prima facie evidence of brain dysfunction. Instead, there is a need to document that behavioral dysfunction observed on a test is related to brain pathologies and not to other sources of variability such as experiential, socioeducational, or emotional factors. As Fletcher and Taylor (1984) noted, there is no simple relationship between the degree or extent of brain involvement and the degree of behavioral disorder among children with brain pathology. This fallacy is often embedded in the language employed by the child neuropsychologist such that descriptions of behavioral dysfunctions are equated inferentially to etiology (developmental delay) or to diagnosis (brain damage) (Hartlage & Telzrow, 1986).

Boll (1983) cautioned against several other persistent misconceptions in the field of child neuropsychology. One misconception suggests that there are certain predictable characteristics of brain-damaged children rather than recognizing that the overriding effect of brain damage on psychological functioning is to increase the variability of behavior. A second misconception asserts that brain damage in children causes characteristic hyperactive motor behavior rather than recognizing that changes in simple, complex, and integrated motor skills may occur in many but not all neurologic disorders, including psychiatric/behavioral disorders without evidence of neurologic abnormality (Tramontana & Hooper, 1989).

Still another misconception asserts that perceptual dysfunctions are the major difficulties produced by brain damage in children. This misconception fails to recognize that no single pattern of neuropsychological deficits is characteristic of brain damage in children. A final misconception is that brain damage causes serious emotional disturbance. This misconception ignores the complex interplay between intrapersonal factors (age, type of lesion), interpersonal factors (family, school environment), and adaptational abilities that can lead to the same spectrum of emotional and conduct disorders seen in non-brain-damaged children (Taylor & Fletcher, 1990). Although many of these misconceptions were based in the use of single-test behavioral indices of brain pathology, they continue to persist in part because of the need for more comprehensive data on the developmental effects of brain lesions in children.

Summary

In its present state, the typical approach to assessment of children for the presence of neuropsychological dysfunction involves the collation of data from developmental/clinical history with data derived from a battery of neuropsychological tests. On the basis of a quantitative analysis of the test data and to a lesser extent an analysis of the fit between qualitative aspects of test performance with known clinical subtypes as well as with historical data and presenting symptoms, the child neuropsychologist then can proceed by a process of primary inference to relate test data to brain function and further, by secondary inference, assign the individual child to a classification group.

The context of the primary or secondary inferential process in child neuropsychology is influenced by several critical factors that include the lack of a consistently employed neurologic model of brain development to relate to behavioral data; the differential effects of lesions according to age at insult; type and etiology of lesion on a developing brain; the need for better descriptive data on a wide variety of clinical populations in developmental neuropathologies; and the need for better specification of quantitative as well as qualitative aspects of normal and abnormal behavior. In the absence of substantive knowledge of the influence of such critical factors, inferential models in child neuropsychology are still primarily descriptive in nature. The beginning emergence of an integration of description and adequate neuropsychological tests (Friedes, 1985; Rourke, 1995) with classification schemes should facilitate prescriptions for remediation and better understanding of the effects of intervention on the remediation of neurobehavioral deficits resulting from neurologic pathologies in infancy, childhood, and adolescence.

References

Adams, R. D., & Victor, M. (1977). *Principles of neurology.* New York: McGraw–Hill.

Bakker, D. J. (1984). The brain as a dependent variable. *Journal of Clinical Neuropsychology, 6,* 1–16.

Barkley, R. A. (1994). The assessment of attention in children. In G. R. Lyon (Ed.), *Frames of reference for the assessment of learning disabilities* (pp. 69–102). Baltimore: Paul H. Brookes.

Baron, I. S., Fennell, E. B., & Voeller, K. J. K. (1995). *Pediatric neuropsychology in a medical setting.* London: Oxford University Press.

Bauer, R. M. (1994). The flexible battery approach to neuropsychological assessment. In R. Vanderploeg (Ed.), *Clinician's guide to neuropsychological assessment* (pp. 259–290). Hillsdale, NJ: Lawrence Erlbaum.

Berg, R. A., & Linton, J. C. (1989). Neuropsychological sequelae of chronic medical disorders. In C. R. Reynolds & E. Fletcher-Janzen (Eds.), *Handbook of clinical child neuropsychology* (pp. 107–127). New York: Plenum Press.

Boll, T. J. (1983). Neuropsychological assessment of the child: Myths, current status, and future prospects. In C. E. Walker & M. C. Roberts (Eds.), *Handbook of clinical child psychology* (pp. 186–208). New York: Wiley–Interscience.

Boll, T. J., & Barth, J. (1981). Neuropsychology of brain damage in children. In S. B. Filskov & T. J. Boll (Eds.), *Handbook of clinical neuropsychology* (Vol. I, pp. 418–452). New York: Wiley–Interscience.

Bolter, J. F., & Long, C. J. (1985). Methodological issues in research in developmental neuropsychology. In L. C. Hartlage & C. F. Telzrow (Eds.), *The neuropsychology of individual differences* (pp. 42–59). New York: Plenum Press.

Bornstein, R. A., King, G., & Carroll, A. (1983). Neuropsychological deficits in Gilles de la Tourette's syndrome. *Journal of Nervous and Mental Diseases, 17,* 497–502.

Brunswick, E. (1956). *Perception and the representative design of psychological experiments.* Berkeley: University of California Press.

Chadwick, O., & Rutter, M. (1983). Neuropsychological assessment. In M. Rutter (Ed.), *Developmental neuropsychiatry* (pp. 181–212). New York: Guilford Press.

Christensen, A. L. (1975). *Luria's neuropsychological investigation.* New York: Spectrum.

Clark, C. M. (1984). Statistical models and their application in clinical neuropsychological research and practice. In S. B. Filskov & T. J. Boll (Eds.), *Handbook of clinical neuropsychology* (Vol. II, pp. 577–605). New York: Wiley–Interscience.

Cronbach, L. J., Rajaratnam, N., & Gleser, G. C. (1963). Theory of generalizability: A liberalization of reliability theory. *British Journal of Statistical Psychology, 16,* 137–163.

Damasio, A. R., & Maurer, R. G. (1978). A neurological model for childhood autism. *Archives of Neurology, 35,* 777–786.

Dean, R. S. (1986). Foundation and rationale for neuropsychological bases of individual differences. In L. C. Hartlage & C. F. Telzrow (Eds.), *The neuropsychology of individual differences* (pp. 8–39). New York: Plenum Press.

Denckla, M. B. (1979). Childhood learning disabilities. In K. Heilman & E. Valenstein (Eds.), *Clinical neuropsychology* (pp. 535–573). London: Oxford University

Fennell, E. B. (1994). Issues in child neuropsychological assessment. In R. Vanderploeg (Ed.), *Clinician's guide to neuropsychological assessment* (pp. 165–184). Hillsdale, NJ: Lawrence Erlbaum.

Fletcher, J. M., & Taylor, H. G. (1984). Neuropsychological approaches to children: Towards a developmental neuropsychology. *Journal of Clinical Neuropsychology, 6,* 39–56.

Freides, D. (1985). Desirable features in neuropsychological tests. *Journal of Psychopathology and Behavioral Assessment, 7*(4), 351–364.

Golden, C. J. (1989). The Nebraska Neuropsychological Children's Battery. In C. R. Reynolds & E. Fletcher-Janzen (Eds.), *Handbook of clinical child neuropsychology* (pp. 193–204). New York: Plenum Press.

Goodglass, H. (1986). The flexible battery in neuropsychological assessment. In T. Incagnoli, G. Goldstein, & C. J. Golden (Eds.), *Clinical application of neuropsychological test batteries* (pp. 121–134). New York: Plenum Press.

Hammond, K. R., Hursch, C. J., & Todd, F. J. (1964). Analyzing the components of clinical inference. *Psychological Review, 71,* 438–456.

Hartlage, L. C., & Telzrow, C. F. (1986). *Neuropsychological assessment and intervention with children and adolescents.* Sarasota, FL: Professional Resource Exchange.

Heilman K., & Valenstein, D. (1993). *Clinical neuropsychology* (3rd ed.). London: Oxford University Press.

Holt, R. R. (1968). Editor's foreword. In D. Rapaport, M. M. Gill, & R. Schafer, *Diagnostic psychological testing.* New York: International Universities Press.

Hursch, C. J., Hammond, K. R., & Hursch, J. L. (1964). Some methodological considerations in multiple-cue probability studies. *Psychological Review, 71,* 42–60.

Hynd, G. W., Obrzut, J. E., Hayes, F., & Becker, M. G. (1986). Neuropsychology of childhood learning disabilities. In D. Wedding, A. M. Horton, & J. Webster (Eds.), *The neuropsychology handbook: Behavioral and clinical perspectives* (pp. 456–485). Berlin: Springer.

Incagnoli, T., Goldstein, G., & Golden, C. J. (Eds.). (1986). *Clinical application of neuropsychological test batteries.* New York: Plenum Press.

Ivinskis, A., Allen, S., & Shaw, E. (1971). An extension of Wechsler Memory Scale norms to lower age groups. *Journal of Clinical Psychology, 26,* 354–357.

Kail, R. (1984). *The development of memory in children.* San Francisco: Freeman.

Kinsbourne, M., & Warrington, E. K. (1963). The developmental Gerstmann syndrome. *Archives of Neurology, 8,* 490–501.

Landy, F. J. (1986). Stamp collecting versus science: Validation as hypothesis testing. *American Psychologist, 41,* 1183–1192.

Lezak, M. D. (1995). *Neuropsychological assessment* (3rd ed.). London: University Press.

Luria, A. R. (1973). *The working brain.* New York: Basic Books.

Lyon, G. R. (Ed.). (1994). *Frames of reference for the assessment of learning disabilities.* Baltimore: Paul H. Brookes.

Maurer, R. G., & Damasio, A. R. (1982). Childhood autism from the point of view of behavioral neurology. *Journal of Autism and Developmental Disorders, 12,* 211–221.

Meehl, P. E. (1957). When shall we use our heads instead of the formula? *Journal of Counseling Psychology, 4,* 268–273.

Meehl, P. E. (1960). The cognitive activity of the clinician. *American Psychologist, 15,* 19–27.

Menkes, J. H. (1990). *Textbook of child neurology* (4th ed.). Philadelphia: Lea & Febinger.

Morris, R., Blashfield, R., & Satz. P. (1986). Developmental classification of reading-disabled children. *Journal of Experimental and Clinical Neuropsychology, 8,* 371–392.

Netley, C., & Rovet, J. (1983). Relationships among brain organization, maturation rate, and the development of verbal and nonverbal ability. In S. Segalowitz (Ed.), *Language functions and brain organization* (pp. 245–266). New York: Academic Press.

Pirozzolo, F. J., Campanella, D. J., Christensen, K., & Lawson-Kerr, K. (1981). Effects of cerebral dysfunction on neurolinguistic performance in children. *Journal of Consulting and Clinical Psychology, 49*(6), 791–806.

Platt, J. R. (1964). Strong inference. *Science, 146,* 347–353.

Popper, K. R. (1959). *The logic of scientific discovery.* New York: Harper.

Rasmussen, T., & Milner, B. (1977). The role of early left-brain injury in determining lateralization of cerebral speed functions. *Annals of the New York Academy of Sciences, 299,* 355–369.

Reitan, R. M., & Davison, L. A. (1974). *Clinical neuropsychology: Current status and applications.* Washington, DC: Winston.

Reynolds, C. R. (1989). Measurement and statistical problems in neuropsychological assessment of children. In C. R. Reynolds & E. Fletcher-Janzen (Eds.), *Handbook of clinical child neuropsychology* (pp. 147–166). New York: Plenum Press.

Reynolds, C. R., & Fletcher-Janzen, E. (Eds.). (1989). *Handbook of clinical child neuropsychology.* New York: Plenum Press.

Ross, D. M., & Ross, S. A. (1992). *Hyperactivity: Current issues, research and theory* (2nd ed.). New York: Wiley–Interscience.

Rourke, B. P. (1983). Reading and spelling disabilities: A developmental neuropsychological perspective. In U. Kirk (Ed.), *Neuropsychology of language, reading, and spelling* (pp. 209–234). New York: Academic Press.

Rourke, B. P. (1995). *Syndrome of nonverbal learning disabilities.* New York: Guilford Press.

Rourke, B. P., & Adams, K. M. (1984). Quantitative approaches to the neuropsychological assessment of children. In R. M. Tarter & G. Goldstein (Eds.), *Advances in clinical neuropsychology* (Vol. 2, pp. 79–108). New York: Plenum Press.

Rourke, B. P., Bakker, D. J., Fisk, J. L., & Strang, J. D. (1983). *Child neuropsychology: An introduction to theory, research and clinical practice.* New York: Guilford Press.

Rourke, B. P., Fisk, J. L., & Strang, J. D. (1986). *Neuropsychological assessment of children: A treatment oriented approach.* New York: Guilford Press.

Rutter, M. (Ed.). (1983). *Developmental neuropsychiatry.* New York: Guilford Press.

Satz, P., & Fletcher, J. M. (1980). Minimal brain dysfunction: An appraisal of research concepts and methods. In H. E. Rie and E. D. Rie (Eds.), *Handbook of minimal brain dysfunction: A critical review* (pp. 669–714). New York: Wiley.

Satz, P., & Morris, R. (1981). Learning disability subtypes: A review. In F. J. Pirozzolo & M. Wittrock (Eds.), *Neuropsychological and cognitive process in reading* (pp. 109–141). New York: Academic Press.

Segalowitz, S. (Ed.). (1983). *Language functions and brain organization.* New York: Academic Press.

Segalowitz, S. J., & Gruber, F. A. (Eds.). (1977). *Language development and neurological theory.* New York: Academic Press.

Shafer, S. Q., Shaffer, D., O'Connor, P. A., & Stokman, C. J. (1983). Hard thoughts on neurological soft signs. In M. Rutter (Ed.), *Developmental neuropsychiatry* (pp. 133–143). New York: Guilford Press.

Shaffer, D., O'Connor, P. A., Shafer, S. Q., & Prupis, S. (1983). Neurologic "soft signs": Their origins and significance for behavior. In M. Rutter (Ed.), *Developmental neuropsychiatry* (pp. 144–163). New York: Guilford Press.

Spellacy, F., & Peter, B. (1978). Dyscalculia and elements of the developmental Gerstmann syndrome in school children. *Cortex, 14,* 197–208.

Spreen, O., Risser, A. T., & Edgell, D. (1995). *Developmental neuropsychology.* New York: Oxford.

Stein, D. G., Rosen, J. F., & Butters, N. (Eds.). (1974). *Plasticity and recovery of function in the central nervous system.* New York: Academic Press.

Tarter, R. E., & Edwards, K. L. (1986). Neuropsychological batteries. In T. Incagnoli, G. Goldstein, & C. J. Golden (Eds.), *Clinical application of neuropsychological test batteries* (pp. 135–153). New York: Plenum Press.

Taylor, H. G., & Fletcher, J. M. (1990). Neuropsychological assessments of children. In G. Goldstein & M. Hersen (Eds.), *Handbook of psychological assessment* (pp. 228–255). New York: Pergamon Press.

Taylor, H. G., & Schatschneider, C. (1992). Child neuropsychological assessment: A test of basic assumptions. *The Clinical Neuropsychologist, 6,* 259–275.

Tramontana, M. G., & Hooper, S. R. (1987). Discriminating the presence and pattern of neuropsychological impairment in child psychiatric disorders. *International Journal of Clinical Neuropsychology, 9,* 111–119.

Tramontana, M. G., & Hooper, S. R. (1989). Neuropsychology of child psychopathology: In C. R. Reynolds & E. Fletcher-Janzen (Eds.), *Handbook of clinical child neuropsychology* (pp. 87–106). New York: Plenum Press.

Van der Vlugt, H. (1979). Aspects of normal and abnormal neuropsychological development. In M. S. Gazzaniga (Ed.), *Handook of behavioral neurobiology* (Vol. 2, pp. 99–117). New York: Plenum Press.

van Santen, J. P. H., Black, L. M., Wilson, B. C., & Risucci, D. A. (1994). Modeling clinical judgment: A reanalysis of data from Wilson and Risucci's paper "A model for clinical-qualitative classification: Generation I: Application to language-disordered preschool children." *Brain and Language, 46,* 469–481.

Waber, D. P., & Holmes, J. M. (1985). Assessing children's copy of productions of the Rey–Osterrieth complex figure. *Journal of Clinical and Experimental Psychology, 7,* 264–280.

Wiggins, J. S. (1973). *Personality and prediction: Principles of personality assessment.* Reading, MA: Addison–Wesley.

Witelson, S. F. (1977). Early hemisphere specialization and interhemisphere plasticity: An empirical and theoretical review. In S. Segalowitz & F. A. Gruber (Eds.), *Language development and neurological theory* (pp. 213–287). New York: Academic Press.

Woods, B. T., & Teuber, H. L. (1973). Early onset of complementary specialization of cerebral hemispheres in man. *Transactions of the American Neurological Association, 98,* 113–117.

II

Neuropsychological Diagnosis

11

Halstead–Reitan Neuropsychological Test Batteries for Children

NANCY L. NUSSBAUM AND ERIN D. BIGLER

The purpose of this chapter is to review the children's version of the Halstead–Reitan neuropsychological test batteries for children. The Halstead–Reitan Neuropsychological Test Battery for Children 9 to 14 years of age (Reitan & Davison, 1974) and the Reitan–Indiana Test Battery for Children ages 5 through 8 (Reitan, 1969) are two children's batteries based on the adult version of the Halstead–Reitan (Reitan & Wolfsun, 1985). These two batteries will be discussed in terms of their development and validity. This discussion will be followed by a description of the measures, their administration, scoring, and the functional domains they are purported to measure. Finally, the interpretation of test results obtained from the Halstead–Reitan and the Reitan–Indiana will be discussed.

The Halstead–Reitan Neuropsychological Test Battery for Older Children (9 to 14) and the Reitan–Indiana Neuropsychological Test Battery for Younger Children (5 to 8) are two of the most commonly used neuropsychological test batteries for children. These batteries were developed by Ralph Reitan based on the adult version of the Halstead–Reitan Neuropsychological Test Battery (Halstead, 1947; Reitan & Davison, 1974; Reitan & Wolfsun, 1985). The children's batteries include modifications and a downward extension of the adult Halstead–Reitan, as well as the addition of some supplementary measures not included in the adult version (see Table 1).

NANCY L. NUSSBAUM • Austin Neurological Clinic, Austin, Texas 78705. ERIN D. BIGLER • Department of Psychology, Brigham Young University, Provo, Utah 84602; and LDS Hospital, Salt Lake City, Utah 84143.

The reason for the development of the Halstead–Reitan and the Reitan–Indiana was to standardize a battery of measures to assess various aspects of brain functioning in children. The major theoretical basis of the Halstead–Reitan and the Reitan–Indiana is the proposition that behavior has an organic basis. Thus, performance on behavioral measures can be used to assess brain functioning. Obviously, in order to infer brain functioning based on behavioral measures, it was necessary to validate these measures on children with known brain damage.

Validation Studies

The validation of the Halstead–Reitan for children was first reported by Reed, Reitan, and Klove (1965) for 9- to 15-year-old children with known brain damage, and by Klonoff, Robinson, and Thompson (1969) for 5- to 9-year-old children. These studies demonstrated the validity of using neuropsychological variables from the Halstead–Reitan to differentiate brain-damaged from non-brain-damaged children. Subsequently, numerous studies have shown the discriminant validity of the Halstead–Reitan and the Reitan–Indiana in separating children with known brain damage from non-brain-damaged children (Boll, 1974; Reitan, 1974; Selz, 1981; Selz & Reitan, 1979a,b). For example, Boll (1974) matched 27 brain-damaged children with 27 normal children on the basis of age, sex, race, and handedness. Significantly poorer performance by the brain-damaged group was reported for

TABLE 1. Subtests of the Halstead–Reitan Neuropsychological Test Batteries for Children

Halstead battery[a] (9–14 years)	Reitan–Indiana battery[a] (5–8 years)
Category test	Category test
Tactual performance test	Tactual performance test
Fingertapping test	Fingertapping test
Speech sounds perception test	—
Seashore rhythm test	—
Trail-making test, A & B	Marching test
Strength of grip test	Strength of grip test
Sensory perceptual exam	Sensory perceptual exam
Tactile finger localization test	Tactile finger localization test
Fingertip number writing test	Fingertip symbol writing test
Tactile form recognition test	Tactile form recognition test
Aphasia screening test	Aphasia screening test
	Color form test
	Progressive figures test
	Matching pictures test
	Target test
	Matching figures and matching V's test
	Drawing of star and concentric squares

[a] The Wechsler Intelligence Scale for Children-Revised (Wechsler, 1974), the Wide Range Achievement Test-Revised (Jastak & Wilkinson, 1984), and the Lateral Dominance Test (Harris, 1947) are often included in the comprehensive neuropsychological evaluation of children.

finger oscillation (dominant and nondominant), the tactual performance test (dominant, nondominant, and both hands), finger recognition (dominant), fingertip number writing (dominant and nondominant), Seashore Rhythm Test, and Speech Sounds Perception Test. Similar results were found by Reitan (1974) in a study with children aged 5 to 8, matched for age and sex. Furthermore, in a study of children with questionable rather than definite neurological impairment, it was found that a neuropsychological test battery correctly identified the presence or absence of impairment, even when the initial subjective clinical impressions did not suggest deficits (Tsushima & Towne, 1977). Also, in a more recent study (Nici & Reitan, 1986) using intellectual, achievement, and neuropsychological measures, it was found that measures of motor functioning and general neuropsychological abilities were the best discriminators of 9- to 14-year-old brain-damaged children versus non-brain-damaged children.

It should be added that although the Reitan–Indiana and the Halstead–Reitan were originally developed to assess brain damage in children, they also have been used extensively to evaluate various aspects of purely behavioral functioning. As such, in general clinical practice, the assessment of functional aspects of behavior may be the most widely used application of these measures. Through the use of the Reitan–Indiana and the Halstead–Reitan, a great deal of information can be obtained concerning certain aspects of sensory functioning, motor abilities, auditory processing, attention, spatial abilities, memory, visuospatial abilities, visuomotor abilities, conceptual processing, sequential processing, and language functioning. Therefore, although the Reitan–Indiana and the Halstead–Reitan are often used in the evaluation of organic dysfunction in children, they also have a great deal of clinical utility as measures of behavioral competencies in children. In regard to this use of the Reitan–Indiana and the Halstead–Reitan to assess behavioral functioning, Fletcher and Taylor (1984) proposed that the greatest clinical utility of these instruments is in their usefulness in defining the ability structure of the child. They argued that the widest clinical application of the children's neuropsychological batteries is related to the clinical sensitivity of these measures to the child's behavioral strengths and weaknesses.

In particular, the HRNB has been found to be useful in the diagnosis of learning disabilities (LD) and in defining strengths and weakness within the LD population. For example, the HRNB is being used more as an adjunct to traditional psychoeducational measures, such as the Wechsler intelligence scales. In a study examining the incremental validity of the HRNB to the WISC-R in an LD sample, it was found that HRNB increased the variability accounted for in academic measures from 16 to 30% (Strom, Gray, Dean, & Fischer, 1987). This suggests that there was a significant amount of unique variance contributed by the HRNB. Similarly, a study by Shurtleff, Fay, Abbott, and Berninger (1988) found that cognitive and HRNB variables were not redundant, and that inclusion of both improved educational assessment. Also, in terms of predictive validity, it was found that the Seashore Rhythm Test appeared to be a useful tool in detecting young children who showed early signs of reading impairment (McGivern, Berka, Languis, & Chapman, 1991).

In summary, as can be seen from the previous discussion, the Reitan–Indiana and the Halstead–Reitan have a wide variety of clinical applications. These test batteries can be useful in the behavioral assessment of children with known brain damage, as well as in the evaluation of the ability structure of the child without known brain damage. In the next section, types of behaviors measured and the administration and scoring of the Halstead–Reitan and the Reitan–Indiana will be discussed in greater detail.

Subtests from the Halstead–Reitan Neuropsychological Test Battery for Children Ages 9 through 14

Normative data for the measures included in the Halstead–Reitan have been developed by Spreen and Gaddes (1969) and Knights and Norwood (1980).* Also, Spreen and Strauss (1991) present normative data for children for a number of subtests from the Halstead–Reitan. See Tables 2 and 3 for an example of a raw score conversion table, in which raw scores are converted to standard scores ($X = 100$, SD $= 15$) using normative data.

Category Test

Description. This test includes 168 items presented visually to the child. The child must respond by selecting a number (1, 2, 3, or 4) that corresponds with the visual stimulus. Feedback is given on each item regarding the correctness or incorrectness of the response.

Scoring. The child's raw score is the total of errors made. Normative data are also available for each of the six subtests of the category test (Knights & Norwood, 1980).

Domain Measured. The category test is a measure of concept formation. The child must abstract principles related to number concepts, spatial position, and unusualness of the stimuli. There also is a memory component involved in the last subtest of this measure.

Tactual Performance Test

Description. On this test, the child is required to complete a six-figure form board while blindfolded. The test is carried out first with the dominant hand, then the nondominant hand, and finally with both hands. Next, the board is removed and the child is asked to draw from memory the shapes and their correct locations.

Scoring. The child's raw score is the amount of time taken with the dominant, nondominant, and both hands. The total time is the sum of the trials with the dominant, nondominant, and both hands. Also, the memory raw score is the total number of blocks recalled, and the location raw score is the number of blocks reproduced in their correct locations.

Domain Measured. The tactual performance test is a measure of tactile, motor, spatial, and memory functioning.

Fingertapping Test

Description. This test requires a child to tap a mounted key as quickly as possibly with the index finger of the dominant and nondominant hand. Five trials are given for each hand.

Scoring. The child's raw score is the average of the five scores from the dominant and nondominant hand.

Domain Measured. This task is a measure of fine motor speed and coordination.

Speech Sounds Perception Test

Description. On this test, the child must discriminate nonsense words presented on a tape recorder. The child is given four choices to select from and must underline the correct stimulus.

Scoring. The child's raw score is the total number of items correct out of 30.

Domain Measured. Auditory discrimination, sound–symbol matching, and attentional abilities are assessed on this task.

Seashore Rhythm Test

Description. The child is presented pairs of rhythms on a tape recorder and must discriminate whether they are the same or different.

Scoring. The child's raw score is the total number of items correct out of 30.

Domain Measured. This test is a measure of nonverbal auditory perception, attention, and concentration.

*Address for normative data: Dr. Robert M. Knights Psychological Consultants, Inc., 52 Hopewell Ave., Ottawa, Ontario K15 2Y8, Canada.

TABLE 2. Finger Oscillation—Dominant Hand[a]

	Electric tapper			Manual tapper			
Age[b]	6	7	8	9	10	11	12
X	30.9	33.6	37.9	34.3	37.7	38.9	41.3
SD	3.27	3.93	5.45	4.37	4.98	5.57	5.47
Raw score							
20	*	*	*	*	*	*	*
21	55	*	*	*	*	*	*
22	59	56	56	58	*	*	*
23	64	60	59	61	56	57	*
24	68	63	62	65	59	60	*
25	73	67	64	68	62	63	55
26	78	71	67	72	65	65	58
27	82	75	70	75	68	68	61
28	87	79	73	78	71	71	64
29	91	82	76	82	74	73	66
30	96	86	78	85	77	76	69
31	100	90	81	89	80	79	72
32	105	94	84	92	83	81	74
33	110	98	87	96	86	84	77
34	114	102	89	99	89	87	80
35	119	105	92	102	92	89	83
36	123	109	95	106	95	92	85
37	128	113	98	109	98	95	88
38	133	117	100	113	101	98	91
39	137	121	103	116	104	100	94
40	142	124	106	120	107	103	96
41	146	128	109	123	110	106	99
42	151	132	111	126	113	108	102
43	**	136	114	130	116	111	105
44	**	140	117	133	119	114	107
45	**	144	120	137	122	116	110
46	**	**	122	140	125	119	113
47	**	**	125	144	128	122	116
48	**	**	128	**	131	125	118
49	**	**	131	**	134	127	121
50	**	**	133	**	137	130	124
51	**	**	136	**	140	132	126
52	**	**	139	**	143	135	129
53	**	**	141	**	**	137	132
54	**	**	144	**	**	141	135
55	**	**	**	**	**	143	137
56	**	**	**	**	**	**	140
57	**	**	**	**	**	**	143
58	**	**	**	**	**	**	**
59	**	**	**	**	**	**	**
60	**	**	**	**	**	**	**

[a]Standard scores ($X = 100$, SD $= 15$) were calculated based on the normative data developed by Spreen and Gaddes (1969). *, standard score greater than three standard deviations below the mean; **, standard score greater than three standard deviations above the mean.

[b]Six- to eight-year-old norms are for the electric fingertapper; 9- to 12-year-old norms are for the manual fingertapper.

TABLE 3. Right Hand[a]

	Fingertip symbol writing				Fingertip number writing					
Age	5	6	7	8	9	10	11	12	13	14
X errors	6.00	3.50	2.70	2.05	4.36	3.25	2.75	2.00	0.50	0.50
SD	3.00	2.50	2.00	1.50	3.73	3.01	2.00	1.00	0.55	0.40
Raw score										
0	130	121	120	121	117	116	121	130	113	119
1	125	115	113	111	113	111	113	115	86	81
2	120	109	105	101	109	106	106	100	59	**
3	115	103	98	91	105	101	98	85	**	**
4	110	97	90	81	101	96	91	70	**	**
5	105	91	83	71	97	91	83	55	**	**
6	100	85	75	61	93	86	76	**	**	**
7	95	79	68	**	90	81	68	**	**	**
8	90	73	60	**	86	76	61	**	**	**
9	85	67	**	**	82	71	**	**	**	**
10	80	61	**	**	78	66	**	**	**	**
11	75	55	**	**	74	61	**	**	**	**
12	70	**	**	**	70	56	**	**	**	**
13	65	**	**	**	66	**	**	**	**	**
14	60	**	**	**	62	**	**	**	**	**
15	55	**	**	**	58	**	**	**	**	**

[a]Standard scores ($X = 100$, SD = 15) were calculated based on the normative data developed by Knights and Norwood (1980). **, standard score greater than standard deviations below the mean.

Trails A

Description. On this test, the child must connect circles containing the numbers 1 through 15 as quickly as possible.

Scoring. The child's raw score is the number of seconds taken to complete the task, and the number of errors made.

Domain Measured. This task includes components measuring visual perception, motor speed, sequencing skills, and symbol recognition.

Trails B

Description. This test requires the child to connect alternating letters (A to G) and numbers (1 to 8).

Scoring. As in Trails A, the child's raw score is the number of seconds taken to complete the task, and the number of errors made.

Domain Measured. Trails B measures visual perception, motor speed, sequencing skills, and symbol recognition. It also is a measure of simultaneous processing and cognitive flexibility.

Strength of Grip Test

Description. The child's grip strength is measured using a dynamometer adjusted for hand size. Three alternating trials are allowed for the dominant and nondominant hand.

Scoring. A mean raw score is obtained for each hand.

Domain Measured. Differential hand strength is assessed by this measure.

Sensory Perceptual Exam

Tactile, auditory, and visual perception are measured by this task.

Tactile Perception. The child is asked to close the eyes and to report whether the right hand, left hand, right face, or left face is being lightly touched. Following unilateral trials to determine whether the child can perceive unilateral stimulation, bilateral trials are randomly interspersed with unilateral trials. Bilateral trials include the stimulation of both hands and the contralateral stimulation of the hand and face, the so-called double simultaneous stimulation (DSS) procedure. (In addition, we have found it useful to include ipsilateral hand/face trials. This appears to require more sensitive tactile discrimination.)

Scoring. A raw score for each body side is calculated by summing the total number of errors made on unilateral and bilateral trials. (Ipsilateral errors are not included in this raw score when converting raw scores to standard scores.)

Domain Measured. Differential tactile perception is measured by this task.

Auditory Perception. The examiner lightly rubs his or her fingers together by the child's right ear, left ear, or both ears. The child is asked to close his or her eyes and report where the sound is coming from. Following unilateral trials to determine whether the child can perceive unilateral stimuli, bilateral trials are randomly interspersed with unilateral trials. Bilateral stimulation constitutes the DSS procedure for auditory stimulation.

Scoring. A raw score for each ear is calculated by summing the total number of errors made on unilateral and bilateral trials.

Visual Perception. The child's visual fields are tested by quadrant. Then the child is asked to report peripheral, unilateral, and bilateral single movements by the examiner at eye level, above eye level, and below eye level. Bilateral stimulation constitutes the DSS procedure for visual stimulation.

Scoring. A raw score for the right and left visual fields are calculated by summing the total number of errors made on unilateral and bilateral trials.

Domain Measured. Differential visual perception in the right and left visual fields is measured by this task.

Tactile Finger Localization Test

Description. With the child observing, the examiner numbers the child's fingers. The child must then close his or her eyes and report the number of the finger being stimulated.

Scoring. The raw score is the sum of the errors made on each hand.

Domain Measured. This test is a measure of tactile perception, tactile localization, and attention for each body side.

Fingertip Number Writing Test

Description. The child watches while the examiner traces the numbers 3, 4, 5, and 6 on the palm of the child's hand. The child is then asked to close his or her eyes and report the number written in a set order on the fingertips of the right and left hands.

Scoring. The raw score is the sum of the errors made on each hand.

Domain Measured. Aspects of complex tactile perception and concentration are assessed by this task for each body side.

Tactile Form Recognition Test

Description. The child places a hand through an opening in a board, and the examiner places either a small cross, triangle, square, or circle in the child's hand without the child seeing what object has been placed there. The child must then point to the correct object on the board with the other hand. The task is carried out twice with each hand.

Scoring. The raw score is the sum of errors made with each hand, and the number of seconds taken to identify the object with the right and the left hand.

Domain Measured. This test is a measure of attention, tactile perception, and reaction time for each body side.

Aphasia Screening Test

Description. This test includes 32 items requiring naming, copying, spelling, reading, writing, repeating, verbal comprehension, and right/left discrimination.

Scoring. Selz and Reitan (1979b) developed a scoring system for the items from the Aphasia Screening Test.

Domain Measured. The Aphasia Screening Test is a useful screening measure for dyspraxia (both spelling and constructional), dysnomia, dysgraphia, dyslexia, dyscalculia, ideational dyspraxia, expressive aphasia, receptive aphasia, dysarthria, visual dysgnosia, auditory dysgnosia, and right/left disorientation.

Subtests from the Reitan–Indiana Neuropsychological Test Battery for Children 5 through 8

The Reitan–Indiana (Reitan, 1969) is a downward extension of the Halstead–Reitan Neuropsychological Test Battery (see Reitan & Wolfsun, 1985) developed for children 5 to 8 years of age. The modifications discussed below were necessary because of the developmental differences found between younger and older children (Boll, 1981; Reitan & Davison, 1974). In addition, as in the older children's battery, normative data for measures included in the Reitan–Indiana have been developed by Spreen and Gaddes (1969) and Knights and Norwood (1980).

Category Tests

Description. The number of test items was reduced to 80 items in five categories. On the first subtest the child is required to identify colors by selecting a corresponding lever. The following four subtests involve principles of size, shape, color, or memory.

Scoring. See the previous description of scoring for the Category Test.

Domain Measured. Nonverbal reasoning, learning, memory, and concept formation are assessed by this task.

Tactual Performance Test

Description. The same six-figure form board employed in the older children's battery is used on this test, but the board is presented horizontally. (See the previous discussion of the tactual performance test for a more detailed description of the task, the scoring, and the abilities measured.)

Fingertapping Test

Description. The same procedure is used with younger children, as was described for older children, except that an electric fingertapping device is used to compensate for the younger child's poorer fine motor coordination. (The scoring and domain measured are the same as described previously.)

Speech Sounds Perception Test, Seashore Rhythm Test, Trails A and B

These tests are not components of the younger children's battery.

Marching Test

Description. On this test the child is required to follow a sequence of circles connected by lines up a page, by touching each circle as quickly as possible.

Scoring. The raw score is the number of errors and time taken to complete the task.

Domain Measured. This test is a measure of upper extremity gross motor functioning and coordination.

Strength of Grip

This test remains unchanged from the older children's battery.

Sensory–Perceptual Exam (SPE)

The tactile and auditory tasks of the SPE remain unchanged. Only a minor modification of the visual task has been made requiring that visual stimulation be presented at eye level only. In addition, if the young child has difficulty verbally reporting the body part touched or the side of stimulation (i.e., right, left), he or she is allowed to point to or raise the hand on the side of stimulation.

Tactile Finger Localization. The procedure for this task remains unchanged from the older children's battery.

Fingertip Symbol Writing. This task is very similar to the Fingertip Number Writing Test from the older children's battery. The child is required to close his or her eyes and report which symbols (X's and O's) are written on the child's fingertips. (See the older children's battery for a description of the scoring procedure and the domain measured.)

Tactile Form Recognition. The procedure for this task remains unchanged from the older children's battery.

Aphasia Screening Test

Description. Some items were deleted or simplified for the younger children. Items included in this test require the child to write, copy simple geometric figures, identify pictures, read letters and simple words, carry out simple mathematical functions, identify body parts, and identify right/left body side.

Scoring. Knights and Norwood (1979) developed a scoring system for the younger children's version of the Aphasia Screening Test.

Domain Measured. This is a screening instrument for constructional dyspraxia, dysgraphia, dyslexia, dyscalculia, right/left disorientation, receptive aphasia, expressive aphasia, visual dysgnosia, and body dysgnosia.

Color Form Test

Description. A board is presented with different colored geometric shapes. The child must alternate between touching shapes and colors selectively attending to one aspect of the stimulus (e.g., color), while ignoring the other (e.g., shape).

Scoring. The child's raw score is the total number of errors made and the amount of time taken to complete the task.

Domain Measured. This test is a measure of attention, ability to inhibit, visual screening, cognitive flexibility, and upper extremity gross motor coordination.

Progressive Figures Test

Description. The child is presented a sheet of paper on which are printed eight large geometric shapes (e.g., circle), with a smaller shape (e.g., square) inside. The child must use the small inside figure as a cue for moving to the outside shape of the next figure.

Scoring. The child's raw score is the total number of errors made and the amount of time taken to complete the task.

Domain Measured. This test measures visual perception, motor speed, cognitive flexibility, attention, and concentration.

Matching Pictures Test

Description. The child must match pictures beginning with identical pictures and progressing to matching pictures from more general categories.

Scoring. The raw score is the total correct out of a possible 19.

Domain Measured. This test is a measure of visual discrimination, reasoning, and categorizing skills.

Target Test

Description. The child is shown an 18-inch card with nine dots printed on it, and is given a sheet with the same dot configuration. The examiner taps out a design on the stimulus card and the child must draw the design on the response test.

Scoring. The raw score is the number of items correct.

Domain Measured. Visual/spatial memory is measured by this task.

Matching Figures and Matching V's Test

Description. On the Matching Figures Test the child must match figures printed on blocks with figures printed on a card. The figures become progressively more complex. The matching V's task requires the child to match V's that vary in the width of the angle.

Scoring. The raw score is the number of errors and time taken to complete the task.

Domain Measured. This test is a measure of visual perception and reaction time.

Drawing of Star and Concentric Squares

Description. The child must copy figures of varying complexity.

Scoring. The raw score is the number of errors and time taken to complete the task.

Domain Measured. This test is a measure of visual perception, fine motor coordination, and constructional praxis.

Interpretation of Children's Performance on Neuropsychological Batteries

In the past, a number of approaches have been applied to the interpretation of children's performance on neuropsychological tasks (Fletcher & Taylor, 1984; Reitan & Davison, 1974; Rourke, Bakker, Fisk, & Strang, 1983; Selz, 1981; Teeter, 1986). These various approaches and their limitations will be discussed below.

Level of Performance

In this approach, the child's level of performance on neuropsychological measures is compared with normative data, such as the norms developed by Spreen and Gaddes (1969) and Knights and Norwood (1980). If the child's performance falls significantly below (e.g., two standard deviations below the mean) what would be expected for her or his age, then a deficit is diagnosed in the particular area measured by the neuropsychological task. For example, on the fingertapping test, the mean performance for a 9-year-old is 34.3 (SD = 4.37) (Spreen & Gaddes, 1969) for the dominant hand. Using the level-of-performance approach, if a 9-year-old obtained a score of 25, fine motor speed with the dominant hand would be interpreted as impaired.

There are a number of disadvantages to relying solely on this method for the interpretation of children's neuropsychological test performance. First, because of the large variability in normal children's performance on neuropsychological measures, it is often difficult to interpret the individual child's scores. For example, the mean performance for an 8-year-old on the Tactual Performance Test (dominant hand) is 5.71 min but the standard deviation of 6 min is greater than the mean (Knights & Norwood, 1980)! If a two-standard-deviation cutoff is adhered to for interpreting a deficient level of performance on this task, the child would be required to continue for over 17 min in order to diagnose impaired performance. Another problem that is encountered when using only the level of performance to interpret children's neuropsychological performance is the tendency to yield a large number of false positives. This is largely because so many factors other than impairment can negatively influence a child's performance (e.g., motivation, attention, frustration tolerance) (Rourke et al., 1983).

Pathognomonic Signs

The pathognomonic signs (e.g., hemiplegia, aphasia, hemisensory deficit) approach refers to the identification of specific deficits that are not com-

monly seen in normal individuals. For example, articulation errors on the Aphasia Screening Test could be interpreted as an aphasic "sign." Again, one of the limitations of this approach would be the large variability see in the normal population. For example, because of the wide variation in the development of language abilities in children, it is often quite difficult to interpret specific errors made by the individual child. There may be a tendency to interpret as abnormal an isolated error made by the child.

Conversely, it has also been found that the sole use of the pathognomonic signs approach has a tendency to yield a large number of false negatives. For example, Boll (1974) found that 26 of 35 children with known brain damage were misclassified as normal when the sign approach was used to classify objects. One reason for this is that such conditions as infantile hemiplegia may show considerable plasticity and recovery of function (see Bigler & Naugle, 1985), and their neuropsychological test performance may not conform with what would be expected with a more recently acquired brain lesion.

Patterns of Performance

In this approach, the relationship among performance on neuropsychological measures is examined. If large discrepancies are noted, then strengths and weaknesses are interpreted. For example, a child who does very well on the Speech Sounds Perception Test and the verbal items from the Aphasia Screening Test, but who performs poorly on the constructional tasks of the Aphasia Screening Test and poorly on the Tactual Performance Test Memory and Locations subtests, may be interpreted as having adequate auditory processing but deficits in the area of nonverbal, visual/spatial functioning.

This approach is of limited use in the interpretation of neuropsychological performance of very young children and children with severe disabilities (Rourke et al., 1983). However, it has been used quite extensively in the subgrouping of children with LD (Nussbaum & Bigler, 1986; Rourke, 1984).

Comparison of Right and Left Body Sides

This approach compares the relative performance of one body to the other on motor and sensory–perceptual tasks. For example, a large discrepancy between the right (dominant) and the left (nondominant) hand on the fingertapping test, with the right-hand score less than the left-hand score, may indicate impairment in left-hemisphere functioning. However, once again, because of the wide variability in the performance of normal children, discrepancies between performance on the right and left body sides may often be difficult to interpret for the individual child. This is especially true of the younger child.

Multiple Inferential Approach

Boll (1974, 1981) proposed a multiple inferential approach to the interpretation of children's neuropsychological performance because of the limitations of the isolated use of the approaches discussed previously. In the multiple inferential method, the complementary use of level of performance, pathognomonic signs, pattern analysis, and right/left comparisons is employed in the interpretation of neuropsychological performance. This approach minimizes the limitations that are encountered when these methods are used in isolation.

Rules Approach

The rules approach developed by Selz and Reitan (1979b) also combines a number of inferential methods in the interpretation of children's neuropsychological performance. The rules are based on the four methods of inference discussed earlier: level of performance, pathognomonic signs, pattern analysis, and right/left differences.

The rules were initially developed and validated as an objective system for classifying children as normal, learning disabled, or brain damaged. They consist of a four-point scoring system in which 37 aspects of neuropsychological performance are rated on a scale from 0 (normal to excellent performance) to 3 (very abnormal performance). For example, a child who made nine or more errors on the Tactile Finger Recognition task would receive a score of 3 (impaired) using the rules system. In summary, the rules approach is an attempt at providing an objective system to measure the degree of impairment in the neuropsychological performance of children.

Biobehavioral Approach

The biobehavioral approach is another method that has been proposed for the interpretation of chil-

dren's neuropsychological performance (Taylor & Fletcher, 1990). In this model, there are four basic factors that differentiate child neuropsychological assessment from other types of child assessment.

First, neuropsychological evaluation involves the assessment of four types of variables: (1) the manifest form of the disability or *presenting complaint* [e.g., the impulsive behavior of the child suspected of having attention deficit/hyperactivity disorder (ADHD)]; (2) the *cognitive* and *psychosocial* characteristics (data from formal measures of attention, emotional functioning, and so on) of the child; (3) the *environmental, sociocultural, and historical* variables (e.g., classroom setting, home setting); (4) the *biological and genetic* variables (e.g., parental history of ADHD, maternal prenatal alcohol use).

Second, it is recognized that although the manifest disability is at least partially based on weaknesses in basic neurocognitive functioning, these interact with other child characteristics and environmental influences. The extent to which these cognitive weaknesses result in the manifest disability is influenced by these other factors, which may either intensify or mute the disability.

Third, although there is often a high degree of covariation among skills, an increased amount of variability is often characteristic of many children with disabilities. Thus, it is important to analyze the child's assessment profile in terms of strengths and weaknesses in order to understand how they are expressed in the manifest form of the disability. For example, a child who has ADHD and an auditory processing disorder may have even greater attentional problems in a noisy environment.

Fourth, although there are some childhood disorders and manifest disabilities that have very strong neurological influences (e.g., learning difficulties in a child with hydrocephalus), one also must take into account environmental factors. When interpreting neuropsychological data, the relevance of the central nervous system can only be determined by taking into account both biological limitations and environmental variables.

This model avoids the tenuous inference involved in the interpretation of direct brain–behavior relationships in children using behavioral data. Rather, the biological or neurological substrate is seen as influencing the manifest disability by imposing limits on the basic behavioral competencies of the child. Additional moderator variables, such as the family system and the educational setting, are also taken into consideration.

Furthermore, the relationship between performance on neuropsychological measures and the manifest disability is not seen as causal but instead as correlational. Thus, performance on neuropsychological measures is used to clarify various functional aspects of the child's manifest disability. For example, the ADHD child's performance on neuropsychological measures can help to determine the degree of cognitive impulsivity present in the disorder. In this example the functional aspects of the child's performance would be stressed in the interpretation of the neuropsychological data. Also the importance of interpreting neuropsychological data in a developmental context is emphasized in this model.

Normative Analysis of Halstead–Reitan Neuropsychological Tests for Children

Recently, Findeis and Weight (1995) presented metanorms for several of the child neuropsychological tests from the Halstead–Reitan batteries. Using these normative data, presented in Table 4 and Figure 1, the clinician can examine a child's performance on a given test in comparison with other children of similar age. This approach is different from Reitan's initial one, which was a "cutoff" approach (Reitan, 1974). The "cutoff" approach viewed brain dysfunc-

tion more as a dichotomy—either present or absent. However, more contemporary views of brain dysfunction are from a perspective of a continuum. By using Table 4 and Figure 1 in this chapter, a given child's performance can be compared with normative standards and the coherence or discrepancy from those standards documented. For the clinician, this table and the figures that follow may be extremely useful.

Summary

In summary, the Halstead–Reitan and the Reitan–Indiana were developed by Reitan (Reitan & Davison, 1974) based on the adult version of the Halstead–Reitan Neuropsychological Test Battery (Reitan & Wolfsun, 1985). Since the initial modifications of the Halstead–Reitan Neuropsychological Test Battery, a great deal of work has been done in developing normative data (Knights & Norwood, 1980; Spreen & Gaddes, 1969) and interpretive models (Fletcher & Taylor, 1984; Obrzut & Hynd, 1986) for the children's neuropsychological batteries. In this chapter the various measures included in the Halstead–Reitan and the Reitan–Indiana were reviewed. A description of each measure was given, as well as a brief discussion of

TABLE 4. Metanorms for Neuropsychological Test Performance by Age: Metameans (Meta-SD)

Metanorms for Reitan–Indiana and Halstead–Reitan Neuropsychological Test Batteries: Ages 5–14

Subtest	5	6	7	8	9	10	11	12	13	14
Category Test	27.40	26.00	20.56	12.35	53.56	46.58	40.88	35.12	36.29	30.81
(errors—ages 5–8 (80 items), 9–14 (168 items)	(9.1)	(12.7)	(8.9)	(6.7)	(17.4)	(18.6)	(16.3)	(16.0)	(16.4)	(12.0)
Finger Oscillation,	29.39	29.87	33.67	36.40	34.01	37.52	40.72	41.36	44.64	44.38
DH (taps per 10 seconds)	(4.2)	(3.3)	(4.6)	(4.6)	(4.1)	(5.4)	(4.8)	(5.4)	(5.2)	(6.8)
Finger Oscillation,	26.32	27.22	30.01	32.03	30.31	34.04	35.06	36.66	39.64	40.67
NDH (taps per 10 seconds)	(4.6)	(3.3)	(3.9)	(3.8)	(3.3)	(4.8)	(4.8)	(4.1)	(4.7)	(6.1)
Grip Strength, DH	8.27	9.13	11.60	12.48	14.74	17.14	19.45	22.92	26.65	36.50
(klgs)	(1.9)	(2.2)	(2.3)	(2.6)	(1.9)	(2.7)	(3.4)	(3.5)	(4.7)	(3.0)
Grip Strength, NDH	7.53	8.41	10.56	11.47	14.12	16.09	18.86	21.65	25.40	32.48
(klgs)	(1.9)	(2.2)	(2.1)	(2.3)	(1.9)	(2.3)	(3.2)	(4.3)	(4.9)	(4.6)
Tactual Performance	6.47	5.93	5.17	4.15	4.36	3.67	3.15	3.20	2.44	NA
Test, DH (minutes)—ages 5–8 (6 blocks), 9–14 (10 blocks)	(3.1)	(3.1)	(2.7)	(2.2)	(2.4)	(1.7)	(1.4)	(1.6)	(0.8)	

(*continued*)

TABLE 4. (*Continued*)

Metanorms for Reitan–Indiana and Halstead–Reitan Neuropsychological Test Batteries: Ages 5–14

Subtest	5	6	7	8	9	10	11	12	13	14
Tactual Performance	5.24	4.74	3.66	3.13	3.08	2.73	2.17	2.20	1.61	NA
Test, NDH (minutes)	(3.1)	(2.8)	(1.9)	(3.1)	(1.7)	(1.6)	(0.9)	(1.4)	(0.9)	
Tactual Performance	3.80	3.11	1.98	1.68	1.28	1.27	1.13	1.03	0.80	
Test, Both Hands	(2.6)	(2.1)	(1.2)	(1.1)	(0.7)	(0.7)	(0.6)	(0.5)	(0.3)	
(minutes)										
Tactual Performance	15.50	13.83	10.98	8.79	8.80	7.66	6.36	6.13	4.90	NA
Test, Total Time	(5.6)	(6.8)	(4.5)	(3.8)	(4.1)	(3.3)	(2.3)	(2.6)	(1.5)	
(minutes)										
Tactual Performance	2.47	3.06	4.15	4.44	4.40	4.48	4.53	4.77	5.04	NA
Test, Memory	(1.8)	(1.5)	(1.2)	(1.2)	(1.2)	(1.2)	(1.1)	(0.8)	(0.9)	
(correct)										
Tactual Performance	1.10	1.80	2.69	3.22	3.00	3.07	3.07	3.75	3.00	NA
Test, Location	(1.1)	(1.5)	(1.7)	(1.7)	(1.6)	(1.5)	(1.6)	(1.5)	(1.3)	
(correct)										

Metanorms for the Halstead–Reitan Neuropsychological Test Battery for Older Children (Ages 9–14)

Subtest	9	10	11	12	13	14
Trail Making Test, Part A (seconds)	25.09 (9.4)	21.04 (5.9)	18.87 (6.2)	17.19 (5.8)	16.00 (5.7)	NA
Trail Making Test, Part B (seconds)	54.77 (20.0)	49.80 (20.0)	41.20 (15.6)	37.14 (14.1)	32.73 (10.9)	NA
Trail Making Test, Total Time (seconds)	79.85 (28.9)	70.84 (30.4)	60.07 (20.3)	54.33 (22.6)	48.73 (10.3)	NA
Speech Sounds Perception (errors)	7.23 (4.7)	6.58 (3.3)	5.36 (2.6)	5.50 (2.9)	5.04 (1.3)	NA
Seashore Rhythm Test (correct)	14.23 (5.5)	18.85 (6.3)	19.10 (6.3)	19.66 (5.3)	20.85 (4.9)	19.43 (5.4)

Metanorms for the Reitan–Indiana Neuropsychological Test Battery for Younger Children (Ages 5–8) (Individual Performance Tests)

Subtest	5	6	7	8
Matching Figures (seconds)	41.30 (13.7)	30.70 (9.7)	23.82 (9.0)	21.07 (7.8)
Matching Figures (errors)	0.48 (0.9)	0.40 (0.8)	0.21 (0.6)	0.15 (0.5)
Matching V's (seconds)	52.39 (26.5)	40.22 (16.9)	32.31 (12.6)	28.72 (11.5)
Matching V's (errors)	2.58 (1.9)	1.91 (1.7)	1.29 (1.6)	1.08 (1.3)
Star (correct)	3.72 (3.1)	6.03 (2.6)	7.17 (1.4)	7.82 (1.4)
Star (seconds)	29.63 (23.1)	23.43 (17.1)	19.71 (17.4)	17.65 (9.4)
Concentric Squares (seconds)	37.48 (21.4)	33.24 (14.8)	32.29 (18.1)	30.22 (15.6)
Concentric Squares (correct)	2.21 (2.2)	2.75 (2.3)	4.26 (2.8)	5.10 (2.5)
Progressive Figures (seconds)	96.12 (57.4)	73.43 (50.4)	51.74 (31.0)	41.50 (21.4)
Target Test (correct)	7.36 (3.28)	9.60 (3.6)	13.63 (2.5)	12.89 (2.53)
Marching Test, DH (seconds)	29.51 (10.4)	23.77 (6.6)	20.91 (8.0)	18.22 (6.1)
Marching Test, NDH (seconds)	33.67 (10.8)	28.28 (9.1)	23.77 (7.5)	21.07 (6.5)
Marching Test, DH (errors)	1.95 (1.8)	1.79 (2.0)	1.23 (1.5)	0.92 (1.2)
Marching Test, NDH (errors)	3.86 (2.6)	3.32 (2.5)	2.84 (2.3)	2.20 (1.9)
Marching Pictures (correct)	15.48 (3.2)	18.40 (4.3)	19.98 (1.1)	21.75 (2.6)
Color Form (seconds)	44.61 (0.3)	32.00 (19.1)	28.34 (12.0)	19.58 (8.9)
Color Form (errors)	2.31 (2.6)	0.86 (1.4)	0.43 (0.9)	0.33 (0.9)

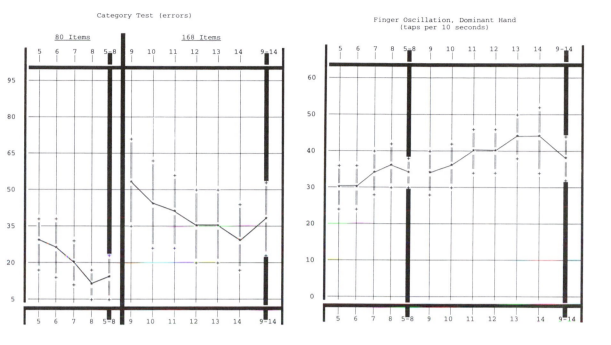

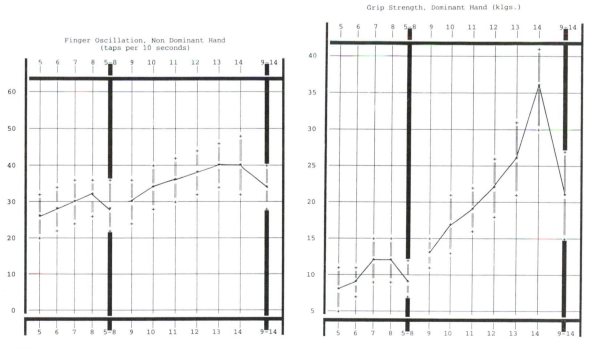

FIGURE 1. Mean and standard deviation performance by age on each of 15 neuropsychological variables; *, mean; +, standard deviation.

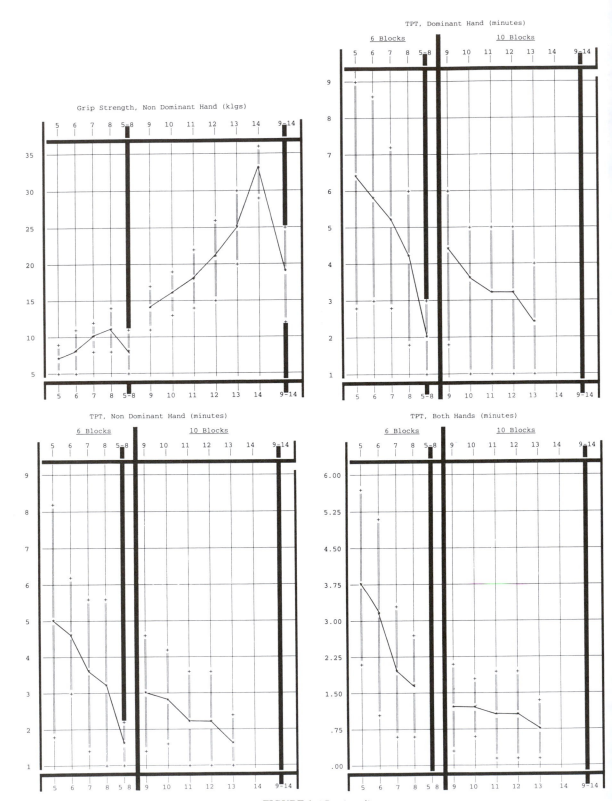

FIGURE 1. (*Continued*).

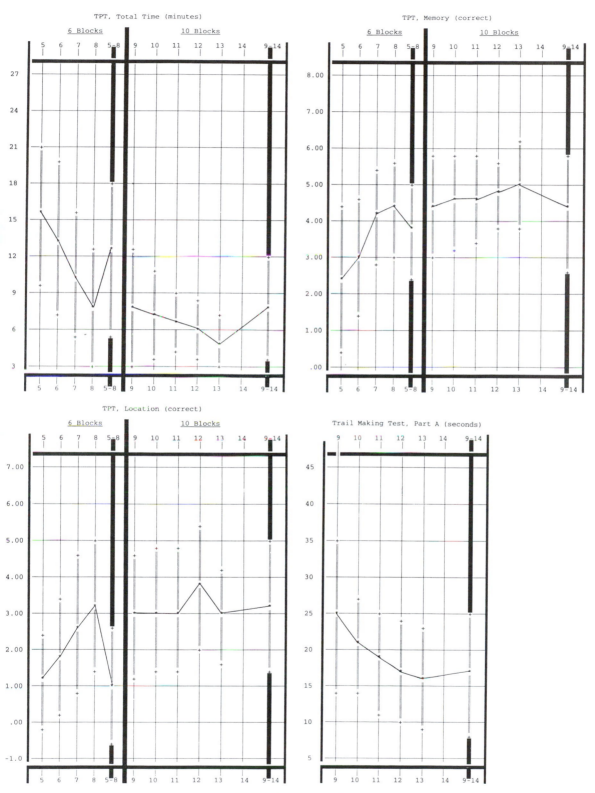

FIGURE 1. (*Continued*).

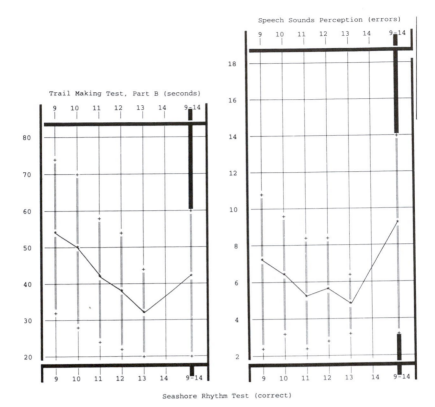

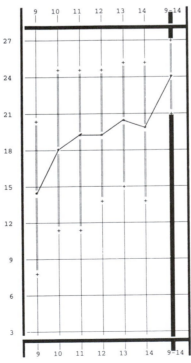

FIGURE 1. (*Continued*).

scoring and domains measured by the various tests. Finally, a number of approaches to the interpretation of children's neuropsychological performance were reviewed.

References

Bigler, E. D., & Naugle, R. I. (1985). Case studies in cerebral plasticity. *Clinical Neuropsychology, 7,* 12–23.

Boll, T. J. (1974). Behavioral correlates of cerebral damage in children age 9–14. In R. M. Reitan & L. A. Davison (Eds.), *Clinical neuropsychology: Current status and applications.* Washington, DC: Winston.

Boll, T. J. (1981). The Halstead–Reitan Neuropsychological Battery. In S. Filskov & T. J. Boll (Eds.), *Handbook of clinical neuropsychology.* New York: Wiley–Interscience.

Findeis, M. K., & Weight, D. G. Meta-norms for two forms of neuropsychological test batteries for children (under review).

Fletcher, J. M., & Taylor, H. G. (1984). Neuropsychological approaches to children: Towards a developmental neuropsychology. *Journal of Clinical Neuropsychology, 6*(1), 39–56.

Halstead, W. C. (1947). *Brain and intelligence: A quantitative study of the frontal lobes.* Chicago: University of Chicago Press.

Harris, A. J. (1947). *Harris test of lateral dominance, manual of directions for administration and interpretation.* New York: Psychological Corporation.

Jastak, S., & Wilkinson, G. J. (1984). *The Wide Range Achievement Test-Revised.* Wilmington, DE: Jastak.

Klonoff, H., Robinson, J. C., & Thompson, G. (1969). Acute and chronic brain syndromes in children. *Developmental Medicine and Child Neurology, 11,* 198–213.

Knights, R. M., & Norwood, J. A. (1979). *Neuropsychological test battery for children: Examiners' manual.* Ottawa: Knights Psychological Consultants.

Knights, R. M., & Norwood, J. A. (1980). *Revised smooth normative data on the neuropsychological test battery for children.* Ottawa: Knights Psychological Consultants.

McGivern, R. F., Berka, C., Languis, M. L., & Chapman, S. (1991). Detection of deficits in temporal pattern discrimination using the Seashore Rhythm Test in young children with reading impairments. *Journal of Learning Disabilities, 24*(1), 58–62.

Nici, J., & Reitan, R. M. (1986). Patterns of neuropsychological abilities in brain-disordered versus normal children. *Journal of Consulting and Clinical Psychology, 54,* 542–545.

Nussbaum, N. L., & Bigler, E. D. (1986). Neuropsychological and behavioral profiles of empirically derived subgroups of learning disabled children. *International Journal of Clinical Neuropsychology, 8,* 82–89.

Obrzut, J. E., & Hynd, G. W. (Eds.). (1986). *Child neuropsychology* (Vol. II). New York: Academic Press.

Reed, H. B. C., Reitan, R. M., & Klove, H. (1965). Influence of cerebral lesions on psychological test performances of older children. *Journal of Consulting Psychology, 29,* 247–251.

Reitan, R. M. (1969). *Manual for administration of neuropsychological test batteries for adults and children.* Indianapolis, IN: Author.

Reitan, R. M. (1974). Psychological effects of cerebral lesions in children of early school age. In R. M. Reitan & L. A. Davison (Eds.), *Clinical neuropsychology: Current status and applications.* Washington, DC: Winston.

Reitan, R. M., and Davison, L. A. (Eds.). (1974). *Clinical neuropsychology: Current status and applications.* Washington, DC: Winston.

Reitan, R., & Wolfsun, D. (1985). *The Halstead–Reitan Neuropsychological Test Battery: Theory and clinical interpretation.* Tucson, AZ: Neuropsychology Press.

Rourke, B. P. (Ed.). (1984). *Subtype analysis of learning disabilities.* New York: Guilford Press.

Rourke, B. P., Bakker, D. J., Fisk, J. L., & Strang, J. D. (1983). *Child neuropsychology: An introduction to theory, research and clinical practice.* New York: Guilford Press.

Selz, M. (1981). Halstead–Reitan Neuropsychological Test Battery for Children. In G. W. Hynd & J. E. Obrzut (Eds.), *Neuropsychological assessment and the school-aged child: Issues and procedures.* New York: Grune & Stratton.

Selz, M., & Reitan, M. (1979a). Neuropsychological test performance of normal, learning-disabled and brain-damaged older children. *Journal of Nervous and Mental Disease, 167,* 298–302.

Selz, M., & Reitan, M. (1979b). Rules for neuropsychological diagnosis: Classification of brain function in older children. *Journal of Consulting and Clinical Psychology, 47,* 258–264.

Shurtleff, H. A., Fay, G. E., Abbott, R. D., & Berninger, V. W. (1988). Cognitive neuropsychological correlates of academic achievement: A levels of analysis assessment model. *Journal of Psychoeducational Assessment, 6* (3), 298–308.

Spreen, O., & Gaddes, W. (1969). Developmental norms for fifteen neuropsychological tests for ages 6 to 15. *Cortex, 5,* 171–191.

Spreen, O., & Strauss, E. (1991). *A compendium of neuropsychological tests.* London: Oxford University Press.

Strom, D. A., Gray, J. W., Dean, R. S., & Fischer, W. E. (1987). The incremental validity of the Halstead–Reitan Neuropsychological Battery in predicting achievement for learning-disabled children. *Journal of Psychoeducational Assessment, 5*(2), 157–165.

Taylor, H. G., & Fletcher, J. M. (1990). Neuropsychological assessment of children. In G. Goldstein & M. Hersen (Eds.), *Handbook of psychological assessment.* New York: Pergamon Press.

Teeter, P. A. (1986). Standard neuropsychological batteries for children. In J. E. Obrzut & G. W. Hynd (Eds.), *Child neuropsychology* (Vol. II). New York: Academic Press.

Tsushima, W. T., & Towne, W. S. (1977). Neuropsychological abilities of young children with questionable brain disorders. *Journal of Consulting and Clinical Psychology, 45,* 757–762.

Wechsler, D. (1974). *Wechsler Intelligence Scale for Children-Revised.* New York: Psychological Corporation.

12

The Nebraska Neuropsychological Children's Battery

CHARLES J. GOLDEN

Beginning in the mid-1970s, there was increasing interest in the application of the theories and assessment procedures developed by the Russian neurologist A. R. Luria. Luria's theories integrated sophisticated analysis of the way in which the brain is organized in the individual client along with a series of assessment procedures and rehabilitation techniques that were attractive to the newly developing area of clinical neuropsychology. Among these interests were the adaptation of Luria's testing procedures for U.S. audience.

Adaptation of Luria's work was hampered by the need to translate Luria's open-ended, qualitative evaluations into a more standardized format consistent with U.S. approaches to psychological assessment (as contrasted to neurological assessment techniques). For children, this was first attempted by Lawrence Majovski in an unpublished manuscript. Majovski had studied with Luria shortly before Luria's death and so was intimately familiar with his approach.

The Luria–Nebraska Children's Battery was an amalgamation of some of Majovski's work along with terms and procedures selected from the adult version of the Luria–Nebraska. Following completion of this first test for 8- to 12-year-olds, Golden and his associates embarked on a decade-long study to develop a second form, initially the LNNB-3, which integrated the adult and child versions to pro-

duce a more comprehensive single battery applicable from ages 5 through adulthood.

The present chapter will focus on the development of these tests and most directly on the issues around neuropsychological assessment and interpretation in children using these tests. Specifically, it will look at several issues: (1) the process of development of the original battery; (2) a description of the original battery with a brief review of current research; (3) methods of interpreting the original test battery; and (4) current research studies (on the LNNB-3) aimed at improving the test battery and extending its usefulness to lower ages.

Development of the Battery

The original development of the battery was begun by administering the adult LNNB to children from ages 5 to 12. It was discovered that children 8 and up could do a majority of the procedures used in the adult battery. It was also found that those items in general corresponded to those that one would expect from Luria's theories on brain development. It was also found that below age 8, drastic changes were needed in the battery content to have a useful test. Thus, it was initially decided to develop a test down to age 8.

Similarly, it was found that 13- and 14-year-olds could perform adequately on the adult battery (which was originally intended to extend down to age 15). At the 12-year-old level, children began to show difficulties with the adult battery (although above-average 12-year-olds can also perform normally). Thus, it was decided that the adult battery

CHARLES J. GOLDEN • Center for Psychological Services, Nova Southeastern University, Fort Lauderdale, Florida 33314.

could be used down to age 13 and that the new children's battery should aim at ages 8 to 12. A battery for younger children was postponed until completion of this work and is described in the last section of this chapter.

Items were deleted from the adult battery that appeared to be too difficult for initial normative youngsters in this age range. When possible, similar but easier items were substituted. We were also privileged to consult with Dr. Lawrence Majovski who was working on developing a qualitative approach to the assessment of children based on his studies with Luria. We were able to adapt and add several additional items and areas of examination to the test from his suggestions. This initial work consisted of three successive versions of the test that were evaluated on groups of normal and impaired children until the fourth and published version was completed.

Description of the Battery

The final version of the children's battery consisted of 11 basic scales (as for the adult battery) and 149 procedures. However, most of these procedures consist of numerous items so that the actual number of items exceeds 500. Administration takes about $1\frac{1}{2}$ to 3 hours depending on levels of cooperation and levels of impairment.

This version was given to 125 children. The group consisted of 25 normal children at each of five age levels: 8, 9, 10, 11, and 12. Performance norms were developed on each procedure and scale based on the performance of this group. The first task was the development of scale scores for each item. It was decided to have different scale scores for each age group on each item so that scores for a given individual could be directly compared. For each procedure, a score of 0 was set to mean a performance within one standard deviation of the mean score for the age group. A score of 1 represented a performance between one and two standard deviations below the mean, and a score of 2 represented scores more than two standard deviations below the mean.

Each item of the test was assigned to 1 of the 11 basic scales. Originally, this was done on the basis of our experience with the adult battery and on our theoretical belief of where items should load. From this assignment, scale raw scores were calculated by adding up the scaled score on each procedure to yield a total raw score. Procedures were then correlated with each of the raw scores to ensure that procedures correlated highest with the scale they were assigned to, so that items could be recognized when necessary.

After final scale assignments were determined, scale T scores were generated by first calculating the means and standard deviations of each of the original 125 normal subjects. An ANOVA for each scale score by age indicated no significant differences between the scale mean scores for each age group, and F tests indicated no significant differences among group variances. As a result, the conversion of scale raw scores to T scores was done on the basis of all 125 subjects rather than for each age group alone.

Each of the 11 scales is multifactorial in structure. This was done for several reasons. First, each scale was conceived not as covering a specific skill but rather as a domain of skills in a given area (such as motor function). Second, this allowed the test to yield stable test scores (which is related to the number of items on the scale as well as the individual stabilities of the items) with fewer items in each skill area. This has the positive effect of allowing for a broader coverage of skills in a reasonable period of time. This has the drawback, however, of not covering any one area in as much detail as possible. This is remedied by simply following the LNNB with specifically selected testing in areas in which more information is needed after examining the LNNB performance, and by using qualitative observations to enrich the data generated by quantitative analysis alone.

The original test scales (which are described in detail later) were labeled Motor, Rhythm, Tactile, Visual, Receptive, Expressive, Reading, Writing, Arithmetic, Memory, and Intelligence. In addition to the basic scales, the 149 items were factor analyzed in a population of 719 brain-damaged and normal children. The resulting factors were impressive in that few of the factor scales used items from multiple scales, suggesting that item placement was essentially correct. Some factor scales simply repeated what the regular scales already yielded, and some failed to achieve reasonable stability. Those scales that were both stable and yielded new information were kept for further study.

A second analysis involved the factor analysis of each scale alone. Many of the resultant factors duplicated factors found in the first analysis and were discarded, as were factors that were insufficiently stable. At the end of this process, 11 additional scales were derived, 2 of which were cross scale factors and 9 of which were intrascale. For each of these 11 scales, T scores were derived on the basis of the performance of 240 normal children in the overall sample.

The 11 factors were briefly described as: (1) academic achievement, the largest cross scale factor including reading, writing, arithmetic, and expressive items; (2) spatial organization, the second major cross scale factor; (3) purposeful unspeeded movement; (4) motor speed; (5) drawing quality; (6) drawing time; (7) rhythm perception and reproduction; (8) basic tactile function; (9) basic receptive language skills; (10) repetition; and (11) abstract verbal skills.

For those readers interested in the details of general research on the battery, the test manual (Golden, 1986) offers the most complete and detailed account of this work. Other reviews may be found in Plaisted, Gustavson, Wilkening, and Golden (1983). In general, research has examined the ability of the test to discriminate between brain-damaged and normal subjects (with hit rates of about 86%), and other studies have examined correlations between the LNNB and such tests as the PIAT and the WISC-R. As reported in the test manual, this work has generally confirmed the validity of the LNNB scales. Other work has evaluated the effectiveness of the test with such groups as children who are learning disabled or who have epilepsy.

Interpretation

Of prime importance with any test battery are the methods of interpreting the battery. This is especially important with the LNNB-C for many because the process is often different from the procedures used with other tests. In interpreting the LNNB-C, little confidence is placed in formal interpretations of elevations on individual scales, a major reason being that these are clearly not homogeneous scales with many items intended to measure just one ability but rather a domain of abilities. As a result, a single interpretation of an elevation on any particular scale would be ludicrous and possibly lead to obscure diagnostic errors. Thus, pattern analysis of the scales and items, combined with a qualitative analysis of the test performance, is the major approach to interpreting scale profiles.

Levels of Interpretation

When interpreting the LNNB-C, or other similar batteries, it is important to be aware that the many levels on which the battery can be interpreted depend on the needs, as well as the skill and knowledge, of the user. While the LNNB-C has clear rules for classifying children derived from research and clinical practice, the major goal of the battery is an analysis of the way in which the child functions cognitively and the implications for rehabilitation or educational planning.

As a consequence, the first two levels of analysis are considered preliminary to a full analysis consisting of all of the steps outlined below. The first level is primarily concerned with ascertaining whether significant brain injury exists in a given child. The test can determine the probability of such a classification, although the concept of "brain injury" in children is complicated by the difficulty of differentiating genetic and early developmental disorders from brain damage. Luria's theories emphasize that the organization of the brain in the child is as sensitive to environment as it is to the structure of the brain. Thus, environmental factors, especially when extreme, can lead to conditions that appear very similar to brain injury. When there is a high likelihood of brain damage, children must be referred for a more sophisticated evaluation of the data. On the other hand, because most children are seen initially by nonneuropsychologists, this level of practice is quite important to determine which children should be referred for further evaluation.

The second level of interpretation involves simple description of what the child can and cannot do, without drawing any conclusions or reaching any integrative statements. This level is enhanced by the qualitative analysis of the data. The qualitative or process analysis requires an identification of the basic reasons why an individual erred in a given item as well as any unusual ways in which the person got specific items right. The LNNB-C includes 66 qualitative categories that are used to classify specific performance on each item as well as extratest behavior. The latter application is especially important as the battery is designed to generate a large number of conditions for the child to react to, which can yield abundant behavior and insights far beyond the basic quantitative score. Thus, the examiner is encouraged not only to score the items but to observe and test for why items were missed.

This step is enhanced by the test standardization that allows flexibility in administration in many areas. This flexibility is limited within each scale by the specific quantitative purpose of the scale (e.g., receptive language items cannot be repeated when misunderstood, expressive speech items can be repeated). This procedure allows the examiner to search for methods that maximize the child's accuracy and effectiveness. By noting these methods within the qualitative scoring and in general observation, the process of giving the test can yield valuable rehabilitative cues.

The third level of interpretation takes the second level to the next logical step: identification of the probable underlying causes of the child's overall behavior. This step requires extensive understanding of the various brain–behavior relationships. The interpretation process generally evolves from a theoretical orientation of how the brain functions and the ways in which information is processed through the central nervous system.

Finally, the fourth level of interpretation involves the integration of all findings and conclusions into a description of how the brain of the individual is functioning. This is a difficult task in most cases, because the result of brain damage is affected by a variety of factors. In many cases, this last level of interpretation concerns the understanding of basic underlying deficits rather than simply determining location. Our goal is not to understand location *per se,* but rather the functional localization of a disorder, i.e., how does it affect the ability of the brain to function in a normal manner? By an analysis of the functional localization we develop a map of the child's strengths and weaknesses.

In general, there has been too much emphasis in neuropsychology on localization of lesions to the exclusion of understanding the individual being tested. Physical localization of a lesion can be generated from detailed functional analysis, but in most cases this is an academic rather than a useful exercise (the exceptions to this lie primarily in the forensic arena and occasionally in identifying an unsuspected acute lesion). Actual physical localization in children is complicated by the fact that early lesions can dramatically change the normal organization of the brain so that the normal relationships between function and location are severely disrupted.

The study of function allows us to generate testable hypotheses about the child's cognitive behavior as a whole. By testing these hypotheses we gradually develop a fully integrated analysis of how the individual child functions neuropsychologically, which allows us to understand the child as an individual. This information *must* be integrated with personality, family, environmental, and social data before a complete and fully formed picture can emerge. In too many cases, unfortunately, the analy-sis is never completed to this level, which lessens the value of the neuropsychological data.

Identifying Brain Damage

Use of the Critical Level

Adjusting for Age. The first step in identifying when a profile is statistically abnormal and likely to be indicative of brain damage is based on establishing a valid critical level for the child. The critical level represents the highest LNNB-C score that can be considered normal for the battery. In contrast to some other tests, this cutoff level is variable with the LNNB-C, and is adjusted for age.

Identifying Deviant Scores. Once the critical level has been established using the appropriate formulas, determining the probability of brain damage is relatively simple. The number of scales on the battery that exceed the critical level is counted, yielding the number of abnormal scores. The scores that are considered at this point are the basic clinical scales (C1 through C11). *In general, three or more scores above the critical level are thought to be indicative of brain damage, whereas zero or only one elevated scale suggests the probable absence of brain damage.* If the critical level has been chosen correctly, the accuracy of this decision is about 75 to 85% of all cases. The likelihood increases as the number of elevations increase. Other rules may be applied to further refine the assessment at this level, especially in borderline cases.

Interpreting Scale Patterns

Factors Affecting Scale Interpretation

It is important to recognize that injuries in any part of the brain can potentially affect the scores on any of the scales of the battery. This reflects the relatively homogeneous content of the scales with respect to secondary skills that are measured in conjunction with the primary skill as denoted by the scale label. Despite this caution, hypotheses may be generated from individual scales and overall patterns of scores if proper caution is used in recognizing the wide ranges of factors that affect the neuropsychological performance on a given scale. For example, a child may have such severe expressive language problems that any item that requires any verbal response, no matter how simple, may be missed. Similarly, severe receptive language problems may make it impossible to adequately communicate instructions to the child. Although the administrative procedures attempt to minimize the effects of these disorders, in some cases it is not possible to eliminate these factors. Similarly, children with severe peripheral deficits or brain stem injuries may appear to have more severe cognitive injuries than are actually present. These problems are unfortunately common to all standardized tests. To an extent, the identification of these factors through the qualitative scoring is possible, although interpretation of these indices is not as well established as for the quantitative scores.

Other factors that cause changes in scale elevations as well as overall patterns include a wide variety of neurological factors. One of the most important factors is the duration of the brain disorder, and whether or not it is still present. In general, the acute disorders, i.e., those that are continuing, will affect LNNB-C scores much more significantly than will disorders from which the child has had 3 to 6 months or more to recover.

The size of the lesion must be considered along with the question of chronicity. In individuals with disorders that resolve themselves without structural damage to the brain, LNNB-C scores will return essentially to normal, reflecting the child's recovery of all major skills. The examiner should nevertheless be alert to specific items, even on normal scales, that the child may fail to adequately perform and that may reflect residual damage. It is important to notice these factors, as they are often useful in explaining specific problems the child may be having that were not noticed before the damage occurred, as well as in designing specific rehabilitation training.

Another important aspect is the location of the damage. Brain damage in each hemisphere is expressed very differently on the pattern of scores, as is brain damage in different locations within a single hemisphere. In general, the LNNB-C is more sensitive to the disruptive effects of left hemisphere lesions.

The cause of the brain dysfunction also represents a major problem with respect to the battery's results. Brain dysfunction may be caused by a wide range of problems: from overt structural damage to metabolic disorders and idiopathic problems that have no clear genesis. In general, those disorders that destroy brain tissue cause much more damage to the brain and therefore cause more highly signif-

icant deviations on the LNNB-C battery. Disorders such as idiopathic epilepsy, which may not have a clear structural focus or clear cause, may produce relatively little damage.

A final consideration is the premorbid level of the individual. Specifically, an individual with higher skills prior to a given brain injury will have higher skills afterward than would a person with overall lower initial cognitive skills; the person with higher cognitive skills can more easily reorganize brain function to adapt to the loss in specific areas. An individual who is extremely intelligent prior to an injury may show only motor and sensory signs with relatively few cognitive deficits in the abnormal range even after a significant injury, because the person's skills have simply been reduced from above average to average. In these cases, one must be sensitive again to the pattern of items missed by the child that may indicate brain dysfunction. One obvious problem with children is that we may not have an idea of what the "premorbid" level was.

For the reasons discussed above, interpretation of the LNNB-C typically focuses more on scale patterns and on intrascale variability than on interpretation of scale elevations *per se*. Scale patterns have the advantage of allowing the user to make deductions about the reason a given scale was impaired. For example, in profiles in which C5 (Receptive Speech) is the highest score, one can hypothesize that deficits on other scales may be attributed to the loss in receptive skills. As with any other procedure, this leads only to hypotheses, but can offer valuable insights in attempting to understand the child's basic underlying deficits. The major patterns on the LNNB-C are discussed below in the context of the highest scale among the basic clinical scales.

Developmental Issues in Interpretation. Another substantial problem in interpretation is the role of developmental issues. There are several major problems that must be recognized when the test is interpreted. All of these problems stem from the fact that children's brains are not fully developed until midway in their teenage years. Thus, there is a difference in what brain skills can be affected at given ages and in the long-term impact of such injuries when the injury occurs at different developmental stages. It is not the purpose of this chapter to review theories of brain development, but such issues must be considered in the interpretation of any child neuropsychology battery. Even with these limitations, one can examine scale patterns to generate hypotheses. Each hypothesis that is generated must be tested against the actual patterns of items in the scales and the qualitative data on how the items were performed. The scale pattern serves only to generate hypotheses that must be checked against more detailed analysis of the child's performance on the individual items.

Clinical Scales

C1 (Motor Functions). The C1 scale is one of the most complex scales on the LNNB-CR. A wide variety of motor skills reflect both right and left hemisphere performance. The first three items involve simple movements of the hands. These items are especially sensitive to disorders in or near the posterior frontal lobe. In many cases, evidence of lateralized motor disorders may be detected by examining the raw scores on these items.

Items 21 through 32 assess construction dyspraxia. Items that are performed very poorly often reflect severe spatial disorganization characteristic of injuries to the right hemisphere or to the left parietal area. Drawings that are accurate but done slowly may simply reflect motor dysfunction of the dominant hand and the opposite cerebral hemisphere (or, sometimes, compulsiveness).

Because of the nature of the items on the C1 scale, it tends to be sensitive to many different types of brain dysfunction. Primary sensitivity is to sections of the posterior frontal lobe, but lesions of the temporal and parietal lobes, as well as the anterior frontal lobe, will also cause significant elevations in the score. However, extreme elevations (scores exceeding 80T) will usually only be caused by lesions in the motor system.

Elevations on the C1 scale are best interpreted relative to elevations on C3 (Tactile Functions). When C1 is elevated but C3 is not, this is suggestive of difficulties with motor tasks. This comparison can be very useful in initially localizing a deficit in the anterior–posterior dimension. Clients displaying pure parietal lobe dysfunction will rarely achieve a C1 score above 60T, although specific items involving kinesthetic feedback will be most frequently missed. On examination, the items on the battery will usually show a clear pattern in these posterior injuries that is highly effective in localizing a given disorder.

When both of these scales (C1 and C3) are highly elevated, generalized impairment of motor and sensory areas is suggested, but this is often in the context of diffuse deficits. If only these four scales are affected, then peripheral disorders affecting motor and sensory skills need to be considered, as well as the possibility of subcortical diseases.

C2 (Rhythm). The C2 scale is much more simply organized than the C1 scale. Item 35 involves the analyses of groups of tones. The child must compare two groups of tones, saying whether one is higher or lower. Items 36 through 38 require the child to reproduce tones. Whereas the initial items involve the perception of tonal qualities, these latter items involve the expression of tonal relationships.

Items 39 and 40 involve the evaluation of acoustic signals. The child must identify the number of beeps in groups of sounds. The last two items in the C2 scale deal with the perception and reproduction of rhythm. Item 41 measures the ability of the child to reproduce rhythmic patterns. This item requires both the perception of rhythmic patterns and the reproduction of sounds, usually using the dominant hand. The item can be missed by individuals with deficits in either hemisphere. Item 42 asks the child to make a series of rhythms from verbal commands. The combination of verbal and rhythmic content on this item also makes it sensitive to injuries in either hemisphere.

Of all of the basic clinical scales, C2 is the most sensitive to disorders of attention and concentration. When giving these items to such individuals, it is often useful for the examiner to stop the administration between the stimuli in each item and not go on to the next item until the individual's attention has been secured. Because there are usually only two choices in each item, items cannot be repeated. Consequently, it is important to ensure that the first administration is carried out as accurately as possible.

When elevations of the C2 scale are the highest in the profile, they are most often associated with right hemisphere injuries that are usually more anterior than posterior. This is especially true when the highest scales are some combination of C2, C9 (Arithmetic), and C10 (Memory). However, this same pattern may be seen in left anterior lesions as well, although in those cases it is accompanied by at least subtle, if not gross, deficits in some form of verbal skills. When the C2 deficit is combined with C4 (Visual Functions) scale elevation, then the lesion may be either anterior or posterior, with a more posterior lesion being more likely with higher elevations on C4.

C3 (Tactile Functions). Items 43 through 56 involve different levels of cutaneous sensation. Individuals must identify where they are touched, how hard they are touched, and so forth. Injuries to the anterior parietal area will cause significant elevations on this scale as will injuries to the middle parietal areas that Luria (1973) designated as the "secondary area" of the parietal lobe. Individuals with damage in and around the angular gyrus may have particular problems with verbal/tactile items. The last two items on the C3 scale involve the stereognostic perception. Individuals with old injuries to the parietal lobe on either side may have difficulty meeting the time requirements.

Profiles with highest scores on the C3 scale are interpreted in conjunction with the relative standings on the C1 scale. If C3 is greatly elevated over C1, then this points to a posterior lesion. This generally remains true even when the C1 scale equals the C3 scale, especially if the C1 deficits arise from construction difficulty and sequencing rather than motor paralysis.

Deficits may be related to an inability to concentrate, which should also result in inconsistent behavior, or to an inability to integrate and identify all stimuli. In the latter case, the deficit will have a similar effect but will also show up as a rule in other naming and identification tasks while causing less difficulty in purely spatial tasks. When the deficit is purely spatial, such as in profiles with C3 and C4 (Visual Functions) elevations, the injury is likely to be right parietal–occipital, although this pattern may also reflect subcortical involvement of one or both hemispheres. When naming is strongly involved, left parietal deficits should be considered. All such hypothesized localizations assume a normally dominant left hemisphere. Such patterns can be changed significantly by mixed or right hemisphere dominance for speech.

C4 (Visual Functions). The C4 scale evaluates a range of visual functions. Items 59 and 60 ask the child to identify objects by viewing either an object itself or a picture of an object. The person need not identify the object by name but rather can describe function or indicate recognition in other ways. Despite this, naming must be considered a component of these items. If the child is not able to do these items, later items on the battery that are more sensitive to right hemisphere function may be missed simply because of left hemisphere involvement. Thus, interpretation of the scale must depend on the child's performance on the simple, initial items.

Later items require a great deal more visual–spatial perception than do these first two items, although naming is still required. Item 61 presents pictures that are difficult to perceive. Item 62 presents objects that overlap one another and that the child with poor visual–spatial skills has difficulty identifying. Item 63 examines the ability to determine that two figures are mirror-image versions of one another. Item 64 is a modification of items from the Raven Progressive Matrices (Raven, 1960). It is also a strong measure of visual–spatial organization and right hemisphere function. Item 65 involves spatial rotation without any speech components. Individuals may point to the correct answer or circle it as necessary (or say it if this is not possible). Poor performance on this task is suggestive of impairment of visual–spatial skills.

Profiles in which the C4 scale is highest, in combination with any secondary scale, generally reflect impairment in the right hemisphere or the occipital areas of the left hemisphere. The C4 scale can be elevated in other left hemisphere injuries, but rarely will it be the highest scale overall. In right hemisphere injuries, deficits on only more complex visual tasks suggest either a mild parietal involvement or injury to anterior areas. These lesions are usually accompanied by elevation on the C1 scale suggestive of right hemisphere lesions. Subcortical lesions that interfere with visual processing can also cause patterns suggestive of right hemisphere injury, as can severe peripheral visual problems.

C5 (Receptive Speech). C5 items evaluate the ability of the child to understand receptive speech, from simple phonemic analysis to the understanding of complex sentences with inverted English grammar. Items 66 through 71 concern the understanding of simple phonemes. For items 66 through 70, the individual hears simple phonemes and must then repeat or write them. It is important to note if individuals are able to either say or write phonemes but not to do both.

Item 71 tests the ability to understand phonemes spoken at different levels of pitch. It is not unusual for individuals with significant damage in the right temporal area to miss this item. Items 72 through 77 involve the understanding of simple words and sentences. The child must do relatively simple tasks of naming, pointing, and identifying, and must define simple words. The intent of these items is simply to ensure that the child is hearing correctly and interpreting correctly what is said to her or him.

Beginning with item 78 and continuing through the end of this scale to item 83, the individual is given increasingly more difficult instructions. These items assess the child's ability to understand and to perform or answer as requested.

All of these items can be affected by damage to the left hemisphere, but several items can also be affected by right hemisphere dysfunction. For example, item 79 requires some spatial orientation on the part of the child. If the child appears to understand the sentence but disrupts the spatial requests made, the possibility of right hemisphere dysfunction must be suspected.

When this scale is highest, as well as significantly elevated above the critical level by at least 15 points, deficits are usually associated with left hemisphere injury. Lesser elevations, caused by difficulty with the more complex items, can occur as the highest scale in right anterior injuries. This can be especially true in mild elevation combinations of C5 and C10 (Memory), C5 and C2 (Rhythm), C5 and C4 (Visual Functions), C5, C11 (Intellectual Processes), and C9 (Arithmetic). In the most significant elevations, however, left hemisphere involvement is generally indicated.

An important caveat in evaluating speech in children without a history of normal language achievement is differentiating between problems related to environment and nonneurological physical factors and those related to brain-based deficits. One common problem is the child with hearing difficulties resulting from multiple infections requiring tubes or infections that caused partial or complete deafness. In these children, language abnormalities may simply reflect an inadequate chance to develop the relevant skills. Similar problems arise from backgrounds with inadequate verbal stimulation. It is very difficult to differentiate between deficits related to a poor premorbid history and those related solely to brain damage.

C6 (Expressive Speech). The C6 scale evaluates the individual's ability to repeat simple phonemes and words and to generate automatic as well as more complex speech forms. Initial items simply require the repetition of sounds or words spoken by the examiner. Beginning with item 89, the child must repeat the same list of words and sounds by reading them rather than hearing them. If an individual is able to pass either one of these sections, significant expressive speech deficits are not present. For example, the individual who is able to read but not to receive auditory information will be able to do the second section. Inversely, the child who is unable to read will be able to do only the first section. Therefore, one must carefully examine the pattern of answers to see if the errors are confined to one modality or the other.

Beginning with item 93, the child must repeat increasingly more difficult sentences. Item 94 examines the ability to name from a description rather than from a visual presentation of the object. Items 95 through 98 ask individuals to count and say the days of the week, first forward and then backward, all a form of automatic speech. Items 99 through 104 evaluate the ability to produce speech spontaneously under three conditions: after looking at a picture, after hearing a story, and after being given a topic to discuss. If other items on this scale are performed without difficulty, and yet the child experiences problems with these items, there is the possibility of low intelligence. The final section involves complex systems of grammatical expression; the child must fill in words that are missing in a sentence or make up a sentence from words that are given to the child.

In general, C6 scores are sensitive to injuries in the left hemisphere only. It is rare to see a high C6 score in individuals with unilateral right hemisphere injuries. Exceptions to this are individuals who had difficulty reading prior to their injury, or whose disorders have somehow interfered with auditory perception or have had generalized effects (e.g., pressure effects from a tumor). However, examination of the patterns of the items on the battery can easily eliminate these possibilities. In the absence of these types of conditions, elevation on the C6 scale, especially above a score of 70T, is almost always indicative of a left hemisphere injury.

Very mild C6 elevations may be associated with right hemisphere lesions, with the major errors occurring in the last items of the scale (spontaneous speech, sequencing, and fill-in terms). One assumption underlying interpretation of all of the language scales is that the child was originally fluent in English, as all of the current research is based on native-born speakers.

C7 (Writing). The C7 scale evaluates the ability to analyze words phonetically in English and then to do copying of increasing difficulty. Initially, children are asked to copy simple letters, then combinations of letters and words, and then write their first and last names. They are then asked to write sounds, words, and phrases from dictation.

In general, disorders of writing localize to the temporal–parietal–occipital area, especially in and around the angular gyrus of the left hemisphere. However, specific disorders may indicate problems in other areas. For example, the ability to write from written material but not from auditory material suggests a specific lesion in the temporal lobe. Conversely, the ability to write from dictation but not from written material suggests a lesion in the occipital or occipital–parietal areas of the cerebral cortex.

If the child is, in general, able to write but has difficulty forming letters and changing from one letter to another, there could be a problem in kinesthetic feedback in which the child mixes up letters that are formed by similar motor movements. If the child is unable to write at all because of paralysis, this, of course, is suggestive of a lesion in the motor strip area of the posterior frontal lobe. Finally, if the child writes at an angle to the page, suggesting some spatial problems, and has no other writing disorders, this can be related to right hemisphere dysfunction. Lack of the ability to read or write one's name is often indicative of a general dementia or, in some cases, a disorder of automatic writing that may occur with injuries in both hemispheres.

Motor writing errors are generally associated with the hemisphere opposite the child's normal writing hand, although care must be taken in injuries that cause the child to change writing hands. In these cases, writing may remain poor but reflects an injury in the ipsilateral hemisphere. Motor writing problems may arise simply as a result of motor problems reflecting the functions of the motor areas of the brain, but may also arise in injuries involving kinesthetic and tactile feedback. Motor writing deficits in which the writing itself is motorically intact but spatially disrupted (at large angles to the horizontal, or where words are written over one another) may reflect injuries to the right (or spatially dominant) hemisphere.

C8 (Reading). The C8 scale closely parallels the C7 scale. The child is asked to generate sounds from letters that the examiner reads aloud. This generally measures the ability of the child to show integration of letters and auditory analysis functions of the temporal and parietal areas of the left hemisphere. The child is then asked to name simple letters, read simple sounds, and read simple words and letter combinations that have meaning. Finally, the child must read entire sentences as well as paragraphs. If the child is able to read simple words but not entire sentences or paragraphs, possible injuries include disorders of visual scanning that make it impossible for the child to grasp more than one word at a time.

Generally, deficits on the C8 scale, in a child who could read prior to an injury, are almost always associated with a left hemisphere injury, usually posterior. The exceptions to this are deficits that occur because of spatial disruption (inability to follow a line, which shows most clearly in the paragraph reading) or neglect of the left side (which should be corrected by the examiner if the test is administered correctly). Both suggest right hemisphere dysfunction. However, we are not justified in making such conclusions in an individual who never was able to read unless there is other evidence to confirm a given injury.

C9 (Arithmetic). The C9 scale is the most sensitive of all of the LNNB-C scales to educational deficits. Even in normally educated individuals, this is the scale most likely to appear in a severely pathological range when there is, in fact, no damage.

This scale starts with the child simply writing down numbers from dictation in both Arabic and Roman numerals. Several items have been employed to identify the spatial dysfunctions that are possible. The child is asked to write 17 and 71, 69 and 96. Thereafter, the scale requires the person write down numbers of increasing complexity. As numbers become more complex, it is possible to see if the child places the numbers in the correct sequence, again looking for possible spatial deficits that can be caused by right hemisphere or left occipital–parietal dysfunction. In the next section, the child is asked to compare numbers, an operation that is basic to the left occipital–parietal area. In items 124 and 125, the child is asked to do simple arithmetic problems. These are problems that most individuals can probably do from memory. The last item is the presentation of serial 3s.

The C9 scale appears to be potentially sensitive to lesions in all parts of the brain, as well as to preexisting deficits common to about 20% or more of the normal population whose performance is well below grade level expectations.

C10 (Memory). The C10 scale is basically involved with short-term memory functions. The first items on C10 look at the ability of the child to memorize a list of seven simple words and to predict his or her performance. Items 129 through 131 involve immediate sensory trace recall. The items test word memory and visual memory.

Items 132 and 133 involve simple verbal memory under two conditions of interference. Several difficulties in short-term memory are seen in these items. Finally, item 135 is a measure of the individual's ability to associate the verbal stimulus with a picture. This item can be interfered with by either left or right hemisphere dysfunction and is sensitive to high-level disturbances in memory skills.

Overall, the C10 scale is most sensitive to verbal dysfunction because of its importance in a majority of the items. However, nonverbal dysfunction caused by right hemisphere lesions will show up in a moderately elevated C10 score of about 60T, with a pattern of missing the nonverbal items. It is always important to look at the pattern of the items missed before venturing the hypothesis of a possible etiology.

C11 (Intellectual Processes). The items in C11 should be differentiated from items in a standard intelligence test. All of the items on this scale have been selected because they are able to discriminate between brain-damaged and normal subjects. Thus, rather than giving a level of intelligence that can be associated with a child's learning history, the items tend to give a functional intellectual level.

Initial items in the scale involve the understanding of thematic pictures. The first item asks the child to interpret a picture in her or his own words; items 137 and 138 ask the individual to put pictures into a series that makes sense, similar to the items in Picture Arrangement. Item 139 asks the child to tell what is comical or absurd about certain pictures. Deficits of visual scanning can also be seen in individuals who are not able to appreciate the complexity of a picture and who, thus, tend to focus on one area. Item 140 requires the child interpret a story. Items 141 and 142 ask for similarities. Item 141 involves simple concept formations and definitions; items 142 and 143 call for comparisons and differences between objects in much the same way as do items on the Similarities subtest of the Wechsler Adult Intelligence Scale (WAIS). Performance in this area is further evaluated by items 144 through 146, in which the child must find the logical relationships between specific objects and the groups to which they belong. The last items on the scale, items 147 through 149, involve simple arithmetic problems very similar to those seen on the WISC-R Arithmetic subtest.

Overall, the C11 scale is highly sensitive to disorders in both hemispheres but is most sensitive to disorders in the left hemisphere. Injuries in the parietal lobes will cause maximum dysfunction. The determination of laterality, however, must be made by investigating specific items to judge whether those initial items that are right hemisphere oriented suggest adequate visual interpretation skills. If these skills appear to be intact, then the scale is likely to be reflecting a left hemisphere dysfunction alone. If these are the only items missed on the scale, the possibility of isolated right frontal dysfunction must be seriously considered.

The C11 scale score correlates about 0.7 with WISC-R Full Scale IQ. However, this scale, because of its flexibility in administration, may yield higher IQ estimates in individuals with impairment in expressive or receptive speech skills. Although the scale can reflect impairment in either hemisphere, a high elevation combined with C2 (Rhythm), C4 (Visual Functions), C10 (Memory), and C9 (Arithmetic) generally points to right hemisphere dysfunction, whereas elevations combined with C6 (Expressive Speech), C8 (Reading), and C7 (Writing) indicate left hemisphere damage.

Qualitative Analysis

The LNNB-C lends itself to a qualitative analysis along with the quantitative analysis discussed in this chapter. The consideration of the qualitative factors becomes the next step in the diagnostic process. Here, the interest is not in whether a child got a certain score on a certain item but rather *how* that score was achieved. One of the great advantages of this battery is that the same test procedures lend themselves to both quantitative and qualitative analyses. Although it is possible to interpret the battery from only one method or the other, the use of only one technique does not take full advantage of the possibilities within the battery nor does it yield the maximum amount of useful information in any given case.

In scoring qualitative errors, there is a wide range of possibilities aimed at gaining a better understanding of the "why" behind a child's error. Qualitative analysis can also aid in the evaluations of responses that are correct in terms of the quantitative scoring but still unusual, such as the child who reads a word on the C8 scale but stutters in pronouncing it, or the child who can describe an object and its uses on the C4 scale but is unable to give its name.

The disadvantage of qualitative inferences is the lack of formal scoring criteria and reliability across examiners. At present, there is no way in which such problems can be completely eliminated, but there are ways in which such problems can be minimized. The Qualitative Scoring Summary allows the user to score over 60 categories of qualitative observations that can be made during administration of the battery. The presence of such a scoring system emphasizes the need for intelligent observation on the part of the user. The effectiveness of the system is directly related to the effectiveness of the observer/tester as well as her or his active participation in the testing procedure. Interpretation of this information requires a detailed understanding of the ways in which the brain functions.

It is very important that the clinician learn to observe and record the child's approach to the items, especially if that approach differs from those seen in the normal child. (The examiner must have adequate experience with normals to make this comparison.) This should be done even if the examiner does not understand the meaning of the behavior or its significance. Sometimes the significance becomes clear after the quantitative analysis is completed, or it may become clear on consultation with one's supervisor or a consultant. By doing this on a systematic basis, the user will begin to appreciate the meaning of the child's behavior and to develop the ability to perform such analyses independently.

After a qualitative analysis has been made, it should be integrated with the quantitative analysis. It is our strong belief that neither form of data is inherently "superior" in any given case. In some cases, the qualitative data help to explain inconsistencies that cannot be resolved in the quantitative results. In other cases, the quantitative data suggest an alternate approach to an observation that clears up in the interpretation of a qualitative aspect of behavior. Only when the two sets of data have been integrated has a fully effective initial evaluation been completed.

Personality

Another important aspect of the analysis is to identify the personality factors playing a role in the child's behavior. Personality, as much as cognition, is derived from the brain. Indeed, those functions we label as personality may be the only things impaired in a given disorder. Evidence is increasing that personality is as much a function of biology as it is of environment, although both are absolutely necessary. Evaluation of personality comes from testing (e.g., Rorschach, CAT, PIC), observation, as well as clinical interaction.

Prior History

Even at this point, there still remains another step in the diagnostic process, namely, the reconciliation of the conclusions of the above techniques

with the history. This can be done in two ways: (1) knowing the history when the case begins and considering it throughout the diagnostic process or (2) analyzing the case with a minimum of information and checking the detailed history afterward. (Doing any case completely blind is not recommended.) Both techniques have their drawbacks. If too much history is known, one may be so biased that the inconsistencies between the history and data are overlooked or deemed unimportant.

History includes information about medical status but also social information, family information, school proceedings, social situation, and environmental inputs. In current language, this is a holistic approach that recognizes that everything we are and experience interact to produce our behaviors, successes, and failures. Only such a holistic approach is adequate for maximum understanding.

Historical information and the conclusions made available by others prior to the neuropsychological assessment may be right or wrong. A lesion may exist as reported, or may not. The child's developmental history may be accurate or may contain serious errors. The relative accuracy of information does depend on the source of that information as well as its nature. In all cases, however, it is important to double-check all such information.

Consequently, our bias suggests working from a basic history for important aspects that concern the validity of testing. In the evaluating process, we treat conclusions from the data as simply hypotheses to be confirmed or discarded. This leaves the clinician more flexibility to take his or her data seriously and to learn from those data all that is possible. If, at the end, discrepancies are found between history and neuropsychological findings, the clinician should investigate the history and the findings for errors that may cause this discrepancy, and look for conditions outside neuropsychology that may have affected one or the other source of data. It should also be recognized that conclusions are working conclusions, open to revision at any time when events suggest that the conclusions are inadequate. This allows us to work closer toward "perfection" although it is unlikely we will ever achieve that.

New Research Approaches

The LNNB-3 has been in development for approximately 10 years. It represents a major expansion of the children's battery along with an integration with the adult battery to create a single test that can be given from age 5 through adulthood. The LNNB-3 was developed by integrating the items of the existing Luria-based tests, and augmenting these items with an additional 1000 items covering such areas as complex visual–spatial skills, nonverbal complex auditory discrimination, speeded repetition, new memory items, nonverbal intelligence, problem solving, complex receptive language skills, and reading comprehension. Easier items and more complex items were added to existing scales. These items were culled from the existing literature and identified as potential areas not currently on the test.

This battery of items was subjected to a factor analysis that initially identified a solution of some 33 to 38 factors which accounted for over three-fourths of the total variance. Because the test was intended to be used serially to track recovery and change, scales that were found to have poor test–retest reliability were eliminated. These generally represented tests that require surprise to work properly. As a result, when given a second time scores often change dramatically except in severe injuries. While such tests can be a valuable component of an analysis, they are less appropriate for a battery such as this.

Other scales were found to be simple and hard versions of the same scale. For example, a basic arithmetic (e.g., number identification, simple counting), and a complex arithmetic (multiplication, division, basic algebra) were combined into a single scale. The resulting test had some 29 scales and 1200 items. Further evaluation eliminated items that were redundant and tightened up the longer scales, leaving overall approximately 1000 items. Four scales were condensed to two, leaving a final tally of 27 scales.

The 27 scales were a mixture of original LNNB scales [e.g., Non-verbal Comprehension (Rhythm), Arithmetic, Writing, Oral Reading, Spelling, Intelligence] with minor modifications, subscales of the original scales (e.g., Bilateral motor coordination, drawing skills, simple and complex Tactile scales), and completely new scales (e.g., Visual–Intellectual skills, Speeded Repetition, Repetition, Reading Comprehension, Verbal List Learning, Nonverbal List Learning).

The resulting test was also organized so that items are ranked in order of difficulty on most of the scales. Within these scales, only items appropriate to the client's level of performance can be administered, saving considerable time. Equipment was kept minimal to allow easy administration in all potential settings including bedside or in a client's home. Overall, the test takes less than 150 minutes, similar to the earlier versions of the battery. In normals and individuals with specific focal injuries, the test can be given in as little as an hour, yet appears to yield large amounts of valuable information. The test is also designed to be modular, allowing clinicians to give only part of the test and allowing for the development of new scales in the future.

Test Description

The test consists of 27 internally consistent and factorially sound scales that each yield individual item scores, scale scores, and qualitative scores.

1. Motor Coordination. This scale evaluates bilateral and unilateral motor speed and coordination. It consists of 11 items, some of which are taken from the LNNB-C and some of which are new items. All items allow for practice and demonstration.

2. Purposeful movements. This scales examines the accuracy of motor movements and the inability to modify them according to specific instructions and commands. These items range from imitating specific actions without the actual materials (such as pretending to comb your hair) to performing motor movements inconsistent with initial expectations or contrary to what a model is doing. Most of these items come from previous versions of the LNNB.

3. Drawing. This scale examines basic drawing skills from simple tracing to Greek crosses. Mazelike items are included for younger children. About half of these items are found on previous versions of the LNNB.

4. Nonverbal auditory processing. This is the analysis of tonal and rhythmic items, all of which are only slight modifications of earlier versions of the LNNB.

5. Nonverbal sound interpretation. These are all new items measuring the ability to recognize the direction of a sound, the meaning of sounds (such as the sound of a typewriter), and the role of inflection in emotional sounds.

6. Tactile discrimination. These are the basic items taken from earlier versions of the test involving the detection of the movement of stimuli, the location, and the firmness along with basic stereognosis items. All are administered with the client's eyes closed or blindfolded.

7. Complex Tactile Pattern Recognition. This scale tests the ability to detect shapes, letters, and

numbers written on one's wrist with the client's eyes closed. These items are taken from previous versions of the LNNB.

8. Visual identification. This scale consists of the basic items of the LNNB Visual scales combined with both simpler and more complex items including detecting hidden pictures, facial recognition, visual closure, visual identification, and visual matching. The scale does not require significant verbal or motor responses.

9. Visual–Spatial. These items measure visual–spatial relationships ranging from simple jigsaw puzzles, Raven's matrices-type items, line orientation, and time reading to simple visual rotation skills. Some of these items are found on older versions of the LNNB.

10. Visual–Intellectual. Visual intellectual analysis comprises more complex visual items that require intellectual as well as spatial and identification skills. This includes rotating objects 180 degrees, identifying visual similarities and differences, and connect-the-dot tasks similar to the Trail Making Test. These items are new.

11. Phonemic Discrimination. Partially taken from previous versions of the LNNB, these items measure the discrimination of basic sounds and words using only auditory cues. Items range in difficulty from recognizing "bye-bay-boe" to discriminating between "relieve" and "relief." All items allow either verbal or pointing responses.

12. Repetition. Mostly taken from earlier versions of the LNNB, these items require simple repetition of words such as "the" and "see" through "participate" and "discretionary." An oral response is required.

13. Speeded repetition. This is a new subtest. Clients must quickly repeat words and phrases ranging from "papa" to "Patty picked a pail of pretty posies."

14. Auditory Comprehension. This scale examines the ability to follow basic commands that require pointing to pictures or simple manipulation (like the Token Test). Items range in complexity from simple, easily discriminated pictures (like a horse) to items that illustrate more complex concepts ("A boy is riding his bicycle and waving his hand"). Over half of these items are new.

15. Complex auditory discrimination. These represent complex auditory commands that generally require recognition of more subtle grammatical constructs and sentence structure. These items generally are found on earlier versions of the LNNB.

16. Naming. These items require basic naming including body parts, pictures, and colors. About 70% come from previous versions of the LNNB.

17. Expressive Speech. These items cover speech (not including naming or repetition) from automatic speech (reciting the alphabet), completing sentences, making up sentences, word generation (such as things that start with the letter "t"), and making up sentences with specific words. About half of the items are new.

18. Motor writing. This scale examines aspects of motor writing from copying to writing from dictation. About 30% of the items are new. Items on this scale are measured only for the quality of writing *per se* and not for the accuracy of spelling.

19. Spelling. Using the items of scale 18, this scale measures the adequacy of spelling regardless of the quality of handwriting. For clients who cannot write or whose writing is illegible, the client may spell out loud or indicate letters on an optional letter sheet by pointing.

20. Reading Recognition. This is mostly derived from the old LNNB Reading scale, covering basic letter identification, matching, and reading words (and one sentence) at different levels of complexity. It is shorter than but similar to the WRAT Reading and PIAT Reading Recognition scales.

21. Reading Comprehension. This is a new scale organized like the PIAT Reading Comprehension scale. The client reads sentences of increasing complexity and must select the correct picture that corresponds to the sentence.

22. Arithmetic. Very similar to the original LNNB Arithmetic but expanded with a variety of new items, this scale measures everything from number recognition through square roots in 35 items.

23. Figural Memory. This is a new subtest. The targets consist of eight nonsense drawings that the client is shown for 20 seconds. The client is then shown a page of 20 figures in which the correct figures are randomly embedded. As the examiner points to each figure on the test page, the client must say whether each item was in the target group. The client is allowed up to four learning trials with retesting after each trial. After a delay of 30–40 minutes, the client is again retested for retention.

24. Serial Auditory List Learning. This is also a new subtest. The targets consist of a list of 12 words read to the client. After each trial, there is a free recall phase followed by a recognition phase where the correct words are embedded in a longer list of 26.

There are up to four trials, and a delayed recall after 30–40 minutes using only the recognition phase.

25. Stroop. This is a shortened form of the Stroop Color and Word Test and consists of three pages. Page 1 measures the ability to read color words (red, green, and blue). The second page measures the ability to name color patches (also red, green, and blue). The third page measures the ability to name color patches (such as the color red) when it is written in a distractor word (such as *blue*). The test requires the suppression of a basic tendency to read the word rather than name the color. The ability to suppress this basic tendency is a measure of the client's control over cognitive processes.

26. General Intelligence and Orientation. This scale incorporates some elements of basic mental status examinations along with intellectual items found on standard tests of intelligence. Items include basic information about the client (e.g., name), similarities and difference type items, verbal arithmetic, the ability to generalize, comparisons, opposites, categorization, vocabulary, and visual orientation and analysis. About half of the items are new.

27. Intellectual Analysis and Integration. These items consist of a variety of picture interpretation and analysis tasks including visual incongruities, picture arrangement tasks, and picture analysis. This scale is a mixture of previous and new items as well as adapted items.

Scoring

Scoring for each item ranges from right/wrong to points based on how deviant the performance is from an arbitrary normal standard. Scores are totaled to yield scale scores. Earlier versions of the LNNB may also be extracted with good reliability when required (with the exception of the old Memory scale). The test may also be used to generate IQ estimates and scores on other commonly used tests. Total scores can be compared with expected scores for normals, much as is done with previous versions of the LNNB.

However, the greatest emphasis remains on an analysis of test patterns both within and between scales. Of great importance as well are the qualitative scales that measure the incidence of 66 qualitative categories throughout the test administration. These categories are grouped into ten major areas:

1. Dysarthria. These represent the scores that measure basic speech dysfluency. These include articulation, paraphasias, simplification and substitutions, slurring, and stuttering. All of these categories represent mispronunciation of words, except for some paraphasias which may represent substitutions of words for one another (such as hat for dress).

2. Expressive Language. These categories are generally disorders of oral speech, although they may have cognitive rather than motor etiologies. These categories include circumlocution, dropping of articles, impoverished speech, jargon, naming disorder, oral language absence, prosody, spelling, stiff speech, and vocal quality. In each case, errors on speech items or general cognitive items can be more precisely defined by using these categories or others as appropriate.

3. Motor. These categories measure disorders of motor functions (other than motor speech). These include associated movements, involuntary movements, macrographia, micrographia, midline failure, motor awkwardness, motor writing, paralysis, stiff motor movements, torque, and tremors.

4. Peripheral Impairment. These categories identify when peripheral injuries to the limbs, face, or spinal cord cause defects on the tests which may not be related to "brain" function *per se*. For example, we need to identify when errors on visual items are caused by inability to see the items clearly.

5. Receptive Language. These items identify when problems in the understanding of language interfere with test performance (which potentially includes all items since all have some form of instructions). The categories include auditory discrimination, failure to comprehend instructions, grapheme recognition, and letter–number recognition.

6. Self-cueing. These categories evaluate when the client uses some external aid to help solve a problem. These include gestural and visual cueing, postural cueing, repetition, and verbal cueing. These all identify circumstances where clients cannot work things out "in their head."

7. Self-monitoring. These are very important categories where there may be profound functional effects but only mild concrete cognitive effects. These categories include additional responses (where they give a right answer plus additional information), anticipation, automatic phrases, confusion, context confabulation, description, elaboration, emotional responses, impulsivity, irrelevant associations, perseveration, self-correction, and sequence errors. All of these categories represent instances where clients cannot monitor or control their behavior so as to conform to the requests of the

item even though they may still get a correct answer in some cases. It is entirely possible that a brain injury may be restricted to these and related categories alone with minimal objective findings.

8. Speed. These categories identify problems related to response latency (taking too long to begin) and time delay (getting the right answer but in an excessive time period).

9. Sustained Performance. These are important indicators about how well the client can maintain a level of function over time. These clients may be characterized as individuals who do well for a period of time and then do poorly. Their performance depends less on the item content than on when the item is presented in the course of the test. It is important to discriminate between those clients who do poorly because of cognitive dysfunction and those who do poorly for problems in sustained attention: Both may be injured but the necessary rehabilitation is quite different. These categories include attention difficulties, fatigue, and impersistence.

10. Visual–Spatial. These include a variety of disorders related to basic spatial orientation, e.g., counting errors, echopraxia, number spatial impairment, omission, reversal, right–left disorientation, rotations, unilateral neglect, and visual focusing.

These general categories and the 66 individual categories allow the clinician a great deal of flexibility in identifying the underlying cause of a client's problems. Consistent with Luria's own testing and theoretical approach, this extends the information that can be gathered from simply doing a basic objective scoring of items. By using them within a quantitative context, we can generate both types of information enhancing the value and strength of the overall evaluation.

Interpretation

Interpretation is basically similar to the earlier versions of the test, with an emphasis on a multilevel, integrationist, holistic approach to both testing and interpretation. Although diagnoses can be generated from the test, the biggest emphasis is on understanding the individual's underlying issues and problems and how these affect day-to-day function. The new version of the test enhances the range of information gathered and thus permits both recreation of the information generated by the earlier tests as well as new information to better understand the underlying neuropsychological performance.

Conclusions

The Luria–Nebraska Children's Battery is a test that evaluates a wide range of skills aimed at assessing the neuropsychological competence of children between the ages of 8 and 12. The battery offers a variety of quantitative and qualitative scores by which to detail the performance of children and to integrate that performance with historical data. The battery has been shown to be highly successful in diagnosis, but does need to be supplemented by other tests when detailed analysis of single areas is necessary or preferable. The battery lends itself to interpretation on a variety of levels. Thus, it can be useful to people with varying backgrounds provided caveats on use are followed carefully. The test is in the process of being updated and extended down to ages 5 through adult. The new test offers a large number of advantages and extensions to the previous battery in a variety of areas.

References

Golden, C. J. (1986). *Manual for the Luria–Nebraska Neuropsychological Battery: Children's Revision.* Los Angeles: Western Psychological Services.

Plaisted, J. R., Gustavson, J. L., Wilkening, G. N., & Golden, C. J. (1983). The Luria–Nebraska Neuropsychological Battery—Children's Revision: Theory and current research findings. *Journal of Clinical Child Psychology, 12,* 13–21.

Raven, J. C. (1960). *Guide to the Standard Progressive Matrices.* London: Lewis.

13

Applications of the Kaufman Assessment Battery for Children (K-ABC) in Neuropsychological Assessment

CECIL R. REYNOLDS, RANDY W. KAMPHAUS,

BECKY L. ROSENTHAL, AND JENNIFER R. HIEMENZ

The Kaufman Assessment Battery for Children (K-ABC) (Kaufman & Kaufman, 1983a) is now a widely accepted and used, individually administered clinical test of intelligence and achievement for use with preschoolers and young children. There is research guidance regarding the use of the K-ABC with samples of Asian children (Ishikuma, Moon, & Kaufman, 1988; Mardell-Czudnowski, 1995), correlations between K-ABC scores and heart rate (Kaufman, Eller, & Applegate, 1990), the utility of the K-ABC with samples suffering from depression (Kaufman, Grossman, & Kaufman, 1994) and autism (Allen, Lincoln, & Kaufman, 1991), investigation of K-ABC short forms (Kaufman & Applegate, 1988), and commentary and inclusion of the K-ABC in reference works on neuropsychological testing (e.g., Spreen & Strauss, 1991).

The K-ABC is likely well known and researched for many reasons, including the fact that it was developed from a theoretical framework that to a large degree reflects a coalescence of the work of Luria and Vygotsky, and U.S. researchers with interests in cerebral specialization as interpreted and integrated by Alan and Nadeen Kaufman. The K-ABC is thus of continuing interest to clinical child neuropsychologists. This chapter attempts to update the reader regarding the use of the K-ABC in a neuropsychological framework by (1) reviewing the theoretical framework of the K-ABC and describing its conceptual and empirical relationship to neuropsychology, (2) reviewing the literature regarding the use of the K-ABC with neurologically impaired samples, and (3) providing an overview of techniques for rehabilitation of academic disturbances as viewed from the K-ABC model.

Theoretical Framework

The K-ABC intelligence scales are based on a model of sequential and simultaneous information processing. The theoretical underpinnings of the processing model were gleaned from a convergence of research and theory in a variety of areas including both neuropsychology and cognitive psychology. The neuropsychological theory employed by the Kaufmans was distilled from two lines: the information processing approach of Luria (e.g., Luria, 1966) and the cerebral specialization work done by Sperry (1968, 1974), Bogen (1969), Kinsbourne (1975), and Wada, Clarke, and Hamme (1975).

CECIL R. REYNOLDS • Department of Educational Psychology, Texas A&M University, College Station, Texas 77843. RANDY W. KAMPHAUS AND JENNIFER R. HIEMENZ • Department of Educational Psychology, University of Georgia, Athens, Georgia 30602. BECKY L. ROSENTHAL • Intermediate Educational Cooperative, Du Page, Illinois 60510

TABLE 1. Definitions of the Two Types of Mental Processing That Underlie the K-ABC Intelligence Scales from the K-ABC Manual and from Several Theoretical Perspectives[a]

Source	Labels for process	Definitions
K-ABC: Kaufman & Kaufman (1983a)	Sequential	Places a premium on the serial or temporal order of stimuli when solving problems.
	Simultaneous	Demands a gestaltlike, frequently spatial, integration of stimuli to solve problems with maximum efficiency.
Cerebral specialization: Nebes (1974) (summarizing model of Bogen, Levy-Agresti, and Sperry)	Analytic/propositional/left hemisphere	Sequentially analyzes input, abstracting out the relevant details to which it associates verbal symbols in order to more efficiently manipulate and store the data.
	Synthetic/appositional/right hemisphere	Organize and treat data in terms of complex wholes, being in effect a synthesizer with a predisposition for viewing the total rather than the parts.
Luria/Das: Das, Kirby, & Jarman (1979)	Successive	Processing of information in a serial order. The important distinction between this type of information processing and simultaneous processing is that in successive processing the system is not totally surveyable at any point in time. Rather, a system of cues consecutively activates the components.
	Simultaneous	The synthesis of separate elements into groups, these groups often taking on spatial overtones. The essential nature of this sort of processing is that any portion of the result is at once surveyable without dependence on its position in the whole.
Cognitive psychology: Neisser (1967)	Sequential/serial	Viewed as a constructive process, it constructs only one thing at a time. The very definitions of "rational" and "logical" also suggest that each idea, image, or action is sensibly related to the preceding one, making an appearance only as it becomes necessary for the aim in view.
		A spatially serial activity is one that analyzes only a part of the input field at any given moment . . . On the other hand *sequential* refers to the manner in which a process is organized; it is appropriate when the analysis consists of successive, interrelated steps.
	Parallel/multiple	Carries out many activities simultaneously, or at least independently.

[a]From Kaufman (1984). Reprinted with permission.

Table 1 reviews the various theories and definitions that influenced K-ABC development most strongly.

Lurian Theories

Luria's theory was of paramount importance in the formulation of the Kaufmans' approach to assessing intelligence with the K-ABC. This seems only appropriate given the stature of Luria's theory. "Alexander R. Luria's theory of higher cortical functioning has received international acclaim. His conceptual schemes of the functional organization of the brain are probably the most comprehensive currently available" (Adams, 1985, p. 878). Much of Luria's work grew from earlier writings of Sechenov (translation, 1965) and Vygotsky (trans-

lation, 1978). Majovski (1984), who studied with Luria in Russia for several years near the end of Luria's life, evaluated the K-ABC regarding its relevance to Luria's approach with children and to child neuropsychology in general, and gave the scale high marks.

Luria defined mental processes in terms of two sharply delineated groups, simultaneous and successive, following Sechenov's suggestions. The first process involves the integration of elements into simultaneous groups. He further qualified Sechenov's original meaning, indicating that simultaneous processing meant the synthesis of successive elements (arriving one after the other) into simultaneous spatial schemes whereas successive processing meant the synthesis of separate elements into successive series. These qualifications are crucial in seeing the match between the various subtests of the K-ABC mental processing scales and this processing dichotomy. For those not fluent with the K-ABC, Figure 1 provides a listing of the various subtests and a brief description of each.

In the K-ABC the Kaufmans define these processes in a manner similar to Luria and provide a standardized assessment of these functions. Simultaneous processing here refers to the mental ability of the child to integrate input simultaneously to solve a problem correctly. Simultaneous processing frequently involves spatial, analogic, or organizational abilities (Kaufman & Kaufman, 1983b) as well as problems solved through the application of visual imagery. The Triangles subtest on the K-ABC (an analogue of Wechsler's Block Design task) is a prototypical measure of simultaneous processing. To solve these items correctly, one must mentally integrate the components of the design to "see" the whole. Such a task seems to match up nicely with Luria's qualifying statement of synthesis of separate elements (each triangle) into spatial schemes (the larger pattern of triangles, which may form squares, rectangles, or larger triangles). Whether the tasks are spatial or analogic in nature, the unifying characteristic of simultaneous processing is the mental synthesis of the stimuli to solve the problem, independent of the sensory modality of the input or the output.

Sequential processing, on the other hand, emphasizes the arrangement of stimuli in sequential or serial order for successful problem solving. In every instance, each stimulus is linearly or temporally related to the previous one (Kaufman & Kaufman, 1983b) creating a form of serial interdependence within the stimulus. The K-ABC includes sequential processing subtests that tap a variety of modalities. The Hand Movements subtest involves visual input and a motor response; the Number Recall subtest involves auditory input with a response involving the auditory output channel only; Word Order involves the visual channel for input and an auditory response. Therefore, the mode of presentation or mode of response is not what determines the scale placement of a task, but rather it is the *mental processing demands* of the task that are important (Kaufman & Kaufman, 1983b). By providing systematic variation of modality of input and modality of response, the K-ABC provides a clinical vehicle for locating intact complex functional systems as well as specifying where any potential breakdown may have occurred in a faulty functional system.

Mental Processing Scale

Sequential Processing Scale

Hand Movements (ages 2½–12½ years)*: Imitating a series of hand movements the same sequence as the examiner performed them

Number Recall (ages 2½–12½): Repeating a series of digits in the same sequence as the examiner said them

Word Order (ages 4–12½):Touching a series of pictures in the same sequence as they were named by the examiner, with more difficult items employing a color-interference task

Simultaneous Processing Scale

Magic Window (ages 2½–4): Identifying a picture that the examiner exposes by moving it past a narrow slit or "window," making the picture only partially visible at any one time

Face Recognition (ages 2½–4)*: Selecting from a group photograph the one or two faces that were exposed briefly in the preceding photograph

Gestalt Closure (ages 2½–12½): Naming the object or scene pictured in a partially completed "inkblot" drawing

Triangles (ages 4–12½)*: Assembling several identical triangles into an abstract pattern that matches a model

Matrix Analogies (ages 5–12½)*: Selecting the picture or abstract design that best completes a visual analogy

Spatial Memory (ages 5–12½)*: Recalling the placement of pictures on a page that was exposed briefly

Photo Series (ages 6–12½)*:Placing photographs of an event in chronological order

Achievement Subtests

Expressive Vocabulary (ages 2½–4):Naming the object pictured in a photograph

Faces & Places (ages 2½–12½): Naming the well-known person, fictional character, or place pictured in a photograph or illustration

Arithmetic (ages 3–12½): Answering a question that requires knowledge of math concepts or the manipulation of numbers

Riddles (ages 3–12½): Naming the object or concept described by a list of three characteristics

Reading/Decoding (ages 5–12½): Naming letters and reading words

Reading/Understanding (ages 7–12½): Acting out commands given in written sentences

FIGURE 1. K-ABC subtests. Asterisks denote subtests that also make up the nonverbal scale.

Qualitative evaluation of a child's performance on the K-ABC can be most useful in such instances and can lead to more effective rehabilitation plans.

No one with an intact brain uses only a single type of information processing to solve problems. These two methods of information processing are constantly interacting (even in the so-called split-brain following commissurotomy, the two hemispheres of the brain often "whisper" to each other even if they cannot talk), although one approach will often take a lead role in processing. Which method of processing takes the lead role can change according to the demands of the problem or, as is the case with some individuals, persist across problem type [i.e., forming what Das, Kirby, and Jarman (1979) refer to as habitual modes of processing]. In fact, any problem can be solved through either method of processing. In most cases, one method is clearly superior to another. It is the latter case that makes the K-ABC a valuable tool—the two mental processing scales are *primarily,* not exclusively, measures of sequential or simultaneous processing. Pure scales, i.e., scales measuring only one process, do not exist. Careful observation of a child's performance, which should be the order of the day during any evaluation, will be particularly important to any neuropsychological assessment or neuropsychological interpretation of K-ABC test results; observation in many cases will be a primary source of information regarding which mental processes a child invoked on any given task, regardless of its scale.

An equally important component of the K-ABC is the Achievement Scale. This scale measures abilities that serve to complement the intelligence scales. Performance on the achievement scales is viewed as an estimate of children's success in the application of their mental processing skills to the acquisition of knowledge from the environment (Kaufman, Kamphaus, & Kaufman, 1985). This scale contains measures of what have been identified traditionally as verbal intelligence, general information, and acquired school skills. Keeping in mind that it is not possible to separate entirely *what* you know (achievement) from *how well* you think (intelligence), the Kaufmans attempted to differentiate the two variables better than traditional measures of intelligence. From a clinical neuropsychological standpoint, the K-ABC allows one to assess information processing skills without as much contamination from prior learning. Measurement of children's academic skills, however, is a traditional component of the comprehensive neuropsycholog-

ical assessment. The inclusion of the Achievement Scale in the K-ABC affords the opportunity to observe the application of processing skills to complex learning tasks, to assess functional academic levels, and to estimate long-term memory ability. For a thorough review of interpretation of the K-ABC Achievement Scale, see Kamphaus and Reynolds (1987).

Majovski (1984) noted the high degree of "fit" between Luria's theory and the K-ABC" and recommended that the test be used as an integral part of the neuropsychological battery for children (see Spreen & Strauss, 1991). The K-ABC is not, under any circumstance, a complete or substitute battery for a comprehensive neuropsychological assessment; it is a good complement to nearly any choice of neuropsychological instruments. Majovski found the K-ABC particularly useful in contrasting problem-solving skills with acquisition of facts and in evaluating how a child solves a particular problem.

When young children (below age 6) are being assessed, the K-ABC is the test of choice for measuring intellectual skill for the neuropsychologist. The K-ABC mental processing subtests are child oriented and much briefer but with comparable reliability to its major competitor, the Wechsler Preschool and Primary Scale of Intelligence-Revised (WPPSI-R; Wechsler, 1989). For assessing mental processes, the K-ABC seems far superior to other measures of intelligence since it is far less dependent on prior learning and exposure to the mainstream Anglo culture (e.g., see Kamphaus & Reynolds, 1987). When assessing the intellectual processes of nonnative English speakers, the independence of the K-ABC intelligence subscales is particularly important so as not to confound cultural experiences and cultural dependency of test items with neuropsychological processing (e.g., see Ardila, Roselli, & Puente, 1994). There is a growing body of literature to show the appropriateness of the K-ABC across a broad range of U.S. ethnic minorities (e.g., Fan, Willson, & Reynolds, in press; Ishikuma *et al.,* 1988; Kamphaus & Reynolds, 1987; Mardell-Czudnowski, 1995).

Cerebral Specialization Theories

Support for use of the K-ABC in the context of neuropsychological assessment also comes from a variety of sources in cerebral specialization research. In a comprehensive review of research concerning the lateralization of human brain functions, Dean (1984) concluded that the K-ABC was well suited to clinical use and in research with children. Research evidence to be reviewed in a subsequent section provides additional but still tentative support for Dean's conclusion.

It has been proposed that sequential and simultaneous processing are lateralized to the left and right hemispheres, respectively (e.g., Obrzut, 1991; Reynolds, 1981a; Sperry, 1974; Sperry, Gazzaniga, & Bogen, 1969; Spreen, Risser, & Edgell, 1995; Springer & Deutsch, 1989). Many other dichotomies have been suggested. Some find research on cerebral specialization difficult to coalesce. Indeed, the many seeming contradictions in the results of cerebral specialization studies have prompted at least one leading researcher to remark thus: "[To] say that the field of hemispheric specialization is in a state of disarray and that the results are difficult to interpret is an understatement. The field can best be characterized as chaotic" (Tomlinson-Keasey & Clarkson-Smith, 1980, p. 1). On the other hand, reviews by Dean (1984) and Reynolds (1981b) have noted some consistencies.

For the vast majority of individuals, the left cerebral hemisphere appears to be specialized for linguistic, propositional, serial, and analytic tasks and the right hemisphere for more nonverbal, appositional, synthetic, and holistic tasks (Bever, 1975; Bogen, 1969; Gazzaniga, 1970; Harnad, Doty, Goldstein, Jaynes, & Krauthamer, 1977; Kinsbourne, 1978; Schwartz, Davidson, & Mear, 1975; Segalowitz & Gruber, 1977). One will find in the literature a large number of studies of hemispheric specialization attempting to provide anatomical localization of performance on specific, yet higher-order, complex tasks. Much of the confusion in the literature stems from the apparently conflicting data of many of these studies. However, the dynamic functional localization principle of Luria, and knowledge that any specific task potentially can be performed through any of the brain's processing modes, should give some insight into the conflicting results that appear in the literature. In this regard, it is most important to remember that cerebral hemispheric asymmetries of function are *process-specific* and not stimulus-specific. Shure and Halstead (1959) noted early in this line of research that manipulation of stimuli was at the root of hemispheric differences, a notion that is well supported by current empirical research (e.g., Ornstein, Johnstone, Herron, & Swencionis, 1980) and thought (e.g., Reynolds, 1981a,b). The confusion of the content and sensory modality through which stimuli are presented with the process by which they are ma-

nipulated, particularly in the secondary and tertiary regions of each lobe of the neocortex, seems to be at the root of the chaos. How information is manipulated while in the brain is not dependent on its modality of presentation and not necessarily on its content, though the latter may certainly be influential. The *variation in content* and *method of presentation* of the tasks that make up the three scales of the K-ABC allow one to tease out any modality or content effects that might nevertheless occur for a specific child, though clearly the emphasis of the K-ABC is on process, not content.

We think that a process-oriented explanation provides a better organizing principle than does a focus on content. The "content-driven" attempts at explaining hemispheric differences fail to recognize the possibilities for processing any given set of stimuli or particular content in a variety of processing modes. Bever (1975) emphasized this point and elaborated on two modes of information processing that are of interest here because of their similarity to simultaneous and successive cognitive processes.

According to Bever (1975), cerebral asymmetries of function result from two fundamental lateralized processes: holistic and analytic processing. Lateralization of these two methods of information processing is necessary because the two processes are incompatible and cannot coexist in the same physical space. Analytic processing appears analogous to successive processing and is lateralized, in most individuals, to the left hemisphere. Holistic processing is analogous to simultaneous processing and is typically lateralized to the right hemisphere.

The K-ABC also taps most of the functions identified by Dean (1984) in his review of the cerebral specialization literature, with the exceptions of depth, haptic, and melodic perceptions. These skills are assessed by other traditional neuropsychological batteries, although such tasks are virtually nonexistent for the very young child. Careful observation may still provide insight into neuropsychological processing deficits especially if one pays particular attention to the manner in which errors are made. Qualitative and quantitative data are complementary, not interchangeable; the intelligent testing philosophy of Kaufman (1979b) is just as crucial to neuropsychological assessment as to any other area of clinical evaluation.

Das *et al.* (1979) do not agree that simultaneous and successive processing are represented in the right and left hemispheres, respectively, but rather believe that each mode of processing is prominently represented in both hemispheres. According to Bever's

(1975) line of reasoning, this is an impossible state of affairs in the normally functioning human brain. Additionally, the hemispheric-lateralization literature is consistent with the notion of a successive-processing left hemisphere and simultaneous-processing right hemisphere relationship. Das *et al.* (1979) have developed their theory exclusively on the basis of group data, yet they attempt to discredit hemispheric lateralization of cognitive processing by calling on anecdotal individual case data. Hardly anyone would contend that hemispheric specialization for cognitive processing is the same in every individual. However, this seems to be the requisite state of affairs for Das *et al.* to accept the hypothesis of lateralization of simultaneous and successive processing. This hardly seems necessary. The sheer weight of evidence at present (cited later in this chapter) indicates that, for the vast majority of individuals, the lateralization of simultaneous and successive processes is to the right and left hemispheres, respectively.

Children may also form habitual modes of information processing that detract from efficiency in learning new material or in solving novel problems (Reynolds, 1981a). This would be one explanation of large sequential–simultaneous score differences that should also be explored, perhaps through protocol analysis or some related technique during a limits-testing type of procedure. Children who attempt to solve sequential tasks using simultaneous processing approaches or vice versa are likely to have academic as well as behavioral problems. In any event, a problem is evident when this occurs, one that needs more detailed study for the individual child in order to explain the reason for this persistent approach. Normally functioning individuals appear to be able to use the two modes of information processing separately or in conjunction with one another or possibly shift at will depending on the type of information to be processed (Gazzaniga, 1974, 1975), although such decisions are more likely to be made at an unconscious level in interaction between the stimuli to be processed and the child's preferred processing approach. At the highest level of function, the two modes of processing operate in a complementary manner, achieving maximal interhemispheric integration of processing or, in Bogen, Dezure, Tenhouten, and Marsh's (1972) terminology, "cerebral complementarity." For example, right hemisphere function (simultaneous processing) is important in contributing to letter and word recognition during the formative stages of learning to read. It is a more complex function handled primarily through successive process-

ing in the intermediate learning stage, because of its linguistic nature. Highly skilled readers who have mastered the component skills of reading and have made it an automatic function demonstrate extensive use of both processes in reading (Cummins & Das, 1977).

When first learning to read, successive processing is most important and many children with difficulties in learning to read have problems in this area (Cummins & Das, 1977). This is also consistent with the findings of higher Wechsler Performance than Verbal IQ in most groups of reading-disabled children. Performance IQ is almost certainly more closely related to the simultaneous processing of information than to successive processing whereas the converse relationship holds for Verbal IQ, the latter being a language task as is reading. Most (though certainly not all) young children with reading and language-related problems have greater difficulty with sequential processing (Kamphaus & Reynolds, 1987; Obrzut, 1991).

The traditional verbal–nonverbal distinction between the two hemispheres, although partially accurate, is likely an overcharacterization and simplification of hemispheric differences (Dean, 1984). Hemispheric differences seem more related to the method by which information is processed than to the specific modality of presentation (Brown & Hécaen, 1976; Dean, 1984; Reynolds, 1981a,b). The K-ABC seems to be the best available measure of intelligence to quantify this bimodal functioning. Although specific neural substrates related to K-ABC performance remain to be detailed, the scale appears useful as a tool to gain insight into the relative efficacy of the two hemispheres.

Specific Neuropsychological Research Using the K-ABC

The amount of neuropsychological research devoted to the K-ABC is limited at present, but the few studies available are generally supportive of its role in adding useful information to general neuropsychological batteries. Studies relating the K-ABC to the child forms of the Halstead–Reitan Neuropsychological Battery are noticeably absent from the literature and are certainly needed. Such studies are a necessary component of any comprehensive assessment of the utility of the K-ABC to determine how it precisely fits into the neuropsychological assessment process. Several studies are available relating the

K-ABC to the Luria–Nebraska Neuropsychological Battery-Children's Revision (LNNB-CR) and several have compared the K-ABC and WISC-R with relatively well-defined samples of neurologically impaired or medically involved children. In fact, some recent studies have used the K-ABC as a criterion measure for comparing the results of medical interventions. Other studies have looked at use of the K-ABC alone with neurologically impaired children.

Correlation with the Luria–Nebraska Scales

Of particular importance to understanding how the K-ABC might contribute to neuropsychology, clinically as well as in the research setting, is understanding how the K-ABC is related to existing neuropsychological scales. To be useful in neuropsychological assessment, the K-ABC should be related to existing measures, but not so closely that its use is merely redundant with preexisting scales. Although no data are available relating the K-ABC to the Halstead–Reitan techniques, several studies have been reported comparing the K-ABC with the LNNB-CR. The first report was by Snyder, Leark, Golden, Grove, and Allison (1983).

Snyder et al. (1983) evaluated 46 elementary school children (ages 8–12½) who had been referred for a variety of learning difficulties. All children were administered the K-ABC, WISC-R, and LNNB-CR as described in Golden (1978). Correlations between the K-ABC and LNNB-CR ranged from −0.001 (LNNB-CR Writing Scale with K-ABC Simultaneous) to −0.64 (LNNB-CR Intelligence with K-ABC Sequential and MPC). The LNNB-CR Intelligence scale correlated highest of all LNNB-CR scales with the K-ABC global scales (SIM −0.54, SEQ −0.64, MPC −0.64, Nonverbal −0.51, ACH −0.26). Correlations with the LNNB-CR are negative in direction because high scores on the LNNB-CR are indicative of increasingly high levels of pathology, i.e., the LNNB-CR is scored negatively, not positively as are most mental tests such as the K-ABC. In a stepwise multiple regression, from three to five LNNB-CR scales were required to maximize the prediction of each of the K-ABC scales. The pattern of relationships is much as one would anticipate. After the intelligence scale, the *visual and the motor scales contributed the greatest to the prediction of the Simultaneous scale;* for the Sequential scale, following intelligence, the *Rhythm and the Receptive Speech scales were the best predictors of performance.* The MPC and

K-ABC Nonverbal scales showed the same pattern as the Simultaneous scale, and not surprisingly because these scales overlap so much with the Simultaneous scale. The K-ABC ACH scales correlated from −0.50 to −0.58 with the school-related scales of the LNNB-CR (e.g., Expressive Language, Reading). In the multiple regression, academic skills again dominated prediction of the ACH scales. The K-ABC mental processing scales also were related significantly to each WISC-R IQ in this study; correlations ranged from 0.35 between SEQ and PIQ to 0.72 between the MPC and FSIQ and the Nonverbal and FSIQ. The K-ABC ACH scale correlated 0.66 with FSIQ, 0.77 with VIQ, but only 0.28 with PIQ. After examining the overall pattern of correlations in the study, Snyder et al. concluded that the relationships revealed were "basically consistent" with the model of intelligence on which the K-ABC was based and the theoretical perspective of Luria in particular. Snyder et al. also concluded that the K-ABC provides additional information, beyond the WISC-R and LNNB-CR, that should be useful to the clinical neuropsychologist. We agree. The pattern of correlations as well as the magnitude of correlations is encouraging. The K-ABC is clearly related to children's neuropsychological function as determined by the LNNB-CR, but not so much that K-ABC scores are simply redundant with other neuropsychological test results; the K-ABC apparently has something to add. Another recent study supports this conclusion.

In a similar study with a larger sample (65 children), Leark, Snyder, Grove, and Golden (1983) provide more detailed information. Table 2 displays the correlation matrix between the K-ABC global scales and the subscales of the LNNB-CR. Several interesting patterns emerge here. The LNNB-CR subscales that are known to be the most sensitive to brain impairment (Pathognomonic and Intellectual) are clearly the most closely related to performance on all of the K-ABC global scales in the Leark et al. study. However, there is very little overlap in item content from these scales to the K-ABC and yet the K-ABC seems sensitive to deficits in cortical functioning, at least at the level of the higher information-processing functions of the brain. The SEQ–SIM distinction and the separate Achievement scale of the K-ABC receive support from the pattern of correlations in Table 2 as well. The school-related subscales of the LNNB-CR correlate considerably higher with the K-ABC ACH scale than with the mental processing scales. Clear differentiations occur elsewhere as well. When evalu-

TABLE 2. Correlations between K-ABC Global Scales and Luria–Nebraska Neuropsychological Battery-Children's Revision Summary Scale ($N = 65$)[a]

Luria–Nebraska scale	Correlation with K-ABC global scale				
	Sequential processing	Simultaneous processing	MPC	Achievement	Nonverbal
Motor	−0.382	−0.424	−0.456	−0.242	−0.481
Rhythm	−0.405	−0.132	−0.282	−0.370	−0.199
Tactile	−0.115	−0.320	−0.270	−0.221	−0.321
Visual	−0.252	−0.498	−0.461	−0.192	−0.489
Receptive	−0.515	−0.355	−0.482	−0.600	−0.427
Expressive	−0.323	−0.154	−0.260	−0.614	−0.259
Writing	−0.324	−0.144	−0.248	−0.539	−0.246
Reading	−0.210	−0.060	−0.066	−0.618	−0.012
Arithmetic	−0.307	−0.152	−0.258	−0.607	−0.202
Memory	−0.471	−0.300	−0.427	−0.629	−0.356
Intelligence	−0.567	−0.570	−0.645	−0.439	−0.599
Pathognomonic	−0.598	−0.469	−0.606	−0.642	−0.656
Left	−0.171	−0.379	−0.335	−0.222	−0.352
Right	−0.075	−0.319	−0.244	−0.091	−0.301

[a]Adapted from Leark *et al.* (1983).

ating correlations with the LNNB-CR Rhythm scale, one sees that the SEQ scale is significantly related to the Rhythm scale ($r = -0.40$) whereas the SIM scale is not ($r = -0.13$). A similar pattern is observed for the LNNB-CR Receptive Speech scale. Additionally, the K-ABC Nonverbal scale is more highly correlated with the LNNB-CR Motor scale than is any other K-ABC scale. The Nonverbal and the SIM scales are more closely related to the LNNB-CR Visual scale than is the SEQ scale. Most of these relationships are intuitively obvious but their actual occurrence, especially given the moderate magnitude of the relationships, is certainly encouraging with respect to potential contributions of the K-ABC to neuropsychological assessment and research.

Relationships with Other Neuropsychological and Neurological Test Results

Several early studies have related the K-ABC to other neuropsychologically based scales and to hard evidence of neurological impairment. Much more is needed but progress is evident in these few studies.

Telzrow, Redmond, and Zimmerman (1984) examined test score patterns of children classified into Boder's three subtypes of dyslexia—dysphonetics, dyseidetics, and mixed. Telzrow *et al.* attempted to determine whether the WISC-R or the K-ABC would be more closely aligned with Boder's neuropsychological classification of reading disorders. WISC-R scores were grouped into Bannatyne's four categories of neuropsychological functions, as these groupings (Verbal Conceptualization, Sequencing, Spatial, and Acquired Knowledge) seem most clearly related to various schemes for regrouping the Wechsler subtests to Boder's diagnostic categories. The children could not be differentiated on the basis of their Bannatyne patterns on the WISC-R. Boder's subtypes were randomly distributed across Bannatyne's suggested patterns. On the K-ABC a significant relationship ($p < 0.01$) occurred between Boder classification and the pattern of Sequential–Simultaneous score differences on the K-ABC. In particular, Boder's dysphonetic dyslexics were far more likely to display a SIM greater than SEQ pattern than were the other diagnostic groups. Though Telzrow *et al.* used a small sample ($N = 23$), the results are impressive with large effect sizes. The pattern of K-ABC results was precisely in keeping with predictions of underlying neuropsychological deficits in Boder's classification scheme. A follow-up study with a second sample showed similar results with one major difference (Telzrow, Century, Harris, & Redmond, 1985).

In the latter study, 27 children with reading disorders were compared according to their performance on the WISC-R and the K-ABC, just as in the previous study. In the Telzrow *et al.* (1985) work, considerable consistency was found among the K-ABC, WISC-R, and the Boder results. Three-quarters of the dyslexic children who displayed a Bannatyne WISC-R pattern of Spatial greater than Sequential also showed a K-ABC pattern of Simultaneous greater than Sequential scores. In each case, it was the dysphonetic reading-disabled children who showed the higher Spatial and Simultaneous scores. Results with dyseidetic children are less clear on this point, most likely because of the small number of reading-disabled children showing this particular problem. The results of these two studies, considered in concert, though ambiguous with regard to the WISC-R, provide support for the use of the K-ABC in evaluating children with neuropsychologically related reading problems.

Hooper and Hynd (1985) also examined the utility of using the K-ABC in differential diagnosis of developmental dyslexia according to Boder's subtypes. Their sample consisted of 30 normal readers and 87 reading-disabled students (two or more grade levels below their grade placement). On the basis of the Boder Reading–Spelling Pattern test, 32 of the reading-disabled students were classified as "nonspecific" (significantly low achievement in reading, but reading and spelling pattern typical of normal readers), and 55 were classified as dyslexics. Of the dyslexics, 30 were classified as dysphonetics, 5 as dyseidetics, and 20 as alexics. Evaluation of the performance of all of these children on the K-ABC indicated the discriminatory value of the Sequential Processing scale but not the Simultaneous Processing scale in terms of Boder's subtypes. Normal readers scored significantly higher than all of the reading-disabled subtypes on the Sequential Processing scale. Sequential/Simultaneous discrepancies, however, did not discriminate between the subtypes of dyslexia. The small number of dyseidetics in the study may have contributed to this outcome. When combined with the results of Telzrow *et al.* (1985), Hooper and Hynd's results provide support for the simultaneous > sequential pattern in dyslexia (particularly dysphonetic subtype) but the importance of the simultaneous < sequential pattern in dyslexia (as it may apply to dyseidetics) is much less clear. Hooper and Hynd note, "It would be of interest to examine the discriminant validity of the K-ABC with empirically, as opposed to clinically, derived subgroups of developmental dyslexia."

In a conceptually related work, Dietzen (1986), using dichotic listening tasks to assess hemispheric specialization, found a positive correlation between the K-ABC simultaneous processing scores and hemispheric specialization for nonverbal processing for 75 children of low SES. Dietzen reported a significant positive relationship between sequential processing on the K-ABC and degree of hemispheric specialization for verbal information in this same sample.

Additional studies have added to our knowledge through the use of physical evidence of neurological damage and relating it to the K-ABC results. Morris and Bigler (1985) investigated whether the K-ABC SEQ and SIM scales can be related to left and right hemisphere functioning and whether the K-ABC is better able to indicate neuropsychological deficits than the WISC-R. In this study, 79 children ages 6 to 12 years were administered the WISC-R, the K-ABC, and several neuropsychological measures of left and right hemisphere functioning. Neurological data, including EEGs and CAT scans, were also available. Neuropsychological test scores were collapsed into two composite scores for each subject, right hemisphere (RH) and left hemisphere (LH). Twenty-five children who were right-handed and neurologically impaired were divided into three groups according to their K-ABC scores: SIM > SEQ, SEQ > SIM, and SIM = SEQ. A one-way MANOVA revealed a significant difference among these groups on the RH and LH scores ($p < 0.05$) but not for WISC-R groups using VIQ–PIQ differences for classification ($p = 0.41$). Further analyses revealed that the key to understanding these differences was the inability of the WISC-R to detect RH dysfunction. Whereas both scales seemed to pick up LH dysfunction, only the K-ABC could diagnose RH problems at a statistically significant level. These results also are consistent with lateralization of sequential and simultaneous processing of the left and right hemispheres, respectively, giving evidence also consistent with the findings of Leark *et al.* (1983).

Shapiro and Dotan (1985) provided a replication along the lines of the Morris and Bigler (1985) study, though their sample size ($N = 27$) makes statistical comparisons less relevant. The pattern of Shapiro and Dotan's results is most interesting, however. These researchers compared two groups of children with neurological impairment defined as focal versus nonfocal on the K-ABC and on the Wechsler scales. All had neurological examinations and most had EEGs or CAT scans or both. Two groups were formed. The nonfocal group was determined to be children with normal examinations with the exception of soft neurological signs that were not unilateral in nature. Most of these 13 children were diagnosed as ADD, LD, BD, or developmentally delayed. The 14 children in the focal group had lateralized deficits on the neurological examination and a focal abnormality on the EEG or structural damage on the CAT scan. The nonfocal group contained 10 males and 3 females (a typical occurrence) and the focal group, 7 males and 7 females. Of particular interest here, Verbal–Performance IQ differences on the Wechsler scales were not related to the presence of focal neurological findings.

> However . . . one finds that of the eight children with significantly lower sequential than simultaneous score, six had predominantly left hemisphere findings. The two children with right-hemisphere findings were non-right-handers. Of the six children with significantly lower simultaneous scores, four showed right hemisphere findings. Of the two with left hemisphere findings, one was left-handed and the other had primarily left occipital findings with some visual impairment. (Shapiro & Dotan, 1985, p. 6)

The K-ABC Simultaneous scale should always show considerable impairment for children with visual problems.

Even with the small sample size available, highly significant ($p < 0.005$) relationships occurred between left-brain focal findings and lower sequential than simultaneous scores and focal right-brain problems and lower simultaneous than sequential scores. Shapiro and Dotan noted that the relationship was stronger for males than for females. They concluded in part that "the lack of relationship of verbal/performance discrepancies on the Wechsler tests to neurological findings may reflect the lack of homogeneity of function in those scales as compared to the K-ABC" (p. 7). These results and the subsequent conclusions are clearly in accordance with the results of Morris and Bigler and the two studies by Telzrow et al.

Taken as a whole, empirical results available thus far are impressive in their support of the potential of the K-ABC in contributing to the tasks of the neuropsychologist. Not only does the K-ABC model appear useful, but the psychometric integrity of the K-ABC lends the scale to other theoretical approaches, thus avoiding the fate of the inadequately developed ITPA. The K-ABC seems to be related, even at this early stage in its career, to neuropsychological functioning both theoretically and empirically. The moderate but consistent relationships with other neuropsychological batteries bode well for its use, indicating that it does provide additional

or at least distinctive information. It also seems more closely related to recent neuropsychological models of higher cognitive processes than the Wechsler series. The Wechsler series is much more researched at this point, however, and we should proceed cautiously with the K-ABC; existing data are very promising and dictate that research should continue full speed ahead.

Research with Pediatric Samples

Recent research has also been done with certain pediatric samples using the K-ABC to differentiate among the cognitive effects of various types of neurologically related pathology, including children with sickle-cell disease and children who were prenatally exposed to alcohol. Brown, Buchanan, et al. (1993) examined the effects on cognitive ability of the various types of sickle-cell disease, as compared with a control group of their healthy siblings. Sickle-cell disease is a chronic, hereditary disease that is most commonly found in African Americans in the United States, with an incidence rate of 1 in about 400 or 500 (Brown, Armstrong, & Eckman, 1993). Three types of sickle-cell disease exist: homozygous HbSS, also known as sickle-cell anemia, in which the child has both abnormal genes for hemoglobin S; heterozygous HbSC, in which the child has one gene for hemoglobin S and hemoglobin C; and heterozygous HbS-thalassemia, in which the child has one gene for hemoglobin S and one gene for thalassemia. In all of these cases, the child actually presents the symptoms of sickle-cell disease, although in HbSS type the symptoms are more severe, more frequent, and may occur earlier (Brown, Armstrong, & Eckman, 1993). A child may also be a carrier of the sickle-cell trait, but may not show symptoms of the disease, and has the genotype of HbSA. Normal children who do not carry the gene for sickle-cell disease have the genotype HbAA (Brown, Buchanan, et al., 1993).

Brown, Buchanan, et al. (1993) hypothesized that children with sickle-cell disease would perform worse on cognitive and achievement measures than their healthy siblings (who were matched on race, SES, sex, and as closely as possible on age), and that children with the homozygous condition (HbSS) should do worse than those with the heterozygous conditions, as all other symptoms showed that pattern. Children selected for the sickle-cell disease group (SCD) had been diagnosed with SCD but had no history of neurological disease and none were on narcotic analgesics, which have been shown to have some effect on reaction time (Brown, Buchanan, et al., 1993). The K-ABC was chosen as the measure of cognitive ability in this study because it is less dependent on prior learning than the Wechsler series and features minimal use of verbal content. This latter feature was particularly critical in this study as most of the children in the sample came from low-SES backgrounds, and it has been demonstrated that low-SES children are at a disadvantage on tests that tap verbal ability (Brown, Buchanan, et al., 1993). The K-ABC Reading Decoding and Arithmetic Achievement subtests were included so that the researchers could see the application of the child's processing skills to complex learning tasks, assess the child's functional academic level, and estimate long-term memory ability. No effect was found for SCD type on cognitive ability or academic achievement in this study. However, hemoglobin level was shown to be a significant predictor of cognitive ability ($R^2 = 0.10, p < 0.03$) and K-ABC Achievement Composite ($R^2 = 0.12, p < 0.04$). As expected, the SCD children showed normal overall cognitive ability, but with specific deficits in sustained attention, concentration, and reading decoding that were not found in their healthy siblings (Brown, Buchanan, et al., 1993). Thus, the K-ABC was useful in identifying cognitive processing problems that were not identified by neurological assessment techniques.

In another study, Coles et al. (1991) compared the cognitive ability and achievement of children who had been prenatally exposed to alcohol with those who had not, using the K-ABC as the criterion measure. The K-ABC was chosen for use with this population because its subtests tap specific cognitive functions in which children with neurological impairment are likely to be deficient, and also because it provides local norms for low-SES children, which comprised the majority of the sample (Coles et al., 1991). Three groups were compared: those whose mothers drank heavily throughout pregnancy, despite an educational intervention during the second trimester; those whose mothers drank heavily through the second trimester but then had stopped for the remainder of the pregnancy; and those whose mothers had abstained from alcohol for the entire pregnancy and did not drink afterwards. The results of this study indicate that both alcohol-exposed groups had significantly lower scores than those who were not exposed, with the "continued to drink" group scoring lowest on all but one subtest. There were significant deficits in sequential processing, achievement, and the Mental Processing Composite in the alcohol-exposed groups, espe-

cially when patterns of current drinking were controlled. Sequential processing was affected more than Simultaneous processing, but the children in the "stopped drinking" group performed about the same as the children in the "never drank" group on sequential processing. The results of this study suggest that children whose mothers continued to drink throughout pregnancy suffer from deficits in short-term memory, or encoding. The crucial brain structure involved in learning and memory, the hippocampus, has been shown to be especially susceptible to the effects of alcohol (e.g., Korsakoff's syndrome, which is a memory deficiency common in people who consume excessive amounts of alcohol). Therefore, third-trimester exposure to alcohol may affect hippocampal development, which may in turn lead to deficits in ability to encode visual or auditory information. The K-ABC achievement tests also indicated that there were significant deficits in math skills and in reading decoding of words and letters in both alcohol-exposed groups, which supports these results. Coles et al. (1991) hypothesize that prenatal alcohol exposure does create deficits in cognitive development and later in academic achievement, but that the children whose mothers stopped drinking in the third trimester may experience a "recovery" in cognitive development and other areas during that time of fetal development. Both of these studies indicate the utility of the K-ABC for use in identifying processing problems in various pediatric samples, but there is much room for future research in this area.

A study by Donders (1992) suggests caution when using the K-ABC as a measure of cerebral impairment. The subjects of this study were 43 consecutive patients at a regional rehabilitation hospital. The children ranged in age from 6 to 12 years and none of them had suffered previous CNS dysfunction or displayed evidence of psychopathology. All children were administered both the K-ABC and WISC-R within a year after their initial injury. The children's initial status in the emergency room was classified as severe (using the Glasgow Coma Scale) in 27 cases and mild in 16 cases. The sample included 32 males and 11 females. In all cases the K-ABC scored slightly higher than the WISC-R. The mean WISC-R FSIQ for the total sample was 89.33 whereas the MPC was 92.88. Based on these findings Donders (1992) concluded that "the K-ABC appears to be no more sensitive to diffuse cerebral impairment than the WISC-R" (p. 228). An alternative interpretation of these results is that the K-ABC is no more sensitive than the WISC-R to the presence of diffuse CNS dysfunction and no less sensitive.

Clinical Neuropsychological Applications of the K-ABC

The general field of clinical neuropsychology is seen by many as a set of tests and related techniques for relating observed, quantifiable behavior to the integrity of an individual's functional neurological organization and structure. The efficacy of these techniques in the diagnosis and remediation of learning disturbances has been well documented over the last decade (e.g., Bradley, Battin, & Sutter, 1979; Gaddes, 1981; Golden, 1978; Hartlage, 1982; Hartlage & Reynolds, 1981; Knight & Bakker, 1980; Reitan & Davison, 1974; Rourke & Orr, 1977; Spreen & Strauss, 1991). It is not surprising, then, that many individuals believe that to become a successfully functioning clinical neuropsychologist, it is only necessary to master the technical skills involved in the administration and scoring of tests like the Halstead–Reitan Neuropsychological Test Battery. Such thinking is a gross oversimplification of the profession and function of clinical neuropsychology.

Much more than being a set of techniques, the principal tool of neuropsychology is the paradigm it offers for viewing and interpreting individual test data. Without the provision of a strong paradigm, clinical neuropsychology could not have progressed to the point of applicability and generalizability that has emerged today. As with other areas and subspecialties of psychology, several competing paradigms and theories exist in clinical neuropsychology, and any one of these may be the most appropriate for interpreting data for any single child (e.g., Ayers, 1974; Das et al., 1979; Luria, 1966; Pribram, 1971; Reynolds, 1981b; Tarnopol & Tarnopol, 1977; Wittrock, 1980). It is thus crucial to achieve an understanding of the various neuropsychological models of higher-order human information processing in order to be effective in translating test results into meaningful educational programs, i.e., teasing out the aptitude × treatment interaction for a single individual. The relationship of the K-ABC to a particular neuropsychological model, Vygotsky's Zones of Proximal Development, will be explored in some detail later in this chapter.

Contemporary neuropsychological theories of the intellect and its function are presented in a number of sources (e.g., Das et al., 1979; Joseph, 1990; Kolb & Whishaw, 1985; Luria, 1966; Pribram, 1971; Reynolds, 1981a; Spreen et al., 1995; Springer & Deutsch, 1989; Wittrock, 1980) and will not be reviewed further here. Well-grounded, empirically evaluated theoretical models of neurological function enable one to make specific predictions about how children will perform under a given set of learning circumstances. Of course, one will not always be correct; but a good theory from which to work allows the psychologist to narrow the number of alternative hypotheses (methods of remediation) considerably. Without a viable set of theories, one would be a completely stimulus-bound technician relying entirely on trial-and-error experience and more or less shooting in the dark whenever encountering a child with a set of behavioral nuances and test scores not previously seen.

The neuropsychological approach proffered here and by the K-ABC generally is one that matches up cognitive neuropsychological strengths with methods of presenting and acquiring information that rely most heavily on these strengths. Neuropsychological strengths in a child's ability spectrum may be in traditional areas of ability like linguistic processing or in a particular cognitive/learning style. Cognitive and/or learning styles are now being more fully explored but seem almost certainly to be tied strongly to the underlying neuropsychological integrity, development, and preferences of the individual (Guyer & Friedman, 1975; Reynolds, 1980, 1981a,b).

Of course, merely detecting cerebral dysfunction (or minimal brain dysfunction or minimal brain damage) is not a very useful exercise from an educational or rehabilitative perspective. It is the accurate description of the dysfunction (an integral part of diagnosis) leading to an educational program to enhance the child's acquisition of skills in a subject matter area that is of significance. The K-ABC and the WISC-III provide excellent instruments for determining a baseline standard of general mental ability against which to compare other, more specific scales, during the process of ipsative test score interpretation. The multidimensional scaling of these tests also makes them amenable to a variety of neuropsychological interpretive strategies (Hartlage, 1982; Kaufman, 1979a) despite the K-ABC's reliance on Luria's approach. As Hartlage (1982) has discussed, one can compare the functional integrity of the left and right temporal lobes through the Similarities versus Picture Arrangement contrast, or left and right parietal lobe function by contrasting the child's performance on Arithmetic and Block Design. Knowing that Arithmetic significantly exceeds Block Design or even that the child's left parietal lobe function presents as superior to right parietal lobe function is of little import in and of itself. Rather, the inferences that can be drawn from such a finding are the important focal point of the evaluation, and can be turned toward the design of educational programs.

Certain cognitive skills tend to cluster together within an individual's overall functional level. Neuropsychological and certain other approaches to assessment allow one to make inferences about skills that have not actually been evaluated by knowing the correlates of these skills. Look–say, whole word, configurational approaches to reading seem to be moderated much more by the posterior right parietal lobe in coordination with sections of the right occipital and temporal lobes than in the left hemisphere counterparts of these structures. Knowing that these structures in the right hemisphere function more effectively (efficiently or at a higher level) thus gives rise to the designation of a method for teaching reading to the child in question that can capitalize on the identified neuropsychological strengths. Additionally, there is no reason why behavioral methods cannot be employed as motivational strategies in such programs. The neuropsychological interpretation of many common psychological tests can generate good hypotheses for choosing a particular method of instruction, and operant psychology or one of its variants can assist in promoting the student's interest in and learning through the specified method.

The K-ABC, designed with such approaches in mind, *a priori*, should help in such models. It can also offer information on the intact nature of a variety of processes for young children that are poorly tapped by most existing scales. Extensions of tasks such as Hand Movements, Word Order, and Spatial Memory can be useful tools rather than methods of testing. Attention seems to be to the area of cognitive rehabilitation of deficit skills most influenced by cognitive retraining and such an addition of teaching tasks can prove useful. The K-ABC is a nice fit to Reynolds's (1981b) approach, an approach that has been elaborated and integrated with cognitive and behavioral models (Reynolds, 1986).

Vygotsky's Zones of Proximal Development

Vygotsky (translation, 1978) has offered another neuropsychologically related concept that may be amenable to assessment with the K-ABC, with some modification in the standardized administration procedures. Vygotsky espoused what continues to be a widely held "truth" even today as regards children's learning. "A well known and empirically established fact is that learning should be matched in some manner with the child's developmental level" (Vygotsky, 1978, p. 85). Hunt (1961) in his now-classic volume concurred and conceptualized this concept in part as the "problem of the match." Although true for normally developing children, such a match may be absolutely crucial for promoting the development of children with an immature or traumatized central nervous system.

In formulating the concept of zones of proximal development (ZPD), Vygotsky rejected what he considered to be the three primary alternative developmental theories of learning (learning broadly defined, as it should be, and not restricted to school learning). The first rejected theory centers on the assumption that processes of child development are independent of learning, which is considered an external process, not an activity involved in development. Accordingly, learning uses the achievements of development in acquisition of new knowledge rather than providing impetus for modifying the course of development. Vygotsky classified Piagetian theory under this theoretical rubric. The second rejected approach are theories assuming that learning *is* development, approaches that reduce development to a simple accumulation of all possible responses by the child. The third rejected theoretical proposition is based on a combination of the two prior positions, in which development is based on two different but related processes, maturation, which depends on the development of the central nervous system, and learning, also considered here as a developmental process. In this apparently reciprocal relationship, maturation makes new learning possible, which then stimulates and pushes forward the maturation process. The latter is the approach that led educators in the past to conclude that the study of certain subjects (e.g., Latin) was of great value for mental development. Vygotsky framed the concepts of ZPD to provide a more adequate view of the relationship between learning and development. This concept can lead us to better cognitive retraining and rehabilitation programs for children who have resisted more traditional approaches.

In determining and using ZPDs, two developmental levels must first be established. The first is the child's current, *actual level of development.* Vygotsky viewed this level as that already completed as a level determined by rigidly administered, standardized measures of intelligence and achievement. It is the level determined by what children can do on their own. The second level of development to determine is the level the child can achieve if an adult or more advanced, accomplished peer provides help through demonstration, asking leading questions, or actual collaboration leading the child to discover the answer. It is the difference between these two levels that is important to use here, and that difference is the ZPD. ZPD is "the distance between actual developmental level as determined by independent problem solving and the level of potential development as determined through problem solving under adult guidance or in collaboration" (Vygotsky, 1978, p. 86). The upper limit of the ZPD today becomes the actual developmental level of tomorrow. The fundamental principles of ZPD are the basis for the approaches taken by Feuerstein, Haywood, Campione, and others to cognitive assessment and cognitive training though some key differences exist (see Reynolds, 1986, for a brief review).

In neuropsychological work in particular, it can be of help to apply this principle in rehabilitation efforts and the K-ABC is structured in such a way as to give the best available assessment of the ZPD. Typically, the ZPD is determined by contrasting scores on the same test under standardized versus nonstandardized limit-testing procedures. The requirement of initial testing under standardized procedures confounds the latter. The use of two different tests is confounded by differences in normative samples and other technical differences between the scales (e.g., see Reynolds, 1984, 1986, for discussions of these problems). The structure of the K-ABC offers a good solution to these problems.

The first developmental level, independent problem solving, can be determined from administration of the K-ABC Achievement scale or preferably from the more restricted Verbal Intelligence scale described in the text *Clinical and Research Applications of the K-ABC* (Kamphaus & Reynolds, 1987), the latter being more appropriate in this instance because it does invoke considerable reasoning skills and is so much akin to Cattell's concept of crystallized intelligence. The second level of development can be ascertained perhaps more accurately with the K-ABC Mental Processing scales than with any other currently available technique, but only through the use of a nonstandard administration.

To assess the second developmental level, administer the K-ABC mental processing subtests using the following procedures:

1. Begin all children with the sample item just as directed for the standardized administration.
2. Use the teaching item of the K-ABC as instructed with the following exception: If the child determines the solution to the problem with help or simple repetition, then give credit for successful completion of the item. If you must give the child the correct answer rather than lead him or her to develop a correct response, do not assign passing credit. Under these conditions it is permissible to give strategies and practice trials on subtests that are heavily memory dependent such as Hand Movements or Number Recall.
3. After the sample and teaching items, continue to use the teaching procedures whenever a child misses an item when administered under standardized conditions. Give credit for the item as above, i.e., whenever you can lead the child to the correct response, but do not assign credit when you must demonstrate or recite the correct response.
4. Continue administration of each subtest until the child fails to obtain credit on two consecutive items (a ceiling we have estimated to be appropriate based on the growth curves of the various mental processing subtests and the length of time available for testing) *when assistance has been provided by the examiner.*
5. Compute the raw and scaled scores for the mental processing subtests and the MPC just as though a standardized administration had been conducted.

This procedure obviously does not allow one to report standard scores for the MPC or other K-ABC mental processing scales. The Verbal Intelligence scale (Kamphaus & Reynolds, 1987) or Achievement scale can be reported as needed, however. The difference between the MPC, as derived above, and the Verbal or Achievement scale approximates the child's ZPD, and is thus easily quantified for research purposes. On a more practical level, it provides relatively clear guidance in developing short-term and intermediate goals for cognitive rehabilitation programs. The next step in the developmental process is revealed through assessment of the ZPD, the near point in development. In cognitive retraining it is certainly important to know which skills are most likely to be responsive to rehabilitation efforts at specific points on the retraining process. Again the ZPD provides clues. Individual subtests as well as subscales of the MPC can be contrasted with the regularly obtained Verbal Intelligence Composite or Achievement scale score to ascertain areas needing greater attention or even in the evaluation process to determine what progress has been made and in what areas. Given the uneven nature of progress in development and cognitive rehabilitation, the latter can be useful in determining where next to focus rehabilitative efforts.

This assessment can be repeated periodically as well. By this conceptualization, we are constantly seeking to move children forward to a level that is within their reach by constantly reassessing the child's reach so that we continue the "match" (à la Hunt, 1961) between development and learning. This can be a useful guide for learning-disabled children and mentally retarded children as well and is certainly not restricted to children with neuropsychological problems, and is an approach that seems, at least at this stage, similar to approaches proposed by Haywood and Switzky (1986) (but see also Reynolds, 1986).

Implications for Educational Rehabilitation

One of the goals for the K-ABC was to develop a children's intelligence test that yields scores that can provide guidance to educational interventions (Kaufman & Kaufman, 1983b). Chapter 7 of the *K-ABC Interpretive Manual* provides a framework for educational intervention.

The Kaufmans support a strength model of remediation as opposed to deficit-centered ability training models (approaches focusing on the remediation of underlying cognitive processing deficiencies rather than the specific behavioral deficit), which have permeated much of past and present special education practice. Findings in neurology, genetics, and related areas have repeatedly suggested major limitations of the deficit model (e.g., Adams & Victor, 1977; Hartlage, 1975; Hartlage & Givens, 1981; Hartlage & Hartlage, 1973a,b, 1978). Viewed from contemporary neuropsychological models, the deficit approach to remediation is doomed to failure, as it takes damaged or dysfunctional areas of the brain and focuses training specifically on these areas. Not only does knowledge of neurology predict failure for such efforts (Kolb & Whishaw, 1985), but evaluations of these approaches have also found them to be quite ineffectual in the remediation of learning problems

(e.g., Glass & Robbins, 1967; Levine, Brooks, & Shonkoff, 1980). One need not embrace localizationist approaches to the diagnosis and descriptive etiology of learning problems, however, in order to employ the neuropsychological model. Most current neuropsychological models do not subscribe to strict localizationist approaches, but rather employ dynamic localization concepts similar to that of Luria (1966, 1970). The paramount discovery thus far, however, is that deficit approaches to remediation do not seem to be very effective. Such approaches have been criticized as being potentially harmful to the child as well (Hartlage & Reynolds, 1981).

A more meaningful, efficacious approach to a child's learning problems is provided by adopting a strength model of remediation. The strength model is based on abilities that are sufficiently intact so as to subserve the successful accomplishment of the steps in the educational program, so that the interface between cognitive strengths (rather than weaknesses) determined from the assessment and the intervention strategy is the cornerstone of meaningfulness for the entire diagnostic-intervention process. Placed in the language of Luria's neuropsychological model of intelligence, it is necessary to locate an intact complex functional system capable of taking over and moderating the learning process needed to acquire the academic skills in question.

The K-ABC philosophy is reflected in the attitude that the best remedial program for a child who cannot read is to teach the child to read, but to do so using methods and materials optimally related to the child's best information-processing skills. The focus is clearly on direct instruction in the child's area of academic deficit allowing children to exploit their preference for processing in a particular way. The structure of the K-ABC provides theoretical guidance to this admittedly muddy area of educational research and practice, guidance that is sorely needed (see Reynolds, 1981b), and guidance that is focused on instruction, not peripheral activities.

The K-ABC provides a clear model for using neuropsychological data and theories to make inferences regarding important aptitudes for the individual learner. A model for matching neuropsychological aptitudes to treatment approaches that is nicely complemented by the K-ABC has been presented by Hartlage and Telzrow (1983). Their model teaches "circumvention" of dysfunctional areas of the brain to develop compensatory (not remedial) skills and then to capitalize on the child's strengths. Hartlage and Telzrow's approach is very much in line with the K-ABC philosophy and may be useful particularly to the neuropsychologist in designing rehabilitation approaches from K-ABC results, thus expanding the potential utility of the K-ABC in clinical application in neuropsychology.

While the K-ABC approach to remediation is congruent with other intuitively appealing models, a caveat is in order. Much of the work on so-called "strength" models of remediation is theoretical rather than empirical. This state of affairs is not surprising given the nature of remediation research which is laborious and difficult to conduct with adequate controls. At this point some small-scale studies, essentially pilot in nature, support the strength model (Kaufman & Kaufman, 1983b) while a recent study of six children does not (Good, Vollmer, Creek, Katz, & Chowdhri, 1993). These findings leave the clinician to his or her own devices when designing intervention plans based wholly or in part on K-ABC results, and the resulting effectiveness of such plans depends largely on the clinician's acumen as opposed to science.

Summary

We have much to learn about the neurological substrates that underlie performance on the K-ABC. Yet research thus far suggests that there is a great deal of support for the continued use and exploration of the K-ABC as a tool in the neuropsychological and educational assessment of children. Very much remains to be done. The results of the studies available to date suggest that the K-ABC will continue to show evidence of utility in helping neuropsychologists gain a better picture of children's brain–behavior relationships, leading to improved rehabilitation programs. We must, of course, keep in mind the tenuous nature of localization in the $2\frac{1}{2}$- to $12\frac{1}{2}$-year-old group, the age group addressed by the K-ABC, but also one of the most perplexing and demanding age groups of all those encountered by the clinical neuropsychologist. The K-ABC is particularly interesting in the evaluation of school-age children with learning disabilities, a majority of whom demonstrate special problems with memory and sequential recall (see also Reynolds & Bigler, 1993), and come to the attention of the neuropsychologist.

References

Adams, K. (1985). Review of the Luria–Nebraska Neuropsychological Battery. In J. V. Mitchell (Ed.), *Ninth mental measurement yearbook.* Lincoln, NE: Buros Institute of Mental Measurements.

Adams, R. D., & Victor, M. (1977). *Principles of neurology.* New York: McGraw–Hill.

Allen, M. H., Lincoln, A. J., & Kaufman, A. S. (1991). Sequential and simultaneous processing abilities of high-functioning autistic and language impaired children. *Journal of Autism and Developmental Disorders, 21,* 483–502.

Ardila, A., Roselli, M., & Puente, A. (1994). *Neuropsychological evaluation of the Spanish speaker.* New York: Plenum Press.

Ayers, A. J. (1974). *Sensory integration and learning disorders.* Los Angeles: Western Psychological Services.

Bever, T. G. (1975). Cerebral asymmetries in humans are due to the differentiation of two incompatible processes: Holistic and analytic. In D. Aaronson & R. Reiber (Eds.), *Developmental psycholinguistics and communication disorders.* New York: New York Academy of Sciences.

Bogen, J. E. (1969). The other side of the brain: Parts I, II, and III. *Bulletin of the Los Angeles Neurological Society, 34,* 73–105, 135–162, 191–203.

Bogen, J. E., Dezure, R., Tenhouten, W., & Marsh, J. (1972). The other side of the brain, IV. *Bulletin of the Los Angeles Neurological Society, 37,* 49–61.

Bradley, P. E., Battin, R. R., & Sutter, E. G. (1979). Effects of individual diagnosis and remediation for treatment of learning disabilities. *Clinical Neuropsychology, 1,* 25–31.

Brown, J. W., & Hécaen, H. (1976). Lateralization and language presentation. *Neurology, 26,* 183–189.

Brown, R. T., Armstrong, F. D., & Eckman, J. R. (1993). Neurocognitive aspects of pediatric sickle cell disease. *Journal of Learning Disabilities, 26*(1), 33–45.

Brown, R. T., Buchanan, I., Doepke, K., Eckman, J. R., Baldwin, K., Goonan, B., & Schoenherr, S. (1993). Cognitive and academic functioning in children with sickle cell disease. *Journal of Clinical Child Psychology, 22*(2), 207–218.

Coles, C. D., Brown, R. T., Smith, I. E., Platzman, K. A., Erickson, S., & Falek, A. (1991). Effects of prenatal alcohol exposure at school age: I.) Physical and cognitive development. *Neurotoxicology & Toxicology, 13,* 1–11.

Cummins, J., & Das, J. P. (1977). Cognitive processing and reading difficulties: A framework for research. *Alberta Journal of Educational Research, 23,* 245–256.

Das, J. P., Kirby, J. R., & Jarman, R. F. (1979). *Simultaneous and successive cognitive processes.* New York: Academic Press.

Dean, R. S. (1984). Functional lateralization of the brain. *Journal of Special Education, 8,* 239–256.

Dietzen, S. R. (1986). *Hemispheric specialization for verbal sequential and non-verbal simultaneous information processing styles of low income 3 to 5 years olds.* Doctoral dissertation, Washington State University.

Donders, J. (1992). Validity of the Kaufman Assessment Battery for Children when employed with children with traumatic brain injury. *Journal of Clinical Psychology, 48,* 225–229.

Fan, X., Willson, V. L., & Reynolds, C. R. (in press). Assessing the similarity of the construct structure of the K-ABC for black and white children from 7 to $12\frac{1}{2}$ years in age. *Journal of Psychoeducational Assessment.*

Gaddes, W. H. (1981). An examination of the validity of neuro-psychological knowledge in educational diagnosis and remediation. In G. W. Hynd & J. E. Obrzut (Eds.), *Neuropsychological assessment of the school-aged child: Issues and procedures.* New York: Grune & Stratton.

Gazzaniga, M. S. (1970). *The bisected brain.* Englewood Cliffs, NJ: Prentice–Hall.

Gazzaniga, M. S. (1974). Cerebral dominance viewed as a decision system. In S. Dimond & J. Beaumont (Eds.), *Hemisphere functions in the human brain.* London: Halstead Press.

Gazzaniga, M. S. (1975). Recent research on hemispheric lateralization of the human brain: Review of the split brain. *UCLA Educator, 17,* 9–12.

Glass, G. F., & Robbins, M. P. (1967). A critique of experiments on the role of neurological organization in reading performance. *Reading Research Quarterly, 3,* 5–52.

Golden, C. J. (1978). *Diagnosis and rehabilitation in clinical neuropsychology.* Springfield, IL: Thomas.

Good, R. H., Vollmer, M., Creek, R. J., Katz, L., & Chowdhri, S. (1993). Treatment utility of the Kaufman Assessment Battery for Children: Effects of matching instruction and student processing strength. *School Psychology Review, 22,* 8–26.

Guyer, B. L., & Friedman, M. P. (1975). Hemispheric processing and cognitive styles in learning disabled and normal children. *Child Development, 46,* 658–668.

Harnad, S., Doty, R. W., Goldstein, L., Jaynes, J., & Krauthamer, G. (Eds.). (1977). *Lateralization in the nervous system.* New York: Academic Press.

Hartlage, L. C. (1975). Neuropsychological approaches to predicting outcome of remedial educational strategies for learning disabled children. *Pediatric Psychology, 3,* 23–28.

Hartlage, L. C. (1982). Neuropsychological assessment techniques. In C. R. Reynolds & T. B. Gutkin (Eds.), *The handbook of school psychology.* New York: Wiley.

Hartlage, L. C., & Reynolds, C. R. (1981). Neuropsychological assessment and the individualization of instruction. In G. W. Hynd & J. E. Obrzut (Eds.), *Neuropsychological assessment of the school-aged child: Issues and procedures.* New York: Grune & Stratton.

Hartlage, L. C., & Telzrow, C. F. (1983). The neuropsychological basis of educational intervention. *Journal of Learning Disabilities, 16,* 521–528.

Hartlage, P. L., & Givens, T. S. (1981). Common neurological problems of school age children. In C. R. Reynolds & T. B. Gutkin (Eds.), *The handbook of school psychology.* New York: Wiley.

Hartlage, P. L., & Hartlage, L. C. (1973a). Comparison of hyperlexic and dyslexic children. *Neurology, 23,* 436–437.

Hartlage, P. L., & Hartlage, L. C. (1973b). *Dermatoglyphic markers in dyslexia.* Paper presented at the meeting of the Child Neurology Society, Nashville.

Hartlage, P. L., & Hartlage, L. C. (1978). Clinical consultation to pediatric neurology and developmental pediatrics. *Journal of Clinical Child Psychology, 12,* 52–53.

Haywood, H. C., & Switzky, H. N. (1986). The malleability of intelligence: Cognitive process as a function of polygenic–experiential interaction. *School Psychology Review, 15,* 245–255.

Hooper, S. R., & Hynd, G. W. (1985). Differential diagnosis of subtypes of developmental dyslexia with the Kaufman Assessment Battery for Children (K-ABC). *Journal of Clinical Child Psychology, 14,* 145–152.

Hunt, J. M. (1961). *Intelligence and experience.* New York: Ronald Press.

Ishikuma, T., Moon, S., & Kaufman, A. S. (1988). Sequential–simultaneous analysis of Japanese children's performance on the Japanese McCarthy scales. *Perceptual and Motor Skills, 66,* 355–362.

Joseph, R. (1990). *Neuropsychology, neuropsychiatry, and behavioral neurology.* New York: Plenum Press.

Kamphaus, R. W., & Reynolds, C. R. (1987). *Clinical and research applications of the K-ABC.* Circle Pines, MN: American Guidance Service.

Kaufman, A. S. (1979a). *Intelligent testing with the WISC-R.* New York: Wiley–Interscience.

Kaufman, A. S. (1979b). Cerebral specialization and intelligence testing. *Journal of Research and Development in Education, 12,* 96–197.

Kaufman, A. S. (1984). K-ABC and controversy. *Journal of Special Education, 18*(3), 409–444.

Kaufman, A. S., & Applegate, B. (1988). Short forms of the K-ABC mental processing and achievement scales at ages 4 to 12½ years for clinical and screening purposes. *Journal of Clinical Child Psychology, 17,* 359–369.

Kaufman, A. S., Eller, B. F., & Applegate, B. (1990). An investigation of somatic anxiety and intelligence in children using the Kaufman-ABC and Apple IIe program measuring heart rate. *Perceptual and Motor Skills, 70,* 387–394.

Kaufman, A. S., Grossman, I., & Kaufman, N. L. (1994). Comparison of hospitalized depressed patients and matched normal controls on tests that differ in their level of cognitive complexity. *Journal of Psychoeducational Assessment, 12,* 112–125.

Kaufman, A. S., Kamphaus, R. W., & Kaufman, N. L. (1985). The Kaufman Assessment Battery for Children (K-ABC). In C. S. Newark (Ed.), *Major psychological assessment instruments.* Boston: Allyn & Bacon.

Kaufman, A. S., & Kaufman, N. L. (1983a). *Kaufman Assessment Battery for Children (K-ABC) administration and scoring manual.* Circle Pines, MN: American Guidance Service.

Kaufman, A. S., & Kaufman, N. L. (1983b). *K-ABC interpretive manual.* Circle Pines, MN: American Guidance Service.

Kinsbourne, M. (1975). Cerebral dominance, learning, and cognition. In H. R. Myklebust (Ed.), *Progress in learning disabilities.* New York: Grune & Stratton.

Kinsbourne, M. (1978). Biological determinants of functional bisymmetry and asymmetry. In M. Kinsbourne (Ed.), *Progress in learning disabilities.* New York: Grune & Stratton.

Knight, R. M., & Bakker, D. J. (1980). *Treatment of hyperactive and learning disordered children: Current research.* Baltimore: University Park Press.

Kolb, B., & Whishaw, I. Q. (1985). *Fundamentals of human neuropsychology* (2nd ed.). San Francisco: Freeman.

Leark, R. A., Snyder, T., Grove, T., & Golden, C. J. (1983, August). *Comparison of the K-ABC and standardized neuropsychological batteries: Preliminary results.* Paper presented at the annual meeting of the American Psychological Association, Anaheim, CA.

Levine, M. D., Brooks, R., & Shonkoff, J. P. (1980). *A pediatric approach to learning disorders.* New York: Wiley.

Luria, A. R. (1966). *Human brain and psychological processes.* New York: Harper & Row.

Luria, A. R. (1970). The functional organization of the brain. *Scientific American, 18,* 266–268.

Majovski, L. V. (1984). The K-ABC: Theory and applications for child neuropsychological assessment and research. *Journal of Special Education, 18,* 266–268.

Mardell-Czudnowski, C. (1995). Performance of Asian and white children on the K-ABC: Understanding information processing differences. *Assessment, 2,* 19–29.

Morris, J. M., & Bigler, E. (1985, January). *An investigation of the Kaufman Assessment Battery for Children (K-ABC) with neurologically impaired children.* Paper presented at the annual meeting of the International Neuropsychological Society, San Diego.

Nebes, R. D. (1974). Hemispheric specialization in commissurotomized man. *Psychological Bulletin, 81*(1), 1–14.

Neisser, V. (1967). *Cognitive psychology.* New York: Appleton-Century-Crofts.

Obrzut, J. E. (1991). Hemispheric activation and arousal asymmetry in learning disabled children. In J. Obrzut & G. Hynd (Eds.), *Neuropsychological foundations of learning disabilities.* (pp. 179–198). New York: Academic Press.

Ornstein, R., Johnstone, J. Herron, J., & Swencionis, C. (1980). Differential right hemisphere engagement in visuospatial tasks. *Neuropsychologia, 18,* 49–64.

Pribram, K. (1971). *Languages of the brain.* Englewood Cliffs, NJ: Prentice-Hall.

Reitan, R., & Davison, L. A. (1974). *Clinical neuropsychology: Current status and applications.* Washington, DC: Winston.

Reynolds, C. R. (1980, July). *The neuropsychological basis of intelligence and a reconceptualization of dominance.* Invited address to the Utah State University Conference on Brain Research and Teaching, Logan.

Reynolds, C. R. (1981a). The neuropsychological basis of intelligence. In G. Hynd & J. Obrzut (Eds.), *Neuropsychological assessment and the school-aged child: Issues and procedures.* (pp. 87–124). New York: Grune & Stratton.

Reynolds, C. R. (1981b). Neuropsychological assessment and the habilitation of learning: Considerations in the search for the aptitude × treatment interaction. *School Psychology Review, 10,* 343–349.

Reynolds, C. R. (1984). Critical measurement issues in learning disabilities. *Journal of Special Education, 18,* 451–476.

Reynolds, C. R. (1986). Transactional models of intellectual development, yes. Deficit models of process remediation, no. *School Psychology Review, 15,* 256–260.

Reynolds, C. R., & Bigler, E. D. (1993). *Manual for the Test of Memory and Learning.* Austin, TX: PRO-ED.

Rourke, B. P., & Orr, R. R. (1977). Prediction of the reading and spelling performances of normal and retarded readers: A four-age follow-up. *Journal of Abnormal Child Psychology, 5,* 9–20.

Schwartz, G. E., Davidson, R. J., & Mear, F. (1975). Right hemisphere lateralization for emotion in the human brain: Interactions with cognition. *Science, 190,* 286–288.

Sechenov, I. (1965). *Reflexes of the brain.* Cambridge, MA: MIT Press. (Original work published in 1863.)

Segalowitz, S. J., & Gruber, F. A. (Eds.). (1977). *Language development and neurological theory.* New York: Academic Press.

Shapiro, E. G., & Dotan, N. (1985, October). *Neurological findings and the Kaufman Assessment Battery for Children.* Paper presented at the National Association of Neuropsychologists, Philadelphia.

Shure, G. H., & Halstead, W. C. (1959). Cerebral lateralization of individual processes. *Psychological Monographs: General and Applied, 72*(12).

Snyder, T. J., Leark, R. A., Golden, C. J., Grove, T., & Allison, R. (1983, March). *Correlations of the K-ABC, WISC-R, and Luria–Nebraska Children's Battery for exceptional children.* Paper presented at the meeting of the National Association of School Psychologists, Detroit.

Sperry, R. W. (1968). Hemisphere deconnection and unity in conscious awareness. *American Psychologist, 23,* 723–733.

Sperry, R. W. (1974). Lateral specialization in the surgically separated hemispheres. In F. O. Schmitt & F. G. Worden (Eds.), *The neurosciences: Third study program.* Cambridge, MA: MIT Press.

Sperry, R. W., Gazzaniga, M. S., & Bogen, J. E. (1969). Interhemispheric relationships: The neocortical commissures: Syndromes of hemispheric disconnection. In R. Vinken & G. W. Beuyn (Eds.), *Handbook of clinical neurology.* New York: Wiley–Interscience.

Spreen, O., Risser, A. H., & Edgell, D. (1995). *Developmental neuropsychology.* London: Oxford University Press.

Spreen, O., & Strauss, E. (1991). *A compendium of neuropsychological tests.* London: Oxford University Press.

Springer, S., & Deutsch, G. (1989). *Left brain, right brain.* New York: Wilt Freeman.

Tarnopol, L., & Tarnopol, M. (1977). Introduction to neuropsychology. In L. Tarnopol & M. Tarnopol (Eds.), *Brain function and reading disabilities.* Baltimore: University Park Press.

Telzrow, C. F., Century, E., Harris, B., & Redmond, C. (1985, April). *Relationship between neuropsychological processing models and dyslexia subtypes.* Paper presented at the National Association of School Psychologists, Las Vegas.

Telzrow, C., Redmond, C., & Zimmerman, B. (1984, October). *Dyslexic subtypes: A comparison of the Bannatyne, Boder, and Kaufman models.* Paper presented at the annual meeting of the National Academy of Neuropsychologists, San Diego.

Tomlinson-Keasey, C., & Clarkson-Smith, L. (1980, February). *What develops in hemispheric specialization?* Paper presented at the meeting of the International Neuropsychological Society, San Francisco.

Vygotsky, L. S. (1978). *Mind in society* (M. Cole, V. John-Steiner, S. Scribner, & E. Souberman, Eds.). Cambridge, MA: Harvard University Press.

Wada, J., Clarke R., & Hamme, A. (1975). Cerebral hemisphere asymmetry in humans. *Archives of Neurology, 37,* 234–246.

Wechsler, D. (1989). *Wechsler Preschool and Primary Scale of Intelligence-Revised.* San Antonio, TX: The Psychological Corporation.

Wittrock, M. C. (1980). *The brain and psychology.* New York: Academic Press.

14

Utilizing a Neuropsychological Paradigm for Understanding Common Educational and Psychological Tests

RIK CARL D'AMATO, BARBARA A. ROTHLISBERG,
AND ROBERT L. RHODES

The field of psychology has long been marked by philosophical diversity and theoretical movements devoted to the investigation of individual differences (D'Amato & Rothlisberg, 1992). Scores of single paradigm assessment approaches designed to provide appropriate diagnosis and treatment of individual difficulties have come to the forefront, only to be eclipsed later by rival viewpoints or theoretical perspectives (e.g., psychoanalysis, behaviorism). Throughout this procession of philosophies and theories, countless numbers of educational and psychological tests have been administered and interpreted in an effort to better understand the abilities and needs of the individuals in question. The purpose of this chapter is to help consolidate available information and provide an integrative approach to the neuropsychological interpretation of common measures.

This chapter is designed to be of special assistance to practitioners who work with children and young adults and who, perhaps more than any other

members of the field, have seen the greatest amount of emphasis placed on the assessment of individual differences. Currently, over 4,300,000 children living within the United States have been referred, assessed, and placed into special education programs. Of these children, more than half receive services as a result of a learning disability or other concern related to an inability to profit from instruction (U.S. Department of Education, 1993). This staggering number of children bring with them the myriad possibilities of potential hypotheses regarding the etiology and prognosis of their individual conditions.

As assessment specialists, psychologists must quickly and accurately wade through the cumulative data available about the child in order to select the most viable of alternative hypotheses to explain the findings. The strategy the practitioner uses to accomplish this task must, of necessity, be based on well-grounded, empirically validated theories of behavior. Only through the use of a theoretical framework are specific predictions regarding performance under a given set of ecological circumstances made possible (Dean, 1985a,b, 1986a; Rothlisberg, 1992). Unfortunately, no single diagnostic paradigm or theory has proven sufficient to fully explain the vagaries of behavior (D'Amato & Rothlisberg, 1992). Psychoanalytically, behaviorally, and biologically based as well as other theoretical positions have been continually challenged not only to describe behavior, but also to provide

RIK CARL D'AMATO • Division of Professional Psychology, University of Northern Colorado, Greeley, Colorado 80639-0001. BARBARA A. ROTHLISBERG • Department of Educational Psychology, Ball State University, Muncie, Indiana 47306. ROBERT L. RHODES • School Psychology Program, Special Education/Communication Disorders Department, New Mexico State University, Las Cruces, New Mexico 88003-8001.

effective interventions for the population whom they serve (D'Amato & Dean, 1989b; Gutkin & Reynolds, 1990). Prepackaged programs dealing with psycholinguistic or visual–motor training, and sensory integration have typically failed to meet the demands of this challenge. Gradually, the field has acknowledged that the effective use of assessment procedures is reliant on a theoretical foundation that allows the incorporation of information from multiple data sources and environments in such a manner as to increase the amount of effective and appropriate interventions generated.

Why Consider a Neuropsychological Perspective?

Neuropsychology represents a view thought to be important for assessment, pedagogy, and the development of intervention-related hypotheses (Hartlage & Telzrow, 1986; Whitten, D'Amato, & Chittooran, 1992). Serving as a conscious and continuing attempt to look both inward, at the brain, and outward, at behavior, it is the goal of neuropsychology to integrate both the biological and social/behavioral aspects of functioning (Lezak, 1983; Reitan, 1989).

Numerous authors have advocated for a neuropsychological interpretation of traditional assessment measures (e.g., Chittooran, D'Amato, Lassiter, & Dean, 1993; D'Amato, Gray, & Dean, 1988), with many arguing that school psychologists should receive training in neuropsychology (D'Amato, Hammons, Terminie, & Dean, 1992). A major impetus behind this approach is the number of children with learning problems, as well as behavior problems, who have been found to have some degree of cerebral impairment (D'Amato, Dean, Rattan, & Nickell, 1988; Gaddes & Edgell, 1994; Selz & Wilson, 1989). A neuropsychological view of data allows for the consideration of a wider spectrum of functions and has been shown to improve the differential diagnosis of learning problems both between and within groups of students (D'Amato & Dean, 1988; Das, Naglieri, & Kirby, 1994; Hynd & Obrzut, 1981). Of particular utility is the amount of information generated regarding the neuropsychological functions on which learning is predicated (e.g., sensory perceptions, motor functions). Overall, it appears that the information provided by a neuropsychological perspective facilitates a better understanding of etiology, which, in turn, may result in

an increased ability to rehabilitate existing problems, or prevent future difficulties (Dean, 1985a, 1986a,b; Whitten et al., 1992).

It is important to note that many of the measures routinely administered by psychologists (e.g., Wechsler Intelligence Scales, Minnesota Multiphasic Personality Inventory 2) are included as part of the neuropsychological examination (Kelly & Dean, 1990). The neuropsychological interpretation of these measures may differ greatly, however, from the traditional psychological interpretation of performance. More specifically, the neuropsychological interpretation of these measures is based on research that has examined the relation of the specific test utilized and the functional integrity of the brain, rather than on research that has focused on school-based outcomes (Dean, 1979, 1986c; Jortner, 1965).

Approaches to Neuropsychological Assessment

The field of neuropsychology began with a focus on adults with brain damage and the intriguing relation between site of damage and behavioral outcome (Dean, 1985a, 1986a,c). With this in mind, a considerable data base developed relating specific tests or procedures to areas of cerebral damage in adults. The emphasis was often on localization, lateralization, and lesion detection. Not surprisingly then, while neuropsychologists have become experts in studying relations between damaged areas of the mature brain and overt behavior, the educational relevance of how to teach individuals with brain damage has not been well understood, particularly among children (D'Amato, 1990; D'Amato & Dean, 1987; D'Amato & Rothlisberg, 1996; Telzrow, 1990). This relates to the fact that many tests and procedures are simply downward extensions of adult batteries, with little relevance offered for the educational enterprise, and with little acknowledgment given to the developmental variations seen in the immature nervous system. Indeed, the developmental aspects of brain injury are only now becoming clear, increasing the complexity of the evaluation process and leading to a new view of educational and psychological testing. Thus, the thrust of this chapter will be to address commonly used educational and psychological instruments from a neuropsychological perspective and focus on those tests or assessment areas that hold the greatest promise for intervention (D'Amato, 1990;

D'Amato & Rothlisberg, 1996; Rothlisberg, 1987; Telzrow, 1986).

Quantitative Standardized Approaches

Like psychology in general, assessment techniques and related methods have reflected different psychological paradigms (D'Amato & Rothlisberg, 1992). In Britain and North America, the most popular approach to neuropsychological assessment has been a standardized battery-based quantitative approach that offers data-based psychometric scores used to make actuarial predictions (Dean, 1986a; Kelly & Dean, 1990). This atheoretical approach stresses short-term client involvement, where deficits are measured accurately with structured assessment techniques (Reitan, 1989). Thus, clinicians carefully consider a variety of scores that are viewed as products (like summative scores), as opposed to a focus on the process. The assemblage of standardized tests is generally held constant for everyone, to evaluate a set variety of functions for all individuals. If ten brain functions are deemed important, then all patients would be tested with a core standardized battery that covers those ten primary areas.

Practitioners from the quantitative camp who have administered an invariant battery to all of their patients have developed an impressive data base and have become experts in evaluating the meaning of those tests. A typical battery with a strong educational focus may include the Bender Visual–Motor Gestalt Test, the Wechsler Intelligence Scale for Children-III (WISC-III), the Woodcock–Johnson Achievement Battery, a finger tapping test, a grip strength test, a parent behavior rating scale, a teacher behavior rating scale, a self-report personality measure, a memory test, a review of school records, and a clinical interview. Some comprehensive neuropsychological batteries like the Halstead–Reitan Neuropsychological Test Battery also fall under this quantitative paradigm. This systematic method of data collection is consistent with most batteries of tests used by psychologists in the public schools. In fact, some public laws require that areas like intelligence, achievement, and processing skills be evaluated, parents be interviewed, and students be observed in school, if students are to receive special services like those offered for children with learning disabilities or traumatic brain injuries (D'Amato & Rothlisberg, 1996).

Unfortunately, one obvious difficulty with this approach relates to the cost-effectiveness of such a system. Although a certain number of functions need to be evaluated with everyone, rarely do practitioners have the time to evaluate areas that do not appear compromised. The quantitative approach also has been criticized for its emphasis on differential diagnosis, its easy link to localization of cerebral dysfunction, its product orientation, and its lack of utility in linking assessment data to intervention development (D'Amato, 1990). The strength most evident from this view relates to the impressive standardized and normative foundation that many of the tests used in this area enjoy.

Qualitative Clinical Approaches

In an attempt to evaluate people in an individualized fashion, Luria and his colleagues (Luria, 1966, 1970; Luria & Majovski, 1977) offered a qualitative approach to neuropsychological assessment focusing on the clinical interaction and process to provide a comprehensive understanding of the individual. Here, each student is uniquely evaluated with a comprehensive set of what the untrained eye has seen as informal, clinical measures. Luria (1966, 1973) organized a dynamic, interactive assessment process that culminates in an understanding of the patient's functional systems. The qualitative approach has been popular in European and Asian countries (Kelly & Dean, 1990). This approach utilizes extensive long-term client involvement to offer what is essentially a case-study analysis. While the major areas traditionally covered in a qualitative evaluation seem comprehensive (e.g., investigations of motor functions, expressive speech, writing, reading; see Hynd & Semrud-Clikeman, 1990), this view does not rely on standardized batteries or clear comparisons to normative populations. Instead, the selection of tests utilized follows significant clinical patient–practitioner interactions. For example, Luria (1970) described a detailed method of examining mathematical functions. He began by asking the subject to read numbers, then measured whether the subject understood the relation between numbers, and the quantities associated with numbers. Next, Luria evaluated whether the subject could read and then write one-digit numbers accurately. Finally, automatic number skills were explored. Many additional steps could be utilized to capture the subject's understanding of mathematical processes (as cited in Gaddes, 1985). Luria's procedure demonstrated how neuropsychological data can be gleaned from work samples, informal tests, criterion-based measures, and clinical interactions. While the focus of this chapter is not centered on qualitative assessment, such an approach offers much for practicing psychologists or neuropsychologists. All evaluations should utilize qualitative information from the student under consideration, as well as information from peers, classroom teachers, other school personnel, and parents. Information considered should include cognitive and academic data, and social and emotional information, together with how the student interacts with others including his or her teacher (e.g., Leu & D'Amato, 1994).

The qualitative perspective has been faulted because of its subjective foundation, its use of process-based interactions, use of case reports, and emphasis on clinical impressions. The ability to evaluate the reliability and validity of the qualitative approach has been problematic. However, its obvious strengths relate to how the practitioner understands the process the patient displays in areas of difficulty and this can have clear and obvious links to intervention.

An Integrative Flexible Battery Model

Basic Assumptions

To combat the respective weaknesses of the quantitative and qualitative approaches, an integrative model of assessment is proposed to aid practitioners in utilizing common tests to better understand the neuropsychological functioning of children and youth. This model, designed to be comprehensive in scope, is based on a multitrait, multisource, multisetting assessment strategy (Kaufman, 1990; Merrell, 1994). Stated simply, it encourages exploration of the totality of the individual's behavioral repertoire—including intellectual functioning, academic functioning, and social/emotional functioning through quantitative and qualitative interviews, observations, and tests. Such an approach should consider the views of parents, family members, friends, and teachers (Knoff, 1990; Sachs, 1991; Savage & Wolcott, 1994). Formal tests provide the needed quantitative data whereas interviews, observations, and informal measures offer the qualitative information necessary for a complete profile.

The Flexible Battery Approach

This integrative model is based on a contemporary understanding of the evaluation process (Kamphaus, 1993; Knoff, 1990; Sattler, 1992). Kaufman (1979, 1990) has argued that the focus of any assessment should be on the *person* being assessed, not on the *test* being used; that the goal of any examination is to be better than the tests that were used; that information collected only represents illustrative samples of behavior (and is not meant to be exhaustive); that tests are meant to be administered and interpreted individually; and finally that tests are to be used to generate hypotheses of potential help to the person being evaluated. With this as a backdrop, we offer the flexible battery approach. Although it is clear that all individuals need to be evaluated in the eight areas displayed in Table 1, the selection of tests utilized to evaluate these abilities will vary greatly because of the unique needs of the individual—considered in tandem with the reason for referral.

In the neuropsychological area, common age expectations can be misleading, and must be cautiously scrutinized in light of the developmental abilities of the child or adolescent. For example, an individual who has sustained a traumatic brain injury and is reportedly functioning at grade level may in actuality exhibit specific skill deficits that are at variance with what has been observed in the classroom, and these deficits may interfere with continued educational progress (Begali, 1994). Stated differently, the child may be compensating in ways that are not recognizable by teachers (D'Amato & Rothlisberg, 1996). For instance, some children will benefit from a multiple-choice format, which decreases memory requirements, while others will be overwhelmed with the number of choices available in such a situation. Telzrow (1989) and others have advocated for determining the essential and nonessential features of a measure before considering its use (Kaufman, 1990; Sattler, 1992; Savage & Wolcott, 1994). From this view, tests can be utilized if modifications are made to nonessential features opposed to essential features. A case in point may be a child who is not able to point to a template, but could signal verbally without violating the intent of the measure. Indeed, consideration should be given to the type of response required, and alternate responses accepted if they do not violate the integrity of the measures being used. Such modifications may be necessary if valid and reliable instruments are not available in the areas to be evaluated.

Areas the Evaluation Should Encompass

The eight key areas that best reflect a comprehensive, developmentally appropriate examination are displayed in Table 1: (1) perceptual/sensory functions, (2) motor functions, (3) intelligence/cognitive abilities, (4) attention/learning/

TABLE 1. Areas to Be Formally and Informally Assessed in Neuropsychological Evaluations[a]

Perceptual/sensory	Communication/language skills
Visual	Receptive vocabulary
Auditory	Expressive vocabulary
Tactile–kinesthetic	Speech/language
Integrated	Written language
Motor functions	Academic achievement
Strength	Preacademic skills
Speed	Academic skills
Coordination	Reading decoding
Lateral preference	Reading comprehension
Intelligence/cognitive abilities	Arithmetic facts
Verbal functions	Arithmetic calculation
Language skills	Social studies
Concepts/reasoning	Language arts
Numerical abilities	Science
Integrative functioning	Personality/behavior
Nonverbal functions	Adaptive behavior
Receptive perception	Daily living
Expressive perception	Development
Abstract reasoning	Play/leisure
Spatial manipulation	Environmental/social
Construction	Parental/siblings
Visual	Family/community
Integrative functions	Student coping/tolerance
Attention/learning/processing	Interpersonal style
Visual processing	Educational/classroom environment
Motoric processing	Learning environment
Auditory processing	Peer/community reactions
Spatial processing	Teacher/staff knowledge
Linguistic/verbal processing	Student competencies
Simultaneous processing	Teacher/staff reactions
Sequential processing	
Memory/learning	

[a]Adapted from D'Amato and Rothlisberg (1996).

processing capacity, (5) communication/language skills, (6) academic achievement, (7) personality/behavior functioning, and (8) the educational/classroom environment. All of these areas should be considered both formally and informally. Direct observations and interviews with the individual and family members are vital components in evaluating any individual's performance in these areas. Behavior rating scales and self-report measures, a review of records, and a collection of work samples should also be among the methods used to collect information (Lezak, 1983; Sattler, 1992; Telzrow, 1986). As demonstrated in Table 2, a variety of testing instruments are appropriate in all areas discussed. The practitioner must take responsibility for carefully matching the student with potential assessment options—after considering the distinct features of the instruments and the unique needs of the student.

The Evaluation–Intervention Link

The development of appropriate interventions from neuropsychological data has a long history replete with many difficulties. For decades many neuropsychologists have focused on the documentation of deficits (e.g., visual–spatial problems) with interventions geared to reduce the effects of or compensate for the deficit areas (e.g., visual–motor training). Another great body of research probes the relation of behavior change to specific areas of brain insult (Lezak, 1983; Wedding, Horton, & Webster, 1986). Although it may be of interest to realize that a child suffered frontal lobe damage in an

TABLE 2. Common Instruments and Procedures Used to Evaluate Neuropsychological Constructs

Perceptual/sensory
  Child and classroom observations
  Developmental history
  Goldman–Fristoe–Woodcock Test of Auditory Discrimination
  Mental status examination
  Motor-Free Visual Perception Test
  Vision and hearing screening
  Wepman's Auditory Discrimination Test
Motor (fine and gross)
  Bender Visual–Motor Gestalt Test
  Detroit Tests of Learning Aptitude-3 (Motoric Composite)
  Developmental Test of Visual–Motor Integration
  K-ABC Nonverbal Scale (e.g., Hand Movements subtest)
  McCarthy Scales of Children's Abilities (Motor Scale)
  WISC-III (Block Design, Object Assembly, Coding subtests)
Intelligence/cognitive
  Battelle Developmental Inventory
  Bayley Infant Intelligence Test (2nd ed.)
  Das–Naglieri Cognitive Assessment System
  Differential Ability Scales
  Kaufman Adolescent and Adult Intelligence Test
  Kaufman Assessment Battery for Children
  McCarthy Scales of Cognitive Ability
  Wechsler Adult Intelligence Scale-Revised
  Wechsler Intelligence Scale for Children (3rd ed.)
Academic achievement
  Differential Ability Scales
  Kaufman Assessment Battery for Children
  Kaufman Test of Educational Achievement
  Key Math Diagnostic Arithmetic Test-Revised
  Peabody Individual Achievement Test-Revised
  Wechsler Individual Achievement Test
  Woodcock–Johnson Psycho-Educational Battery-
    Revised: Achievement
  Woodcock Reading Mastery Test-Revised

Communication/language skills
  Bracken Basic Concept Scale
  Peabody Picture Vocabulary Test-Revised
  Revised Token Test
  Test of Adolescent Language
  Test of Language Development
  Test of Written Language
Attention/learning/processing
  Children's Auditory Verbal Learning Test
  Detroit Tests of Learning Ability-3
  Test of Memory and Learning
  Test of Nonverbal Intelligence-2
  Wechsler Memory Scale-Revised
  Wide Range Assessment of Memory and Learning
Personality/behavior
  Behavior Assessment System for Children
    Parent Rating Scales
    Self-Report of Personality
    Teacher Rating Scales
  Burks' Behavior Rating Scales
  Clinical Interview with Child or Adolescent
  Family Environment Scale
  Home Visit and Family/Parent Interview
  Kinetic Family or School Drawings
  Minnesota Multiphasic Personality Inventory-2
  Multidimensional Self Concept Scale
  Personality Inventory for Children
  Piers–Harris Revised Children's Manifest Anxiety Scale
  Revised Children's Manifest Anxiety Scale
  Sentence Completion Tests
  Vineland Adaptive Behavior Scales
  Wishes and Fears Interview
Educational/classroom environment
  Classroom Environment Scale
  Classroom observations
  School Social Behavior Scales
  Sociograms
  Teacher interviews
  The Instructional Environment Scale

automobile accident last summer, that an infant has general cerebral impairment caused by anoxia at birth, or that an adolescent has right parietal damage (and seizures) as a result of surgery, this causative information relating to individuals' difficulties offers little, if any, direction for the uninitiated regarding rehabilitation. All practitioners must select data-gathering approaches that offer information deemed directly relevant for understanding the educational and life needs of these children.

The *hypothesis-testing* approach is offered as a heuristic guide for understanding individual students. Practitioners evaluate the data generated

from individuals examined, and begin to problem solve concerning the abilities the student displays. Many have argued for strength-based approaches (Hartlage & Telzrow, 1983; Reynolds, 1981, 1986) as opposed to a focus on student weaknesses. Hypotheses based on the data can be utilized to develop student profiles concerning environmental stimulation, endurance and stamina, instructional tactics, organizational abilities, and an evaluation of resulting student feelings given the profile exhibited (D'Amato & Rothlisberg, 1996). Most evaluations traditionally focus exclusively on the area where students display deficiencies (e.g., in reading decoding or mathematical computations; D'Amato & Dean, 1987); a flexible neuropsychological approach to assessment for intervention must consider both how and why students best process information (D'Amato, 1990; Whitten *et al.*, 1992). For example, students who vary on modality strength profiles may require different teaching strategies to accommodate student learning styles (e.g., independent workbook tasks versus chalkboard work) (Leu & D'Amato, 1994). In addition, each student may exhibit a preferential hemispheric processing style (e.g., simultaneous or sequential processing) (Dean, 1986a,c). An evaluation must also consider if the individual would profit from compensatory teaching methods (used to circumvent a deficit) or remedial instruction (geared to address and improve an academic weakness) (Gaddes & Edgell, 1994; Telzrow, 1986). The answers to these questions offer the foundation for the development of a broad-based rehabilitation program.

Interview and Generation of Assessment Plan

Developmental History

Any assessment of function would be incomplete without the compilation of a comprehensive developmental history. Information regarding prenatal, perinatal, and postnatal development should be gathered through a combination of structured interviews and the administration of more formalized measures like the Maternal Perinatal Scale (Gray, Dean, & Rattan, 1987). Significant deviations from normal developmental patterns may indicate potential areas of difficulty that warrant further investigation. Current medical issues and a gross observation of perceptual and motor functioning are also of interest during this contact. Knowledge of the individual's perception and motor skills, current health status, and physical limitations is essential for the formulation of an appropriate assessment battery. This same information should later be integrated in the interpretation of results.

Perceptual/Sensory and Motor Functions

Perceptual and motor functions form the basis of children's understanding of the world and their response to it. Therefore, differences in these primary areas may portend difficulties in other areas of functioning. For example, the reproduction of a vi-

sual stimulus in response to a request involves both perceptual discrimination and fine motor development, as well as the ability to integrate visual, tactile, and auditory skills. Therefore, inadequate performance in copying geometric designs developed to assess these skills may stem from: a misperception, or faulty interpretation of the input information; problems in executing the fine motor response, or output; and/or difficulties integrating the input and output, otherwise known as integrative or central processing difficulties. Other variables that contribute to poor performance include poor motivation, maturational delays, limited development, neurological impairment, sensory deprivation, and other handicaps or illnesses, including fatigue, stress, and injury (Sattler, 1992). The following sections will offer information on representative tests that are used to evaluate these processes.

Perceptual/Sensory Functions

Perception of stimuli is a complex process involving many different aspects of brain functioning (Lezak, 1983). The assessment of these functions is useful in determining the extent to which visual, auditory, and tactile–kinesthetic information is received and integrated.

The Motor-Free Visual Perception Test (MFVPT). Structure: A 36-item measure assessing five facets of visual perception—spatial relations, visual discrimination, figure-ground, visual closure, and visual memory. The MFVPT is intended for children 4 to 8 years of age.

The MFVPT is designed to assess visual perception in the school-age population. The child is required to pick the correct response from four options arranged in a multiple-choice format (Reynolds & Kamphaus, 1990). The MFVPT is used when the results from measures such as the Bender leave the clinician uncertain as to whether difficulties displayed are the result of visual and/or motor concerns. Clinical observations and other methods of data collection may also prove inconclusive regarding the etiology of performance difficulties. The MFVPT can offer information essential for the differential diagnosis of motor versus visual processing problems. However, when used in isolation of other measures or techniques, the MFVPT offers information regarding visual processing difficulties but is unable to rule out motor concerns.

Practical Implications. Assesses perception without the confounding motor component present in popular visual–motor integration measures. Thus, the MFVPT can offer important diagnostic and rehabilitation information.

Motor Functions

Motor dysfunctions that are best explored using a neuropsychological paradigm are fine motor in nature (those that occur despite the appearance that the person moves normally through space) (Lezak, 1983). Numerous paper-and-pencil tests have been developed to assess motor functions as they relate to visual motor integration. Two of the most popular measures for this purpose are the Bender Visual–Motor Gestalt Test and the Developmental Test of Visual–Motor Integration.

Developmental Test of Visual–Motor Integration. Bender Visual–Motor Gestalt Test (Bender). Structure: Individually administered test containing nine geometric figures that the child copies. While historically this test was seen as a general measure of organicity, it is more appropriately used as a measure of visual–motor skills. Standard scores are provided in the developmental scoring system for children aged 5–0 to 11–11.

Most commonly known as the Bender, this measure is perhaps the best known and most widely used visual–motor assessment procedure available today (Bender, 1938; Reynolds & Kamphaus, 1990). As a component of a comprehensive assessment battery, performance on the Bender has long been thought to reveal visual–motor difficulties that may be associated with cerebral impairment (Sattler, 1992). Traditionally used to assess an individual's constructional praxic skills, the Bender provides an evaluation of motor integration employed in the execution of complex learned movements (Hartlage & Golden, 1990). The information generated through this process may then be compared with levels of performance across other measures of functioning. Contrary to once-common practice, the Bender is inappropriate as a test of brain damage. In fact, the very idea of a single screening instrument having the potential for evaluating the complex nature of the brain has proven to be naive at best (D'Amato, 1990).

Alternate uses of the Bender include its administration as a memory test and then as a copying test. This dual administration process can be employed to assess different mental functions (short-term visual memory and visual perception) that utilize the same modalities in perception and task execution (Sattler, 1992). An additional technique available when interpreting Bender performance is to have the child compare the figure that he or she produced with the corresponding stimulus design. If the child is unable to recognize obvious differences between the two designs, a perceptual deficit may be involved. Likewise, if the child is able to detect differences between the two figures, but is unable to make them alike, motor involvement may be influencing performance (Hartlage & Golden, 1990). In the personality area, performance on the Bender may also be used to develop hypotheses regarding impaired performance caused by poor planning, impulsivity, or compulsivity. Extremely large or small figures, heavily reinforced lines, and second attempts are examples of the item reproduction difficulties that are thought to indicate emotional concerns on the part of the individual.

Practical implications: The Bender provides information relevant to visual–motor skills and visual–motor integration. Results from this measure can be useful in evaluating prereading, reading, and penmanship concerns, and other areas requiring the input and output of information. However, since the Bender does not differentiate between visual and motor components of performance, it is not practical for use if isolated from other measures.

The Developmental Test of Visual–Motor Integration (VMI). Structure: Involves copying a sequence of 24, increasingly complex, geometric figures. The VMI may be administered in either an individual or a group setting and requires a relatively short administration time. It is designed primarily for ages 4 through 13.

The VMI was first published in 1967 and is now in its third edition. Because the VMI does not require a verbal response, it has been used to assess visual–motor processes among non-English-speaking children (Brand, 1991; Frey & Pinelli, 1991). The VMI is also frequently employed when investigating the reliability and validity of other tests of visual–motor integration, such as the Bender, self drawing tasks, progressive matrices, and neuropsychological tests (Goldstein, Smith, & Waldrep, 1986; Palisano & Dichter, 1989). The most common use of the VMI, however, seems to be in assisting with the diagnosis of children who are suspected of having visual–motor difficulties related to learning problems.

The VMI offers several advantages as a tool for assessment and is widely used in psychological evaluation and research. The major advancements in the 1989 revised VMI include more explicit scoring criteria and the expansion of the scoring system to a total of 50 points. This expansion was intended to provide for a finer differentiation of individual performance, particularly with respect to older children. From a neuropsychological perspective, the VMI differs from the Bender on two variables: age range and level of planning required (Hartlage & Golden, 1990). First, the age range of the VMI is more extensive than that of the Bender. Whereas the Bender has limited application to children under 5, the VMI is able to be used in the assessment of children younger than 2. Second, unlike the Bender in which the child is allowed to copy the stimulus design on any section of the paper, the VMI requires the design to be placed within a predesignated area. This restriction omits analysis of planning, but does allow for the evaluation of visual–motor integration in a structured format.

Practical implications: The VMI allows for relatively fine differentiation of individual performance on tasks requiring visual–motor integration. The age range and structured format of the measure render the VMI applicable to a wide range of children.

Cognitive/Intellectual Functioning

Aptly described as a cornerstone of the testing movement, intelligence tests predate efforts to efficiently measure neuropsychological constructs (Kamphaus, 1993). Ability tests probably are considered among the most acceptable types of measurement currently available because of their public aura of infallibility born from society's expectations of the tests' capability to gauge the true intellectual level of individuals. Unfortunately, the tests cannot live up to their public persona; they are simply tools that measure the individual's status as the person compares to others who have engaged in the same task. However, available intelligence measures do still provide the most valid test of skill when they are used to help predict the future performance of the individual in educational contexts and can provide insight into preferred processing style.

Intelligence testing is a useful adjunct to standard neuropsychological testing. Neuropsychological instruments try to evaluate one or more of the areas of sensory or motor skills, language processing, visual–spatial skills, memory and learning, attention, and abstract reasoning (Taylor, 1988). Cognitive/intellectual instruments arguably assess these same constructs/areas and thus may offer valuable corroborative data in the overall profile of the individual's performance. In fact, some researchers have found information from intelligence tests to add a unique element to that discerned from standard neuropsychological tests (D'Amato, Gray, & Dean, 1988; Dean & Gray, 1990). However, interpretation of an individual's performance on intelligence tests is complicated by the fact that no two ability tests conceive of intelligence in exactly the same way or include items that measure only one capacity at a time. Instead, tests that purport to measure the broad construct of intellect can differ substantially from one another and be made up of items that tap multiple skills (Kamphaus, 1993; Kaufman, 1979). In general, children who have experienced some form of neuropsychological dysfunction or damage display general cognitive impairment; specific profile subtypes on intelligence tests have not been found (Kamphaus, 1993).

Although tests of cognitive skill cannot provide a ready means of interpreting performance and selecting intervention options, careful analysis of all aspects of the tests (i.e., formal and informal observations) can provide a starting point for integration with other data sources using a neuropsychological framework. Practitioners should be encouraged to go beyond the superficial aspects of the tests (e.g., the global scores) when building hypotheses and interpreting assessment findings (Kaufman, 1979). Review of the test features—in terms of theoretical orientation, subtest construction, and item characteristics, modality of presentation and response—can be helpful clues to understanding children's performance. For the instruments discussed, such features will be addressed.

Battelle Developmental Inventory (BDI). Structure: Five domains incorporating 24 subdomains are assessed in making up the Total Battery score. The domains (and associated subdomains) are as follows—Personal-social (Adult Interaction, Expression of Feeling-Affect, Self-Concept, Peer Interactions, Coping, Social Role); Adaptive (Attention, Eating, Dressing, Personal Responsibility, Toileting); Motor (Muscle Control, Body Coordination, Locomotion, Gross Motor, Fine Muscle, Perceptual Motor, Fine Motor); Communication (Receptive, Expressive); and Cognitive (Perceptual Discrimination, Memory, Reasoning and Academic Skills, Conceptual Development). The BDI was normed for individuals from birth to 8 years.

The BDI was designed as a means of evaluating the government's Handicapped Children's Early Education Program (Kamphaus, 1993; Salvia & Ysseldyke, 1991). As such, it is functionally oriented to provide a profile of developmental strengths and weaknesses suitable for generating individualized programs for children at risk (Snyder, Lawson, Thompson, Stricklin, & Sexton 1993). Items were chosen based on existing infant and preschool measures to provide a comprehensive view of early functioning.

The BDI and other measures of early cognitive performance have a difficult job in trying to explain the factors potentially relevant for later success. Goodman (1990) decries the state of infant testing and the lack of predictive power for the instruments currently used. The rudimentary nature of infant behavior and the lack of agreement as to the structure of intelligence (i.e., its continuity versus its discontinuity) lessen the influence that information about infant behavior can provide (Lewis, Jaskir, & Enright, 1986). However, for diagnostic purposes and for gauging the needs of these youngest learners, the press for assessment of behaviors will continue.

The BDI is unique in that it addresses the idea that infant and preschool behavior can be conceived of as mutlifaceted. It depends on parent interview, observation, and structured assessment in the collection of data; however, its length and formal administrative procedure may make it difficult for examiners to accurately survey the child's functioning. For instance, Bailey, Vandiviere, Dellinger, and Munn (1987) found that teachers trained to administer the BDI needed multiple sessions to complete the assessment and made many computational errors in scoring the test. Adaptations (of procedures) for impaired youngsters were only partially successful and the restricted range of scores (Developmental Quotients below 65 must be extrapolated) lessened the BDI's value for children with severe delays.

Additionally, the BDI has suffered from norming difficulties that led to the recalibration of its norms in 1988 and still is criticized for the wide age ranges used in developing the norms (Kamphaus, 1993). Because infants grow and develop rapidly, it is disheartening that up to almost 2 years of age, the BDI uses 6-month age spans to convert raw into standard scores (McLinden, 1989); thereafter, age spans of 12 months are used. Likewise, it has been suggested that the BDI may have gaps in its survey of skills for some scales and a limited score range for some domains (Bracken, 1987; McLinden, 1989). As mentioned earlier, a Developmental Quotient of 65 is the lowest attainable, necessitating a computational correction for children below this level.

The BDI has proved to correlate moderately well with the Bayley Scales of Infant Development, suggesting that it is an appropriate measure for assessing a young child's status (Boyd, Welge, Sexton, & Miller, 1989; Johnson, Cook, & Kullman, 1992). However, caution has been advised by Snyder et al. (1993) in viewing the domains measured by the test as discrete; instead of five domains, they found three emerging from their study of children with disabilities. Questions addressing social, communicative, and cognitive domains may be more related than originally thought. The slow differentiation of skills into separate domains may be a function of the developmental process.

Practical implications: Although the BDI has not resolved all of the questions concerning appropriate assessment of early development, its attempt at multidimensional evaluation and its functional approach to intervention strategies make it an inviting addition to traditional assessment methodology. By acknowledging that infant behavior can be viewed in a diversified fashion and grouped in what some see as neuropsychological domains, the BDI opens the door to a next generation of development of conceptions of early intelligence.

Bayley Scales of Infant Development (Bayley). Structure: Three components make up the Bayley: a Motor Scale, a Mental Scale, and the Infant Behavior Record. The Bayley was normed for individuals 2 to 30 months of age. Recently, the Bayley II has been made available. It has the same three components but its age range has been extended from 1 to 42 months.

The Bayley is arguably the finest normreferenced instrument available to assess the cognitive and motor status of infants and toddlers (Kamphaus, 1993; Whatley, 1987). It attempts to look at the infant's sensorimotor functioning, rudimentary communication, and problem-solving abilities as well as the child's early fine and gross motor capacities. The measure is based on Bayley's research with infants and her belief that, at best, a picture of current functioning relative to other infants is our best way of understanding the progress of very young children. Moreover, infants may display idiosyncratic rates of skill attainment based on their characteristics and the environments to which they are exposed (Bendell-Estroff, Greenfield, Hogan, & Claussen, 1989). Consequently, the Bayley provides the infant with the opportunity to experience a range of tasks in a rather fluid format to determine how each child's pattern of performance compares with that commonly found.

The Bayley used much smaller age ranges when developing the normative information on the test than did the BDI; items up to the 6-month level are normed at 2-week intervals, with 1-month intervals thereafter. Materials include those designed to be attractive to young children. Unfortunately, although the Bayley offers a selection of different types of activities to its examinees, it does not provide subtest or subdomain scores for different aspects of motor or mental functioning (Whatley, 1987). Such global assessment may make it difficult to develop interpretive statements and treatment plans for the children served. Likewise, lack of commonality of tasks at different age levels causes difficulties in tracking the growth of sensorimotor development.

Lately, measures such as the Bayley have been criticized for their lack of predictive power and a new contender for evaluating infant skills has emerged. Habituation, or the decrement in attentive behavior to a familiar stimulus, has been proposed as a better predictor of ability than sensorimotor measures like the Bayley (Kamphaus, 1993). Butterbaugh (1988) reviewed the comparison between sensorimotor and these proposed recognition tests (like the Fagan Test of Infant Intelligence; Fagan, 1984) and cautioned that low to moderate reliabilities and other psychometric considerations may prohibit a clear understanding of how habituation tasks work with infants with disabilities. Such concern was seconded by Kamphaus (1993) who noted that such alternate measures have not improved on the predictive power of the Bayley and assess only a very narrow range of information-processing capacity.

Practical implications: The Bayley provides to the examiner the psychometric sophistication and control that ensures the most reliable estimate of infant behavior currently available. It is supported by decades of research. Although it does not allow for explanation of different domains of cognitive function, it does provide the youngster an opportunity to display progressive growth in its series of skills.

Differential Ability Scales (DAS). Structure: Two levels with cluster scores for all ages except lower preschool. A General Conceptual Ability (GCA) score is computed based on level subtests. Preschool includes lower (ages 2 years, 6 months to 3 years, 5 months) and upper (3 years, 6 months to 5 years, 11 months) levels. GCA is made up of Block Building, Verbal Comprehension, Picture Similarities, and Naming Vocabulary for the Lower Preschool Level while cluster scores, Verbal (Verbal Comprehension, Naming Vocabulary) and Nonverbal (Picture Similarities, Pattern Construction, Copying) as well as an Early Number Concepts subtest appear for the Upper Preschool Level. At the

School-Age Level, GCA is defined by three clusters: Verbal (Word Definitions, Similarities), Nonverbal Reasoning (Matrices, Sequential and Quantitative Reasoning), and Spatial (Recall of Designs, Pattern Construction). The DAS was normed for children from $2\frac{1}{2}$ to 17 years. It also includes diagnostic subtests [Recall of Digits, Recall of Objects—Immediate and Delayed, Speed of Information Processing (school-age only), Matching Letter-Like Forms (preschool only), Recognition of Pictures (preschool only)] for both levels and Achievement tests (Basic Number Skills, Spelling, Word Reading) for the school-age level.

The DAS is based on the British Ability Scales and is unique in that it can promote itself as a "full-service" test. The DAS has two distinct levels, preschool (2 years, 6 months to 5 years, 11 months) and school-age (6 years to 17 years, 11 months) made up of core subtests related strongly to "g," i.e., general ability. In addition, several diagnostic tests and a brief achievement screener are available if the examiner wishes to examine different aspects of performance. Packaging different components of performance within one scale with common norms across ability and achievement may make analysis of examinee responses clearer and more clinically relevant (Elliott, 1990).

One aspect of interest in the structure of the core battery is the acknowledgment of the developmental changes occurring in intellectual skills during the early years of life. The lower preschool level provides only a general conceptual ability scale, reflecting the lack of differentiation of ability present among the very young. The upper preschool version offers verbal and nonverbal components whereas the school-age version includes verbal, nonverbal, and spatial clusters. Unfortunately, the DAS is not based on a particular model of intelligence, so the tendency may be to shift interpretive schemes with each case. Also, since clusters are made up of only two subtests, one may be limited in the breadth of options or measures of behavior; performance is either equivalent across subtests in a cluster or one subtest proves to be significantly higher in score than its partner.

The authors have found the DAS to be an appealing test to individuals of all ages—suggesting that motivation to perform is less a problem than with some other instruments. In fact, the preschool level of the DAS may be the most physically attractive measure for this population. Colorful objects, pictures, and an item format based on item sets rather than common basal and ceiling rules engage examinees in the items covered. Teaching items that allow the examiner to offer feedback and the alternate untimed method of administration for the Pattern Construction provide options in examiner technique unlike those of other tests. Language demands may be less than those for the Stanford–Binet IV and the WISC-III in that simple phrases or one-word responses may suffice to answer vocabulary or similarity items. In terms of neuropsychological principles, the DAS may be viewed as fitting under a verbal/nonverbal dichotomy, with nonverbal skills including both nonverbal reasoning and spatial clusters at the school-age level. However, depending on the examinee, even the nonverbal tasks may involve verbal mediation. For instance, even Recall of Designs, where the individual must remember and reproduce a line drawing, is aided when the child can attach a verbal label to the design. This is also a factor in Matrices and Sequential and Quantitative Reasoning where concept formation can be facilitated through verbal rehearsal of cues.

Diagnostic subtests available for the DAS can be useful adjuncts to the core battery. Both Recall of Digits and Recall of Objects involve the use of verbal labels to determine success; however, Recall of Objects includes a delayed component which may indicate the degree of incidental learning under way when the individual is rehearsing the items seen on the card. Similarly, at the preschool level, Matching Letter-Like Forms and Recognition of Pictures may anticipate the child's need to be aware of the spatial orientation of letters and shapes and attend to meaningful detail.

Practical implications: The DAS is designed to offer the examiner a broad array of assessment options. Including both a preschool and school-age level, the addition of diagnostic and achievement tests affords the examiner ways of exploring hypotheses about learning difficulties. The core subtests basically describe verbal versus visual–spatial–numerical reasoning, while the diagnostic subtests explore auditory and visual short-term recall as well as processing speed. The engaging items available may make the measure very attractive to preschoolers in particular.

Kaufman Adolescent and Adult Intelligence Test (KAIT). Structure: Two scales—Crystallized (Definitions, Auditory Comprehension, Double Meanings) and Fluid (Rebus Learning, Logical Steps, Mystery Codes)—make up the Core Battery. Although a Composite score is available, it is only suggested for interpretation if there is no significant difference between Crystallized and Fluid scales.

The Expanded Battery adds the subtests Famous Faces (alternate, Crystallized Scale), Memory for Block Designs (alternate, Fluid Scale), and Rebus Delayed Recall and Auditory Delayed Recall (Measures of Delayed Recall). A Mental Status Examination is also provided. The KAIT was normed for individuals 11 to 85 years of age.

The KAIT (Kaufman & Kaufman, 1993) is among the newest of intelligence tests available and is in direct competition with the WAIS-R for assessment of the adult population. However, unlike the WAIS-R, the KAIT has attached to it a strong theoretical direction that unites classical views of crystallized and fluid abilities with the abstract reasoning abilities associated with Piaget's concept of formal operations (Kaufman & Kaufman, 1993). Whereas one would expect the KAIT to be congruent in design to the Kaufman Assessment Battery for Children (K-ABC), the two Kaufman tests are not extensions of one another. In fact, Kaufman (1993) illustrated this point in a factor-analytic study that compared the KAIT with the K-ABC. The fluid components of the K-ABC are defined by measures of simultaneous and sequential processing; however, planning and formal operational features are believed to address fluid abilities on the adult scale. Kaufman defends the shift in his theoretical orientation by ascribing the differences in the tests to the different reasons behind testing in childhood and adulthood. Although the K-ABC presumes to assess crystallized ability through a separate achievement scale and reserves fluid tests as those that best represent cognitive potential, the KAIT sees the mature individual as a functional composite of both problem-solving abilities and the rich store of experiences to which the person has been exposed. This broadened view, integrated with some novel subtest formats, could provide examiners with a new perspective of intellectual performance for the adult.

In a way, the structure of the KAIT is somewhat deceiving. A cursory preview of the materials may suggest a simple measure that takes little time to administer. Actual practice and administration of the KAIT will disavow that notion. Adolescents and adults will be challenged by the apparently modest stimuli to uncover the relations between concepts. To generate the most complete picture of the adolescent or adult, both the core and expanded battery sections must be administered. The expanded battery may provide the best picture of learning among its examinees because the instrument includes what it considers to be measures of immediate, long-term, and remote memory. Rebus Delayed Recall and Auditory Delayed Recall will test out the examinee's ability to retrieve information learned recently and Famous Faces involves retrieval of past experiences. Certainly, informal observations of examinee strategies to handle the various situations will add clinical insight about the individual's approach to problems.

Even though the KAIT seeks to provide a comprehensive view of functioning that is relevant to understanding both fluid and crystallized ability, caution should be exercised if one is tempted to embrace the measure without additional validity studies supportive of the KAIT's structure and intent. The authors noted that marginal performance by individuals of limited ability could still result in Fluid and Crystallized Scale scores higher than expected based on measures with the Wechsler Adult Intelligence Scale-Revised (WAIS-R) or WISC. That is, several subtests did not appear to have adequate floors to allow for the range of abilities possible. Likewise, the assumption that all individuals have access to formal operational thinking may be unfounded. Although concrete operational thought has been found in a variety of cultural settings, formal operational thought is not considered to be universal and has been estimated to be attained by only a portion of the adult populations in technological societies. Therefore, expectations that the skills needed to solve the items of the KAIT tap into formal operational thought may be better explained by some other component of mature reasoning.

In terms of a neuropsychological orientation to the task, the KAIT may at this point defy easy analysis. The breakdown of subtests into measures of classic fluid and crystallized ability suggests that the subtests given over to crystallized skills are analogous to those found in the WAIS that tap predominantly verbal knowledge and those designated as fluid hold the strongest connection to WAIS performance items. Indeed, the subtle novelty of the subtests of the KAIT may require openness to new problem-solving situations even when the response involves retrieving verbal information from memory. Likewise, the fluid subtests may tap logical or purportedly left-hemisphere functions (Logical Steps), simultaneous or purportedly right-hemisphere functions (Memory for Block Designs), and integrative functions (Mystery Codes). It seems that, in nearly every task, a verbal organizational strategy could aid in problem solution. Given the innovative item types, however, individuals who are operating at more concrete levels of reasoning or who have ex-

perienced significant trauma may be unable to understand the questions with enough clarity to respond.

Practical implications: The KAIT is unique in that it seeks to examine the complexity of mature cognition through the combined use of crystallized/fluid distinctions and presence of formal operational thought. At this point, however, linkages between fluid and crystallized abilities and hemispheric function cannot be clearly stated. Formal operational skills tested may help to describe frontal lobe function, but the neuropsychological relations in the test have yet to be delineated.

Kaufman Assessment Battery for Children (K-ABC). Structure: Two scales—Sequential Processing (Hand Movements, Number Recall, Word Order) and Simultaneous Processing (Magic Window, Face Recognition, Gestalt Closure, Triangles, Matrix Analogies, Spatial Memory Photo Series)—make up the Mental Processing Composite score. A separate Achievement scale (Expressive Vocabulary, Faces and Places, Arithmetic, Riddles, Reading/Decoding, Reading/Understanding) is included. The K-ABC was normed for children $2\frac{1}{2}$ to $12\frac{1}{2}$ years old.

The K-ABC, designed to assess the cognitive functioning of children aged $2\frac{1}{2}$ to $12\frac{1}{2}$, is based on the neuropsychological premise of problem-solving associated with the Luria–Das model of simultaneous and sequential processing (Das, Kirby, & Jarman, 1979; Luria, 1980). Actually, the full model incorporates the three units of the brain: arousal, simultaneous and sequential processes, and planning; however, the K-ABC only directs its attention at the aspects of the second unit—that which explains the underlying organizational processes used for solving unique problems. Sequential processing involves the use of temporal or serial aspects of the problem whereas simultaneous uses the gestaltlike or spatial aspects of tasks to describe the way in which a learner deals with a learning situation. Overlaid on the issue of processing style is that of crystallized and fluid intellectual abilities. Hence, the K-ABC seeks to address sequential versus simultaneous processing using fluidlike tasks and equates crystallized abilities with the conception of academically related content. The resultant component scores of mental processing and achievement rework the previous verbal/performance dichotomy so prevalent in views of ability into one that distinguishes fund of knowledge from strategy choice. The K-ABC was the first mainstream ability test to tie its utility to neuropsychologically grounded theory.

The separate simultaneous and sequential scales of the mental processing composite of the K-ABC propose that the learner must exhibit that particular processing style when completing the subtests within each scale. Use of simultaneous or sequential processing is believed to be independent of modality of presentation. Unfortunately, the K-ABC has had difficulty providing proof that its view of processing style can be relevant for intervention. Soon after publication of the test, a great deal of activity tried to establish the linkage of the simultaneous/sequential processing to academic behavior (e.g., see Rothlisberg, 1989) but when straightforward connections between processing and academic skill development did not materialize, interest in the test waned (Chattin & Bracken, 1989). It may be that the novel theoretical orientation of the test and its limited verbal requirements made the K-ABC too discrepant from practitioner notions of intelligence as to make it appear a less viable option than other scales. Nevertheless, comparisons with other measures of ability offer evidence that the K-ABC measures similar constructs to those assessed by the WISC-R and SBIV.

Practical implications: The K-ABC was one of the first major assessment tools to define its structure in terms of a specific theoretical orientation. Conceiving of intelligence as involving the simultaneous and sequential fluid processing strategies, the K-ABC sought to offer a closer match between diagnosis and intervention. Sequential skills were tied to left-hemisphere, step-by-step analysis, whereas simultaneous abilities were purported to tap right-hemisphere strengths. A separate achievement scale offers comparison between problem-solving and acquired components of functioning.

Stanford–Binet Intelligence Scale, 4th Edition (SBIV). Structure: Four Area scores—Verbal Reasoning (Vocabulary, Comprehension, Absurdities, Verbal Relations), Quantitative Reasoning (Quantitative, Number Series, Equation Building), Abstract/Visual Reasoning (Pattern Analysis, Copying, Matrices, Paper Folding and Cutting), and Short-Term Memory (Bead Memory, Memory for Sentences, Memory for Digits, Memory for Objects)—make up the Composite standard age score. The SBIV was normed for individuals 2 to 23 years of age.

The SBIV is the latest revision in the test's venerable history. Earlier versions of the instrument were organized according to an age scale format and provided a single or composite score to characterize cognitive skill. In addition, the Stanford–Binet had a unique adaptive format that allowed examiners to route the examinee through items and skills considered to be indicative of intellectual performance at various age levels. Functional in nature, the early versions of the Stanford–Binet gave examiners the luxury of a wide age range for testing and item groupings that often piqued younger children's interest while challenging children of higher capabilities.

In its latest form, the SBIV has dramatically modified its format, and in essence re-created itself from the ashes of its earlier versions—to the dismay of many (e.g., see Canter, 1990; Vernon, 1987; Wersh & Thomas, 1990). Now, a point scale or discrete subtest format has replaced the age levels of the past. The SBIV also was constructed to measure aspects of a hierarchical model of intelligence incorporating the Crystallized–Fluid types of ability supported by Cattell and Horn (Horn & Cattell, 1966). By eliciting information in four areas of ability as well as still providing a composite score, the SBIV's interpretive power would seem to be enhanced. Unfortunately, the test's goals of providing a clearer picture of individual performance have not been realized (Kamphaus, 1993; Sattler, 1992).

Interpretation using the SBIV is complicated by the fact that the area scores have not been convincingly validated by a host of factor-analytic studies (Laurent, Swerdlik, & Ryburn, 1992). In fact, Sattler (1992) disputes the conception of the area scores and proposes the use of factor scores in their stead. Suffice it to say, the confusion over the underlying structure of the test has made it less applicable for neuropsychological use. Furthermore, disputes over aspects of administration have caused the SBIV to be used less often by school psychologists than other available tests (Chattin & Bracken, 1989).

Kamphaus (1993) reports that the verbal and abstract/visual reasoning areas of the test appear to be fairly robust and similar to the verbal/performance scales of the Wechsler series. However, several cautions must be given for the SBIV. First, quantitative and memory areas do not appear to be consistent across the age span of the test and so should not be thought of as unified groupings. The Quantitative subtest seems to be particularly weak at the younger age levels where a different item type is used (dice) and may be likened to a computational task rather than a reasoning task. In a similar vein, the memory subtests do not appear to measure a unified construct but appear to be more dependent on other reasoning skills than anticipated. For example, Bead Memory appears to be less a memory task at elementary ages than a strategic exercise.

The child must recall not only sequence of color, but shape and orientation as well. Given the number of salient features, it is no wonder that it is sometimes linked with the abstract reasoning area.

Moreover, the SBIV seems to have insufficient floor and ceiling levels. Young children with moderate to severe levels of disability will not be able to complete even the simplest items on some subtests, yet the score ranges available may actually exaggerate their skill levels. Similarly, gifted children may not obtain ceilings on many subtests. The suggested solution for the attenuated range of scores is to list performance as "estimated"; however, having such estimated scores can complicate the types of interpretation available.

Finally, interpretive schemes appear at best unclear, given the uncertainty of the structure of the test. Although Kamphaus (1993) suggests that the verbal and abstract/visual reasoning areas are interpretable in their present form, Sattler (1992) provides a modified factor approach that necessitates recalculation of scores and consultation with a host of tables for interpretive suggestions. The complications involved with administering, scoring, and interpreting the SBIV do not bode well for its acceptance as an adjunct to neuropsychological findings.

Practical implications: Designed to support a hierarchical model of intelligence, the structural integrity of the SBIV has not lived up to its hypothesized ideal. Difficulties in administration, scoring, and interpretation have cast doubts on the overall utility of the SBIV for analysis from any neuropsychological perspective. If used, the most salient aspects, verbal versus nonverbal/visualization areas, may be thought of as analogous to verbal versus performance breakdowns.

Wechsler Adult Intelligence Scale-Revised (WAIS-R). Structure: Two scales—Verbal (Information, Digit Span, Vocabulary, Arithmetic, Similarities, Comprehension) and Performance (Picture Completion, Picture Arrangement, Digit Symbol, Block Design, Object Assembly)—make up the Full Scale Score. The WAIS-R was normed for individuals 16 to 74 years of age.

Until recently uncontested in the area of assessment of adult intelligence, the WAIS-R brings to the measure of ability a rich history of clinical and research findings (Bornstein, 1987). The WAIS-R is the last installment in the measurement of adult ability by David Wechsler himself, who managed to shape a generation's conception about psychometric intelligence. Kaufman (1990) provides a comprehensive overview of the contributions made by Wechsler to the field of adult testing with the WAIS-R and its predecessors; anyone interested in a full accounting of the test and its influence should read that resource. Here, only a sketch of the test and its relevance will be provided.

The WAIS-R, and the WAIS before it, have been used as an integral part of neuropsychological testing (e.g., see Goldstein, Katz, Slomka, & Kelly, 1993; Moore *et al.,* 1990, 1992; Russell, 1987). As such, each subtest has been analyzed and reviewed as to the unique contributions it makes to the neuropsychological battery. In some cases, an individual's WAIS-R profile is interpreted relative to the three-factor structure of the measure, Bannatyne's categorization, fluid versus crystallized skill, or a host of other configurations (Kaufman, 1990). In any case, interpretive strategies must take into account the match between performance on the WAIS-R and other documented evidence.

Perhaps one of the greatest contributions that Wechsler made to the study of intelligence was his recognition of the importance of nonverbal abilities in the evaluation of cognitive skill. Today, the basis of much of interpretation is grounded in the appearance of verbal/performance splits in an individual's protocol. Verbal skills such as vocabulary, understanding of similarity of concept, and comprehension of social situations may be resilient in the face of cerebral insult. At the same time, the spatial or fluid skills associated with construction tasks such as Block Design or with fine motor control tasks such as Digit Symbol may not be spared. In any event, clinicians' familiarity with the WAIS-R makes it a trusted addition to any assessment situation.

In the study of adolescents, however, one quirky aspect of the WAIS-R must be noted. As Kaufman (1990) details, the norms of the WAIS-R for adolescents 16–19 years of age are "questionable" with inadequate floors available for several of the subtests and lower subtest reliabilities than with older age groups. Because the target population for this discussion intersects this very problematic range for the WAIS-R, caution is warranted when applying interpretive strategies to this "youngest" age group of the test.

Practical implications: The WAIS-R is the adult measure to which all others are compared. Offering an extensive age range as well as an impressive research base relative to neuropsychological testing, the WAIS-R differentiation between verbal and performance abilities along with related neuropsychological interpretive strategies are among the most widely known in the world.

Wechsler Intelligence Scale for Children, 3rd Edition (WISC-III). Structure: Two scales—Verbal (Information, Vocabulary, Arithmetic, Similarities, Comprehension) and Performance (Picture Completion, Picture Arrangement, Coding, Block Design, Object Assembly)—make up the Full Scale Score. In addition, a supplemental verbal subtest (Digit Span) and two performance subtests (Symbol Search, Mazes) are available. The WISC-III was normed for individuals 6 to 16 years old. The WISC-III was conormed with the Wechsler Individual Achievement Test.

The WISC-III is the latest version of the highly successful Wechsler series. Created as a clinical tool and as a downward extension of Wechsler's adult measure, the WISC has been embraced as the instrument of choice for the assessment of children's ability by school practitioners and neuropsychologists alike (Chattin & Bracken, 1989). Unfortunately, questions remain about the third edition's comparability to the WISC-R in terms of neuropsychological utility. Some researchers have complained that the WISC-III offers only a cosmetic upgrading of the WISC-R, without necessarily recapturing its ability to measure cognitive skills.

As with all of the Wechsler series, the major division among WISC-III subtests is between verbal and performance measures. Kaufman (1979) provided a rich framework from which to analyze examinee performance on the WISC-R and made much of the meaning of verbal/performance splits and subtest consistency. One component of analysis well known to those familiar with the WISC-R was the importance of the third factor, Freedom from Distractibility, made up of Arithmetic, Coding, Digit Span and sometimes, Information. Children with learning disabilities would often show a preference for performance tasks over verbal tasks and have particular problems with the subtests of the third factor. Unfortunately, although the subtests of the WISC-III purportedly were designed to measure cognitive abilities in the same way as the WISC-R, subtle changes in item types and administrative procedure have acted to modify the results the WISC-III provides.

Aspects of the WISC-III's scores are currently being made available (see e.g., Kamphaus & Platt, 1992; Naglieri, 1993). One of the greatest changes in test structure appears to be the dissolution of the third factor (Kamphaus, 1993). When the test constructors added a 13th subtest, Symbol Search, to clarify the existence and nature of the WISC-R's third factor, they instead splintered it into two separate components known now as freedom from distractibility (Arithmetic and Digit Span) and perceptual speed (Coding and Symbol Search). Such a reconfiguration could just as likely pick up the auditory versus the visual nature of these processing tasks. The result of the four-factor structure on the interpretation of the test has yet to be decided, but this change, as well as modifications in the factor loadings of other subtests (e.g., Picture Arrangement and the perceptual organization factor) make the translation of test scores tenuous at best.

Practical implications: As with the WAIS-R, this latest revision of the WISC has the strength of many years of acceptance on its side as the premiere measure of intellectual functioning in childhood. The WISC-III continues to offer a clinically relevant overview of intelligence, but the expected associations between test scores and academic performance may need to be modified in accord with the changing psychometric nature of the test. Children who have experienced some sort of trauma will typically exhibit a depression of scores with the performance scale more adversely affected than the verbal scores.

Academic Achievement

Although some would hold that there is little difference in the measure of ability and the measure of achievement (Anastasi, 1988), it would seem that the operationalization of the two areas allows for a comparison of more generic problem-solving and verbal tasks to those directly involved in scholastic performance. Thus, the measure of ability may be conceived of as attempting to address the concept of underlying skills or capacities, whereas the measure of achievement is tied to the notion of the individual's facility in applying those faculties in a functional way to master real-world skills. For the purposes of this discussion, several norm-referenced instruments will be used to represent the area. Although it could be argued that alternate methods to norm-referenced assessment are preferable (i.e., curriculum-based), the availability of a standard normative context allows for comparison of skills across a wide variety of curricular contexts.

The broad-based tests listed all have a similar organizational structure. For example, measures of a particular area, such as reading, are typically divided into basic skill (reading recognition) and some form of applied skill (reading comprehension) so that variation in the aspects of that academic task can be noted. The difference between instruments often lies in the method by which they obtain their information (i.e., whether visual–motor or oral responses are required).

Peabody Individual Achievement Test-Revised (PIAT-R). Structure: Five subtest scores (General Information, Reading Recognition, Reading Comprehension, Mathematics, Spelling) are provided in addition to the Total Reading and Total Test scores. A Written Expression and optional Written Language score also are available. The PIAT-R was normed for individuals 5 to 18 years old.

The PIAT-R has been regarded as a well-developed instrument by reviewers (Williams & Vincent, 1991). It is made up of five subtests and does what few other achievement tests do, namely, it provides a composite achievement score. The utility of such a score is puzzling, however, as it averages the child's performance over disparate academic categories and essentially hides performance discrepancies. Of greater benefit to the practitioner will be subtest scores based on specific content.

The PIAT-R is different from other tests in that it includes a larger pictorial component in its item types, letting children avoid the need for verbal reply, and instead expecting them to point at the correct answer (out of four) for reading, spelling, and mathematics items. Because the task demands for recognition of information do not appear to be the same as for recall, this response format may aid children with retrieval difficulties or those who have developed some background knowledge of the area in question. It should be noted, however, that this response-type advantage may not give a good indication of the expectations for student performance in the classroom where recall and more integrated answers are the norm.

One aspect of the PIAT-R that is of great benefit to the evaluator is the inclusion of the Written Expression subtest. Previously, when spelling skill was used to assess the written language area, children who could manage to spell words in isolation may have been perceived as being able to translate those spelling skills into fully developed written discourse. Unfortunately, this estimation of writing skill may have complicated the student's ability to have written language deficits recognized. On the PIAT-R, students above the second grade are asked to create a story for one of two pictures. This writing experience allows the examiner to begin to evaluate ability in terms of organization, grammar, and development of ideas. This testing situation more closely approximates classroom activities in writing than do the other subtests.

Practical implications: The PIAT-R is a well-constructed instrument that requires less oral language and makes greater use of recognition as a response type than other achievement tests. The inclusion of a written expression subtest begins to address the notion of a continuum of skills in written discourse beyond spelling.

Wechsler Individual Achievement Test (WIAT). Structure: Four composites—Language (Oral Expression, Listening Comprehension), Writing (Written Expression, Spelling), Reading (Basic Reading Skill, Reading Comprehension), and Math (Mathematics Calculation, Mathematics Reasoning)—make up the battery. Basic Reading, Mathematics Reasoning, and Spelling can also be used as a screener. The WIAT was normed for children 5 to 19 years old.

The WIAT is unique in that its subtests were designed to reflect major aspects of the definition of learning disabilities; hence, oral expression, listening comprehension, and written expression will sound familiar to those well versed in classification criteria. Unfortunately, it should be noted that little agreement as to the key elements of the definition exists so that specific aspects of the WIAT may relate to artifacts of our difficulties in understanding the nature of learning disorders. Be that as it may, the WIAT matches others of its genre in its basic structure and intent. It samples basic academic skill areas through the use of two tests per area and provides composite scores for reading, writing, language, and mathematics.

Although it appears to match the PIAT-R in its inclusion of a Written Expression subtest, the most distinctive parts of the WIAT are the Listening Comprehension and Oral Expression components of this instrument. Listening Comprehension requires that the child listen to a paragraph and then respond orally to questions. The ability to understand orally presented material in an educational setting cannot be underestimated. Yet, although care has been taken to minimize the effect of the knowledge base on the child's ability to answer, it is possible in several instances to take educated guesses and receive credit for the items in this subtest. In contrast, Oral Expression appears to be different than any other subtest from competing achievement tests. Given a task, this subtest looks at the child's capacity to describe in an organized fashion the steps needed to complete an activity, recognize relations between objects, and take another person's perspective. This type of activity would seem to be extremely difficult if a nonverbal disability existed that interfered with the interpretation of social perspective taking or if the pragmatic aspects of speech were underdeveloped.

Practical implications: The WIAT attempts to measure aspects of academic skill unaccounted for by other instruments. The addition of a language component may afford practitioners a greater capacity to compare components of language function. The purported relation of test construction and scoring to the educational category of learning disability may also prove attractive in a clinical setting.

Woodcock–Johnson Tests of Achievement-Revised (WJTA-R). Structure: Two batteries are included. The Standard Battery is divided into four broad areas: Reading (Letter-Word Identification, Passage Comprehension), Mathematics (Calculations, Applied Problems), Written Language (Dictation, Writing Samples), and Broad Knowledge (Science, Social Studies, Humanities) and allows for scores for each subtest and area. A Supplemental Battery also is available to expand the Standard Battery coverage. It includes Word Attack, Reading, Vocabulary, Quantitative Concepts, Proofing, and Writing Fluency subtests. Employing one or more of the supplemental subtests gives the examiner the option of computing additional areas of achievement such as Basic Reading Skills and Reading Comprehension. The WJTA-R is normed for individuals 2 to 95 years old.

Concerns have been raised as to the functional aspects of the WJTA-R and to its effectiveness in identifying young children at risk (Webster, 1991); however, as expected, its basic structure is similar to those achievement tests mentioned above. What the WJTA-R does provide that the others do not is a higher degree of flexibility in the types of norm-referenced data collected. With the inclusion of the supplemental battery, academic areas such as reading or mathematics can be approached from more than a single direction. For example, four subtests looking at different aspects of reading can be included if the examiner so chooses. In addition, a broad knowledge category is included that requires the recall of factual information from the areas of science, social studies, and the humanities. The Broad Knowledge Cluster allows the examiner to compare whether aspects of the basic skills measured in the other portions of the scale may have influenced the student's ability to perform well in specific content areas.

Unlike the PIAT-R, the WJTA-R is similar to the WIAT in its oral language demands and in its requirement for the recall (rather than the recognition) of information. However, it varies in its structure from the other two scales in its requirements for written language. Instead of composing a single story, the standard battery of the WJTA-R samples a student's sentence construction ability in a graded set of items. Early items refer to specific picture descriptions while later items attempt to measure more complex writing requirements. However, although measurement of the unity and organization of a single story may be lost, a broader range of writing situations may be sampled with this approach.

Practical implications: The WJTA-R may be the most versatile of the norm-referenced individual achievement tests. This measure includes a broad knowledge area and a supplemental battery, providing practitioners with flexibility in the sampling of achievement-related behavior. In addition to covering more areas, the WJTA-R also features an extended age range.

Communication/Language Skills

When attempting to assess the potential for cerebral dysfunction, communication and language skills are prime candidates for analysis. A comprehensive assessment should include an analysis of receptive vocabulary and the ability to analyze and integrate information presented in a verbal format, since a common difficulty among children experiencing traumatic brain injury is a decreased capacity to coordinate the social aspects of language. Instruments useful for this purpose (in addition to the diagnostic information gained through the clinical evaluation of language-based measures of general intelligence and achievement) include the Bracken Basic Concept Scale, the Test of Written Language, and the Test of Language Development. Importantly, speech–language therapists frequently contribute significantly to this area through the multidisciplinary process. In many cases, they serve as critical team leaders, when individuals have lost or nearly lost the ability to communicate clearly. Despite this, clinicians considering this key skill may choose to utilize the following instrument to gain a clearer picture of receptive language.

Peabody Picture Vocabulary Test-Revised (PPVT-R). Structure: Two forms, each of which includes 175 picture plates designed to measure receptive vocabulary. Although normed for individuals $2\frac{1}{2}$ years of age through adulthood, the PPVT-R is most appropriate for a school-age population.

The PPVT-R is one of the most frequently used measures of receptive language because it addresses the development of vocabulary in a relatively brief and flexible way (Kamphaus, 1993). The PPVT-R is untimed and requires the examinee to select from each plate of four pictures the one that best represents the target word. The test requires no reading ability, nor is the ability to point or provide an oral response essential (Shea, 1989). Starting and stopping points for the PPVT-R are determined by both the individual's chronological age and basal and ceiling requirements.

Research focusing on the PPVT-R indicates that it can be successfully used as a predictor of intelligence and achievement as well as a diagnostic indicator of children who are at risk and who may have difficulty communicating (Shea, 1989). The PPVT-R can also help to establish the level of verbal understanding children have when expressive language is not required. Comparing such receptive skills with those expressive skills needed for other tests may help in developing hypotheses about the qualitative nature of verbal performance and in framing potential treatment.

Practical implications: The PPVT-R is frequently the instrument of choice for the assessment of receptive vocabulary. The PPVT-R's wide range of applicable age groups and the absence of reading and motor requirements are especially beneficial for work with children with limited intellectual and physical abilities. This test covers an important area that is critical for intervention development.

Learning/Memory/Processing

Generally, three approaches have been utilized when evaluating how students preferentially process information. The first approach, seen as the traditional test approach, utilizes established measures (like the WISC-III) with the practitioner seeking to understand information processing through an analysis of common test results such as reviewing global scores, subtests, and clusters of subtests (Kaufman, 1979, 1990). The second view of information processing, regarded as the informal approach, considers classroom data, observations, checklists, and learning style inventories to understand how students learn. From this view, students who seem to profit most from visual clues may be seen as visual learners, and might be taught utilizing overheads, visual diagrams, and worksheets. The final approach to understanding processing stems from the administration and analysis of the many unique measures that have been offered as learning style, memory, or processing tests. This approach is seen as the nontraditional test approach.

These specialized measures of performance in learning, memory, or processing do not fall neatly within the traditional domains of intelligence, achievement, or neuropsychological processing. These tests, including the Detroit Tests of Learning Aptitude-3 (Detroit), the Children's Auditory Verbal Learning Test, the Boder Test of Reading–Spelling Patterns, the Wechsler Memory Scale-Revised, the Wide Range Assessment of Memory and Learning, the Test of Memory and Learning (TOMAL), and others can offer valuable information concerning how children deal with information. Although practitioners have used these instruments to document student strengths and weaknesses, diagnose learning problems, and chart the course of disorders, these instruments offer more practical information concerning rehabilitation or program planning than for diagnostic activities. Whereas all of these tests have been helpful in different circumstances, space does not permit reviews of these instruments. One measure that has a long history in the evaluation of processing styles is the Detroit. This measure may be the most popular processing instrument available in special education today. The Detroit has been especially helpful when evaluating children who have suffered traumatic brain injuries. The TOMAL, the most recently developed of the instruments listed, will be discussed as a measure representative of the contributions that tests in this domain offer for delineating student skills.

Test of Memory and Learning (TOMAL). Structure: Four Core Indexes including Verbal Memory, Nonverbal Memory, Composite Memory, and Delayed Recall are provided. Supplementary Indexes include Learning, Attention and Concentration, Sequential Memory, Free Recall, and Associative Recall. Subtests include Memory for Stories, Facial Memory, Word Selective Reminding, Visual Selective Reminding, Object Recall, Abstract Visual Memory, Digits Forward, Visual Sequential Memory, Paired Recall, Memory-for-Location, Manual Imitation, Letters Forward, Digits Backwards, Letter Backwards. The TOMAL was standardized for children ages 5 through 19.

The TOMAL is, perhaps, the most reliable measure available to evaluate child and adolescent memory. The evaluation of memory has long been a staple in the neuropsychological testing arena. Indeed, an understanding of memory and related learning processes is critical in all areas of neuropsychology including working with students who display learning disabilities, traumatic brain injuries, or psychiatric disabilities. The TOMAL boasts many unique features, including a great variety of memory indexes (Reynolds & Bigler, 1994). Although some of the subtests appear similar to other memory measures, some unique features of the test include a learning index where teaching is permissible (similar to some K-ABC subtests), a sequential memory index, and an attention and concentration index. Delayed recall subtests are also available and are offered as an evaluation of forgetting or memory decay. It is possible to compare the examinee's own personal learning curve with a standardized learning curve.

The test is easy to administer and generally user friendly. For example, directions are clear and many memory comparisons are readily utilized by virtue of the side-by-side layout of the measure. Unfortunately, the black-and-white templates do not seem engaging for young children. The TOMAL appears to hold promise for evaluating neuropsychologically impaired children and youth.

Practical implications: The recent release of this instrument makes it intriguing but at the same time difficult to evaluate. Clearly, a comprehensive instrument is needed in this area because memory is intrinsic to all learning. Measures in the memory area have typically suffered from psychometric and clinical difficulties and no single measure has gained prominence in the field. The TOMAL seems psychometrically sound with several unique features that are clinically relevant.

Personality Variables

Cognitive and educational data cannot be interpreted and evaluated without considering the context of the individual's interpersonal and social abilities (Dean, 1985b, 1986a; Gaddes, 1985). Because the goal of neuropsychology is to integrate internal and behavioral aspects of functioning, a comprehensive neuropsychological evaluation would be incomplete without consideration of personality and social adaptation. To accomplish data collection in this area, direct observation of the child, interviews with involved parties (e.g., parents, teachers), and formal and informal surveying of behavior, personality, and daily functioning are required. The individual's view of educational competencies, cognitive abilities, recent difficulties and failures, peer relations, family relations, and important life events should be the focus of inquiry. In short, the individual's world needs to be

evaluated and understood. This is especially important if a recent accident (e.g., traumatic brain injury) or new or changed diagnosis has been offered. In order to fully explore this domain, both objective and projective measures of personality will offer complementary insights. Objectively scored measures allow for a normative comparison of the individual's functioning, and the inclusion of projective devices provides information regarding the unconscious motives behind behavior (Knoff, 1986; Lanyon & Goodstein, 1982). The inclusion of both avenues of evaluation also serves as a safeguard against biased information (i.e., faking good or faking bad). Therefore, measures included in this section represent a sample of the instruments and techniques that address the complex area of personal development through both objective and projective formats. See Table 2 for a more complete listing of measures available for the assessment of personality variables.

Piers–Harris Children's Self-Concept Scale (Piers–Harris). Structure: The Piers–Harris is a self-report questionnaire designed to assess how children and adolescents feel about themselves. Six cluster scales provide information concerning behavior, intellectual and school status, physical appearance, anxiety, popularity, and life satisfaction. An overall assessment of self-concept is provided. The Piers–Harris was developed for individuals 8 to 18 years old.

The Piers–Harris, in contrast to projective measures, evaluates the conscious self-perceptions/self-concept of the individual. This measure defines self-concept as a relatively stable set of attitudes reflecting both a description and an evaluation of one's own behavior and attributes. Through the use of the Piers–Harris the practitioner is able to directly access the child's view of him- or herself in various situations and settings, rather than relying on interpretive inference.

The individual's responses to the questions of the Piers–Harris allow for the evaluation of both general and specific dimensions of self-concept. The six separate cluster scales provide for a detailed interpretation of the individual's self-perception. The normative information gathered from this measure serves to round out the clinical hypotheses developed through the use of other measures.

Practical implications: The Piers–Harris is a wide-band measure that offers insight into the individual's perception of her or his strengths and difficulties. The breadth of information gathered through this measure provides an overview of all major areas of a child's life. However, because of the use of one respondent, results are not adequate for differential diagnosis.

The Personality Inventory for Children (PIC). Structure: The PIC is a multidimensional, objective measure typically completed by a parent of the child. Three measures of informant response style, an adjustment scale, and 12 clinical scales are computed. Four factor scales are also included to clarify diagnosis in individual cases. The PIC was designed to assess the functioning of individuals from preschool to adolescence.

The PIC is perhaps the most clinically useful actuarial measure available for a school-age population (Lachar, Kline, & Boersma, 1986). An adult who is knowledgeable about the child (typically a parent) completes the inventory items. Results from this measure are then used to identify domains that may relate to specific behavioral problems. The individual's PIC profile may also be compared with the profiles of children exhibiting similar traits in order to predict behaviors and patterns of behavior.

The measures of informant response style included (e.g., Lie, Frequency, and Defensiveness Scales) are designed to assist in determining the validity of results. The Adjustment Scale is a general screening measure of poor psychological adjustment and may assist in identifying children in need of further psychological assessment. The first 3 of the 12 clinical scales (Achievement, Intellectual, and Development) provide information regarding the cognitive status of the individual. The remaining clinical scales evaluate such areas as somatic concerns, depression, family relations, delinquency, withdrawal, anxiety, psychosis, hyperactivity, and social skills (Lachar, 1990).

The PIC offers actuarially based information regarding the behavioral functioning of the child when included as part of a comprehensive battery. The information gathered from a parent or guardian is unique in comparison with that provided by a teacher or self-report. This information may then be used to evaluate situation-specific behaviors and parental perception of difficulties. The PIC also seems to be a promising instrument for characterizing the behavioral sequelae of a head injury, for following the course of a disorder, and for examining personality correlates in light of development of a rehabilitation program (Hynd & Willis, 1988; Knoff, 1986).

Practical implications: The PIC assesses the parent's or guardian's view of individual functioning across various settings and demands. Results pro-

vide empirical analysis of a child's behavior, affect, ability, and family functions. The great variety of scales included in the PIC allows for a more detailed description of behavior than is typically provided by parent report measures. The clinical specificity of this measure offers the neuropsychological evaluation an actuarial component important in the diagnosis and treatment of individual difficulties.

The Behavior Assessment System for Children (BASC). Structure: The BASC provides an actuarially based approach to the evaluation of behavior. This measure includes a structured developmental history, a self-report inventory, a parent rating scale, and a teacher rating scale. The BASC scales are designed for use with children and adolescents 4 to 18 years old.

The BASC is one of the most innovative and comprehensive rating scales available (Reynolds & Kamphaus, 1992). It is a multimethod, multidimensional approach to evaluating the behavior and self-perceptions of children and adolescents. The multimethod feature of the BASC is found in the five separate components available for use: a structured developmental history, a self-report scale completed by the child, rating scales for both parents and teachers, and a form for recording and classifying observed classroom behavior. The multidimensional feature of the BASC is found in the numerous aspects of behavior and personality measured, including adaptive and clinical dimensions.

Perhaps the most clinically useful aspect of the BASC, in comparison with other instruments such as the PIC, is the provision of information from three separate sources: child, parent, and teacher. The Self-Report of Personality, the Parent Rating Scales (PRS), and the Teacher Rating Scales provide information from multiple points of reference and across multiple settings. The Self-Report of Personality assesses the respondent's level of clinical maladjustment, school maladjustment, depression, sense of inadequacy, and personal adjustment. The PRS evaluates the individual's actions toward others, actions toward self, attention problems, withdrawal, and adaptive skills. The Teacher Rating Scales include the areas evaluated by the PRS as well as specific school-related concerns such as study skills and learning problems. Overall, the inclusion of information from multiple points of reference provides for a more complete and balanced picture of the current functioning and concerns of the child in question.

Practical implications: A clear strength of the BASC is the inclusion of information from the perspective of the individual, the parent, and the teacher.

The analysis of behavioral information from multiple sources and settings should be of great utility to practitioners of neuropsychology. Overall, the BASC integrates a variety of perspectives that are often lacking in traditional neuropsychological evaluations.

Vineland Adaptive Behavior Scales (VABS). Structure: Each of the three versions of the VABS (Interview Edition, Survey Form; Interview Edition, Expanded Form; and the Classroom Edition) measures adaptive behavior across four separate domains: Communication, Daily Living Skills, Socialization, and Motor Skills. The Maladaptive Behavior domain is provided as an optional area in the Survey and the Expanded Form. An Adaptive Behavior Composite, a combination of the four adaptive behavior domains, provides an overall analysis of personal and social sufficiency. The VABS measures adaptive skill across the age range of birth to adulthood.

The VABS is designed to assess the living skills of individuals through the report of a parent, caregiver, or teacher. The current form of the VABS is a revision of the Vineland Social Maturity Scale (Doll, 1935). Each of the four adaptive behavior domains is composed of subdomains that provide specific information regarding the individual's ability to function within his or her environment. The Communication domain contains Receptive, Expressive, and Written subdomains, examining what the individual understands, says, reads, and writes. The Daily Living Skills domain evaluates the individual's ability to independently eat, dress, perform household tasks, and use time, money, and job skills through the Personal, Domestic, and Community subdomains. The Socialization domain includes the three subdomains of Interpersonal Relationships, Play and Leisure Time, and Coping Skills, examining how the individual acts with others, plays, uses leisure time, and demonstrates responsibility and sensitivity to others. Finally, the Motor Skills domain evaluates how the individual uses arms and legs for movement, and hands and fingers to manipulate objects through the Gross and Fine subdomains (Harrison, 1990; Kamphaus, 1993).

The original Vineland was characterized by a limited normative sample and inadequate support for reliability and validity. In order to combat this weakness, great care was taken to ensure the technical adequacy of the VABS (Harrison, 1990). The VABS provides standardized evaluation of behavioral status in those situations in which the individual is unable to consistently respond to evaluation questions or tasks. This measure is most typically used in school psychology evaluations considering the real-life performance of children suspected of or diagnosed as having limited intellectual capacity. In neuropsychology, the VABS may be used following traumatic brain injuries, degenerative disorders, or other cerebral impairments to document the loss or return of adaptive behaviors (Lezak, 1983). In fact, the VABS can be one of the most beneficial instruments available to help develop rehabilitation plans for impaired individuals.

Practical implications: The VABS considers life skills to a greater degree than any measure previously discussed. The information provided by the VABS is important in discerning what tasks the individual is capable of performing independently. In addition to the evaluation of living skills related to limited intellectual capacity, the VABS is also of use in determining the skills of children following neuropsychological impairment.

The Thematic Apperception Test (TAT). Structure: The TAT is a projective test consisting of 31 cards, with 30 cards depicting various scenes and people, and 1 card being blank. Specific male/female, children, adolescent, and adult issues are presented. Typically, 10 cards that relate to the issues thought to be faced by the individual are selected for use.

The TAT was the first widely used thematic technique. Developed by Murray (1938, 1943), the TAT was designed to facilitate the psychoanalytic exploration of an individual's dominant drives, emotions, traits, and conflicts. By identifying significant needs, presses, and themes, the inhibited and unconscious personality characteristics of the individual were thought to be brought to the surface. Through the use of projective interpretation, the TAT offers insight into the etiology of behavior, and allows for a better understanding of the issues presented by the individual in question (Bellak, 1993). Few personality tests provide the depth of insight relative to the child's view of the world. This wide-band, open-ended technique offers data regarding how the individual responds to authority, popularity, male/female roles, dominant personality traits, and familial relationships.

The validity and reliability of the TAT have been difficult to establish because of the open-ended, free-response nature of the measure, and limited avenues through which to validate inferences (Knoff, 1986). In an effort to address this difficulty, a number of quantitative scoring methods have been established. Although these methods have aided practitioners in developing a more normative approach to interpretation, the clinical use of the TAT often remains rather informal and idiosyncratic

(Lanyon & Goodstein, 1982). A distinct advantage of including the TAT as part of a comprehensive assessment battery is the opportunity it provides for examining the individual's ability to organize and maintain ideas (Lezak, 1983). Practitioners operating from a neuropsychological paradigm are able to evaluate the individual's verbal behavior. Those individuals with cerebral impairment are more likely to use fewer words and ideas in telling the stories, tend to take longer to respond to the stimuli, are more likely to describe the picture than make up a story, and may present inflexible, concrete responses to the various cards (Lezak, 1983). An alternate administration technique is to have the individual write her or his response to each pictorial card. The written product may then be used to compare verbal and written response styles.

Practical implications: The TAT enables individuals to relate their thoughts and feelings through a free-response, open-ended technique. In comparison to other personality measures, this measure does not limit the individual to a set choice of responses. The projective nature of the measure is useful in alleviating response sets resulting from social constraints. The TAT allows for a thorough analysis of verbal behavior, as well as a glimpse into the individuals' view of their world.

Conclusions

Because neuropsychological assessment is geared to treat all manifestations of behavior as related to the functional integrity of the central nervous system, it follows that the tests commonly ascribed to psychological and educational functioning can provide a wealth of information to that enterprise. The strength of the flexible battery view of assessment as proposed here lies in its adaptability to clinical need. By integrating knowledge of brain function with the overt aspects of behavior detailed by formal and informal techniques, the clinician can gain a balanced picture of individuals in their interactions with various environmental systems. The domains of a behavior discussed here have offered insight into the breadth of evaluation available to probe the diverse nature of cognition, affect, and action. Once the practitioner identifies the assessment needs of the individual child, and a decision is made as to the components most relevant for exploring the dimensions of behavior, the process can begin. It is only through the quality of the data obtained that the effectiveness of potential intervention strategies can be gauged. To this end, this chapter intended to give the practitioner a range of assessment options from which to make wise choices.

References

Anastasi, A. (1988). *Psychological testing* (6th ed.). New York: Macmillan Co.

Bailey, D. B., Jr., Vandiviere, P., Dellinger, J., & Munn, D. (1987). The Battelle Developmental Inventory: Teacher perceptions and implementation data. *Journal of Psychoeducational Assessment, 3,* 217–226.

Begali, V. (1994). The role of the school psychologists. In R. C. Savage & G. F. Wolcott (Eds.), *Educational dimensions of acquired brain injury* (pp. 453–474). Austin, TX: Pro-Ed.

Bellak, L. (1993). *The TAT, CAT, and SAT in clinical use* (5th ed.). Boston: Allyn & Bacon.

Bendell-Estroff, D., Greenfield, D. B., Hogan, A. E., & Claussen, A. H. (1989). Early assessment of sensorimotor and cognitive development in high-risk infants. *Journal of Pediatric Psychology, 14,* 549–557.

Bender, L. (1938). A Visual Motor Gestalt Test and its clinical use. *American Orthopsychiatric Association Research Monograph,* No. 3.

Bornstein, R. A. (1987). The WAIS-R in neuropsychological practice boon or bust. *The Clinical Neuropsychological, 1,* 185–190.

Boyd, R. D., Welge, P., Sexton, D., & Miller, J. H. (1989). Concurrent validity of the Battelle Developmental Inventory: Relationship with the Bayley Scales in young children with known or suspected disabilities. *Journal of Early Intervention, 13,* 14–23.

Bracken, B. A. (1987). Limitations of preschool instruments and standards for minimal levels of technical adequacy. *Journal of Psychoeducational Assessment, 4,* 313–326.

Brand, H. J. (1991). Correlation for scores on revised tests of visual–motor integration and copying test in a South African sample. *Perceptual and Motor Skills, 73,* 225–226.

Butterbaugh, G. J. (1988). Selected psychometric and clinical review of neurodevelopmental infant tests. *The Clinical Neuropsychologist, 2,* 350–364.

Canter, A. (1990). A new Binet, an old premise: A mismatch between technology and evolving practice. *Journal of Psychoeducational Assessment, 8,* 443–450.

Chattin, S. H., & Bracken, B. A. (1989). School psychologists' evaluation of the K-ABC, McCarthy Scales, Stanford–Binet IV, and WISC-R. *Journal of Psychoeducational Assessment, 7,* 112–130.

Chittooran, M. M., D'Amato, R. C., Lassiter, K., & Dean, R. S. (1993). Factor structure of psychoeducational and neuropsychological measures with learning disabled children. *Psychology in the Schools, 30,* 109–118.

D'Amato, R. C. (1990). A neuropsychological approach to school psychology. *School Psychology Quarterly, 5,* 141–160.

D'Amato, R. C., & Dean, R. S. (1987). Psychological assessment reports, individual education plans, and daily lesson plans: Are they related? *Professional School Psychology, 2,* 93–101.

D'Amato, R. C., & Dean, R. S. (1988). School psychology practice in a department of neurology. *School Psychology Review, 18,* 416–420.

D'Amato, R. C., & Dean, R. S. (Eds.). (1989a). *The school psychologist in nontraditional settings: Integrating clients, services, and settings.* Hillsdale, NJ: Erlbaum.

D'Amato, R. C., & Dean, R. S. (1989b). The past, present, and future of nontraditional school psychology. In R. C. D'Amato & R. S. Dean (Eds.), *The school psychologist in nontraditional settings: Integrating clients, services, and settings* (pp. 185–209). Hillsdale, NJ: Erlbaum.

D'Amato, R. C., Dean, R. S., Rattan, G., & Nickell, K. A. (1988). A study of psychological referrals for learning-disabled children. *Journal of Psychoeducational Assessment, 6,* 118–124.

D'Amato, R. C., Gray, J. W., & Dean, R. S. (1988). A comparison between intelligence and neuropsychological functioning. *Journal of School Psychology, 26,* 283–292.

D'Amato, R. C., Hammons, P. F., Terminie, T. J., & Dean, R. S. (1992). Neuropsychological training in American Psychological Association-accredited and nonaccredited school psychology programs. *Journal of School Psychology, 30,* 175–183.

D'Amato, R. C., & Rothlisberg, B. A. (1996). How education should respond to students with traumatic brain injuries. *Journal of Learning Disabilities, 29,* 670–683.

D'Amato, R. C., & Rothlisberg, B. A. (Eds.). (1992). *Psychological perspectives on intervention: A case study approach to prescriptions for change.* New York: Longman.

Das, J. P., Kirby, J. R., & Jarman, R. F. (1979). *Simultaneous and successive processes.* New York: Academic Press.

Das, J. P., Naglieri, J. A., & Kirby, J. R. (1994). *Assessment of cognitive processes.* Boston: Allyn and Bacon.

Dean, R. S. (1979). Cerebral laterality and verbal–performance discrepancies in intelligence. *Journal of School Psychology, 17,* 145–150.

Dean, R. S. (1985a). Neuropsychological assessment. In J. D. Cavenar, R. Michels, H. K. H. Brodie, A. M. Cooper, S. B. Guze, L. L. Judd, G. L. Klerman, & A. J. Solnit (Eds.), *Psychiatry* (pp. 1–16). Philadelphia: Lippincott.

Dean, R. S. (1985b). Foundation and rationale for neuropsychological bases of individual differences. In L. C. Hartlage & C. F. Telzrow (Eds.), *The neuropsychology of individual differences: A developmental perspective* (pp. 7–39). New York: Plenum Press.

Dean, R. S. (1986a). Perspectives on the future of neuropsychological assessment. In B. S. Plake & J. C. Witt (Eds.), *Buros–Nebraska series on measurement and testing: Future of testing and measurment* (pp. 203–241). Hillsdale, NJ: Erlbaum.

Dean, R. S. (1986b). Neuropsychological aspects of psychiatric disorders. In J. E. Obrzut & G. W. Hynd (Eds.), *Child neuropsychology* (Vol. 2, pp. 10–34). New York: Academic Press.

Dean, R. S. (1986c). Lateralization of cerebral functions. In D. Wedding, A. M. Horton, & J. S. Webster (Eds.), *The neuropsychology handbook: Behavioral and clinical perspectives* (pp. 80–102). Berlin: Springer-Verlag.

Dean, R. S., & Gray, J. W. (1990). Traditional approaches to neuropsychological assessment. In C. R. Reynolds & R. W. Kamphaus (Eds.), *Handbook of psychological and educational assessment of children* (pp. 371–388). New York: Guilford Press.

Doll, E. A. (1935). A genetic scale of social maturity. *American Journal of Orthopsychiatry, 5,* 180–188.

Elliott, C. D. (1990). *Differential Ability Scales: Introductory and technical handbook.* San Antonio, TX: The Psychological Corporation.

Fagan, J. F. (1984). The relationship of novelty preferences during infancy to later intelligence and later recognition memory. *Intelligence, 8,* 339–346.

Frey, P. D., & Pinelli, B. (1991). Visual discrimination and visuomotor integration among two classes of Brazilian children. *Perceptual and Motor Skills, 72*(3), 847–850.

Gaddes, W. H. (1985). *Learning disabilities and brain function: A neuropsychological approach* (2nd ed.). Berlin: Springer-Verlag.

Gaddes, W. H., & Edgell, D. (1994). *Learning disabilities and brain function* (3rd ed.). Berlin: Springer-Verlag.

Goldstein, D. J., Smith, K. B., & Waldrep, E. E. (1986). Factor analytic study of the Kaufman Assessment Battery for Children. *Journal of Clinical Psychology, 42,* 890–894.

Goldstein, G., Katz, L., Slomka, G., & Kelly, M. A. (1993). Relationships among academic, neuropsychological, and intellectual status in subtypes of adults with learning disability. *Archives of Clinical Neuropsychology, 8,* 41–53.

Goodman, J. F. (1990). Infant intelligence: Do we, can we, should we assess it? In C. R. Reynolds & R. W. Kamphaus (Eds.), *Handbook of psychological and educational assessment of children: Intelligence and achievement* (pp. 183–208). New York: Guilford Press.

Gray, J. W., Dean, R. S., & Rattan, G. (1987). Assessment of perinatal risk factors. *Psychology in the Schools, 24,* 15–21.

Gutkin, T. B., & Reynolds, C. R. (Eds.). (1990). *The handbook of school psychology* (2nd ed.). New York: Wiley.

Harrison, P. L. (1990). Mental retardation: Adaptive behavior assessment, and giftedness. In A. S. Kaufman (Ed.), *Assessing adolescent and adult intelligence* (pp. 533–585). Boston: Allyn & Bacon.

Hartlage, L. C., & Golden, C. J. (1990). Neuropsychological assessment techniques. In T. B. Gutkin & C. R. Reynolds (Eds.), *The handbook of school psychology* (pp. 431–457). New York: Wiley.

Hartlage, L. C., & Telzrow, C. F. (1983). The neuropsychological bases of educational intervention. *Journal of Learning Disabilities, 16,* 521–528.

Hartlage, L. C., & Telzrow, C. F. (Eds.). (1986). *The neuropsychology of individual differences: A developmental perspective.* New York: Plenum Press.

Horn, J. L., & Cattell, R. B. (1966). Refinement and test of the theory of fluid and crystallized general intelligence. *Journal of Educational Psychology, 57,* 253–270.

Hynd, G. W., & Obrzut, J. E. (Eds.). (1981). *Neuropsychological assessment and the school-age child: Issues and procedures.* New York: Grune & Stratton.

Hynd, G. W., & Semrud-Clikeman, M. (1990). Neuropsychological assessment. In A. S. Kaufman (Ed.), *Assessing adolescent and adult intelligence* (pp. 638–695). Boston: Allyn & Bacon.

Hynd, G. W., & Willis, W. G. (1988). *Pediatric neuropsychology.* New York: Grune & Stratton.

Johnson, L. J., Cook, M. J., & Kullman, A. J. (1992). An examination of the concurrent validity of the Battelle Developmental Inventory as compared with the Vineland Adaptive Scales and the Bayley Scales of Infant Development. *Journal of Early Intervention, 16,* 353–359.

Jortner, S. (1965). A test of Hovey's MMPI scale for CNS disorders. *Journal of Clinical Psychology, 21,* 285.

Kamphaus, R. W. (1993). *Clinical assessment of children's intelligence.* Boston: Allyn & Bacon.

Kamphaus, R. W., & Platt, L. O. (1992). Subtest specificities for the WISC-III. *Psychological Reports, 70,* 899–902.

Kaufman, A. S. (1979). *Intelligent testing with the WISC-R.* New York: Wiley.

Kaufman, A. S. (1990). *Assessing adolescent and adult intelligence.* Boston: Allyn & Bacon.

Kaufman, A. S. (1993). Joint exploratory factor analysis of the Kaufman Assessment Battery for Children and the Kaufman Adolescent and Adult Intelligence Test for 11- and 12-year-olds. *Journal of Clinical Child Psychology, 22,* 355–364.

Kaufman, A. S., & Kaufman, N. L. (1993). *Manual: Kaufman Adolescent and Adult Intelligence Test.* Circle Pines, MN: American Guidance Service.

Kelly, M. D., & Dean, R. S. (1990). Best practices in neuropsychology. In A. Thomas & J. Grimes (Eds.), *Best practices in school psychology—II* (pp. 491–506). Washington, DC: National Association of School Psychologists.

Knoff, H. M. (1986). *The assessment of child and adolescent personality.* New York: Guilford Press.

Knoff, H. M. (1990). Best practices in personality assessment. In A. Thomas & J. Grimes (Eds.), *Best practices in school psychology—II* (pp. 547–562). Washington, DC: National Association of School Psychologists.

Lachar, D. (1990). Objective assessment of child and adolescent personality: The Personality Inventory for Children (PIC). In C. R. Reynolds & R. W. Kamphaus (Eds.), *Handbook of psychological and educational assessment of children* (pp. 298–323). New York: Guilford Press.

Lachar, D., Kline, R. B., & Boersma, D. C. (1986). The Personality Inventory for Children: Approaches to actuarial interpretation in clinic and school settings. In H. M. Knoff (Ed.), *The psychological assessment of child and adolescent personality* (pp. 273–308). New York: Guilford Press.

Lanyon, R. I., & Goodstein, L. D. (1982). *Personality assessment* (2nd ed.). New York: Wiley.

Laurent, J., Swerdlik, M., & Ryburn, M. (1992). Review of validity research on the Stanford–Binet Intelligence Scale: Fourth Edition. *Psychological Assessment, 4,* 102–112.

Leu, P. W., & D'Amato, R. C. (1994). *Right children, wrong teachers? Using an ecological assessment for placement decisions.* Paper presented at the 26th Annual Convention of the National Association of School Psychologists, Seattle, WA.

Lewis, M., Jaskir, J., & Enright, M. K. (1986). The development of mental abilities in infancy. *Intelligence, 10,* 331–354.

Lezak, M. D. (1983). *Neuropsychological assessment* (2nd ed.). London: Oxford University Press.

Luria, A. R. (1966). *Higher cortical functions in man.* New York: Basic Books.

Luria, A. R. (1970). *Traumatic aphasia, its syndromes, psychology and treatment.* The Hague: Mouton.

Luria, A. R. (1973). *The working brain.* Harmondsworth: Penguin Books.

Luria, A. R. (1980). *Higher cortical functions in man* (2nd ed.). New York: Basic Books.

Luria, A. R., & Majovski, L. V. (1977). Basic approaches used in American and Soviet clinical neuropsychology. *American Psychologist, 32,* 959–968.

McLinden, S. E. (1989). An evaluation of the Battelle Developmental Inventory for determining special education eligibility. *Journal of Psychoeducational Assessment, 7,* 66–73.

Merrell, K. W. (1994). *Assessment of behavioral, social, and emotional problems.* New York: Longman.

Moore, A. D., Stambrook, M., Gill, D. D., Hawryluk, G. A., Peters, L. C., & Harrison, M. M. (1992). Factor structure of the Wechsler Adult Intelligence Scale-Revised in a traumatic brain injury sample. *Canadian Journal of Behavioral Science, 25,* 605–614.

Moore, A. D., Stambrook, M., Hawryluk, G. A., Peters, L. C., Gill, D. D., & Hymans, M. M. (1990). Test–retest stability of the Wechsler Adult Intelligence Scale-Revised in the assessment of head-injured patients. *Psychological Assessment, 2,* 98–100.

Murray, H. A. (1938). *Explorations of personality.* London: Oxford University Press.

Murray, H. A. (1943). *Thematic Apperception Test manual.* Cambridge, MA: Harvard University Press.

Naglieri, J. A. (1993). Pairwise and ipsative comparisons of WISC-III IQ and index scores. *Psychological Assessment, 5,* 113–116.

Palisano, R. J., & Dichter, C. G. (1989). Comparison of two tests of visual–motor development used to assess children with learning disabilities. *Perceptual and Motor Skills, 68,* 1099–1103.

Reitan, R. M. (1989). A note regarding some aspects of the history of clinical neuropsychology. *Archives of Clinical Neuropsychology, 4,* 385–391.

Reynolds, C. R. (1981). Neuropsychological assessment and the habitation of learning: Considerations in the search for the aptitude × treatment interaction. *School Psychology Review, 10,* 343–349.

Reynolds, C. R. (1986). Transactional models of intellectual development, yes. Deficit models of process remediation, no. *School Psychology Review, 15,* 256–260.

Reynolds, C. R., & Bigler, E. D. (1994). *Test of memory and learning*. Austin, TX: Pro-Ed.

Reynolds, C. R., & Kamphaus, R. W. (Eds.). (1990). *Handbook of psychological and educational assessment of children*. New York: Guilford Press.

Reynolds, C. R., & Kamphaus, R. W. (1992). *Behavior Assessment System for Children manual*. Circle Pines, MN: American Guidance Services.

Rothlisberg, B. A. (1987). Assessing learning problems: How to proceed once you know the score. In R. S. Dean (Ed.), *Introduction to assessing human intelligence: Issues and procedures* (pp. 207–227). Springfield, IL: Thomas.

Rothlisberg, B. A. (1989). Processing styles, reading performance and the Kaufman Assessment Battery for Children. *Journal of Psychoeducational Assessment, 7,* 304–311.

Rothlisberg, B. A. (1992). Integrating psychological approaches to intervention. In R. C. D'Amato & B. A. Rothlisberg (Eds.), *Psychological perspectives on intervention: A case study approach to prescriptions for change* (pp. 190–198). New York: Longman.

Russell, E. W. (1987). Neuropsychological interpretation of the WAIS. *Neuropsychology, 1,* 2–6.

Sachs, P. R. (1991). *Treating families of brain-injury survivors*. Berlin: Springer-Verlag.

Salvia, J., & Ysseldyke, J. E. (1991). Assessment of infants, toddlers, and preschool children. In J. Salvia & J. E. Ysseldyke (Eds.), *Assessment* (5th ed., pp. 465–494). Boston: Houghton Mifflin.

Sattler, J. M. (1992). *Assessment of children* (3rd ed., revised). San Diego: Sattler.

Savage, R. C. & Wolcott, G. F. (Eds.). (1994). *Educational dimensions of acquired brain injury*. Austin, TX: Pro-Ed.

Selz, M. J., & Wilson, S. L. (1989). Neuropsychological bases of common learning and behavior problems in children. In C. R. Reynolds & E. Fletcher-Janzen (Eds.), *Handbook of clinical child neuropsychology* (pp. 129–145). New York: Plenum Press.

Shea, V. (1989). Peabody Picture of Vocabulary Test-Revised. In C. S. Newmark (Ed.), *Major psychological assessment instruments* (Vol. II, pp. 271–283). Boston: Allyn & Bacon.

Snyder, P., Lawson, S., Thompson, B., Stricklin, S., & Sexton, D. (1993). Evaluating the psychometric integrity of instruments used in early intervention research: The Battelle Developmental Inventory. *Topics in Early Childhood Special Education, 13,* 216–232.

Taylor, H. G. (1988). Neuropsychological testing: Relevance for assessing children's learning disabilities. *Journal of Consulting and Clinical Psychology, 56,* 795–800.

Telzrow, C. F. (1986). The science and speculation of rehabilitation in developmental neuropsychological disorders. In L. C. Hartlage & C. F. Telzrow (Eds.), *The neuropsychology of individual differences: A developmental perspective* (pp. 271–307). New York: Plenum Press.

Telzrow, C. F. (1989). Neuropsychological applications of common educational and psychological tests. In C. R. Reynolds & E. Fletcher-Janzen (Eds.), *Handbook of clinical child neuropsychology* (pp. 227–245). New York: Plenum Press.

Telzrow, C. F. (1990). Management of academic and educational problems in traumatic brain injury. In E. D. Bigler (Ed.), *Traumatic brain injury* (pp. 251–272). Austin, TX: Pro-Ed.

U.S. Department of Education. (1993). *Digest of educational statistics*. Washington, DC: Office of Educational Research and Improvement.

Vernon, P. E. (1987). The demise of the Stanford–Binet Scale. *Canadian Psychology, 28,* 251–258.

Webster, R. E. (1991). Review of the Woodcock–Johnson Psycho-Educational Test Battery-Revised. In D. J. Keyser & R. C. Sweetland (Eds.), *Test critiques* (Vol. 10, pp. 804–815). Kansas City, MO: Test Corporation of America.

Wedding, D., Horton, A. M., & Webster, J. S. (Eds.). (1986). *The neuropsychology handbook: Behavioral and clinical perspectives*. Berlin: Springer-Verlag.

Wersh, J., & Thomas, M. R. (1990). The Stanford–Binet Intelligence Scale: Fourth Edition; observations, comments and concerns. *Canadian Psychology, 31,* 190–193.

Whatley, J. L. (1987). Review of the Bayley Scales of Infant Development. In D. J. Keyser & R. C. Sweetland (Eds.), *Test critiques* (Vol. 6, pp. 38–47). Kansas City, MO: Test Corporation of America.

Whitten, C. J., D'Amato, R. C., & Chittooran, M. M. (1992). The neuropsychological approach to intervention. In R. C. D'Amato & B. A. Rothlisberg (Eds.), *Psychological perspectives on intervention: A case study approach to prescriptions for change* (pp. 112–136). New York: Longman.

Williams, R. E., & Vincent, K. R. (1991). Review of the Peabody Individual Achievement Test-Revised. In D. J. Keyser & R. C. Sweetland (Eds.), *Test critiques* (Vol. 8, pp. 557–562). Kansas City, MO: Test Corporation of America.

15

Clinical Neuropsychological Assessment of Child and Adolescent Memory with the Test of Memory and Learning

CECIL R. REYNOLDS AND ERIN D. BIGLER

Memory complaints seem ubiquitous in the clinical practice of neuropsychology. Nearly every central nervous system (CNS) disorder associated with disturbances of higher cognitive functions has memory disturbance in some form noted as a common complaint (see, for example, reviews of disorders and their assessment in Baron, Fennell, & Voeller, 1995; Cullum, Kuck, & Ruff, 1990; Cytowic, 1996; Gillberg, 1995; Knight, 1992; Lezak, 1995; Mapou & Spector, 1995; Reeves & Wedding, 1994). In cases of traumatic brain injury (TBI), memory disturbances are the most common of all patient complaints (Cronwall, Wrightson, & Waddell, 1990; Golden, Zillmer, & Spiers, 1992; Reeves & Wedding, 1994). Individuals between 10 and 20 years old account for a majority of cases of TBI with males outnumbering females by about 3 to 1 in acquired brain injuries during this time, with motor vehicle accidents the most common cause of TBI (Goldstein & Levin, 1990). TBI produces the least predictable forms of memory loss with the exception of increased forgetting curves. However, as research becomes more sophisticated, disturbances of memory and learning are being discovered elsewhere as well. In childhood medical disorders as well as in a variety of neu-

ropsychiatric disturbances, memory is often compromised along with acquisition of new material. Table 1 lists the most frequent childhood disorders in which memory and learning are likely to be compromised and should thus be assessed.

Memory is almost always one focus of cognitive rehabilitation or retraining as well (Prigatano, 1990). However, recovery of memory functions post-TBI is less predictable than improvements in more general aspects of intellectual function, likely, at least in part, because of the disturbances of attention and concentration that typically accompany TBI. Problems with memory are some of the most persistent sequelae of TBI. While some forms of memory tasks are suppressed in functional and organic disorders (e.g., immediate recall), other memory tasks provide very good discrimination between psychiatric disorders such as depression and TBI and other CNS insult (e.g., delayed recall or forgetting).

Given the ubiquitous nature of memory in daily affairs, particularly during the school-age years, and the importance of memory in evaluating the functional and the physiological integrity of the brain, it is surprising that comprehensive assessment of memory in children and adolescents is a recent phenomenon. This seems particularly odd given the plethora of such tasks available for adults dating from at least the 1930s.

To some extent memory assessment with children and adolescents must have been viewed as important since the earliest of modern intelligence tests (the 1907 Binet) and even the venerable

CECIL R. REYNOLDS • Department of Educational Psychology, Texas A&M University, College Station, Texas 77843.
ERIN D. BIGLER • Department of Psychology, Brigham Young University, Provo, Utah, 84602; and LDS Hospital, Salt Lake City, Utah 84143.

**TABLE 1. Most Frequent Childhood Disorders in Which Memory and Learning
Are Likely to Be Compromised**

Attention deficit-hyperactivity disorder	*In utero* toxic exposure (e.g.,	anencephaly, microcephaly,
Autism and other developmental	cocaine babies, fetal alcohol syndrome)	callosal dysgenesis)
disorders	Juvenile Huntington's disease	Neurofibromatosis
Cancer (especially brain tumors,	Juvenile parkinsonism	Prader–Willi syndrome
lung cancer, parathyroid tumors,	Kidney disease/transplant	Rett's syndrome
leukemia, and lymphoma)	Learning disability	Schizophrenia
Cerebral palsy	Lesch–Nyhan disease	Seizure disorders
Down syndrome	Liver disease/transplant	Tourette's syndrome
Endocrine disorders	Major depressive disorder	Toxic exposure (e.g., lead,
Extremely low birth weight	Meningitis	mercury, CO)
Fragile X	Mental retardation	Traumatic brain injury
Hydrocephalus	Myotonic dystrophy	Turner's syndrome
Hypoxic–ischemic injury	Neurodevelopmental	Williams syndrome
Inborn errors of metabolism	abnormalities affecting	XXY syndrome
(e.g., PKU, galactosemia)	brain development (e.g.,	XYY syndrome

Wechsler Scales, in their various children's versions, all included one or two brief assessments of immediate recall. Still, the major texts on child neuropsychology of the 1970s and 1980s (e.g., Bakker, Fisk, & Strang, 1985; Hynd & Obrzut, 1981) do not discuss assessment of memory despite the finding that 80% of a sample of various clinicians who perform testing noted memory as an important aspect of the assessment of cognitive and intellectual functions (Snyderman & Rothman, 1987). By 1995 (e.g., Rourke, Bakker, Fisk, & Strang, 1993), assessment of memory function in children is discussed in key textbooks and its relation to various medical (e.g., Baron *et al.,* 1995) and neuropsychiatric disorders (e.g., Gillberg, 1995) routinely included in major works on child neuropsychology.

Dorothea McCarthy, the noted psycholinguist, was aware of the importance of memory and included a memory index on the then-innovative McCarthy Scales of Children's Abilities (McCarthy, 1972). Koppitz (1977), another pioneer in assessment of children, noted the need for a more detailed evaluation of children's memory functions and devised the four-subtest Visual–Aural Digit Span Test (VADS; Koppitz, 1977). The VADS quickly became popular with school psychologists, among whom Koppitz was well known because of her work in childhood assessment with the Bender–Gestalt Test and human figure drawings, but was not adopted among neuropsychologists. The VADS is relatively narrow, assessing only sequential memory for digits but altering modality of input and output. No real attempt at developing a comprehensive assessment of children's memory appears until the introduction of the Wide Range Assessment of Memory and Learning (WRAML) for ages 5 through 17 by Sheslow and Adams (1990).

The WRAML was born of the frustration and dissatisfaction of its authors in not having a sound, comprehensive measure of memory functioning in children (Sheslow & Adams, 1990). The WRAML consists of nine subtests divided equally into three scales, Verbal Memory, Visual Memory, and Learning, followed by a brief delayed recall to assess rapidity of decay of memory (i.e., forgetting). The WRAML was a substantial improvement over existing measures of memory for children but still provided a limited sample of memory and learning tasks. To increase the breadth and depth of analysis of memory function from the preschool years through the high school years (ages 5 to 20), Reynolds and Bigler (1994a) developed the Test of Memory and Learning (TOMAL).

After a brief review of the basic neurobiology of memory, this chapter turns to a description of the TOMAL and its clinical interpretation. The TOMAL is featured for assessment of children's memory because "this measure is the most comprehensive of its kind . . . and will undoubtedly be a useful tool for assessing memory functioning in children and adolescents in many clinical, research, and educational settings" (Ferris & Kamphaus, 1995). The variety of well-normed, reliable subtests available on the TOMAL provides examiners with the maximum flexibility in evaluating various referral questions with the choice of the most comprehensive of assessments available as well, with good reliability and specificity of measurement for individual subtests.

Basic Neurobiology of Memory

Attention leaves tracks or traces within the brain that become memory. Memory, as commonly thought of, is the ability to recall some event or information of various types and forms. Biologically, memory functions at two broad levels, one at the level of the individual cell and the other at a systemic level. With the creation of memories, changes occur in individual cells (e.g., see Cohen, 1993; Diamond, 1990; Scheibel, 1990), including alterations in cell membranes and synaptic physiology.

At a systems level, there exists a division of sorts in the formation of memory and memory storage. There is considerable evidence for distributed storage of associative memory throughout the cortex, and which may even occur in a statistical function (Cohen, 1993). At the same time, there is evidence for more localized storage of certain memories and localized centers for the formation of memory and in classical and operant conditioning.

The medial aspect of the temporal lobe, particularly the hippocampus and its connecting fibers within the other limbic and paralimbic structures, is particularly important in development of associative memory. The limbic system (with emphasis on the posterior hippocampal regions) also mediates the development of conditioned responses and some patients with posterior hippocampal lesions may not respond to operant paradigms absent one-to-one reinforcement schedules. Damage to the medial temporal lobe and its connecting fibers or to the midline structures of the diencephalon typically results in the difficulties in formation of new memories (anterograde amnesia), but may also disrupt recently formed memories preceding the time of injury (retrograde amnesia). Various regions within the limbic and paralimbic structures have stronger roles in formation of certain types of memory, and simple conditioned memories may occur at a subcortical level. Through all of the interactions of these systems, related mechanisms of attention, particularly in the brain stem and

the frontal lobes, are brought to bear and will influence memory formation directly and indirectly. Memory is a complex function of the interaction of brain systems (with unequal contributions) and damage to one or more of many structures may impair the ability to form new memories.

In right-handed individuals there is a tendency for damage to the left temporal lobe and adjacent structures to affect verbal and sequential memory most strongly. Damage to the cognate areas of the right hemisphere affects visual and spatial memory more adversely.

Through distributive storage of memory, the entire brain participates in memory functioning. The recall of well-established memories tends to be one of the most robust of neural functions while the formation of new memories, sustained attention, and concentration tend to be the most fragile of neural functions. Neurological dysfunction of most types is associated with a nonspecific lessening of memory performance along with disruptions of attention and concentration, but with greater consequence when temporolimbic, brain stem, or frontal lobe involvement occurs. However, a variety of psychiatric disturbances, especially depression, may also supress fragile anterograde memory systems and a careful analysis of memory, forgetting, affective states, history, and comprehensive neuropsychological testing may be necessary before one can conclude that memory disturbances are organic in origin.

TOMAL

The TOMAL is a comprehensive battery of 14 memory and learning tasks (10 core subtests and 4 supplementary subtests) normed for use from ages 5 years 0 months 0 days through 19 years 11 months 30 days. The 10 core subtests are divided into the content domains of verbal memory and nonverbal memory that can be combined to derive a Composite Memory Index. A Delayed Recall Index is also available that requires a repeat recall of the first four subtests' stimuli 30 minutes after their first administration.

As noted above, memory may behave in unusual ways in an impaired brain and traditional content approaches to memory may not be useful. The TOMAL thus provides alternative groupings of the subtests into the Supplementary Indexes of Sequential Recall, Free Recall, Associative Recall, Learning, and Attention and Concentration. These Supplementary Indexes were derived by having a group of "expert" neuropsychologists sort the 14 TOMAL subtests into logical categories (Reynolds & Bigler, 1994b). To provide greater flexibility to the clinician, a set of four purely empirically derived factor indexes representing Complex Memory, Sequential Recall, Backward Recall, and Spatial Memory have been made available as well (Reynolds & Bigler, 1996). (The derivation of these empirical indexes is described in detail later in this chapter.)

Table 2 summarizes the names of the subtests and summary scores, along with their metric. The TOMAL subtests are scaled to the familiar metric of

TABLE 2. Core and Supplementary Subtests and Indexes Available for the TOMAL

	M	SD
Core subtests		
Verbal		
Memory for Stories	10	3
Word Selective Reminding	10	3
Object Recall	10	3
Digits Forward	10	3
Paired Recall	10	3
Nonverbal		
Facial Memory	10	3
Visual Selective Reminding	10	3
Abstract Visual Memory	10	3
Visual Sequential Memory	10	3
Memory for Location	10	3
Supplementary subtests		
Verbal		
Letters Forward	10	3
Digits Backward	10	3
Letters Backward	10	3
Nonverbal		
Manual Imitation	10	3
Summary scores		
Core indexes		
Verbal Memory Index (VMI)	100	15
Nonverbal Memory Index (NMI)	100	15
Composite Memory Index (CMI)	100	15
Delayed Recall Index (DRI)	100	15
Supplementary indexes (expert derived)		
Sequential Recall Index (SRI)	100	15
Free Recall Index (FRI)	100	15
Associative Recall Index (ARI)	100	15
Learning Index (LI)	100	15
Attention Concentration Index (ACI)	100	15
Factor scores (empirically derived)		
Complex Memory Index (CMFI)	100	15
Sequential Recall Index (SRFI)	100	15
Backwards Recall Index (BRFI)	100	15
Spatial Memory Index (SMFI)	100	15

mean equaling 10 and a standard deviation of 3 (range 1 to 20). Composite or summary scores are scaled to a mean of 100 and standard deviation of 15. All scaling was done using the method of rolling weighted averages and is described in detail in Reynolds and Bigler (1994b).

TOMAL Subtests

The ten core and four supplementary TOMAL subtests require about 60 minutes for a skilled examiner if the delayed recall subtests are also administered. The subtests were chosen to provide a comprehensive view of memory functions and, when used in toto, provide the most thorough assessment of memory available (Ferris & Kamphaus, 1995). The subtests are named and briefly described in Table 3.

The TOMAL subtests systematically vary the mode of presentation and response so as to sample verbal, visual, motoric, and combinations of these modalities in presentation and in response formats. Multiple trials to a criterion are provided on several subtests, including selective reminding, so that learning or acquisition curves may be derived. Multiple trials [at least five are necessary according to Kaplan (1996) and the TOMAL provides up to eight] are provided on the selective reminding subtests to allow an analysis of the depth of processing. In the selective reminding format (wherein examinees are reminded only of stimuli "forgotten" or unrecalled), when items once recalled are unrecalled by the examinee on later trials, problems are revealed in the transference of stimuli from working memory and immediate memory to more long-term storage. Cueing is also provided at the end of certain subtests to add to the examiner's ability to probe depth of processing.

Subtests are included that sample sequential recall (which tends strongly to be mediated by the left hemisphere, especially temporal regions; e.g., see Lezak, 1995) and free recall in both verbal and visual formats to allow localization; purely spatial memory tasks are included that are very difficult to confound via verbal mediation to assess more purely right hemisphere functions.

Well-established memory tasks (e.g., recalling stories) that also correlate well with school learning are included along with tasks more common to experimental neuropsychology that have high (e.g., Facial Memory) and low (e.g., Visual Selective Reminding) ecological salience; some subtests employ highly meaningful material (e.g., Memory for

TABLE 3. Description of TOMAL Subtests

Core

Memory for Stories. A verbal subtest requiring recall of a short story read to the examinee. Provides a measure of meaningful and semantic recall and is also related to sequential recall in some instances.

Facial Memory. A nonverbal subtest requiring recognition and identification from a set of distractors: black-and-white photos of various ages, males and females, and various ethnic backgrounds. Assesses nonverbal meaningful memory in a practical fashion and has been extensively researched. Sequencing of responses is unimportant.

Word Selective Reminding. A verbal free-recall task in which the examinee learns a word list and repeats it only to be reminded of words left out in each case: tests learning and immediate recall functions in verbal memory. Trials continue until mastery is achieved or until eight trials have been attempted: sequence of recall unimportant.

Visual Selective Reminding. A nonverbal analogue to WSR where examinees point to specified dots on a card, following a demonstration of the examiner, and are reminded only of items recalled incorrectly. As with WSR, trials continue until mastery is achieved or until eight trials have been attempted.

Object Recall. The examiner presents a series of pictures, names them, has the examinee recall them, and repeats this process across four trials. Verbal and nonverbal stimuli are thus paired and recall is entirely verbal, creating a situation found to interfere with recall for many children with learning disabilities but to be neutral or facilitative for children without disabilities.

Abstract Visual Memory. A nonverbal task. AVM assesses immediate recall for meaningless figures when order is unimportant. The examinee is presented with a standard stimulus and required to recognize the standard from any of six distractors.

Digits Forward. A standard verbal number recall task. DSF measures low-level rote recall of a sequence of numbers.

Visual Sequential Memory. A nonverbal task requiring recall of the sequence of a series of meaningless geometric designs. The ordered designs are shown followed by a presentation of a standard order of the stimuli and the examinee indicates the order in which they originally appeared.

Paired Recall. A verbal paired-associative learning task is provided by the examiner. Easy and hard pairs and measures of immediate associative recall and learning are provided.

Memory for Location. A nonverbal task that assesses spatial memory. The examinee is presented with a set of large dots distributed on a page and asked to recall the locations of the dots in any order.

Supplementary

Manual Imitation. A psychomotor, visually based assessment of sequential memory where the examinee is required to reproduce a set of ordered hand movements in the same sequence as presented by the examiner.

Letters Forward. A language-related analogue to common digit span tasks using letters as the stimuli in place of numbers.

Digits Backward. This is the same basic task as Digits Forward except the examinee recalls the numbers in reverse order.

Letters Backward. A language-related analogue to the Digits Backward task using letters as the stimuli instead of numbers.

Stories) while some use highly abstract stimuli (e.g., Abstract Visual Memory).

Aside from allowing a comprehensive review of memory function, the purpose for including such a factorial array of tasks across multiple dimensions is to allow a thorough, detailed analysis of memory function and the source of any memory deficits that may be discovered. The task of the neuropsychologist demands subtests with great specificity and variability of presentation and response and that sample all relevant brain functions in order to solve the complex puzzle of dysfunctional brain–behavior relationships. Kaufman (1979) first presented a detailed model for analyzing test data in a comprehensive format (later elaborated, Kaufman, 1994) that likens the task of the clinician to that of a detective. The thoroughness, breadth, and variability of the TOMAL subtests, coupled with their excellent psychometric properties, make the TOMAL ideal for use in an "intelli-

gent testing" model and particularly in the analysis of brain–behavior relationships associated with memory function.

Standardization

The TOMAL was standardized on a population-proportionate stratified (by age, gender, ethnicity, socioeconomic status, region of residence, and community size) random sample of children throughout the United States. Standardization and norming was conducted for ages 5 up to 20. Details of the standardization and specific statistics on the sample are provided in Reynolds and Bigler (1994b).

Reliability

The TOMAL subtests and composite indexes show excellent evidence of internal consistency reliability. Reynolds and Bigler (1994b) report coefficient alpha reliability estimates that routinely exceed 0.90 for individual *subtests* and 0.95 for composite scores. Stability coefficients are typically in the 0.80s.

Validity

Reynolds and Bigler (1994b) review a series of prepublication studies that demonstrate evidence for the validity of the TOMAL as a measure of memory functioning. The TOMAL scores correlate around 0.50 with measures of intelligence and achievement, indicating the TOMAL is related to but not the same as these measures. Measures of intelligence typically correlate with one another around 0.75 to 0.85 and with measures of achievement around 0.55 to 0.65.

Since publication of the TOMAL, several studies have provided evidence of convergent and divergent validity of the TOMAL subtests as measures of various aspects of memory by examining patterns of correlations among TOMAL subtests and the Rey Auditory Verbal Learning Test and the Wechsler Memory Scale-Revised. The verbal components of the TOMAL correlate well with these measures but the nonverbal sections are relatively independent (Barker *et al.*, 1994; Mueller *et al.*, 1994; Russo *et al.*, 1994). The TOMAL nonverbal subtests, unlike a number of other purportedly visual and nonverbal memory tests, are difficult to encode verbally, making the TOMAL nonverbal subtests more specific and less contaminated by examinees' attempts at verbal mediation. On the nonverbal or visual memory portions of existing memory batteries, examiners should expect larger differences across tests than on verbal memory measures.

Validity is a complex concept related to the interpretation of scores on tests and many approaches to the question of meaning of performance on tests such as the TOMAL are appropriate. Case studies, group comparisons, and views of the internal structure of tests all add to this knowledge. We next turn to the internal structure of the TOMAL.

Factor Structure of the TOMAL

Reynolds and Bigler (1996) provide extended information on the factor structure of the TOMAL and the derivation of the empirically derived *factor indexes* noted in Table 2. Using the method of principal factors with Varimax and Promax rotations,

the correlation matrix for all 14 TOMAL subtests was examined. Factors were extracted for three age groupings (5–8, 9–12, and 13–18) and were found to be consistent across age levels. The analyses reviewed below are based on the full sample of 1342 children. It is worthy of note that those analyses are based on normal, nonreferred children and that factor analyses do not always demonstrate the same results with exceptional samples, especially samples with CNS dysfunction (e.g., see review material by Kamphaus & Reynolds, 1987). The following is based substantively on the presentation by Reynolds and Bigler (1996).

The two-factor solutions of the TOMAL did not support the division of the subtests into a verbal and a nonverbal scale. Clearly the structure of the TOMAL is more complex than is represented by these two groupings. There is a general factor present, much as with the intellectual factor, g, but weaker, that nevertheless supports the use of a composite score such as the CMI with normal populations. Tables 4 and 5 show the two-factor Varimax and Promax results for the TOMAL when these factors are forced.

The unconstrained, exploratory factor analyses are also given in Tables 4–6. The use of the criteria for factor extraction recommended by Reynolds (1982) including an examination of scree plots across age, absolute value of the eigenvalues, and the psychological meaningfulness of each statistically viable solution indicated the possibility that three-, four-, and five-factor solutions had the potential to be the most appropriate alternative. A visual inspection of each of these solutions indicated that the four-factor factor solution best met the criteria given by Reynolds (1982) and essentially made the most psychological sense. The first and strongest factor appearing in the Promax solution appears to be a reflection of overall memory skills that perhaps represents more complex memory tasks and cuts across all modalities and memory processes. This first factor is designated primarily by the large loadings of Memory for Stories, Word Selective Reminding, Object Recall, Paired Recall, Facial Memory, and Visual Selective Reminding.

The second factor emphasizes sequential recall and attention and is composed principally of large loadings by Digits Forward, Letters Forward, Visual Sequential Memory, and Manual Imitation. The third factor consists of Digits Backward and Letters Backward, pointing clearly to the need for separate scaling of backward and forward memory span tasks. Backward digit recall is known to be a more

TABLE 4. Two- and Four-Factor Promax Solutions of TOMAL Subtests

Subtest	Subtest g_m[c]	FAC specificity[d]	Two-factor solution[a]		Four-factor solution[a]			
			FAC ONE	FAC TWO	FAC ONE	FAC TWO	FAC THREE	FAC FOUR
Memory for Stories	0.53	0.56	0.17	0.45	0.37	0.05	0.19	0.19
Word Selective Reminding	0.59	0.46	0.01	0.67	0.73	0.08	0.03	0.13
Object Recall	0.55	0.51	0.05	0.58	0.57	0.08	0.01	0.01
Digits Forward	0.64	0.45	0.71	0.00	0.03	0.74	0.05	0.06
Paired Recall	0.55	0.48	0.03	0.67	0.68	0.05	0.07	0.04
Letters Forward[b]	0.68	0.40	0.78	0.03	0.01	0.76	0.10	0.03
Digits Backward[b]	0.63	0.59	0.64	0.06	0.06	0.10	0.63	0.01
Letters Backward[b]	0.64	0.46	0.72	0.00	0.02	0.13	0.66	0.07
Facial Memory	0.39	0.66	0.02	0.47	0.37	0.01	0.08	0.24
Visual Selective Reminding	0.45	0.69	0.06	0.45	0.33	0.01	0.04	0.29
Abstract Visual Memory	0.54	0.60	0.14	0.49	0.32	0.01	0.03	0.39
Visual Sequential Memory	0.55	0.61	0.28	0.34	0.26	0.38	0.13	0.18
Memory for Location	0.31	0.68	0.24	0.12	0.06	0.00	0.09	0.44
Manual Imitation[b]	0.61	0.57	0.59	0.09	0.02	0.38	0.15	0.29

[a]Largest loading is underscored.
[b]Supplementary subtest.
[c]First unrotated factor loading, taken to represent a general memory factor.
[d]Subtest specific variance, using median values across age.

highly g-loaded task than forward digit recall and is likely to be more demanding mentally (e.g., see Jensen & Figueroa, 1975). The fourth factor, as seen in Table 4, is composed of Abstract Visual Memory and Memory for Location. This factor seems to tap spatial memory more strongly than other tasks. The four-factor Varimax solution provides the same results, essentially, but once again shows stronger secondary loadings of the various subtests than was true with the Promax solution. Both solutions

TABLE 5. Two- and Four-Factor Varimax Solutions of TOMAL Subtests

Subtest	Two-factor solution[a]		Four-factor solution[a]			
	FAC ONE	FAC TWO	FAC ONE	FAC TWO	FAC THREE	FAC FOUR
Memory for Stories	0.29	0.48	0.42	0.12	0.25	0.29
Word Selective Reminding	0.21	0.65	0.68	0.20	0.14	0.02
Object Recall	0.21	0.57	0.57	0.19	0.11	0.13
Digits Forward	0.68	0.21	0.21	0.69	0.23	0.09
Paired Recall	0.16	0.64	0.64	0.11	0.15	0.08
Letters Forward[b]	0.74	0.20	0.19	0.72	0.28	0.13
Digits Backward[b]	0.63	0.25	0.22	0.32	0.60	0.18
Letters Backward[b]	0.68	0.21	0.16	0.35	0.63	0.23
Facial Memory	0.12	0.45	0.39	0.08	0.02	0.27
Visual Selective Reminding	0.19	0.45	0.37	0.12	0.07	0.32
Abstract Visual Memory	0.27	0.54	0.40	0.13	0.14	0.43
Visual Sequential Memory	0.37	0.41	0.36	0.38	0.05	0.26
Memory for Location	0.26	0.18	0.06	0.10	0.14	0.43
Manual Imitation[b]	0.59	0.27	0.17	0.45	0.28	0.38

[a]Largest loading is underscored.
[b]Supplementary subtest.

TABLE 6. Three-Factor Promax and Varimax Solutions

Subtest	Varimax[a]				Promax[a]		
	FAC ONE	FAC TWO	FAC THREE		FAC ONE	FAC TWO	FAC THREE
Memory for Stories	0.20	0.43	0.31		0.05	0.38	0.25
Word Selective Reminding	0.24	0.67	0.01		0.10	0.70	0.12
Object Recall	0.16	0.58	0.09		0.08	0.58	0.00
Digits Forward	0.72	0.23	0.05		0.78	0.05	0.11
Paired Recall	0.16	0.64	0.10		0.00	0.66	0.00
Letters Forward[b]	0.76	0.21	0.10		0.82	0.00	0.06
Digits Backward[b]	0.54	0.19	0.37		0.51	0.01	0.28
Letters Backward[b]	0.58	0.14	0.42		0.55	0.06	0.34
Facial Memory	0.06	0.42	0.21		0.08	0.43	0.16
Visual Selective Reminding	0.12	0.40	0.27		0.02	0.39	0.22
Abstract Visual Memory	0.15	0.44	0.39		0.02	0.40	0.35
Visual Sequential Memory	0.35	0.40	0.15		0.27	0.33	0.05
Memory for Location	0.12	0.10	0.41		0.02	0.02	0.43
Manual Imitation[b]	0.50	0.21	0.37		0.45	0.04	0.28

[a]Largest loading is underscored.
[b]Supplementary subtest.

demonstrate clearly that the TOMAL is factorially complex and indicate that it measures multiple components of memory. The content-driven division into verbal and nonverbal memory indexes and the various expert-derived supplementary indexes described in Reynolds and Bigler (1994b) may be supplemented further for some children by the groupings discovered in these analyses.

Table 6 presents the three-factor Promax and Varimax solutions. The three-factor solutions suggest common factors across the Varimax and Promax rotations but once again the Promax solution seems more distinctive in nature. When three factors are extracted, the first factor is quite similar to the second factor derived in the four-factor solution and consists primarily of tasks such as letter and digit recall that require intense concentration and sequential recall. Manual Imitation loads on this factor as well, but carries a large secondary loading on the third factor where it is paired once again with Memory for Location. The second factor appears to be much the same in the three-factor solution as the first factor that appeared when two- and four-factor solutions are examined and is a factor made up of more complex memory tasks. Essentially, the three-factor solution presents a singlet as a third factor although Digits and Letters Backward tend to gravitate toward this factor which is defined by Memory for Location and may indicate that there is indeed a spatial component to backward memory

span (via the use of visualization strategies) as has been suspected by many clinicians. The four-factor solution, as can be seen, however, provides significantly greater clarity than the three-factor solution. A five-factor solution was also examined and was not viable.

Overall, these results suggest that memory as evaluated on the TOMAL is more process driven than content driven. Although the verbal–nonverbal memory distinction is useful clinically and may be more viable with clinical populations, especially those with TBI or highly localized space-occupying lesions, when memory function is examined in normal individuals, process appears to be more salient than item content or modality of presentation. It will be extremely useful in the future to conduct large-sample factor analyses of a broad-based set of memory tasks such as is available on the TOMAL using a clearly defined neurologically impaired sample. A large-sample analysis with a more heterogeneous group of learning-disabled children would also be quite informative in understanding the structure of memory and its role in learning problems among such populations.

Subtest Specificities

Subtest-specific variance can be derived from factor analysis as well and represents the proportion of variance of a subtest that is specific to the subtest (not shared with other variables) and that is also reliable. Table 4 lists the subtest specificities of the 14 TOMAL subtests as determined by subtracting the squared multiple correlation of all other subtests with the subtest in question from the reliability of the subtest (using the median value given in Reynolds & Bigler, 1994b, Table 5.1). A specificity value of 0.25 has been considered appropriate to support interpretation of an individual subtest score (e.g., see Kaufman, 1979).

The values reported in Table 4 reflect quite high specificities relative to measures of intelligence and achievement, which tend to be more highly interrelated. In all cases, the TOMAL subtests show specificity of 0.40 or higher and each specificity value exceeds the error variance ($1 - r_{xx}$) of the subtest. The TOMAL subtests thus demonstrate more than adequate specificity to support their interpretation as reflecting variation in an individual skill or component of memory when performance on a subtest deviates at a statistically significant level from the mean level of performance on the primary factor underlying the scale to which it is assigned. Procedures for making the latter determination are presented in the TOMAL Manual (Reynolds & Bigler, 1994b) and are also available through automated interpretation (Stanton, Reynolds, & Bigler, 1995).

Factor Indexes

The four-factor Promax solution offers an alternative approach to interpretation of the TOMAL, one that appears more process oriented than content oriented as the TOMAL was originally offered. To be useful clinically, however, standard scores for the various factors must be derived and normative tables provided.

Table 7 presents normative tables for the factors derived from the factor analysis described earlier. The derivation of the scores, or factor indexes, has been described previously. To use Table 7, it is necessary to sum the scaled scores for the subtests as follows:

- Complex Memory Factor Score (CMF) = Memory for Stories + Word Selective Reminding + Object Recall + Paired Recall + Visual Selective Reminding + Facial Memory
- Sequential Recall Factor Score (SRF) = Digits Forward + Letters Forward + Visual Sequential Memory + Manual Imitation

- Backwards Recall Factor Score (BRF) = Digits Backward + Letters Backward
- Spatial Memory Factor Score (SMF) = Abstract Visual Memory + Memory for Location

Scaled scores for the subtests must be used. The sum of scaled scores, the "factor score," is then converted to a factor index with a mean of 100 and a standard deviation of 15 by Table 7. The leftmost column provides the appropriate factor index for the sum of scaled scores, the factor score, in the table beneath the factor score headings.

The Appendix provides a form that may be reproduced and used to calculate the TOMAL factor indexes.

Reliability of the Empirically Derived Factor Indexes

Table 8 provides internal consistency reliability data for the four TOMAL factor indexes at 1-year age intervals, calculated as noted previously. All of these values fall above 0.90 except for the Spatial Memory Factor Index at the youngest age, 5 years, where it has a reliability coefficient of 0.85. Nearly all of the values are between 0.94 and 0.99 with median values of 0.95 for the Complex Memory Factor Index, and 0.94 for the Spatial Memory Factor Index. These reliability coefficients are quite comparable to the TOMAL Core Indexes and Supplementary Indexes described in the TOMAL Manual (Reynolds & Bigler, 1994b).

These factor indexes are thus highly reliable and add to the armamentarium of the clinician seeking to understand individual cases. How the subtests of the TOMAL will be understood best for each case encountered requires individualized interpretation; however, these scales have strong empirical support and their fit to the child's or adolescent's performance should be examined early in the interpretive process.

Cross-Ethnic Stability of Factor Indexes

When using tests outside the majority group in a population, one is always concerned about making common interpretations of performance. Black–white differences on various aptitude measures are well documented, well known, and are present on many neuropsychological measures. This has led to claims of cultural bias in diagnostic psychological testing with blacks. Very little re-

TABLE 7. Conversion Tables for Deriving Standard Score Index for Empirically Derived Factors on the TOMAL

Factor Index[a]	Sum of scaled scores				
	Complex Memory Factor Score[b] (CMFI)	Sequential Recall Factor Score[c] (SRFI)	Backwards Recall Factor Score[d] (BRFI)	Spatial Memory Factor Score[e] (SMFI)	Percentile
160+	112	76	40	40	>99
159	111	—	—	—	>99
158	—	75	—	—	>99
157	110	74	39	39	>99
156	109	—	—	—	>99
155	108	73	—	—	>99
154	107	—	38	38	>99
153	106	72	—	—	>99
152	105	71	—	—	>99
151	104	—	37	37	>99
150	103	70	—	—	>99
149	—	—	—	—	>99
148	102	69	36	36	>99
147	101	68	—	—	>99
146	100	—	—	—	>99
145	99	67	35	35	>99
144	98	—	—	—	>99
143	97	66	—	—	>99
142	—	65	34	34	>99
141	96	—	—	—	>99
140	95	64	—	—	>99
139	94	—	33	33	>99
138	93	63	—	—	99
137	92	62	—	—	99
136	91	—	32	32	99
135	90	61	—	—	99
134	—	60	—	—	99
133	89	59	31	31	99
132	88	—	—	—	99
131	87	58	—	—	98
130	86	—	30	30	98
129	85	57	—	—	97
128	84	56	—	—	97
127	—	—	29	29	97
126	83	55	—	—	96
125	82	—	—	—	95
124	81	54	28	28	95
123	80	53	—	—	94
122	79	—	—	—	93
121	78	52	27	27	92
120	77	—	—	—	91
119	—	—	—	—	90
118	76	51	26	26	89
117	75	50	—	—	87
116	74	—	—	—	86
115	73	49	25	25	84
114	72	—	—	—	82
113	71	48	—	—	81
112	—	47	24	24	79

(continued)

TABLE 7. (*Continued*).

111	70	—	—	—	77
110	69	46	—	—	75
109	68	—	23	23	73
108	67	45	—	—	70
107	66	44	—	—	68
106	65	—	22	22	65
105	64	43	—	—	63
104	—	—	—	—	61
103	63	42	21	21	58
102	62	41	—	—	55
101	61	—	—	—	53
100	60	40	20	20	50
99	59	—	—	—	47
98	58	39	—	—	45
97	—	38	19	19	42
96	57	—	—	—	39
95	56	37	—	—	37
94	55	—	18	18	35
93	54	36	—	—	32
92	53	35	—	—	30
91	52	—	17	17	27
90	51	34	—	—	25
89	50	—	—	—	23
88	—	33	16	16	21
87	49	32	—	—	19
86	48	—	—	—	18
85	47	31	15	15	16
84	46	—	—	—	14
83	45	30	—	—	13
82	44	29	14	14	12
81	—	—	—	—	10
80	43	28	—	—	9
79	42	—	13	13	8
78	41	27	—	—	7
77	40	26	—	—	6
76	39	—	12	12	5
75	38	25	—	—	5
74	37	—	—	—	4
73	—	24	11	11	3
72	36	23	—	—	3
71	35	—	—	—	3
70	34	22	10	10	2
69	33	—	—	—	2
68	32	21	—	—	1
67	31	20	9	9	1
66	—	—	—	—	1
65	30	19	—	—	1
64	29	—	8	8	<1
63	28	18	—	—	<1
62	27	17	—	—	<1
61	26	—	7	7	<1
60	25	16	—	—	<1
59	24	—	—	—	<1
58	—	15	6	6	<1
57	23	14	—	—	<1
56	22	—	—	—	<1
55	21	13	5	5	<1

TABLE 7. (*Continued*).

54	20	—	—	—	<1
53	19	12	—	—	<1
52	18	11	4	4	<1
51	—	—	—	—	<1
50	17	10	—	—	<1
49	16	—	3	3	<1
48	—	9	—	—	<1
47	15	8	—	—	<1
46	14	—	2	2	<1
45	13	7			<1
44	12	—			<1
43	11	6			<1
42	—	5			<1
41	10	—			<1
40	8–9	4			<1

[a]Index scores $X = 100$, SD = 15.
[b]Sum of scaled scores: Memory for Stories + Word Selective Reminding + Object Recall + Paired Recall + Visual Selective Reminding + Facial Memory.
[c]Sum of scaled scores: Digits Forward + Letters Forward + Visual Sequential Memory + Manual Imitation.
[d]Sum of scaled scores: Digits Backward + Letters Backward.
[e]Sum of scaled scores: Abstract Visual Memory + Memory for Location.

search has been done with neuropsychological measures and the cultural test bias hypothesis particularly relative to the plethora of bias research on intelligence tests (e.g., see Reynolds, 1995).

Reynolds and Bigler (1994b) report item-level bias studies of the TOMAL indicating that individual test items on the TOMAL function in highly similar ways for blacks and for whites. The question of the stability of the TOMAL factor indexes across race for blacks and whites arises as well. Research on intelligence tests reports comparability of factor structures across race for most major tests (Reynolds, 1995). There is but one such study of memory batteries, a study of the TOMAL by Mayfield and Reynolds (in press).

Mayfield and Reynolds (in press) analyzed the factor structure of the TOMAL separately for blacks and whites using the model of Reynolds and Bigler (1996) and recommendations of Reynolds (1982) for comparing factor-analytic results across groups.

Tables 9 and 10 present the rotated four-factor solutions for the Promax and Varimax rotations, respectively, as derived separately for blacks and for whites by Mayfield and Reynolds (in press). These factors represent factors similar to those proposed by Reynolds and Bigler (1996) for the combined sample. The coefficients of congruence (r_c) indicate that, regardless of the method of rotation (oblique or orthogonal), the latent structure of children's mem-

TABLE 8. Coefficient Alpha Reliability Estimates (Decimals Omitted) Based on Equally Weighted Composites Used to Derive TOMAL Factor Indexes

	Age															
Factor index	5	6	7	8	9	10	11	12	13	14	15	16	17	18	19	Mdn[a]
Complex Memory Factor Index (CMFI)	95	95	95	95	95	94	96	96	95	95	96	94	95	95	95	95
Sequential Recall Factor Index (SRFI)	98	98	98	98	98	98	98	98	98	98	98	98	97	98	97	98
Backwards Recall Factor Index (BRFI)	92	98	97	97	97	97	98	98	98	98	98	99	99	98	96	97
Spatial Memory Factor Index (SMFI)	85	94	95	94	93	96	96	96	95	95	91	91	95	94	96	94

[a]Median value across age.

TABLE 9. Four-Factor Promax Solution for Blacks and Whites[a]

	g_m[d]		Factor 1[b]		Factor 2[b]		Factor 3[b]		Factor 4[b]	
Subtest	Black	White	Black	White	Black	White	Black	White	Black	White
Memory for Stories	0.74	0.45	0.59	0.35	<u>0.80</u>	0.41	0.55	0.19	0.22	<u>0.45</u>
Word Selective Reminding	0.68	0.59	0.60	0.35	<u>0.66</u>	<u>0.70</u>	0.45	0.30	0.23	0.15
Object Recall	0.72	0.53	0.65	0.28	<u>0.69</u>	<u>0.61</u>	0.53	0.29	0.13	0.23
Digits Forward	0.78	0.58	0.74	0.49	0.47	0.33	<u>0.80</u>	<u>0.72</u>	0.16	0.27
Paired Recall	0.47	0.58	0.28	0.35	<u>0.64</u>	<u>0.66</u>	0.26	0.29	0.38	0.24
Letters Forward[c]	0.82	0.65	<u>0.82</u>	0.55	0.51	0.39	0.72	<u>0.78</u>	0.21	0.27
Digits Backward[c]	0.81	0.59	<u>0.90</u>	<u>0.70</u>	0.52	0.37	0.54	0.47	0.21	0.18
Letters Backward[c]	0.74	0.57	<u>0.87</u>	<u>0.72</u>	0.48	0.31	0.36	0.51	0.29	0.34
Facial Memory	0.54	0.42	0.37	0.21	<u>0.65</u>	<u>0.48</u>	0.36	0.18	0.32	0.30
Visual Selective Reminding	0.47	0.43	0.35	0.21	0.40	<u>0.47</u>	0.28	0.25	<u>0.63</u>	0.27
Abstract Visual Memory[c]	0.70	0.52	0.57	0.31	0.54	<u>0.50</u>	<u>0.59</u>	0.28	0.46	<u>0.50</u>
Visual Sequential Memory	0.53	0.54	0.33	0.30	0.40	<u>0.53</u>	<u>0.66</u>	0.46	0.34	0.17
Memory for Location	0.40	0.26	0.24	0.21	0.29	0.14	0.41	0.17	<u>0.53</u>	<u>0.45</u>
Manual Imitation[c]	0.82	0.45	<u>0.73</u>	<u>0.44</u>	0.59	0.27	<u>0.73</u>	0.38	0.38	0.42
Coefficient of Congruence	0.98		0.98		0.96		0.94		0.91	
Salient Variable Similarity Index[e]	1.00		1.00		0.96		0.88		0.78	

[a]Modified from Mayfield and Reynolds (in press).
[b]Largest loading is underscored.
[c]Supplementary subtests.
[d]First unrotated factor loading, taken to represent a general memory factor.
[e]Where salience ≥ 0.20.

ory, at least as assessed by the TOMAL, is constant for blacks and whites. The values of s (Cattell's salient variable similarity index) for each comparison are also statistically significant in each case bolstering the argument for comparability of the latent structure of the TOMAL for these two ethnic groups. The designation of each factor continues to be reasonable as suggested in prior research as well: Factor 1, Complex Memory; Factor 2, Sequential Recall; Factor 3, Backwards Recall; and Factor 4, Spatial Memory.

The general memory factor, designated from the first unrotated factor, reveals a strong overall tendency of these memory tasks to trend in a constant direction although the "g" of memory is less powerful than the general factor associated with intelligence. This also supports the distinction of memory from intelligence although the two surely overlap (Reynolds & Bigler, 1994b). The large value of r_c (0.98) and maximal value of s (1.00) show that this general memory factor is constant across race as are the four rotated factors (see Tables 9 and 10).

The values of r_c all exceed 0.90 for the Promax solution with values of 0.94, 0.93, 0.84, and 0.83 (for factors 1–4, respectively) for the Varimax solution and s is significant for each pair of factors. Although the values of r_c for factors 3 and 4 of the

Varimax solution are below 0.90, they are very close to this value and the Varimax solution is a poorer fit overall to the data than the Promax solution in the combined samples (Reynolds & Bigler, 1996); s is significant in each case. The strong fit across groups of the Promax solution and the reasonably good fit of an inferior solution support a consistent view of these factors across groups.

The consistency of the factor structure of the TOMAL across race for blacks and for whites indicates the test materials are perceived and reacted to in a highly similar manner for these two groups. Consistent interpretation of performance across race on the TOMAL is thus supported and changes in interpretation as a function of race do not appear to be appropriate based on current results.

Forward versus Backward Recall

One new feature of the TOMAL is the allowance of contrasts, in scaled score form, of forward and backward recall. Often, forward and backward recall are combined into a single score such as on the Wechsler Digit Span tasks. This is inappropriate and will mask important neurologic and diagnostic information (Ramsay & Reynolds, 1995;

TABLE 10. Four-Factor Varimax Solution for Blacks and Whites[a]

Subtest	Factor 1[b]		Factor 2[b]		Factor 3[b]		Factor 4[b]	
	Black	White	Black	White	Black	White	Black	White
Memory for Stories	0.36	0.21	<u>0.68</u>	0.32	0.28	0.01	0.11	<u>0.38</u>
Word Selective Reminding	0.43	0.18	<u>0.53</u>	<u>0.68</u>	0.18	0.12	0.13	−0.01
Object Recall	0.48	0.09	<u>0.55</u>	<u>0.58</u>	0.27	0.14	0.03	0.10
Digits Forward	<u>0.60</u>	0.25	0.18	0.16	<u>0.60</u>	<u>0.65</u>	0.12	0.14
Paired Recall	0.07	0.17	<u>0.61</u>	<u>0.63</u>	0.04	0.10	0.28	0.09
Letters Forward[c]	<u>0.69</u>	0.29	0.22	0.21	0.46	<u>0.69</u>	0.16	0.13
Digits Backward[c]	<u>0.84</u>	<u>0.60</u>	0.25	0.21	0.20	0.27	0.11	0.17
Letters Backward[c]	<u>0.83</u>	<u>0.61</u>	0.23	0.13	−0.01	0.31	0.22	0.20
Facial Memory	0.16	0.05	<u>0.57</u>	<u>0.45</u>	0.15	0.04	0.23	0.21
Visual Selective Reminding	0.19	0.04	0.24	<u>0.43</u>	0.05	0.13	<u>0.59</u>	0.18
Abstract Visual Memory[c]	0.38	0.10	0.32	<u>0.42</u>	0.35	0.11	<u>0.40</u>	0.41
Visual Sequential Memory	0.12	0.08	0.21	<u>0.47</u>	<u>0.58</u>	0.36	0.30	0.04
Memory for Location	0.07	0.08	0.21	0.04	0.28	0.09	<u>0.52</u>	<u>0.43</u>
Manual Imitation[c]	<u>0.55</u>	0.28	0.31	0.14	0.46	0.25	0.32	<u>0.34</u>
Coefficient of Congruence	0.94		0.93		0.84		0.83	
Salient Variable Similarity Index[d]	0.80		0.90		0.67		0.71	

[a]Modified from Mayfield and Reynolds (in press).
[b]Largest loading is underscored.
[c]Supplementary subtests.
[d]Where salience ≥ 0.20.

Reynolds, in press). Following a review of 27 relevant articles, Ramsay and Reynolds (1995) concluded that forward and backward memory span tasks should be treated separately. While forward memory span has strong attentional and sequential demands, backward memory span appears to have spatial and/or transformative element not apparent in forward memory span.

Reynolds (in press) examined this issue specifically with the TOMAL, which contains a variety of forward and backward recall tasks. The TOMAL has six different sequential recall tasks, four for-

TABLE 11. Six-Variable Varimax and Promax Two-Factor Solutions of Sequential Memory Tasks

Subtest	Varimax solution		Promax solution	
	Factor 1	Factor 2	Factor 1	Factor 2
Digits Forward	0.70	0.31	0.73	0.05
Letters Forward	0.71	0.38	0.71	0.13
Digits Backward	0.32	0.67	0.06	0.71
Letters Backward	0.32	0.69	0.07	0.69
Visual Sequential Memory	0.42	0.20	0.43	0.04
Manual Imitation	0.42	0.39	0.33	0.29

ward ordered (Digits Forward, Letters Forward, Visual Sequential Memory, and Manual Imitation) and two backward ordered (Digits Backward and Letters Backward). An examination of these sequential recall tasks (described in Table 2 and in Reynolds & Bigler, 1994b, in greater detail) independent of other measures of memory is useful in determining whether backward and forward recall tasks on the TOMAL should be combined into a single score. The analyses of Reynolds and Bigler (in press) are presented below examining these subtests and the two digit recall and two letter recall subtests to determine whether multiple factors are present and if so whether they conform to a forward–backward division. Reynolds (in press) analyzed all six sequential recall tasks and the four digit and letter recall tasks separately. For all six sequential tasks, he found that a two-factor solution was most appropriate. Table 11 presents the Varimax and Promax rotated solutions reported therein. In both cases it is clear that the forward and backward recall tasks form two factors. Manual Imitation is the only task to load nearly equally on the two tasks arguing for the salience of imagery on this task, a finding echoed in the results of analyses of the K-ABC where a similar task (Hand Movements) shifts from high loadings on a sequential scale below age 5 to a simultaneous scale at older ages (see Kamphaus &

TABLE 12. Four-Variable Varimax and Promax Two-Factor Solutions of Sequential Memory Tasks

Subtest	Varimax solution		Promax solution	
	Factor 1	Factor 2	Factor 1	Factor 2
Digits Forward	0.70	0.31	0.73	0.04
Letters Forward	0.70	0.38	0.71	0.12
Digits Backward	0.32	0.66	0.09	0.68
Letters Backward	0.33	0.67	0.09	0.69

TABLE 13. Zero-Order Pearson Correlations for Digits and Letters Forward and Backward

Subtest	Letters Forward	Digits Backward	Letters Backward
Digits Forward	0.70	0.44	0.43
Letters Forward		0.47	0.50
Digits Backward			0.65

Reynolds, 1987, for a review and discussion). The Promax solution is the most distinctive of the two solutions but both argue strongly for a two-factor interpretation of these six tasks as forward recall and backward recall.

When the four most similar tasks, except for order of recall (forward versus backward), were examined, Reynolds (in press) again found that a two-factor solution was best. Table 12 presents the Varimax and Promax rotated solutions. There is no mistaking the clarity of the patterns evident in these loadings. The two forward memory span tasks clearly break apart from the backward memory span tasks, with the Promax solution once again the most distinctive.

These patterns are clearly evident in the correlation matrix for the digit span and letter span tasks seen in Table 13. Digits Forward correlates at a statistically significantly higher level ($p < 0.001$) with Letters Forward ($r = 0.70$) than with Digits Backward ($r = 0.44$). Digits Forward correlates about equally well with Letters Backward ($r = 0.43$). Digits Backward correlates at a statistically significantly higher level ($p < 0.001$) with Letters Backward ($r = 0.65$) than with Letters Forward ($r = 0.47$).

Based on these correlations, it is known that 25 to 30% of normal children will show at least a one standard deviation (3 scaled score points) difference between their scores on Digits Forward versus Digits Backward and on Letters Forward versus Letters Backward. Nearly half or a normal sample will show a scaled score difference of two or more points. Thus, statistically significant dif-

TABLE 14. Mean and Standard Deviations of Subtest[a] Performance on the TOMAL for Black and for White Children from the Standardization Sample

Subtest	Mean		Standard deviation		
	Black	White	Black	White	D[c]
Memory for Stories	10.10	10.02	2.94	3.06	−0.03
Word Selective Reminding	9.90	10.00	3.00	3.03	0.03
Object Recall	10.13	9.96	3.30	2.97	−0.06
Digits Forward	10.09	9.99	3.18	3.00	−0.03
Paired Recall	9.96	10.00	3.00	3.00	0.01
Letters Forward[b]	10.17	9.97	3.51	2.88	−0.07*
Digits Backward[b]	9.97	9.98	3.30	2.97	−0.00
Letters Backward[b]	10.09	9.97	3.69	2.88	−0.04
Facial Memory	10.12	9.95	3.33	2.94	−0.05
Visual Selective Reminding	9.96	9.99	3.93	3.00	0.01
Abstract Visual Memory[b]	9.97	9.99	3.03	3.00	0.01
Visual Sequential Memory	10.14	9.99	3.30	2.91	−0.05
Memory for Location	9.90	10.00	2.73	3.03	0.03
Manual Imitation[b]	10.13	9.98	3.54	2.94	−0.06

[a]Mean = 10; SD = 3.
[b]Supplementary subtests.
[c]Difference expressed as a function of the white sample standard deviation: (white mean − black mean)/white standard deviation.
*$p \leq 0.02$; all other differences, $p \geq 0.08$.

ferences in forward and backward memory span are relatively common in scaled score terms and should not be overinterpreted when scaled separately just as they should not be ignored by simply viewing a composite of forward and backward memory span as the difference in the two is potentially informative for many patients, especially those with TBI or CHI.

When the current results are considered in the context of various theoretical works such as that of Jensen (1980; Jensen & Figueroa, 1975), and Kaufman and Kaufman (1983) and the review and reanalyses of Ramsay and Reynolds (1995), there seems to be little justification for continuing the practice of summing raw scores on forward and backward memory span tasks. Indeed, this practice is clearly not necessary to enhance reliability of the measurements as might be argued. Reynolds and Bigler (1994a) report reliability coefficients (coefficients alpha) for the six tasks noted above of greater than 0.92. Collapsing these variables routinely without making separate scores available is likely to mask useful information as is clear from the clinical studies of patients reviewed but also now in multiple factor-analytic studies (e.g., Reynolds & Bigler, 1996) of large samples of normal individuals. This break between forward and backward memory span is enhanced in certain minority populations as well (e.g., Jensen & Figueroa, 1975; Mayfield & Reynolds, in press).

While combining forward and backward memory span may be useful at times (e.g., Smyth & Scholey, 1994; Vanderploeg, Schinka, & Retzlaff, 1994), the evidence now seems overwhelming that separate scaled scores for forward and for backward memory span tasks should be provided routinely on any standardized assessment. This practice will facilitate clinical practice and research applications concerning the differential meaning of performance on the two tasks. Current evidence seems to support forward span tasks as being simpler, perhaps verbally oriented, and strongly sequential while backward memory span invokes more complex processes that require transformations not necessary with forward memory span. Backward recall may also invoke, for many individuals, visuospatial imaging processes even for ostensibly verbal material such as letters. Potential differences in the attentional demands or components of these two types of tasks deserve additional study as well. Forward memory span measures may have a stronger attentional component

than backward recall measures, which are more highly correlated with general intelligence and require cognitive transformation, an element missing from rote, forward recall. Surprisingly much remains to be done to understand the distinction between forward and backward memory span and what it means both clinically and to theories of brain–behavior relationships, but it is clear the tasks are sufficiently different to be assessed separately for clinical purposes, and are so presented on the TOMAL.

Delayed Recall

Delayed recall, asking an examinee to recall previously exposed material after some period of time of engagement in other tasks, is a routine component of the psychiatric mental status examination. It has been a part of the major memory batteries for over 50 years and there is a delayed recall (although briefer than on other tests) component to the Tactual Performance Test of the Halstead–Reitan Neuropsychological Test Battery.

Delayed recall on the TOMAL requires the examinee to recall stimuli from the first four subtests administered (two verbal, two nonverbal), 30 minutes after testing has been initiated. The Delayed Recall Index (DRI) acts as a measure of forgetting. Most examinees will score within about ten points of their Composite Memory Index (CMI) on the TOMAL. The *manual* also contains values for assessing the significance of the difference between DRI and CMI and this is checked automatically by the TOMAL computer scoring program.

DRI scores significantly below the CMI are often an indication of an organically based disturbance of memory. Memory scores can be suppressed by various psychiatric disturbances, especially depression; however, in these disorders, delayed recall is relatively preserved. In some research (e.g., Grossman, Kaufman, Mednitsky, Scharff, & Dennis, 1994), depressed patients actually score higher on delayed recall than immediate recall. This has been attributed to motivation. Whenever DRI exceeds CMI to a significant degree, level of effort on immediate recall should be evaluated carefully. DRI allows the clinician to explore a variety of hypotheses about depth of processing (especially in conjunction with selective reminding which may show more intermediate forgetting if examinees forget on later trials material

TABLE 15. Test of Memory and Learning (TOMAL) Results for Mary 5

Name:	Mary 5			
Gender:	Female			
Grade:	12			
Date of birth:	09/23/76			
Test date:	07/01/94			
Age:	17 years, 9 months			

	Raw score	Scaled score	%ile rank	Classification
Verbal subtests				
Memory for Stories (MFS)	49	11	63	Average
Word Selective Reminding (WSR)	76	9	37	Average
Object Recall (OR)	46	6	9	Low average
Digits Forward (DF)	55	8	25	Average
Paired Recall (PR)	28	11	63	Average
Letters Forward (LF)	21	3	1	Very deficient
Digits Backward (DB)	31	9	37	Average
Letters Backward (LB)	21	8	25	Average
Nonverbal subtests				
Facial Memory (FM)	32	12	75	Average
Visual Selective Reminding (VSR)	62	13	84	Above average
Abstract Visual Memory (AVM)	36	11	63	Average
Visual Sequential Memory (VSM)	36	12	75	Average
Memory for Location (MFL)	21	13	84	Above average
Manual Imitation (MI)	52	12	75	Average
Delayed recall scores				
Memory for Stories (MFSD)	40	9	37	Average
Facial Memory (FMD)	11	10	50	Average
Word Selective Reminding (WSRD)	11	11	63	Average
Visual Selective Reminding (VSRD)	8	11	63	Average

	Sum of scaled scores	Memory Index	%ile rank	90% C.I.	Classification
Composite indexes					
Verbal Memory Index (VMI)	45	93	32	85–101	Average
Nonverbal Memory Index (NMI)	61	115	84	107–123	Above average
Composite Memory Index (CMI)	106	104	61	98–110	Average
Delayed Recall Index (DRI)	41	102	55	88–116	Average
Attention/Concentration Index	40	86	18	78–94	Low average
Sequential Recall Index	35	92	30	78–106	Average
Free Recall Index	42	103	58	89–117	Average
Associative Recall Index	22	106	65	95–117	Average
Learning Index	39	98	45	84–112	Average

	Difference	Significance level	Frequency of difference
Global scale comparisons			
VMI vs NMI	−22	0.01	12.7
VMI vs DRI	−9	0.05	51.9
NMI vs DRI	13	0.01	38.8
CMI vs DRI	2	NS	83.1

TABLE 15. (*Continued*).

	Difference	Significance level
Ipsative comparisons		
Memory for Stories vs mean VMI score	2.0	NS
Word Selective Reminding vs mean VMI score	0.0	NS
Object Recall vs mean VMI score	−3.0	0.01
Digits Forward vs mean VMI score	−1.0	NS
Paired Recall vs mean VMI score	2.0	NS
Facial Memory vs mean NMI score	−0.2	NS
Visual Selective Reminding vs mean NMI score	0.8	NS
Abstract Visual Memory vs mean NMI score	−1.2	NS
Visual Sequential Memory vs mean NMI score	−0.2	NS
Memory for Location vs mean NMI score	0.8	NS

recalled correctly on earlier trials), forgetting, and motivation.

Ethnic Differences in Mean Levels of Performance

As noted earlier, black–white differences in mean level of performance are well documented on IQ tests and average, over different tests and nearly 100 years of data collection, about one standard deviation (Jensen, 1980). Memory tests behave quite differently. Mayfield and Reynolds (in press) calculated mean levels of performance separately for blacks and whites on all 14 subtests of the TOMAL. Table 14 reports the essential results of their findings. A multivariate analysis of variance revealed a single significant difference with blacks scoring higher than whites on Letters Forward by 0.07 standard deviation—statistically significant, but of no real clinical significance. Variations in profiles of blacks then cannot be related reasonably to artifacts of the test and most likely reflect real variations in memory for individual children.

Interpretive Strategies

The TOMAL manual reviews a basic top-down interpretive strategy that mimics Kaufman's (1979, 1994) basic philosophy of intelligent testing and that requires integration of history and other test data. The additional information presented here and in other papers cited throughout this chapter supplement the strategies given by Reynolds and Bigler

(1994b), who also provide data on within-test scatter and the relationship of the TOMAL to the major intelligence scales and to achievement tests as well.

Brief Case Examples

Mary 5

This patient was involved in a motor vehicle accident on April 7, 1992. She was a passenger in an auto traveling at excessive speed when it struck a telephone pole. Her initial Glascow Coma Score was rated at 12 with loss of consciousness and post-traumatic amnesia lasting 7 to 10 days. Injuries included a closed head injury, laceration of the right frontal temporal area, as well as fractures of the

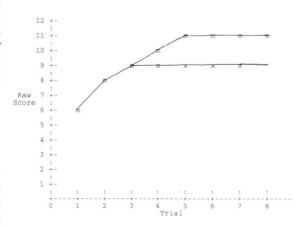

FIGURE 1. Jason 7's TOMAL learning curve on Word Selective Reminding. Top curve (m) is curve of standardization sample and lower curve (x) is Jason 7's curve.

TABLE 16. Test of Memory and Learning (TOMAL) Results for Jason 7

Name: Jason 7
Gender: Male
Grade: 5
Date of birth: 07/30/82
Test date: 10/27/94
Age: 12 years, 2 months

	Raw score	Scaled score	%ile rank		Classification
Verbal subtests					
Memory for Stories (MFS)	31	7	16		Low average
Word Selective Reminding (WSR)	70	8	25		Average
Object Recall (OR)	54	9	37		Average
Digits Forward (DF)	55	9	37		Average
Paired Recall (PR)	24	9	37		Average
Letters Forward (LF)	23	6	9		Low average
Digits Backward (DB)	18	8	25		Average
Letters Backward (LB)	12	7	16		Low average
Nonverbal subtests					
Facial Memory (FM)	34	15	95		Superior
Visual Selective Reminding (VSR)	48	8	25		Average
Abstract Visual Memory (AVM)	24	9	37		Average
Visual Sequential Memory (VSM)	16	7	16		Low average
Memory for Location (MFL)	4	4	2		Deficient
Manual Imitation (MI)	13	5	5		Deficient
Delayed recall scores					
Memory for Stories (MFSD)	31	8	25		Average
Facial Memory (FMD)	12	11	63		Average
Word Selective Reminding (WSRD)	7	8	25		Average
Visual Selective Reminding (VSRD)	5	8	25		Average

	Sum of scaled scores	Memory Index	%ile rank	90% C.I.	Classification
Composite indexes					
Verbal Memory Index (VMI)	42	89	23	82–96	Low average
Nonverbal Memory Index (NMI)	43	90	25	83–97	Average
Composite Memory Index (CMI)	85	89	23	84–94	Low average
Delayed Recall Index (DRI)	35	92	30	78–106	Average
Attention/Concentration Index	35	79	8	72–86	Deficient
Sequential Recall Index	27	78	7	64–92	Deficient
Free Recall Index	37	95	37	81–109	Average
Associative Recall Index	16	88	21	78–98	Low average
Learning Index	34	90	25	76–104	Average

	Difference	Significance level	Frequency of difference
Global scale comparisons			
VMI vs NMI	−1	NS	89.2
VMI vs DRI	−3	NS	78.5
NMI vs DRI	−2	NS	85.2
CMI vs DRI	−3	NS	78.5

TABLE 16. (*Continued*).

	Difference	Significance level
Ipsative comparisons		
Memory for Stories vs mean VMI score	−1.4	NS
Word Selective Reminding vs mean VMI score	−0.4	NS
Object Recall vs mean VMI score	0.6	NS
Digits Forward vs mean VMI score	0.6	NS
Paired Recall vs mean VMI score	0.6	NS
Facial Memory vs mean NMI score	6.4	.01
Visual Selective Reminding vs mean NMI score	−0.6	NS
Abstract Visual Memory vs mean NMI score	0.4	NS
Visual Sequential Memory vs mean NMI score	−1.6	0.05
Memory for Location vs mean NMI score	−4.6	0.01

Note: Mean of Verbal Memory Index scaled scores = 8.40; mean of Nonverbal Index scaled scores = 8.60.

clavicle and right pubic ramus. Acute CT imaging noted left intracranial hemorrhage and surrounding edema in the deep left frontal area.

Prior to the accident, the patient was in good health. She recently graduated from high school with a GPA of 3.3. Currently, the patient is in trade school to become an ophthalmology assistant. Her current functioning probably reflects a decrease from premorbid performance.

Current difficulties include labile behaviors and mood. She is noted to have twitching in her sleep, episodic unresponsiveness with staring, and episodes of hypersomnia. Given these difficulties, the patient is probably experiencing a posttraumatic seizure disorder.

Table 15 summarizes the TOMAL scores obtained by Mary 5 some 27 months postaccident and in a format obtained from the TOMAL computer scoring program. Verbal Memory is clearly impaired relative to nonverbal memory as might be anticipated from the left temporal horn dilation seen on follow-up MRI scans. Attention/Concentration Index and Sequential Recall are also depressed relative to other scores. When her factor indexes are consulted, we note the following scores:

CMFI	102
SRFI	92
BRFI	91
SMFI	112

Tasks that tend to emphasize right hemisphere functions are relatively preserved as reflected in her SMFI of 112 and NMI of 115. Language-related and sequential recall tasks are more impaired and the combination of language and sequential as reflected in her Letters Forward performance (scaled score of 3 versus 8 on Letters Backward) is particularly adversely impacted. Memory then shows an overall decline from expected premorbid levels but with increasingly adverse effects on language and sequential tasks especially with decreased associative or contextual potential. Her WAIS-R scores showed limited variability (VIQ = 89, PIQ = 98, FSIQ = 92 with a subtest range of 5 to 11) and reflect only a general decline in intellectual skill. WRAT-3 scores showed reading of 107, spelling of 104, and math of 112. Word fluency was notably impaired. Her TOMAL learning curves showed great inconsistency across trials reflecting considerable variability in attentional processes.

Jason 7

This patient was seen to assess potential problems with ADHD and learning difficulties. Jason 7's WISC-III performance showed a VIQ = 100, PIQ = 113, and FSIQ = 107 with subtest scores having a below-average range of scatter (from 9 to 13) and no distractibility pattern evident. On the TOMAL, however, his Attention/Concentration Index of 79 reveals considerable impairment of these processes that may also be producing depressed memory performance overall. His TOMAL subtest scores range from a low of 5 to a high of 15 with his greatest difficulty on immediate and sequential recall tasks that highlight attention. Consistent with his eventual diagnosis of ADHD, Figure 1 shows an example learning curve from his Word Selective Reminding performance demonstrating the rapid

TABLE 17. Test of Memory and Learning (TOMAL) Results for Marie 6

Name: Marie 6
Gender: Female
Grade: 6
Date of birth: 12/28/81
Test date: 05/18/94
Age: 12 years, 4 months

	Raw score	Scaled score	%ile rank		Classification
Verbal subtests					
Memory for Stories (MFS)	8	1	1		Very deficient
Word Selective Reminding (WSR)	18	1	1		Very deficient
Object Recall (OR)	27	1	1		Very deficient
Digits Forward (DF)	12	1	1		Very deficient
Paired Recall (PR)	24	9	37		Average
Letters Forward (LF)	6	1	1		Very deficient
Digits Backward (DB)	7	4	2		Deficient
Letters Backward (LB)	5	2	1		Very deficient
Nonverbal subtests					
Facial Memory (FM)	2	1	1		Very deficient
Visual Selective Reminding (VSR)	0	1	1		Very deficient
Abstract Visual Memory (AVM)	29	10	50		Average
Visual Sequential Memory (VSM)	12	6	9		Low average
Memory for Location (MFL)	1	1	1		Very deficient
Manual Imitation (MI)	7	2	1		Very deficient

	Sum of scaled scores	Memory Index	%ile rank	90% C.I.	Classification
Composite indexes					
Verbal Memory Index (VMI)	13	49	<1	42–56	Very deficient
Nonverbal Memory Index (NMI)	19	58	<1	51–65	Very deficient
Composite Memory Index	32	51	<1	46–56	Very deficient
Delayed Recall Index					
Attention/Concentration Index	10	45	<1	38–52	Very deficient
Sequential Recall Index	10	50	<1	36–64	Very deficient
Free Recall Index	13	55	<1	41–69	Very deficient
Associative Recall Index	10	70	2	60–80	Deficient
Learning Index	12	53	<1	39–67	Very deficient

	Difference	Significance level	Frequency of difference
Global scale comparisons			
VMI vs NMI	−9	0.05	49.9

	Difference	Significance level
Ipsative comparisons		
Memory for Stories vs mean VMI score	−1.6	NS
Word Selective Reminding vs mean VMI score	−1.6	NS
Object Recall vs mean VMI score	−1.6	NS
Digits Forward vs mean VMI score	−1.6	0.05
Paired Recall vs mean VMI score	6.4	0.01
Facial Memory vs mean NMI score	−2.8	0.05
Visual Selective Reminding vs mean NMI score	−2.8	0.01
Abstract Visual Memory vs mean NMI score	6.2	0.01
Visual Sequential Memory vs mean NMI score	2.2	0.05
Memory for Location vs mean NMI score	−2.8	0.01

Note: Mean of Verbal Memory Index scaled scores = 2.60; mean of Nonverbal Index scaled scores = 3.80.

flattening of the acquisition curve so common in clinical work with these children. Once information is learned, it stays with Jason 7, but his attention wanes readily.

Marie 6

This patient was referred for a neuropsychological evaluation in an attempt to gain information to improve her school situation. This 12-year-old female has a static encephalopathy associated with viral encephalitis with onset in December 1987. She suffers from intractable epilepsy which is not fully controlled by any medication regime. Currently, she is taking Mysoline, Tegretol, and Tranxene. Surgical interventions have been ruled out because of diffuse and multifocal abnormalities.

Socially, she represents a large management problem causing classroom disruptions. She is immature for her age, has delayed social skills, and has difficulty staying on task. She attends school for approximately 3 hours a day. During testing she was oriented only to person and evidenced numerous mannerisms, repetitive noises as well as inappropriate jocularity. There were periods of time when she was quite lucid and others when she was loud and defiant. Testing was completed in short segments and discontinued unless there was evidence of adequate attention.

Testing found that this child is significantly neurologically impaired with involvement of all areas of functioning. Her WISC-III indicated a VIQ = 57, PIQ = 59, and FSIQ = 54. Her scaled score range was from 1 to 8 (Picture Arrangement). Table 17 shows her TOMAL results. They are quite consistent with her WISC-III and other neuropsychological testing results with the exception of notable areas of strength or preservation of skills on Paired Recall and Abstract Visual Memory. Clearly, approaches that invoke her intact skills in these areas are more likely to promote academic success than approaches aimed at remediation of her weaknesses in most areas of processing. Development of association strategies in acquisition of reading skills through techniques such as rebus reading and progressing to language experience techniques will be far more successful than phonics and purely ortho-

Appendix: Calculation Aid for Computing TOMAL Factor Indexes

Subtest	Scaled score
Memory for Stories	_____
Word Selective Reminding	_____
Object Recall	_____
Paired Recall	_____
Visual Selective Reminding	_____
Facial Memory	_____
Factor score (sum of scaled scores)	_____
Complex Memory Factor Index	_____(CMFI)
Digits Forward	_____
Letters Forward	_____
Visual Sequential Memory	_____
Manual Imitation	_____
Factor score (sum of scaled scores)	_____
Sequential Recall Factor Index	_____(SRFI)
Digits Backward	_____
Letters Backward	_____
Factor score (sum of scaled scores)	_____
Backwards Recall Factor Index	_____(BRFI)
Abstract Visual Memory	_____
Memory for Location	_____
Factor score (sum of scaled scores)	_____
Spatial Memory Factor Index	_____(SMFI)

Note: After computing the sum of scaled scores for each factor, locate the factor score in Table 7, under the appropriate head. To locate the factor index, read to the extreme left column. The corresponding percentile rank may be found in the far right column of Table 7. This form may be copied and used as necessary. (From Reynolds & Bigler, 1996.)

graphic techniques. Building on the development of strategies for finding associations would also be crucial to long-term success.

Conclusion

Memory assessment has much to offer the clinician when viewing the neuropsychological processing of children and adolescents, especially those with CNS compromise. The TOMAL is the most detailed and comprehensive of approaches and allows for a careful look at how children are processing and learning information as well.

We have much to learn about memory in children and especially about the use of delayed recall indices that have proven so valuable with adults. Current work is focused on delineating diagnostic and remedial implications of test results and are promising. The ubiquitous nature of memory in daily life and memory complaints in CNS compromise makes clinical assessment of memory crucial to the tasks of the neuropsychologist.

References

Bakker, D. J., Fisk, J. L., & Strang, J. D. (1985). *Child neuropsychology.* New York: Guilford Press.

Barker, L. H., Mueller, R. M., Russo, A. A., Lajiness-O'Neill, R., Johnson, S. C., Anderson, C., Norman, M. A., Sephton, S., Primus, E., Bigler, E. D., & Reynolds, C. R. (1994, November). *The Word Selective Reminding subtest of the Test of Memory and Learning (TOMAL): A concurrent and construct validity study using the Rey Auditory Verbal Learning Test (RAVL) and the Wechsler Memory Scale-Revised WMS-R.* Paper presented at the annual meeting of the National Academy of Neuropsychology, Orlando.

Baron, I. S., Fennell, E. B., & Voeller, K. K. S. (1995). *Pediatric neuropsychology in the medical setting.* London: University Press.

Cohen, R. A. (1993). *The neuropsychology of attention.* New York: Plenum Press.

Cronwall, D., Wrightson, P., & Waddell, P. (1990). *Head injury: The facts.* London: Oxford University Press.

Cullum, M., Kuck, J., & Ruff, R. M. (1990). Neuropsychological assessment of traumatic brain injury in adults. In E. Bigler (Ed.), *Traumatic brain injury* (pp. 129–163). Austin, TX: PRO-ED.

Cytowic, R. E. (1996). *The neurological side of neuropsychology.* Cambridge, MA: MIT Press.

Diamond, M. C. (1990). Morphological cortical changes as a consequence of learning and experience. In A. Schiebel & A. Wechsler (Eds.), *Neurobiology of higher cognitive function.* New York: Guilford Press.

Ferris, L. M., & Kamphaus, R. W. (1995). Review of the Test of Memory and Learning. *Archives of Clinical Neuropsychology, 10*(6).

Gillberg, C. (1995). *Clinical child neuropsychiatry.* London: Cambridge University Press.

Golden, C. J., Zillmer, E., & Spiers, M. (1992). *Neuropsychological assessment and intervention.* Springfield IL: Thomas.

Goldstein, F. C., & Levin, H. S. (1990). Epidemiology of traumatic brain injury: Incidence, clinical characteristics, and risk factors. In E. Bigler (Ed.), *Traumatic brain injury* (pp. 51–67). Austin, TX: PRO-ED.

Grossman, I., Kaufman, A. S., Mednitsky, S., Scharff, L., & Dennis, B. (1994). Neurocognitive abilities for a clinically depressed sample versus a matched control group of normal individuals. *Psychiatry Research, 51,* 231–244.

Hynd, G., & Obrzut, J. (1981). *Neuropsychological assessment of the school-aged child: Issues and procedures.* New York: Grune & Stratton.

Jensen, A. R. (1980). *Bias in mental testing.* New York: The Free Press.

Jensen, A. R., & Figueroa, R. (1975). Forward and backward digit span interaction with race and IQ: Predictions from Jensen's theory. *Journal of Educational Psychology, 67,* 882–893.

Kamphaus, R. W., & Reynolds, C. R. (1987). *Clinical and research application of the K-ABC.* Circle Pines, MN: American Guidance Service.

Kaplan, E. (1996, March). Discussant. Symposium presented at the annual meeting of the National Association of School Psychologists, Atlanta.

Kaufman, A. S. (1979). *Intelligent testing with the WISC-R.* New York: Wiley–Interscience.

Kaufman, A. S. (1994). *Intelligent testing with the WISC-3.* New York: Wiley–Interscience.

Kaufman, A. S., & Kaufman, N. L. (1983). *Kaufman Assessment Battery for Children: Interpretive manual.* Circle Pines, MN: American Guidance Service.

Knight, R. G. (1992). *The neuropsychology of degenerative brain diseases.* Hillsdale, NJ: Erlbaum.

Koppitz, E. M. (1977). *The visual aural digit span test.* New York: Grune & Stratton.

Lezak, M. D. (1995). *Neuropsychological assessment* (3rd ed.). London: Oxford University Press.

McCarthy, D. (1972). *McCarthy Scales of Children's Abilities.* San Antonio, TX: The Psychological Corporation.

Mapou, R. L., & Spector, J. (Eds.). (1995). *Clinical neuropsychological assessment.* New York: Plenum Press.

Mayfield, J. W., & Reynolds, C. R. (in press). Black–white differences in memory test performance among children and adolescents. *Archives of Clinical Neuropsychology.*

Mueller, R. M., Russo, A. A., Barker, L. H., Lajiness-O'Neill, R., Johnson, S., Anderson, C., Norman, M. A., Sephton, S., Primus, E., Bigler, E. D., & Reynolds, C. R., (1994, November). *Memory testing and memory for sentences: Concurrent and construct validity of the Test of Memory and Learning (TOMAL) utilizing the Wechsler Memory Scale-Revised (WMS-R).* Paper presented at the annual meeting of the National Academy of Neuropsychology, Orlando.

Prigatano, G. P. (1990). Recovery and cognitive retraining after cognitive brain injury. In E. Bigler (Ed.), *Traumatic brain injury* (pp. 273–295). Austin, TX: PRO-ED.

Ramsay, M. C., & Reynolds, C. R. (1995). Separate digit tests: A brief history, a literature review, and a reexamination of the factor structure of the Test of Memory and Learning (TOMAL). *Neuropsychology Review, 5*(3), 151–171.

Reeves, D., & Wedding, D. (1994). *The clinical assessment of memory.* Berlin: Springer-Verlag.

Reynolds, C. R. (1982). Methods for detecting construct and predictive bias. In R. Berk (Ed.), *Handbook of methods for detecting test bias* (pp. 199–227). Baltimore: Johns Hopkins University Press.

Reynolds, C. R. (1995). Test bias and the assessment of intelligence and personality. In D. Saklofske & M. Zeidner (Eds.), *International handbook of personality and intelligence* (pp. 545–573). New York: Plenum Press.

Reynolds, C. R. (in press). Forward and backward memory span should not be combined for clinical analysis. *Archives of Clinical Neuropsychology.*

Reynolds, C. R., & Bigler, E. D. (1994a). *Test of Memory and Learning.* Austin, TX: PRO-ED.

Reynolds, C. R., & Bigler, E. D. (1994b). *Manual for the Test of Memory and Learning.* Austin, TX: PRO-ED.

Reynolds, C. R., & Bigler, E. D. (1996). Factor structure, factor indexes, and other useful statistics for interpretation of the Test of Memory and Learning (TOMAL). *Archives of Clinical Neuropsychology, 11*(1), 29–43.

Rourke, B. P., Bakker, D. J., Fisk, J. L., & Strang, J. D. (1983). *Child neuropsychology.* New York: Guilford Press.

Russo, A. A., Barker, L. H., Mueller, R., Lajiness-O'Neill, R., Johnson, S. C., Anderson, C. V., Norman, M. A., Sephton, S., Primus, E., Bigler, E. D., & Reynolds, C. R. (1994, November). *Memory and digit span: Concurrent and construct validity of the Test of Memory and Learning (TOMAL) using the Wechsler Memory Scale-Revised (WMS-R).* Paper presented at the annual meeting of the National Academy of Neuropsychology, Orlando.

Scheibel, A. B. (1990). Dendritic correlates of higher cognitive function. In A. Scheibel & A. Wechsler (Eds.), *Neurobiology of higher cognitive function.* New York: Guilford Press.

Sheslow, D., & Adams, W. (1990). *Wide Range Assessment of Memory and Learning.* Wilmington, DE: Jastak Associates.

Smyth, M. M., & Scholey, K. A. (1994). Interference in immediate spatial memory. *Memory and Cognition, 22,* 1–13.

Snyderman, M., & Rothman, S. (1987). Survey of expert opinion on intelligence and aptitude testing. *American Psychologist, 42,* 137–144.

Stanton, H. C., Reynolds, C. R., & Bigler, E. D. (1995). *PROSCORE: Computer Scoring System for the Test of Memory and Learning.* Austin, TX: PRO-ED.

Vanderploeg, R. D., Schinka, J. A., & Retzlaff, P. (1994). Relationships between measures of auditory verbal learning and executive functioning. *Journal of Clinical and Experimental Neuropsychology, 16,* 243–250.

16

Assessment of Behavior and Personality in the Neuropsychological Diagnosis of Children

MARGARET SEMRUD-CLIKEMAN, RANDY W. KAMPHAUS, PHYLLIS ANNE TEETER, AND MELANIE VAUGHN

For many clinicians, behavior and personality have been traditionally evaluated by assessing behavior patterns and interpolating these behaviors as reflecting underlying personality variables (Martin, 1988). Behavior has been defined as the *what* a child does with personality defined as the *why* the child does what he or she does. Behaviors can be quantified and graphed fairly easily, whereas personality variables are more difficult to measure and are generally described qualitatively. Such differentiation is artificial and the boundaries between these concepts become blurred when observing a child. For the purposes of this chapter, behavior will be conceptualized as the outward expression of inner experience and personality will be viewed as the overarching principle encompassing behavior. Personality, therefore, is the constant principle across situations whereas behaviors may vary depending on situational characteristics (Martin, 1988). A discussion of distinctions between the concepts of behavior and personality is beyond the

scope of this chapter. The interested reader is referred to further discussions by Martin (1988) and Lewis and Miller (1990).

Historically, behavioral and personality disorders have been the purview of psychology and psychiatry; however, recent conceptualizations of childhood disorders have emerged from neuropsychiatry.

> Although there is considerable disagreement about just what neuropsychiatry comprises, fundamental to any definition is the indelible inseparability of brain and thought, of mind and body, and of mental and physical. Neuropsychiatry spans these interrelationships to enlarge understanding of cognitive, emotional, and behavioral function and dysfunction. (Yudovsky & Hales, 1989, p. 363)

On the other hand, neuropsychology focuses on broad brain–behavior relationships, which generally include investigation into how brain function/dysfunction affects the cognitive–intellectual, memory, psychomotor, perceptual, and attentional functions of children. Although neuropsychologists frequently study neurodevelopmental (e.g., learning disorders), traumatic brain injury, and central nervous system disease processes, the overlap between neuropsychiatric and neuropsychological disorders is quite extensive. Recently, neuropsychologists have advocated for a transactional framework for investigating childhood disorders, where personality and resulting behav-

MARGARET SEMRUD-CLIKEMAN • Department of Neurology, University of Minnesota Medical School, Minneapolis, Minnesota 55455. RANDY W. KAMPHAUS AND MELANIE VAUGHN • Department of Educational Psychology, University of Georgia, Athens, Georgia 30602. PHYLLIS ANNE TEETER • Department of Educational Psychology, University of Wisconsin–Milwaukee, Milwaukee, Wisconsin 53201.

iors are viewed as an integration of learned and biologically predisposed variables (Teeter & Semrud-Clikeman, 1995). In such a transactional, neuropsychological approach the interplay of biogenetic and environmental factors with the maturation and development of the central nervous system is considered (Teeter & Semrud-Clikeman, 1995). Similarly, Achenbach (1990) suggests that childhood psychopathology should be conceptualized as a combination of "microparadigms" including neuropsychological, cognitive–behavioral, psychodynamic theory, and family systems which are then formed into a "macroparadigm." The assessment of the child's support system, prior developmental history and behavior, social and emotional development, as well as neuropsychological deficits provides a comprehensive and useful picture for the understanding of the whole child and for the subsequent development of appropriate interventions.

The purpose of this chapter is to discuss common behavioral and psychiatric disorders of childhood from a neuropsychological–neuropsychiatric viewpoint. The first part of this chapter will review various disorders from a neuropsychological–neuropsychiatric viewpoint. The neurobiological contributions, the associated behaviors frequently noted with common disorders of children referred for neuropsychological assessment, and the impact of neurobehavioral deficits on development are discussed. The second section of this chapter will discuss psychosocial and behavioral measures for evaluation of neuropsychiatric and psychological disorders of childhood. Finally, guidelines for incorporating behavior and personality assessment in neuropsychological evaluations are presented.

Neuropsychology of Emotions

Although the brain has a defined neuroanatomy at birth, the myelination of axons, the formation of synaptic connections, and the arrangement of these into synapses begins in infancy and continues into adolescence with the environment effecting changes in neuroanatomy (Teeter & Semrud-Clikeman, 1995). Such neurodevelopment generally corresponds to the emergence of complex human behaviors. Childhood disorders (i.e., obsessive–compulsive disorder, attention deficit hyperactivity disorder, and Tourette's syndrome) may involve neurodevelopmental abnormalities for regulation when the brain is overproducing and then

pruning the axonal–synaptic processes (Cook & Leventhal, 1992). Moreover, disorders in childhood rarely affect an isolated function (e.g., language, motor, or cognitive processes) because interference in the developmental process of one brain region will affect the development of other areas as well. (Reitan & Wolfson, 1985; Tranel, 1992).

An example of the interplay between systems and resulting behavior following faulty development or traumatic injury is discussed by Bear (1983). Bear details the relationship between temporofrontal (ventral system) and parietofrontal functions (dorsal system), and psychological behavior in adults. The ventral temporofrontal systems (inferotemporal visual cortex to limbic structures to orbital frontal structures) are thought to assist in the storage of associations made between visual and emotional processes, the evaluation of basic drives, and the development of response strategies to environmental stimulation. Bear (1983) hypothesizes that damage to temporal or orbital prefrontal regions interferes with the ability to access previously learned emotional responses including the ability to utilize social restraint. When this system is dysfunctional, an individual may engage in aggressive (or sexual) responses to the environment with little or no regard for learned consequences. Damage in any part of this functional network results in discrete emotional and behavioral deficits. The inferior parietal lobe to limbic system to dorsolateral frontal cortex is involved in the activation of emotions, and lesions to this region result in apathy of neglect.

Through an integration of the findings from numerous studies (Dimond, Farrington, & Johnson, 1976; Geschwind, 1965; Heilman, Schwartz, & Watson, 1978), Bear hypothesizes that the cognitive processing functions of the left hemisphere are related to reflective and rigid or stereotypic responding. Conversely, the right hemisphere is thought to be particularly suited for incidental learning as well as the addition of affective qualities to cognitions in order to provoke emotional responses, recognize threats, and initiate goal-directed responses. The temporo-frontal portions of the right hemisphere have been implicated in memory functioning, discrimination of vocal intonations, identification of facial expressions, and the ability to decode and assign emotional meaning to perceptions (Semrud-Clikeman & Hynd, 1990).

Although several studies have addressed the neuropsychological basis of emotions in adults, the research base for understanding the neuropsychology of emotions in children is sparse. Measuring childhood emotions and their development is confounded by maturational variations, environmental influences, and the onset of injury on the developing brain.

Fletcher and Taylor (1984) conceptualize developmental neuropsychology as the study of how moderator variables (i.e., including environmental and social factors) can influence the basic competencies/deficits present in a child. In this model the central nervous system is viewed as just one of several influences on the developing child. Therefore, developmental neuropsychology focuses on the sequence in which skills are developed and how these skills change with each developmental stage. Fletcher and Taylor (1984) further suggest a need to focus on how a deficit interferes with or disrupts normal development instead of focusing on localization of deficient brain areas. Thus, if we are interested in assessing how brain function affects behavior and personality, it is important to: (1) determine the effects of damage or dysfunction on behavioral and psychosocial functioning and (2) determine how moderator variables (e.g., intelligence, therapeutic interventions, social support) affect the overall adjustment of the child.

Childhood Psychopathology from a Neuropsychological–Neuropsychiatric View

Studies investigating children with psychopathology have looked for cognitive and/or neuropsychological patterns across different types of psychiatric disturbance. Results from recent research suggest that many psychiatric disorders may well have an underlying organic etiology (Dean, 1986). There is mounting evidence that diagnoses previously considered to be functional in origin may, in fact, be organically based. Further, it is believed that organic and environmental components interact with development and that each variable, in turn, affects the other variable.

Difficulty in differentiating between functional and organic etiology for diagnosis is found in child and adolescent samples (Dean, 1985, 1986). A study by Hertzig (1982) found that roughly a third of an adolescent sample with a history of psychiatric disorders also possessed neurological impairments. Another study found 60% of child and adolescent psychiatric patients to have neuropsychological deficits (Tramontana, Sherrets, & Golden, 1980). The duration of the psychiatric disorder predicted the severity of neuropsychological

dysfunction. For example, when the duration of the psychiatric disorder exceeded 2 years, there was a higher probability of neuropsychological disorder. In addition, complex cognitive and perceptual abilities were the most severely affected.

In summary, the frequent distinction that is made between psychiatric and organic syndromes may be erroneous. Historically, such a distinction was based on the assumption that psychiatric disorders were the result of psychosocial influences. In contrast, organic disorders have been ascribed to biological influences. Mounting evidence from new technology allowing for the visualization of the brain suggests that biochemical and structural neurological abnormalities are present in many psychiatric disorders (Andreasen, Olsen, Dennert, & Smith, 1982; Semrud-Clikeman, Hynd, Novey, & Eliopulos, 1991; Zametkin *et al.*, 1990). Neurochemical differences have also been found in patients with affective disorders (Jarvik, 1977), as well as some forms of schizophrenia (Andreasen *et al.*, 1982). As a result of this new body of evidence, Dean (1986) suggests that the "organic–functional distinction for mental disorders" is better understood as a continuous and not as an all-or-none phenomenon (p. 95). Thus, a combined view of child psychological disorders utilizing a neuropsychological–neuropsychiatric interface would be most informative and lead to a more comprehensive understanding for these diagnoses. The following section reviews influences of various neuroanatomical structures on behavioral functions.

The Role and Development of Frontal Lobes in Children

One of the regions implicated in several childhood disorders is the frontal lobe. In order to more fully understand its role in childhood dysfunction, it is important to first discuss normal frontal lobe development. Studies have recently focused on the neurodevelopment of cognitive abilities in an effort to determine when specific brain areas become functionally operational in children. These studies have focused on the frontal lobes in children because attentional and behavioral control, planning, flexibility, and self-monitoring (executive functions) have been attributed to this area. The frontal lobes are also thought to play a prominent role in the control of human emotions in adults (Bear, 1983; Grafman, Vance, Weingartner, Salazar, & Amin, 1986).

The frontal lobes are a large and heterogeneous anatomical structure that makes up one-third of the cerebral cortex (Stuss, 1992). The frontal lobes are richly connected to almost all of the other parts of the central nervous system (Stuss & Benson, 1984). The myelination of the frontal lobes takes place throughout development (Dennis, 1991).

Some suggest that the frontal lobes of children begin to develop between the ages of 4 and 7 years (Luria, 1973); others suggest that development begins in adolescence and continues up to about age 24 (Golden, 1981). Current research suggests that children and even infants exhibit behaviors thought to be mediated by the frontal lobes much earlier than previous estimates (Bell & Fox, 1992; Dawson, 1994). Thatcher (1992) found in an EEG study that there are continuous and discontinuous growth processes which show growth spurts in the early postnatal period and again after puberty. Such growth spurts are characterized by increases in the amount of neural connections between the frontal lobes and other portions of the brain. Thatcher suggests that the growth spurt in the right frontal pole, which occurs at about age $4\frac{1}{2}$ years, corresponds with the ability to take another person's perspective. Such a correlation between brain maturation and psychological processes suggests that there is a direct relationship between anatomy and function.

Frontal lobe development is thought to involve a hierarchical, dynamic, and multistage process (Case, 1992; Thatcher, 1992). A study by Becker, Isaac, and Hynd (1987) supports this hypothesis. Becker *et al.* (1987) found that 10- and 12-year-olds had mastered the capability of inhibiting motor responses, of remembering the temporal ordering of visual designs, of using strategies for memory tasks, and of attending to relevant details and ignoring distracting stimuli. All of these skills are thought to be mediated by the frontal lobes. In contrast, 6-year-olds had more difficulty inhibiting motor responses and had trouble remembering the order of designs. Therefore, a developmental shift for 8-year-olds occurs that allows for inhibition of motor response. Moreover, while children at all age levels were able to verbalize directions, they were not always able to inhibit perseverative responding until about age 8. In contrast, older children (10- and 12-year-olds) displayed verbal and nonverbal strategies that aided their performance.

Similarly, Passler, Isaac, and Hynd (1985) found a developmental progression through stages requiring mastery of some frontal-mediated tasks at 6 and at 8 years of age, whereas other tasks were not mastered by the age of 12. These findings suggest that the greatest period of development for frontal lobe functioning occurs between the ages of 6 and 8, with continued growth beyond age 12 for more complex skills. Although basic research is useful for building a neurodevelopmental model for children, research with psychiatric populations can provide further information concerning the relationship between personality, behavior, and neuropsychological functioning.

Evidence from Childhood Psychopathology

Frontal lobe dysfunction has been found in children with various behavioral and psychological difficulties; however, frontal lobe dysfunction does not appear to be specific to one particular disorder. For example, a study that compared children with diagnoses of externalizing (i.e., ADD, conduct disorder), internalizing (i.e., anxiety, depression), and comorbid psychopathology found frontal lobe dysfunction in all of these disorders (Kusche, Cook, & Greenberg, 1993). Children with these diverse disorders performed more poorly on neuropsychological measures thought to be implicated in frontal lobe functioning.

From initial reports it appears that the frontal lobe is charged with the modulation of behavior and is heavily implicated in "functional" and psychiatric disorders of childhood. Evidence from children with traumatic brain injury (TBI) also sheds light on our understanding of the neuropsychological basis of behavior and personality.

Evidence from TBI

Although brain injury in adults frequently produces highly focal damage, childhood behavioral disorders are hypothesized to be a result of neurodevelopmental disorders in an otherwise healthy brain rather than caused by lesions or degenerative disorders (Cook & Leventhal, 1992). The question of whether early damage to the developing brain has a better prognosis than later damage is currently under debate.

Marlowe (1992) discussed a case study of a boy who experienced a focal prefrontal injury at age 3. Neuropsychological evaluations at 5 and 6 indicated that the injury at 3 disrupted the acquisition of executive and emotional control. Behavioral changes after the accident included emotional lability, difficulty falling asleep, and increase in impulsivity, agitation, and aggression. Although no decrease in intelligence scores was found, the boy experienced difficulty in school on tasks thought to be prefrontally based (i.e., self-regulation, planning and carrying out a strategy). Another study by Mateer and Williams (1991) investigated four children with nonfocal frontal lobe injuries in childhood. Maladaptive social behaviors were present in all four. Three main areas were found to be impacted: self-regulation, attention, and the ability to carry out plans. These difficulties were present despite normal intellectual, linguistic, and perceptual functioning. Welsh, Pennington, and Groisser (1991) also found that intelligence tests are not related to frontal lobe damage.

Thus, these investigations lead one to believe that frontal lobe dysfunction may be responsible for social adjustment difficulties in children. Particular problems are found in self-regulation and planning. These behaviors are frequently implicated in childhood disorders. Frontal lobe damage seems to result in difficulty in executive planning and strategic behaviors, as well as interference with or loss of previously learned skills. It is not clear whether frontal lobe damage inhibits, alters, or halts the process of continuing development. What is known is that age of injury has an important role in the severity of the injury on later development.

Age of Injury. Age plays a role not only in brain development but also in outcome following trauma. Injuries prior to age 8 have been found to produce more severe cognitive deficiencies than injuries after age 10 (Brink, Garrett, Hale, Woo-Sam, & Nickel, 1970; Woo-Sam, Zimmerman, Brink, Uyehara, & Miller, 1970). Woods (1980) found that children injured in the first year of life tend to have severe verbal and nonverbal deficits, and children injured after age 1 show more lateralized effects from the injury. Left-hemisphere damage between the ages of 5 and 12 often produces transitory aphasia, and adultlike aphasia is seen with left-hemisphere damage after age 16 (Boll & Barth, 1981).

Reading Difficulties following TBI. Reading deficits are sequelae of some forms of TBI (Klonoff, Low, & Clark, 1977; Schaffner, Bijur, Chadwick, & Rutter, 1980). Neurodevelopmental processes, particularly in the left planum temporale, have been implicated in reading difficulty in dyslexic children (Galaburda, 1991). Over time, reading deficits can depress overall verbal intelligence, vocabulary attainment, and verbal comprehension abilities of children (Stanovich, 1993).

Thus, brain trauma at an early age, as well as neurodevelopmental disorders resulting in reading deficits, may reduce the overall ability for children to acquire basic knowledge across the life span.

Swanson (1982, 1993) asserts that previously acquired information influences a child's ability to encode, process, and utilize new information. Reitan and Davison (1974) have argued that early damage to the immature, developing brain can have serious long-term effects. It may be that the longer the brain is "normal," the greater is its capacity to increase the richness and complexity of the knowledge base which is ultimately related to new learning.

Since brain damage appears to have its greatest effect on new learning (Hebb, 1942), young children, who by definition have less accumulated knowledge and experience, would experience difficulty with new learning. Severe deficiencies may not show up until later years when cognitive flexibility and independent thinking are required for learning and social-psychological functioning. These findings coupled with knowledge gained about the effect of frontal lobe damage on social functioning indicate that children with head injuries may well evidence behavioral difficulties that significantly affect their adjustment. Even mild head injury has been implicated in behavioral difficulties that may appear to be functionally based (Boll, 1983). Functional differences between the two hemispheres are important factors affecting emotional, behavioral, and psychosocial adjustment in children.

The Role of the Right and Left Hemispheres

Differences between the two hemispheres appear early in life, and these functional asymmetries may underlie variations in behavior (Teeter & Semrud-Clikeman, 1995). Goldberg and Costa (1981) describe the basic anatomical differences between the hemispheres related to the ratio of gray matter to white matter: the left hemisphere has greater gray matter than white and the right hemisphere has more white than gray matter. These structural differences may relate to the capacity of each hemisphere to deal with complex and novel information in social-psychological situations.

Anatomical asymmetries are present at birth, and functional differences in the processing of emotional stimuli appear early in life. For example, the right hemisphere appears central to the discrimination of facial expressivity and emotional tone; and the left hemisphere is more reactive to emotional stimuli, especially in younger children (9-year-olds). It has been hypothesized that as the right hemisphere matures, it has a modulating effect on the more reactive left hemisphere (Heller, 1990).

Adult research suggests that damage to the left hemisphere results in depression and catastrophic reactions, whereas damage to the right produces abnormal emotional reactions (e.g., euphoria or indifference) (Kolb & Whishaw, 1990). The extent to which these patterns hold true for children needs further investigation.

In a report of clinical case studies, Teeter (1989) found that children with signs of significant depression demonstrate various profiles depending on the hemisphere involved. For example, a child (CA = 10-5 years) with a right frontal pattern showed: left-handed tactual deficits; left-handed motor weaknesses; poor nonverbal reasoning abilities; visual–perceptual deficits; and abnormal EEG findings (bilateral anterior regions). Behavioral and psychological problems were noted as: dysthymia, impulsivity, disinhibition, social imperception, and suicidal ideation. Conversely, a child (CA = 9-8 years) with a left frontal lobe pattern displayed: right-handed motor weaknesses; tactile imperception; auditory sequential memory problems; verbal reasoning weaknesses; lower verbal IQ; and abnormal EEG ratings of a diffuse nature. In this instance, the child demonstrated anxiety, denial of emotions, isolation from peers, dysphoria, and inappropriate affect. Further examination revealed abnormal dexamethasone suppression results. The extent to which right frontal regions are involved with attention to social cues, execution of social interaction skills, and control over the left frontal regions for the appropriate expression of emotions in children with depression needs further study.

In summary, the apparent ratio of activation between the right and left hemispheres appears important—such that the right hemisphere might inhibit or modulate the left. Maturation of later-developing interhemispheric regions (i.e., corpus callosum) may also play a role in the control and modulation of emotional processes. Kolb and Whishaw (1990) suggest that differences between the front/back (anterior/posterior) quadrants are as essential as right–left differences in the control of human emotions. Further, it must be noted that controversy over whether the two hemispheres operate in autonomous, interactive, or domain-specific ways when it comes to complex behaviors still remains (Teeter & Semrud-Clikeman, 1995).

The following section discusses different types of psychopathology from a functional organizational approach utilizing a combined neuropsychological–neuropsychiatric and personality paradigm.

Externalizing Disorders of Childhood

Externalizing disorders are defined as those behaviors involving aggression, inattention, overactivity, and antisocial behavior. These problems are often classified as disruptive behavior disorders in infancy, childhood, and adolescence (APA, 1994). Behavior problems affect academic achievement in an age-dependent way. A strong correlation exists between delinquent behavior and underachievement for adolescents (Hinshaw, 1992). Further, early learning problems have also been found to be highly related to later psychopathology (Pianta & Caldwell, 1990). Two externalizing disorders—ADHD and conduct disorders—are briefly reviewed from a neuropsychological–neuropsychiatric point of view.

ADHD

Frick and Lahey (1991) suggest that it is important to differentiate primary symptoms from associated problems in children with ADHD. These authors state that the main variables involved in ADHD are those of inattention/disorganization and motor hyperactivity/impulsivity. Associated behaviors are poor academic achievement, problematic peer relationships, and low self-esteem. Such behaviors often cloud the diagnostic picture and have led clinicians to believe that they are part of the disorder. Further studies have attempted to separate out correlated symptoms from the main area of difficulty (Frick & Lahey, 1991; Pennington, 1991).

There appear to be significant differences in social competence between children who are overactive with inattention and those with inattention without overactivity. Children with ADHD plus aggressive behavior have been found to be less popular, more disliked, and more likely to be rejected by their peers (Atkins & Pelham, 1991). Although these children do not evidence skill deficits, they do experience difficulty in carrying out their intentions in a social situation. In contrast, children with ADD and withdrawn behaviors are often isolated and seem to lack needed social skills (Hynd et al., 1991). These children also appear to be at higher risk for mood disorders including anxiety and depression (Hynd et al., 1991; Milich & Landau, 1989).

Thus, children with ADHD with comorbid externalizing or internalizing disorders appear to be at risk for poor academic achievement and for the development of concurrent psychopathology. It is currently unclear whether these developmental disorders with co-occurring psychopathology are mutually independent or whether they are interrelated; that is, it is possible that having one disorder (i.e., ADHD) makes one vulnerable for the development of another disorder (e.g., conduct disorder or oppositional defiant disorder). However, ADHD children are at risk for the development of psychopathology. The outcome for children with ADHD and conduct disorder has been found to be the poorest compared with any other childhood disorder (Moffitt & Henry, 1989). Early aggressive tendencies plus neuropsychological delays in early childhood have been found to be highly predictive of delinquent behavior in adolescence, and criminal behavior in adulthood (Moffitt & Silva, 1988).

Executive function deficits have been found in children with ADHD particularly when overactivity and comorbid aggressive behaviors are present. These deficits were found on measures thought to evaluate planning, inhibition, and divided attention (Gorenstein, Mammato, & Sandy, 1989). In support of these behavioral findings, brain scanning techniques have found lowered metabolism in the prefrontal brain regions on sustained attention tasks in both children and adults with ADD (Lou, Henriksen, & Bruhn, 1984; Zametkin et al., 1990). This finding serves to demonstrate a possible relationship between brain function and the resulting behavior. Moreover, given the negative impact of deficient executive functions on day-to-day functioning, brain differences coupled with problematic behavior and difficulty in learning from experience may often result in feelings of lowered self-esteem and self-efficacy.

Biederman et al. (1992; Biederman, Newcorn, & Sprich, 1991) have found that children with ADHD have a tendency to develop affective disorders in about 30% of cases. Moreover, children with ADHD tend to have parents and/or siblings who evidence ADHD or affectively based psychopathology. In addition, ADHD continues into adulthood for approximately 50% of subjects perhaps as a result of their difficulty in developing compensatory techniques. For the adolescent or adult with ADHD, continuing difficulty with the law, substance abuse problems, difficulty holding a job, and problems with interpersonal relationships also occur (Biederman & Steingard, 1989).

It is reasonable to speculate that there is an interaction between genetics and environment which affects how ADHD is manifested (Teeter & Semrud-Clikeman, 1995). It may well be that a biological predisposition interacts with environmental variables (e.g., parental psychopathology, parenting styles) to foster the development of a more severe type of ADHD. Thus, children with ADHD who have parents with ADHD may be at highest risk for the disorder to appear and for comorbid disorders to also be present.

Conduct Disorder

Children with conduct disorder appear to have significantly lower intelligence than non-conduct-disordered children (Nieves, 1991; Semrud-Clikeman, Hynd, Lorys, & Lahey, 1993). Conversely, higher intelligence may mitigate against the development of delinquent behavior in high-risk children, as well as in adults (Kandel et al., 1988; White, Moffitt, & Silva, 1989). Most studies have found language-related deficits in adolescents with conduct disorders, which may suggest involvement of the left hemisphere (Moffitt, 1992). Adult males diagnosed as conduct disordered have also been found to have poorer verbal processing skills, with less language lateralization than adults without conduct disorder (Hare & Connoly, 1987). In contrast to left-hemisphere involvement found in conduct disorder, some researchers have suggested that chronic delinquents may show impairment in right frontal regions (Yeudall, Fromm-Auch, & Davies, 1982). Further, Teeter and Smith (1993) found that severely emotionally disturbed children with conduct-related disorders (e.g., severe physical aggression and sexual-acting out) had lower verbal intelligence, and significantly weaker nonverbal reasoning abilities. Thus, determining the extent to which clear-cut lateralizing signs are present may not be as important as determining the types of associated neuropsychological deficits (i.e., language and reasoning problems), and assessing their effect on later psychosocial and emotional development.

Studies with delinquents have yielded equivocal findings about the nature and extent of neuropsychological deficits that are present (Appellof, 1986; Berman & Siegal, 1976). It may be that these equivocal findings are a result of different levels of violent and nonviolent behaviors reported in children across various studies (Linz, Hynd, Isaac, & Gibson, 1988). Delinquents with aggressive behavioral difficulties have been found to perform poorly on measures of receptive language skills (Linz *et al.,* 1988). These children may experience difficulty understanding the consequences of their actions and thus are unable to mediate their behaviors appropriately.

A study using linear structural equations found that poor school achievement in middle elementary school and adolescence is predicted by disruptive behaviors in first grade (Tremblay, Masse, Perron, & Leblanc, 1992). In this study, academic difficulties were found in both first and fourth grade. However, when first-grade disruptive behaviors were used as a covariate, the relationship between first- and fourth-grade achievement and delinquency at age 14 diminished. These findings suggest that the primary foci of intervention strategies need to be placed on early behavioral control, as well as on academic acquisition.

Thus, it would appear that a child with a predisposition to develop a conduct disorder with co-occurring poorly developed language skills has a higher risk factor for developing significant antisocial behavior as an adolescent and as an adult. The contribution each variable has to the ultimate development of an "antisocial personality disorder" is unknown at this time. Reasoning problems may also play a role in the development and progression of conduct-related disorders. Moreover, which variables are correlated and which are causative is currently under investigation. Nonetheless, it appears that intervention strategies need to address the cognitive, reasoning, and language deficits that have been linked to delinquent behavior and conduct disorder as well.

Internalizing Disorders of Childhood

Although some believe that internalizing disorders in children are more closely related to brain dysfunction than are externalizing disorders (Tramontana & Hooper, 1989), there is a paucity of published research to support this hypothesis. Moreover, this picture is complicated by the finding that internalizing disorders such as depression have been found to co-occur with disruptive behaviors (Semrud-Clikeman & Hynd, 1991). As mentioned previously, approximately 30 to 40% of ADD children also experience depression and/or anxiety disorders (Biederman *et al.,* 1991). Moreover, ADD children have a significantly higher tendency to have parents with diagnoses of anxiety disorder and/or depression than do normal children or chil-

dren with other psychiatric diagnoses. Thus, it is often difficult to obtain a sample of children with only internalizing symptomatology and research that has done so is rare (Kusche *et al.,* 1993).

Childhood Depression

Based on extensive investigation of depression, Weinberg suggests that the following criteria be applied when diagnosing children and adolescents: "depressed mood; self-deprecatory ideation; aggressive behavior; sleep disturbance; change in school performance; diminished socialization; change in attitude toward school; somatic complaints; loss of usual energy; and, change in appetite/weight" (Emslie, Kennard, & Kowatch, 1995, p. 43). Further distinctions should be made concerning the type of depression, including differentiating major depressive disorder, minor depressive disorder, dysthymic disorder, and bipolar disorder.

Cognitive and sensorimotor dysfunction associated with right-hemisphere processes have been found to frequently occur in children with depression (Brumback, 1988). Moreover, a much lower incidence of left-hemisphere dysfunction was found with approximately 10% showing this type of lateralization compared with 50 to 66% with right-hemisphere dysfunction, and 30% of depressed children showing bilateral dysfunction. Support for the hypothesis of right-hemisphere involvement in depression comes from studies that have reported poor performance on the Wechsler Intelligence Scale for Children-Revised (WISC-R) subtests of Block Design, Coding, and Digit Span (Kaslow, Rehm, & Siegel, 1984; Wechsler, 1974). These WISC-R subtests are thought to be sensitive to right-hemisphere function (Teeter, 1986). Conversely, these children performed at an average level on measures thought to be sensitive to left-hemisphere function, such as the Vocabulary subtest of the WISC-R, or Trails A and B of the Reitan batteries (Reitan & Wolfson, 1995).

Performance and verbal intelligence quotients are not generally depressed as a whole, but over time depression does have a negative effect on the child's performance on these measures (Emslie *et al.,* 1995). Further, depressed children often show poor academic achievement (Kovacs & Goldston, 1991) and possess cognitive distortions on initial admittance into psychiatric hospitals (Tems *et al., 1993*).

Environmental factors also play a role in childhood depression, and may well shape the development of physiological processes (Dawson, Hessl, &

Frey, in press). The percentage of persons with major depression who have been found to have family members with depression is six times greater than those without depression (Downey & Coyne, 1990). Twin studies have found a 65% concordance rate for affective disorders for monozygotic twins versus 14% for dizygotic twins. While this finding suggests a genetic risk factor for depression, environment and biology may interact in this disorder. Mothers who are depressed may interact differently with their children and an insecure attachment may occur (Quay *et al.,* 1985). Such insecure attachment has been found to be a significant risk factor in the development of childhood depression (Cummings & Cicchetti, 1990).

Dawson, Grofer-Klinger, Panagiotides, Hill, & Spieker (1992) found that infants of mothers with depression had more activation in the right versus left frontal lobe even when placed in neutral conditions. This is considered to be an atypical pattern of activation, and is also found in subjects who are in remission for depressive symptoms (Henriques & Davidson, 1990). What is not clear is whether the patterns of brain activity are the consequence of the environmental impact of a depressed episode or episodes or if a biologically mediated depressive tendency is present. Thus, depression, as with many other disorders, appears to have multiple facets that likely interact to produce the syndrome.

Childhood Anxiety

Anxiety disorders have not been as extensively studied from a neuropsychological perspective as other disorders of childhood. Performance difficulties have been found in anxious children on the WISC-R, including Digit Span, Arithmetic, and Coding (Kaufman, 1979; Strauss, 1991). Dependent behavior coupled with signs of motor clumsiness, associated movements, and/or fine motor delays appear to be high risk factors for the development of long-term problems in children with anxiety and withdrawal (Shaffer *et al., 1985).*

Anxiety disorders have been found to be highly comorbid with ADHD (Biederman *et al.,* 1991) and depression (Brumback, 1988). The neuropsychological differences between children with comorbid internalizing and externalizing disorders (i.e., conduct disorder and anxiety or depression) and those with co-occurring internalizing disorders (i.e., anxiety and depression) have not been investigated. Children with various comorbid psychiatric disorders may well present differences behaviorally

as well as neuropsychologically. Further research is needed in this area to more fully determine characteristics that are unique to each combination of diagnosis.

Conclusions

Children with internalizing and externalizing psychiatric disorders appear to present with both functional–behavioral and neuropsychological–organic markers. These domains are intertwined and are difficult to separate out. It seems safe to conclude that children who have more than one disorder are more likely to be referred for assessment and are more likely to demonstrate severe types of psychopathology and neuropsychological dysfunction. For example, Kusche *et al.* (1993) evaluated neuropsychological differences among children with internalizing-only, externalizing-only, and mixed symptoms. They found that while all groups performed more poorly than a control group, the mixed symptom group showed the most severe and widespread deficits. The internalizing-only group was the closest to the control group and showed the least amount of neuropsychological impairment; the externalizing-only group showed moderate amounts of impairment. Unfortunately, parental psychopathology was not evaluated in this study so that contributing familial–environmental factors could not be ascertained.

Many of the personality assessment measures evaluating a child's behavior utilize parent report, and therefore it is reasonable to speculate that parental psychpathology may be related not only to the child's behavior but also to parental report. Given the relationship between neuropsychological measures and environmental correlates reported in most of the studies of childhood disorders, it is important to be cognizant of these influences when assessing a child. The following section discusses methods for assessment of children's behavioral and psychosocial difficulties.

Specific Assessment Methods

The technology for assessing behavioral/emotional problems in neurologically impaired children and adolescents has lagged behind the methods available for assessing other domains of functioning, including intelligence and academic achievement (Martin, 1988). Fortunately, this lag in innovation is beginning to abate somewhat as evidenced by the pace of publication of new instruments with improved psychometric properties (Kamphaus & Frick, 1996).

In this section a brief overview of available personality/behavioral assessment methodology is provided. Although not an exhaustive list, the focus will be on increasingly popular methods of parent and teacher ratings of child behavior. The reader is referred to other resources for detailed information regarding peer assessment methods, self-ratings, history-taking schemes, structured diagnostic schedules, projective techniques, observations, and other methods (e.g., see Kamphaus & Frick, 1996).

The assessment of behavioral/personality constructs is emphasized as opposed to specific isolated behaviors, which is consistent with the expressed purpose of most of the instrumentation that will be reviewed. Thus, an overview of specific behavioral assessment (i.e., molecularly defined behaviors) for intervention planning is not offered. The utility of assessing constructs or dimensions of behavior that have broader implications for case conceptualization, diagnosis, and treatment planning for neurologically impaired children will be explored.

Although a broad introduction to each measure will be presented, a detailed analysis of reliability and validity evidence is beyond the scope of this review. An analysis of important strengths and weaknesses of each measure is provided in an effort to assist clinicians in selecting and using specific instruments. The content of each scale is also reflected in tabular format.

Parent Rating Scales

Children who are referred for psychological or neuropsychological evaluations do not always demonstrate sufficient reading or oral expression skills for self-report purposes, which has led to the increasing popularity of parent rating scales (Lachar, 1990). Parent ratings of child behavior possess additional advantages, including ease and brevity of assessment and cost efficiency in the evaluation process. The minimal time involved in obtaining parent ratings makes it easy to collect parental information about child behavior problems or assets. Parent rating scales also provide a method for obtaining broad-based assessment of the child's problems as well as her or his assets. Although unstructured interviews may allow the clinician to carefully evaluate a specific area of the child's functioning, other important behavior problems may be

missed (Witt, Heffer, & Pfeiffer, 1990). Furthermore, the parental perspective, regardless of its validity, is often of value when conceptualizing a case. Given the importance of parental influences on child behavior, parent perceptions of behavior problems, in particular, should routinely be collected for neurologically involved children and adolescents.

Although parent rating scales are helpful, they are not interchangeable. With the seemingly exponential growth of such measures, psychologists have to make many decisions about the utility of various measures. This chapter attempts to aid the clinical neuropsychologist in the process of test selection by providing an overview of a variety of recently developed scales. Particular attention is devoted to defining the strengths and weaknesses of each measure.

Further, discussion will be limited to a coverage of multidomain/multisyndrome/omnibus measures as opposed to the universe of single domain/syndrome measures that are designed to measure specialized traits (e.g., ADHD symptoms only). An omnibus measure is preferred for most assessment purposes in order to ensure that comorbidity of other disorders is not overlooked (Kamphaus & Frick, 1996). A review of the strengths and weaknesses of five popular parent rating scales follows.

Behavior Assessment System for Children Parent Rating Scales (BASC-PRS) (Reynolds & Kamphaus, 1992)

The BASC-PRS is part of the larger BASC system that was published concurrently with a teacher and self-report rating method among other components (Reynolds & Kamphaus, 1992). Although the BASC-PRS is relatively new, and there is a lack of independently published research, early reviews have been favorable (e.g., Sandoval & Echandia, 1994).

The BASC-PRS has three separate forms that are composed of similar items and scales spanning the preschool (4–5 years), child (6–11 years), and adolescent (12–18 years) age ranges. The PRS allows the clinician to take a broad sampling of the child's behavior in home and community settings (see Table 1).

Initial reports indicate that the BASC-PRS: (1) possesses strong psychometric properties (Adams & Drabman, 1994; Jones & Witt, 1994); (2) has a large number of scales that may be useful for differential diagnosis (e.g., attention problems

Table 1. Overview of Parent and Teacher Rating Scales and Scale Content

Parent Rating Scales

BASC Parent Rating Scales (BASC-PRS; Reynolds & Kamphaus, 1992)	Adaptability, Aggression, Anxiety, Attention Problems, Atypicality, Conduct Problems, Depression, Hyperactivity, Leadership, Social Skills, Somatization, Withdrawal
Child Behavior Checklist (CBCL; Achenbach, 1991)	Aggressive Behavior, Delinquent Behavior, Anxious/Depressed, Somatic Complaints, Social Problems, Attention Problems, Thought Problems, Withdrawn
Conners' Parent Rating Scales (CPRS; Conners, 1989)	The Conners'-93 includes Conduct Disorder, Anxious–Shy, Restless–Disorganized, Learning Problem, Psychosomatic, Obsessive–Compulsive, Antisocial, and Hyperactive–Immature scales. The Conners'-48 provides Conduct Problem, Learning Problem, Psychosomatic, Impulsive–Hyperactive, and Anxiety scales.
Devereux Scales of Mental Disorders (DSMD; Naglieri, LeBuffe, & Pfeiffer, 1994)	Internalizing Composite: Anxiety Scale (Anx), Depression Scale (Dep), Critical Pathology Composite: Autism Scale (Aut), Acute Problems Scale (AP), Externalizing Composite: Conduct Scale (Con) (ages 13–18 only), Delinquency Scale (Del) (ages 13–18 only), Attention Scale (Att) (ages 5–12 only)
Personality Inventory for Children-Revised (PIC-R, Wirt, Lachar, Klinedinst, & Seat, 1990)	Lie Scale (L), Frequency Scale (F), Defensiveness Scale (DEF), Adjustment Scale, Achievement Scale (ACH), Intellectual Screening Scale (IS), Development Scale (DVL), Depression Scale (D), Family Relations Scale (FAM), Delinquency Scale (DLQ), Withdrawal Scale (WDL), Anxiety Scale (ANX), Psychosis Scale (PSY), Hyperactivity Scale (HPR), Social Skills Scale (SSK)

Teacher Rating Scales

Behavior Assessment System for Children— Teacher Rating Scales (BASC-TRS; Reynolds &; Kamphaus, 1992)	Aggression, Hyperactivity, Conduct Problems, Anxiety, Depression, Somatization, Attention Problems, Learning Problems, Atypicality, Withdrawal, Adaptability, Leadership, Social Skills, Study Skills
Child Behavior Checklist-91—Teacher's Report Form (TRF, Achenbach, 1991).	Withdrawn, Somatic Complaints, Anxious/Depressed, Social Problems, Thought Problems, Attention Problems, Delinquent Behavior, Aggressive Behavior
Comprehensive Behavior Rating Scale for Children (CBRSC; Neeper, Lahey, & Frick, 1990)	Three scales focus on learning problems and cognitive and cognitive processing (Reading Problems, Cognitive Deficits, Sluggish Tempo), three scales are related to attention deficits and motor hyperactivity (Inattention–Disorganization, Motor Hyperactivity, Daydreaming), and one scale each assesses conduct problems (Oppositional–Conduct Disorders), anxiety (Anxiety), and peer relations (Social Competence)
Conners' Teacher Rating (CTRS; Conners, 1989)	Attention, Hyperactivity, Conduct, & Anxiety—39 items (Conduct, Hyperactivity, & Attention—28 items)
Devereux Behavior Rating Scale— School Form (DBRS-SF; Naglieri, LeBuffe, & Pfeiffer, 1993)	Interpersonal Problems, Inappropriate Behaviors/Feelings, Depression, & Physical Symptoms/Fears—40 items.

versus hyperactivity, and anxiety versus depression) (Adams & Drabman, 1994); (3) provides useful validity indexes (Adams & Drabman, 1994); and (4) possesses adaptive scales, such as social skills and leadership (Adams & Drabman, 1994). With regard to the inclusion of adaptive scales, Jones and Witt (1994) observed that "by delineating positive as well as negative behaviors, the BASC may be more useful than other similar scales in identifying target alternative behaviors for intervention."

Areas that need to be addressed in future revisions/development of the BASC-PRS are: (1) the lack of interpretive information in the manual; (2) the highly structured response format does not allow parents to provide additional detail about their responses; (3) forms for children aged 2 and 3 are not available; (4) the hand score answer sheets can be unwieldy for the new user (Adams & Drabman, 1994); (5) cross informant comparisons are not as readily made as is the case for the Achenbach; and

(6) the computer scoring program may be of more use to the clinician than the researcher because fields for research information (e.g., an ID number) are not included (Hoza, 1994). However, the BASC-PRS appears to possess many strengths that increase its utility for assessing children who are referred to many clinicians (Sandoval & Echandia, 1994).

Child Behavior Checklist (CBCL)
(Achenbach, 1991)

The CBCL has long been considered one of the premier parent rating scale measures of child psychopathology (Merrell, 1994). This scale is the product of an extensive research effort and it has a distinguished history of research usage (Kamphaus & Frick, 1996). The CBCL, like the BASC and other new scales, is composed of a comprehensive system of scales including teacher rating, self-report, and classroom observation measures. The newest version of the CBCL (Achenbach, 1991) has an extended age range of 4 through 18 years. The CBCL is considered to be an essential component of the child assessment process (Achenbach, 1991).

The CBCL includes both behavior problem and "competence" scales that assess Activities, Social, and School competencies (see Table 1). The use of the CBCL is fostered by a large research base that continues to provide evidence of differential validity for many of the scales, and a collection of journal articles that provide further interpretive guidance. The considerable familiarity clinicians have with the CBCL also increases its utility.

Despite its strengths, some weaknesses in the CBCL have been noted including: (1) a lack of empirical profile typing that has been validated against external criteria (Kline, 1994); (2) considerable item overlap of scales, which may hinder the interpretation of individual scales as measuring distinct entities; (3) a lack of construct differentiation among some clinical scales, which makes differential diagnosis more difficult (e.g., hyperactivity versus inattention) and may even hinder differential diagnosis; and (4) some items may be better suited to clinical rather than school settings because of the severity of some of the behaviors assessed (Merrell, 1994).

In summary, the CBCL continues to be widely used by child clinicians. The continuing development of the CBCL research base should ensure its popularity well into the future (Kamphaus & Frick, 1996).

Conners' Parent Rating Scales (CPRS)
(Conners, 1989)

The CPRS is a widely used behavior rating scale that was primarily used for research purposes until it was commercially published in 1989. The scale was designed to be "used to characterize the behaviors of a child and compare them to levels of appropriate normative groups" (Conners, 1989, p. 3). Parent forms are designed for ages 3 through 17; and two parent forms are available, a 93- and a 48-item version.

One advantage of the CPRS is that it does constitute a multirater system that includes both teacher and parent forms. Another strength is that its response forms can be quickly completed by parents and scored by clinicians. It does, however, possess some noteworthy weaknesses such as: (1) items are worded negatively, which may inadvertently encourage a response set; (2) reliability and validity evidence is limited; and (3) few details regarding norming and scaling are available. In fact, Kamphaus and Frick (1996) question whether the CPRS (93- and 48-item forms) can be used as norm-referenced measures by concluding:

> They may be useful for pre- and post-testing purposes in drug studies but their diagnostic usage is compromised by little evidence to support the adequacy of the norm referenced scores. Consequently, until further evidence of psychometric integrity is offered the T-scores yielded should be considered suspect unless they are corroborated by other sources. Merrell (1994) reinforces this opinion by observing that, 'The size of the CPRS-48 norm population is relatively small, and the geographic and racial composition of the norm sample is so limited that the generalizability of the norm-based scores should be questioned.' (p. 81)

Aman (1994) further expresses reservations about the use of the CPRS with children who have diagnoses of cognitive or mental retardation. He concludes:

> The first is that hyperactivity may not manifest itself identically in children with and without mental retardation. For example, two groups found that both classic attention deficit item types and noncompliance items tend to cluster onto one factor in those with mental retardation . . . , whereas this is not the case in normal IQ children. The second reservation is that teachers have complained that aspects of the Conners Scales are not relevant to the handicapped children they teach. Items like 'appears to lack leadership' may be examples. The success of the Conners scales cannot be denied, and there is merit in using a stan-

dard instrument to bridge the work with children who are and are not mentally retarded. With time, however, this field must find its own identity, and it is hoped that the Conners scales will either be validated for this population or that investigators will begin to use tools that are. (p. 7)

So, while the CPRS may have a role to play in medication monitoring, it may be less useful to the clinician in the initial assessment and diagnosis of children with particular behavioral/personality problems.

Devereux Scales of Mental Disorders (DSMD) (Naglieri, LeBuffe, & Pfeiffer, 1994)

The new version of the Devereux is designed for children between the ages of 5 and 18. Although the DSMD is somewhat unique in that *either* parents or teachers may serve as raters, current evidence of the equivalence of the DSMD with both parents and teachers is not available (Riccio, 1995). The DSMD is intended to "indicate whether a child or adolescent is experiencing or is at risk for an emotional or behavioral disorder."

Although the DSMD items were created using both rational and empirical means with special attention given to sampling DSM-IV symptoms, this instrument only assesses problem behaviors and excludes the measurement of adaptive skills. The DSMD possesses a modern normative base which increases confidence in the obtained scores, a practical test length, and a helpful manual. Of particular importance is the fact that high reliability coefficients are reported for the three composite scores.

Potential weaknesses of the DSMD are: (1) a relatively limited number of scales (six), which creates greater opportunity to overlook important problems; (2) an absence of a computer scoring option at the time of this writing; and (3) a lack of validity scales. Further research and development with the DSMD will help determine its long-term utility.

Personality Inventory for Children-Revised (PIC-R) (Wirt, Lachar, Klinedinst, & Seat, 1990)

The PIC is one of the oldest and best known of all parent rating scales. In fact, much of the early development work completed on the PIC took place in the 1950s and 1960s. The PIC is the longest of the scales available—the full scale includes 420 items—for use with parents of children between the ages of 3 and 16 .

Some of the PIC-R strengths include: (1) a thorough updated manual by Lachar (1990) that summarizes important validity studies; (2) a large collection of research studies; and (3) a manual that includes interpretive guidance. Weaknesses of the PIC-R may include: (1) excessive test length; (2) outdated normative sample; and (3) excessive item overlap between scales, which calls into question the degree to which each scale can be interpreted as measuring a unique construct.

Although it is the first of its genre, the PIC-R suffers in comparison with more recently developed measures. Unlike the BASC, CBCL, Conners, and DSMD, for example, the PIC-R has not developed complementary teacher rating scales. In addition, the lack of modern norms is a noteworthy problem that detracts from interpretive confidence.

While parental perceptions about the child are important, it is also critical to assess the perceptions of the child's teacher(s) in a comprehensive assessment. Frequently the kinds of problems that children have are manifested in the classroom or in social situations with the child's peer group; thus, the teacher's perceptions can be helpful for understanding the nature and extent of the child's problems. A select list of teacher rating scales is briefly reviewed.

Teacher Ratings

It has not always been customary for clinicians to use teacher ratings as centerpieces of the assessment of child and adolescent social/emotional functioning (Kamphaus & Frick, 1996). There are several reasons, however, why teacher ratings should be part of the evaluation of all school-age children. Among the most important reasons is that schooling constitutes much of the child's daily activity. In some ways the school is a metaphor for the workplace. Schooling is as important for the child evaluation as occupational issues are for adult assessment. Second, it is important to note how a child responds to the demands to sit still, participate in group activities, complete assignments, and engage in other activities required in academic and social settings in the school. Finally, it can be valuable to understand how a child responds to schooling at different stages of development. The demands of schooling change considerably from grade to grade which produces many opportunities for a mismatch between the child's strengths and weaknesses and the demands of the environment.

Clinicians are increasingly recognizing the importance of obtaining teacher ratings for screening, intervention design, treatment evaluation, and diagnostic purposes. As children with brain injuries are increasingly integrated into the regular schooling process, teacher ratings will be essential, particularly for monitoring the progress of these children.

The following section is a presentation and discussion of some of the newly available and widely used teacher rating scales.

Behavior Assessment System for Children—Teacher Rating Scales (BASC-TRS) (Reynolds & Kamphaus, 1992)

The BASC-TRS was designed to gather information regarding a child's observable behaviors and then place this information in the context of other data obtained in the overall BASC system (e.g., self-report scale, parent rating scales, classroom observation system) (Kamphaus & Frick, 1996). Many aspects of the BASC-TRS are comparable to its companion parent form (PRS) including: (1) comparable age ranges; (2) separate levels for preschool (4–5), elementary school (6–11), and middle/high school (12–18) children; (3) four-point scales to describe the frequency of occurrence of the behavior, ranging from "Never" to "Almost Always"; (4) different numbers of items for the three forms: 109, 148, and 138 items for the preschool, elementary school, and middle/high school versions, respectively; and (5) inclusion of items that were chosen to measure multiple aspects of a child's personality and behavior, including both positive (adaptive) and pathological (clinical) dimensions.

The BASC-TRS possesses many assets (Sandoval & Echandia, 1995) including: coordination with other components of a multimethod, multi-informant system; item content covering important domains of classroom behavioral and emotional functioning; and excellent sampling from a large national normative group on which norm-referenced scores are based. These apparent strengths allow the clinician to make norm-referenced interpretations of scores with confidence.

An area that needs to be considered when using the BASC-TRS is that the norm sample is smaller in the adolescent age range, especially at ages 14–18. In addition, few studies of the use of the BASC in clinical populations have been published to date. In summary, selection of the BASC-TRS in

conjunction with the BASC-PRS provides the clinician with valid measures of teacher and parent perceptions of the child's behavior.

Child Behavior Checklist-91—Teacher's Report Form (TRF) (Achenbach, 1991)

The TRF is part of a multi-informant system that has a long and prominent history for assessing children's emotional and behavioral functioning (Kamphaus & Frick, 1996). The CBCL is a widely used rating scale system, and the dimensions of functioning covered by these scales are often considered the "standard" by which the content of other rating scales is judged. The 1991 revision of the TRF includes many psychometric improvements from the original version of TRF; however, the item content remains virtually unchanged in the revision. The content of the TRF was designed to be analogous to the original parent-completed CBCL, which explicitly attempted to be atheoretical in the development of the item pool.

The use of the TRF is supported by a large research literature showing correlations between CBCL scales and important clinical criteria, especially for the externalizing scales. Obtained scores on the TRF are also based on a national normative sample that is geographically and ethnically representative of the population.

The clinician is advised that the normative sample excludes children who have received mental health or special education services and, therefore, cannot be considered fully representative of the general population. In addition, the TRF utilizes normalized T-scores instead of linear conversions which may serve to normalize otherwise lawfully skewed distributions of scores (see Kamphaus & Frick, 1996, for a discussion of scaling methods). The TRF is also limited in the number of child competencies that can be assessed. Thus, when choosing the methods to use, the clinician must keep these considerations in mind.

Comprehensive Behavior Rating Scale for Children (CBRSC) (Neeper, Lahey, & Frick, 1990)

The CBRSC is a 70-item teacher rating scale designed to assess the classroom functioning of children aged 6 to 14. Teachers rate 70 behaviors on a 5-point scale based on whether the child exhibits the behavior "Not at all" (1), to "Very Much" (5). Unlike most of the other rating scales reviewed in this chapter, the CBRSC is not part of a multi-informant assessment system, and it targets a more limited age range of children. However, while these two factors limit its usefulness in situations, the CBRSC possesses content that is uniquely suited for assessing the classroom adjustment of elementary aged children.

The CBRSC Reading Problems and Cognitive Deficits scales correlate with standardized achievement and intelligence measures, and thus make these scales good screeners for children with learning problems who might warrant a more comprehensive academic evaluation. Also, CBRSC items closely correspond to DSM diagnostic criteria particularly for ADHD as four of the nine scales seem relevant to the assessment of attentive/hyperactive. Further the Inattention–Disorganization and Motor Hyperactivity scales are related to the Hyperactive and Combined Types of ADHD as specified in the DSM-IV (APA, 1994).

The CBRSC, however, does not have analogous rating scales for parents or other informants to aid in a multi-informant assessment, and the age range of the CBRSC is limited to 6- to 14-year-olds. Also, a lack of information on the socioeconomic status of the children in its general normative sample may limit the use of its norm-referenced scores. Additional validity studies of the CBRSC are also needed. Thus, the CBRSC may be considered as part of a comprehensive battery when these issues are properly weighed in individual cases.

Conners' Teacher Rating Scales (CTRS)
(Conners, 1989)

The CTRS is a well-known research instrument that was published commercially in 1989 by Multi-Health Systems, Inc. The CTRS-39 (39 items) describes behaviors that are scored on a four-point frequency scale ranging from "Not at all" (0), to "Very Much" (3). The CTRS-39 was the original scale published in 1969 (see Table 1). It has been normed for use with children between the ages of 4 and 12. The CTRS-28 is a 28-item version of the CTRS that includes three scales (see Table 1). For both versions of the CTRS there is a 10-item scale, labeled the Hyperactivity Index, composed of the "ten items most sensitive to drug effects" (Conners, 1989, p. 2) in the treatment of childhood hyperactivity.

Although the Hyperactivity Index does possess clinical utility, the CTRS is hampered by some glaring psychometric inadequacies. For example, both forms of the CTRS were normed only for

English-speaking Canadian schoolchildren, thus calling into question the accuracy of its norm referenced scores for U.S. children. The CTRS item content is also limited primarily to the assessment of disruptive behavior problems to the exclusion of adaptive skills and internalizing problems. Thus, the CTRS is probably inappropriately classified as an omnibus rating scale.

Devereux Behavior Rating Scale—School Form (DBRS-SF) (Naglieri, LeBuffe, & Pfeiffer, 1993)

The DBRS-SF is a revision of the Devereux rating scales published in the 1960s by the Devereux Foundation (Spivack & Spotts, 1966; Spivack, Spotts, & Haimes, 1967). The DBRS-SF is a brief measure containing two 40-item forms, one for children (ages 5–12) and a second for adolescents (ages 13–18). Based on their occurrence in the previous 4 weeks, items are rated on a five-point frequency scale ranging from "Never" to "Very Frequently." The DBRS-SF was designed to be completed by either a parent or a teacher.

The DBRS-SF possesses acceptable reliability indexes and its scores are based on an extensive normative base. Evidence is presented in the manual that the scales can discriminate between emotionally disturbed children and nonhandicapped children. The main weakness of the DBRS-SF is its item content. The DBRS-SF measures a very limited range of behavioral domains with a noteworthy absence of externalizing behaviors. This situation is unfortunate given that teachers are most adept at providing information regarding externalizing problems. Also, there is a significant lack of items relating to symptoms of inattention and motor hyperactivity.

Conclusions Regarding Parent and Teacher Rating Scales

There has been a substantial improvement in the technology available to the child neuropsychologist who assesses behavioral and emotional functioning. This situation is welcome news given that we are well aware of the need to assess these behavioral domains (Prigatano, 1992).

Clinical neuropsychologists may use the large armamentarium of parent and teacher rating scales in concert with other measures to assess the numerous sequelae associated with TBI. Prigatano (1992), for example, provides a useful review of some of the postmorbid difficulties associated with various

TABLE 2. Behavioral/Emotional Disturbances Associated with TBI[a]

Irritability
Agitation
Belligerence
Anger
Violence
Impulsiveness
Restlessness
Inappropriate social responses
Emotional lability
Hypersensitivity to noise or distress
Anxiety
Suspiciousness
Delusions
Paranoia
Mania
Aspontaneity
Sluggish
Loss of interest or drive
Fatigue
Depression
Immature behavior
Helplessness
Poor insight

[a]Adapted from Prigatano (1992).

childhood disorders that require assessment (see Table 2). Some of these problems, and others, are conveniently assessed with the newer parent and teacher methods described above.

The manner in which the behaviors associated with TBI are measured depends in part on the characteristics present. However, a combination of parent and teaching rating scales, self-report measures, observational formats, and clinical interviews will afford methods for broad-based evaluation.

Integrating Psychological–Behavioral Assessment Findings into Neuropsychological Evaluation Results

Clinical child neuropsychologists historically have focused on investigation of the brain–behavior relationship in children, with special attention to cognitive, memory, language, visual–spatial, sensory–perceptual, reasoning, alertness, and motor functions. Recent integrated, transactional conceptualizations of child neuropsychology call for the inclusion of methods to identify associated psychosocial and behavior problems that may ac-

company brain-related disorders or disease processes (Teeter & Semrud-Clikeman, 1995). In order to fully appreciate the manner in which neuropsychological dysfunction affects the psychosocial and behavioral functioning of children, several guidelines are recommended. As the assessment process should ultimately assist in the determination of appropriate interventions, clinicians may want to consider the following when assessing childhood disorders, and when subsequently designing and implementing intervention plans.

Identify Neuropsychological Assets and Deficits

It is critical to fully assess the child's neuropsychological assets and deficits, and to determine their impact on the psychosocial and behavioral functioning in the home and school setting. In an effort to appreciate the effects of neuropsychological dysfunction on behavior, the following deficit patterns need to be assessed.

First, does the child have intact or dysfunctional frontal lobe systems? The extent to which disinhibition (motor and attentional), poor planning and execution of plans, inflexibility and rigidity, inadequate language and verbal skills, and impaired reasoning strategies are affecting the child's overall adjustment should be ascertained. These behaviors affect the child's social interaction patterns and acceptance by age peers.

Second, does the child have intact temporal lobe association regions? Temporal lobe impairment often results in significant memory deficits, an inability to analyze affective qualities of stimuli, and trouble recognizing nonverbal social cues. Memory deficits may significantly impair the child's ability to learn and profit from experience. The extent to which the child is plagued by temporal association region deficits may affect the manner in which social and emotional problems are manifested. Differences in right- and left-hemisphere systems should also be assessed, and deficits may affect the manner in which verbal and nonverbal information is perceived and remembered.

Third, does the child have neurodevelopmental disorders affecting sensory–perceptual systems? For example, children with tactile defensiveness often recoil from touch and are not easily soothed as infants. Children with these deficits may have displayed temperamental difficulties as infants, and may not have established firm emotional bonds. These neurological sensitivities may result in bonding and attachment problems with the primary caretaker (i.e., the mother), which may persist into early childhood and adolescence. In other instances, children with significant psychomotor delays or weaknesses may avoid physical-play activities, such as bicycle riding, swimming, baseball, soccer, basketball, and tennis, to name a few. The extent to which avoidance isolates the child from her or his peers is of concern. These physical activities are a significant part of the early socialization of childhood. When children withdraw from play activities and become isolated from peers, depression is a likely outcome.

Fourth, does the child have a particular pattern of neuropsychological deficits and assets? A number of syndromes have been described that appear to have a fairly reliable set of neuropsychological asset/deficit patterns, associated psychosocial, academic, and behavioral features, and relatively consistent developmental course (e.g., nonverbal learning disabilities). It is critical to ascertain the child's capacity to develop compensatory skills, and the child neuropsychologist is advised to identify potential strengths and assets that can be used in the intervention phase of treatment.

Finally, to what extent do basic neuropsychological assets/deficits affect the psychosocial and behavioral functioning of the child? While causal relationships are difficult to determine, a number of childhood disorders do have rather predictable clusters of neuropsychological problems that interfere with normal adjustment. (See the discussion of specific disorders at the beginning of the chapter.) While assessing the functional neuropsychological status of children is critical, it is also important to identify comorbid psychiatric and learning problems in children.

Identify Comorbid Disorders

It is imperative to obtain a total picture of the child's functional and dysfunctional systems—neuropsychological, psychosocial, behavioral, and academic. Thus, the clinician must determine the presence of comorbid disorders when assessing the child, and when developing intervention programs. For example, are psychological disorders also present with neuropsychological symptoms? Are externalizing, internalizing, or combined disorders obvious? Do learning disabilities interfere with the child's overall functional capacity? Do parental psychopathology and family stress or dys-

function exacerbate the child's problems? The extent to which associated features, full-blown syndromes or disorders, and/or environmental stress are identified may significantly increase intervention outcomes. When these important features are ignored, children with neuropsychological-based disorders are often unable to adequately profit from treatment programs.

Further, it is important to note that neuropsychological deficits are more likely to be present in children with chronic and severe forms of psychopathology. In summary, the presence of comorbid disorders may affect the child's ability to profit from interventions, to remember past experiences, and to anticipate consequences of their behavior—all of which are related to positive intervention and developmental outcomes.

Identify the Developmental Course of the Disorder

The process of neuropsychological assessment and determination of associated psychosocial and behavioral features should consider developmental issues. The clinician should be well versed in the developmental course of various childhood brain-related and neuropsychiatric disorders of childhood. It is also important to determine/ascertain: (1) which behaviors are expected to improve with little or no interventions? (2) which behaviors are likely to increase without interventions? (3) which behaviors may improve when other behaviors are targeted for intervention? (4) which behaviors, if left untreated, are likely to produce other more serious disorders?

Answers to these questions are critical for setting treatment priorities. Although the developmental course of some disorders of childhood (e.g., ADHD) has been described (Barkley, 1990; Teeter, in preparation), other disorders are not well delineated (e.g., depression and anxiety). Further, very little research has been conducted on how specific deficits affect other behaviors over time. There are a few exceptions. For example, a causal link has been established between early aggression and later achievement deficits. However, the extent to which early intervention targeting aggression may reduce subsequent academic problems needs to be investigated. It may also be helpful to determine if interventions in verbal–language and reasoning deficits also assist in improving the long-term prognosis of children with conduct-related problems. This is certainly a rich area for future research.

Identify Child Competencies

Identification of the child's unique assets, interests, and competencies should be explored. By describing the child's strengths and incorporating these into intervention plans, the clinician may help to avoid the cycle of low self-esteem that often accompanies long-term school failure, social isolation, and/or rejection that many children with problems experience. Levine (1993, 1994) advocates for "demystification" processes in treatment programs that specifically address the children's knowledge and perceptions about their own disorders. Thus, measures that assist in the identification of assets as well as deficits should be utilized by the clinician. The newly developed BASC system for parents, teachers, and the child seems perfectly well suited to this end. Interview and observational techniques also provide information about what the child excels at, or "feels at home" doing. These can be powerful factors to increase self-esteem and motivation in children with various disorders.

Identify Ecological Factors

Child neuropsychologists are advised to incorporate ecologically valid assessment and intervention methods when treating children with various disorders. With this in mind, three factors seem pertinent. First, understanding the child's social, cultural, and family context is important. Resources available to the family, psychological as well as economic, should be assessed. Intervention plans should be developed with these assets/limitations in mind. Second, selection of ecologically valid, empirically based intervention strategies is recommended. Numerous behavioral, psychosocial, and cognitively based interventions have proven effective for children with behavior and personality disorders (Semrud-Clikeman, 1995). Pharmacotherapy may also be warranted for some disorders of childhood (Teeter & Semrud-Clikeman, 1995). Third, intervention plans should include strategies for parents and teachers. Although we may not always be able to change the neuropsychological profile of a child, we may effect significant change in the child's adjustment by modifying parenting strategies, coping skills, learning environments, and classroom management techniques. Thus, careful evaluation and planning for the school and home environment is essential.

References

Achenbach, R. (1991). Conceptualizations of developmental psychopathology. In M. Lewis & S. Miller (Eds.), *Handbook of developmental psychopathology* (pp. 3–13). New York: Plenum Press.

Adams, C. D., & Drabman, R. S. (1994). BASC: A critical review. *Child Assessment News, 4*(1), 1–5.

Aman, M. G. (1994). Instruments for assessing treatment effects in developmentally delayed populations. *Assessment in Rehabilitation and Exceptionality, 1,* 1–19.

American Psychiatric Association. (1994). *Diagnostic and statistical manual of mental disorders* (4th ed.). Washington, DC: Author.

Andreasen, N. C., Olsen, S. A., Dennert, J. W., & Smith, M. R. (1982). Ventricular enlargement in schizophrenia: Relationship to positive and negative symptoms. *American Journal of Psychiatry, 139,* 297–302.

Appellof, E. (1986). Prefrontal lobe functions in juvenile delinquents (Wisconsin Card Sorting Test). *Dissertation Abstracts International, 46*(9), 3206B.

Atkins, M. S., & Pelham, W. E. (1991). School-based assessment of attention deficit–hyperactivity disorder. *Journal of Learning Disabilities, 24,* 197–204.

Bear, D. M. (1983). Hemispheric specialization and the neurology of emotions. *Archives of Neurology, 40,* 195–202.

Becker, M., Isaac, W., & Hynd, G. W. (1987). Neuropsychological development of nonverbal behaviors attributed to "frontal lobe" functioning. *Developmental Neuropsychology, 3,* 275–298.

Bell, M. A., & Fox, N. A. (1992). The relations between frontal brain electrical activity and cognitive development during infancy. *Child Development, 63,* 1142–1163.

Berman, A., & Siegal, A. (1976). Adaptive and learning skills in juvenile delinquents: A neuropsychological analysis. *Journal of Learning Disabilities, 9*(9), 51–58.

Biederman, J., Faraone, S. V., Keenan, K., Benjamin, J., Krifcher, B., Moore, C., Sprich-Buckminster, S., Ugaglia, K., Jellinek, M. S., Steingard, R., Spencer, T., Norman, D., Kolodny, R., Kraus, I., Perrin, J., Keller, M. B., & Tsuang, M. T. (1992). Further evidence for family-genetic risk factors in attention deficit hyperactivity disorder. *Archives of General Psychiatry, 49,* 728–738.

Biederman, J., Newcorn, J., & Sprich, S. (1991). Comorbidity of attention deficit hyperactivity disorder with conduct, depressive, anxiety, and other disorders. *American Journal of Psychiatry, 148,* 564–577.

Biederman, J., & Steingard, R. (1989). Attention deficit hyperactivity disorder in adolescents. *Psychiatric Annals, 19,* 587–596.

Boll, T. J. (1983). Minor head injury in children: Out of sight but not out of mind. *Journal of Clinical Child Psychology, 12,* 74–80.

Boll, T. J., & Barth, J. T. (1981). Neuropsychology of brain damage in children. In S. B. Filskov & T. J. Boll (Eds.), *Handbook of clinical neuropsychology* (pp. 86–99). New York: Wiley.

Brink, J., Garrett, A., Hale, W., Woo-Sam, J., & Nickel, V. (1970). Recovery of motor and intellectual function in children sustaining severe head injuries. *Developmental Medicine and Child Neurology, 12,* 565–571.

Brumback, R. A. (1988). Child depression and medically treatable learning disability. In D. L. Molfese & S. J. Segalowitz (Eds.), *Brain lateralization in children: Developmental implications* (pp. 463–505). New York: Guilford Press.

Case, R. (1992). The role of the frontal lobes in the regulation of cognitive development. *Brain and Cognition, 20,* 51–73.

Conners, C. K. (1989). *Conners' Rating Scales.* Toronto: Multi-Health Systems.

Cook, E. H., & Leventhal, B. L. (1992). Neuropsychiatric disorders of childhood and adolescence. In S. C. Yudofsky & R. E. Hales (Eds.), *Textbook of neuropsychiatry* (pp. 639–662). Washington, DC: American Psychiatric Press.

Cummings, E. M., & Cicchetti, D. (1990). Toward a transactional model of relations between attachment and depression. In M. T. Greenberg, D. Cicchetti, & E. M. Cummings (Eds.), *Attachment in the preschool years: Theory, research, and intervention* (pp. 339–374). Chicago: University of Chicago Press.

Dawson, G. (1994). Development of expression and emotion regulation in infancy: Contributions of the frontal lobe. In G. Dawson & K. Fischer (Eds.), *Human behavior and the developing brain* (pp. 346–379). New York: Guilford Press.

Dawson, G., Grofer-Klinger, L., Panagiotides, H., Hill, D., & Spieker, S. (1992). Frontal lobe activity and affective behavior of infants of mothers with depressive symptoms. *Child Development, 63,* 725–737.

Dawson, G., Hessl, D., & Frey, K. (in press). Environmental influences on early-developing biological and behavioral systems related to risk for affective disorder. *Development and Psychopathology.*

Dean, R. S. (1985). Neuropsychological assessment. In J. D. Cavenar, R. Michels, H. K. H. Brodie, A. M. Cooper, S. B. Guze, L. L. Judd, G. L. Klerman, & A. J. Solnit (Eds.), *Psychiatry* (pp. 219–231). Philadelphia: Lippincott.

Dean, R. S. (1986). Neuropsychological aspects of psychiatric disorders. In J. Obrzut & G. W. Hynd (Eds.), *Child neuropsychology* (Vol. 2, pp. 83–112). New York: Academic Press.

Dennis, M. (1991). Frontal lobe function in childhood and adolescence: A heuristic for assessing attention regulation, executive control, and the intentional states important for social discourse. *Developmental Neuropsychology, 7,* 327–358.

Dimond, S. J., Farrington, L., & Johnson, P. (1976). Differing emotional responses from right to left hemispheres. *Nature, 261,* 690–692.

Downey, G., & Coyne, J. (1990). Children of depressed parents: An integrative view. *Psychological Bulletin, 108,* 50–76.

Emslie, G. J., Kennard, B. D., & Kowatch, R. A. (1995). Affective disorders in children: Diagnosis and management. *Journal of Child Neurology, 10,* s42–s49.

Fletcher, J., & Taylor, H. (1984). Neuropsychological approaches to children: Towards a developmental neuropsychology. *Journal of Clinical Neuropsychology, 6,* 39–56.

Frick, P., & Lahey, B. B. (1991). Nature and characteristics of attention deficit hyperactivity disorder. *School Psychology Review, 20,* 163–173.

Galaburda, A. (1991). Anatomy of dyslexia: Argument against phrenology. In D. Duane & D. Gray (Eds.), *The reading brain: The biological basis of dyslexia* (pp. 119–131). Parkton, MD: York Press.

Geschwind, N. (1965). Disconnection syndromes in animals and man. *Brain, 88,* 237–294.

Goldberg, E., & Costa, L. D. (1981). Hemisphere differences in the acquisition and use of descriptive systems. *Brain and Language, 14,* 144–173.

Golden, C. (1981). The Luria–Nebraska Children's Battery: Theory formulation. In G. W. Hynd & J. Obrzut (Eds.), *Neuropsychological assessment and the school-aged child* (pp. 277–302). New York: Grune & Stratton.

Gorenstein, E. E., Mammato, C. A., & Sandy, J. M. (1989). Performance of inattentive–overactive children on selected measures of prefrontal-type function. *Journal of Clinical Psychology, 45,* 619–632.

Grafman, J., Vance, S., Weingartner, H., Salazar, A., & Amin, D. (1986). The effects of lateralized frontal lobe lesions on mood regulation. *Brain, 109,* 1127–1148.

Hare, R. D., & Connoly, J. F. (1987). Perceptual asymmetries and information processing in psychopaths. In S. A. Mednick & T. E. Moffitt (Eds.), *Biology and antisocial behavior* (pp. 169–198). London: Cambridge University Press.

Hebb, D. O. (1942). The effect of early and late brain injury on test scores, and the nature of normal adult intelligence. *Proceedings of the American Philosophical Society, 85,* 275–292.

Heilman, K. M., Schwartz, H. D., & Watson, R. T. (1978). Hypoarousal in patients with neglect syndrome and emotional indifference. *Neurology, 29,* 229–232.

Heller, W. (1990). The neuropsychology of emotion: Developmental patterns and implications for psychopathology. In N. Stein, B. Leventhal, & T. Trabasso (Eds.), *Psychological and biological approaches to emotion* (pp. 167–214). Hillsdale, NJ: Erlbaum.

Henriques, J., & Davidson, R. (1990). Regional brain electrical asymmetries discriminate between previously depressed subjects and healthy controls. *Journal of Abnormal Psychology, 99,* 22–31.

Hertzig, M. E. (1982). Stability and change in nonfocal neurologic signs. *Journal of the American Academy of Child Psychiatry, 21,* 231–236.

Hinshaw, S. P. (1992). Externalizing behavior problems and academic underachievement in childhood and adolescence: Causal relationships and underlying mechanisms. *Psychological Bulletin, 111,* 127–155.

Hoza, B. (1994). Review of the Behavior Assessment System for Children. *Child Assessment News, 4*(1), 5, 8–10.

Hynd, G. W., Lorys, A. R., Semrud-Clikeman, M., Nieves, N., Huettner, M. I. S., & Lahey, B. B. (1991). Attention deficit disorder without hyperactivity (ADD/WO): A distinct behavioral and neurocognitive syndrome. *Journal of Child Neurology, Supplement,* 17–25.

Jarvik, M. E. (1977). *Psychopharmacology in the practice of medicine.* New York: Appleton–Century–Crofts.

Jones, K. M., & Witt, J. C. (1994). Rating the ratings of raters: A critique of the Behavior Assessment System for Children. *Child Assessment News, 4,* 10–11.

Kamphaus, R. W., & Frick, P. J. (1996). *Clinical assessment of child and adolescent personality and behavior.* Boston: Allyn & Bacon.

Kandel, E., Mednick, S. A., Kirkegaard-Sorenson, L., Hutchings, B., Knop, J., Rosenberg, R., & Schulsinger, F. (1988). I.Q. as a protective factor for subjects at high risk for antisocial behavior. *Journal of Consulting and Clinical Psychology, 56,* 224–226.

Kaslow, N., Rehm, L., & Siegel, A. (1984). Social-cognitive and cognitive correlates of depression in children. *Journal of Abnormal Child Psychology, 12,* 605–620.

Kaufman, A. S. (1979). *Intelligent testing with the WISC-R.* New York: Guilford Press.

Kline, R. B. (1994). New objective rating scales for child assessment, I. Parent- and teacher-rating informant inventories of the Behavior Assessment System for Children: the Child Behavior Checklist, and the Teacher Report Form. *Journal of Psychoeducational Assessment, 12,* 289–306.

Klonoff, H., Low, M. D., & Clark, C. (1977). Head injuries in children: A prospective five year follow-up. *Journal of Neurology, Neurosurgery, and Psychiatry, 40,* 1211–1219.

Kolb, B., & Whishaw, I. (1990). *Fundamentals of human neuropsychology* (3rd ed.). San Francisco: Freeman.

Kovacs, M., & Goldston, D. (1991). Cognitive and social development of depressed children and adolescents. *Journal of the American Academy of Child and Adolescent Psychiatry, 30,* 388–392.

Kusche, C. A., Cook, E. T., & Greenberg, M. T. (1993). Neuropsychological and cognitive functioning in children with anxiety, externalizing, and comorbid psychopathology. *Journal of Clinical Child Psychology, 22,* 172–195.

Lachar, D. (1990). Objective assessment of child and adolescent personality: The Personality Inventory for Children. In C. Reynolds & R.W. Kamphaus (Eds.), *Handbook of psychological and educational assessment of children: Personality, behavior, & context* (pp. 298–323). Boston: Allyn & Bacon.

Levine, M. (1993). *Developmental variation and learning disorders.* Cambridge, MA: Educators Publishing Service.

Levine, M. (1994). *Educational care: A system for understanding and helping children with learning problems at home and in school.* Cambridge, MA: Educators Publishing Service.

Lewis, M., & Miller, S. M. (1990). *Handbook of developmental psychology.* New York: Plenum Press.

Linz, T., Hooper, S. R., Hynd, G. W., Isaac, W., & Gibson, D. (1990). Frontal lobe functioning in conduct disordered juveniles: Preliminary findings. *Archives of Neuropsychology, 5,* 411–416.

Lou, H. C., Henriksen, L., & Bruhn, P. (1984). Focal cerebral hypoperfusion in children with dysphasia and/or attentional deficit disorder. *Archives of Neurology, 41,* 825–829.

Luria, A. R. (1973). *The working brain.* New York: Basic Books.

Marlowe, W. (1992). The impact of a right prefrontal lesion on the developing brain. *Brain and Cognition, 20,* 205–213.

Martin, R. P. (1988). *Personality and behavior assessment.* New York: Guilford Press.

Mateer, C. A., & Williams, D. (1991). Effects of frontal lobe injury in childhood. *Developmental Neuropsychology, 7,* 359–379.

Merrell, K. W. (1994). *Assessment of behavioral, social, and emotional problems: Direct and objective methods for use with children and adolescents.* New York: Langman.

Milich, R., & Landau, S. (1989). The role of social status variables in differentiating subgroups of hyperactive children. In L. M. Bloomingdale & J. Swanson (Eds.), *Attention deficit disorder: Current concepts and emerging trends in attentional and behavioral disorders of childhood* (Vol. 5, pp. 1–16). Elmsford, NY: Pergamon Press.

Moffitt, T. E. (1992, April). *The neuropsychology of conduct disorder.* Paper presented at the NIMH workshop on Conduct Disorders, Washington, DC.

Moffitt, T. E., & Henry, B. (1989). Neuropsychological assessment of executive functions in self-reported delinquents. *Development and Psychopathology, 1,* 105–118.

Moffitt, T. E., & Silva, P. A. (1988). IQ and delinquency: A direct test of the differential detection hypothesis. *Journal of Abnormal Psychology, 97,* 330–333.

Naglieri, J. A., LeBuffe, P. A., & Pfeiffer, S. I. (1993). *Devereux Behavior Rating Scales-School Form.* New York: The Psychological Corporation.

Naglieri, J. A., LeBuffe, P. A., & Pfeiffer, S. I. (1994). *Devereux Scales of Mental Disorders.* New York: The Psychological Corporation.

Neeper, R., Lahey, B. B., & Frick, P. J. (1990). *Comprehensive behavior rating scale for children.* New York: The Psychological Corporation.

Nieves, N. (1991). Childhood psychopathology and learning disabilities: Neuropsychological relationships. In J. E. Obrzut & G. W. Hynd (Eds.), *Neuropsychologcial foundations of learning disabilities* (pp. 113–146). San Diego: Academic Press.

Passler, M., Isaac, W., & Hynd, G. W. (1985). Neuropsychological behavior attributed to frontal lobe functioning in children. *Developmental Neuropsychology, 1,* 349–370.

Pennington, B. F. (1991). *Diagnosing learning disorders.* New York: Guilford Press.

Pianta, R. C., & Caldwell, C. B. (1990). Stability of externalizing symptoms from kindergarten to first grade and factors related to instability. *Development and Psychopathology, 2.*

Prigatano, G. P. (1992). Personality disturbances associated with traumatic brain injury. *Journal of Consulting and Clinical Psychology, 60,* 360–368.

Quay, H. C., Peterson, D. R., Radke-Yarrow, M., Cummings, E., Kuczynski, L., & Chapman, M. (1985). Patterns of attachment in two- and three-year-olds in normal families and families with parental depression. *Child Development, 56,* 884–893.

Reitan, R. M., & Davison, L. (1974). *Clinical neuropsychology: Current status and applications.* New York: Wiley.

Reitan, R. M., & Wolfson, D. (1985). *Neuroanatomy and neuro-pathology: A clinical guide for neuropsychologists.* Tucson, AZ: Neuropsychology Press.

Reitan, R. M., & Wolfson, D. (1995). Category test and trail-making test as measures of frontal lobe functions. *Clinical Neuropsychologist, 9,* 50–56.

Reynolds, C. R., & Kamphaus, R. W. (1992). *Behavior Assessment System for Children (BASC).* Circle Pines, MN: AGS.

Riccio, C. R. (1995). Review of the Devereux Scales of Mental Disorders. *Child Assessment News, 5,* 4.

Sandoval, J., & Echandia, A. (1994). Behavior assessment system for children. *Journal of School Psychology, 32*(4), 419–425.

Schaffner, D., Bijur, P., Chadwick, O., & Rutter, M. (1980). Head injury and later reading disability. *Journal of the American Academy of Child Psychiatry, 19,* 592–610.

Semrud-Clikeman, M. (1995). *Child and adolescent therapy.* Boston: Allyn & Bacon.

Semrud-Clikeman, M., & Hynd, G. W. (1990). Right hemispheric dysfunction in nonverbal learning disabilities: Social, academic, and adaptive functioning in adults and children. *Psychological Bulletin, 107,* 196–209.

Semrud-Clikeman, M., & Hynd, G. W. (1991). Assessment of depression. *International Journal of School Psychology, 12,* 275–298.

Semrud-Clikeman, M., Hynd, G. W., Lorys, A. R., & Lahey, B. B. (1993). Differential diagnosis of children with ADD/H and ADD/with co-occurring conduct disorder: Discriminant validity of neurocognitive measures. *School Psychology International, 14,* 361–370.

Semrud-Clikeman, M., Hynd, G. W., Novey, E. S., & Eliopulos, D. (1991). Dyslexia and brain morphology: Relationships between neuroanatomical variation and neurolinguistic tasks. *Learning and Individual Differences, 3,* 225–242.

Shaffer, D., Schoenfeld, I., O'Conner, P. A., Stokman, C., Trautman, P., Shafer, S., & Ng, S. (1985). Neurological soft signs. *Archives of General Psychiatry, 42,* 342–351.

Spivack, G., & Spotts, J. (1966). *Devereux child behavior rating scale.* Devon, PA: The Devereux Foundation.

Spivack, G., Spotts, J., & Haimes, P. E. (1967). *Devereux adolescent behavior rating scale.* Devon, PA: The Devereux Foundation.

Stanovich, K. E. (1993). The construct validity of discrepancy definitions of reading disability. In G. R. Lyon, D. B. Gray, J. F. Kavanagh, & N. A. Krasnegor (Eds.), *Better understanding learning disabilities: New views from research and their implications for education and public policies* (pp. 273–308). Baltimore: Paul H. Brookes.

Strauss, C. S. (1991). Anxiety disorders of childhood and adolescence. *School Psychology Review, 19,* 142–157.

Stuss, D. (1992). Biological and psychological development of executive functions. *Brain and Cognition, 20,* 8–23.

Stuss, D., & Benson, F. (1984). *The frontal lobes.* New York: Raven Press.

Swanson, H. L. (1982). A multidimensional model for assessing learning-disabled student's intelligence: An information-processing framework. *Learning Disabilities Quarterly, 5,* 312–326.

Swanson, H. L. (1993). Learning disabilities from the perspective of cognitive psychology. In G. R. Lyon, D. B. Gray, J. F. Kavanagh, & N. A. Krasnegor (Eds.), *Better understanding learning disabilities: New views from research and their implications for education and public policies* (pp. 199–228). Baltimore: Paul H. Brookes.

Teeter, P. A. (1986). Standard neuropsychological batteries for children. In J. Obrzut & G. W. Hynd (Eds.), *Child neuropsychology: Clinical practice* (Vol. 2, pp. 187–228). New York: Academic Press.

Teeter, P. A. (1989). Childhood depression: A contrast in neuropsychological profiles. *Archives of Clinical Neuropsychology, 4,* 115.

Teeter, P. A. (in press). *Interventions for children and adolescents with attention deficit hyperactivity disorders.* New York: Guilford Press.

Teeter, P. A., & Semrud-Clikeman, M. (1995). Integrating neurobiological, psychosocial, and behavioral paradigms: A transactional model for the study of ADHD. *Archives of Clinical Neuropsychology, 10,* 433–461.

Teeter, P. A., & Semrud-Clikeman, M. (1996). *Child clinical neuropsychology: Assessment and interventions for neuropsychiatric and neurodevelopmental disorders for childhood.* Boston: Allyn & Bacon.

Teeter, P. A., & Smith, P. L. (1993). WISC-III and WJ-R: Predictive and discriminant validity for students with severe emotional disturbance. *Journal of Psychoeducational Assessment, WISC-III Monograph,* 113–124.

Tems, C. L., Stewart, S., Skinner, J. R., & Hughes, C. W. (1993). Cognitive distortions in depressed children and adolescents: Are they state dependent? *Journal of Clinical Child Psychology, 23,* 316–326.

Thatcher, R. W. (1992). Cyclic cortical reorganization during early childhood. *Brain and Cognition, 20,* 24–50.

Tramontana, M. G., & Hooper, S. R. (1989). Neuropsychology of child psychopathology. In C. R. Reynolds & E. Fletcher-Janzen (Eds.), *Handbook of clinical child neuropsychology* (pp. 87–106). New York: Plenum Press.

Tramontana, M. G., Sherrets, S. D., & Golden, C. J. (1980). Brain dysfunction in youngsters with psychiatric disorders: Application of Selz–Reitan rules for neuropsychological diagnosis. *Clinical Neuropsychology, 2,* 118–123.

Tranel, D. (1992). Functional neuroanatomy: Neuropsychological correlates of cortical and subcortical damage. In S. C. Yudofsky & R. E. Hales (Eds.), *Textbook of neuropsychiatry* (pp. 57–88). Washington, DC: American Psychiatric Press.

Tremblay, R. E., Masse, B., Perron, D., & Leblanc, M. (1992). Early disruptive behavior, poor school achievement, delinquent behavior, and delinquent personality: Longitudinal analyses. *Journal of Consulting & Clinical Psychology, 60,* 64–72.

Wechsler, D. (1974). *Manual for the Wechsler Intelligence Scale for Children-Revised.* New York: The Psychological Corporation.

Welsh, M. C., Pennington, B. F., & Groisser, D. B. (1991). A normative-developmental study of executive function: A window of prefrontal function in children. *Developmental Neuropsychology, 7,* 131–149.

White, J. L., Moffitt, T. E., & Silva, P. A. (1989). A prospective replication of the protective efforts of IQ in subjects at high risk for juvenile delinquency. *Journal of Consulting and Clinical Psychology, 57,* 719–724.

Wirt, R. D., Lachar, D., Klinedinst, J. K., & Seat, P. S. (1990). *Personality Inventory for Children—1990 edition.* Los Angeles: Western Psychological Services.

Witt, J. C., Heffer, R. W., & Pfeiffer, J. (1990). Structured rating scales: A review of self-report and informant rating processes, procedures, and issues. In C. R. Reynolds & R. W. Kamphaus (Eds.), *Handbook of psychological and educational assessment of children: Personality, behavior and context* (pp. 364–394). New York: Guilford Press.

Woods, B. T. (1980). The restricted effects of right-hemisphere lesions after age one: Wechsler test data. *Neuropsychologia, 18,* 65–70.

Woo-Sam, J., Zimmerman, I. L., Brink, J. A., Uyehara, K., & Miller, A. R. (1970). Socioeconomic status and post-traumatic intelligence in children with severe head injuries. *Psychological Reports, 27,* 147–153.

Yeudall, L., Fromm-Auch, D., & Davies, P. (1982). Neuropsychological impairment in persistent delinquency. *Journal of Nervous and Mental Disease, 170,* 257–265.

Yeudofsky, S. C., & Hales, R. E. (1989). When patients ask . . . What is neuropsychiatry? *Journal of Neuropsychiatry & Clinical Neurosciences, 1,* 362–365.

Zametkin, M. D., Nordahl, T. E., Gross, M., King, A. C., Semple, W. E., Rumsey, J., Hamburger, S., & Cohen, R. M. (1990). Cerebral glucose metabolism in adults with hyperactivity of childhood onset. *New England Journal of Medicine, 323,* 1361–1366.

17

Neuroimaging in Pediatric Neuropsychology

ERIN D. BIGLER, DAVID E. NILSSON, ROBERT B. BURR, AND
RICHARD S. BOYER

Of all of the advances in clinical neuroscience, the advent of brain imaging represents one of the most significant, particularly for assessment of pediatric neurologic disorders. Prior to brain imaging, only inferences of structural brain integrity could be made from behavior, development, and standard physical neurologic examinations of the child. These measures continue to be important in the diagnostic process, but now the brain can be viewed *in vivo*. This chapter will overview some major categories where brain imaging provides critical information relative to brain structure and function in pediatric neuropsychology. First is a basic review of some underlying assumptions in pediatric neuroimaging, followed by an overview of some major childhood categories wherein neuroimaging provides useful diagnostic information that can be integrated with neuropsychological assessment and/or consultation. We feel that it is critical for neuropsychologists to have more familiarity with neuroimaging procedures and interpretation in the assessment, development of treatment strategies, and clinical feedback involving parents, school, and

other healthcare professionals. For more detailed exposition of pediatric neuroimaging *per se,* the reader is referred to Barkovich (1995), Osborn and Boyer (1994) and Wolpert and Barnes (1992).

Basic Assumptions

Basic anatomy as revealed by magnetic resonance (MR) imaging or computerized tomography (CT) is influenced by the age of the child. The brain of the neonate, while having a full complement of neurons and basic structural organization, lacks specific development, particularly in myelination. Thus, the distinct boundaries normally seen between white and gray matter in the mature brain take time to develop (see Figure 1). What may be normal at one stage may be abnormal at a later stage, if proper development does not occur.

Another basic assumption is that the pathologies that afflict the infant and child brain typically are not the same as those observed in adult disorders. For example, the age-related dementias of adulthood (e.g., Alzheimer's disease) develop after a lengthy "normal" stage of maturity, whereas degenerative diseases of childhood develop in a brain that may be "normal" only for a short period of time (e.g., adrenoleukodystrophy, see Figure 2) or never normal (e.g., Rett syndrome). In the latter case, whatever development occurs does so only in the context of degenerative changes. A case of childhood degenerative disorder is presented in Figure 2.

ERIN D. BIGLER • Department of Psychology, Brigham Young University, Provo, Utah 84602; and LDS Hospital, Salt Lake City, Utah 84143.   DAVID E. NILSSON • Neurology, Learning and Behavior Center, Salt Lake City, Utah 84102; and Primary Children's Medical Center, Provo, Utah 84113.
ROBERT B. BURR • Neurology, Learning and Behavior Center, and Department of Neurosurgery, University of Utah Medical Center, Salt Lake City, Utah 84102.   RICHARD S. BOYER • Department of Medical Imaging, Primary Children's Medical Center, Salt Lake City, Utah 84113.

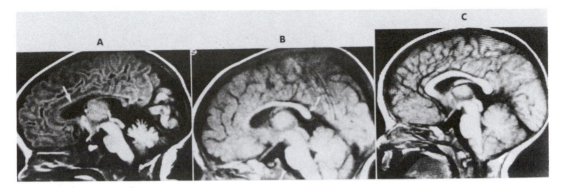

FIGURE 1. Myelination of the brain as depicted by changes in MR white matter signal intensity in the developing brain at (A) 21 days, (B) 4 months, and (C) 9 months. For brain myelination, the corpus callosum is the prototype structure to view, particularly in the midsagittal plane, because it is so readily differentiated from the surface of the cingulate gyrus, a gray matter structure. As depicted in A, initially the corpus callosum (arrow) is not well myelinated and therefore no distinct signal difference exists between white and gray matter. As myelination proceeds, signal intensity differences become evident (B), particularly at the level of the splenium, which has begun to thicken (curved arrow). By 9 months (C), myelination is distinct with clear differentiation of the corpus callosum from cingulate cortex. Although rapid changes in myelination occur during the first years of life, myelination continues into adolescence (see Jernigan & Tallal, 1990). (Adapted from Wolpert & Barnes, 1992.)

Another basic tenet is that there are a host of genetic and brain maldevelopment syndromes, often expressed *in utero,* that result in malformed brains. As with the congenital degenerative disorders, these children begin life with an abnormal brain. In contrast to fatal degenerative diseases of childhood, children who survive with developmental errors of brain structure have subsequent development regulated by a statically damaged brain. As such, development may be abnormal to varying degrees, depending on the characteristics of the neurologic compromise and genetic endowment of the individual child. A prototype of this is congenital hydrocephalus (see Figure 3). The child shown was born with hydrocephalus. Although he was shunted, massive hydrocephalus was present. Nonetheless, he did acquire language skills and upper extremity coordinated movement. As of this writing, he is not ambulatory and displays a host of neurodevelopmental sequelae.

An extension of this tenet applies to any acquired neurologic injury that occurs in childhood. When such an injury occurs in adulthood, the injury is superimposed on an already fully mature brain. However, in pediatric brain injury, the injury is superimposed on a developing nervous system. Such injury typically imposes, at a minimum, a developmental arrest at the time of injury, often accompanied by a loss in level of function before "recovery" proceeds. Thus, "recovery" proceeds at a pace where already acquired developmental stages again have to be attained and built upon. In the recovery process, even when the child attains a previous level of function, all future function acquired and developmental progression is superimposed on a damaged/dysfunctional brain, which probably alters capacity and scope of recovery. When the brain of a child is damaged, there is usually a shift in the progression of development that is reflected either in delay or an absence in acquisition of that developmental skill. In some situations, the earlier the injury occurs, the greater is the disruption. In summary, when a childhood brain injury occurs in an otherwise normal brain, there is typically some arrest of development and from that point on, what may be "normal" development proceeds within the context of a damaged brain.

The intent of this chapter is to overview the general field of neuroimaging in pediatric neuropsychology and how neuroimaging findings relate to neuropsychological findings. The major clinical syndromes of cerebral trauma, vascular disease, neoplastic disease, congenital abnormalities, and developmental disorders will be reviewed. A host of profound congenital abnormalities and degenerative diseases exist, but will not be reviewed here because these children typically are so severely impaired or rarely live beyond infancy, that they are infrequently seen by a neuropsychologist.

Types of Brain Imaging

The two most common methods for brain imaging are CT and MR imaging. Both forms of

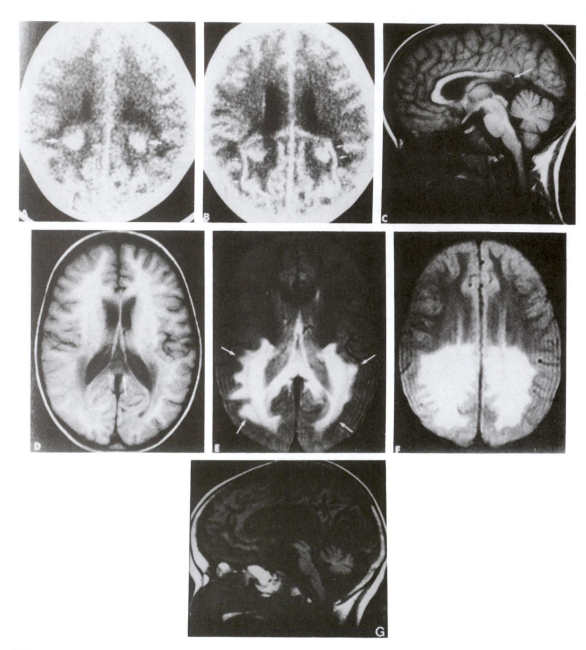

FIGURE 2. (A) Nonenhanced CT scan indicating low-density areas bilaterally in the periatrial white matter with central high-density areas (arrows) in a 5-year-old male with adrenoleukodystrophy. (B) Contrast-enhanced CT at approximately the same level demonstrating enhancement of the margins of the low-density areas (arrows). (C, D) T1-weighted sagittal and axial scans of a different 6-year-old male demonstrating areas of low signal intensity in the splenium of the corpus callosum (arrows) with axial T2-weighted images (E, F) displaying areas of high signal intensity in the white matter bilaterally. These images were adapted from Wolpert and Barnes (1992). A comment should be made about the differences in nomenclature between interpreting CT and MR images. In CT the image is based on a density measure related to the passage of an "X-ray" beam. "Dark" means less dense, "light" means more dense. Thus, the convention in CT imaging is to have bone depicted as white and CSF as black. Intermediate on this gray scale is brain parenchyma, which will be dark gray for white matter and light gray for gray matter. Because white matter is generated by myelinated fibers and myelinated fibers have high water content, white matter structures are less dense than gray; hence, in CT imaging the lighter shade of gray. MR imaging is based on an entirely different principle, namely, that molecules spin with a particular orientation. If a radio frequency wave is passed through the brain, nuclei emit characteristic radio waves that can be detected. Different molecules emit energy at different frequencies and this can be influenced by the parameters of the magnetic field and how it is pulsed. By utilizing sophisticated computer programs, images of the brain can be generated by detecting the different radio frequencies emanating from different tissues. Thus, in MR imaging the nomenclature uses the concept of "signal intensity" for the particular weighting of the image. In E and F the bright signal of the posterior regions

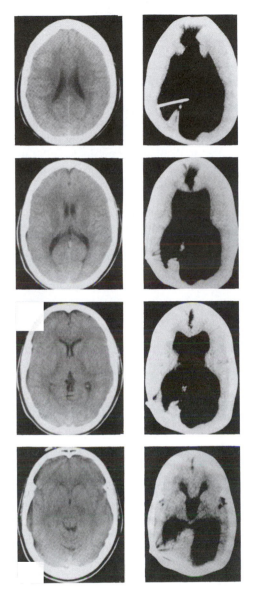

brain imaging are commonly used in pediatric neuroimaging. Although an older technology than MR imaging, advances in computer technology have resulted in excellent gross brain imaging with CT. Accordingly, CT imaging continues to be extensively used and, in some situations, preferred over MR imaging. For example, CT imaging can be accomplished very quickly and in some situations not as influenced by movement artifact as MR, which can be a particular problem with children. CT imaging is excellent in detecting bone abnormalities and fractures and can be used in the presence of most life support devices. It is likewise sensitive enough to detect acute hemorrhagic lesions. However, CT imaging simply does not provide the image detail that can be achieved by MR. For viewing gross brain pathology, such as that depicted in Figure 3 (i.e., hydrocephalus), CT is quite adequate. But as can be seen in Figure 4, which compares CT with MR in a case of a ruptured congenital aneurysm, it is obvious that MR imaging provides a more refined assessment of brain anatomy than CT.

Visual display from CT and MR is displayed on a gray scale. For CT imaging bone is represented as white, CSF as dark, and gray and white matter as intermediate with gray matter being lighter because of greater density than white, which is represented as dark gray.

Unlike CT imaging, which is based on tissue density, MR imaging is based on the physical characteristics of atomic nuclei. By capitalizing on the predictable nature of atomic nuclei in a magnetic field and applying a short-wave radio frequency (RF) pulse to produce a resonance signal that can be quantified and computerized, various tissues can be differentiated. This process is particularly sensitive to water content in tissue, hence the ability to readily differentiate brain from bone, CSF from brain, and white from gray matter, as each has characteristic properties of water that distinguish it from all other tissues. Such distinctions also aid in clinical differentiation of pathological conditions. For example, T1-weighted MR images depict fat or subacute hemorrhage as bright or white and black represents CSF. On T2-weighted images, fat ap-

FIGURE 3. (Right) Hydrocephalus in a 5-year-old depicted by CT imaging and (left) normal scans at similar levels. Note the massive expansion of the ventricular system.

of the brain reflects greater water content. Thus, even though the abnormality is discussed in terms of a "bright" signal or increased "signal intensity," in the case of adrenoleukodystrophy, the abnormality is really an indication of degenerative changes in the tissue. The other important feature of this figure is that the anterior aspects of brain development in these individuals appear to be normal. The degenerative changes associated with adrenoleukodystrophy typically develop in a brain that initially shows normal development. In contrast, the sagittal view of the brain presented in G depicts whole brain degeneration in a 6-year-old female with GM$_1$ gangliosidosis. Note the widening of all cerebral and cerebellar sulci and shrunken appearance of the brain stem.

pears gray, iron black, and CSF white. A proton density-weighted image enhances the distinction between gray and white matter. These different types of weightings and their utility in distinguishing various aspects of brain anatomy are represented in Figure 4.

Single photon emission computed tomography (SPECT) imaging is another procedure that may be performed with children (see Figure 5). SPECT imaging provides a means by which uptake of a radiolabeled substance is measured which provides an index of metabolic function through the distribution of regional cerebral blood flow at the time of injection. Both CT and MR primarily present information that reveals brain anatomy and structure, without much information about function. In contrast, SPECT imaging provides some information about metabolic integrity of the brain. For example, the child in Figure 6 sustained a significant crush injury to the head when he fell and was run over by a vehicle. He sustained massive skull and facial bone fractures and neuropsychologically displayed persistent problems in the domain of learning and memory. MR imaging demonstrated right temporal horn dilation, which can be a sign of trauma-induced temporal lobe atrophy. However, the surrounding tissue of the temporal horn appears "normal," without particular evidence of a "lesion." To assist in neurodiagnostic differentiation, SPECT imaging was performed, which revealed abnormal metabolic uptake (i.e., hypoperfusion) in the right temporal lobe region. This case demonstrates the confluence of two imaging methods with neuropsychological information that coalesce to form a rather straightforward conclusion: this child's right temporal lobe was significantly compromised by this injury. Further details of traumatic injury to the brain will be provided below.

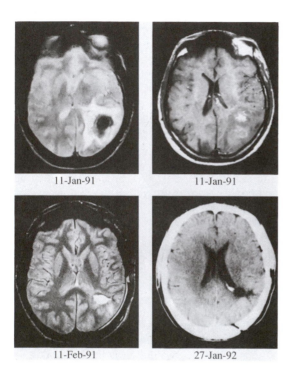

11-Jan-91   11-Jan-91

11-Feb-91   27-Jan-92

FIGURE 4. Rupture of a congenital aneurysm in the left temporal-parietal region as displayed with different MR weightings at different times in comparison with CT. (Upper left) Axial T2-weighted image showing focal area of hemorrhage (black, circular structure) surrounded by edema (white). (Upper right) T1-weighted image at a slightly higher level in the brain depicting midline shift of the ventricular system, which can also be observed in the T2-weighted image. Note the T1 image highlights the ventricle but the hemorrhage and surrounding edema are not as readily differentiated. (Lower left) Mixed-weighted MR scan depicting bright signal in the posterior periatrial white matter of the left hemisphere. Clinically, at this time postrecovery the patient has a prominent dyslexia and dyscalculia. The parameters of this lesion have remained quite identical to those depicted here, as the patient has been imaged several times since the 1991 cerebrovascular accident. (Lower right) CT scan performed almost 1 year postinjury. In addition to permanent changes in reading and mathematical ability, this patient developed epilepsy. Note the slight asymmetry of the ventricular system with posterior extension into the region of encephalomalacia where tissue has infarcted.

Clinical Syndromes

There are a variety of major childhood clinical syndromes where neuroimaging studies are routinely performed on the child, who will ultimately benefit from neuropsychological consultation and/or testing. For the purposes of this overview, four of the most common syndromes are presented: cerebral trauma, cerebrovascular disease, neoplastic disease, and developmental abnormalities. For more exhaustive treatises on pediatric neuroimaging and the multitude of clinical syndromes possible, the reader is referred to Greenberg (1995), Grossman and Yousem (1994), Kucharczyk, Moseley, and Barkovich (1994), Osborn (1994), and Wolpert and Barnes (1992). For each clinical syndrome presented below, case studies will be presented that provide additional information on the integration of neuroimaging and neuropsychological findings in formulating

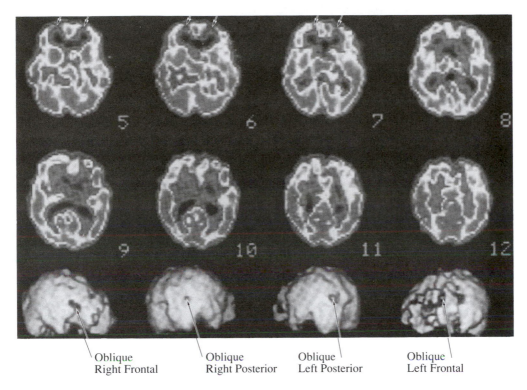

Oblique   Oblique   Oblique   Oblique
Right Frontal   Right Posterior   Left Posterior   Left Frontal

FIGURE 5. SPECT imaging of TBI. This patient sustained a closed head injury in a motor vehicle accident. MR imaging demonstrated no significant structural abnormality. However, neuropsychological studies demonstrated changes in level of executive function and personality/temper changes. Such neurobehavioral findings can be associated with damage/dysregulation at the level of the frontal lobes (see Bigler, 1988). SPECT imaging was recommended to more thoroughly explore this problem. As might be predicted by the neuropsychological studies, SPECT imaging demonstrated perfusion abnormalities in the frontal region of the brain (see arrows). In SPECT imaging, since cortical cell bodies are located on the brain surface, at rest it is expected that cortical gray will display a uniform activation pattern, with no gaps or abnormal regions of high or low uptake. Here, eight axial images (5–12) taken at different levels are presented which depict uneven and/or absent cortical perfusion in the left frontal region of the brain (see arrows). The row of three-dimensional images at the bottom demonstrates generally "smooth" areas which represent uniform regions of cerebral activation in the lateral and posterior regions of the brain, In contrast, in the frontal region, particularly in the left frontal area, the activation pattern is very irregular, demonstrating perfusion abnormalities.

diagnoses, outlining treatment, and prognosticating about outcome.

Cerebral Trauma

Over the past several decades, pediatric head injury has remained one of the top causes of mortality and morbidity in children (Goldstein & Levin, 1990). Cerebral trauma may result in focal lesions, such as contusions, or more generalized injury, such as diffuse axonal injury (DAI) or shearing (Bigler, 1990). Since DAI, by definition, likely damages white matter (i.e., axonal level) disproportionately to gray, this represents a particularly adverse consequence for children, since they have incomplete myelination. In a variety of studies with adult TBI victims, it has been demonstrated that significant white matter changes occur following head injury (see Figure 7; Anderson & Bigler, 1995a,b; Bigler et al., 1994; Gale, Burr, Bigler, & Blatter, 1993; Gale, Johnson, Bigler, & Blatter, 1994, 1995a,b; Johnson, Bigler, Burr, & Blatter, 1994). In these studies it has been demonstrated that white matter changes are often accurately reflected in ventricular change, particularly evidenced by ventricular expansion and corpus callosum atrophy (see Figure 7).

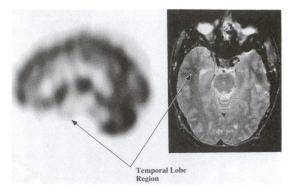

FIGURE 6. MR imaging demonstrating temporal horn dilation in the right temporal lobe and reduced perfusion in the region of the right temporal lobe in this adolescent male with a history of TBI. Such findings suggest localized area of damage/dysfunction in response to trauma.

An example of trauma-induced disrupted white matter development in a child is presented in Figures 8 and 9. This injury occurred in a 6-week-old, restrained infant riding in the back seat of his parent's vehicle that at excessive speed (both vehicles > 55 mph) collided head-on with another vehicle. According to witnesses at the scene, the infant did not appear to have lost consciousness, but did display diminished responsiveness. At the emergency room the child was described as lethargic, with possible bulging fontanel (possible brain edema), but the examination results were otherwise normal. He was hospitalized and observed for approximately 36 hours. Out of parental concern, a CT scan was performed several days postinjury, the results of which were interpreted as "normal." Subsequent to the injury, the child displayed developmental delays, particularly in aspects of motor skills acquisition, along with hyperactivity and short attention span. Because of these developmental delay problems, follow-up MR imaging was obtained, which demonstrated ventricular dilation and corpus callosum thinning. The presumption in this child's MR imaging studies, when compared with the CT findings shortly after injury, was that this child likely sustained DAI caused by shear/strain action from the abrupt cessation of movement. DAI subsequently resulted in a disruption of the normal myelination process postinjury. The ultimate expression of this injury was in the form of significant white matter volume decrease with corresponding ventricular volume increase as depicted in Figures 8 and 9.

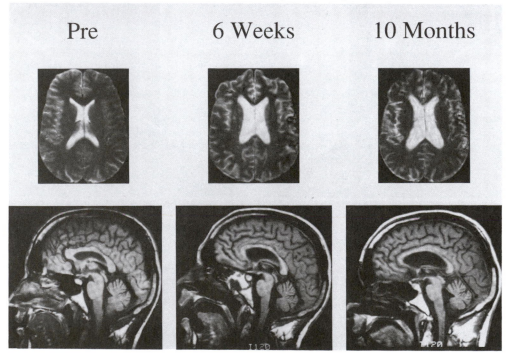

FIGURE 7. Series of MR scans depicting ventricular dilation postinjury (middle and right frames) in a patient for whom a preinjury MR scan (left) had been obtained. Note also the thinning of the corpus callosum. Ventricular expansion posttrauma is considered to be related to trauma-induced white matter degeneration.

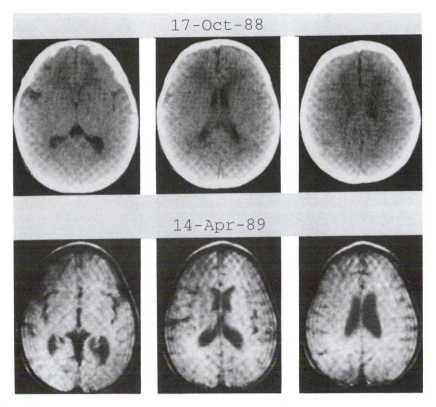

17-Oct-88

14-Apr-89

FIGURE 8. (Top) CT imaging several days post-closed head injury in a 6-week-old male. The CT scan was interpreted as being within normal limits, although aspects of the ventricular system were considered to be generous in size. Note the lack of distinct differentiation between white and gray matter structures, which is normal for this age. (Bottom) MR imaging performed approximately 6 months postinjury, indicating expansion of the ventricular system. Image quality is limited because of motion artifact, a common problem with infants and children. See Figure 9.

Another example of DAI is provided in Figure 10. This case demonstrates the utility of using the day-of-injury (DOI) scan for comparison of trauma-induced structural changes in brain morphology. This child sustained a significant closed head injury with loss of consciousness. DOI imaging demonstrates nonspecific edema and a small hemorrhagic lesion just lateral to the right lateral ventricle in the apex of the internal capsule. Imaging 3 weeks later demonstrates increased ventricular size and a density change in the region where the acute hemorrhagic lesion occurred. In studies examining the ventricle-to-brain ratio (VBR), a measure of ventricular volume divided by brain volume, a normal ratio typically is 1.5 with a standard deviation of 0.5. In this child, the DOI VBR was 0.56, nearly two standard deviations below normal (see Bigler, Johnson, Jackson, & Blatter, 1995; Blatter *et al.*, 1995), a reflection of the severity of the acute edema. Three weeks postinjury, VBR is recorded at 3.67, over three standard deviations from normal. This type of ventricular expansion is considered to be a form of hydrocephalus *ex vacuo,* ventricular expansion that occurs as parenchymal wasting develops (see Blatter *et al.,* 1997). Also, note greater prominence of the interhemispheric fissure and cortical sulci, which likely would not be present if this were an active outward-expanding hydrocephalus (compare with Figure 3). Thus, the ventricular dilation related to DAI occurs "passively" in response to the loss of brain parenchyma. In Figure 10 the DOI and follow-up scans were CT. Typically the DOI scan is CT, but follow-up scans are most often MR imaging. Even though they are different imaging modalities, DOI CT scanning can be compared with follow-up MR scans as depicted in Figure 11. A number of studies have demonstrated a relationship between trauma- induced ventricular expansion and neuropsychological outcome. These studies essentially demonstrate that increased ventricular size

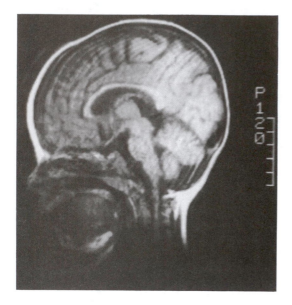

FIGURE 9. Sagittal MR of the same patient seen in Figure 8. Note the thinning of the corpus callosum.

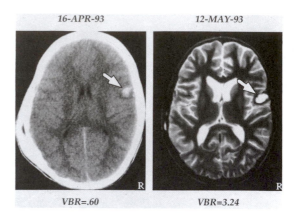

VBR=.60   VBR=3.24

FIGURE 11. CT imaging in cerebral trauma in a child. (Left) Axial CT scan obtained on the day of injury (DOI) demonstrating generalized cerebral edema and an acute hemorrhagic cortical contusion. (Right) Comparison MR scan obtained approximately 3½ weeks postinjury. Note the prominence of the ventricular system on the MR scan. VBR comparisons are presented below each scan. See Bowen *et al.* (1997).

is associated with more severe brain injury and worse neuropsychological outcome (see Gale *et al.,* 1995a,b).

Cerebrovascular Disease

Anderson, Wolpert, and Kayle (1992) outline four major types of vascular disease in children: (1) arteritis and arteriopathies, (2) infarction, (3) vascular malformations and aneurysms, and (4) angiodysplasias. As with adult vascular disorders, the key feature in vascular disease with children is the relationship of the vascular territory affected and neuropsychological outcome. For example, in Figure 12 a large cystic formation has developed in the region of the middle cerebral artery where a large infarction developed. The nature of the infarction was idiopathic. The child was first noted not to be moving the right upper extremity and at about 15 months other motor skills were delayed. At this age the child was scanned, with the results depicted in Figure 12. At age 3 when last seen clinically, this child displayed prominent right-side hemiplegia (upper extremity more affected than the lower) and delayed language. This scan depicts many classic abnormalities observed with vascular lesions. Note the overall asymmetry of the head, with the left side of the skull smaller than the corresponding unaffected right side. Early in brain/cranial development, skull development is stimulated by the developing, expanding

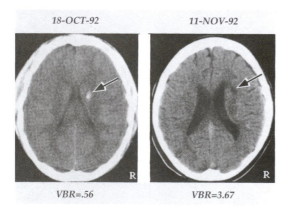

VBR=.56   VBR=3.67

FIGURE 10. CT imaging in cerebral trauma in a child. (Left) Axial CT scan obtained on the day of injury (DOI) demonstrating generalized cerebral edema and hemorrhagic lesion in the superior aspect of the internal capsule just lateral to the head of the caudate nucleus. Cerebral edema is manifested by indistinct boundaries between gray and white matter and compression of the lateral ventricles. (Right) Axial CT imaging at approximately the same level as on the DOI scan obtained 3 weeks postinjury. Follow-up imaging demonstrates ventricular enlargement, more prominent cortical sulci, and residual density change in the position of the DOI hemorrhagic lesion. Expansion of the ventricle is the typical response of the atrophic process following trauma. Comparison VBR values are presented below each scan. See text for discussion of the significance of the VBR values. See Bowen *et al.* (1997).

A

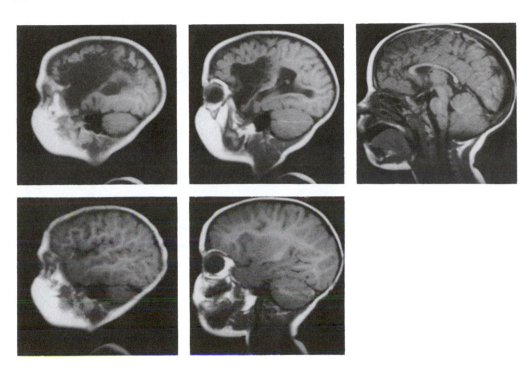

FIGURE 12. MR studies from a 3-year-old with mild right-side hemiplegia but normal language development. Note the large cystic formation (porencephaly) of the lesion in the left hemisphere that follows the distribution of the left middle cerebral artery. (A) Sagittal, (B) coronal, and (C) axial views are presented.

brain. In response to the expanding brain, skull size develops in dynamic proportion to brain expansion. Accordingly, if a hemisphere does not grow normally, the ipsilateral skull will not expand normally. In some cases lateralized skull size differences may correspond to underlying failure of brain growth.

Another classic abnormality present in this brain is the marked asymmetry of the cerebral peduncle. Note the prominent atrophy of the left cerebral peduncle relative to the normal configuration of the right peduncle. This type of atrophy occurs when the influence of a distal site results in wasting of projection fibers; in this case the corticospinal tract projecting from ipsilateral motor cortex in the region of the left motor strip has been completely damaged. This results in a downstream atrophy of the corticospinal projection fibers that pass through the peduncle, resulting in peduncular atrophy. The same principle is at play in the atrophy of the left thalamus, except thalamic atrophy is related more to the retrograde loss of the sensory afferent because

those fibers no longer have a terminus in parietal cortex, thereby degenerating back to the thalamus with associated cell body loss. This case also demonstrates the principle of ventricular expansion that passively occurs as brain parenchyma wastes away. Note the marked asymmetry of the ventricular system wherein the right lateral ventricles are perfectly normal in contrast to the expanded left.

The clinical significance of these types of lesions in infants and children represents something of an enigma in pediatric neuropsychology. If such a substantial lesion were to occur in the left hemisphere of a mature brain, it would most likely result in a dense hemiplegia and aphasia. In contrast, when last examined this child demonstrated only a mild right-side hemiplegia and only a 3- to 6-month language delay. The reason why such lesions often do not have such a profound effect in children is related to plasticity factors that result in nontraditional language areas taking over function. Typically the type of plasticity exemplified by the

B

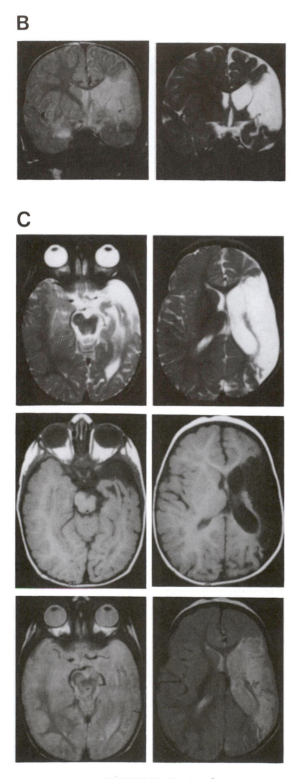

C

FIGURE 12. (*Continued*).

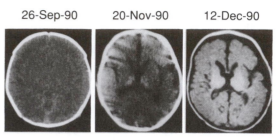

FIGURE 13. Anoxic brain injury. (Left) This neonate sustained a severe anoxic injury as a complication of a very traumatic birth and delivery. This scan, taken on the day of birth, exhibits extensive edema as the ventricular system cannot be identified nor any cortical sulcal patterns. With the passage of time, significant brain atrophy develops.

case in Figure 12 only occurs when the injury is unilateral and either *in utero* or early in life.

The case just presented in Figure 12 represents the classic picture of cerebral infarction. The case previously presented in Figure 4 depicts an initial hemorrhagic lesion with surrounding edema as a consequence of a ruptured aneurysm. Figure 4 also presents contrasting MR image acquisition weightings demonstrating the manner in which different tissues and pathologic states can be differentiated, using the MR technique. One important pathologic consequence to point out in the initial image sequence in Figure 4 is the midline shift and surrounding edema, a consequence related to hemorrhagic pressure effects. In this pathologic state, the pressure effects collapse the ventricle typically on the side of the lesion where the greatest hemispheric pressure effects occur. However, note that the follow-up CT scan done a year later demonstrates posterior ventricular asymmetry. The ventricle has expanded into the territory of the lesion as a passive increase in ventricle volume fills the void of brain tissue loss. The location of this hemorrhagic lesion (the aneurysm was most likely congenital) was in the posterior left temporoparietal region, which in this college educated young adult male was the dominant left hemisphere. The location of this lesion resulted in an acquired dyslexia and dyscalculia.

Since anoxic injury occurs either as a failure of vascular supply (e.g., ischemia) to a particular region or as a disruption in the level of oxygenated blood (e.g., secondary to carbon monoxide poisoning), anoxic injuries are often covered under the heading of vascular disorders. Figure 13 presents sequential scan data from a child who experienced significant anoxia at birth. In this case the anoxic injury was severe, re-

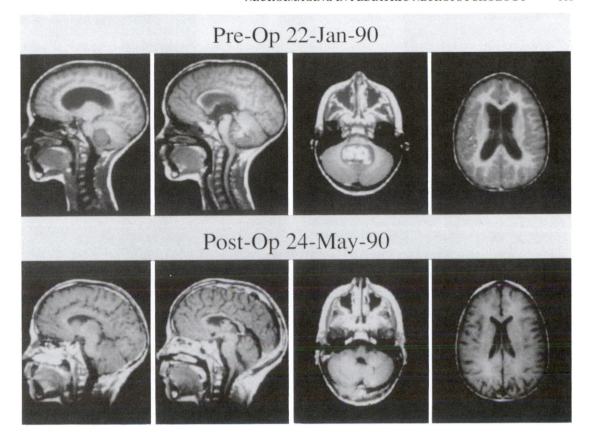

FIGURE 14. Pre and postoperative MR scans taken from a child with cerebellar tumor. (Top) Preoperatively, the location and size of the tumor have resulted in brain stem compression and an obstructive hydrocephalus, manifested by ventricular dilation. (Bottom) Postoperatively, MR imaging demonstrates excellent neurosurgical results with complete tumor resection and return to normal size of the ventricular system.

sulting in generalized brain atrophy. Typically, when atrophic changes are as prominent and disseminated as in this case, clinical outcome is poor. In this child, neuropsychological studies demonstrated generalized cognitive deficits, with intellectual levels in the moderate range of mental retardation and mild-moderate spastic quadriparesis. In the more mature brain, anoxic injury tends to have both nonspecific as well as specific effects (see Hopkins *et al.,* 1995). The nonspecific effects are often noted in terms of generalized atrophy of the brain, whereas the specific effects may be observed in subcortical degeneration, specifically the hippocampus and basal ganglia.

Neoplastic Disease

A host of neoplastic diseases may affect the child's brain. The neuropsychological relevance of a brain tumor is typically related to the type of tumor, location, secondary tumor effects (e.g.,

edema, vascular compromise), and any untoward effects from treatment (e.g., radiation necrosis). Typically, the child with a brain tumor is seen by a neuropsychologist after the diagnosis of tumor has already been made, and most often after surgical and radiation therapies have been implemented. Thus, in tumor cases the neuropsychologist typically will have extensive brain imaging studies and information before neuropsychological consultation and/or testing is initiated. Obviously, neuropsychological sequelae associated with brain tumors depend on a host of factors, particularly the stage of tumor development or treatment and the age of the child. For example, Figure 14 depicts a child with a large cerebellar tumor that has produced localized mass effect at the cerebellar level and an obstructive hydrocephalus. Postoperatively, MR imaging demonstrates excellent resolution of the hydrocephalus and complete surgical resection of the tumor mass.

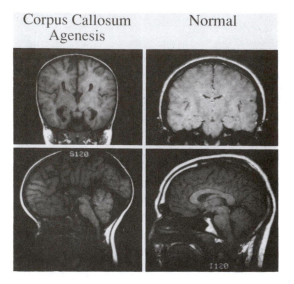

Corpus Callosum   Normal
Agenesis

FIGURE 15. (Left) Congenital agenesis of the corpus callosum and (right) normal callosal development. Note in both the coronal (top, left) and sagittal (bottom, left) views the complete absence of the corpus callosum.

Congenital and Developmental Abnormalities

The feat of cerebral embryogenesis is remarkable. The rapid growth of the fetal brain combined with the shear complexity of neuronal migration and integration represents many developmental stages wherein normal brain development may be disrupted. For example, as the cerebral cortex forms, commissural fibers interconnecting the evolving cerebral hemispheres also develop.

Disruption of this process can result in either a malformation of the corpus callosum or its absence. Such a case is presented in Figure 15, which depicts sagittal and coronal MR scan findings in a child with congenital callosal agenesis. Note in this case that the cerebral hemispheres appear to develop normally, but with complete absence of the corpus callosum. Interestingly, some children with callosal agenesis do not have clinically significant disconnection syndromes (see Bigler, 1988). These children reflect the effect of early brain plasticity that reroutes hemispheric integration through vertical integration (i.e., hemispheric information integrated vertically wherein information may ascend/descend and "cross over" at brain stem/cerebellar level and ascend/descend in the contralateral system by similar pathways) and intact noncallosal interhemispheric structures (e.g., anterior commissure).

Another common problem associated with maldevelopment of the brain occurs in hydrocephalus. A variety of developmental aberrations and acquired problems can result in hydrocephalus. Figure 3 displays CT data of a case of congenital hydrocephaly with considerable brain maldevelopment. In such cases, structural changes are generalized and affect all regions of the brain, but particularly cortical development.

Conclusions

Modern era neuroimaging has brought with it an opportunity to perform *in vivo* studies of pediatric neurologic disorders and utilize that information in the context of neuropsychological consultation and assessment (Bigler, 1991). However, the pediatric brain poses several major problems from the perspective of integrating neuroimaging information with clinical outcome (Bigler, 1995, 1996). Early lesions often are not predictive of outcome because of plasticity of nondamaged regions taking over function and individual differences. Thus, a particular lesion may appear impressive in its size and location by neuroimaging standards, but the immature brain "develops around" the lesion, such that the lesion no longer is predictive of outcome. Often such lesions occur very early *in utero* or early in life and are unilateral. In children who sustain lateralized injury to the brain after age 5 to 7, there is a greater likelihood that the more traditional relationships between brain and behavior will be observed. For example, had the infarction depicted in Figure 12 occurred in a 12-year-old rather than a neonate, it is likely that significant receptive language deficits would be present, which were not present in this child whose lesions likely developed *in utero*. Regardless of when the lesion occurs in development, other developmental consequences may not be appreciated until later stages in development.

Another concluding point is that bilateral and/or diffuse lesions typically have more significant impact on neurobehavioral function than do unilateral lesions. In traumatic brain injury, where the lesions often are nonspecific and diffuse, the size of the ventricular system is a good indicator of the severity of injury. Similarly, trauma-induced ventricular expansion is negatively correlated with neuropsychological outcome. Such relationships also exist with degenerative disorders. As atrophic responses occur in brain parenchyma, ventricular size increases to fill the void left by brain volume loss. Lastly, it needs to be stated that not all "brain damage" is going to be detected by contemporary neuroimaging methods. A host of pathological states exist beneath the threshold of current neuroimaging methods.

References

Anderson, C. V., & Bigler, E. D. (1995a). The role of caudate nucleus and corpus callosum atrophy in trauma-induced anterior horn dilation. *Brain Injury, 8*, 565–569.

Anderson, C. V., & Bigler, E. D. (1995b). Ventricular dilation, cortical atrophy, and neuropsychological outcome following traumatic brain injury. *Journal of Neuropsychiatry and Clinical Neurosciences, 7*(1), 42–48.

Anderson, M. L., Wolpert, S. M., & Kayle, E. M. (1992). Vascular diseases and trauma. In S. M. Wolpert & P. D. Barnes (Eds.), *MRI in pediatric neuroradiology* (pp. 177–203). St. Louis: Mosby.

Barkovich, A. J. (1995). *Pediatric neuroimaging* (2nd ed.). New York: Raven Press.

Bigler, E. D. (1988). *Diagnostic clinical neuropsychology.* Austin: University of Texas Press.

Bigler, E. D. (1990). *Traumatic brain injury.* Austin, TX: Pro-Ed Publishers.

Bigler, E. D. (1991). Neuropsychological assessment, neuroimaging and clinical neuropsychology: A synthesis. *Archives of Clinical Neuropsychology, 6*, 113–132.

Bigler, E. D. (1995). Advances in brain imaging with children and adults. In M. G. Tramontana & S. R. Hooper (Eds.), *Advances in child neuropsychology.* (pp. 44–83). Berlin: Springer-Verlag.

Bigler, E. D. (1996). Bridging the gap between psychology and neurology: Future trends in pediatric neuropsychology. In E. S. Batchelor & R. S. Dean (Eds.), *Pediatric neuropsychology* (pp. 27–54). Boston: Allyn & Bacon.

Bigler, E. D., Burr, R. B., Gale, S., Norman, M., Kurth, S., Blatter, D., & Abildskov, T. (1994). Day of injury CT scan as an index to pre-injury brain morphology. *Brain Injury, 8,* 231–238.

Bigler, E. D., Johnson, S. C., Jackson, C., & Blatter, D. D. (1995). Aging, brain size, and IQ. *Intelligence, 21*(1), 109–119.

Blatter, D. D., Bigler, E. D., Gale, S. D., Johnson, S. C., Anderson, C., Burnett, B. M., Parker, N., Kurth, S., & Horn, S. (1995). Quantitative volumetric analysis of brain MRI: Normative database spanning five decades (16–65). *American Journal of Neuroradiology, 16*, 241–251.

Blatter, D. D., Bigler, E. D., Gale, S. D., Johnson, S. C., Anderson, C. V., Burnett, B. M., Ryser, D. K., Macnamara, S., & Bailey, B. (1997). MRI based brain and CSF quantification following traumatic brain injury: Correlation with neuropsychological outcome. *American Journal of Neuroradiology* (in press).

Bowen, J. M., Clark, E., Bigler, E. D., Gardner, M., Nilsson, D., Gooch, J. & Pompa, J. (1997). Childhood traumatic brain injury: Neuropsychological status at time of hospital rehabilitation discharge. *Developmental Medicine and Child Neurology, 39* (in press).

Gale, S. D., Burr, R. B., Bigler, E. D., & Blatter, D. D. (1993). Fornix degeneration and memory in traumatic brain injury. *Brain Research Bulletin, 32*, 345–349.

Gale, S. D., Johnson, S. C., Bigler, E. D., & Blatter, D. D. (1994). Traumatic brain injury and temporal horn enlargement correlates with tests of intelligence and memory. *Neuropsychiatry, Neuropsychology, and Behavioral Neurology, 7*, 160–165.

Gale, S. D., Johnson, S. C., Bigler, E. D., & Blatter, D. D. (1995a). Nonspecific white matter degeneration following traumatic brain injury. *Journal of the International Neuropsychological Society, 1*, 17–28.

Gale, S. D., Johnson, S. C., Bigler, E. D., & Blatter, D. (1995b). Trauma-induced degenerative changes in brain injury: A morphometric analysis of three patients with preinjury and postinjury MR scans. *Journal of Neurotrauma, 12*(2), 151–158.

Goldstein, F. C., & Levin, H. S. (1990). Epidemiology of traumatic brain injury: Incidence, clinical characteristics, and risk factors. In E. D. Bigler (Ed.), *Traumatic brain injury: Mechanisms of damage, assessment, intervention, and outcome* (pp. 51–67). Austin, TX: Pro-Ed.

Greenberg, J. O. (1995). *Neuroimaging.* New York: McGraw–Hill.

Grossman, R. I., & Yousem, D. M. (1994). *Neuroradiology: The requisites.* St. Louis: Mosby.

Hopkins, R. O., Gales, S. D., Johnson, S. C., Anderson, C. V., Bigler, E. D., Blatter, D. D., & Weaver, L. K. (1995). A case study in review: Severe anoxia with and without concomitant brain atrophy and neuropsychological impairments. *Journal of the International Neuropsychological Society, 1*, 501–509.

Jernigan, T. L., & Tallal, P. (1990). Late childhood changes in brain morphology observable with MRI. *Developmental Medicine and Child Neurology, 32*, 379–385.

Johnson, S. C., Bigler, E. D., Burr, R. B., & Blatter, D. D. (1994). White matter atrophy, ventricular dilation, and intellectual functioning following traumatic brain injury. *Neuropsychology, 8*, 307–315.

Kucharczyk, J., Moseley, M., & Barkovich, A. J. (1994). *Magnetic resonance neuroimaging.* Boca Raton, FL: CRC Press.

Osborn, A. G. (1994). *Diagnostic neuroradiology.* St. Louis: Mosby.

Osborn, A. G., & Boyer, R. S. (1994). Brain development and congenital malformations. In A. G. Osborn (Ed.), *Diagnostic neuroradiology* (pp. 3–113). St Louis: Mosby.

Wolpert, S. M., & Barnes, P. D. (1992). *MRI in pediatric neuroradiology.* St. Louis: Mosby.

18

Psychophysiological Evaluation of Neuropsychological Disorders in Children

THALÍA HARMONY

Introduction

In recent years important advances have been made in the analysis of processes that are affected in different groups of children with cognitive deficits. For example, developmental disorders of language (dysphasia) and reading (dyslexia) had been viewed as distinct clinical syndromes, although more recent research findings have suggested a clear link between these developmental learning disabilities. First, longitudinal studies have demonstrated that children with language disorders are at very high risk for developing reading disabilities. Second, neuropsychological profiles specifically focused on the areas of phonological disorders and specific temporal processing deficits appear to be quite similar for children with developmental language and reading disorders (Tallal, Galaburda, Llinás, & von Euler, 1993).

A specific temporal processing disorder that may underlie both the phonological and neuropsychological deficits has been proposed for children with dyslexia and language impairments (for a review see Tallal *et al.,* 1993), and the notion of a developmental lag can appropriately be used with respect to "poor readers" (Stanovich, 1986). It is frequently observed that many children with mild reading deficits show significant improvement with age, whereas severe reading impairments in childhood tend to persist into adolescence and adulthood (Rayner & Pollatsek, 1989; Rutter, 1978). Attention deficit disorders, with and without hyperkinesia, have been clearly identified as independent from developmental learning disabilities, although in some children reading disabilities and attention deficit disorders may coexist (Harter, Anllo-Vento, & Wood, 1989; Holcomb, Ackerman, & Dykman, 1985).

An extremely important factor that should be taken into consideration during the evaluation of these cognitive disorders in children is the sociocultural environment. We have demonstrated that children with clear sociocultural disadvantages, coming from marginal urban areas or poor rural environments, have an EEG developmental pattern different from that of other populations (Harmony *et al.,* 1988; Harmony, Marosi, Díaz de León, Becker, & Fernández, 1990a). Satz, Taylor, Friel, and Fletcher (1978) observed that socioeconomic status was a more potent predictor of subsequent reading failure than any of their behavioral measures. Recently, Spear-Swerling and Sternberg (1994) have emphasized the role of sociocultural factors in their model of reading disabilities.

Another aspect frequently found in children with neuropsychological disorders is the presence of antecedents of risk factors, such as perinatal asphyxia and low birth weight. Harmony, Marosi, Díaz de León, Becker, and Fernández (1990a, b) reported abnormal values of variables obtained by EEG frequency analysis in these cases. In some cases these antecedents may be related to the presence of small brain infarcts observable in computed tomography (CT) scans (Fernández-Bouzas *et al.,* 1991). For this reason it is desirable to obtain a CT or MRI in cases with personal antecedents of a biological risk factor.

THALÍA HARMONY • Neurosciences Research Program, ENEP Iztacala, National University of Mexico, Mexico City 03710, Mexico.

The objective of this chapter is to discuss procedures that explore psychological processes by measuring different physiological variables. The study of brain electrical activity in humans allows the exploration of two fundamental levels of function: a very basic one, which provides information about the functional and anatomical integrity of the nervous system, and a second one, which explores higher cognitive activity. We shall review results obtained through these procedures that have provided deeper knowledge of the different processes affected in children with neuropsychological disorders.

Developmental Learning Disabilities

Poor Readers

"Poor readers," or less skilled readers, are defined as children who are reading between 1 and 2 years below their expected level. Such children make up about 10% of the school population. When IQ differences are controlled, it appears that good and poor readers differ primarily in terms of short-term memory for linguistic information and in the ability to code information phonetically in short-term memory (for a review see Rayner & Pollatsek, 1989). Silva et al. (1995), using a computerized reading skill test composed of ten different types of tasks (naming, reading comprehension, picture naming, syntactic tasks, phonological categorization tasks, and visual perception tasks), observed that syntactic tasks, consisting of the ordering of words to complete a sentence, differentiated less skilled readers from normal readers better than other tasks. They concluded that, because the participation of working memory is needed to perform the syntactic tasks, the deficit observed may be related to a decreased capacity for short-term memory, according to the capacity theory of language comprehension advanced by Just and Carpenter (1992).

Based on behavioral studies accessing vocabulary, phonological awareness, general name retrieval ability, decoding skill, word recognition speed, and the ability to use context to speed word recognition, Stanovich (1988) showed that the profiles of skilled third-grade readers and less skilled fifth-grade readers were quite similar. Based on the findings of Stanovich and some other authors, it has been proposed that less skilled readers may suffer from some type of developmental lag.

Using EEG frequency analysis, many authors have shown that absolute and relative power in the delta and theta bands (the slow EEG bands) decrease with age, while alpha relative power increases (Gasser, Verleger, Bacher, & Stroka, 1988; Harmony et al., 1990b; John et al., 1980; Matousek & Petersén, 1973). Therefore, an increase in delta and theta power, with a concomitant decrease in alpha power, seems to be related to an immature EEG pattern. EEG spectrum analysis during rest conditions has yielded conflicting results with respect to the presence of differences between children with reading disabilities. Such contradictory results may be related to differences in sample selection, differences in relation to age range, or differences in the subtyping of reading disabilities. It appears that, whereas children with dyslexia have no differences in their EEG during resting conditions when compared with children without dyslexia (Fein et al., 1986; Yingling, Fein, Galin, Peltzman, & Davenport, 1986), less skilled readers do. Ahn et al. (1980) and John et al. (1983) described an abundance of delta and theta power during rest in specific learning disabilities. Harmony, Hinojosa, Marosi, Becker, Fernández, Rodriguez, Reyes, & Rocha (1990) analyzed EEG in three groups of children, according to their performance on a reading–writing test. Children from group 1 had adequate performance according to age and grade; children from group 2 had below-level performance with minor difficulties; and children from group 3 had below-level performance with severe difficulties. Children from groups 2 and 3 had more diffuse theta absolute power and relative power and less alpha relative power than group 1. Children from group 3 also had a higher amount of delta in frontotemporal leads than the other two groups. These results led the authors to conclude that the diffuse increase of theta and decrease of alpha may be related to a maturational lag, but that in group 3 children frontotemporal delta power reflected an underlying dysfunction in these areas.

However, subsequently, in a longitudinal quantitative EEG study of the same groups of children, we observed that children with mild and severe difficulties on the test had a maturational spurt of their EEG between the ages of 10 and 13. Figure 1 shows the mean value of theta absolute power for the first and second sessions in the three groups of children in the 10/20 International monopolar leads. The age of the children during the first session was $9.0 + 1.6$ years; the second recording was carried out 3 years later. A greater decrease of theta absolute power between sessions was observed in children from groups 2 and 3 than in children from group 1. Figure 2 shows mean theta relative power EEG maps for

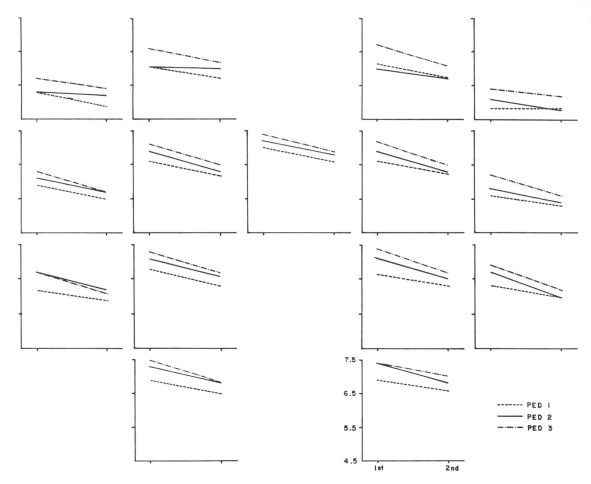

FIGURE 1. Mean values of theta absolute power in the three performance groups for the first and second sessions. PED 1: adequate performance according to age and grade; PED 2: below-level performance with minor difficulties; PED 3: below-level performance with severe difficulties. Each graph corresponds to a different monopolar lead of the 10/20 system. First column: F7, T3, T5. Second column: F3, C3, P3, O1. Third column: Cz. Fourth Column: F4, C4, P4, O2. Fifth column: F8, T4, T6. A greater decrease of theta absolute power between sessions may be observed in children from groups 2 and 3 than in children from group 1. (From Harmony *et al.*, 1995.)

each group in each session. Greater changes may be observed in children with mild and severe problems on the reading and writing test. Our quantitative EEG (qEEG) results agree with the hypothesis of a maturational lag in children with mild and severe problems in reading up to the age of 10. Afterwards, a maturational spurt caused less skilled readers to almost reach grade level by the age of 13 (Harmony *et al.*, 1995).

On the other hand, we have reported a higher correlation between higher delta and theta power in the EEG at rest, and the number of incorrect responses, the reaction times in a selective visual

attention task and in a memory task in normal children. Figure 3 shows the significant correlations observed between reaction times in the memory task and relative power in delta and alpha bands in the various leads. Lower alpha and higher delta values were correlated with longer reaction times (Harmony *et al.*, 1992). We have therefore postulated that slow EEG may be the underlying cause for cognitive deficiencies.

To investigate this hypothesis, in our laboratory Fernández (Fernández *et al.*, 1994) has been performing a series of experiments with skilled and less skilled readers, recording EEG during different

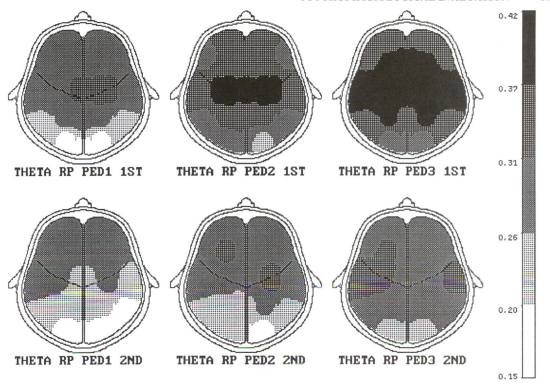

FIGURE 2. Distribution of mean theta relative power in the leads of the 10/20 system in the same groups as in Figure 1. Upper row: first session; bottom row: second session. During the first session, groups 3 and 2 had a higher amount of theta relative power than group 1; however, during the second session, these differences almost disappeared. (From Harmony *et al.*, 1995.)

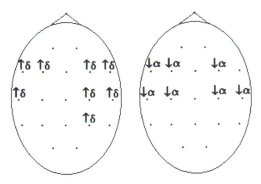

FIGURE 3. Significant correlations between reaction time in the short-term memory task and EEG delta (left) and alpha (right) relative power. Longer reaction times were highly correlated with higher values of delta and lower values of alpha relative power in the EEG at rest.

mental tasks: a Continuous Performance Task and a memory task using Sternberg's paradigm. Preliminary results show that the EEG *previous* to the presentation of the stimulus is slower when incorrect responses are given than when correct responses are obtained. Figure 4 shows EEG maps of absolute power in the delta, theta, alpha, and beta bands of EEG recorded before presentation of stimuli. The upper row shows EEG maps when the response was correct; the lower row, EEG maps when the response was incorrect. More delta and less alpha absolute power are observed in the EEG previous to the incorrect responses.

Other quantitative EEG measures, such as coherence, have also provided results suggesting that a different pattern of EEG maturation exists in learning-disabled children. Coherence is a measure of covariation of the spectra of two EEG signals. High coherences between EEG signals have been interpreted as evidence of a structural and functional connection between cortical areas underlying the recording electrodes. Marosi *et al.* (1992) observed that the maturation of EEG coherences in skilled readers was characterized by an increase in coherence values with age between vertex and the posterior regions and by a decrease with age in the

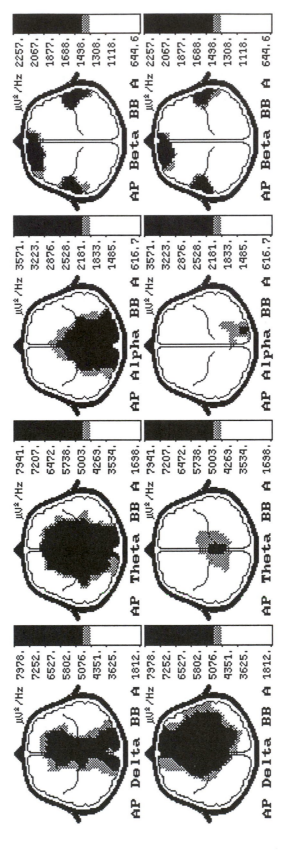

FIGURE 4. Distribution of delta, theta, alpha, and beta absolute power of the EEG previous to stimuli presentation. Upper line: correct responses; bottom line: incorrect responses. Higher delta and lower alpha absolute power may be observed in the EEG previous to the incorrect responses than in the EEG previous to the correct responses.

coherences of frontal interconnections. Decreased frontal coherences with age may be related to an increase in cortical differentiation (Thatcher, Krause, & Hrybyk, 1986). Children with learning disabilities showed a different pattern of EEG coherence maturation, demonstrating that age affects the coherence of skilled and less skilled readers in a differential way.

The comparison of coherence values between three groups of children with different performances on a reading and writing test showed that between the ages of 7 and 9, children with below-average performance showed higher coherences in the delta, theta, and beta bands and lower coherences in the alpha band. However, in older children (9 to 11 years old), while the same tendency was observed, significant differences between groups were obtained only in the delta band. In this age range, the significant group differences were almost entirely in interhemispheric coherences, whereas in the youngest group the significant differences were observed in both intrahemispheric and interhemispheric coherences. These results also suggest that less skilled readers have a developmental spurt of EEG coherences at age 9 (Marosi *et al.,* 1995).

Another important aspect in the evaluation of less skilled readers' EEG is the presence of paroxysmal activity in the EEG. Paroxysmal activity is defined as a group of waves that appear and disappear abruptly; it is clearly distinguished from background activity by different frequency, morphology, and amplitudes. Spikes, multispike complexes, sharp waves, spike and slow-wave complexes, and paroxysmal slow waves are recognized as the fundamental patterns. In normal children, such activity is rarely observed (Petersén, Selldén, & Eeg-Olofsson, 1975), whereas in various groups of children with cognitive impairments, a significantly higher proportion of paroxysmal activity has been described (Hughes, 1971; Lezny, Provasnik, Jirasek, & Komarek, 1977; Murdoch, 1974). Becker, Velasco, Harmony, Marosi, and Landazuri (1987) reported more paroxysmal (25%) and atypical (39%) EEG activity in children with learning disabilities than in normal controls. The presence of paroxysmal EEG discharges, even in persons not considered to have epilepsy, may in fact produce subtle clinical phenomena. In 1939, using a simple reaction time task during EEG recording, Schwab showed that apparently subclinical discharges may be accompanied by subtle decreases in cognitive function. Many subsequent investigators have confirmed the occurrence, in patients with subclinical discharges, of a momentary

cognitive deficit, to which Aarts, Binnie, Smith, and Wilkins (1984) gave the name *transitory cognitive impairment* (TCI). Binnie, Channon, and Marston (1990) have pointed out that paroxysmal activity may produce learning disabilities through disruption of longer-term processes of elaboration, storage, and retrieval, and by a prolonged or permanent reduction in the brain's capacity to react adaptively to incoming information.

The presence of TCI was also demonstrated by Binnie (1993) in children with benign epilepsy characterized by rolandic spikes. He demonstrated TCI using a test of short-term memory for spatial material. In this group of children, behavioral or cognitive problems such as dyslexia, speech delay, underachievement, and inattentiveness were reported. Binnie (1993) concluded that it might be expected that all children with TCI would have behavioral or cognitive difficulties. The practical implication of this finding was that subclinical EEG discharges that produce TCI could be ameliorated by the use of medication to suppress epileptiform EEG activity. Binnie was the first to present such evidence under controlled conditions.

Alvarez, Pérez-Avalo, and Morenza (1992) assessed the effect of paroxysmal activity in the performance of a psychological task in two groups of children: nine epileptic children who attended a special education school, and nine learning-disabled children without clinical diagnosis of epilepsy. In each of the groups, TCI could be demonstrated in three children. In a recent report, the same group of authors administered, in a counterbalanced design, three variants of a Continuous Performance Test in which visual stimuli had to be classified according to color, semantic, or phonological criteria. TCI was found in a significant proportion of nonepileptic learning-disabled children. The tasks in which TCI was present differed from one child to another. Thus, the paroxysmal activity apparently interfered with different mental processes in different children (Alvarez, Morgades, Pérez-Avalo, Rojas, & Díaz-Comas, 1994).

In conclusion, EEG recordings and qEEG may be very useful in the evaluation of less skilled readers. The presence of paroxysmal activity suggests the possibility of TCI affecting the cognitive functions of the child. Controlled experiments have not yet been carried out using anticonvulsive medication in nonepileptic children with TCI, but such applications remain a possibility.

qEEG has shown an abnormal pattern of EEG maturation in less skilled readers. The higher amount of delta and theta power in these children below the age of 10 may also explain the cognitive deficits observed. The increase of delta and theta power during rest has been correlated with more incorrect responses and prolonged reaction times in visual selective attention and short-term memory tasks. More impressive, however, are results showing that the presence of slow waves during the presentation of a stimulus during a Continuous Performance task is highly correlated with incorrect responses, in both skilled and less skilled readers. These results support the old hypothesis of Grey Walter (1959) suggesting that EEG rhythms may signal an internal clock for brain processing.

On the other hand, qEEG results support the hypothesis of a maturational lag in less skilled readers. In a longitudinal study, we were able to show that children with mild or severe problems on a reading and writing test experience an EEG developmental spurt at age 10, approaching normality 2 or 3 years later (Harmony et al., 1995).

Children with Language Impairment (LI) and Reading Disabilities (RD)

We shall follow Tallal's concept (1987) in considering developmental dysphasia and dyslexia as the same syndrome. Recent formulations of the underlying deficits in this syndrome have focused on three major areas: (1) deficits in the ability to rapidly integrate presented nonlanguage auditory stimuli (Tallal, Miller, & Fitch, 1993); (2) deficits in the functioning of the transient visual system (Galaburda & Livingstone, 1993; Lovegrove, 1993); and (3) deficits in verbal short-term memory (Baddeley, 1979; Vellutino, 1983).

According to Tallal et al. (1993), the dysfunction of higher-level speech processing, which is necessary for normal language and reading development, may result from difficulties in the processing of basic sensory information entering the nervous system in rapid succession (within milliseconds). They provided data showing that this deficit affects processing in multiple sensory modalities, as well as motor output within the millisecond time frame. They linked these basic temporal integration deficits to specific patterns of speech perception and speech production deficits in children with LI. They also suggested that these basic temporal deficits cause a cascade of effects, starting with disruption of the normal development of the phonological system. These phonological processing deficits result in a subsequent failure to learn to speak and read normally. That is, for Tallal et al., both language and reading problems have their basis in deficiently established phonological processing and decoding.

Neville, Coffey, Holcomb, and Tallal (1993) recorded auditory evoked responses (AERs) to a standard tone of 1000 Hz and to a target tone of 2000 Hz, with different interstimulus intervals in a group of normal children and a group of children with LI. They observed significant differences between groups only when the children with LI were split into two subgroups based on their behavioral performance on the rapid sequencing subtest of the Tallal Repetition Test. Only those children scoring between 0 and 16 who were classified as "low" rep showed AERs of lower amplitude in the N140 component following the shortest interval and in N260 and N440 components for all intervals. The authors concluded that in some children with LI/RD, reduced and slowed activity within primary and association auditory areas contributed to their language impairment. The fact that the subsequent responses, N260 and N440, were also reduced to all interstimulus intervals suggested that auditory sensory processing may be abnormal even at moderate rates of stimulus presentation in a subset of children with LI/LD.

Other very interesting results that show abnormal auditory processing in children with LI/RD are those of Lang, Korpilahti, Holopainen, and Sillänpää (1993). They analyzed the mismatch negativity (MMN) in a group of dysphasic children. The MMN component appeared when a deviant tone was presented embedded in a series of tones (Näätänen, Gaillard, & Mantysalo, 1978). The deviant tones were characterized by a different pitch or a different duration relative to the standard tones. The MMN seems to reflect a neural mismatch process triggered by a sensory input from a deviant stimulus at the presence of a neural trace of the frequent (standard) stimuli. This process serves as an automatic, preconscious change-detection mechanism that initiates a sequence of brain events that lead to an attention switch to a stimulus change when some threshold is exceeded (Näätänen, Paavilainen, Tiitinen, Jiang, & Alho, 1993). In children with dysphasia, MMN is significantly attenuated especially to pitch difference and has a somewhat different scalp distribution than in normal children. These results indicate that dysphasia might, at least partially, be the result of a functional disturbance in the preattentive auditory discrimination stage and the echoic memory (Lang et al., 1993).

With regard to deficits in visual processing in subjects with dyslexia, although it was a common clinical assumption that reading disability was not attributable to visual deficits, since the early 1970s recordings of visual evoked responses (VERs) have shown that children with dyslexia display amplitude attenuation of these responses (Cohen, 1980; Conners, 1971; Preston, Guthrie, & Childs, 1974) and greater variability of VERs in parietal areas (Harmony, 1989; Harmony & Díaz de León, 1982). In recent years, Lovegrove (1993) has proposed a theory to explain dyslexia on the basis of deficits in the transient visual system. Information is transmitted from the eye to the brain via a number of separate parallel pathways or channels. The different channels transmit their information at different rates and respond differently to different rates of temporal change. Some channels are sensitive to very rapidly changing stimuli and others to stationary or slow-moving stimuli, and two subsystems have been proposed within the visual system: the transient and sustained systems. The transient system is highly sensitive to contrast, most sensitive to low spatial and high temporal frequencies, with fast cellular and parvocellular systems of the visual pathways often being equated with the transient and sustained systems, respectively.

Lovegrove (1993) used measures of low-level visual processing as visible persistence, which is measured by the temporal separation required for distinguishing between two presentations. Flicker fusion rate, which is the fastest rate at which a contrast reversal of a stimulus can be seen, led to the observation that approximately 75% of children with dyslexia showed reduced transient system sensitivity, but did not differ from controls in the functioning of the sustained vision system. Galaburda and Livingstone (1993) analyzed the brains of five dyslexic subjects and five nondyslexics, observing that the magnocellular layers of the lateral geniculate nuclei were more disorganized in the dyslexic brains, thereby supporting the hypothesis of a deficit in the transient visual system.

VERs to pattern reversal stimuli are of smaller amplitude in children with RD (May, Lovegrove, Martin, & Nelson, 1991; Mecacci, Sechi, & Levi, 1983; Solan, Sutija, Ficarra, & Wurst, 1990). Neville et al. (1993), in the same sample of children with LI/RD mentioned above, reported that children with LI had smaller amplitudes of P150 and P350, and longer latency of N230. These findings are further evidence for the proposed deficits in visual processing in dyslexia.

The third set of underlying deficits that have been postulated for the explanation of LI/RD in children are those related to short-term memory. It is assumed that short-term memory plays a role in reading (Baddeley, 1979). Strong theoretical evidence for a link between linguistic coding and reading disability has been provided by Torgesen (1985) and Vellutino (1983). These authors pointed out the importance of language processes for reading in general and, in particular, the vulnerability of decoding processes to deficiencies in encoding abilities.

Event-related potentials (ERPs) can be used for chronometric analysis of cognitive processes (McCarthy & Donchin, 1981) yielding information not available from behavioral measures, and therefore offering the possibility of investigating the cognitive processing required for reading. Among the most frequent components of the ERPs studied is P300. This is an endogenous positive wave with a latency of 300 ms or greater, and is typically elicited by rare target stimuli in a detection task. In selective attention tasks, when the signal is correctly detected the ERP shows a large P300 component that does not appear when targets are missed. P300 seems to be related to stimulus evaluation processes and to be independent of response selection and execution processes. It is the activation of a unique processor, a subroutine, with a specific function, that is indicated by the appearance of P300. Any stimulus, once identified and categorized, is thought to initiate two processes, one concerned with response selection, the other with what might be called "context updating," which depends in turn on stimulus evaluation. If the unexpected happens, the model of the operating context must be revised. Donchin, Ritter, and McCallum (1978) hypothesized that this context revision is manifested by P300. Because context updating involves the activation of working memory, P300 has also been related to processing of stimuli in memory. Posner (1978) proposed that the higher-level process responsible for the generation of P300 is conscious attention. A large P300 would indicate that the subject was focusing a substantial amount of available attentional resources on the stimulus event, while a small or nonexistent P300 would indicate that these resources were unavailable or diverted elsewhere.

A common finding has been smaller P300 responses in children when using a language-related task (Barner, Lamm, Epstein, & Pratt, 1994; Erez & Pratt, 1992; Lovrich & Stamm, 1983; Ollo & Squires, 1982; Taylor & Keenan, 1990). Holcomb et al. (1985) reported a dissociation of findings between children with RD and those with ADD using words and symbols as stimuli: children with ADD had lower amplitudes of P300 in both conditions. However, RD and control groups were better differentiated by the amplitude of P300 when word stimuli were contrasted with nonlinguistic symbols. Because symbols elicited larger P300 than words in children with RD, whereas the two kinds of stimuli elicited equivalent amplitudes in controls, the results were interpreted as displaying a selective deficit in the group with RD when processing word stimuli. Using a spatial task, Harter *et al.* (1989) found a greater enhancement of N100 and reduced P300 in children with RD. However, the effects of RD on ERP did not vary as a function of ADD, indicating that these two disorders are distinct. These authors concluded that children with RD, while deficient in their ability to select a target stimulus—as indexed by smaller P300 component—nevertheless had enhanced spatial attention abilities. However, Stelmack, Saxe, Noldy-Cullum, Campbell, and Armitage (1989), using word recognition memory tasks in normal and RD groups, found differences in P200 but not in P300.

Another very interesting component of the ERPs is N400, which typically has a peak latency of 400 ms and a broad scalp distribution, although it is usually largest at more posterior sites. Semantic manipulations, such as presenting a target word following an appropriate context versus an inappropriate context, modulates the amplitude of N400. N400 are larger for words after an inappropriate context (Kutas & Hillyard, 1980). Figure 5 shows mean average ERPs from a normal group of 10-year-old children, to appropriate versus inappropriate sentence final words.

As N400 amplitude is strongly negatively correlated with word frequency, semantic context, and controlled processing, it is reasonable to assume that it indexes processes invoked by the integration of a word into context (Brown & Hagoort, 1993; Holcomb & Neville, 1990; Kutas & Hillyard, 1984; Rugg & Doyle, 1992). Holcomb, Coffey, and Neville (1992) recorded subjects aged 5–26 as they listened to and read sentences that ended either with an appropriate and highly expected or a semantically inappropriate word. ERPs to sentence final words displayed effects of contextual priming in both modalities, in all age groups. An important finding was that there were significant reductions in semantic priming effects with age. The results suggest that as children acquire better language skills, they rely less on semantic context for language comprehension.

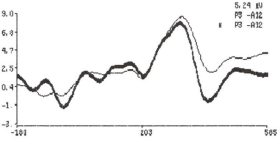

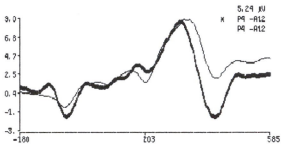

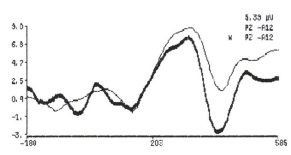

FIGURE 5. Grand average ERP to final words of sentences in normal children for P3, P4, and Pz leads. Thicker line: incongruent ending. Thinner line: congruent ending. Negativity downwards. A major negative wave (N400) may be observed to the incongruent endings.

Neville *et al.* (1993), in the same paper studying children with LI/RD quoted above, found that N400 enhancement to semantic anomalies tended to be longer than in control children, although they did not reach significance ($p < 0.08$). The authors interpreted this result to indicate that the auditory and visual sensory processing deficits observed in this group of children led to compensatory increases in the effect required to integrate words into context and a greater reliance on context for word recognition than in control subjects. However, less skilled readers did not show this effect: in our laboratory, Rodríguez did not find significant differences in N400 amplitude or latency between a group of skilled readers and a group of less skilled readers (Rodríguez *et al.*, 1994).

The final conclusion of the Neville *et al.* (1993) study of the auditory and visual recovery cycles and the N400 (in the same group of children with LI/RD) was that multiple factors contribute to the emergence of language-processing deficits, and that these deficits are heterogeneous across populations of children with LI/RD.

There have also been several studies searching for EEG differences in dyslexia. Recordings of EEG at rest have shown that when subjects with "pure dyslexia" are selected, qEEG variables are normal (Fein *et al.*, 1986; Yingling *et al.*, 1986).

Using the topographic mapping of EEG and sensory evoked responses during rest and during different tasks (reading and recall, listening to speech, memorization and recall of geometric figures, listening to music, forming associations between geometric forms and nonsense words), Duffy and McAnulty (1985) found the following significant differences between normal control subjects and subjects with dyslexia ranging in age from 10 to 12 years old: (1) group differences were better demonstrated during EEG activated tasks than during resting states; (2) EEG differences between groups were largely anterior; (3) although the classical left temporal and parietal speech regions were prominent as a locus of dyslexic versus normal differences, a between-group difference was also found in frontal regions, with more alpha activity in frontal regions in the dyslexics during active states. The abundance of alpha activity was interpreted by Duffy and McAnulty as a tendency toward inactivity or functional "idleness" (Gevins *et al.*, 1979), or as a lack of electrophysiological responsiveness to different experimental situations. Lower alpha and beta 2 responsiveness was also reported by Ortiz, Exposito, Miguel, Martin-Loeches, and Rubia (1992) in a group of children with dysphonemic dyslexia during an auditory phonemic discrimination task. A significantly smaller change in theta power between oral and silent reading has been observed in subjects with dyslexia by Galin *et al.* (1992). What all of these studies have in common is a decreased responsiveness of EEG during different active states, which may reflect cognitive differences between children with versus without RD.

ADD

Subjects with ADD are by definition individuals with attentional problems. Sometimes cognitive problems are associated with ADD. However, using ERPs, it has been shown that reading disabilities and ADD are distinct disorders (Harter *et al.*, 1989; Holcomb *et al.*, 1985). It is generally accepted that P300 amplitude between targets and nontargets is smaller in ADD using auditory or visual stimuli (Holcomb *et al.*, 1985; Loiselle, Stamm, Maitinsky, & Whipple, 1980; Satterfield, Schell, Nicholas, & Backs, 1988). In a recent report, Satterfield, Schell, and Nicholas (1994) analyzed the ERPs from 36 hyperkinetic ADD and 35 normal 6-year-olds to auditory and visual stimuli in a two-choice discrimination task. When normal subjects paid attention to stimuli in a given modality, enhanced N200 and P300 responses (as compared with responses to nonattended stimuli) were found for auditory and visual target stimuli. In contrast, when subjects with ADD attended, little or no enhanced negative responses were found in either modality, and P300 responses were found only to visual target stimuli. Auditory N100, N200, and P300 and visual N200 to attended target stimuli were significantly reduced in subjects with ADD versus controls. No between-group differences were found for responses to nontarget stimuli. The authors concluded that the lack of enhancement of brain response to attended stimuli reflects deficits in cognitive processes essential to the discrimination of novel and important stimuli (as reflected by small N200 responses), and deficits in cognitive processes—thought to be crucial to memory and learning (as reflected by small P300 responses)—in young males with hyperkinetic ADD.

Satterfield *et al.* proposed two alternate hypotheses to explain these deficits: (1) Selective triggering of the noradrenergic neurotransmitter systems by novel stimuli results in a release of noradrenaline at widespread cortical terminals. This release enhances signals in the brain systems engaged by exogenous attended sensory stimuli (Tucker & Williamson, 1984). A deficit in triggering of the adrenergic system could underlie the abnormally small N200 and P300 responses in subjects with ADD. (2) Children with hyperkinetic ADD have abnormal cerebral blood flow (Lou, Henriksen, Bruhn, Borner, & Nielsen, 1989) and adults with a history of hyperactivity in childhood have an abnormally low cerebral metabolism (Zametkin *et al.*, 1990). Because neuronal activity is linked to brain metabolism, when subjects with ADD are engaged in a task that requires a fair amount of sustained attention and effort, the system fails because they have a deficiency in energy pools or allocation of energy in the case of a special demand.

The implication of these ERP findings is very clear: Males with hyperkinetic ADD have no abnormally large responses to the to-be-ignored stimuli, but do have abnormally small responses to the attended stimuli. Therefore, it no longer seems logical to isolate hyperactive children in order to facilitate their learning. Satterfield's results suggest that learning and performance of children with ADD should be enhanced on tasks in which the relevant information is highly salient.

Another element of the practical importance of ERPs in the study of hyperkinetic ADD is their use in the evaluation of medication. In two different sessions, one before treatment and the second after a drug dose, it is possible to reach conclusions as to whether a particular child will respond to pharmacological treatment. In "responders," amphetamines and methylphenidate produced improvement of the ERP measures toward normalization (Halliday, Callaway, & Naylor, 1983; Klorman *et al.*, 1983; Prichep, Sutton, & Hakerem, 1976; Saletu, Saletu, Simeon, Viamontes, & Itil, 1975).

Childhood Autism

From a neurophysiological point of view, studies on infantile autism have been conducted in an effort to show defects in information processing and defects in mechanisms of orienting to novel stimulation. Because of serious problems in obtaining the cooperation of these children, technical difficulties are frequent and for this reason some studies have been carried out during unmedicated sleep. On the other hand, it is often difficult to state the role played respectively by autism and by mental deficit.

Studies of BAERs in children with autism have yielded contradictory results. Sohmer and Student (1978) observed an increase in latency of all waves and a prolonged transmission time, which have also been reported by Skoff, Mirsky, and Turner (1980) and by Rosemblum *et al.* (1980). Although these results *per se* do not clarify the question as to whether this functional deviation was caused by a specific lesion of the auditory pathways or was a sign of diffuse brain damage, Sohmer and Student concluded that a diffuse lesion was the most probable explanation. However, Rumsey, Grimes, Pikus, Duara, and Ismond (1984) did not find differences in BAER characteristics in their study of 25 children and adults with pervasive developmental disorders, including autism, versus sex- and age-matched controls.

Martineau, Garreau, Barthelemy, and Lelord (1984) measured amplitude and latencies of peak N100, P200, and P300 to sound alone and to paired sound and light stimuli in 18 normal and 15 children with autism. Latencies of AERs to sound alone were smaller in children with autism than in normal controls. P300 amplitude was also larger in the autistic group to sound alone. Pairing sound with light, latencies had few modifications but the amplitude of all peaks increased in controls and diminished in children with autism. P300 showed greater variability in children with autism. This finding agrees with that of Novick, Vaughan, Kurtzberg, and Simon (1980), who examined the standard deviation of the mean ERP in children with autism and found considerable variability.

Another approach to the study of infantile autism has been followed by Courchesne, Lincoln, Kilman, and Galambos (1985) based on the clinical observation that individuals with autism do not orient to normal information in a normal fashion. VERs and AERs to stimuli requiring simple classification decisions and ERPs to unexpected, novel information, presented without forewarning the subjects, were analyzed in a group of ten nonretarded subjects with autism between 13 and 25 years old. Two conditions were studied in each session of AERs and VERs: no task condition, where children simply looked at or listened to these stimuli, and a task or performance condition where they pressed a button at the occurrence of target stimuli intermixed with unexpected, novel stimuli and also with expected, familiar stimuli. In the task condition, auditory stimuli evoked AERs of smaller amplitude in autistic subjects to novel sounds in vertex, to target (N100, P300) and nontarget sounds (N100, P300) in frontal regions. In the visual modality the autistic group had smaller VER amplitudes at the frontal sites to novels and targets. The results suggested: (1) nonretarded subjects with autism may have a limited capacity to process novel information—they are neither hypersensitive to novel information nor misperceive it as nonnovel and insignificant; (2) classification of simple visual information may be less impaired than auditory; and (3) with the exception of only one latency difference, visual and auditory ERP abnormalities do not seem to reflect maturational delay.

This study was performed in high-functioning subjects with autism to permit the analysis of the relationship between neurophysiological variables and information processing not confounded by mental retardation, poor attention, poor cooperation, and low performance capacity. The results supported the findings of Martineau *et al.* (1984) and Novick *et al.* (1980) in relation to a decreased

P300 to auditory stimuli in subjects with autism, which reflects that some particular aspects of information processing are abnormal in autism. Such replicability across laboratories, designs, and quantification approaches gives support to the hypothesis that long-latency ERP components associated with cognitive processing could prove valuable in determining the neurobiological dysfunction of autism (Courchesne *et al.*, 1985). On the other hand, Courchesne *et al.* did not find the striking changes, in the AERs and VERs, during nontask conditions, that have been reported by others. Such differences may relate to the fact that children with autism may display a pattern of ERP abnormalities different from that of adolescents and young adults with autism.

References

Aarts, J. H. P., Binnie, C. D., Smith, A. M., & Wilkins, A. J. (1984). Selective cognitive impairment during focal and generalised epileptiform EEG activity. *Brain, 107,* 293–308.

Ahn, H., Prichep, L., John, E. R., Baird, H., Trepetin, M., & Kaye, H. (1980). Developmental equations reflect brain dysfunction. *Science, 210,* 1259–1262.

Alvarez, A., Morgades, R., Pérez-Avalo, M. C., Rojas, J., & Díaz-Comas, L. (1994). Transient cognitive impairment in learning disabled children. *7th International Congress of Psychophysiology,* Thessaloniki, Greece.

Alvarez, A., Pérez-Avalo, M. C., & Morenza, L. (1992). Neuropsychological assessment of learning disabled children with paroxysmal EEG activity. *New Issues in Neurosciences, 4,* 40–75.

Baddeley, A. (1979). Working memory and reading. In P. A. Kolers, M. E. Wrolstal, & H. Bonoma (Eds.), *Processing of visible language* (Vol. 1). New York: Plenum Press.

Barner, A., Lamm, O., Epstein, R., & Pratt, H. (1994). Brain potentials from dyslexic children recorded during short-term memory tasks. *International Journal of Neuroscience, 74,* 227–237.

Becker, J., Velasco, M., Harmony, T., Marosi, E., & Landazuri, M. (1987). Electroencephalographic characteristics of children with learning disabilities. *Clinical Electroencephalography, 18,* 93–101.

Binnie, C. D. (1993). Significance and management of transitory cognitive impairment due to subclinical EEG discharges in children. *Brain & Development, 15,* 23–30.

Binnie, C. D., Channon, S., & Marston, D. (1990). Learning disabilities in epilepsy. Neurophysiological aspects. *Epilepsia, 31*(Suppl. 4), 19.

Brown, C., & Hagoort, P. (1993). The processing nature of the N400: Evidence from mask priming. *Journal of Cognitive Neuroscience, 5,* 34–44.

Cohen, J. (1980). Cerebral evoked potentials in dyslexic children. In D. A. Otto (Ed.), *Multidisciplinary perspectives in event-related brain potential research.* Washington, DC: EPA 600/977–043.

Conners, C. K. (1971). Cortical visual evoked response in children with learning disorders. *Psychophysiology, 7,* 418–428.

Courchesne, E., Lincoln, A., Kilman, B. A., & Galambos, R. (1985). Event-related brain potentials correlates of the processing of novel visual and auditory information in autism. *Journal of Autism and Developmental Disorders, 15,* 55–76.

Donchin, E., Ritter, W., & McCallum, W. C. (1978). Cognitive psychophysiology: The endogenous components of the ERP. In E. Callaway, P. Tueting, & S. Koslow (Eds.), *Event-related brain potentials in man* (pp. 349–411). New York: Academic Press.

Duffy, F. H., & McAnulty, G. B. (1985). Brain electrical activity mapping (BEAM): The search for a physiological signature of dyslexia. In F. H. Duffy & N. Geschwind (Eds.), *Dyslexia. A neuroscientific approach to clinical evaluation* (pp. 105–123). Boston: Little, Brown.

Erez, A., & Pratt, H. (1992). Auditory event-related potentials among dyslexic and normal-reading children: 3CLT and midline comparisons. *International Journal of Neuroscience, 63,* 247–264.

Fein, G., Galin, D., Yingling, C. D., Johnstone, J., Davenport, L., & Herron, J. (1986). EEG spectra in dyslexic and control boys during resting conditions. *Electroencephalography and Clinical Neurophysiology, 63,* 87–97.

Fernández, T., Silva, J., Harmony, T., Yáñez, G., Marosi, E., Guerrero, V., Rodríguez, M., Bernal, J., & Reyes, A. (1994). Children's EEG characteristics previous to the presentation of the stimulus related with the performance in mental tasks. *7th International Congress of Psychophysiology,* Thessaloniki, Greece.

Fernández-Bouzas, A., Malacara, F., Ramírez, H., Harmony, T., Becker, J., Marosi, E., Rodríguez, M., & Reyes, A. (1991). Computer tomography in children with electrophysiological abnormalities. *International Journal of Neurosciences, 56,* 247–254.

Galaburda, A., & Livingstone, M. (1993). Evidence for a magnocellular defect in developmental dyslexia. In P. Tallal, A. M. Galaburda, R. R. Llinas, & C. von Euler (Eds.), *Temporal information processing in the nervous system: Special reference to dyslexia and dysphasia* (pp. 70–82). New York: New York Academy of Sciences.

Galin, D., Raz, J., Fein, G., Johnstone, J., Herron, J., & Yingling, C. (1992). EEG spectra in dyslexic and normal readers during oral and silent reading. *Electroencephalography and Clinical Neurophysiology, 82,* 87–101.

Gasser, T., Verleger, R., Bacher, P., & Stroka, L. (1988). Development of the EEG of school-age children and adolescents. I. Analysis of band power. *Electroencephalography and Clinical Neurophysiology, 69,* 91–99.

Gevins, A. S., Zeitlin, G. M., Doyle, J. C., Yingling, C. D., Schaffer, R. E., Callaway, E., & Yeager, C. L. (1979). Electroencephalogram correlates of higher cortical functions. *Science, 203,* 655–667.

Halliday, R., Callaway, E., & Naylor, H. (1983). Visual evoked potential changes induced by methylphenidate in hyperactive children: Dose/response effects. *Electroencephalography and Clinical Neurophysiology, 55,* 258–267.

Harmony, T. (1989). Psychophysiological evaluation of children's neuropsychological disorders. In C. R. Reynolds & E. Fletcher-Janzen (Eds.), *Handbook of clinical child neuropsychology* (pp. 265–290). New York: Plenum Press.

Harmony, T., Alvarez, A., Pascual, R., Ramos, A., Marosi, E., Díaz de León, A. E., Valdés, P., & Becker, J. (1988). EEG maturation in children with different economic and psychosocial characteristics. *International Journal of Neurosciences, 41,* 103–113.

Harmony, T., & Díaz de León, A. E. (1982). Visual evoked responses in children with learning disorders. *Second International Evoked Potential Symposium,* Cleveland, Ohio.

Harmony, T., Hinojosa, G., Marosi, E., Becker, J., Fernández, T., Rodríguez, M., Reyes, A., & Rocha, C. (1990). Correlation between EEG spectral parameters and an educational evaluation. *International Journal of Neurosciences, 54,* 147–155.

Harmony, T., Marosi, E., Becker, J., Rodríguez, M., Reyes, A., Fernández, T., Silva, J., & Bernal, J. (1995). Longitudinal quantitative EEG study in children with different performance on a reading-writing test. *Electroencephalography and Clinical Neurophysiology, 95,* 426–433.

Harmony, T., Marosi, E., Becker, J., Reyes, A., Rodríguez, M., Bernal, J., Hinojosa, G., & Fernández, T. (1992). Correlación entre el análisis de frecuencias del EEG y el rendimiento en pruebas de atención selectiva y memoria en niños. *Revista Latina de Pensamiento y Lenguaje, 1,* 96–103.

Harmony, T., Marosi, E., Díaz de León, A. E., Becker, J., & Fernández, T. (1990a). Effect of sex, psychosocial disadvantages and biological risk factors on EEG maturation. *Electroencephalography and Clinical Neurophysiology, 75,* 482–491.

Harmony, T., Marosi, E., Díaz de León, A. E., Becker, J., & Fernández, T. (1990b). Analysis of electroencephalographic maturation. In E. R. John, T. Harmony, L. Prichep, M. Valdés, & P. Valdés (Eds.), *Machinery of the mind* (pp. 360–375). Boston: Birkhauser.

Harter, M. R., Anllo-Vento, L., & Wood, F. B. (1989). Event-related potentials, spatial orienting and reading disabilities. *Psychophysiology, 26,* 404–421.

Holcomb, P. J., Ackerman, P. T., & Dykman, R. A. (1985). Cognitive event-related brain potentials in children with attention and reading deficits. *Psychophysiology, 22,* 656–667.

Holcomb, P. J., Coffey, S. A., & Neville, H. J. (1992). Visual and auditory sentence processing: A developmental analysis using event-related brain potentials. *Developmental Neuropsychology, 8,* 203–241.

Holcomb, P. J., & Neville, H. J. (1990). Auditory and visual semantic priming in lexical decision: A comparison using event-related brain potentials. *Psychobiology, 19,* 286–300.

Hughes, J. R. (1971). Electroencephalography and learning disabilities. In H. R. Myklebust (Ed.), *Progress in learning disabilities* (Vol. 2). New York: Grune & Stratton.

John, E. R., Ahn, H., Prichep, L., Trepetin, M., Brown, D., & Kaye, H. (1980). Developmental equations for the electroencephalogram. *Science, 210,* 1255–1258.

John, E. R., Prichep, L., Ahn, H., Easton, P., Friedman, J., & Kaye, H. (1983). Neurometric evaluation of cognitive dysfunctions and neurological disorders in children. *Progress in Neurobiology, 21,* 239–290.

Just, M. A., & Carpenter, P. A. (1992). A capacity theory of comprehension: Individual differences in working memory. *Psychological Review, 99,* 122–149.

Klorman, R., Salzman, L., Bauer, L., Coons, H., Borgstedt, A., & Halpen, W. (1983). Effects of two doses of methylphenidate in cross-situational and borderline hyperactive children's evoked potentials. *Electroencephalography and Clinical Neurophysiology, 56,* 169–185.

Kutas, M., & Hillyard, S. A. (1980). Reading senseless sentences: Brain potentials reflect semantic incongruity. *Science, 207,* 203–205.

Kutas, M., & Hillyard, S. A. (1984). Brain potentials during reading reflect word expectancy and semantic association. *Nature (London), 307,* 161–163.

Lang, A. H., Korpilahti, P., Holopainen, I., & Sillänpää, M. (1993). Abnormal frequency and duration mismatch negativity in dysphasic children. *XIII International Congress of EEG and Clinical Neurophysiology,* Vancouver, British Columbia.

Lezny, L., Provasnik, K., Jirasek, J., & Komarek, L. (1977). The value of EEG, specially of hyperventilation test in learning disability. *Activitas Nervosa Superior, Praha, 19,* 263–264.

Loiselle, D. L., Stamm, J. S., Maitinsky, S., & Whipple, S. C. (1980). Evoked potentials and behavioral signs of attentive dysfunctions in hyperactive boys. *Psychophysiology, 17,* 193–201.

Lou, H. C., Henriksen, L., Bruhn, P., Borner, H., & Nielsen, J. B. (1989). Striatal dysfunction in attention deficit and hyperkinetic disorder. *Archives of Neurology, 46,* 48–52.

Lovegrove, W. (1993). Weakness in the transient visual system: A causal factor in dyslexia? In P. Tallal, A. M. Galaburda, R. R Llinas, & C. von Euler (Eds.), *Temporal information processing in the nervous system: Special reference to dyslexia and dysphasia* (pp. 57–69). New York: New York Academy of Sciences.

Lovrich, D., & Stamm, J. (1983). Event-related potential and behavioral correlates of attention in reading retardation. *Journal of Clinical Neuropsychology, 4,* 343–365.

McCarthy G., & Donchin, E. (1981). A metric for thought: A comparison of P300 latency and reaction time. *Science, 211,* 77–80.

Marosi, E., Harmony, T., Becker, J., Reyes, A., Bernal, J., Fernández, T., Rodríguez, M., Silva, J., & Guerrero, V. (1995). Electroencephalographic coherences discriminate between children with different pedagogical evaluation. *International Journal of Psychophysiology, 19,* 23–32.

Marosi, E., Harmony, T., Sánchez, L., Díaz de León, A. E., Becker, J., Rodríguez, M., Reyes, A., Bernal, J., & Fernández, T. (1992). Maturation of EEG coherence in normal and learning disabled children. *Electroencephalography and Clinical Neurophysiology, 83,* 350–357.

Martineau, J., Garreau, B., Barthelemy, C., & Lelord, G. (1984). Evoked potentials and P300 during sensory conditioning in autistic children. *Annals of the New York Academy of Sciences, 425,* 362–369.

Matousek, M., & Petersén, I. (1973). Frequency analysis of the EEG in normal children and adolescents. In P. Kellaway & I. Petersén (Eds.), *Automation of clinical electroencephalography* (pp. 75–102). New York: Raven Press.

May, J. G., Lovegrove, W. J., Martin, F., & Nelson, P. (1991). Pattern-elicited visual evoked potentials in good and poor readers. *Clinical Vision Science, 6,* 131–136.

Mecacci, L., Sechi, E., & Levi, S. (1983). Abnormalities of visual evoked potentials by checkerboard in children with specific reading disability. *Brain and Cognition, 2,* 135–143.

Murdoch, B. D. (1974). Changes in the electroencephalogram in minimal cerebral dysfunction: A controlled study over 8 months. *South African Medical Journal, 48,* 606–610.

Näätänen, R., Gaillard, A. W. K., & Mantysalo, S. (1978). Early selective-attention effect reinterpreted. *Acta Psychologica, 4,* 313–329.

Näätänen, R., Paavilainen, P., Tiitinen, H., Jiang, D., & Alho, K. (1993). Attention and mismatch negativity. *Psychophysiology, 30,* 436–450.

Neville, H. J., Coffey, S. A., Holcomb, P. J., & Tallal, P. (1993). The neurobiology of sensory and language processing in language-impaired children. *Journal of Cognitive Neuroscience, 5,* 235–253.

Novick, B., Vaughan, H. G., Kurtzberg, D., & Simon, R. (1980). An electrophysiological indication of auditory processing defects in autism. *Psychiatric Research, 3,* 107–115.

Ollo, C., & Squires, N. (1982). Event related potentials in learning disabilities. In R. Q. Cracco & I. Bodis Wollner (Eds.), *Evoked potentials: Frontiers of neuroscience* (Vol. 3, pp. 475–512). New York: Liss.

Ortiz, T., Exposito, F. J., Miguel, F., Martin-Loeches, M., & Rubia, F. J. (1992). Brain mapping in dysphonemic dyslexia: In resting and phonemic discrimination conditions. *Brain and Language, 42,* 270–285.

Petersén, I., Sellden, U., & Eeg-Olofsson, O. (1975). The evolution of the EEG in normal children and adolescents from 1 to 21 years. *Handbook of Electroencephalography and Clinical Neurophysiology, 6B,* 31–68.

Posner, M. (1978). *Chronometric explorations of mind.* Hillsdale, NJ: Erlbaum.

Preston, M. S., Guthrie, J. T., & Childs, B. (1974). Visual evoked responses in normal and disabled readers. *Psychophysiology, 11,* 452–457.

Prichep, L., Sutton, S., & Hakerem, G. (1976). Evoked potentials in hyperkinetic and normal children under certainty and uncertainty: A placebo and methylphenidate study. *Psychophysiology, 13,* 419–428.

Rayner, K., & Pollatsek, A. (1989). *The psychology of reading.* Englewood Cliffs, NJ: Prentice–Hall.

Rodríguez, M., Harmony, T., Bernal, J., Yáñez, G., Silva, J., Fernández, T., Galán, L., Rodríguez, H., Marosi, E., Guerrero, V., & Reyes, A. (1994). N400 in poor readers. *7th International Congress of Psychophysiology,* Thessaloniki, Greece.

Rosemblum, S. M., Arick, J. R., King, D. A., Stubbs, E. G., Young, N. B., & Pelson, R. O. (1980). Auditory brainstem evoked responses in autistic children. *Journal of autism and developmental disorders, 10,* 215–225.

Rugg, M., & Doyle, M. (1992). Event-related potentials and recognition memory for low- and high-frequency words. *Journal of Cognitive Neuroscience, 4,* 69–79.

Rumsey, J. M., Grimes, A. M., Pikus, A. M., Duara, R., & Ismond, D. R. (1984). Auditory brainstem responses in pervasive developmental disorders. *Biological Psychiatry, 19,* 1403–1418.

Rutter, M. (1978). Prevalence and types of dyslexia. In A. L. Benton & D. Pearl (Eds.), *Dyslexia: An appraisal of current knowledge.* London: Oxford University Press.

Saletu, B., Saletu, M., Simeon, J., Viamontes, G., & Itil, T. M. (1975). Comparative symptomatological and evoked potential studies with d-amphetamine, thioridazine and placebo in hyperkinetic children. *Biological Psychiatry, 10,* 253–275.

Satterfield, J. H., Schell, A. M., & Nicholas, T. (1994). Preferential neural processing of attended stimuli in attention-deficit hyperactivity disorder and normal boys. *Psychophysiology, 31,* 1–10.

Satterfield, J. H., Schell, A. M., Nicholas, T., & Backs, R. W. (1988). Topographic study of auditory event-related potentials in normal boys and boys with attention-deficit disorder with hyperactivity. *Psychophysiology, 25,* 591–606.

Satz, P., Taylor, H. G., Friel, J., & Fletcher, J. M. (1978). Some developmental and predictive precursors of reading disabilities: A six year follow-up. In A. L. Benton & D. Pearl (Eds.), *Dyslexia: An appraisal of current knowledge.* London: Oxford University Press.

Schwab, R. S. (1939). A method of measuring consciousness in petit-mal epilepsy. *Journal of Nervous and Mental Disorders, 89,* 690–691.

Silva, J., Harmony, T., Bernal, J., Fernández, T., Rodríguez, M., Reyes, A., Marosi, E., Yañez, G., Guerrero, V., Rodríguez, H., & Rodríguez, M. (1995). Comparación entre las habilidades en la lectura de dos grupos con diferente desempeño académico. *Revista Latina de Pensamiento y Lenguaje, 3*(1), 65–82.

Skoff, B. F., Mirsky, A. F., & Turner, D. (1980). Prolonged brain-stem transmission time in autism. *Psychiatric Research, 2,* 157–166.

Sohmer, H., & Student, M. (1978). Auditory nerve and brain stem evoked response in normal, autistic, minimal brain dysfunction and psychomotor retarded children. *Electroencephalography and Clinical Neurophysiology, 44,* 380–388.

Solan, H. A., Sutija, V. G., Ficarra, A., & Wurst, S. A. (1990). Binocular advantage and visual processing in dyslexic and control children measured by visual evoked potentials. *Optometry and Vision Science, 67,* 105–110.

Spear-Swerling, L., & Sternberg, R. J. (1994). The road not taken: An integrative theoretical model of reading disability. *Journal of Learning Disabilities, 27,* 91–122.

Stanovich, K. E. (1988). Explaining the differences between the dyslexic and the garden-variety poor reader: The phonological-core variable-difference model. *Journal of Learning Disabilities, 21,* 590–604.

Stelmack, R., Saxe, B. J., Noldy-Cullum, N., Campbell, K. B., & Armitage, R. (1989). Recognition memory for words and event-related potentials: A comparison of normal and disabled readers. *Journal of Clinical and Experimental Psychology, 10,* 185–200.

Tallal, P. (1987). *Developmental language disorders.* Interagency Committee on learning disabilities—Report to the U. S. Congress.

Tallal, P., Galaburda, A. M., Llinás, R. R., & von Euler, C. (Eds.). (1993). *Temporal information processing in the nervous system: Special reference to dyslexia and dysphasia* (Annals of New York Academy of Sciences, vol. 62). New York: New York Academy of Sciences.

Tallal, P., Miller, S., & Fitch, R. S. (1993). Neurobiological basis of speech: A case for the preeminence of temporal processing. In P. Tallal, A. M. Galaburda, R. R. Llinás, & C. von Euler (Eds.), *Temporal information processing in the nervous system: Special reference to dyslexia and dysphasia* (Annals of the New York Academy of Sciences, vol. 62, pp. 27–47). New York: New York Academy of Sciences.

Taylor, M. J., & Keenan, N. K. (1990). Event related potentials to visual and language stimuli in normal and dyslexic children. *Psychophysiology, 27,* 318–327.

Thatcher, R. W., Krause, P. J., & Hrybyk, M. (1986). Cortico-cortical associations and EEG coherence: A two-compartmental model. *Electroencephalography and Clinical Neurophysiology, 64,* 13–145.

Torgesen, J. K. (1988). Studies of children with learning disabilities who perform poorly on memory span task. *Journal of Learning Disabilities, 18,* 350–357.

Tucker, D. M., & Williamson, P. A. (1984). Asymmetric neural control systems and human self regulation. *Psychological Review, 91,* 185–215.

Vellutino, F. R. (1983). Childhood dyslexia: A language disorder. In H. R. Myklebust (Ed.), *Progress in learning disabilities* (Vol. V, pp. 135–176). New York: Grune & Stratton.

Walter, G. W. (1959). Intrinsic rhythms of the brain. In J. Field (Ed.), *Handbook of physiology: Sec. I* (pp. 279–298). Washington, DC: American Physiological Society.

Yingling, C. D., Fein, G., Galin, D., Peltzman, D., & Davenport, L. (1986). Neurometrics does not detect "pure" dyslexics. *Electroencephalography and Clinical Neurophysiology, 63,* 426–430.

Zametkin, A. J., Nordahl, T. E., Gross, M., King, C. A., Semple, W. E., Rumsey, J., Hamberger, M. S., & Cohen, R. M. (1990). Cerebral glucose metabolism in adults with hyperactivity of childhood onset. *New England Journal of Medicine, 323,* 1361–1366.

19

Neuropsychological Assessment of Spanish-Speaking Children and Youth

ANTONIO E. PUENTE, MARIA SOL MORA, AND
JUAN MANUEL MUNOZ-CESPEDES

Introduction

Manolito had been crying since the day the social service department placed him in the second grade. He had been born about 8 years earlier in Central America in a one-room hut with no flooring, electricity, or running water. After a complicated labor of 3 days, he was "black and blue all over" and began to cry only several days after delivery. Although he had been "slow," he adapted well to life in the rural village; well, that is, until his parents decided to pursue a "better" life in the United States. After several years of migrating from one state to another and from one labor camp to another, his parents had settled for several months in a county with an aggressive social service department. As a consequence, he was placed in a school for the first time. Not knowing English, Manolito was referred to a school psychologist for testing in English. The diagnosis that was reached by this professional was retardation, probably organically caused by such factors as the delivery. Special education classes were the next stop for this maladapted child. Manolito's case is not only not unusual but occurring with

increasing frequency. This chapter addresses some of the major issues in the neuropsychological assessment of children such as Manolito.

The Hispanic population of the United States is one of the fastest growing segments of this nation. Terman (1916), in his early work on intelligence, had noticed not only the large number of Hispanics but their fertility rates as well. Combined with the increasing immigration of Central and South Americans to the United States, present Hispanic Americans are poised to become the largest ethnic-minority group in the United States by the early part of the 21st century.

A second issue is that of the complexity of the Hispanic person. Whereas one could argue that African Americans are different, if nothing else because of racial background (see Helms, 1992), most African Americans do speak and understand English, and their recent ancestors can be traced for several generations to the United States. The opposite is true for Hispanics. Indeed, most Hispanics have immigrated recently to the United States. Specifically, they represent one of the most recent waves of immigration to this country. Thus, the issue of being a minority is compounded with unusual isolation from linguistic and cultural perspectives.

Review of ethnic-minority research in the United States has traditionally focused on the plight of the African American. The seminal works of Jones (1994) and Cross (1994) stand as excellent examples of these scholarly efforts. Further, whenever ethnic minorities have traditionally been

ANTONIO E. PUENTE • Department of Psychology, University of North Carolina at Wilmington, Wilmington, North Carolina 28406.   MARIA SOL MORA • University of North Carolina at Wilmington, Wilmington, North Carolina 28406; and Universidad de San Francisco, Quito, Ecuador. JUAN MANUEL MUNOZ-CESPEDES • Departmento de Psicologia Basica (Procesos Cognitivas), Universidad Compluterse de Madrid, 28223 Madrid, Spain.

considered in research paradigms, the operational definitions of ethnic minorities have been African American. There is no question that more knowledge and sensitivity are needed to understand African Americans. However, it is extremely important to realize that ethnic minorities mean just that, ethnic minorities. Unfortunately, relatively little research has been directed to understanding all underrepresented groups, especially the largest and youngest of all U.S. ethnic groups, Hispanics.

A fourth issue is that of scientifically (not politically) correct neuropsychology. At the very least, neuropsychologists should be concerned about these issues from an ethical standpoint. The American Psychological Association ethical and testing standards dictate that sociocultural variables must be explicitly considered when assessing individuals from different cultures. Also, a neuropsychology of North Americans, or for that matter Anglo-Saxons, is a neuropsychology with serious limitations. For example, if broad-based sampling from all segments of the population to be understood is a requirement for valid test construction and interpretation, then understanding people from all backgrounds must be a prerequisite. Finally, the brain is not immune to variables such as education, culture, and language. Indeed, too little is known about the effects of these critical sociocultural variables. Numerous authors (e.g., Anastasi, 1976; Ardila, Roselli, & Puente, 1994; Myers, Echemendia, & Trimble, 1991; Puente, 1990) have addressed these issues. Unfortunately, these concerns have not become standard in neuropsychological knowledge, theory, and practice.

The purpose of this chapter is to add to the breadth and scope of this important volume by focusing on the neuropsychological assessment of Hispanic children and youth. First, these children represent the largest growing segment of ethnic minorities in the United States (Statistical Abstract, 1995). Second, unlike some other minority groups (e.g., African Americans), they possess not only a different sociocultural background but also different communication strategies and language (e.g., Dupont, Ardila, Roselli, & Puente, 1992). Third, most of the research traditionally has focused on African Americans and, hence, this group has been less well understood. Finally, in understanding the demands of this unique situation, neuropsychologists will be able to better address the unique aspects of nonbiological (e.g., culture) variables in clinical neuropsychology and brain function (e.g., Puente & McCaffrey, 1992).

Psychosocial Variables

There is much more to neuropsychology than neurological concerns. In Puente and McCaffrey's (1992) volume and in the works of Ardila (1995), among others, the importance of nonbiological, or sociocultural concerns, has been raised. This section provides a background and rationale for the inclusion of these variables.

Demographic Characteristics

The United States is a diverse country populated by an unprecedented variety of ethnic and racial groups. For example, in 1994, over 8% of the population was born outside the country, a level matched only during the early immigration into the country during the first part of this century (Statistical Abstract, 1995). Of those emigrating to the United States, a larger group (especially relative to the first part of this century) comes from Spanish-speaking countries.

At the very least, this group should be studied and understood simply because of their existence, especially as they comprise a large and growing segment of the population. In 1990, the United States Bureau of the Census estimated that there were 22.4 million Hispanics in this country. Further, the population is increasing at such a rapid rate that Hispanics will surpass African Americans as the largest group of ethnic minorities by the year 2025 (Statistical Abstract, 1995). Interestingly, worldwide there are almost as many Spanish speakers as English speakers. According to the World Population Data Sheet (1986–1990), there were 300 million Spanish speakers and 350 million English speakers. Also, the United States contains the fifth largest group of Spanish speakers in this world. This is particularly interesting in light of recent Congressional attempts to make English the official language of the United States.

Future projections reflect even more startling statistics. Hispanics are extremely fertile; they tend to be younger and more family oriented, relative to other ethnic groups (including Anglo-Saxons). As an illustration of how complex this problem might become, by 1992, over half of those under the age of 30 living in the Southwest United States were Hispanic (Statistical Abstract, 1995).

Cultural Variables

Linguistic equivalence has generated only minimal attention where Hispanic children are concerned. It should be obvious that equivalence cannot exist unless precepts of a construct are communicated in a language that is equally comprehensible to both groups. Several studies (Bernal, 1990; Cauce & Jacobson, 1980; Figueroa, 1983; Helms, 1992) have reported that language is a major contributing factor in performance on cognitive ability tests and that some items do not, in fact, have the same linguistic meaning across ethnic groups.

Language usage differs according to the cultural and subcultural background and strongly correlates with the subject's educational level. Often test instructions are given in "formal" language. Hispanic children and youth with limited education find it very difficult to follow such specific and rigid instructions (Ardila, 1995).

The reader is directed to works by Puente and colleagues for additional information regarding the importance of this particular variable (e.g., Ardila, Roselli, & Puente, 1994; Dupont *et al.,* 1992; Perez-Arce & Puente, 1996) in understanding how the Spanish language mediates and affects neuropsychological assessment.

Culture is the other defining variable in this equation. Although there is no universally accepted definition of culture in U.S. psychology, the term refers to learned or acquired behaviors and to traits that are attributable to the socialization experiences resulting from membership in a particular system or institution within a society. Sue and Sue (1990), for example, have suggested that culture "consists of all those things that people have learned to do, believe, value, and enjoin their history. It is the totality of ideas, beliefs, skills, tools, customs and institutions into which each member of a society is born."

Culture prescribes what should be learned and at what age that behavior or knowledge should be learned. Consequently, different cultural environments lead to the development of different patterns of abilities (Harris, 1990; Jones, 1991). Cultural and ecological variables play a role in developing different cognitive styles (Berry, 1979). Further, cultures cannot easily be equated. Cultural equivalence in testing becomes a difficult concept to integrate successfully because some cognitive abilities do not operate similarly for different ethnic groups.

Helms (1992) has provided an interesting cognitive perspective of what it means to be African American. Unfortunately, such a concise description has not been provided for Hispanics. The following should be considered an initial view of cultural issues especially relevant to the Hispanic child and youth.

The obvious demands of the Spanish language quickly segregate the individual from the larger majority group culture. Together with the language barrier come other issues including but not limited to: family values, social interactions, religion, perspective of time, and overall approach to problem-solving. With regard to family values, Hispanics tend to have more intact families than other ethnic groups. Such families tend to reproduce more than average and the nuclear family is usually composed of both parents as well as other siblings. The father is often the symbolic head with the mother being the spiritual, emotional, and nurturing leader. It would not be unusual for the father to appear as omnipotent but in reality the mother would be highly responsible for many of the decisions. Further, family is intended to mean more than the simple nuclear family often referred to in psychological research. This social unit implies aunts, uncles, and cousins (first and second level), with close family friends often being given titles such as "uncle" or "cousin." Independence is replaced with cooperation and family name, pride, and tradition are much more important than singular and material achievement.

Hispanics, in general, and Hispanic children and youth, in particular, are highly social beings. They appreciate the value of friends, social groups, and interactions. They tend to be less competitive across all situations and socioeconomic levels relative to Anglo-Saxon counterparts (Kagan, 1984). Cooperation and long-range relationships and social impressions are often more valued than individual achievement. Further, socialization, a task often given to the schools and peers in the United States, is primarily a task of the extended family (Kagan, 1984).

Even though the standard religious profile of Hispanics is changing, religion remains an influential variable in Hispanic life. One can safely argue that most Hispanics are Catholic but one would have greater confidence in emphasizing spirituality in this group when compared with any other ethnic or majority group. Organized religion, possibly because of the social aspect, is highly popular and similarly influential. For example, major developmental markers are actually celebrated as part of the "sacraments" of the Catholic faith. A child's baptism is the first formal exposure of that child to society. And, of course, this is a cause for major social celebration.

"Mañana" is the stereotypical outcome of questions as to when a problem will be solved. While siestas and mañanas are not typical of Hispanic behavior, time has less importance to the Hispanic. As long as it "gets done," it really does not matter when it gets done. Long-range goals are more focused on a variety of factors, including familial and social ones, and time constraints are less significant a role. People's feelings, social impression formation, and related factors are clearly more a motivating force than how quickly one can reach a measurable and replicable goal. In Hispanic culture, one works to live whereas it might be said in the Anglo culture one lives to work. Finally, although again not just typical of Hispanics, this ethnic group tends to be less educated. This is the case especially for recent immigrants who often lack standard and lengthy educational attainment. Thus, basic literacy skills such as reading, writing, and mathematics are often poorly developed. However, it is important to emphasize that limited education does not imply limited intelligence. Perez-Arce and Puente (1996) argue that adaptive strategies used by Hispanic immigrants would suggest that at least an adequate level of intelligence is exemplified by most immigrants. Literacy skills are not synonymous, although correlated, with successful living.

Immigration and Acculturation

As indicated earlier, almost 10% of the current population of the United States are first-generation immigrants. Of these, the largest segment is not of European ancestry (as was the case during the last immigration boom in the early part of this century). Instead, most immigrants are from south of this country and, thus, are native Spanish speakers.

As early as 1935, the process of adapting psychologically to a new culture was studied by Klineberg, who found that socioeconomic status, language, amount of schooling, and motivation all influenced black children's test performance. Olmedo (1981) suggested that psychological and educational testing of members of linguistic minority groups should take into account the diverse social, political, and economic realities that these groups face. Similarly, Bernal (1977) stated that there is "something" relative to testing situations and tests that affects performance. This "something" included language proficiency, socioeconomic status, motivations, readiness, and understanding of the majority group norms. Barona and Pfeiffer (1992) have suggested that exposure to Anglo-Saxon culture may account for different test scores.

This exposure is probably related to a wide variety of factors including bilingualism, English language proficiency, and actual test-taking expertise. Darcy (1963) stated that bilingualism is more than just knowing two languages, it involves knowing two cultures. Knight and Kagan (1977) reported that with regard to social motivation, children from the United States tended to be focused more on rivalry and superiority when compared with Mexican-American children. In contrast, second-generation Mexican-American children focused more on altruism and equality. Mexican-American children did not view social motivation in a similar fashion as Anglo-Saxon children until the third generation. In summary, it is important to be careful to isolate degree of acculturation from the actual variable in question (e.g., memory) whenever possible. One possible way to accomplish this might be to measure the degree of acculturation. For example, Barona and Miller (1994) have published a brief acculturation scale for use with Hispanic youth.

Educational Attainment

Frequently, educational and cultural variables are not clearly distinguished and are often attributed to cultural or ethnic factors. Whereas test performance between Anglo-Saxon children and other ethnic groups has been readily reported (Reynolds & Brown, 1990; Taylor & Stephen; 1991; Taylor & Ziegler, 1987), such differences may simply be the result of different educational levels. It is often assumed that number of years of schooling are equal, an assumption that carries as its basis clear misunderstanding of different cultural achievements. For example, a college education in Spain typically equals a master's degree in the United States. Further, liberal education, the norm in the United States, is not the norm in other countries. Finally, even if grades could be considered equivalent (e.g., that 9 years of schooling means the same thing in both countries), different subjects are stressed at different times, often in different ways. Hence, educational equivalence between North American and Hispanic educational systems may be a misinterpretation.

Socioeconomic Variables

Investigators and clinicians have often been guilty of either ignoring social class or focusing excessively on the lower socioeconomic stratum when Hispanic test responses are examined. Although it is true that a greater percentage of Hispanic children and youth are poor, it is also true that there is greater socioeconomic variability among Hispanics (Statistical Abstract, 1995). Ardila, Roselli, and Ostrosky (1992) have reviewed the literature on socioeconomic factors and concluded that low socioeconomic status (SES) affects neuropsychological performance. Ardila *et al.* (1994), whose book outlined research on neuropsychological assessment of Spanish speakers, found that non-brain-damaged individuals of lower SES often mimic the performance of highly educated and brain-damaged individuals.

Socioeconomic class might be one of the most uncontrolled variables in research with Hispanics. Some studies have already shown that low SES correlates with lower IQ scores and neuropsychological function (Roselli, 1993; Roselli & Ardila, 1990, 1993; Sandoval, Zimmerman, & Woo-Sam, 1983). In her early and seminal review of the intellectual literature, Darcy (1963) found that when SES was controlled, there were no measurable differences between Hispanic and Anglo-Saxon individuals. Finally, most research with Hispanics has typically used lower SES and primarily from the southwestern United States. Such limitations render prior conclusions of limited generalizability.

Methodological Considerations

Although some data exist outlining neuropsychological performance of Hispanic children and youth, much of the existing literature is plagued with methodological problems. This section attempts to address some of the more critical considerations.

Race and Ethnicity

An important principle underlying neuropsychological assessment of Hispanic children is that of individual variability. One important distinction is that of race and ethnicity. Palmer, Olivarez, Wilson, and Fordyce (1989), Reschly (1978), and Sandoval and Whelan-Mille (1980) have all addressed the issue of bias or prejudice against minority groups. However, in all cases race and ethnicity are not defined. Indeed, in most instances, race and ethnicity are used in similar contexts, including in the methodology. Keachnie (1983) has suggested that race is a basic biological distinction between groups based on physical attributes such as color of skin. Most ethnologists and cross-cultural psychologists

(Brislin, 1988) believe that three major races exist: Caucasian (from the Caucus mountains in Eastern Europe), Negroids (from central Africa), and Mongoloid (from northern China). The latter group is often further subdivided into Asian and American.

Culture is a broader concept that is more focused on behavior (Sue, 1983). Patterns of behavior are fundamentally based on basic beliefs (e.g., life and afterlife) that dictate economic, religious, psychological, and related conduct (Spiro, 1988). It is important to note that cultural beliefs are rarely questioned as they tend to set basic, long-held beliefs about how to conduct oneself, especially in social settings.

Ethnicity could be considered a subset of culture. As with culture it is a concept primarily focusing on behavior although it can include some anatomical variables. Nationality, religion, values, and other psychological and personal constructs are more well defined. For example, each culture (e.g., Western) has numerous ethnic groups (e.g., Jews, Hispanics). Hispanics represent one of the major ethnic groups of the Western culture. However, Hispanics also represent all three races. Further, most Hispanics are of Caucasian ancestry followed by Mongoloid and finally Negroid. It is important to note that Hispanics have long bred interracially in the Caribbean where Caucasian and Negroid races have mixed much like in Central America where the Caucasian and the Mongoloid (American Indian Incas) races have interbred. Thus, while it may be easy to identify native Spanish speakers as "Western" and of the "Hispanic" ethnic group, determining racial background may be much harder. Further, one might speculate that in this case, ethnicity (i.e., Hispanic) may be more of a salient variable in helping predict behavior than race (e.g., Caucasian).

Heterogeneity of Hispanics

Hispanics represent a highly diverse group, maybe more than any other Western-based ethnic group. According to the United States Bureau of the Census (1995), the following subgroups could be classified as depicting Hispanics (in alphabetical order): Cuban, Mexican/Mexican-American/Chicano, Puerto Rican, Hispanic Latin American (e.g., Panamanian, Peruvian, Venezuelan, Ecuadorian, Guatemalan), Spaniard (origin from Spain). Thus, there appear to be five major Hispanic groups, two from the Caribbean, two from Central/South America, and the rest (presumably from

Spain). Assuming that this is an adequate breakdown of Hispanics in the Americas (because similar breakdowns would not apply to Hispanics in Spain; for example, in Spain gypsies would represent one ethnic group), Hispanics represent a very large geographical region. This wide representation may, in turn, have behavioral ramifications.

Some studies have shown that Hispanics do not behave in the same way and that they test differently according to subethnic classification (Laosa, 1975, 1984). Padilla and Ruiz (1973) have suggested that Mexican Americans are a mixture of Spanish and Indian, Puerto Ricans a mixture of Spanish and African, and other Hispanic populations (e.g., Argentineans have more a European origin than anything else).

Sampling and Stratifying

Because of the complexities of defining the different subgroups of Hispanics and the salient variables of socioeconomic and educational variables affecting neuropsychological performance, it would seem that sampling this particular ethnic group would be significantly more difficult than for any other ethnic or majority group.

An obvious starting point would be to carefully stratify according to the five basic subgroups previously identified (Cuban, Mexican/Mexican-American/Chicano, Puerto Rican, Hispanic Latin American, and Spaniard). For some validation studies, it should be remembered that these groups are differentially represented in the population in terms of several issues, primarily total number and geographic representation. Second, careful stratification should be completed based on educational attainment of the subjects. An alternative stratification approach might be to group according to parental educational attainment. Finally, socioeconomic stratification might also be valuable. This might be assessed by a global analysis such as family income (potentially difficult with Hispanics) or according to parental job classification (e.g., managerial, professional; see Barona, Reynolds, & Chastain, 1984, for further information).

One potential manner of stratifying might be to have numerous cells in a 3×3 design where one variable is Hispanic subgroup (e.g., Cuban), educational attainment (e.g., less than grade five), and according to socioeconomic level (e.g., low; the Barona and Reynolds's system). Using parental educational attainment as a marker, children could be grouped into five different categories: grammar school, middle school, high school, college, postgraduate/professional. Of course, if children are used (instead of parents), possibly actual grade attainment would be most accurate. Using the Barona and Reynolds's formula for estimating premorbid intellectual functioning, five groups would be used: unskilled, semiskilled, managerial, professional, and other. Thus, the number of cells in a standardization sample might idealistically reflect a $5 \times 5 \times 5$ design further stratified according to age.

Equivalence

There has been a general failure to develop standards to judge the equivalence of translations across languages or cultures. It is not unusual to have difficulty and even not to find an exact equivalence from one language and culture to another. Bracken and Barona (1991) have addressed this problem and indicated that equivalence is difficult for the following reasons: (1) Test directions are frequently too technical to allow for easy translation; (2) translations are rarely sufficiently perfected to provide equivalent meanings across languages; (3) psychological constructs assessed by translated tests are not universal; (4) context assessed might not be universal; (5) test-taking behaviors and orientation vary across cultures; and (6) there has been a general failure to develop standards to judge equivalence across cultures.

As early as 1934, Sanchez had pointed out that exact equivalence might be impossible. Since that time others have provide empirical evidence to support this contention. For example, Prewitt-Diaz, Rodriguez, and Rivera (1986) studied the predictive validity of the Spanish translation of the Wechsler Intelligence Scale for Children-Revised and the Escala de Inteligencia de Wechsler Para Niños-Revisada. They reported on two studies done in Puerto Rico. The first study was completed with 51 upper elementary school children in Puerto Rico and the Spanish version seemed to be a useful instrument whereas in a bilingual group of 80 students in Connecticut, only the Spanish version was an appropriate predictor for academic achievement.

In another study using Wechsler tests, this time the Spanish and English versions of the Wechsler Adult Intelligence Scale, both versions were administered to a matched sample of English and Spanish speakers as well as bilingual Latinas. In both cases, the Spanish version yielded significantly higher scores. Several researchers, including Velazquez and Callahan (1992) and Malgady,

Rogler, and Costantino (1987), have provided some recommendations to facilitate the production of quality test translations. These include: (1) Test items should consist of simple sentences and pronouns should be avoided; (2) test items should not contain metaphors or colloquialism; (3) the subjunctive mood and passive tense should be avoided in both items and directions.

In addition, phonological and grammatical concerns should also be addressed. Tense and gender are more precisely employed in Spanish than in English. Also, the use of double negatives, common in the English language, should be avoided. In the Luria–Nebraska, a heavily language-based neuropsychological test, certain phonological sounds cannot be directly translated. For example, s-t-o-n-e combines the s and the t, which does not occur in Spanish. Some proverbs, such as "green thumb," simply do not have an equivalent translation. Hence, to simply translate a test without addressing these concerns would produce an invalid test (Candell & Hulin, 1986).

Assessment Approaches

The Spanish-speaking child with a potential brain injury poses more demands than many clinicians are exposed to on a regular basis. Beyond the usual demands of developmental and emotional problems associated with the evaluation of a younger person come a plethora of additional complications. This section, which assumes that the clinician will be aware of the typical demands of a neuropsychological evaluation of children and youth, addresses the additional variables that require special attention.

Family Involvement

Considering the family structure of Hispanics, a child might be viewed more like an extension of the parents than a separate individual. Children are given special status and protection in the Hispanic culture. Turning over a child to a complete stranger, from another cultural and linguistic background, for a period of several hours and possibly over several days is an unusually high demand for the parents. Considering further that the outcome of the evaluation may have a determination not only on the child's future but also on the family's social and financial status makes the evaluation situation even more complex and anxiety provoking.

Hence, family involvement is a must for a successful neuropsychological evaluation. First, education of the rationale and procedures of the evaluation should be undertaken with the parents in the most diplomatic manner possible. Relevance to the future of the child's welfare must be stressed. Care must also be taken to assure the parents of the safety and concern that the test administrator will exhibit on behalf of the child. Permission and generalized feedback should be requested and provided to the parents intermittently as a means of establishing and continuing to build rapport. The parents will provide official sanction and approval for both the evaluation and continued rapport. Once the evaluation is over, care must be taken to provide courteous and diplomatic feedback. Conscious attention to extensive family, cultural, and religious issues must be considered for the evaluation results to have meaning for the child and his or her family.

Translations

When an Anglo-Saxon neuropsychologist is posed with the demands of evaluating a Spanish-speaking child, one of the major hurdles will be in obtaining translated tests. Earlier in this chapter, the issue of test equivalence was discussed. Clearly, it is difficult to equate linguistic, cognitive, and cultural knowledge. Straightforward translations are often incorrect and may introduce as much error as evaluating the child in a nonnative language. A test needs not only to be translated into Spanish but, if at all possible, back-translated into English.

Assuming the test is adequately translated, next comes the question of whether bias exists. Sandoval (1989) suggested that there are two ways to generally determine whether bias exists: external and internal criterion. Bias might be occurring if the test is related to an external criterion at different levels for both the majority and minority groups. In contrast, internal criterion is determined if the two groups, majority and minority, respond to a test in similar fashion. Parameters such as means, standard deviations, reliability coefficient, standard errors, and internal factor structure are different. The importance is to make as certain as possible that the two tests being used are closely matched. If not, care must then be taken to understand and make known those differences.

Further, even if a translation is completed, several other issues remain that need to be addressed. Most translations, even if done correctly, fail to bring to the scientific enterprise adequate norms.

Few translations report corresponding normative data. Mostly Hispanic children are compared with normative data from majority populations. The studies that do report norms (e.g., Peabody) use small samples and inadequate sampling procedures. To date, no study has been published using norms for Spanish speakers residing in separate countries with age and education variables.

Thus, it is not uncommon for a translated test to be used with non-"translated" norms. This mixture is perplexing if not unethical. To complicate matters further, translations also violate copyright laws. Test publishers hold the English and any other language translation of that test. Thus, psychologists using unofficial translations are probably violating copyright laws as well.

Translators

The issue of translators is also critical. Often, the only perceived requirement is simply to have somebody translate the instrument from English to Spanish and the response back to English. Translators are often a more bilingual family member or a paraprofessional from some other department who has a working knowledge of both languages. However, the issue of bilingualism is a difficult one. Dupont, Ardila, Roselli, and Puente (1992) have argued that there are no true bilinguals. Harris, Cullum, and Puente (1995) have published important data on this issue. Segovia-Price and Cuellar (1981) have also reported that symptomatology was reported differently when Hispanics were questioned about their symptoms in Spanish versus in English. Finally, Smart and Smart (1995) have suggested that bilingualism is often associated with "the culture of poverty and academic failure" whereas monolingualism, especially English, is seen as a sign of success in education, commerce, and personal areas.

Probably the most common type of translator is a family member. When family members are used, the complex and dynamic family system is temporarily disrupted. Further, specific and personal emotional issues may pose unusual demands on that situation resulting in clients not revealing personal and potentially disruptive information to the family member. This may particularly arise when the translator does not match the patient in two specific demographic factors, namely, age and gender (Smart & Smart, 1995).

There is growing evidence that training reduces errors in the translation process (Brislin, 1988). This research has fostered the following recommendations by Smart and Smart (1995) for using translators or interpreters:

1. Provide the service in the client's native language.
2. Training should occur with bilingual and bicultural professionals.
3. Bilingual professionals should help train monolingual professionals in the use of interpreters.
4. Translators should assist as cultural consultants.
5. Special attention should be paid to cross-gender situations.
6. Translators and interpreters should become familiar with the type of discipline involved.
7. The introduction of interpreters or translators will probably alter the patient–professional relationship.

Implied in these recommendations are several highly critical issues. Whenever possible the service should be provided by a person knowledgeable in the client's native language and culture. Second, there is more to translating than language. All things being equal, bilingual and bicultural translators are significantly better than either alone. Age and gender issues are critical and some matching to that effect would be valuable. Finally, whenever possible, avoid family members as the translators.

Particularly interesting is the result of a survey by Echemendia, Congett, Harris, Diaz, and Puente (in press). In that study, the authors reported that a large percentage of respondents performed neuropsychological evaluations on Hispanic clients. However, of those, only a small percentage were bilingual. These data strongly suggest that neuropsychologists are not following the guidelines previously discussed.

Premorbid Estimates

Estimating premorbid levels of functioning is an important component of a neuropsychological evaluation. Generally, there are two accepted ways of approaching this problem. First, educational records are obtained and prior educational testing is reviewed. Percentile scores for standardized tests such as the California Achievement Test are used along with actual IQ test scores. Unfortunately, a significant portion of the children being tested by design are not native English speakers and these tests are not given in Spanish. Hence, the validity of those scores is highly variable. Further, these tests are not administered in Latin America and Spain. Thus, such scores are not available if the child is a recent immigrant. The same logic could be used for actual academic grades (e.g., grade point average). Thus, grades alone may not be an adequate variable in predicting premorbid functioning. Also, school records are often extremely difficult to obtain if the client attended school outside the United States.

Considering these complications, an alternative approach might help reduce bias. Using regression formulas (such as the Barona and Reynolds's one) might help reduce the potential misestimation. These formulas use variables such as socio-standing, geographic location, and education to estimate premorbid function. Unfortunately, such formulas have not been explored with people living in other countries and their reliability might be weak when applying such statistical methods.

Interviewing Strategies

Assuming that standard developmental interviewing strategies are applied, the neuropsychologist is faced with the additional obstacle of dealing with a child with language, cultural, and related barriers. Obviously the issues previously discussed in this chapter play a role in the interview process. For example, personal information is less likely to be shared when family members act as the translator. However, it is particularly important to note that the role of the Spanish child and youth is often different than that of the Anglo-Saxon child. Independence, self-assurance, and a sense of curiosity are often fostered qualities in Anglo children, especially middle class. Such attributes are not shared by the Hispanic child and thus the validity of data generated by a strained interview process would be highly variable. Puente (1990) has suggested that interviewing minority group members may require more time than usual. With Hispanic children, interviews spanning 50 to 100% more time would not seem unreasonable. A step of major importance is to focus on rapport building and communication prior to any data gathering. Otherwise the information obtained will result in incomplete or inaccurate data.

Intellectual Assessment

It is well known that intellectual assessment is the most common aspect of both psychological and neuropsychological testing (e.g., Putnam &

DeLuca, 1990). Thus, specific attention to this type of testing is warranted. Perez-Arce and Puente (1996) have provided an overview of intellectual assessment of Hispanics. They report that the traditional measures of the Wechsler Intelligence Scales and the Stanford–Binet have been used more often than any other measures. However, as Kaufman (1979) and others have suggested, standard interpretation of these tests with Hispanic children appears inappropriate.

Numerous researchers (e.g., Kaufman, 1990) have reported that Hispanic children tend to do better on performance measures than verbal ones. Such findings do not seem surprising. First, verbal tests are more loaded on educational and verbal measures, both variables that seem to be generally lower in Hispanic children. Second, Hispanic children, especially immigrants from Central America, have been exposed to performance activities (e.g., visuospatial tasks) probably more frequently than verbal ones in general, even when compared with Anglo-Saxon children.

There is ample evidence, however, that the WISC-R may be generally measuring the same things for different cultural groups. Reschly (1978) compared the factor structures of the WISC-R for Anglo, black, Chicano, and Native American children. The results showed high similarity among groups in terms of the proportion of variance accounted for by a general factor, intelligence. Such results have suggested that the usual interpretation of the Full-Scale IQ as an index of general intelligence appears appropriate for all groups tested. When exploring item difficulty, Sandoval and Whelan-Mille (1980) presented a similar pattern. Item difficulty did not vary among Anglo-American, African-American, and Mexican-American children. Extending these findings to a learning-disabled group, Whitworth (1988) reported that any differences between Anglo and Hispanic learning-disabled children could be explained by limited language proficiency alone.

"Culture"-free intelligence tests, such as the Raven, present an alternative to standard measurement of intellectual abilities. Laosa (1984) examined the performances on various intellectual functions by children from Chicano and non-Chicano white families of diverse home language backgrounds and family sizes. Results revealed ethnic group differences in both the absolute level of performance and the configuration of performance across various ability areas. These ethnic group differences were explained in terms of a combination of effects associated with different cultural backgrounds, where low income level and low educational attainment of the parent accounted for the largest percentage of the variance noted in these findings. Interestingly, the sample of children used for the study was young, ages 2 to 6. Thus, differences in test performance may be formed or imprinted at an extremely young age. Further, factors outside of the child's actual intellectual level, such as parental success, may be extremely critical in determining eventual intellectual performance.

Other Neurocognitive Measures

Two major points need to be considered when addressing other neurocognitive functions. It is often assumed that cognitive measures such as problem-solving may be affected by educational variables, and that such measures as sensory–motor functions are not educationally or culturally bound. There is ample evidence suggesting otherwise. Roselli and Ardila (1990, 1993) have reported that illiteracy affects neuropsychological performance of memory, language, and visuospatial and praxis abilities. Thus, education, among other demographic variables, needs to be careful controlled.

Beyond this, the question remains as to what kinds of neuropsychological assessment can be completed. Again, Roselli and Ardila (1993) reported the use of a standardized battery to measure language, memory, and visuospatial abilities. The battery was administered to 233 normal children between 5 and 12 years of age stratified according to SES and sex. The following tests were used and normative data were presented for each: Boston Naming Test, shortened version of the Token Test, Wechsler Memory Scale, Sequential Verbal Memory Test, and Rey–Osterrieth Complex Figure Test. The reader of this chapter is encouraged to carefully review this paper as a guide for conducting nonintellectual neuropsychological assessment of Hispanic children. Caution should be emphasized, however, in that these are Colombian children whose neuropsychological deficits were not specified.

Summary and Directions

Summary

This has been a difficult chapter to write, in large part because something of this type has not been done before. Hence, one should expect a large number of gaps in possibly the logic and certainly the data supporting the conclusions presented here. However, that first step must be taken, even at the risk of sounding foolish and nonempirical. There is enough evidence in the nonneuropsychological scientific literature and a growing evidence in the clinical neuropsychological literature. Obviously what is sorely needed are empirically based studies. In the meantime, this chapter presents an introduction to the complex issues involving the neuropsychological assessment of the Hispanic child and youth.

Clearly, there is much more to the Spanish-speaking child than language. Culture, education, and socioeconomic variables all play a significant role in determining neuropsychological status of this population. Also, it is very important to understand the difference between race and ethnicity. Further, Hispanics as an ethnic group represent probably as much heterogeneity as any other ethnic group, including Anglo-Saxons. Also, the concept of equivalence is a very complex issue. Language equivalence alone, even as difficult to accomplish as it may be, is insufficient. Cognitive and cultural equivalence must be aspired to even in the face of seemingly impossible to define constructs.

With regard to assessment approaches, the orientation taken in this chapter has been more generalized than specific. For example, there is no table present that outlines the specific intellectual tests. Each of them, whether the Wechsler Scales, the Stanford–Binet, the Peabody, the Kaufman, or even the Raven, presents with unique limitations of its own. These limitations range from inadequate translation to inappropriate norms. Hence, each case must be considered individually, and careful understanding of both the client's need and the restrictions of the test employed is imperative.

Clinical and Research Suggestions

Not much is known about the effects of culture and ethnicity on neuropsychological performance, especially when children and youth are involved. Cummins (1984), McClelland (1973), Puente (1993), and others have called for increased understanding of a psychology of diversity. Obviously, such an understanding would begin in training programs. The incorporation of cultural variables into training curricula seems critical. In addition, specific research needs to be encouraged. Ardila (1995) in a seminal article on cross-cultural neuropsychology suggested the following:

1. Normalization of current basic neuropsy-chological instruments in different cultural contexts
2. The development of new neuropsychological instruments specifically designed for unique situations
3. The analysis of educational and cultural variation test performance
4. The analysis of cognitive disturbance in the case of pathology across differing cultural and educational situations
5. The search for commonality in neuropsychological performance across cultures

Future Directions

Unfortunately, although clinical neuropsychology is experiencing an unprecedented growth (Puente, 1992), the same cannot be said of ethnic issues within the discipline. Indeed, analysis of the Minority Fellowship Program of the American Psychological Association reveals a *decreasing* funding rate over the last several years (J., personal communication). In addition, the ethnicity of those pursuing careers in psychology is for the most part not Hispanic, and over the history of that APA program only one student has received funding to pursue clinical neuropsychology research (out of hundreds of recipients). Further, the recent findings of Echemendia *et al.* (in press) suggest that an increasing number of Hispanic clients are being evaluated for brain dysfunction but unfortunately in a manner not consistent with APA ethical guidelines. Finally, the research base pertaining to ethnic issues in psychology, especially with regard to Hispanics, is eroding (Santos-de-Barona, 1993). The authors hope and anticipate that if a third edition of this volume were to appear at the beginning of the next century, a different story would emerge.

References

Anastasi, A. (1976). *Psychological testing* (6th ed.). New York: Macmillan Co.

Ardila, A. (1995). Directions of research in cross-cultural neuropsychology. *Journal of Clinical and Experimental Neuropsychology, 17,* 143–150.

Ardila, A., & Roselli, M. (1989). Neuropsychological assessment in illiterates; Visuospatial and memory abilities. *Brain and Cognition, 11,* 147–166.

Ardila, A., Roselli, M., & Ostrosky, F. (1992). Sociocultural factors in neuropsychological assessment. In A. E. Puente & R. J. McCaffrey (Eds.), *Handbook of neuropsychological assessment* (pp. 181–192). New York: Plenum Press.

Ardila, A., Roselli, M., & Puente, A. E. (1994). *Neuropsychological evaluation of the Spanish-speaker.* New York: Plenum Press.

Barona, A., & Miller, J. A. (1994). Short Acculturation Scale for Hispanic Youth (SASH-Y): A preliminary report. *Hispanic Journal of Behavioral Sciences, 16,* 155–162.

Barona, A., & Pfeiffer, S. (1992). Effects of test administration procedures and acculturation level on achievement scores. *Journal of Psychoeducational Assessment, 10,* 124–132.

Barona, A., Reynolds, C. R., & Chastain, R. (1984). A demographically based index of premorbid intelligence for the WAIS-R. *Journal of Consulting and Clinical Psychology, 52*(5), 885–887.

Bernal, E., Jr. (1977). Assessment procedures for Chicano children: The sad state of the art. *International Journal of Chicano Studies Research, 8,* 69–81.

Bernal, E. M. (1990). Increasing the interpretative validity and diagnostic utility of Hispanic children's scores on test of achievement and intelligence. In F. C. Serafica, A. Schwebel, R. K. Russell, P. D. Isaac, & L. B. Myers (Eds.), *Mental health of ethnic minorities* (pp. 108–138). New York: Praeger.

Berry, J. W. (1979). Research in multicultural societies: Implications of cross-cultural methods. *Journal of Cross-Cultural Psychology, 10,* 415–434.

Bracken, B., & Barona, A. (1991). State of the art procedures for translating, validating and using psychoeducational tests in cross-cultural assessment. *School Psychology International, 12,* 119–132.

Brislin, R. W. (1988). Increasing awareness of class, ethnicity, culture, and race by expanding on students' own experiences. In I. S. Cohen (Ed.), *The G. Stanley Hall Lecture Series* (Vol. 8, pp. 137–180). Washington, DC: American Psychological Association.

Candell, G., & Hulin, C. (1986). Cross-language and cross-cultural comparisons in scale translations. *Journal of Cross-Cultural Psychology, 17,* 417–440.

Cauce, A. M., & Jacobson, L. (1980). Implicit and incorrect assumptions concerning the assessment of the Latino in the United States. *American Journal of Community Psychology, 8,* 571–586.

Cross, W. E. (1994). Nigrescence theory: Historical and explanatory theory. *Journal of Vocational Behavior, 44*(2), 119–123.

Cummings, J. (1984). *Bilingualism and special education: Issues in assessment and pedagogy.* San Diego: College-Hill Press.

Darcy, N. (1963). Bilingualism and the measurement of intelligence: Review of a decade of research. *The Journal of Genetic Psychology, 103,* 259–282.

Dupont, S., Ardila, A., & Roselli, M., & Puente, A. E. (1992). Neuropsychological assessment in bilinguals. In A. E. Puente & R. J. McCaffrey (Eds.), *Psychobiological factors in clinical neuropsychological assessment* (pp. 193–215). New York: Plenum Press.

Echemendia, R. J., Congett, S. M., Harris, J. G., Diaz, M. L., & Puente, A. E. (in press). Neuropsychology training and practices with Hispanics. *The Clinical Neuropsychologist.*

Figueroa, R. (1983). Test bias and Hispanic children. *The Journal of Special Education, 17,* 431–440.

Harris, J. G., Cullum, M., & Puente, A. E. (1995). Effects of bilingualism on verbal learning and memory in Hispanic adults. *Journal of the International Neuropsychological Society, 1,* 10–16.

Harris, J. L. (1990). Cultural influences on handedness: Historical and contemporary theory and evidence. In S. Coren (Ed.), *Left-handedness: Behavioral implications and anomalies* (pp. 195–258). Amsterdam: North-Holland.

Helms, J. (1992). Why is there no study of cultural equivalence in standardized cognitive ability testing? *American Psychologist, 47*(9), 1083–1101.

Jones, J. (1991). Piercing the veil: Bi-cultural strategies for coping with prejudice and racism. In H. J. Knopke, R. J. Norrell, & R. W. Rogers (Eds.), *Opening doors: Perspectives on age relations in contemporary America.* Tuscaloosa: University of Alabama Press.

Jones, J. M. (1994). Our similarities are different: Toward a psychology of affirmative diversity. In J. M. Jones (Ed.), *Human diversity: Perspectives of people in context* (pp. 27–45). San Francisco: Jossey–Bass.

Kagan, S. (1984). Interpreting Chicano cooperativeness: Methodological and theoretical considerations. In J. L. Martinez & R. H. Mendoza (Eds.), *Chicano psychology* (pp. 289–334). Orlando, FL: Academic Press.

Kaufman, A. S. (1979). WISC-R research: Implications for interpretation. *Journal of School Psychology Review, 8,* 5–27.

Kaufman, A. S. (1990). *Assessing adolescent and adult intelligence.* Boston: Allyn & Bacon.

Keachnie, J. L. (1983). *Webster's new universal unabridged dictionary.* Cleveland, OH: Dorset & Barber.

Klineberg, O. (1935). *Race differences.* New York: Harper.

Knight, G. P., & Kagan, S. (1977). Acculturation of prosocial and competitive behaviors among second- and third-generation Mexican-American children. *Journal of Cross-Cultural Psychology, 8,* 273–284.

Laosa, L. (1975). Bilingualism in the three United States Hispanic groups: Contextual use of language by children and adults in their families. *Journal of Educational Psychology, 67,* 617–627.

Laosa, L. (1984). Ethnic, socioeconomic, and home language influences upon early performance on measures of abilities. *Journal of Educational Psychology, 76,* 1178–1198.

Laosa, L. (1991). The cultural context of construct validity and the ethics of generalizability. *Early Childhood Research Quarterly, 6,* 313–321.

Malgady, R., Rogler, L., & Costantino, X. (1987). Ethnocultural and linguistic bias in mental health evaluation of Hispanics. *American Psychologist, 42*(3), 228–234.

McClelland, D. C. (1973). Testing for competence rather than for "intelligence." *American Psychologist, 3,* 1–14.

McLin Davis, T., & Rodriguez, V. (1979). Comparison of scores on the WAIS and its Puerto Rican counterpart, Escala de Inteligencia Wechsler para Adultos, in an institutionalized Latin American psychiatric population. *Journal of Consulting and Clinical Psychology, 47*(1), 181–182.

Myers, H. F., Echemendia, R. J., & Trimble, J. E. (1991). The need for training ethnic minority psychologists. In H. F. Myers, P. Wohlford, L. P. Guzman, & R. J. Echemendia (Eds.), *Ethnic minority perspectives on clinical training and services in psychology* (pp. 177–182).

Olmedo, E. (1981). Testing linguistic minorities. *American Psychologist, 36*(10), 1078–1085.

Padilla, A., & Ruiz, R. (1973). *Latino mental health.* Rockville, MD: National Institute of Mental Health.

Palmer, D., Olivarez, A., Wilson, V., & Fordyce, T. (1989). Ethnicity and language dominance-influence on the prediction of achievement based on intelligence test scores in nonreferred and referred samples. *Learning Disability Quarterly, 12,* 261–274.

Perez-Arce, P., & Puente, A. E. (1996). Neuropsychological assessment of ethnic-minorities: The case of assessing Hispanics living in North America. In R. Sbordone & C. Long (Eds.), *The ecological validity of neuropsychological testing.* Winter Park, FL: GR St. Lucie Press (pp. 283–300).

Prewitt-Diaz, J., Rodriguez, A. M., & Rivera, D. (1986). The predictive validity of the Spanish translation of the WISC-R (EIWN-R) with Puerto Rican students in Puerto Rico and the United States. *Educational and Psychological Measurement, 46,* 401–407.

Puente, A. E. (1990). Psychological assessment of minority group members. In G. Goldstein & M. Hersen (Eds.), *Handbook of psychological assessment* (pp. 505–520). New York: Pergamon Press.

Puente, A. E. (1992). The status of clinical neuropsychology. *Archives of Clinical Neuropsychology, 7,* 297–312.

Puente, A. E. (1993). Toward a psychology of variance: Increasing the presence and understanding of ethnic minorities in psychology. In T. McGovern (Ed.), *Handbook for enhancing undergraduate education in psychology* (pp. 71–92). Washington, DC: American Psychological Association.

Puente, A. E., & McCaffrey, R. J. (1992). *Handbook of clinical neuropsychology.* New York: Plenum Press.

Putnam, S. H., & DeLuca, J. W. (1990). The TCN Professional Practice Survey: Part I: General practice of neuropsychologists in primary employment of private practice settings. *The Clinical Neuropsychologist, 4,* 199–243.

Reschly, D. (1978). WISC-R factor structure among Anglos, blacks, Chicanos, and Native-American Papagos. *Journal of Consulting and Clinical Psychology, 46*(3), 417–422.

Reynolds, C., & Brown, R. (1990). *Bias in mental testing.* New York: Plenum Press.

Roselli, M. (1993). Neuropsychology of illiteracy. *Behavioural Neurology, 6,* 107–112.

Roselli, M., & Ardila, A. (1990). Neuropsychological assessments in illiterates: Language and praxic abilities. *Brain and Cognition, 12,* 281–296.

Roselli, M., & Ardila, A. (1993). Effects of age, gender, and socioeconomic level on the Wisconsin Card Sorting Test. *The Clinical Neuropsychologist, 7,* 145–154.

Sanchez, G. (1934). Bilingualism and mental measures: A word of caution. *Journal of Social Psychology,* 765–771.

Sandoval, J. (1989). The WISC-R and the internal evidence of test bias with minority groups. *Journal of Consulting and Clinical Psychology, 57,* 919–927.

Sandoval, J., & Whelan-Mille, P. (1980). Accuracy of judgments of WISC-R item difficulty for minority groups. *Journal of Consulting and Clinical Psychology, 48*(2), 249–253.

Sandoval, J., Zimmerman, I. L., & Woo-Sam, J. (1983). Cultural differences on WISC-R verbal items. *Journal of School Psychology, 21,* 49–55.

Santos-de-Barona, M. (1993). The availability of ethnic materials in psychology journals: A review of 20 years of journal publications. *Contemporary Educational Psychology, 18,* 391–400.

Smart, J. F. & Smart, D. W. (1995). The use of translators/interpreters in rehabilitation. *Journal of Rehabilitation,* 14–20.

Spiro, M. E. (1988). Is the Oedipus complex universal? In G. H. Pollock & J. M. Ross (Eds.), *The Oedipus papers, Classics in psychoanalysis monograph 6,* 435–473.

Statistical Abstract of the United States. (1995). U.S. Bureau of the Census: Author.

Sue, D. W., & Sue, D. (1990). *Counseling the culturally different.* New York: Wiley.

Sue, S. (1983). Ethnic issues in psychology: A reexamination. *American Psychologist, 38,* 583–592.

Tamayo, J. (1990). A validated translation into Spanish of the WISC-R Vocabulary subtest words. *Educational and Psychological Measurements, 50,* 915–921.

Taylor, D., & Ziegler, E. (1987). Comparison of the first principal factor on the WISC-R across ethnic groups. *Educational and Psychological Measurement, 47,* 691–694.

Taylor, R. L., & Stephen, B. R. (1991). Patterns of intellectual differences of black, Hispanic and white children. *Psychology in the Schools, 28,* 5–9.

Terman, L. M. (1916). *The measurement of intelligence.* Boston: Houghton Mifflin.

Velazquez, R. J., & Callahan, W. J. (1992). Psychological testing of Hispanic Americans in clinical settings. Overview and issues. In K. F. Geisinger (Ed.), *Psychological testing of Hispanics.* Washington, DC: American Psychological Association.

Whitworth, R. H. (1988). Comparison of Anglo and Mexican American male high school students classified as learning disabled. *Hispanic Journal of Behavioral Sciences, 10,* 127–137.

World Population Data Sheet. (1986–1990). Washington, DC: Population Reference Bureau.

III

Techniques of Intervention

20

Neurocognitive Interventions for Childhood and Adolescent Disorders

A Transactional Model

PHYLLIS ANNE TEETER

Interest in the neuropsychological basis of childhood and adolescent disorders continues to grow (Gaddes & Edgell, 1994; Obrzut & Hynd, 1991; Rourke, 1991), and neurocognitive models for designing effective interventions for treating various disorders show promise (Teeter & Semrud-Clikeman, in press). Technological innovations in computed tomography (CT), magnetic resonance imaging (MRI), single-photon emission computer tomography (SPECT), positron emission tomography (PET), regional cerebral blood flow (rCBF) (Yudofsky & Hales, 1992), and functional magnetic resonance imaging (FMRI) (Binder, personal communication) have transformed our understanding of numerous neuropsychiatric disorders (e.g., attention deficit hyperactivity disorder) and learning disabilities (e.g., dyslexia).

Recent technological advances have had a profound impact on our understanding of childhood disorders. Lewis Judd, M.D., director of the National Institute of Mental Health, stated that "95% of what we know about the brain as it relates to be-

Portions of this chapter are adapted from Teeter, P. A., & Semrud-Clikeman, M. (in press). *Child Clinical Neuropsychology: Assessment and Interventions for Neuropsychiatric and Neurodevelopmental Disorders of Childhood*, Boston. Copyright Allyn & Bacon. Adapted with permission.

PHYLLIS ANNE TEETER • Department of Educational Psychology, University of Wisconsin–Milwaukee, Milwaukee, Wisconsin 53201.

havior has been discovered in the past 5 years" (Yudofsky & Hales, 1992, p. xxii). The fact that this statement was made in 1988 serves to highlight the dramatic scientific advances that have been made in our understanding of brain-related disorders. Further, study of recombinant DNA and complex genetic models of "at-risk" populations has also been important in this effort, stimulating a focus on the biochemistry of neuropsychological functioning (Rourke, 1991). Neurochemical models of human behavior may even begin to overshadow structural, neuroanatomical paradigms in the future (Rourke, 1991). The extent to which these findings advance the science of childhood psychopathology and learning disorders and improve intervention planning is under investigation.

Some argue that advances in neuropsychology have not furthered our knowledge about remedial and treatment programs for brain-related disorders, whereas others indicate that this information can be used as a basis for developing paradigms or models for intervention for childhood disorders (Gaddes & Edgell, 1994; Rourke, 1991, 1994; Teeter & Semrud-Clikeman, in press). Several paradigms have been designed incorporating information about the neuropsychological functioning of children into intervention programs. This chapter explores a number of intervention models and develops a rationale for using a transactional model for understanding and treating learning and neuropsychiatric disorders of childhood. Information about the child's neuropsychological, cognitive, academic, and psychosocial status forms the basis for designing integrated intervention and treatment plans for children and adolescents with brain-related and neurodevelopmental disorders (Teeter & Semrud-Clikeman, in press).

The purpose of this chapter is to review current neuropsychological, neurocognitive, and neurobehavioral paradigms for designing interventions for children with various disorders, including phonological reading disabilities (PRD), nonverbal learning disabilities (NLD), and attention deficit hyperactivity disorders (ADHD). Four models for intervention are discussed in this chapter: (1) the Multistage Neuropsychological Assessment–Intervention Model (Teeter & Semrud-Clikeman in press); (2) the developmental neuropsychological remediation/habilitation framework designed by Rourke (1994); (3) rehabilitation procedures designed by Reitan and Wolfson (1992); and (4) the phenomenological model articulated by Levine (1993, 1994).

Techniques for addressing the cognitive, academic psychosocial, and attentional problems associated with selected disorders of childhood and adolescence are presented. Medications for treating neuropsychiatric disorders of childhood, medication monitoring, consultation with educational staff, and integrated intervention protocols are briefly discussed. Finally, guidelines for collaboration are addressed, including ideas for developing home–school–physician partnerships for treating childhood and adolescent neuropsychiatric, neurodevelopmental, and brain-related disorders.

Theoretical Orientations for the Study of Childhood Disorders

In the past, dichotomies such as "medical" versus "behavioral," "within-child" versus "environmental," and "neuropsychological" versus "psychoeducational" have served as stimuli for controversy and great debate over which orientation or theoretical approach is most relevant (Teeter & Semrud-Clikeman, 1995). Further, some have adopted one approach exclusively in an attempt to diagnose and treat childhood disorders (Teeter & Semrud-Clikeman, in press). Research adopting only one paradigm often oversimplifies the complex interaction of genetic, neurocognitive, psychosocial, and environmental factors that can affect various childhood disorders (Gaddes & Edgell, 1994), including traumatic brain injury (TBI) (Goldstein & Levin, 1990),

ADHD (Barkley, 1990; Weiss & Hechtman, 1993), NLD (Rourke, 1994), and PRD (Teeter & Semrud-Clikeman, in press). With this shortcoming in mind, Teeter and Semrud-Clikeman (1995, in press) developed a transactional paradigm in an effort to assist in the diagnosis and design of intervention programs for children and adolescents with various learning and neuropsychiatric disorders.

Teeter and Semrud-Clikeman (1995) argue that multiple perspectives advance the science of childhood psychopathology and aid in our understanding of cognitive–intellectual development. Neuropsychological functioning should be considered with other cognitive, behavioral, and psychosocial factors for the assessment and intervention of children and adolescents. Diagnostic accuracy and intervention efficacy can also be explored within a developmental framework in a transactional neuropsychological paradigm. Definitions and a brief discussion of the features of a transactional paradigm follow.

Neuropsychological Component

Neuropsychology involves the study of the brain–behavior relationships, with the assumption that there is a causal relationship between brain functioning and behavior (Obrzut & Hynd, 1991). Teeter and Semrud-Clikeman (in press) outline the advantages of incorporating neuropsychology in the study of childhood and adolescent disorders:

> (1) it is a well established science with knowledge relevant to childhood disorders (Gaddes & Edgell, 1994); (2) there is a growing body of evidence suggesting that "behavior and neurology are inseparable" (Hynd & Willis, 1988, p. 5); (3) it provides a means for studying the long-term sequelae of head injury in children (Goldstein & Levin, 1990); (4) it provides a means for investigating abnormalities in brain function that increase the risk for psychiatric disorders in children (Tramontana & Hooper, 1989); and, (5) it provides a means for early prediction and treatment of reading disabilities (Felton & Brown, 1991). (p. 7)

While it is virtually indisputable that all behavior is by the brain (Gaddes & Edgell, 1994), the nature of this relationship is complex and our present knowledge is incomplete, especially in children. However, Gaddes and Edgell (1994) argue that child neuropsychology should not be abandoned because what we do know about the developing brain can be effectively utilized by knowledgeable clinicians. A number of behavioral psychologists have stated that child neuropsychology diverts attention from behavioral techniques with documented treatment validity (Gresham & Gansle, 1992; Reschly & Gresham, 1989), whereas clinical child neuropsychologists consider a broader framework for childhood disorders that includes the interaction of psychosocial, environmental, neurocognitive, biomedical, and neurochemical aspects of behaviors (Teeter & Semrud-Clikeman, in press). The relationships between physiological and psychological systems are of interest; and, within a transactional neuropsychological model, environmental and behavioral factors also must be explored.

Although there have been advances in our understanding of the brain–behavior relations for many childhood disorders, child neuropsychology should not be exclusively employed when assessing and treating children (Gaddes & Edgell, 1994). Further, Levine (1994) argues that even though learning problems may result from neurodevelopmental dysfunctions, including gaps, maturational delays, or differences in how the child's brain is developing, he prefers a model that describes, accurately recognizes, and understands observable phenomena related to learning problems. Behavioral, psychosocial, and cognitive factors are thus important variables affecting both the diagnosis and treatment of children with brain-related disorders.

Behavioral Component

Behavioral approaches typically focus on describing and modifying the antecedents and consequences of behavior. Behavioral assessment and intervention techniques have been found to be valid and effective methods for many disorders of childhood (Kratochwill & Bergan, 1990; Mash & Terdal, 1988; Shapiro, 1989; Shinn, 1989). Behavioral models often incorporate an ecological as well as behavioral analysis, to describe how environmental factors contribute to and maintain learning difficulties in children (Shapiro, 1989). Others incorporate techniques of functional analysis for assessing, treating, and determining treatment efficacy for behavioral, psychosocial, and learning disorders (Kratochwill & Plunge, 1992). However, behavioral approaches can be effectively integrated into neurocognitive models, and child clinical assessment and intervention can be enhanced by this integration.

In other integrated paradigms, Horton and Puente (1986) employed behavioral assessment and intervention techniques with neuropsychological procedures for treating children and adolescents with brain-related disorders. On the surface it may appear that behavioral and neuropsychological paradigms are at odds with one another; however, Teeter and Semrud-Clikeman (in press) argue that important information can be gleaned about a child when these two approaches are integrated. Child neuropsychologists typically consider the influence of environmental factors when investigating numerous problems including: malnutrition and brain development in young children (Cravioto & Arrieta, 1983); changes in brain morphology after intensive behavioral interventions (Hynd, 1992); environmental factors (e.g., school, home, and peer/family interactions) and their effect on recovery of function following brain impairment (Rourke, Bakker, Fisk, & Strang, 1983); the effects of nonneurological factors (e.g., preaccident behavioral, temperamental, and psychosocial problems, and family reactions) when treating psychiatric disorders resulting from TBI (Rutter, Chadwick, & Shaffer, 1983); and applied behavioral intervention strategies for brain-injured children (Gray & Dean, 1989). Rourke (1989) also incorporates an integrated model for investigating the neuropsychological, social–emotional, cognitive, adaptational, behavioral, and academic factors for diagnosing and treating children and adolescents with NLD.

Horton and Puente (1986) advocated for the development of behavioral neuropsychology as a subspeciality within clinical neuropsychology. Behavioral neuropsychology refers to "the application of behavior therapy techniques to problems of organically impaired individuals while using a neuropsychological assessment and intervention perspective" (Horton, 1979, p. 20). Although more research beyond single-subject designs is needed, Horton and Puente (1986) indicate that behavioral interventions have been helpful for disorders resulting from brain injury and learning disabilities.

Psychosocial and cognitive factors are also included in the transactional neuropsychological paradigm developed by Teeter and Semrud-Clikeman (in press) for the assessment and treatment model for childhood and adolescent disorders. The extent to which children with brain-related disorders evidence cognitive, psychological, and social problems will be briefly explored.

Psychosocial and Cognitive Components

Many neuropsychiatric and learning disorders of childhood and adolescence (e.g., ADHD and learning disabilities) have associated psychosocial and cognitive deficits (Teeter & Semrud-Clikeman, in press). Teeter and Semrud-Clikeman (in press) suggest that these factors have a bidirectional relationship, such that cognitive and psychosocial characteristics interact with and can exacerbate disorders with a neuropsychological basis. Further, information about the brain–behavior relationship derived from neuropsychological models can be helpful for understanding the associated features (i.e., behavioral, cognitive, and psychosocial deficits) of ADHD and dyslexia (Semrud-Clikeman & Hynd, 1993; Teeter & Semrud-Clikeman, 1995). Conversely, cognitive abilities (i.e., premorbid intelligence) and psychosocial adjustment affect recovery of functions in children and adolescents sustaining TBI (Bigler, 1990). Thus, the influence of brain function on psychosocial and cognitive functions is transactional in nature and is intricately linked—each influencing and affecting the outcome of treatment programs and intervention plans.

Neurobiological and psychosocial functioning are intricately linked in children with ADHD. Barkley (1990) argues that ADHD is a disorder of dysregulation, which affects inhibition and self-regulation, most likely resulting from impairment in executive functions mediated by the frontal cortex. An inability to inhibit or to regulate one's own behavior can have significant negative consequences in social situations. A number of children with ADHD are described as noncompliant and rebellious (Johnston & Pelham, 1986), and rigid, domineering, irritating, and annoying in social situations (Milich & Landau, 1989). ADHD children with these characteristics are frequently rejected by their peers (Hynd et al., 1991), particularly when they are also aggressive (Milich & Landau, 1989). A transactional model thus provides a framework for investigating whether psychosocial outcomes are related to the primary features of impulsivity, distractibility, and disinhibition, which have been found to have a neurobiological basis (Teeter & Semrud-Clikeman, 1995), or whether these problems are related to secondary personality (i.e., aggression) or environmental factors (i.e., modeling and/or reinforcement history).

Associated cognitive and academic difficulties have also been found in children and adolescents with ADHD, including: school failure (Barkley, 1990) and academic underachievement and learning disabilities (Epstein, Shaywitz, Shaywitz, & Woolston, 1992; Lambert & Sandoval, 1980; Semrud-Clikeman et al., 1992). Further, only a small number of adolescents with ADHD ever finish college (Barkley, 1990). Declines in academic achievement, verbal IQ, and overall psychosocial adjustment may result from difficulties in self-regulation and response inhibition (Barkley, 1990). Thus, the manner in which neurochemical and/or neuropsychological functioning interact with social, psychological, and behavioral functioning in children with ADHD can be more fully investigated within a transactional model (Teeter & Semrud-Clikeman, 1995).

Children with learning disabilities (LD) also demonstrate psychosocial and cognitive deficits that may be associated with underlying dysfunctional neural mechanisms (Teeter & Semrud-Clikeman, in press). For example, LD children with low verbal skills and relatively good visual–spatial abilities demonstrate high rates of depression (Nussbaum, Bigler, & Koch, 1986). Personality function appears related to the neuropsychological assets/deficits observed in this subgroup of LD children (Nussbaum et al., 1986). Further, children with NLD also tend to have high suicide rates (Rourke, Young, & Leenaars, 1989). The neuropsychological assets and deficits (i.e., right hemisphere dysfunction with intact left hemisphere functions) may result in deficient social interaction skills, inappropriate verbal interactions, and poor social adjustment observed in children with NLD (Rourke, 1989).

By gathering data from different paradigms, the clinician can utilize an integrated model for the diagnosis and treatment of children and adolescents (Teeter & Semrud-Clikeman, in press). Thus, when using a transactional neuropsychological paradigm, the clinician would conduct a thorough assessment addressing the pattern of neurocognitive strengths and weaknesses as the first step, and then plan an integrated intervention program for addressing specific problems. By developing interventions within this model, the interaction of environmental–behavioral, psychosocial, and cognitive factors with neuropsychological functioning would result in a more complete clinical study of the child. These various factors are considered when approaching the task of child clinical assessment and intervention planning.

A Transactional Neuropsychological Paradigm for the Assessment and Treatment of Childhood Disorders

Neuropsychological assessment and intervention approaches are strengthened by a careful study of the relationship between brain function and the cognitive, psychosocial, and behavioral characteristics displayed by children with various disorders (Teeter & Semrud-Clikeman, 1995, in press). (See Figure 1.) A transactional model provides a framework for investigating how intact versus impaired neuropsychological systems interact with and limit cognitive–intellectual and psychosocial adjustment in children and adolescents (Teeter & Semrud-Clikeman, in press).

Development and maturation of the brain is influenced by biogenetic as well as environmental factors (e.g., prenatal and postnatal toxins or insults). Subcortical and cortical regions have a bidirectional influence on neural functional systems impacting on the intellectual, reasoning, memory, attentional, and perceptual capacity of the child (Teeter & Semrud-Clikeman, in press). Various functional systems in the brain interact with and influence the expression of the behavioral, psychosocial, and cognitive manifestations of a number of childhood disorders (Teeter & Semrud-Clikeman, in press). Social, family, and school environments

also interact, and can either facilitate or inhibit the development of compensatory and/or coping skills in children with disorders.

A dynamic interaction among the biogenetic, neuropsychological, environmental, cognitive, and psychosocial systems is an essential feature of this transactional model (Teeter & Semrud-Clikeman, in press). Although abnormal neural development can be detrimental, the course and nature of neuropsychiatric and learning disorders are not necessarily inevitable. Effective psychosocial and educational interventions, with modifications in the environment (i.e., home, school, and social environment), can reduce the negative effects of many neuropsychological or biogenetically based disorders (Teeter & Semrud-Clikeman, in press). Further, pharmacotherapy may also be part of treatment programs for some disorders of childhood (e.g., ADHD, depression). Thus, dynamic relationships exist among these variables and should be considered in the clinical assessment and treatment of childhood disorders.

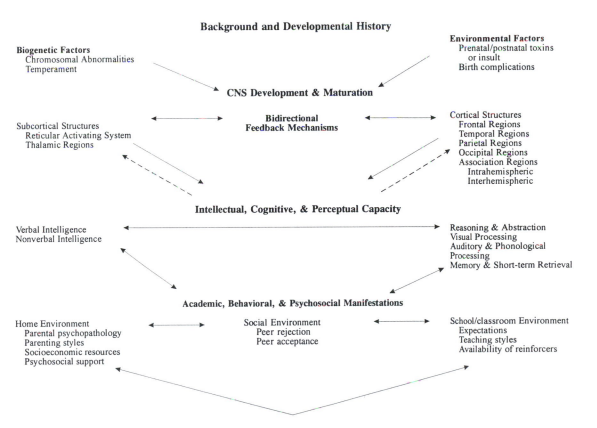

FIGURE 1. Transactional paradigm for understanding neurodevelopmental and neuropsychiatric disorders of childhood. (Adapted with permission from Teeter & Semrud-Clikeman, in press.)

Models Linking Assessment to Interventions

A thorough understanding of the underlying features of a disorder precedes effective intervention; thus, a link between assessment and intervention is critical. Four models are described in the following sections, including: (1) the multistage neuropsychological model developed by Teeter and Semrud-Clikeman (in press); (2) the developmental remediation model developed by Rourke (1994); (3) the REHABIT model designed by Reitan and Wolfson (1992); and (4) the Observable Phenomenon Model developed by Levine (1993, 1994). Table 1 summarizes stages of assessment and intervention planning, and provides a description of the major features of each model.

Each model assumes that comprehensive clinical evaluation precedes intervention plans. A phenomenological model designed by Levine (1993, 1994) is also described. Although Levine's model does not specifically identify the neurodevelopmental mechanisms underlying learning difficulties, it is helpful for determining various observable phenomena (e.g., weak attention controls, reduced remembering, chronic misunderstanding) that affect a child's learning capacity. Levine (1993, 1994) also provides detailed intervention strategies to address various learning problems. These four neuropsychological/neurobehavioral models are discussed in more detail below.

Multistage Neuropsychological Model

Teeter (1992) first presented a multistage neuropsychological model (MNM) for linking neuropsychological assessment to intervention plans. Teeter and Semrud-Clikeman (in press) later expanded the model described below. The MNM uses structured behavioral–observational assessment techniques in the first stage; and if the child's problems do not improve after systematic behavioral interventions, then more extensive cognitive and psychosocial, neuropsychological, and/or neuroradiological evaluation and interventions are considered (Teeter & Semrud-Clikeman, in press). Intervention strategies are developed and implemented after careful assessment and diagnosis at each level of the model. Intervention strategies described in later sections of this chapter can be selected to address the child's specific problems.

Effective interventions may reduce the need for further, more intensive evaluation (e.g., neuropsychological) of the child, particularly when disorders are not severe or chronic in nature (e.g., reading delays versus dyslexia). This requires ongoing and systematic evaluation to determine whether the initial diagnosis and description of the disorder is accurate, and whether the specific intervention plan is effective. Thus, a working diagnostic hypothesis seems reasonable in early assessment–intervention stages. However, for more serious childhood disorders including TBI, CNS diseases, and seizure activity, the clinician may proceed to neuropsychological evaluation and neurodiagnostic examination immediately (Teeter & Semrud-Clikeman, in press).

The eight-stage assessment–intervention model requires expertise from various educational, clinical, and medical professionals. School psychologists and educational professionals typically conduct Stages 1 through 4 assessment–intervention, whereas Stages 5 and 6 usually are conducted by clinical child neuropsychologists outside the school setting (Teeter & Semrud-Clikeman, in press). Pediatric neurologists, neuroradiologists, and pediatricians usually are involved in Stage 7 assessment; and interventions appropriate for Stage 8 may require short-term hospitalization.

Systematic monitoring and modification of intervention plans are required at each stage of the MNM, and accurate diagnosis or problem identification is critical for designing specific intervention strategies (Teeter & Semrud-Clikeman, in press). Periodic evaluation of the treatment plan is essential. This reduces the possibility of continuing to utilize strategies that are not effective. Thus, current assessment of the child's progress is part of effective intervention. (See Teeter & Semrud-Clikeman, in press, for an in-depth discussion of the MNM.)

In summary, the MNM provides guidelines for linking multiple stages of evaluation into intervention plans. Rourke (1994) has also developed a multistage neuropsychological remediation model for children with LD. This model is briefly reviewed next.

Developmental Neuropsychological Remediation/Rehabilitation Model

The Developmental Neuropsychological Remediation/Rehabilitation Model (DNRR) was

TABLE 1. Models for Neuropsychologial Remediation and Rehabilitation: Linking Assessment to Interventions[a]

Models	Stages	Description
MNM (Teeter & Semrud-Clikeman, 1995)[b]	Stage 1: problem identification	Behavioral assessment
	Stage 2: behavioral-based intervention	Self-management
		Contingency management
		Learning strategies
		Peer tutoring
	Stage 3: cognitive child study	Comprehensive cognitive, academic, psychosocial assessment
	Stage 4: cognitive-based intervention	Pattern analysis
		Phonological awareness
		Activating schemata
		Organizational strategies
	Stage 5: neuropsychological assessment	Comprehensive neurocognitive assessment
	Stage 6: integrated neuropsychological intervention	Compensatory skills psychopharmacology
	Stage 7: neurological and neuroradiological assessment	Neurological, CT, MRI
	Stage 8: medical–neurological rehabilitation	Rehabilitation and medical management
DNRR (Rourke, 1994)[c]	Step 1: neuropsychological assets/deficits, academic and psychosocial assessment	Neuropsychological profile
		Ecologically based evaluation
	Step 2: demands of environment	Behavioral, academic, and psychosocial challenges within contextual framework
	Step 3: short and long term	Formulate short- and long-range predictions
		Which deficits will decrease?
		Specific treatment strategies
	Step 4: "ideal" remedial plans	"Ideal" plans
		Monitoring and modification
	Step 5: availability of resources	Therapeutic goals
		Prognosis
		Reduce redundant services
	Step 6: realistic remedial plan	Compare differences between steps 4 and 5
	Step 7: ongoing assessment and intervention	
REHABIT (Reitan & Wolfson, 1992)[d]	Tract A: verbal-language	Materials to increase expressive-receptive skills
	Tract B: abstraction and reasoning	Materials to increase analysis, organization
	Tract C: general reasoning	Materials for general reasoning
	Tract D: visual–spatial	Visual–spatial manipulation sequential skills
	Tract E: visual–spatial and manipulation	

(continued)

TABLE 1. (*Continued*).

Observable Phenomena (Levine, 1993, 1994)	Educational evaluation	Psychoeducational testing, classroom observation and error analysis, identify "breakdown" points, history and interview
	Behavioral and affective evaluation	Assess affective-mood patterns, questionnaires, interviews, personality tests, observation
	Cognitive and developmental	Intelligence tests, neurodevelopmental tests, questionnaires of present and past neurodevelopmental functions and styles
	Environmental assessment	Interview to identify factors in home, consider culture, peer, and community issues
	Medical assessment	Review medical history, physical examination, neurological examination

[a]Adapted with permission from Teeter and Semrud-Clikeman (in press).
[b]Multistage Neuropsychological Model (Teeter & Semrud-Clikeman, in press).
[c]Developmental Neuropsychological Remediation/Rehabilitation Model (Rourke, 1994).
[d]Reitan Evaluation of Hemispheric Abilities and Brain Improvement Training (Reitan & Wolfson, 1992).

designed to address problems experienced by children with LD (Rourke, 1994). However, Rourke's DNRR paradigm provides a useful framework for designing remedial/rehabilitation plans for children with other brain-related childhood disorders (Teeter & Semrud-Clikeman, in press). The DNRR was first described by Rourke *et al.* (1983) and Rourke, Fisk, and Strang (1986).

The DNRR is composed of seven major steps (Rourke, 1994). In Step 1, the clinician assesses the interactions among neuropsychological assets/deficits, LD, academic learning, and psychosocial functioning. Neuropsychological assessment is conducted within an ecological framework. Developmental considerations are investigated at this stage. Step 2 includes assessment of the demands of the environment. The functional status of the child (i.e., neuropsychological) is related to developmental challenges (i.e., behavioral, academic, and psychosocial), and the ecological context of the child (e.g., classroom, social, cultural) (Rourke, 1994).

In Step 3 short- and long-term behavioral predictions are generated. A determination of which deficits are expected to decrease without intervention, and which strategies will be implemented for the other deficits is made. Resources (e.g., family, psychosocial, community) are also assessed during this step. Step 4 involves determining "ideal" short- and long-term remedial plans using information gathered in earlier steps. Ongoing monitoring and modification of the intervention plan is suggested on an "as needed" basis. In Step 5 the availability of remedial resources is assessed, and therapeutic goals, length of intervention, and prognosis of outcome are specified. Clear and specific recommendations at this step may reduce overlap and costs incurred when integrating efforts of the neuropsychologist with those initiated by school professionals. Step 6 requires development of a realistic remedial plan by comparing recommendations developed in Steps 4 and 5. Finally, in Step 7 ongoing neuropsychological assessment is used to modify or clarify intervention plans (Rourke, 1994).

In summary, the DNRR offers an integrated paradigm for the assessment and remediation of LD in children. Further, the DNRR provides a framework for identifying critical factors that should be considered when designing interventions for other disorders as well. Reitan also has described remediation procedures for children with brain-related disorders.

The Reitan Evaluation of Hemispheric Abilities and Brain Improvement Training (REHABIT)

REHABIT was developed for rehabilitating brain-related deficits (Reitan, 1980). REHABIT includes assessment with the Halstead–Reitan test batteries, training with Halstead–Reitan test items, and rehabilitation with special REHABIT materials (Teeter, 1989). The Halstead–Reitan neuropsychological test batteries are used in both the assessment and remediation stages of this program. Neuropsychological evaluations are conducted, and interventions are designed to remediate the child's weaknesses, including abstract, concept formation, and reasoning deficits (Teeter & Semrud-Clikeman, in press).

The REHABIT program includes tracts for training verbal–language deficits, abstract reasoning and logical deficits, visual–spatial problems, and right–left hemisphere deficits (Reitan & Wolfson, 1992). The child's neuropsychological profile is used to design individualized remedial programs (Teeter & Semrud-Clikeman, in press). Difficulty levels can be manipulated, and systematic evaluation is important to monitor the child's progress throughout the remediation program.

More recently, Levine has described a model for addressing learning difficulties in children. The model is reviewed next.

Phenomenological Model for Educational Interventions

Levine (1993, 1994) developed a model based on observing and describing phenomena that are known to interfere with learning and the academic performance of children. The model utilizes neurodevelopmental theory and acknowledges that both the child's brain and his or her environment (i.e., school and home) change over time "in terms of the level and complexity of demands placed on children" (Levine, 1994, p. 2). Levine (1993, 1994) describes 26 observable phenomena that affect a child's performance in the classroom. This model places an emphasis on "observable phenomena," that is, phenomena that are clearly observable when one watches the child perform. For example, it is possible to observe that a child has trouble remembering information when studying for a test or that the child has trouble organizing and planning study time. These phenomena are thus fully described and form the basis for determining intervention strategies.

Although many "observable phenomena" may be neurodevelopmental in nature, resulting from neurochemical/metabolic abnormalities, abnormal or uneven brain growth patterns, or synaptic abnormalities in specific brain regions, not all phenomena result from neurodevelopmental factors (Levine, 1994). Other environmental (e.g., exposure, teaching) or psychosocial factors may account for performance problems. Rather than stressing an investigation into the causes of learning problems, Levine emphasizes recognition and intervention of learning problem(s). Thus, evaluation includes assessment of educational, behavioral/affective, cognitive development, environmental, and medical factors that might affect performance. Levine (1993, 1994) advocates for a descriptive versus a labeling approach when evaluating children. Child assessment may have several levels: parent/teacher informal observation and discussion; consultation from a clinician; multidisciplinary evaluation; and/or further specialized diagnosis.

Once a thorough and comprehensive evaluation has been conducted, the educator and/or clinician can develop a detailed intervention program that specifically addresses the needs of the child. Levine (1993, 1994) describes components of a management plan, involving both parents and teachers, as: (1) demystification; (2) bypass strategies; (3) direct remediation of dysfunctions; (4) direct remediation of skill areas; (5) medical interventions; (6) protection from psychological harm/humiliation and development of pride; and (7) long-term monitoring and child advocacy. These components are briefly described as follows.

Demystification is a process whereby educators and/or clinicians help the child to understand the nature of her or his problems. By helping the child to understand her or his strengths and weaknesses more accurately, fears, frustrations, and negative self-attributions can be modified. Bypass strategies are employed in the classroom to circumvent a child's problems (Levine, 1994). These strategies may include: modifying the amount of time given to take tests; reducing the amount of work that is required; reducing the complexity of information; changing the production/output format (i.e., oral versus examination); changing the evaluation/grading system; and/or using aids (e.g., calculators or word processors). (See Levine, 1994, for more details.)

Direct instruction of observable phenomena is also incorporated into intervention plans. Levine (1993, 1994) provides numerous strategies for attentional, language, memory, production, reasoning, motor, social, and specific academic functions. Techniques that strengthen weaknesses and enhance academic skills are recommended. Medications may also be part of some intervention plans, and when administered, children should be advised of the implications, benefits, and potential side effects. Finally, Levine (1994) describes ways to preserve the child's pride in him- or herself, to protect the child from humiliation, and to facilitate the emergence of healthy self-esteem. Specific intervention strategies are delivered within a collaborative process, where home, school, and physicians work together for the benefit of the child. A long-term commitment is necessary, with ongoing monitoring and advocacy by professionals and parents.

The models described above provide a structure for the assessment, intervention, and management of various childhood disorders. In the following sections, selected neuropsychological, neurocognitive, and neurobehavioral approaches for intervention are described. Aspects of these approaches can be incorporated into assessment–intervention plans for children with various brain-related disorders.

Neuropsychological Orientations for Remediation

Neuropsychological/neurobehavioral intervention orientations are often classified in one of three ways depending on whether the focus is on improving the child's neurocognitive deficits, accessing the child's neurocognitive strengths/assets, or a combination approach addressing both neurocognitive assets and deficits (Teeter, 1989). These three intervention orientations will be briefly reviewed.

Attacking Neurocognitive Deficits

Psycholinguistic training, sensory-integration, perceptual-motor training, or modality training were historically used to strengthen the child's weaknesses (Teeter & Semrud-Clikeman, in press). In general, little improvement in the child's academic performance has been demonstrated with these techniques; however, modest success has been observed in some children with specific problems/

disorders. Specifically, Kavale (1990) reported that children with reading disabilities do improve when given explicit instruction in verbal-comprehension and auditory-perceptual skills. Training in phonological awareness has also proven effective for children with phonological core deficits (Cunningham, 1990). So, in some instances remediation of a child's weakness may be warranted; however, these methods typically utilize approaches where specific processes are taught within the context of reading instruction, and not in isolation.

Teaching to Neurocognitive Strengths

Intervention programs have been designed to access the child's unique neurocognitive strengths and to avoid his or her deficits/weaknesses (Teeter & Semrud-Clikeman, in press). Strength approaches make sense for children with motivational problems (Rourke et al., 1983). Gaddes and Edgell (1994) also cite cases where teaching to the child's intact brain systems might be helpful. For example, interventions accessing intact right hemisphere systems can be successful in improving reading skills in children with bilateral cerebral dysfunction, cognitive retardation, and/or language deficits (Teeter & Semrud-Clikeman, in press).

Combined Treatment Programs

Intervention approaches that address the child's unique neuropsychological assets and deficits, and are primarily compensatory in nature have been advocated by Rourke (1994). Rourke indicates that the age of the child may also help clinicians to determine which orientation should be instituted first. For example, young children with developmental disorders involving the white matter (see discussion on NLD) may improve with intervention methods that attack the child's deficits (Teeter & Semrud-Clikeman, in press). Early intervention in these instances focuses on stimulating intact cortical regions and facilitating gray matter connections (Teeter & Semrud-Clikeman, in press). Conversely, older children with persistent disorders (e.g., NLD) may benefit from compensatory strategies.

Levine (1994) describes a combined intervention model that includes both bypass strategies and methods for improving cognitive-processing, attentional, language, and poor output and adaptational dysfunctions in children. Bypass strategies "circumvent or work around a student's dysfunctions . . . allow the child to continue to acquire skill, knowledge, and a sense of competency" and are "techniques that must be part of the management of every child with significant learning problems" (Levine, 1994, p. 260). However, Levine also describes numerous strategies for remediating or improving specific deficiencies as well. A combined intervention approach seems to provide mechanisms for increasing motivation, self-esteem, and engagement in the learning process, while decreasing the chances of the child falling precipitously below grade level, thus decreasing the probability of school drop-out in later grades.

There is a continued need for conducting research on specific strategies/programs to demonstrate the efficacy of specific intervention approaches. The following sections describe techniques that have been found useful for remediating cognitive–intellectual, academic, and psychosocial problems. The clinician may select specific strategies depending on the child's particular pattern of neurocognitive strengths and weaknesses. First, a number of common childhood disorders are briefly discussed.

Disorders of Childhood: Implications for Remediation

Selected childhood disorders will be briefly reviewed including reading disabilities, NLD, ADD, pervasive developmental delays, seizure disorders, TBI, and childhood brain tumors. Implications for interventions are discussed. Each disorder typically has primary deficits/characteristics (e.g., cognitive, attentional, memory), as well as associated deficits (e.g., academic and psychosocial) that need to be considered when designing intervention programs.

The following discussion highlights major features of each disorder that may need to be targeted for intervention. In later sections, other techniques (e.g., self-management, social skills) will be reviewed.

Reading Disabilities: Phonological Core Deficits

Numerous studies show that phonological awareness deficits are a primary cause of reading deficits (Liberman & Shankweiler, 1985; Mann, 1986; Stanovich, 1986; Wagner & Torgesen, 1987). Phonological awareness is the ability to use the phonemic segments of speech (Tunmer & Rohl, 1991), including the awareness and use of the sound structure of language (Mattingly, 1972). Children with phonological awareness deficits may also demonstrate other language-related deficiencies that appear related to phoneme awareness deficits, including difficulties with: speech perception when listening; naming and vocabulary ability; and short-term memory involving phonetic representations in linguistic tasks (Mann, 1991).

Children with phonological reading disorders (PRD) exhibit a variety of disorders that may be associated with their linguistic problems (Teeter & Semrud-Clikeman, in press). Various studies have shown that linguistic and phonological coding problems are linked to genetic (Olson, Fosberg, Wise, & Rack, 1994) as well as developmental anomalies in the left temporal regions (Semrud-Clikeman, Hynd, Novey, & Eliopulos, 1991). Semrud-Clikeman *et al.* found that slight morphological variations in the left temporal region were related to other language-related deficits including word attack, comprehension, and naming abilities. Table 2 summarizes selected research findings on children with PRD.

Although not every child with PRD demonstrates all of the associated features presented, evidence of an interaction among specific neuropsychological, cognitive, perceptual, memory, academic, and psychosocial problems that accompany reading disabilities is accumulating (Teeter & Semrud-Clikeman, in press).

Intervention Strategies

Remedial techniques that specifically address phonological core deficits are effective for students who are at risk for reading problems and for children with PRD (Byrne & Fielding-Barnsley, 1993; Cunningham, 1990; Iversen & Tunmer, 1993; Molter, 1993; Vellutino & Scanlon, 1987). Reading abilities are significantly increased when phonological awareness training is paired with metacognitive techniques, particularly when contextualized within the child's reading curriculum (Cunningham, 1990).

Motivational and psychosocial disturbances that often occur in children with chronic academic failure may be alleviated with early identification and remediation (Wise & Olson, 1991). Scruggs and Wong (1990) and Wong (1991) provide extensive guidelines for implementing strategy instruction, mnemonic instruction, social skills enhancement, problem-solving processes, and self-recording skills. Thus, intervention techniques for children with PRD should specifically include phonological awareness training within contextual-

TABLE 2. A Summary of Specific Deficits Associated with Reading Disabilities: Phonological Core Deficits (PRD)[a,b]

Biogenetic factors
  40% variance in word recognition is genetic
  h2g = 0.62 phonology/reading deficits
  h2g = 0.22 orthographic/reading deficits

Environmental factors/prenatal/postnatal
  Orthographic deficits related to exposure to print and learning opportunities
  Development of speech and vocabulary related to language acquisition and reading
  Growth spurt in phonemic awareness at 6 years related to reading efforts
  Despite strong heritability of phonological awareness, deficits can be modified

Temperament
  No known correlates

Birth complications
  No known correlates

CNS factors
  White matter dysfunction
  Left temporal anomalies
  Larger plana in right hemisphere
  Symmetrical R/L temporal lobes
  Symmetrical or reversed parieto-occipital regions
  Abnormal asymmetry (R > L) in prefrontal regions
  Abnormal asymmetry in parietal regions

Neuropsychological factors
  Rapid naming
  Abnormal hemispheric lateralization
  Attentional activation of RH interferes with LH verbal processing
  Attentional control mechanisms between hemispheres
  Phonemic hearing, segmenting, and blending

Intellectual	Perceptual	Memory	Attentional
Verbal weaknesses	Phonemic	Digit span	Strong comorbidity of reading
Vocabulary knowledge	Speech	Speech sounds	problems and ADHD
Verbal associations		Word series	Attention to phonemes
Word similarities		Letter strings	
Verbal fluency		Phonetic strategies	
Receptive language			
Expressive language			
Verbal IQ			
Comprehension			

Academic/behavioral	Psychosocial	Family
Motivational problems	Research is sparse	Research is sparse on PRD
Chronic reading problems	RD in general show	Prenatal and postnatal risk factors
Disengaged in learning	internalized disorders (i.e.,	related to general learning and
Spends less time reading	depression)	behavioral problems
Reading and spelling		"Disorganized" and/or poverty, environment more important with age

[a]Adapted with permission from Teeter and Semrud-Clikeman (in press).
[b]PRD, phonological reading disabilities; L and LH, left hemisphere; R and RH, right hemisphere; RD, reading disabilities.

ized reading instruction to increase reading skills. Intervention plans may also include other strategy instruction (e.g., mnemonic, social), based on the child's individual profile.

The extent to which children with PRD require interventions across cognitive, as well as psychosocial domains depends on the individual child. However, these features should be considered when designing treatment programs.

Nonverbal Learning Disabilities

Children with NLD have relatively intact language, reading, and spelling skills and show the most difficulty in the areas of mathematics reasoning and calculation, problem-solving, and basic social-emotional problems (Rourke, 1989). Table 3 presents an overview of the associated features of NLD. The complex set of problems associated with NLD appear related to a pattern of right hemisphere weaknesses (e.g., tactile and visual perception, concept formation, novelty, and complex psychomotor skills), with relative strengths in left hemisphere activities (e.g., phonological skills, verbal abilities, reading, spelling, verbatim memory) (Rourke, 1994). Rourke advocates intervention programs that target both neurocognitive strengths and weaknesses.

Intervention Strategies

Extensive remedial techniques to improve the academic and psychosocial problems experienced

TABLE 3. A Summary of Specific Deficits Associated with Nonverbal Learning Disabilities[a]

Biogenetic factors	Environmental factors/prenatal/postnatal
No known correlates	NLD appear at or soon after birth
	Neurodevelopmental disorder or may be caused by traumatic injury
	Few details on environmental impact

Temperament   Birth complications
No known correlates   No known correlates

CNS factors
    White matter dysfunction
    Intermodal integration (callosal fibers)
    Right hemisphere involvement
Neuropsychological factors
    Bilateral tactile deficits (pronounced on left side)
    Visual–spatial–organizational deficits
    Complex psychomotor deficits
    Oral–motor apraxia
    Concept formation and problem-solving deficits

Intellectual	Perceptual	Memory	Attentional
Concept formation	Visual discrimination	Tactile	Tactile
Strategy generation	Visual detail	Nonverbal	Visual attention
Hypothesis testing	Visual relation	Complex information	Attends to simple, repetitive
Cause–effect relations			verbal material
Little speech prosody			
Formal operational thought			

Academic/behavioral	Psychosocial	Family
Graphomotor	Adapting	Research is sparse
Reading comprehension	Overreliance on rote behaviors	
Mechanical arithmetic	Externalized disorders (i.e., conduct, acting out)	
Mathematical reasoning	Social perception and judgment	
Science	Social interactions skills	
	Social withdrawal or isolation	
	May develop internalized disorders (e.g.,	
	depression, anxiety)	

[a]Adapted with permission from Teeter and Semrud-Clikeman (in press).

by children with NLD are available (Rourke, 1989; Rourke et al., 1983; Rourke, Del Dotto, Rourke, & Casey, 1990; Rourke & Fuerst, 1991). According to Rourke (1994), children with the unique pattern of right hemisphere weaknesses and left hemisphere strengths display a tendency to engage in perseverative or stereotypic responding because they over-rely on information they have previously learned (Teeter & Semrud-Clikeman, in press). Children with NLD often have trouble developing problem-solving strategies and alternative solutions when strategies are ineffective. Typically children with NLD develop verbal compensatory skills, and they actively avoid novel situations. Further, children with NLD do not actively explore their environment because of tactile deficits and delays in early psychomotor skills.

For young children, intensive physiotherapy with sensorimotor integration is necessary to "stimulate the functioning of remaining white matter to the maximum" (Rourke, 1989, p. 130). Compensatory strategies, relying on verbal-language skills, may be considered if intervention is not effective or if it occurs later in childhood. Intervention should focus on academic as well as psychosocial deficits, and should involve the parent. Techniques for increasing social awareness, teaching problem-solving strategies, encouraging generalization of strategies, and improving verbal skills are often included in the intervention plan for children with NLD (Teeter & Semrud-Clikeman, in press). Concrete teaching aids, self-evaluation techniques, and life skills are also used. Methods for improving visual–spatial weaknesses, interpreting competing stimuli, teaching nonverbal behaviors, and providing structure for exploration are described in detail by Rourke (1989).

Further, Rourke (1989) describes techniques for increasing problem-solving skills, generalization of strategies and concepts, appropriate nonverbal skills, accurate self-evaluation, and life skills—preparing for adult life. Because of the very serious psychosocial limitations inherent in the NLD syndrome, Rourke stresses the need for social problem-solving skills, social awareness, structured peer interactions, and parent involvement in the treatment plan. Techniques are also developed to increase the child's exploratory behaviors and interactions with the environment. Rourke's (1989) methods emphasize the need for a step-by-step problem-solving approach, where feedback is provided in a supportive manner. Children are encouraged to "lead with their strong suit," and are also taught more appropriate ways to utilize their relative strengths (i.e., verbal-language skills).

Despite positive findings using single-subject investigations, Rourke (1994) indicates that more systematic research is needed on interventions developed from neuropsychological findings. Studies should specifically address whether interventions should be deficit driven or compensatory in nature. The age of the child also seems to be a critical factor when deciding whether interventions should be deficit driven or compensatory in nature. When deficits result from early white matter disease or dysfunction, Rourke (1994) suggests that remediation might focus on attacking the deficit. However, if the child's problems are identified later in childhood or if NLD persists, compensatory strategies might be the best approach (Teeter & Semrud-Clikeman, in press).

Attention Deficit Hyperactivity Disorder

Children may be identified with primarily hyperactive–impulsive problems, attentional problems, or a combination of the two according to DSM-IV criteria (APA, 1994). The manner in which these characteristics affect academic, behavioral, and psychosocial adjustment has been thoroughly described in numerous publications (see Barkley, 1990; Weiss & Hechtman, 1993). Table 4 summarizes major features and associated characteristics of ADHD.

ADHD appears to have strong genetic linkages (Weiss & Hechtman, 1993), and evidence suggests CNS variation in frontal lobe, corpus callosal, and right hemisphere regions (Teeter & Semrud-Clikeman, 1995). The extent to which these biogenetic factors relate to associated deficits, including executive functions, disinhibition, attentional controls, and self-regulation, is of interest to neuropsychologists (Teeter & Semrud-Clikeman, in press).

This model suggests the need to develop strategies addressing broad domains of academic, behavioral, psychosocial, and family systems interventions.

Intervention Strategies

Intervention programs are typically multifaceted in nature and may include pharmacotherapy, behavioral management, cognitive/academic strategies, social skills building, and parenting and/or family interventions (Barkley, 1990; Teeter &

TABLE 4. A Summary of Specific Deficits Associated with Attention Deficit Hyperactivity Disorder[a]

Biogenetic factors	Environmental factors/prenatal/postnatal
59%–84% MZ	Mulifactorial, polygenetic, cultural, and environmental
29%–33% DZ	transmission seems unlikely
Independent genetic code differs from reading	Poverty, overcrowding, chaotic family style, pollution,
Familial ADD transmitted by single gene	food additives account for very little variance
Single gene has not been isolated, probably	Common environmental factors: 0–30% variance
dopamine receptor gene	
Temperament	Birth complications
Genetic linkage	No known correlates
Activity level	
Distractibility	
Psychomotor activity	
Attentional problems, school competence and	
behavioral problems	

CNS factors
Underactivated frontal lobe
Bilaterally smaller anterior cortex
Reversed asymmetry of anterior cortex (right < left)
Reversed asymmetry of caudate nucleus (left < right)
Reduced metabolic activity in right caudate region
Smaller left caudate nucleus
Right hemisphere deficits (disinhibition of left hemisphere)
Left hemisphere underactivation (Zametkin)
Genu (corpus callosum) smaller
Rostrum and rostral bodies are smaller

Intellectual	Perceptual	Memory	Attentional
Range of IQ		Low verbal	Sustained
Low coding		Less efficient	Selective
			Alternating/divided
Reasoning			
Response inhibition			
Sustained effort			
Complex problem-solving			
Executive functions			
Organization skills			
Academic/behavioral	Psychosocial		Family
Motivational problems	Rejected		Disorder exacerbates
Underachievers	Ignored		Parental psychopathology related to
Comorbid LD	Comorbid INT/EXT		CD/ADHD
Work completion	Comorbid aggression		

[a]Adapted with permission from Teeter and Semrud-Clikeman (in press).

Semrud-Clikeman, 1995). Even when medication is administered, children with ADHD usually require other academic, behavioral, and psychosocial interventions. Studies suggest that attention training (Semrud-Clikeman, 1995), peer tutoring (DuPaul & Stoner, 1994), and contingency management (Barkley, 1990) can be effective intervention strategies for children with ADHD.

It is important to note that a majority of children with ADHD also have comorbid disorders (e.g., oppositional defiant, conduct disorder, LD). When comorbid disorders are present, these problems also need to be addressed in the intervention program. (For detailed information on more specific strategies for children with ADHD, see Barkley, 1990; Teeter, in preparation; Teeter &

Semrud-Clikeman, 1995; and Weiss & Hechtman, 1993.)

Pervasive Developmental Disorders

Autism and pervasive developmental disorders are characterized by deficits in social reciprocity, communication, and cognition (Cook & Leventhal, 1992).

Intervention Strategies

Children with autism often respond to interventions that are similar to strategies used with cognitively delayed children (Teeter & Semrud-Clikeman, in press). Behavioral techniques for reducing stereotypic behaviors and improving communication skills are recommended (Cook & Leventhal, 1992). Fluoxetine and clomipramine are often prescribed to control anxiety and compulsive behaviors in children with autism (Teeter & Semrud-Clikeman, in press). Although behavioral intervention techniques are effective, the long-term prognosis for children with autism remains guarded.

Seizure Disorders

Epilepsy is defined as a chronic disturbance in brain functions that affects perceptions, movements, consciousness, and other behaviors; the term *seizures* refers to individual episodes (Bennett & Krein, 1989). Numerous associated features may be present in children with seizure disorders including: cognitive disabilities (Cook & Leventhal, 1992); psychiatric disturbance (Cook & Leventhal, 1992); academic problems (Pazzaglia & Frank-Pazzaglia, 1976); and social stress related to chronic medical problems (Neppe, 1985). Thus, intervention planning incorporates medical as well as psychosocial techniques.

Intervention Strategies

Anticonvulsant medications (i.e., phenobarbital) are frequently prescribed for children with nonfebrile seizure disorders (Cook & Leventhal, 1992), and require careful monitoring. Side effects (e.g., sedation) may decrease academic performance (Cook & Leventhal, 1992), or increase hyperactivity (Vining, Mellits, Dorsen, *et al.,* 1987) and depression (Brent, Crumrine, Varma, *et al.,* 1987).

In children with intractable seizures, surgical removal of involved brain tissue may be necessary (Teeter & Semrud-Clikeman, in press). In these rare cases, studies demonstrate the resiliency of the developing brain following surgery, wherein intact brain regions compensate for damaged regions. No significant decline in IQ scores was found in children who had undergone surgical removal of the dominant temporal lobes, including the hippocampus and amygdala (Meyer, Marsh, Laws, & Sharbrough, 1986). In another case, Smith, Walker, and Myers (1988) reported that a 6-year-old with perinatal epileptogenic seizures that spread across the hemispheres made remarkable recovery following surgical removal of the right hemisphere. Postsurgical test scores showed average to low-average intellectual abilities. The degree to which cognitive development is affected depends on a number of factors, including the age of the child and the location of the lesion. However, once intact brain regions are freed from the abnormal influences of the lesioned regions, intellectual and cognitive abilities may improve following surgery (Teeter & Semrud-Clikeman, in press).

Traumatic Brain Injury

TBI occurs frequently in childhood (Berg, 1986), because children are at risk for sustaining head injuries from accidents (Hynd & Willis, 1988; Spreen, Tupper, Risser, Tuokko, & Edgell, 1984). (See Bigler, 1990, for an in-depth discussion of the nature and associated features of TBI.) The site of injury, the severity of injury, and the age of the child impact on the types of problems that accompany TBI in children. (See Teeter & Semrud-Clikeman, in press, for an in-depth review of recovery of functions following TBI.) Interventions should be designed to address the specific assets and deficits individual children display following injury.

Intervention Strategies

Child characteristics (i.e., cognitive and personality), family resources, marital stability, and socioeconomic status impact on the child's recovery following TBI (Teeter & Semrud-Clikeman, in press). Developmental history and an assessment of the child's environment must be carefully considered when designing intervention plans (Goldstein & Levin, 1990). Preexisting disorders (e.g., impulsivity–hyperactivity, attentional deficits, social-interaction problems, and academic failure) may be ascertained from teacher reports and a review of educational history (Craft, Shaw, & Cartlidge, 1972). Further, postinjury deficits may reflect premorbid problems, rather than the brain trauma itself (Rutter, 1981). Children with premorbid disorders, including impulsivity and hyperactivity, may have higher injury rates as a result of risk-taking behaviors sometimes associated with these problems (Rutter, 1981).

Guidelines for Educational Services for Students with Traumatic Brain Injury were developed by the Virginia Department of Education (1992), which include intervention plans for developing home–school partnerships. The needs of families and children are addressed in this program (Teeter & Semrud-Clikeman, in press). Assessments, placement decisions, individual educational plans (IEPs) or 504 plans, and strategies for improving the behavioral and academic problems in the classroom should be included in the intervention plan.

Brain Tumors

Brain tumors comprise approximately 20% of malignancies of childhood and are most frequently diagnosed in children between the ages of 3 and 9 years (Carpentieri & Mulhern, 1993). Treatment protocols often include whole-brain radiation, chemotherapy, and/or surgical interventions in the medical treatment protocol of children with brain tumors. About 50–60% of children remain cancer free after 5 years (Carpentieri & Mulhern, 1993). Intervention typically addresses medical, education, and psychosocial domains.

Intervention Strategies

Medical procedures, including surgery, radiation, and chemotherapy, are often employed to reduce the size of the child's brain tumor (Price, Goetz, & Lovell, 1992). Cognitive and neuropsychological symptoms may be relieved once cranial pressure is reduced (Teeter & Semrud-Clikeman, in press). Although medical techniques can produce positive outcomes, pharmacotherapy, psychosocial (i.e., individual and family therapy), and academic support are usually initiated after the child's medical status is stabilized (Teeter & Semrud-Clikeman, in press).

Depending on the nature and type of brain-related disorder, children may require interventions for a variety of problems, including academic, executive functions, and psychosocial adjustment. The following selected strategies and intervention approaches may be employed in individual cases following a comprehensive assessment of the child's assets/deficits. Careful, ongoing monitoring for the effectiveness of these strategies must be included in the intervention plan. Selective classroom and behavioral management techniques are also described.

Interventions for Associated Cognitive–Academic, Psychosocial, Executive Function, and Attentional Problems

Selected strategies for addressing cognitive, academic, executive control, and attentional problems may be utilized for children with various brain-related disorders depending on their individual needs. Careful neuropsychological evaluation, with measures of cognitive, academic, and social–emotional functioning, helps to isolate the child's specific intervention needs. Also, a review of specific techniques that have been previously employed by the teacher or parent should be investigated to determine which strategies have been effective and which have been less successful in individual cases. For those strategies that have proven ineffective, it is important to make sure that the techniques were properly employed and were not prematurely abandoned.

Strategies for Cognitive and Academic Difficulties

Techniques for improving reading, written language, and arithmetic disorders are often employed in remediation programs for children. Strategies for teaching study/organizational skills and social skills training are also sometimes needed. Table 5 reviews selected strategies for addressing these problems.

Depending on the child's pattern of neuropsychological, cognitive, and psychosocial functioning, the clinician may want to consider the specific strategies outlined. Table 5 is not offered as a "one size fits all" approach, because specific techniques should be carefully selected based on results from a comprehensive evaluation and a clear understanding of the child's neuropsychological assets and deficits, and his or her developmental, cognitive,

TABLE 5. Selected Strategies for Addressing Cognitive, Academic, Psychosocial, and Attentional Problems in Children and Adolescents

Disorders	Strategies	References
Reading		
Phonemic awareness	Segmenting, blending, and analyzing sounds	Fox & Routh (1976)
	Phonological recoding, translating letters and letter patterns into phonemes	Iversen & Tunmer (1993)
	Grapheme–phoneme correspondences in word families (e.g., "ight") to teach generalizations	
	Phonemic awareness is contextualized in regular reading lessons	Cunningham (1989)
	Metacognitive strategies	Iversen & Tunmer (1993)
		Cunningham (1989)
Comprehension	"Reciprocal teaching" using predicting, questioning, and clarifying	Palinscar *et al.* (1987)
	"Interactive learning" access and link prior knowledge, "clue lists," and predict relationships	Bos & Van Reusen (1991)
Computer and speech feedback	Speech synthesizer	Wise *et al.* (1989)
Whole language	Strength approach utilizing word recognition with metacognition	Wise & Olson (1991)
	Language activities (reading–writing) linked and literature freely used	
Written language	Cognitive and metacognitive strategies	Bos & Van Reusen (1991)
	Plan, organize, write, edit, and revise "Cognitive Strategy Instruction"	Englert (1990)
	"Self-Instructional Strategy Training"	Graham & Harris (1989)
Mathematics	Cognitive and metacognitive approaches understand the problem, plan solution, carry out solution, and assess accuracy	Montague & Bos (1986)
	Verbal elaboration, written cue cards with rules for problem-solving, and concrete aids	Strang & Rourke (1985)
	Step-by-step problem-solving with feedback	Rourke (1989)
Study and organization	Strategies Intervention Model	Ellis & Lenz (1991)
	Setting priorities, how can task be accomplished, analyzing task, setting goals, monitoring and checking on accomplishments	Ellis & Friend (1991)
Social skills	ACCESS Program	Walker, McConnell, *et al.* (1988)
	ACCEPTS Program	Walker, Holmes, *et al.* (1988)

academic, and social–emotional needs (Teeter & Semrud-Clikeman, in press). Prior to initiating an intervention program, the clinician is advised to conduct a review of the child's educational records and interview the child's teacher. These efforts may reduce the possibility of repeating techniques or strategies that may have failed in the past. Further, it may inform the clinician of pitfalls or behaviors to look out for when attempting certain techniques. Careful observation of the child's performance is also recommended. (See Levine, 1993, 1994, for details on conducting neurobehavioral observations and ratings for children with learning problems.)

Strategies for Reading Disorders

A number of techniques for addressing reading disorders are described, including phonemic awareness training, comprehension strategies, synthesized computer speech, and whole language methods. (See Teeter & Semrud-Clikeman, in press, for a more in-depth review of these techniques.)

Phonological Awareness Training

Phonological coding deficits have been shown to be the strongest predictor of reading disabilities (Wise & Olson, 1991). The following studies report positive effects for teaching children phonemic awareness skills, including: segmenting, blending, and analyzing sounds (Fox & Routh, 1976; Tunmer & Nesdale, 1985; Williams, 1980); preventing phonological awareness deficits in preschool children (Byrne & Fielding-Barnsley, 1993; Lundberg, Frost, & Petersen, 1988); using common sound elements in word families (Iversen & Tunmer, 1993); using words taken from classroom reading lessons (Cunningham, 1989); and incorporating metacognitive techniques showing children how and when to use strategies (Cunningham, 1990; Duffy et al., 1987; Gaskins et al., 1988; Iverson & Tunmer, 1993). Further, grapheme–phoneme correspondences are integrated during reading instruction.

Comprehension Strategies

"Reciprocal teaching" methods have been used to increase comprehension by teaching predicting, questioning, and clarifying strategies (Palinscar, Brown, & Martin, 1987). Maintenance and generalization were demonstrated with these methods (see Wise & Olson, 1991, for a review). "Interactive learning strategies" increase comprehension and vocabulary knowledge utilizing the following steps: (1) identifying the child's prior knowledge about a topic; (2) linking prior knowledge to new information; (3) scanning reading material, to develop "clue lists," "relationship maps," or charts; and (4) predicting relationships across concepts (Bos & Van Reusen, 1991). Teacher–student relationships are a central feature of this program, wherein both work together to enhance and facilitate student learning.

Computer and Speech Feedback

A computerized speech synthesizer (i.e., DECtalk) has been successful in improving phono-logical coding and word recognition skills for children with reading problems (Olson, Foltz, & Wise, 1986). Segmented feedback is presented when the child is unable to read a particular word. The computer highlights and simultaneously "says" the word with the child. Comprehension questions and corrective feedback are also available in this software (Olson et al., 1994; Wise & Olson, 1991).

Whole Language Programs

Whole language incorporates reading into language activities, wherein reading and writing are taught together using the child's literature for reading activities (Teeter & Semrud-Clikeman, in press). Word recognition and metacognitive techniques can also be included in whole language programs (Wise & Olson, 1991). Although still somewhat controversial, some suggest that word decoding can also be incorporated into a whole language curriculum for children who need it (Wise & Olson, 1991).

Strategies for Written Language Disorders

Techniques for written language problems frequently employ metacognitive strategies (Bos & Van Reusen, 1991) to teach students how to plan, organize, write, edit, and revise writing samples (Englert, 1990). Structured curricular programs are available, including the Cognitive Strategy Instruction Writing (Raphael, Kirschner, & Englert, 1986) and Self-Instructional Strategy Training (Graham & Harris, 1987, 1989). Students are taught to identify the main character, where the story takes place, and how the story ends. Self-regulation and self-monitoring techniques are usually stressed, although self-regulation training did not increase performance over the other strategies (Bos & Van Reusen, 1991).

Strategies for Math Disorders

Deficits in math problem-solving have not been viewed as an educational priority until recently (Bos & Van Reusen, 1991). Reasoning ability, metacognitive processing skills, and reading proficiency appear related to deficits in solving word problems (Bos & Van Reusen, 1991). Cognitive and metacognitive approaches wherein students are taught to understand the nature of the problem, plan a solution, carry out the solution, and assess the accuracy of the solution, have been designed to reduce math problem-solving deficits in children (Teeter & Semrud-Clikeman, in press). Strategy instruction has been shown to be effective for math-related difficulties (Montague & Bos, 1986; Smith & Alley, 1981).

Few studies on math LD describe the neuropsychological characteristics of the subjects or the cognitive strategies employed (Fleischner, 1994). In this regard, Fleischner suggests using the Test of Early Mathematics Ability (TEMA-2) or the Diagnostic Test of Arithmetic Strategies to determine information about which strategies might be useful. Further, Rourke (1989) developed a model for describing the neuropsychological characteristics of children with specific deficits in the math area and developed a comprehensive intervention program (Teeter & Semrud-Clikeman, in press). (See Rourke, 1989, for specific details to increase problem-solving and reasoning skills in children with math-related problems.)

Strategies for Deficits in Executive Functions: Planning and Organizational Skills

The Strategies Intervention Model (SIM), developed by the University of Kansas Institute for Research on Learning Disabilities, provides systematic strategy instruction for high school students (Ellis & Lenz, 1991). The SIM program teaches students learning strategies to acquire and store knowledge, and to demonstrate this knowledge (Ellis & Friend, 1991). Effective strategies must be useful, efficient, and memorable, and often include: setting priorities; reflecting on how a task can be attacked and accomplished; and analyzing the task, setting goals, monitoring, and checking to see if goals were accomplished (Ellis & Friend, 1991).

Skills for Success is a structured curriculum to teach students (grades 3–6) study and organization skills (Archer & Gleason, 1989). Reading, organizing and summarizing information, test taking, anticipating test content, how to study, and responding to various test formats are featured (DuPaul & Stoner, 1994). DuPaul and Stoner provide guidelines for organizing materials, using assignment calendars, and steps to organizing and completing a paper. Initial evidence suggests that study and organizational skills are effective procedures for youth with LD (Ellis & Friend, 1991), and warrant further research for children with disorders such as ADHD (DuPaul & Stoner, 1994).

Teachers often comment that organizational, planning, and study skills often impede the performance of children with learning problems. Thus, techniques to increase these academic survival skills may need to be considered to increase the likelihood of school success. Children with various neurodevelopmental or acquired brain-related disorders often evidence problems with social interaction and emotional adjustment. Strategies for addressing these deficits are explored next.

Strategies for Social Skills Deficits

Social skill deficits have been linked to LD (Semrud-Clikeman & Hynd, 1991); school dropout, delinquency, and emotional disturbance (Barclay, 1966); and ADD (Carlson, Lahey, Frame, Walker, & Hynd, 1987). Further, peer rejection resulting from aggression predicts criminal activity in adulthood (Parker & Asher, 1987). This research has prompted the inclusion of social skills deficits in proposed definitions of LD (Bryan & Lee, 1990; Gaddes & Edgell, 1994; Lerner, 1993). Bryan (1991) and Rourke (1994) suggest that interventions plans that focus solely on academic gains and ignore the impact of social skills deficits will limit remediation efforts for many children with LD. The importance of social skills as well as academic competencies is stressed in multifaceted intervention plans.

Bryan (1991) suggests that self-efficacy, self-esteem, attributional thinking, social cognition, comprehension of nonverbal cues and social mores, moral development, social problem-solving, communication skills, and behaviors in the classroom are related to social skills difficulties. These factors have been related to various neuropsychological syndromes associated with right or left hemisphere deficiencies (Semrud-Clikeman & Hynd, 1991). LD children with right hemisphere dysfunction display a variety of problems, including: math weaknesses, visual–spatial and social imperception; motor weaknesses on the left side; verbal reasoning deficits; and social gesturing and communication/language problems (Denkla, 1978, 1983). Conversely, children with abnormal right hemisphere functioning, based on CT scans, EEGs, and neuropsychological measures, had trouble interpreting the emotions of others and expressing appropriate emotions (Voeller, 1986). Increased attentional and hypermotoric behaviors were also found in children with signs of right hemisphere dysfunction.

A number of structured social skills training programs are available, including: the ACCEPTS program for elementary children (Walker, McConnell, *et al.,* 1988) and the ACCESS program for adolescents (Walker, Holmes, Todis, & Horton, 1988). These social skills programs have been shown to be effective for a variety of children with mild to moderate learning and behavior problems (Teeter & Semrud-Clikeman, in press). Further, behavior management is used outside structured sessions to increase generalization of trained skills.

Research investigating the effectiveness of social skills training shows mixed and sometimes disappointing results (Vaghn, McIntosh, & Hogan, 1990). Even when children do show behavioral changes in social interaction skills problems, these improvements are not readily acknowledged or perceived by peers or teachers (Northcutt, 1987). Issues related to generalization of "trained" social skills often do not occur in natural settings.

Vaghn *et al.* (1990) indicate that programs for students with learning problems have been shown to be effective when: (1) LD students obtain part-time versus full-time LD services; (2) LD students are in elementary or high school (middle school students show fewer positive gains); (3) intervention programs include regular class students; (4) programs are individualized; (5) children receive training because of social skills deficits and not placement in LD classes alone; (6) training programs occur over an extended time (average 9 weeks, 23.3 hours) and include follow-up sessions; (7) small groups or one-to-one instruction is utilized; and (8) coaching, modeling, corrective feedback, rehearsal, and strategy instruction are incorporated into the training program.

Intervention programs should address the broader social milieu of the child (La Greca, 1993), and should include high-status or non-problem peers. La Greca recommends using multisystemic intervention models, prevention, peer-pairing and cooperative activities, avoiding cliques and child-picked teams, teacher monitoring, and parental involvement. Friendship building with one or two close friends might buffer the child who is not popular with the larger group (La Greca, 1993). A close friendship might further reduce anxiety, stress, depression, and low self-esteem in children who have been excluded because of social skills problems.

In summary, broader goals should be considered in social skills training where the targeted child, peers, teachers, and parents are included in the social skills intervention plan (Teeter & Semrud-Clikeman, in press).

Classroom and Behavior Management Strategies

Various behavioral management techniques have proven effective for numerous childhood problems (Shapiro, 1989). The literature demonstrating the strengths of behavioral principles is too extensive to review here. (See DuPaul & Stoner, 1994, and Witt, Elliott, & Gresham, 1988, for extensive reviews of token economies, contingency contracting, cost response, and time-out from positive reinforcement.) The following briefly reviews self-management, attention training, home-based contingencies, and peer tutoring.

Self-Management/Self-Control Techniques

Self-management techniques attempt to increase the child's ability to control her or his own behavior and to decrease dependency on the teacher. Lloyd and Landrum (1990) describe the techniques for teaching self-assessment (i.e., observing one's own behavior), self-evaluation (i.e., comparing one's behavior to others), self-recording, and self-reinforcement. (See Table 6.) These techniques can target numerous behaviors, although attending to task has been of major interest (Teeter & Semrud-Clikeman, in press).

Children with learning and behavior disorders from age 4 to adolescence have successfully utilized self-recording techniques to: increase attention to task; decrease behavioral disruption; increase productivity and accuracy; and sustain and complete schoolwork (Lloyd & Landrum, 1990). Self-recording usually employs cuing (e.g., tape-recorded beeps at 1-, 2-, or 3-minute intervals, or kitchen timers that ring every 5 minutes) (Heins, Lloyd, & Hallahan, 1986) and fading of cues (Lloyd & Landrum, 1990).

Home-Based Contingencies

Home-based contingencies, employing daily or weekly teacher notes, reports, or ratings, often supplement school-based token systems (DuPaul & Stoner, 1994). Targeted behaviors may focus on increasing or improving attention, work/homework completion, compliance, and social interactions.

TABLE 6. Selected Classroom and Behavior Management Strategies for Addressing Problems in Children and Adolescents

Strategies	Description	References
Self-management	Self-assessment, self-evaluation, self-recording, and self-reinforcement	Lloyd & Landrum (1990)
Attention training	Self-recording with taped cuing	Heins *et al.* (1986)
Home-based contingencies	Attention training with self-monitoring, and strategic problem-solving	Semrud-Clikeman (1995)
Peer tutoring	Home–school weekly or daily notes target attention, work completion, compliance, and social interactions	DuPaul & Stoner (1994)
	ClassWide Peer Tutoring program dyads, tutor–tutee pairs with specified roles	Greenwood *et al.* (1988)

Teachers provide written comments, the child takes the comments home, and the parent then discusses the child's performance in school, and provides reinforcement depending on school behaviors. Home-based contingencies are increasingly used in schools, and can be very effective (Teeter & Semrud-Clikeman, in press).

Peer Tutoring

Greenwood, Maheady, and Carta (1991) developed peer tutoring techniques for various academic areas, including reading, spelling, and math activities. The class is organized into tutor–tutee pairs who work together on lessons and assignments (Shapiro, 1989). The ClassWide Peer Tutoring (CWPT) program provides systematic and detailed training guidelines for implementing this intervention technique (Greenwood, Delquardi, & Carta, 1988). Academic and behavioral gains for children who have been described as slow learners, learning disabled, and behavioral disordered have been documented (Shapiro, 1989). Recently these techniques were applied to a young child with ADHD and credited with less hyperactivity, increased on-task behavior, and academic gains in math (DuPaul & Henningson, 1993).

The selected techniques may be incorporated into intervention programs for children with various developmental, academic, behavioral, and social problems. Individual assessment and academic planning provides the mechanism for deciding which techniques should be employed (Teeter & Semrud-Clikeman, in press). Intervention techniques are usually used in combination, and must be carefully monitored to determine their impact. Intervention monitoring has been described by DuPaul and Stoner (1994), Shapiro (1989), and Shapiro and Kratochwill (1988).

Childhood disorders may require medical treatments, including psychopharmacology (Pelham, 1993a). The following section briefly reviews pharmacological interventions that are appropriate for a number of childhood and adolescent disorders.

Psychopharmacological Interventions

Although children and adolescents with neurodevelopmental or acquired brain-related disorders may require medication, intervention programs are usually multidimensional in nature. "Appropriate psychosocial and psychoeducational interventions should form a component of treatment for most children with these disorders—even those where pharmacotherapy is helpful" (Pelham, 1993a, p. 161). Medications for major depressive disorders, psychotic disorders, ADHD, Tourette's syndrome, and seizure disorders are briefly discussed. This is not meant to be an exhaustive list of medication options, but serves as an overview emphasizing potential benefits and side effects. Intervention programs for children receiving medication should specify how medications will be monitored, and how teachers, physicians, and parents will communicate about medication efficacy.

Specific Classes of Medication

Green (1991) classified medications as stimulants, antipsychotics, tricyclic antidepressants or monoamine oxidase inhibitors, anxiolytics, and anticonvulsants, depending on their behavioral effects on the CNS. Selected medications for children and adolescents, with potential benefits and side effects, are shown in Table 7. (See Cook & Leventhal, 1992,

TABLE 7. Common Uses, Benefits, and Side Effects of Medications for Neuropsychiatric Disorders of Childhood[a]

Drugs	Common uses	Manifestations	Side effects
Stimulants			
Methylphenidate (Ritalin)	ADHD	75% of children are responders Decreased motor activity, impulsivity, and disruptive behaviors Increased attention Improved socialization Improved ratings (teacher, physician, parent) Increased work completion and accuracy Improved test scores (mazes, PIQ, and visual memory)	Insomnia, appetite loss, nausea, vomiting, abdominal pains, thirst, headaches Tachycardia, change in blood pressure Irritability, moodiness Rebound effects Growth suppression (can be monitored) Lower seizure threshold Exacerbate preexisting tics
Dextroamphetamine (D-amphetamine)	ADHD	Similar to methylphenidate Subdued emotional response Increased reflectivity and ability to monitor self Increased interest level Improved school performance Improved parent ratings (conduct, impulsivity, immaturity, antisocial, and hyperactivity)	Similar to methylphenidate Hallucinations, seizures, and drug-induced psychosis (rare occurrences)
Magnesium pemoline (Cylert)	ADHD	Similar to methylphenidate Improved teacher ratings (defiance, inattention, and hyperactivity) Improved parent ratings (conduct, impulsivity, and antisocial behaviors) Improved test scores (mazes, PIQ, visual memory)	Similar to methylphenidate
Antipsychotics			
Haloperidol (Haldol)	Psychosis Tourette's Autism PDD ADD with CD	Reduces aggression, hostility, negativity, and hyperactivity Reduces psychotic symptoms Reduces Tourette's symptoms Reduces fixations, withdrawal stereotypies, anger, and fidgetiness in autism Increases social responsivity and reality testing in PDD	Behavioral toxicity with preexisting disorders Dystonia (loss of tone in tongue and trunk) Parkinsonian symptoms (tremors, mask face, and drooling) Dyskinesis (mouth, tongue, and jaw) Dose reduction decreases motor side effects Intellectual dulling, disorganized thoughts
Chlorpromazine (Thorazine)	Psychosis Severe aggression, explosiveness, and hyperexcitability in MR children	Reduces hyperactivity Reduces tantrums, aggression, self-injury Not effective for young autistics	Similar to haloperidol Dermatological problems Cardiovascular problems Lowers seizure threshold Endocrinological problems Ophthalmological problems Hematological problems

(continued)

TABLE 7. (*Continued*).

Thioridazine (Mellaril)	Psychosis
	Severe behavior
	  disorders (extreme)
		Reduces hyperactivity
		Improves schizophrenic symptoms
		Similar to Thorazine
			Similar to haloperidol
			Sedation, cognitive dulling,
			  and impaired arousal

Thiothixene (Navane)	Psychosis	Similar to Mellaril	Less sedating than Mellaril
Loxapine succinate (Loxitane)	Psychosis	Similar to Haldol	Similar to Haldol
Fluphenazine HCl (Prolixin, Permitil)	Psychosis		

Pimozide (Orap)	Psychosis
	Tourette's (resistant
	  type)
		Clinical improvement	High doses: death and
			  seizures

Clozapine (Clozaril)	Severe psychosis
	  (resistant type)
		Clinical improvement	Life threatening
			  hypertension, and
			  tachycardia, and EEG
			  changes
			Seizures

Tricyclic antidepressants
Imipramine HCl
  (Tofranil)
	Depression
	Enuresis
	ADHD
	School phobia
		Improves depression (not severe)
		Inhibits bladder muscles
		Reduces hyperactivity
		Reduces separation anxiety
		Improves sleep disorders
			Potentially life-threatening
			  cardiovascular problems
			CNS symptoms (EEG
			  changes, confusion,
			  lowers seizure threshold,
			  incoordination,
			  drowsiness, delusions,
			  and psychosis)
			Blurred vision, dry mouth,
			  and constipation

Nortriptyline HCl
  (Pamelor)
	Depression	Low rate of clinical improvement in
		  children and adolescents
			Withdrawal symptoms

Desipramine HCl
  (Norpramin)
	ADHD
	ADHD with tics
		Improved ratings (parents and
		  teachers Conners)
		Clinical improvement
			Dry mouth, decreased
			  appetite, tiredness,
			  dizziness, insomnia
			EEG changes at high doses

Clomipramine HCl
  (Anafranil)
	Obsessive–compulsive
	  disorders
	Severe ADHD
	Enuresis
	School phobia
		Reduces obsessions
		Reduces school phobia/anxiety
		Reduces aggression, impulsivity, and
		  depressive/affective symptoms
			Withdrawal symptoms
			Seizures
			Somnolence, tremors,
			  dizziness, headaches,
			  sweating, sleep disorder,
			  gastrointestinal problem,
			  cardiovascular effects,
			  anorexia, and fatigue

Monoamine oxidase inhibitors
Fluoxetine HCl (Prozac)
	Depression
	Obsessive–compulsive
		Effective for adults
		Clinical improvement for OCD
			Nausea, weight loss, anxiety,
			  nervousness, sweating,
			  sleep disorder

Bupropion (Wellbutrin)	Depression
	ADHD
		Adolescents 18+ improve
		Improved global ratings not Conners
			Seizures, agitation, dry
			  mouth, insomnia, nausea,
			  constipation, tremors

TABLE 7. (*Continued*).

Anxiolytics			
Chlordiazepoxide (Librium)	Anxiety with hyperactivity and irritability School phobia	Clinical improvement Reduced hyperactivity, fears, enuresis, truancy, bizarreness Decreases emotional overload	Drowsiness, fatigue, muscle weakness, ataxia, anxiety, and depression with high doses
Diazepam (Valium)	Mixed psychiatric DX anxiety and sleep	Improved global ratings Better results for adolescents	Relatively low toxicity
Alprazolam (Xanax)	Anxiety Panic attacks Separation anxiety	Clinical improvements Responders (premorbid personality: shy, inhibited, nervous)	Mild drowsiness
Anticonvulsants			
Phenobarbital	Seizure disorders	Reduces seizures	Lethal at high doses Cognitive impairment, rigidity, and depression
Diphenylhydantoin Sodium (Phenytoin)	Seizure disorders	Reduces tonic–clonic seizures	Cognitive impairment Drug toxicity
Carbamazepine	Seizure disorders Manic–depression	Reduces generalized and tonic–clonic seizures Psychotropic effects	Fewer adverse side effects than other drugs Less cognitive dulling, motoric and affective
Sodium valproate	Seizure disorders	Reduces seizures Petit mal and tonic–clonic	Low cognitive symptoms Relatively nontoxic in adults Rare but potentially fatal hepatoxicity in children

[a]Adapted with permission from Teeter and Semrud-Clikeman (in press). Data from Dubovsky (1992), Green (1991), and Neppe and Tucker (1992).

Green, 1991, and Teeter & Semrud-Clikeman, in press, for in-depth discussions of the interactions among medications, neurotransmitter systems, and neuropsychiatric/neurodevelopmental disorders of childhood.)

Monitoring Medication

Determining whether medication should be administered typically includes comprehensive assessment, and a review of the child's medical, educational, and psychosocial history (Teeter & Semrud-Clikeman, in press). The nature and severity of the child's problem, and the effectiveness of psychosocial and/or behavioral interventions should be considered. Nonmedical interventions for children with severe ADHD, depression, anxiety, and conduct disorders are generally attempted before medication is prescribed. If nonmedical interventions do not sufficiently improve the child's problems, controlled trials of medication may be initiated (Teeter & Semrud-Clikeman, in press).

Baseline data (e.g., ECG, EEG, urinalysis, liver, thyroid, and renal function tests, blood pressure, and serum blood levels) are generally gathered on children receiving antipsychotics, antiepileptics, and antidepressants (Green, 1991). Behavioral data (e.g., rating scales, questionnaires) are also used to measure the benefits/effects of medication.

Response rates to stimulant medications vary considerably from individual to individual (Barkley, 1990; DuPaul & Stoner, 1994; Pelham, 1993a). Thus, careful evaluation using rating scales or home–school notes is important (see Barkley, 1990; DuPaul & Stoner, 1994; Pelham, 1993b). Although a number of scales and procedures are described for children with ADHD, there are fewer scales available for other childhood disorders (Teeter & Semrud-Clikeman, in press).

Ecologically valid behaviors in the classroom and in social situations should be assessed to determine the effects of stimulant medication (Pelham, 1993b). Daily report cards monitoring work completion/accuracy and compliance are helpful in this process (Pelham, 1993b). Ecologically valid assessment of medication effects for depression, anxiety, and conduct-related problems is needed. Specific targeted behaviors (e.g., sadness, panic attacks, or anger outbursts) would be more explicitly defined and monitored on a regular basis (Teeter & Semrud-Clikeman, in press). Further medication monitoring should occur in the child's natural setting (e.g., home and school) and should not be based solely on clinic observations in the doctor's office (Teeter & Semrud-Clikeman, in press). This necessarily increases the need for ongoing home–school–physician communication.

Pharmacological/Behavioral Interventions

Psychopharmacotherapy is rarely employed without other interventions (Teeter & Semrud-Clikeman, in press). Most childhood and adolescent disorders affect multiple areas of adjustment (cognitive, academic, and psychosocial) which are not always improved by medication alone. Pharmacological is often combined with behavioral treatments (e.g., contingency management, home–school notes), individual or group therapy for the child or adolescent, parent training, and family therapy (Teeter & Semrud-Clikeman, in press).

Pelham (1993b) said that "an important result of combined treatments may be that maximal improvement in behavior may be reached without resorting to high dosages of stimulant medication" which also lowers the adverse side effects of medication (p. 220). Carlson, Pelham, Milich, and Dixon (1992) also indicate that combined approaches (i.e., medication with behavioral interventions) complement the shortcomings of either treatment alone, whereas Pelham (1993b) found that combined interventions add incremental effects not found when single interventions are used in isolation for children with ADHD.

Further research investigating combined intervention programs for various childhood disorders is needed. The need for ecologically based medication monitoring increases the need for home–school–physician partnerships. Children requiring medically based interventions need careful monitoring in school and at home. Thus, teachers and parents need to work closely with physicians to coordinate intervention programs and to monitor medication effectiveness. The following section briefly discusses collaborative partnerships.

Home–School–Physician Partnerships

There are numerous reasons why home–school–physician partnerships are important. Teeter and Semrud-Clikeman (in press) include the following reasons: (1) children often are seen by a number of different professionals so that coordination of interventions is required; (2) because of the high cost of medical and psychological services, duplication should be avoided if possible; (3) children on medication require monitoring of their behavior in a natural environment; (4) educational staff working with children with various brain-related diseases or disorders (e.g., brain tumors, TBI) must be knowledgeable about the child's medical, psychosocial, academic, and behavioral needs; and (5) parents and family members may require help from various professionals who must communicate with each other.

Confidentiality is of utmost importance and parental permission is required to obtain and share information (Teeter & Semrud-Clikeman, in press). Further, it is important to have someone act as the coordinator of services when numerous professionals are involved in treatment plans. Parents are often forced into this role, and many are ill-equipped to deal with the demands of coordinator because of the day-to-day stress involved with raising children with significant medical, academic, and/or psychosocial needs. The case coordinator may vary depending on whether the child's problems are primarily educational and/or psychosocial (e.g., ADHD or LD) or medical (i.e., brain tumor or TBI); e.g., school staff may coordinate services in the first instance, and the physician or neuropsychologist may serve in the latter case. The role of case coordinator may also change as the child either improves, recovers, or deteriorates. Nonetheless, if parents are placed in this role by themselves, this may be an extra burden on an already overly taxed family.

Regular communication among all professionals is required, and a set schedule may be needed for initial assessment and intervention planning, and for ongoing monitoring (Teeter & Semrud-Clikeman, in press). Once the child shows improvement or stabilizes medically, follow-up may occur less frequently or at longer intervals (i.e., 6, 12, 18, and 24 months).

Summary and Conclusions

This chapter presented various strategies for developing intervention programs for children with various disorders. A transactional model was discussed, wherein neuropsychological, cognitive, behavioral, and psychosocial factors are considered in the evaluation–intervention process. Intervention strategies for children with neurodevelopmental and acquired brain-related disorders are usually multidimensional in nature. Intervention planning should follow comprehensive evaluation and accurate diagnosis of the child's problems, and should address the full range of the child's neurocognitive, academic, behavioral, and psychosocial needs.

References

American Psychiatric Association. (1994). *Diagnostic and statistical manual of mental disorders* (4th ed.). Washington, DC: Author.

Archer, A., & Gleason, M. (1989). *Skills for school success (grades 3–6).* North Billerica, MA: Curriculum.

Barclay, J. R. (1966). Sociometric choices and teacher ratings as predictors of school dropout. *Journal of Social Psychology, 4,* 40–45.

Barkley, R. A. (1990). *Attention deficit-hyperactivity disorder: A handbook for diagnosis and treatment.* New York: Guilford Press.

Bennett, T. L., & Krein, L. K. (1989). The neuropsychology of epilepsy: Psychological and social impact. In C. R. Reynolds & E. Fletcher-Janzen (Eds.), *Handbook of clinical child neuropsychology* (pp. 19–41). New York: Plenum Press.

Berg, R. A. (1986). Neuropsychological effects of closed-head injury in children. In J. E. Obrzut & G. W. Hynd (Eds.), *Child neuropsychology: Vol. 2. Clinical practice* (pp. 113–135). New York: Academic Press.

Bigler, E. R. (1990). *Traumatic brain injury: Mechanisms of damage, assessment, intervention and outcome.* Austin, TX: PRO-ED.

Bos, C. S., & Van Reusen, A. K. (1991). Academic interventions with learning-disabled students: A cognitive/metacognitive approach. In J. Obrzut & G. W. Hynd (Eds.), *Neuropsychological foundations of learning disabilities* (pp. 659–684). Orlando, FL: Academic Press.

Brent, D. A., Crumrine, P. K., Varma, R. R., Allan, M. A., & Allman, C. (1987). Phenobarbital treatment and major depressive disorder in children with epilepsy. *Pediatrics, 80,* 909–917.

Bryan, T. (1991). Social problems and learning disabilities. In B. Y. L. Wong (Ed.), *Learning about learning disabilities* (pp. 195–229). Orlando, FL: Academic Press.

Bryan, T., & Lee, J. (1990). Social skills training with learning disabled children and adolescents: The state of the art. In T. E. Scruggs & B. Y. L. Wong (Eds.), *Intervention research in learning disabilities* (pp. 263–278). Berlin: Springer-Verlag.

Byrne, B., & Fielding-Barnsley, R. (1993). Evaluation of a program to teach phonemic awareness to young children: A 1-year follow-up. *Journal of Educational Psychology, 85,* 104–111.

Carlson, C. C., Lahey, B. B., Frame, C. L., Walker, J., & Hynd, G. W. (1987). Sociometric status of clinic-referred children with attention deficit disorders with and without hyperactivity. *Journal of Abnormal Psychology, 15,* 537–547.

Carlson, C. C., Pelham, W. E., Milich, R., & Dixon, M. (1992). Single and combined effects of methylphenidate and behavior therapy on the classroom behavior, academic performance, and self-evaluations of children with attention deficit hyperactivity disorder. *Journal of Abnormal Child Psychology, 20,* 213–232.

Carpentieri, S. C., & Mulhern, R. K. (1993). Patterns of memory dysfunction among children surviving temporal lobe tumors. *Archives of Clinical Neuropsychology, 8,* 345–357.

Cook, E. H., & Leventhal, B. L. (1992). Neuropsychiatric disorders of childhood and adolescence. In S. C. Yudofsky & R. E. Hales (Eds.), *The American Psychiatric Press textbook of neuropsychiatry* (2nd ed., pp. 639–662). Washington, DC: American Psychiatric Press.

Craft, A. W., Shaw, D. A., & Cartlidge, N. E. (1972). Head injuries in children. *British Medical Journal, 4,* 200–203.

Cravioto, J., & Arrieta, R. (1983). Malnutrition in childhood. In M. D. Rutter (Ed.), *Developmental neuropsychiatry* (pp. 32–51). New York: Guilford Press.

Cunningham, A. (1989). Phonemic awareness: The development of early reading competency. *Reading Research Quarterly, 24,* 471–472.

Cunningham, A. (1990). Explicit versus implicit instruction in phonemic awareness. *Journal of Experimental Child Psychology, 50,* 429–444.

Denkla, M. B. (1978). Minimal brain dysfunction. In J. S. Chall & A. F. Mirsky (Eds.), *Education and the brain* (pp. 223–268). Chicago: University of Chicago Press.

Denkla, M. B. (1983). The neuropsychology of social-emotional learning disabilities. *Archives of Neurology, 40,* 461–462.

Dubovsky, S. L. (1992). Psychopharmacological treatment in neuropsychiatry. In S. C. Yudofsky & R. E. Hales (Eds.), *The American Psychiatric Press textbook of neuropsychiatry* (2nd ed., pp. 663–702). Washington, DC: American Psychiatric Press.

Duffy, G., Roehler, L., Sivan, E., Rackliff, G., Book, C., Meloth, M., Vavrus, L., Wesselman, R., Putnam, J., & Bassiri, D. (1987). Effects of explaining the reasoning associated with using reading strategies. *Reading Research Quarterly, 22,* 345–368.

DuPaul, G., & Henningson, P. N. (1993). Peer tutoring effects on the classroom performance of children with attention-deficit hyperactivity disorder. *School Psychology Review, 22,* 134–143.

DuPaul, G., & Stoner, G. (1994). *ADHD in the schools: Assessment and intervention strategies.* New York: Guilford Press.

Ellis, E. S., & Friend, P. (1991). Adolescents with learning disabilities. In B. Y. L. Wong (Ed.), *Learning about learning disabilities* (pp. 506–563). Orlando, FL: Academic Press.

Ellis, E. S., & Lenz, B. K. (1991). *The development of learning strategy interventions.* Lawrence, KS: Edge Enterprise.

Englert, C. S. (1990). Unraveling the mysteries of writing through strategy instruction. In T. E. Scruggs & B. Y. L. Wong (Eds.), *Intervention research in learning disabilities* (pp. 186–223). Berlin: Springer-Verlag.

Epstein, M. A., Shaywitz, S. E., Shaywitz, B. A., & Woolston, J. L. (1992). The boundaries of attention deficit disorder. In S. E. Shaywitz & B. A. Shaywitz (Eds.), *Attention deficit disorder comes of age: Toward the twenty-first century* (pp. 197–220). Austin, TX: PRO-ED.

Felton, R. H., & Brown, I. S. (1991). Neuropsychological prediction of reading disabilities. In J. E. Obrzut & G. W. Hynd (Eds.), *Neuropsychological foundations of learning disabilities: A handbook of issues, methods, and practice* (pp. 387–410). San Diego, CA: Harcourt Brace Jovanovich.

Fleischner, J. E. (1994). Diagnosis and assessment of mathematics learning disabilities. In G. R. Lyon (Ed.), *Frames of reference for the assessment of learning disabilities: New views on measurement issues* (pp. 441–458). Baltimore: Paul H. Brookes.

Fox, B., & Routh, D. K. (1976). Phonemic analysis and synthesis as word-attack skills. *Journal of Educational Psychology, 69,* 70–74.

Gaddes, W. H., & Edgell, D. (1994). *Learning disabilities and brain function: A neuropsychological approach* (3rd ed.). Berlin: Springer-Verlag.

Gaskins, I., Downer, M., Anderson, R., Cunningham, P., Gaskins, R., Schommer, M., & the teachers of the Benchmark School. (1988). A metacognitive approach to phonics: Using what we know to decode what you don't. *RASE: Remedial and Special Education, 9,* 36–66.

Goldstein, F. C., & Levin, H. S. (1990). Epidemiology of traumatic brain injury: Incidence, clinical characteristics, and risk factors. In E. D. Bigler (Ed.), *Traumatic brain injury: Mechanisms of damage, assessment, intervention and outcome* (pp. 51–68). Austin, TX: PRO-ED.

Graham, S., & Harris, K. R. (1987). Improving composition skills of inefficient learners with self-instructional strategy training. *Topics in Language Disorders, 7,* 66–77.

Graham, S., & Harris, K. R. (1989). A components analysis of cognitive strategy instruction: Effects on learning disabled student's compositions and self-efficacy. *Journal of Educational Psychology, 81,* 353–361.

Gray, J. W., & Dean, R. S. (1989). Approaches to the cognitive rehabilitation of children with neuropsychological impairment. In C. R. Reynolds & E. Fletcher-Janzen (Eds.), *Handbook of clinical child neuropsychology* (pp. 397–408). New York: Plenum Press.

Green, W. H. (1991). *Child and adolescent clinical psychopharmacology.* Baltimore: Williams & Wilkins.

Greenwood, C. R., Delquardi, J., & Carta, J. J. (1988). *Classwide peer tutoring.* Seattle: Educational Achievement Systems.

Greenwood, C. R., Maheady, L., & Carta, J. J. (1991). Peer tutoring programs in the regular education classroom. In G. Stoner, M. R. Shinn, & H. M. Walker (Eds.), *Interventions for achievement and behavior problems* (pp.

179–200). Silver Spring, MD: National Association of School Psychologists.

Gresham, F. M., & Gansle, K. A. (1992). Misguided assumptions of DSM-III-R: Implications for school psychologists. *School Psychology Quarterly, 7,* 79–95.

Heins, E. D., Lloyd, J. W., & Hallahan, D. P. (1986). Cued and noncued self-recording to task. *Behavior Modification, 10,* 235–254.

Horton, A. M. (1979). Behavioral neuropsychology: Rationale and research. *Clinical Neuropsychology, 1,* 20–23.

Horton, A. M., Jr., & Puente, A. E. (1986). Behavioral neuropsychology in children. In J. E. Obrzut & G. W. Hynd (Eds.), *Child neuropsychology: Vol. 2. Clinical practice* (pp. 299–316). Orlando, FL: Academic Press.

Hynd, G. W. (1992). Misguided or simply misinformed? Comment on Gresham and Gansle's vitriolic diatribe regarding DSM. *School Psychology Quarterly, 7,* 100–103.

Hynd, G. W., Lorys, A. R., Semrud-Clikeman, M., Nieves, N., Huettner, M., & Lahey, B. B. (1991). Attention deficit disorder without hyperactivity: A distinct behavioral and neurocognitive syndrome. *Journal of Child Neurology, 6*(Suppl.), S37–S43.

Hynd, G. W., & Willis, W. G. (1988). *Pediatric neuropsychology.* New York: Grune & Stratton.

Iversen, S., & Tunmer, W. E. (1993). Phonological processing skills and the reading recovery program. *Journal of Educational Psychology, 85,* 112–126.

Johnston, C., & Pelham, W. E. (1986). Teacher ratings predict peer ratings and aggression at 3-year follow-up in boys with attention deficit disorder hyperactivity. *Journal of Consulting and Clinical Psychology, 54,* 571–572.

Kavale, K. (1990). Effectiveness of special education. In T. B. Gutkins & C. R. Reynolds (Eds.), *The handbook of school psychology* (2nd ed., pp. 868–898). New York: Wiley.

Kratochwill, T. R., & Bergan, J. R. (1990). *Behavioral consultation in applied settings: An individual guide.* New York: Plenum Press.

Kratochwill, T. R., & Plunge, M. (1992). DSM-III-R, treatment validity, and functional analysis: Further considerations for school psychologists. *School Psychology Review, 7,* 227–232.

La Greca, A. M. (1993). Social skills training with children: Where do we go from here? Presidential Address. *Journal of Clinical Child Psychology, 22,* 288–298.

Lambert, N. M., & Sandoval, J. (1980). The prevalence of learning disabilities in a sample of children considered to be hyperactive. *Journal of Abnormal Child Psychology, 8,* 33–50.

Lerner, J. (1993). *Learning disabilities: Theories, diagnosis, and teaching strategies* (6th ed.). Boston: Houghton Mifflin.

Levine, M. D. (1993). *Developmental variations and learning disorders.* Cambridge, MA: Educators Publishing Service.

Levine, M. D. (1994). *Educational care.* Cambridge, MA: Educators Publishing Service.

Liberman, I. Y., & Shankweiler, D. (1985). Phonology and the problems of learning to read and write. *Remedial and Special Education, 6,* 8–17.

Lloyd, J. E., & Landrum, T. J. (1990). Self-recording of attending to task: Treatment components and generalization of effects. In T. E. Scruggs & B. Y. L. Wong (Eds.), *Intervention research in learning disabilities* (pp. 235–262). Berlin: Springer-Verlag.

Lundberg, I., Frost, J., & Petersen, O. P. (1988). Effects of an extensive program for stimulating phonological awareness in preschool children. *Reading Research Quarterly, 23,* 267–284.

Mann, V. (1986). Why some children encounter reading problems. In J. Torgesen & B. Wong (Eds.), *Psychological and educational perspectives on learning disabilities* (pp. 133–159). Orlando, FL: Academic Press.

Mann, V. (1991). Language problems: A key to early reading problems. In B. Y. L. Wong (Ed.), *Learning about learning disabilities* (pp. 130–163). Orlando, FL: Academic Press.

Mash, E. J., & Terdal, L. G. (1988). *Behavioral assessment of childhood disorders.* New York: Guilford Press.

Mattingly, I. G. (1972). *Language by ear and eye: The relationship between speech and reading.* Cambridge, MA: MIT Press.

Meyer, F. B., Marsh, W. R., Laws, E. R., & Sharbrough, F. W. (1986). Temporal lobectomy in children with epilepsy. *Journal of Neurosurgery, 64,* 371–376.

Milich, R., & Landau, S. (1989). The role of social status variables in differentiating subgroups of hyperactive children. In L. M. Bloomingdale & J. Swanson (Eds.), *Attention deficit disorder: Current concepts and emerging trends in attentional and behavioral disorders of childhood* (Vol. 5, pp. 1–16). Elmsford, NY: Pergamon Press.

Molter, J. (1993). *The effects of phonemic awareness training on delayed readers.* Unpublished doctoral dissertation, University of Wisconsin–Milwaukee, Milwaukee.

Montague, M., & Bos, C. (1986). The effect of cognitive strategy training on verbal math problem solving performance of learning disabled adolescents. *Journal of Learning Disabilities, 19,* 26–33.

Neppe, V. M. (1985). Epilepsy and psychiatry: Essential links. *Psychiatric Insight, 2,* 18–22.

Neppe, V. M., & Tucker, G. J. (1992). Neuropsychiatric aspects of seizure disorders. In S. C. Yudofsky & R. E. Hales (Eds.), *The American Psychiatric Press textbook of neuropsychiatry* (2nd ed., pp. 397–425). Washington, DC: American Psychiatric Press.

Northcutt, T. E. (1987). The impact of a social skills training program on the teacher–student relationship. *Dissertation Abstracts International, 46,* 1231A.

Nussbaum, N. L., Bigler, E. D., & Koch, W. (1986). Neuropsychologically derived subgroups of learning disabled children: Personality behavioral dimensions. *Journal of Research and Development in Education, 19,* 57–67.

Obrzut, J. E., & Hynd, G. W. (Eds.). (1991). *Neuropsychological foundations of learning disabilities: A handbook of issues, methods, and practice.* San Diego, CA: Harcourt Brace Jovanovich.

Olson, R., Foltz, G., & Wise, B. (1986). Reading instruction and remediation with the aid of computer speech. *Behavior Research Methods, Instruments, and Computers, 18,* 93–99.

Olson, R., Fosberg, H., Wise, B., & Rack, J. (1994). Measurement of word recognition, orthographic, and phonological skills. In G. R. Lyon (Ed.), *Frames of reference for the assessment of learning disabilities: New views on measurement issues* (pp. 243–278). Baltimore: Paul H. Brookes.

Palinscar, A., Brown, A., & Martin, S. (1987). Peer interaction in reading comprehension instruction. *Educational Psychologist, 22,* 231–253.

Parker, J. G., & Asher, S. R. (1987). Peer relations and later personal adjustment: Are low-accepted children at risk? *Psychological Bulletin, 102,* 357–389.

Pazzaglia, P., & Frank-Pazzaglia, L. (1976). Record in grade school of pupils with epilepsy: An epidemiological study. *Epilepsia, 17,* 361–366.

Pelham, W. E. (1993a). Recent developments in pharmacological treatment for child and adolescent mental health disorders. *School Psychology Review, 22,* 158–161.

Pelham, W. E. (1993b). Pharmacotherapy for children with attention deficit-hyperactivity disorder. *School Psychology Review, 22,* 199–227.

Price, T. P., Goetz, K. L., & Lovell, M. R. (1992). Neuropsychiatric aspects of brain tumors. In S. C. Yudofsky & R. E. Hales (Eds.), *The American Psychiatric Press textbook of neuropsychiatry* (2nd ed., pp. 473–498). Washington, DC: American Psychiatric Press.

Raphael, T. E., Kirschner, C. S., & Englert, C. S. (1986). *The impact of text instruction within a process writing orientation on fifth and sixth grade students' comprehension and production of expository text.* Paper presented at the American Educational Research Association, San Francisco.

Reitan, R. M. (1980). *REHABIT–Reitan evaluation of hemispheric abilities and brain involvement training.* Tucson, AZ: Reitan Neuropsychology Laboratory and University of Arizona.

Reitan, R. M., & Wolfson, D. (1992). *Neuropsychological evaluation of older children.* Tucson, AZ: Neuropsychology Press.

Reschly, D. J., & Gresham, F. M. (1989). Current neuropsychological diagnosis of learning problems: A leap of faith. In C. R. Reynolds & E. Fletcher-Janzen (Eds.), *Handbook of clinical child neuropsychology* (pp. 503–519). New York: Plenum Press.

Rourke, B. (1989). *Nonverbal learning disabilities: The syndrome and the model.* New York: Guilford Press.

Rourke, B. (Ed.). (1991). *Neuropsychological validation of learning disabilities subtypes.* New York: Guilford Press.

Rourke, B. (1994). Neuropsychological assessment of children with learning disabilities: Measurement issues. In C. R. Lyon (Ed.), *Frames of reference for the assessment of learning disabilities: New views on measurement issues* (pp. 475–514). Baltimore: Paul H. Brookes.

Rourke, B., Bakker, D., Fisk, J., & Strang, J. (1983). *Child neuropsychology: An introduction to theory, research, and clinical practice.* New York: Guilford Press.

Rourke, B., Del Dotto, J. E., Rourke, S. B., & Casey, J. E. (1990). Nonverbal learning disabilities: The syndrome and a case study. *Journal of School Psychology, 28,* 361–385.

Rourke, B., Fisk, J. L., & Strang, J. D. (1986). *Neuropsychological assessment of children: A treatment-oriented approach.* New York: Guilford Press.

Rourke, B., & Fuerst, D. R. (1991). *Learning disabilities and psychosocial functioning: A neuropsychological perspective.* New York: Guilford Press.

Rourke, B., Young, G. C., & Leenaars, A. A. (1989). A childhood learning disability that predisposes those afflicted to adolescent and adult depression and suicide risk. *Journal of Learning Disabilities, 22,* 169–175.

Rutter, M. (1981). Psychological sequelae of brain damage in children. *American Journal of Psychiatry, 139,* 21–33.

Rutter, M., Chadwick, O., & Shaffer, D. (1983). Head injury. In M. Rutter (Ed.), *Developmental neuropsychiatry* (pp. 83–111). New York: Guilford Press.

Scruggs, T. E., & Wong, B. Y. L. (Eds.). (1990). *Intervention research in learning disabilities.* Berlin: Springer-Verlag.

Semrud-Clikeman, M. (1995, April). *Attention training for children with attentional–hyperactive problems.* Paper presented at the annual meeting of the American Educational Research Association, San Francisco.

Semrud-Clikeman, M., Biederman, J., Sprich-Buckminster, S., Krifcher, B., Lehman, B., Faraone, S. V., & Norman, D. (1992). The incidence of ADHD and concurrent learning disabilities. *Journal of the American Academy of Child and Adolescent Psychiatry, 31,* 439–448.

Semrud-Clikeman, M., & Hynd, G. W. (1991). Specific nonverbal and social skills deficits in children with learning disabilities. In J. E. Obrzut & G. W. Hynd (Eds.), *Neuropsychological foundations of learning disabilities: A handbook of issues, methods, and practice* (pp. 603–630). Orlando, FL: Academic Press.

Semrud-Clikeman, M., & Hynd, G. W. (1993). Assessment of learning and cognitive dysfunction in young children. In J. L. Culbertson & D. J. Willis (Eds.), *Testing young children* (pp. 11–28). Austin, TX: PRO-ED.

Semrud-Clikeman, M., Hynd, G. W., Novey, E. S., & Eliopulos, D. (1991). Dyslexia and brain morphology: Relationships between neuroanatomical variation and neurolinguistic tasks. *Learning and Individual Differences, 3,* 225–242.

Shapiro, E. S. (1989). *Academic skills problems: Direct assessment and intervention.* New York: Guilford Press.

Shapiro, E. S., & Kratochwill, T. R. (1988). *Behavioral assessment in schools: Conceptual foundations and practical applications.* New York: Guilford Press.

Shinn, M. R. (1989). *Curriculum-based measurement: Assessing special children.* New York: Guilford Press.

Smith, A., Walker, M. L., & Myers, G. (1988). Hemispherectomy and diaschisis: Rapid improvement in cerebral functions after right hemispherectomy in a six year old child. *Archives of Clinical Neuropsychology, 3,* 1–8.

Smith, E., & Alley, G. (1981). *The effect of teaching sixth graders with learning disabilities a strategy for solving verbal math problems* (Research Report No. 39). Lawrence: University of Kansas, Institute for Research in Learning Disabilities.

Spreen, O., Tupper, D., Risser, A., Tuokko, H., & Edgell, D. (1984). *Human developmental neuropsychology.* London: Oxford University Press.

Stanovich, K. E. (1986). Matthew effects in reading: Some consequences of individual differences in the acquisition of literacy. *Reading Disability Quarterly, 21,* 360–406.

Strang, J. D., & Rourke, B. P. (1985). Adaptive behavior of children with specific arithmetic disabilities and associated neuropsychological abilities and deficits. In B. P. Rourke (Ed.), *Neuropsychology of learning disabilities: Essentials of subtype analysis* (pp. 302–328). New York: Guilford Press.

Teeter, P. A. (1989). Neuropsychological approaches to the remediation of educational deficits. In C. R. Reynolds & E. Fletcher-Janzen (Eds.), *Handbook of clinical child neuropsychology* (pp. 357–376). New York: Plenum Press.

Teeter, P. A. (1992, March). *Medical and behavioral paradigms: A false dichotomy.* Symposia conducted at the meeting of the National Association of School Psychologists, Washington, DC.

Teeter, P. A. (in preparation). *Interventions for children and adolescents with attention deficit hyperactivity disorders: A developmental perspective.* New York: Guilford Press.

Teeter, P. A., & Semrud-Clikeman, M. (1995). Integrating neurobiological, psychosocial, and behavioral paradigms: A transactional model for the study of ADHD. *Archives of Clinical Neuropsychology.*

Teeter, P. A., & Semrud-Clikeman, M. (in press). *Child clinical neuropsychology: Assessment and interventions for neuropsychiatric and neurodevelopmental disorders of childhood.* Boston: Allyn & Bacon.

Tramontana, M., & Hooper, S. (1989). Neuropsychology of child psychopathology. In C. R. Reynolds & E. Fletcher-Janzen (Eds.), *Handbook of clinical child neuropsychology* (pp. 87–106). New York: Plenum Press.

Tunmer, W. E., & Nesdale, A. R. (1985). Phonemic segmentation skill and beginning reading. *Journal of Educational Psychology, 77,* 417–427.

Tunmer, W. E., & Rohl, M. (1991). Phonological awareness and reading acquisition. In D. Sawyer & B. Fox (Eds.), *Phonological awareness in reading: The evolution of current perspectives* (pp. 1–30). Berlin: Springer-Verlag.

Vaghn, S., McIntosh, R., & Hogan, A. (1990). Why social skills training doesn't work: An alternative model. In T. E. Scruggs & B. Y. L. Wong (Eds.), *Intervention research in learning disabilities* (pp. 263–278). Berlin: Springer-Verlag.

Vellutino, F. R., & Scanlon, D. M. (1987). Phonological coding, phonological awareness, and reading ability: Evidence from a longitudinal and experimental study. *Merrill–Palmer Quarterly, 33,* 321–363.

Vining, E. P. G., Mellits, D., Dorsen, M. M., et al. (1987). Psychologic and behavioral effects of antiepileptic drugs in children: A double-blind comparison between phenobarbital and valproic acid. *Pediatrics, 80,* 165–174.

Virginia Department of Education. (1992). *Guidelines for educational services for children with traumatic brain injury.* Richmond, VA.

Voeller, K. S. (1986). Right hemisphere deficit syndrome in children. *American Journal of Psychiatry, 143,* 1004–1011.

Wagner, R. K., & Torgesen, J. K. (1987). The nature of phonological processing and its causal role in the acquisition of reading skills. *Psychological Bulletin, 101,* 192–212.

Walker, H. M., Holmes, D., Todis, B., & Horton, G. (1988). *The Walker Social Skills Curriculum. The ACCESS Program: Adolescent curriculum for communication and effective social skills.* Austin, TX: PRO-ED.

Walker, H. M., McConnell, S., Holmes, D., Todis, B., Walker, J., & Golden, N. (1988). *The Walker Social Skills Curriculum: The ACCEPTS Program.* Austin, TX: PRO-ED.

Weiss, G., & Hechtman, L. (1993). *Hyperactive children grown up* (2nd ed.). New York: Guilford Press.

Williams, J. P. (1980). Teaching decoding with an emphasis on phoneme analysis and phoneme blending. *Journal of Educational Psychology, 72,* 1–15.

Wise, B. W., & Olson, R. K. (1991). Remediating reading disabilities. In J. E. Obrzut & G. W. Hynd (Eds.), *Neuropsychological foundations of learning disabilities: A handbook of issues, methods, and practice* (pp. 631–658). Orlando, FL: Academic Press.

Wise, B. W., Olson, R. K., Anstett, M., Andrews, L., Terjak, M., Schneider, V., Kostuch, J., & Kriho, L. (1989). Implementing a long-term remedial reading study in the public schools: Hardware, software, and real world issues. *Behavior Research Methods and Instrumentation, 21,* 173–180.

Witt, J. C., Elliott, S., & Gresham, F. (1988). *Handbook of behavior therapy in education.* New York: Plenum Press.

Wong, B. Y. L. (Ed.). (1991). *Learning about learning disabilities.* Orlando, FL: Academic Press.

Yudofsky, S. C., & Hales, R. E. (Eds.). (1992). *The American Psychiatric Press textbook of neuropsychiatry* (2nd ed.). Washington, DC: American Psychiatric Press.

21

The Biofeedback Treatment of Neurological and Neuropsychological Disorders of Childhood and Adolescence

ROBERT L. HODES AND AUSTIN R. WOODARD

Biofeedback is one of several behavioral treatments designed to increase an individual's self-regulation of physiology. It employs instrumentation to provide patients with both immediate and precise information about otherwise occult physiological processes. In clinical settings, biofeedback is typically used in conjunction with other behavioral or medical interventions to reduce the frequency of distressing symptoms or to minimize physical impairments. The mechanisms underlying biofeedback's clinical efficacy are unclear. Different theorists have advanced varying explanations including operant conditioning of discrete physiological responses (Miller, 1969), the learning of a generalized relaxation response (Silver & Blanchard, 1978), and the production of cognitive changes promoting an increased sense of self-control and self-efficacy (Holroyd *et al.*, 1984; Turk, Meichenbaum, & Berman, 1979). Despite these different viewpoints, agreement exists that motivated individuals are able to use biofeedback signals to learn voluntary control over a variety of physiologic parameters.

The popular press has made "biofeedback" almost a household word and the technique has been offered as a potential cure for a myriad of ills of the mind and body. Although many of the early claims were unfounded, biofeedback has earned a well-deserved reputation as an effective treatment for several chronic pain syndromes, psychophysiological complaints, and neuromuscular disorders. In addition, many contemporary clinical applications of biofeedback assume that the self-regulated modification of physiology leads not only to a reduction in physical symptoms, but also to useful behavioral and cognitive changes. For example, the use of EMG biofeedback for children with attention deficit disorders assumes that biofeedback not only prompts a reduction in muscle tension, but also reduces disruptive classroom behavior, improves academic performance, and increases the child's sense of self-control and self-esteem (Braud, 1978; Omizo, 1980a).

Biofeedback with Disorders of Childhood and Adolescence

This chapter reviews the published work on biofeedback training in neurological and neuropsychological disorders of childhood and adolescence. More general reviews of the application of biofeedback in pediatric medicine are provided by Andrasik and Attanasio (1985) and Finley (1983). In the broadest sense, all biofeedback learning studies deal with the modification of neurally controlled phenomena. This chapter is limited to a review of the application of biofeedback technology to the symptoms of neurological disease or neuropsychological dysfunction. In some of these studies, the evidence

ROBERT L. HODES AND AUSTIN R. WOODARD • Department of Neurology, University of Wisconsin–Madison, Madison, Wisconsin 53792-6180.

of neurological dysfunction is unequivocal; in others such evidence is presumptive (Cleeland, 1981). Specific disorders considered include cerebral palsy, epilepsy, neurogenic fecal incontinence, attention deficit hyperactivity disorder, learning disabilities, and migraine headaches. When available, controlled group treatment outcome studies are given emphasis over both controlled and uncontrolled case studies. For each disorder, the literature review emphasizes four basic points relevant to the clinical use of biofeedback. These issues are:

1. Are patients able to learn the desired response?
2. Does physiological self-regulation lead to other clinically relevant changes in either physiology, behavior, or cognition?
3. How effective is biofeedback relative to either control or alternative treatment procedures?
4. Are therapeutic gains maintained over time?

The vast majority of applications of biofeedback have been with adults. Many of the techniques and insights generated by that literature are directly applicable when working with children. For example, the treatment of migraine headaches in children is closely modeled after treatment protocols used with adults (Labbe & Williamson, 1984). However, biofeedback training with children does require attention to several issues, such as varying developmental levels, not typically addressed when working with adult clients (Marcon & Labbe, 1990). The relevancy of these issues to the literature reviewed in this chapter will also be discussed. Finally, this chapter concludes with comments summarizing the current state of knowledge and offering suggestions for future inquiries.

Cerebral Palsy

Of the various abnormalities of muscle tone and movement found in cerebral palsy, spasticity and rigidity have received the most attention from biofeedback clinicians. The essential feature of spasticity is an increased reactivity to an exciting stimulus, most notably rapid stretch. Clinically, this is observed by asking a patient to relax and then passively extending the patient's limb. In normal muscles, no muscular resistance is observed. Spastic muscles, in contrast, reflexively contract to the attempted extension and resist the clinician's efforts (DeBacher, 1983). The degree of resistance is often determined by the velocity of the passive movement and the position of the limb. In rigidity, muscles are almost continuously hypertonic. In contrast to spastic muscles, rigid muscles resist movement throughout their entire range of motion and at slow movement velocities (Adams & Victor, 1977).

Increase in the severity of involuntary movements as a result of environmental stimulation and emotional distress is well known. Based on earlier work with progressive muscle relaxation training in patients with cerebral palsy, Finley, Niman, Standley, and Wansley (1977) employed frontal region EMG biofeedback to produce a generalized state of muscle relaxation and associated emotional calm. The effect of this intervention on motor and speech behavior of four children with cerebral palsy was analyzed employing an ABAB design. All children were able to successfully reduce frontal EMG after an initial 12 training sessions. EMG activity increased during the first reversal phase but only one of the four children was able to reinstitute control during the second treatment period. Similar results were obtained for forearm flexor EMG, where a reduction was observed during the initial training phase, but increases in flexor tension were found during the second training phase. The results were more encouraging for speech and motor skills. All children manifested statistically significant improvement in speech and/or motor measures during initial training. These gains deteriorated during the reversal phase and were reinstituted during the second training phase. Although statistical significance was demonstrated, judgments concerning the clinical significance of performance gains were not provided by the authors.

In a follow-up study, Finley, Etherton, Dickmen, Karimian, and Simpson (1981) studied 15 children with cerebral palsy who primarily manifested spasticity. In this study, the biofeedback was contingent on the combined EMG activity from frontal region and forearm flexor sites. These children also received tangible rewards (e.g., candy, toys) for meeting performance standards involving reductions in both tonic and phasic EMG. For some children, rewards were immediate, while for other children, rewards were given at the end of the training session. The results indicated that children in both groups learned to reduce their combined EMG, but reductions of larger magnitude were found for children receiving immediate reinforcement for performance changes. Data on functional changes in motor behavior were not reported.

Cataldo, Bird, and Cunningham (1978) employed EMG biofeedback to increase neuromuscular control in two children with choreoathetoid cerebral palsy. The first child was given feedback from the right biceps with the effects of biofeedback evaluated with an ABA design. The results suggested that the subject was able to produce muscle relaxation with contingent feedback, and that control deteriorated during the no-feedback phase, but was reinitiated during the final feedback sessions. Although functional motor control was not formally assessed, the authors noted that hospital staff indicated no noticeable changes in adaptive functioning. For the second child, feedback was given from multiple muscle groups using a multiple baseline across behaviors design. The data presented describe appropriate increases or decreases in muscle control that follow the intent of the study design. In addition, muscle control generalized to no-feedback conditions. Finally, the authors reported that anecdotal observations indicated functional improvements in some muscle groups.

In summary, only preliminary data exist on the utility of EMG biofeedback in increasing neuromuscular control in children with cerebral palsy. These initial data suggest that patients are able to learn to reduce undesirable levels of muscle tension. However, no study has demonstrated continued self-regulation of muscle activity during long-term follow-up. In this regard, Seeger and Caudrey (1983) noted that therapeutic gains in gait training made with sensory feedback from a load-sensitive insole were not maintained after a follow-up period of 18–24 months. The available data on the impact of enhanced muscle control on functional activity have been mixed. Greater use of reliable observation methods (e.g., Bird & Cataldo, 1978) or automated recording devices of functional activity (e.g., Seeger, Caudrey, & Scholes, 1981) is clearly indicated.

Finally, it is revealing to compare this early literature on the biofeedback treatment of cerebral palsy with the more extensive literature on the treatment of adult patients with spasticity (e.g., spasticity following strokes). The training of neuromuscular control in children with cerebral palsy has typically taken place while the affected extremity or joint is at rest. This is somewhat surprising given the definition of spasticity as hypertonicity produced by stretch. In greater accordance with this physiological fact, clinicians attempting to reduce spasticity in adult patients (e.g., DeBacher, 1983) typically train muscle control not only while the muscle is at rest, but also during passive and active movement of the muscle and during activation of antagonistic muscle groups. The application of these more sophisticated training procedures with children afflicted with cerebral palsy is indicated.

Epilepsy

Feedback training for various parameters of EEG activity has been used as a method of reducing seizures poorly controlled by medications. Several feedback protocols have been attempted with the patient often required to meet multiple contingencies, such as suppressing slow-wave activity while simultaneously generating increased activity in a faster frequency band. Uniformly, the training period required has been long, often several months. The accumulated evidence from such arduous training suggests that certain individuals with epilepsy can learn "something" that will allow for reduction of seizure frequency (Cleeland, 1981). The reader is cautioned that the research discussed below has generally employed patient populations that include a mixture of both children and adults with epilepsy. Differences in the utility of EEG biofeedback across age ranges have not been systematically evaluated.

The biofeedback treatment of seizures began in the early 1970s. It is rooted in the work by Sterman and others on the sensorimotor rhythm (SMR). This rhythm refers to 12- to 14-Hz activity maximally recorded over the sensorimotor cortex. It was originally identified in the waking EEG of cats, where SMR's most obvious behavioral correlate is immobility and muscular inhibition (Donhoffer & Lissak, 1962; Howe & Sterman, 1972; Roth, Sterman, & Clemente, 1967). Clinical applications of SMR training were initiated when it was observed that cats trained to increase SMR power demonstrated increased threshold for seizures when challenged with a convulsant-producing dose of monomethylhydrazine (Sterman, LoPresti, & Fairchild, 1969). In this way, EEG biofeedback mimicked the therapeutic mechanism of anticonvulsant medications.

Early studies of EEG training attempted to demonstrate its utility for controlling a variety of seizure disorders. Two strategies for producing EEG normalization emerged. One involved the enhancement of intermediate EEG frequencies, such as the SMR, which are thought to inhibit epileptogenic brain activity (Kuhlman, 1978; Seifert & Lubar, 1975; Sterman & Friar, 1972). A second set of strategies involved training patients to suppress the excessive slow-wave activity and/or EEG spikes characteristic of seizure states. This latter training was provided alone (Cott, Pavloski, & Black, 1979) or in combination with biofeedback training to increase either SMR (Finley, 1976; Lubar & Bahler, 1976; Sterman, Macdonald, & Stone, 1974) or beta-range EEG activity (Sterman & Macdonald, 1978; Wyler, Robbins, & Dodrill, 1979). When EEG activity was recorded over the sensorimotor region, these various training procedures produced significant seizure reduction in between 60 and 80% of patients.

The most consistent criticism of these early studies has been the lack of adequate experimental controls. Recent work from the laboratories of Lubar and Sterman has been responsive to this need. Lubar (1982) provided patients with one of three types of EEG normalization training followed by an altered feedback phase where patients were trained to increase epileptiform activity. Training ended with a final EEG normalization period. Dependent measures included self-report of seizure activity and neuropsychological testing. In general, seizure activity paralleled the feedback contingency; five of the eight patients showed clinical improvement during the final treatment phase with an average seizure reduction of 39.7%, while four patients relapsed when epileptiform EEG was reinforced. Because EEG training was provided using double-blind procedures, Lubar's data provide the strongest evidence to date supporting the specific efficacy of biofeedback training in regulating seizure activity. Neuropsychological testing, including the Halstead–Reitan Battery and either the WAIS or WISC, showed little or no change following EEG training, replicating earlier findings of Wyler *et al.* (1979).

Sterman (1982) reported data relevant both to the maintenance of therapeutic gains over time and to the generalization of EEG changes to nonfeedback periods. Fifteen patients with poorly controlled seizures received EEG training to reduce abnormally low (1–5 Hz) and high (20–25 Hz) frequencies while simultaneously increasing intermediate (10–15 Hz) activity. Feedback was also contingent on the absence of high-voltage spiking. For five patients, EEG training was preceded by 6 weeks of symptom self-monitoring, while for a second five patients, 6 weeks of noncontingent (yoked) feedback was provided. The results strongly supported the role of contingent feedback in controlling seizure rates. Seizure reduction only occurred when the EEG normalization feedback contingency was imposed, with 13 of 15 patients reducing seizures by a mean frequency of about 60%. Furthermore, seizure rates were reduced by approximately 42% at follow-up. Finally, Sterman and Shouse (1980) analyzed spectral analyses taken from sleep recordings both before and after EEG conditioning. During periods of maximal clinical improvement, EEG changes showed increased power for intermediate EEG frequencies but decreased power for both low (0–3) and high (20–23) frequency bands. These data suggest that EEG training generalized from the daytime laboratory, when feedback training occurred, to the sleep EEG.

In summary, several investigators have obtained data supporting the utility of biofeedback for the control of a variety of seizure disorders. Even children with mental retardation (e.g., Lubar, 1982) have been able to profit from complicated feedback contingencies to alter their EEG frequency distributions and reduce seizure rate. An evolution in training has occurred with earlier studies of the effects of specific frequency band training (e.g., SMR training) giving way to efforts to produce EEG normalization across multiple frequency bands. Comparisons of different training procedures are just beginning and it is not clear if one approach holds any superiority over the other in producing changes in either seizure rate or neuropsychological functioning. Studies that have compared alternative frequency training procedures have employed small sample sizes, limiting the power of the design to offer reliable recommendations (Lubar, 1982). Similarly, although some data suggest that treatment gains may be maintained over time (Sterman, 1982), the reported sample sizes are too small to allow for a reliable conclusion. As noted by Lubar, "It seems appropriate that wide-scale clinical trials be initiated to determine whether EEG feedback conditioning can become a valuable adjunct in the treatment of epilepsy" (Lubar, 1982).

Fecal Incontinence in Myelomeningocele

Engel, Nikoomanesh, and Schuster (1974) described the first use of biofeedback to treat fecal incontinence in myelomeningocele. As described by these authors and others, biofeedback treatment of fecal incontinence involves the use of three balloon pressure transducers inserted in the patient's anus and rectum. One balloon is placed in the proximal rectum, the second in the internal anal sphincter, and the third in the external anal sphincter. Inflation of the balloon in the rectum stimulated the presence of stool. Pressure measurements from the other two balloons determine muscle tone in the internal and external anal sphincters in response to this rectal distension. By observing the manometric or pressure changes in the three balloons, patients are given feedback concerning these three physiologic activities. Patients use this information to learn to voluntarily produce external anal sphincter contractions that (1) occur in response to rectal distension and (2) outlast the phase of internal sphincter relaxation.

As outlined by Whitehead, Parker, Masek, Cataldo, and Freeman (1981), biofeedback training in myelomeningocele patients usually proceeds in four phases. An initial assessment phase tests the rectosphincteric reflex of the internal anal sphincter, the strength of the voluntary contraction of the external sphincter, and the patient's subjective sensory threshold for rectal distension. In the second phase, patients are trained to make skillful contractions of the external anal sphincter in the absence of rectal distension. If possible, patients are trained to voluntarily contract the external anal sphincter. If this proves too difficult, voluntary contractions of the nearby gluteal muscles may be adequate (Wald, 1981). During this phase, patients are typically given visual feedback in the form of observation of manometric tracings from the external anal sphincter. Verbal and tangible reinforcers are also often employed, especially with younger children. In phase three, patients are trained to make voluntary external sphincter contractions in response to rectal distension. Training often begins with distensions at the level of subjective appreciation and gradually progresses to distensions of increasingly larger amplitude. During this phase, patients observe manometric tracings from all three balloons to aid them in producing sphincter contractions of adequate amplitude, duration, and timing. In the final phase, patients are required to continue to demonstrate skillful control of the external sphincter but without visual feedback and without any cues concerning the onset or duration of rectal distension and internal anal sphincter relaxation.

Uncontrolled case studies (Cerulli, Nikoomanesh, & Schuster, 1979; Shepherd, Hickstein, & Shepherd, 1983; Wald, 1981, 1983; Whitehead et al., 1981) have all found manometric biofeedback to produce clinically significant reductions in fecal soiling in the majority of children treated. Success rates have varied from 46 to 96%. It should be noted that these improvement rates are for children who have invariably failed to achieve continence via more standard medical management. In addition to demonstrating biofeedback's utility, these preliminary data have suggested tentative guidelines for selecting patients who are most likely to benefit from manometric biofeedback training. Wald (1983) observed that patients who benefited from biofeedback had significantly lower thresholds of rectal sensation than did patients who failed to improve. He reported that of the 43% of his sample of children with myelomeningocele who had impaired appreciation of rectal distension, all failed to respond to biofeedback therapy. Shepherd et al. (1983) also found a high incidence of impaired rectal sensation, with 18/22 children assessed as having either subnormal or absent sensation. However, they observed that following behavioral training for continence, previously absent rectal sensation developed in four patients. In those cases, impaired rectal sensation was associated with fecal retention and megarectum. The authors suggested that biofeedback training may be effective for these children following appropriate medical management of their megarectum.

Whitehead and colleagues reported a study comparing biofeedback and behavior modification approaches (Whitehead et al., 1986). After a 2-week baseline period, all subjects received behavior modification training to teach self-initiation of bowel movements. Briefly, this involved regular toileting after meals with reinforcers for successful bowel movements or for accident-free days. In addition, the program used enemas and/or stool softeners under specified conditions to prevent fecal impaction. For one group, biofeedback training was initiated following 1 month of behavior modification training. For a second group, biofeedback training was provided after a 3-month delay.

The results were complex and were interpreted by the authors as suggesting that clinically significant reductions in incontinence occurred primarily during the behavior modification phase of training. The authors also used Markov chain modeling to analyze the separate contributions of behavior modification and biofeedback. This analysis suggested that biofeedback and behavior modification

had differential effects on different types of incontinent states; namely, behavior modification was the only treatment effective in causing patients to move from infrequent incontinence (staining or one accident/day) to continence, whereas biofeedback was more effective than behavior modification for high-frequency (more than once a day) incontinence.

Replicating Wald (1983), children with impaired rectal sensation showed a poor response to biofeedback training. However, these same children were able to improve bowel control with four of these six patients achieving a 75% or greater reduction in episodes of incontinence. This improvement was presumably the result of the addition of behavior modification to these patients' training regimen.

Six-month or longer follow-up data were available on 66% of the patients in the Whitehead *et al.* (1986) study. These data indicated that both the frequency of incontinence and the number of enemas per week were significantly reduced relative to baseline levels. Sphincter strength in patients who previously met a satisfactory training criterion was also well maintained. However, the number of self-initiated bowel movements regressed to pretraining levels.

The results of their experiments led both Shepherd *et al.* (1983) and Whitehead *et al.* (1986) to similar conclusions. Both argued for a partitioning of children with myelomeningocele into two groups based on physiological criteria. In one group, rectal sensation is minimal or absent and augmented reflex activity of the external anal sphincter is present. In this group, chronic constipation and/or megarectum occurs. Whitehead *et al.* (1986) also characterized these patients as being more likely to have spinal cord lesions at L-2 or above. These patients seem to benefit the most from behavior modification combined with medical management to produce regular, complete evacuations of stool from the rectum. The second group is characterized by normal or near-normal rectal sensation, inadequate reflex activity and muscle tone in the external sphincter, and multiple daily bowel movements. These patients benefit the most from biofeedback training to augment the strength of voluntary contractions in the external anal sphincter.

More recently, Loening-Baucke, Desch, and Wolraich (1988) also failed to find a strong effect for biofeedback training. They studied 12 children with myelomeningocele. Patients were randomized to either biofeedback with conventional medical management (stool softeners and scheduled toileting after meals) or manometric biofeedback alone. In addition, these authors used an improved recording device that allowed them to separate pressure in the anal canal from pressure changes caused by muscle squeezing in the buttocks. They failed to find an addictive effect for biofeedback training above and beyond the benefit obtained with their medical management intervention. Further, patients were unable to learn to voluntarily increase anal squeeze pressure when anal pressure was isolated from other contaminating influences.

In conclusion, the early promise of biofeedback training for the modification of fecal incontinence in myelomeningocele has given way to a more modest endorsement. Biofeedback may help a minority of patients improve external sphincter control to a level that leads to fewer soiling episodes. For the majority of children, residual innervation of the external anal sphincter is too sparse to allow biofeedback training to be effective (Bassotti & Whitehead, 1994).

Attention Deficit/Hyperactivity Disorder

Literature reviews of medication treatment studies of children with ADHD indicate that between 70 and 80% of children show a positive response (Barkley, 1977). Improvement of attention-concentration and reduction of impulsive, hyperactive, and disruptive behaviors are the primary therapeutic effects. Social relations may improve reflecting improved compliance with the requests of authority figures and reductions in conflict and aggressive behaviors. Academic achievement may also improve to some extent. Short- and long-term side effects are generally mild when the medication is properly prescribed and monitored. The most common side effects are insomnia and decreased appetite. Long-term side effects are not as well studied. Transient effects on height and weight have been noted. Positive medication treatment effects have not been found to persist after discontinuation of medication therapy.

Because psychostimulant medications are not a panacea for the problems arising from ADHD, other forms of therapy are also usually employed. Behavior therapy and systematic parent training (see Barkley, 1987) are useful adjunctive therapies. Indeed, studies have found that combinations of these treatments are usually superior to either in isolation (see Pelham & Murphy, 1986). These behavior modification techniques are often employed in conjunction with classroom management strategies (e.g., removing classroom distractors, providing a structured classroom routine) that structure the learning environment to accommodate the behavioral and attentional style of the child with ADHD. Behavior modification is clearly effective in changing specific behaviors, such as in-seat behavior or time on task. Unfortunately, generalization to other settings where appropriate contingencies are not in place is often unsatisfactory.

Perhaps because ADHD is regarded by most investigators as a disorder of self-regulation and because of limitations in treatments, some clinicians in the 1970s proposed that biofeedback may provide a useful primary or adjunctive intervention for ADHD. Most investigations of the utility of biofeedback have employed either EMG biofeedback to reduce generalized muscle tension or EEG and SMR biofeedback to promote a brain state associated with inhibited motor activity (Sterman, 1977).

EMG Biofeedback

EMG has been the most frequently used biofeedback technique employed as a treatment for hyperactivity (Lee, 1991). Braud, Lupin, and Braud (1975) are generally credited with first proposing the use of frontal region EMG biofeedback with hyperactive children. Braud's (1978) rationale for the utility of EMG biofeedback was that "hyperactive children are not only overactive but also overly tense. The authors feel that these tension levels could aggravate the symptomatology." Since this initial hypothesis, approximately 23 group outcome studies have been published evaluating frontal region biofeedback in hyperactive children and adolescents.

Numerous group outcome studies (Bhatara, Arnold, Lorance, & Gupta, 1979; Braud, 1978; Christie, DeWitt, Kaltenbach, & Reed, 1984; Connoly, Besserman, & Kirschvink, 1974; Denkowski & Denkowski, 1984; Denkowski, Denkowski, & Omizo, 1983, 1984; Dunn & Howell, 1982; Flemings, 1979; Haight, 1976; Hampstead, 1979; Hughes, Henry, & Hughes, 1980; Jeffrey, 1976; Krause, 1978; Linn & Hodge, 1979; Loux & Ascher, 1980; Moore, 1977; Omizo, 1980a,b; Omizo, Cuberly, Semands, & Omizo, 1986; Omizo & Michael, 1982; Potashkin & Beckles, 1990; Rivera & Omizo, 1980; Shouse & Lubar, 1978; Whitmer, 1977) reported EMG data for patients receiving from 3 to 30 biofeedback training sessions. Reductions in frontal region EMG following biofeedback were regularly found. Further, several studies employed appropriate control procedures allowing the conclusion that the observed reduction in EMG is not the result of habituation across repeated testing occasions.

Four qualifying points need to be made. First, the decision to train a reduction in frontal region EMG makes the implicit assumption that muscle tension is elevated in hyperactive children.

Borkovec and Sides (1979), among others, have argued persuasively that the choice of a relaxation strategy should be matched with the response domains showing excessive levels of arousal. Surprisingly, this assumption has only been confirmed in one study (Braud, 1978) where levels of frontal region EMG during rest were significantly higher in hyperactive than in control children. No other laboratories that we are aware of have replicated this important assumption.

Second, it is often assumed that a reduction of frontal region EMG leads to a generalized state of relaxation at multiple body sites. This state of relaxation ultimately translates into a decrease in overactivity. Unfortunately, none of the studies measured EMG from additional muscle locations. Burish (1983) reviewed the research on frontal region EMG biofeedback in adults and concluded that this type of biofeedback does not reliably produce a generalized reduction in muscle tension or autonomic activity. Although the situation may be different with children, the existing research does not encourage the frequently made assumption that frontal region biofeedback in hyperactivity leads to a generalized relaxation response.

Third, Gargiulo and Kuna (1979) have questioned whether it makes theoretical sense to train reductions in physiological arousal in hyperactive children. Based on the Satterfield and Dawson (1971) finding of hypoarousal in hyperactivity, these authors suggested that relaxation might be an inappropriate regulatory strategy. In support of this, Whitmer (1977) trained one group of hyperactive children to decrease frontal region EMG, but trained a second group to *increase* EMG. Consistent with the underarousal theory, reductions in hyperactive behavior were only found for subjects trained to increase EMG.

Fourth, as Lee (1991) stated, no assumptions can be made that the diagnostic criteria for selecting these "hyperactive" subjects were equivalent across studies. Indeed, although some studies referenced well-recognized diagnostic criteria such as those developed by the American Psychiatric Association or Barkley (1990), many did not. We are aware of only one control group study that compared EMG biofeedback, Ritalin, and nonspecific adult attention (Potashkin & Beckles, 1990). Even in this otherwise important study, it is very unclear how the subjects were diagnosed, other than that they obtained high scores on certain scales of commonly employed behavior rating instruments.

Most but not all cited studies have employed multiple outcome measures in evaluating the utility of biofeedback therapy. Parental and/or teachers' ratings of hyperactive and disruptive behaviors were made in several studies. During treatment, parental questionnaire responses consistently indicated behavioral improvement (Bhatara *et al.*, 1979; Braud, 1978; Connoly *et al.*, 1974; Dunn & Howell, 1982; Hampstead, 1979). In contrast, teachers less consistently noted improvement. Two investigations found no improvement (Bhatara *et al.*, 1979; Denkowski & Denkowski, 1984) whereas several did (Connoly *et al.*, 1974; Haight, 1976; Hampstead, 1979; Hughes *et al.*, 1980; Loux & Ascher, 1980; Moore, 1977; Omizo & Michael, 1982; Omizo & Williams, 1982; Potashkin & Beckles, 1990; Rivera & Omizo, 1980). No follow-up data were reported, except in the Hampstead study, and additional techniques, such as relaxation training and visual imagery, were also provided with EMG biofeedback.

Neuropsychological testing has involved either the Bender Gestalt, the Digit Span and Coding subtests of the WISC-R, or other tests sensitive to attention and impulsivity. In general, the results suggest improved performance on these measures. Braud (1978) found that biofeedback training led to fewer errors on the Bender test and improved scores on the Illinois Test of Psycholinguistic Abilities. No difference between biofeedback subjects and controls was found on Digit Span and Coding. Connoly *et al.* (1974) found improved WISC-R Coding and Mazes scores after biofeedback treatment involving relaxation training and a token system. Dunn and Howell (1982) found that hyperactive subjects improved on the Bender Gestalt and WISC-R subtests following active biofeedback training but not following placebo treatment. Finally, Omizo and Michael (1982) measured both errors and response latency of the Matching Familiar Figures Test. They found decreases in errors and an increase in latency following biofeedback training and concluded that these changes were consistent with decreased inattention and impulsivity in their subjects.

In other response domains, the data are more ambiguous. Academic skills were measured in only two studies (Denkowski *et al.*, 1983; Denkowski & Denkowski, 1984). The former study found improvements in reading vocabulary and comprehension following biofeedback, but similar improvements were not obtained by the same investigators in their second study. The authors attributed this discrepancy to differences in the tests used to measure academic abilities; however, numerous other procedural differences between the studies (such as the number of training sessions and the age of the hyperactive children) may also be important.

Finally, in five studies, Omizo and the Denkowskis and associates assessed a variety of biofeedback-induced changes in either locus of control or self-esteem. These data are important to the hypothesis that biofeedback "may demonstrate to hyperactive children that they have control over their physical behavior and this perception of self-control then generalizes to enable more selective socioeducational behavior" (Denkowski *et al.*, 1983). Four studies assessed locus of control. In two of the four studies, subjects demonstrated increased internality following biofeedback but not following placebo treatment (Denkowski *et al.*, 1983; Omizo, 1980a). Similarly, of the three studies measuring either self-concept or self-esteem, two (Omizo, 1980a,b) found favorable changes, whereas one (Denkowski *et al.*, 1983) obtained no advantage for subjects receiving biofeedback. Hence, the literature is almost evenly split between studies supporting the conclusion that biofeedback produces favorable changes in self-concept and locus of control and negative findings in these areas. Clearly, more research is needed before a confident conclusion can be drawn.

Control procedures varied across the reviewed studies. Braud (1978) employed a no-treatment control group. Bhatara *et al.* (1979) connected control subjects to an inoperative biofeedback unit but provided no other placebo treatment. Omizo (1980a,b) and Denkowski and Denkowski (1984) attached subjects to inoperative equipment and also played for control subjects either neutral tapes or tapes of children's stories. This contrasted to the biofeedback subjects, who listened to relaxation tapes. Denkowski *et al.* (1983) employed a similar procedure but substituted neutral conversations with the children for the neutral tapes. It seems unlikely that any of these control procedures was as credible as biofeedback for either parents or children. Potashkin and Beckles (1990) compared a biofeedback-assisted relaxation group with a Ritalin-only group and another group that was seen for a comparable number of sessions as the biofeedback group but only met to play a table game without any therapeutic intent. The biofeedback group was the only group that improved their ability to reduce EMG readings, although teacher behavior ratings improved for all three groups. The only study that used a potentially credible control procedure was Dunn and Howell (1982). In this study, all children received ten sessions of placebo treatment followed by ten sessions of biofeedback treatment. Relationship and play therapy served as placebo treatments (these indeed had no significant effect on either physiology or hyperactive behaviors). Unfortunately, Dunn and Howell made no attempt to assess the placebo's credibility, and thus it is not known if the placebo treatment prompted the same degree of expectancy for change as did the biofeedback treatment (Borkovec & Nau, 1972). These methodological weaknesses make it impossible to determine the role that the contingent presentation of the biofeedback signal plays in producing the clinical improvement obtained in these research studies.

Three studies compared EMG biofeedback with taped relaxation training. Braud (1978) and Dunn and Howell (1982) obtained comparable improvements in muscle tension, hyperactive behavior, and psychological test data for biofeedback and relaxation. In the Denkowski and Denkowski (1984) study, the results were largely negative for both groups, with one analysis supporting a shift in locus of control toward internality only for subjects receiving relaxation training. Hence, the data do not support the employment of the more expensive biofeedback training over the more cost-effective taped relaxation training.

Since these studies were initial attempts to demonstrate the efficacy of biofeedback, it is not surprising that scant attention was paid to demonstrating the maintenance of change over time. Indeed, this crucial issue was assessed in only one study (Bhatara *et al.*, 1979) and in that case, reductions in hyperactive behaviors, as rated by parents, regressed to pretreatment levels by 12 weeks posttreatment. Clearly, the inclusion of an adequate follow-up period is a prerequisite for all future treatment outcome research in this area.

EEG Biofeedback

No area of biofeedback treatment for children has received more recent media attention and critical scrutiny than the use of EEG biofeedback for the treatment of ADHD. This is interesting and of some concern because of the paucity of actual research in this area. Nall (1973) provided the only controlled group outcome study of EEG biofeedback as a treatment for hyperactivity. In her study, 48 children with hyperkinesis associated with learning disabilities were assigned to either a no-treatment group, contingent alpha biofeedback, or false or noncontingent feedback. Subjects in the latter two groups also received brief relaxation exercises. Her results

suggested little or no difference between the veridical and placebo biofeedback groups. Alpha amplitude increased in 9 of the 16 veridical training subjects and in 7 of the 16 placebo subjects. Measures of hyperkinetic and maladaptive behavior and overall academic achievement did not significantly differ between the biofeedback and control groups following treatment.

More recently, Lubar and his colleagues reported a series of case studies employing an EEG biofeedback contingency designed to train an increase in SMR in the absence of excessive theta wave activity (Lubar & Lubar, 1984; Lubar & Shouse, 1976; Shouse & Lubar, 1979). Lubar's case studies provide strong preliminary support for the efficacy of this form of biofeedback. Five subjects were evaluated with reversal designs and six were evaluated as uncontrolled case studies. Of the 11 subjects, 10 learned to increase SMR and/or beta wave activity while facial EMG and gross motor activity decreased. Observational measures of classroom behavior improved in 8/13 categories for four of the five children for whom these data were available. Electrocortical and to a lesser extent behavioral improvement reversed when the biofeedback contingencies were withdrawn. For six of these children, information was presented on academic test scores and/or school grades. In each case, unspecified "considerable improvements" were reported.

These data suggest that SMR biofeedback warrants an evaluation with a controlled group outcome study or with a larger series of controlled case studies. Since Lubar and his colleagues treated patients with multiple therapies (EEG biofeedback was combined in various studies with medications, academic remediation, and feedback on muscle activity), it will also be necessary to determine the relative contribution of EEG biofeedback. As Barkley (1993) points out, the criteria for diagnosing these children and selecting this treatment need to be clarified. He also comments that the observed parameters of change (SMR, beta wave activity) are markers. What the children are being taught to do and how this can be applied after treatment is completed is entirely unclear. Finally, SMR biofeedback requires a relatively large investment of both human and technological resources and its cost-effectiveness relative to other interventions needs to be addressed.

Children with Learning Disabilities

The treatment of learning disabilities traditionally involves some form of remedial education training, with the specific training methods tailored to the cognitive and academic strengths and weaknesses of the child. Behavior modification principles may also be employed to alter behavior patterns, such as overactivity, which impair the child's ability to profit from educational experiences. Although remediation is often effective, LD children frequently demonstrate a pattern of academic difficulties throughout childhood and adolescence with many individuals showing continued learning problems in adult life (APA, 1994).

As noted above, it is not uncommon for children with hyperactivity to display difficulties in learning, either as a primary neuropsychological problem or secondary to the behavior disruption inherent in hyperactivity. It is not surprising, then, that the biofeedback treatment of learning disabilities closely parallels the treatment of hyperactivity. Both EMG-based relaxation techniques and EEG biofeedback have been employed.

Carter and Russell (1980) reasoned that stress and muscle tension have a debilitating effect on academic attainment in LD children. They speculated that relaxation training would "bring about a cognitive reorganization or integration which allows the recipient to use his abilities more efficiently." To test this, they gave four LD males, aged 8–13, ten sessions of EMG biofeedback from the forearm flexors combined with handwriting training. They were able to demonstrate both a 62% decease in forearm muscle tension and a mean increase of 0.65, 0.68, and 0.53 grade level equivalences in reading, spelling, and arithmetic abilities, respectively.

The authors followed these uncontrolled case studies with two controlled group outcome studies (Carter & Russell, 1985). In the first study, 32 male elementary school LD students were randomly selected for either a combined biofeedback/taped relaxation/handwriting training condition or a no-treatment control group. Each student also completed a test battery measuring intellectual functioning, academic achievement, auditory memory, perceptual motor skills, and handwriting ability. The results demonstrated significantly greater improvement for the experimental group on all measures except the arithmetic subtest of the Wide Range Achievement Test. EMG was only measured for experimental subjects, with those subjects demonstrating a significant reduction in forearm muscle tension following biofeedback/relaxation training. In a replication study, 30 elementary school LD males were randomly selected for either 18 sessions of a similar biofeedback/relaxation/handwriting

training procedure or a no-treatment control group. The results replicated the main findings from the first study, with significantly larger gains made by experimental subjects on all dependent measures except general intelligence and auditory memory. Finally, with an independent group of 20 LD males, the authors obtained significant improvements on both the Tennessee Self-Concept Scale and the Child Behavior Rating Scale. Taken as a whole, the authors suggest that (1) LD children are able to learn to reduce relevant muscle tension levels and (2) these changes are associated with improvement in cognitive abilities, academic achievement, behavioral adjustment, and self-concept.

Omizo and Williams (1982) argued that "relaxation training is effective because the learning-disabled child gains control over his muscle levels, thus improving his ability to perform on visual/perceptual tasks that involve focusing on relevant cues and ignoring irrelevant stimuli." In a controlled outcome study, the authors randomly selected 32 children, aged 8–11, to either three sessions of combined frontal region EMG biofeedback/taped relaxation training or a placebo treatment involving listening to neutral tapes. Significant decreases in frontal region EMG were seen only for subjects in the experimental group. In addition, compared with the control subjects, subjects receiving biofeedback/relaxation training made significantly fewer errors on the Matching Familiar Figures Test and significantly increased their responding latency. These findings were interpreted as reflecting increased attention to task and decreased impulsivity in the relaxation-trained LD pupils. Finally, control and experimental subjects failed to differ on a measure of locus of control, with both groups showing little change from pre- to posttesting.

Unlike the studies previously described, Hunter, Russell, Russell, and Zimmerman (1976) trained a group of LD and normal children regarding digital skin temperature increases. The authors reasoned that temperature feedback would improve academic skills by teaching LD children a "fully attentive, attuned, and stable internal state in which background noise is reduced to a minimum." Hunter and colleagues randomly selected LD and normal children, aged 7–9, to either five sessions of "consistent" temperature feedback or a false feedback "mixed reinforcement" procedure (the success feedback signal followed increases, decreases, and stable temperature patterns). The results demonstrated modest (0.5°F) but statistically reliable increases in skin temperature for both LD and normal children with veridical reinforcement. However, veridical feedback and false feedback LD groups did not vary in improvement on scores on a brief neuropsychological battery.

In summary, EMG and temperature biofeedback training do seem to be associated with increased voluntary control over trained physiology. EMG biofeedback was also associated with desirable changes in behavior and academic achievement, and less consistently with self-report measures of self-concept and locus of control. Unfortunately, the interpretation of these findings is problematic. First, all of the studies combined biofeedback with other training procedures, making it impossible to identify the unique properties of biofeedback training. Second, although the authors all assume that biofeedback leads to a sense of relaxation, no attempt has been made to demonstrate a relaxation response involving multiple response systems. Third, the studies all employed control procedures that may have been inadequate to control for nonspecific treatment effects, such as expectancy for change. As before, treatment credibility was not assessed. Fourth, none of these studies included a follow-up period to determine the stability of behavior change over time. Fifth, the rationale behind the choice of relaxation as a specific intervention for learning disabilities has varied across studies and is poorly articulated at best. Finally, the type and severity of the subjects' learning problems and the methods of identifying these conditions were not well specified. Greater conceptual clarity would aid clinicians in deciding which children with which type of learning disorder might benefit the most from a relaxation-based intervention.

EEG Biofeedback in Learning Disabilities

As noted above, many theories of learning disability assume some underlying neurological dysfunction. Comparison of the EEG of normal and LD children became one way of searching for this. Roberts (1966) demonstrated excessive amounts of slow-wave EEG activity, particularly in the 3- to 4-Hz frequency band, in LD children. More recently, Lubar *et al.* (1985) obtained power spectral fast Fourier analyses of EEG in 69 children with learning disabilities and 34 controls. Among other findings, LD children differed from controls by having significantly more power in theta and low alpha frequency bands, i.e., more slow-wave EEG activity.

Based on these and other observations, it has been suggested that biofeedback techniques might prove useful in training LD children to alter dysfunctional patterns of EEG activity, and that this modification would produce salutary changes in learning and behavior. Gracenin and Cook (1977) gave eight LD children ten sessions of alpha biofeedback. During the last six sessions, subjects were asked to increase alpha while reading. Although statistical analyses were not reported, the authors suggested that four of eight subjects learned to increase alpha amplitude and duration. However, alpha-trained subjects did not differ from no-treatment controls on improvements in oral reading and reading comprehension.

Cunningham and Murphy (1981) hypothesized from earlier research (Murphy, Darwin, & Murphy, 1977) that different types of cognitive tasks (e.g., visuospatial versus verbal) are associated with different patterns of electrocortical arousal. They suggested that LD children may lack the ability to produce these patterns of cortical arousal in a fashion necessary to perform different types of cognitive tasks. Based on this assumption, 24 LD adolescents, ranging in age from 13.1 to 17.9, were assigned to one of three groups: (1) EEG biofeedback to produce a pattern of increased right hemisphere and decreased left hemisphere frequencies, (2) training to decrease EEG frequencies in both hemispheres, and (3) a no-treatment control group. The results were complex and will only be briefly summarized here. First, EEG power data found lower left than right hemisphere cortical arousal across both verbal and nonverbal tasks. These data support theories arguing for left hemisphere hypoarousal in LD children (e.g., Satz, Rardin, & Ross, 1971). In addition, both biofeedback groups displayed decreasing left hemisphere baseline frequencies across sessions. In terms of achievement test data, subjects trained to increase right hemisphere and decrease left hemisphere arousal showed a significant improvement on the Arithmetic subtest of the Wide Range Achievement Test. Other subjects showed no change in arithmetic scores. None of the subjects displayed significant improvement on measures of spelling, reading, or spatial abilities. Finally, a strong correlation ($r = 0.9$) was found between subjects' ability to increase right hemisphere frequencies and improvement on WRAT Arithmetic.

Carter and Russell (1981) reported a single group outcome study on four LD children chosen on the basis of having a WISC-R Verbal IQ score at least 15 points below their Performance IQ (the mean Performance–Verbal discrepancy was 25.34 IQ points). These elementary school-age boys then received 16 sessions of EEG biofeedback training to voluntarily produce either alpha or beta activity coupled with taped relaxation training. Because of equipment problems, the EEG data were not reported. However, posttest data suggested a marked decrease of 14.67 points in the discrepancy between Verbal and Performance IQ with the mean Verbal IQ increasing from 76.3 to 88.7.

Tansey (1984) also reported single group outcome data on six elementary school-age boys with a history of learning disabilities. Unlike the subjects in the previous study, these children varied in the relative strength of their Verbal and Performance IQs. Tansey's subjects received a variable number of biofeedback training sessions to increase bilateral SMR amplitude. Tansey reasoned that many forms of remedial therapy for LD children work by providing external, task-relevant stimulation to the child's sensorimotor cortex. He argued that SMR biofeedback provides for internal cerebral stimulation. Further, by providing bilateral EEG biofeedback, remediation should also occur for learning deficits caused by deficiencies in normal interhemispheric interactions. The results strongly supported the efficacy of SMR biofeedback. First, as a group, SMR amplitude showed a mean increase of 138% above baseline levels. Second, large increases, ranging from 7 to 25 points, were found for all six children in WISC-R Verbal, Performance, and Full-Scale IQ scores. These IQ increments were felt to be much larger than the change that would be expected by maturation alone. Finally, SMR training attenuated the discrepancy between Verbal and Performance IQ scores for the four children with significant pretraining asymmetries in ability levels.

It is premature to offer a reliable opinion as to the utility of EEG biofeedback as a therapy for LD children. In part, this relates to the lack of procedural overlap between the four published articles in this area. However, several observations can be made. First, LD children and adolescents demonstrated reliable changes in physiology from pre- to posttesting. This is remarkable in some respects because it is unclear that these subjects, even though they met criteria set by each examiner, had similar learning problems. Unfortunately, the lack of appropriate control measures makes it impossible to determine if these changes are related to the contingent presentation of the feedback signal, or are caused by other factors, such as confounding treatments, nonspecific treatment effects, or mere instructions to attempt to control EEG. Second, psychoeducational data were limited. The two studies reporting achievement testing found, at best, only minimal changes in academic skills. Also, the absence of appropriate controls makes it difficult to separate the effects of biofeedback training from the influence of both maturation effects and practice effects caused by repeated exposure to tests. Third, none of the studies obtained follow-up data to see if reported benefits of treatment were maintained. Finally, with the exception of the study by Carter and Russell, no attempt was made to sample a group of LD children or adolescents with relatively homogeneous neuropsychological characteristics. Rather, an invariant intervention is assumed to be equally effective for all LD individuals (see Doehring, Hoshko, & Bryans, 1979, and Leslie, Davidson, & Batey, 1985, for criticisms of this strategy in learning disability research in general).

Childhood Migraines

Theories of Migraine

For many years, the vascular hypothesis was the dominant theory of migraine. In this theory, migraine is a two-phase process with an initial period of vasoconstriction followed by a compensatory phase of vasodilation. Cerebral ischemia associated with vasoconstriction was felt to cause the prodromal aura. The pain of migraine was attributed to excessive vasodilation or stretching of the cranial arteries (Fenichel, 1985). Pain was felt to be augmented by the presence of sensitizing peptides released near the cranial arteries and their primary afferents (Saper, 1983).

Recent studies of cerebral blood flow have failed to confirm the vascular theory of migraines (see Saper, Silberstein, Gordon, & Hamel, 1993, or Silberstein, 1992). A consensus is now forming that migraine is more accurately described as a primary disturbance of brain function producing secondary vascular changes. Basic disturbances, perhaps in hypothalamic functioning, initiate a cascade of neuronal events that includes the release of substances such as substance P and calcitonin gene-related peptide (CGRP) in the sensory neurons that innervate the head and face. These peptides produce a neurogenic inflammation of the blood vessels in the head, causing vasodilation and other vascular changes. In addition, these peptides are known to sensitize primary pain afferents. A sensitization mechanism is needed to explain the observation that vasodilation is painful during headaches but not when produced by exercise or by warmth. In summary, the neurogenic hypothesis does not postulate a primary vasoconstrictive phase to initiate a migraine attack; rather, the pain of migraine is felt to be more closely related to sensitization of primary pain afferents than to excessive stretch on blood vessels. (See Saper *et al.*, 1993, for a concise review of the theories of migraine.)

Silberstein (1990) provides recommendations for medication management of pediatric migraine. Treatment typically begins with reassurance, the removal of triggering factors (such as stress, fatigue, or dietary influences), and the use of simple analgesics. If this is not effective, a variety of prescription medications are available. However, the decision to supplement simple analgesics with more powerful medications is one that many physicians and parents are hesitant to make. Antimigraine medications such as dihydroergotamine (for acute migraines) or propranolol (for frequent migraines) often have unpleasant or undesirable side effects. In addition, many physicians are reluctant to prescribe maintenance medications because of concerns about eventual drug dependency or about the unknown effects of long-term use of these medications on children (Hoelscher & Lichstein, 1984). This reluctance has motivated a search for effective, nonpharmacological treatments of childhood migraine.

Biofeedback Treatment of Pediatric Migraine

Early biofeedback interventions for migraines were based on the now-discredited vascular theory of migraines. Sargent, Green, and Walters (1973) developed an intervention where patients were trained to increase skin temperature in their hands. This intervention rested on the assumptions that migraine pain is caused by vasodilation of cranial arteries and that vasodilation is a reaction to a preceding phase of excessive vasoconstriction. These proponents argued that training subjects in peripheral vasodilation (increased digital skin temperature) produces a generalized decrease in sympathetic tone (smooth muscle relaxation) that minimizes the prodromal vasoconstrictive phase and aborts the headache before it starts. Many controlled outcome studies have found this intervention to be very effective in controlling migraines with a 50 to 60% reduction in headache activities in adults following temperature biofeedback treatment (Blanchard & Andrasik, 1987). In hindsight, the efficacy of temperature biofeedback may rely more on its central rather than

peripheral effects although this hypothesis awaits empirical confirmation.

The treatment of childhood migraine with behavioral interventions began in the mid-1970s. The most common intervention was again skin temperature biofeedback combined with autogenic training. Autogenic training is a relaxation method developed around the turn of the century in Germany by Schultz and more recently reintroduced by Luthe (Schultz & Luthe, 1969). The method involves passive concentration on a systematic set of phrases and images suggesting control of physiological responding. The combination of biofeedback and autogenics was popularized by clinicians at the Menninger Foundation who labeled this integrated approach autogenic biofeedback training (Green, Green, Walters, Sargent, & Meyer, 1975).

Although there are many studies of behavioral interventions for childhood headaches (see Andrasik, Blake, & McCarran, 1985, and Duckro & Cantwell-Simmons, 1989, for excellent reviews of this literature), only two group control outcome studies have investigated biofeedback interventions in a pure population of children with migraine. Labbe and Williamson (1984) compared autogenic feedback and a no-treatment control group in 28 children aged 7–16. Autogenic feedback led to significant improvement in headache intensity, frequency, and duration measured posttreatment and at 1-month follow-up. In addition, 93% (13/14) of the patients receiving autogenic feedback reported at least a 50% improvement in their average headache rating. Six-month follow-up data were also available for 8 of the 14 treated patients: 5 were found to be improved or symptom free. In contrast, there were no mean group differences in pre and post ratings of headaches for the control subjects, with only 7 and 14% rating at least a 50% improvement at posttreatment and 1-month follow-up. Finally, across all training sessions, patients were able to produce a statistically significant increase in digital skin temperature while the feedback display was available. However, no differences were found between the treatment and control groups during the pre- and posttreatment self-control assessment. Patients were not able to increase skin temperature in the absence of feedback.

Fentress, Masek, Mehegan, and Benson (1986) evaluated a comprehensive pain management program for childhood migraine. Eighteen children aged 8–12 were randomized to one of three groups: (1) frontal region EMG biofeedback, meditative exercises [similar to Benson's (1975) secular TM], and pain behavior management (operant control of pain behaviors); (2) progressive muscle relaxation, meditative relaxation, and pain behavior management; or (3) a waiting list control group. The data supported clinically significant reductions in headache activity in both treatment groups averaging 60 and 82% across all outcome measures for the biofeedback and relaxation groups, respectively. In contrast, patients in the control group reported a 19% increase in symptoms. These changes were maintained at 1-year follow-up. The authors concluded that the behavioral management of pediatric migraines is very effective, but that frontal region EMG biofeedback does not appear to be an essential component.

These studies encourage the use of behavioral interventions in the treatment of migraine headaches in children. Impressive reductions in headache activity have been found in the two reported group outcome studies with benefits maintained over follow-up. What seems less clear is the specific role that biofeedback plays in contributing to these positive outcomes. In the studies reported, biofeedback is invariably combined with other physiological, cognitive, or behavioral pain management interventions.

Some data suggest that contingent feedback is not a necessary ingredient for producing clinical change. In the Labbe and Williamson (1984) study, trained patients were unable to increase skin temperature at the end of biofeedback training in the absence of a biofeedback display. This finding weakens the argument that specific physiological learning is the mechanism of action for producing therapeutic change. Also, Fentress et al. (1986) found comparable results for the biofeedback and relaxation groups. Perhaps the key factor is the production of a generalized state of relaxation or reduced sympathetic activity and not specific physiological learning related to vasodilation.

Unfortunately, both studies contain flaws that make these interpretations premature. Fentress et al. did not employ the potentially more effective skin temperature biofeedback intervention. In addition, the small group sample size ($n = 6$) limited the power of their study when comparing treatment alternatives. The Labbe and Williamson study does not suffer from these problems. However, they assessed the patients' ability to control skin temperature in a low-arousal context (resting in a recliner). As many migraines emerge in the context of psy-

chosocial stressors, a more relevant test may require the assessment of skin temperature self-regulation during the presentation of an *in vivo* or analogue stressor.

Recent Trends

Despite the limitations of the preceding studies, biofeedback interventions are now commonly employed in the clinical setting and most clinicians see them as potent alternatives to medication management. Recent studies have avoided unresolved issues related to the specificity and mechanisms of biofeedback interventions and have instead looked at issues related to cost-effectiveness and treatment delivery. Clinicians have modified the standard clinic-based biofeedback intervention and have adopted interventions that use detailed treatment manuals, audiotapes, and portable biofeedback monitors to deliver treatment largely in the patient's home setting. These home-based or limited therapist contact treatment protocols share several potential advantages over traditional clinic-based approaches. Physiological learning takes place in a more natural environment, treatment is less expensive, patients develop a greater sense of independence or self-efficacy in the management of their symptoms, and this type of training is much more practical for patients who live a considerable distance from biofeedback or behavioral medicine treatment centers (Nash & Holroyd, 1992).

Three studies have compared home-based and clinic-based treatment of pediatric migraines (Allen & McKeen, 1991; Burke & Andrasik, 1989; Guarnieri & Blanchard, 1990). All three studies found home-based training to be both effective in reducing headache activity and comparable to traditional clinic-based interventions. Burke and Andrasik (1989) found that home-based treatment effects were maintained through a 1-year follow-up period.

The study by Allen and McKeen (1991) is noteworthy for the attempt to identify process variables that predict treatment success when services are delivered in the home environment. In this study, 21 children aged 7–12 participated in home-based autogenic feedback training. Parents were also given guidelines to reduce inadvertent reinforcement of pain behavior (e.g., mandatory attendance at school and regular activities despite headache activity) and to increase adaptive coping with biofeedback skills (e.g., in response to pain, encourage prompt practice of relaxation). Home-based behavioral training was very effective with 87% of the subjects experiencing at least a 70% reduction in headache activity.

Several subanalyses were completed to identify factors that correlated with treatment efficacy. Two are of particular interest. First, Allen and McKeen (1991) replicated an earlier observation that the ability to warm hands prior to biofeedback training is *inversely* correlated with treatment outcome. One interpretation of this finding is that some subjects may already have the ability to generate a relaxation response and that headaches in these subjects are related to some other non-stress-related mechanism (e.g., dietary, operant). In contrast, other subjects may not be able to generate physiological relaxation without specific training and these patients may be uniquely able to profit from biofeedback and other relaxation therapies.

Second, Allen and McKeen (1991) observed that parental noncompliance with behavioral management guidelines was associated with an initial decline in their child's headache activity that was not maintained over time. This treatment failure occurred despite frequent home practice by these children throughout treatment. More persistent effects were found when parents followed behavior management recommendations. The role of parental support has been neglected in most of these outcome studies and Allen and McKeen's results point to the price potentially paid for this neglect.

In conclusion, autogenic biofeedback training appears to be an effective treatment for pediatric migraine. Treatment benefit is maintained over time and occurs even when training is provided with home-based modifications. All studies have applied autogenic biofeedback in the context of multicomponent behavioral pain management training. This reflects our current understanding of headaches and chronic pain as a multidetermined reaction. Documenting the unique benefits of biofeedback may be less important than identifying reliable principles for guiding the clinician when matching treatment components with specific patient variables. Intriguing clues have been identified in some studies (e.g., the relative lack of benefit from autogenic biofeedback for patients who produce large physiological changes even prior to biofeedback training) but the sample sizes

are uniformly small and require replication. Finally, biofeedback clinicians and theorists need to start thinking about their findings in the context of the neurogenic theory of migraines.

General Discussion

Several impressions emerge from this literature review. The findings indicate that children as young as 5 years old are able to learn to control targeted physiology following biofeedback training. It also seems clear that many patients show clinically significant improvements in symptom control following biofeedback interventions. These changes occur despite the fact that biofeedback is often attempted only when patients have not responded to previous medical interventions. Although encouraging, the significance of many of these findings is compromised by numerous methodological shortcomings (see Cleeland, 1981; Cobb & Evans, 1981; Kewman & Roberts, 1983). With the exception of the exemplary programmatic research on the treatment of fecal incontinence and epilepsy, the following problems are common in the studies reviewed in this chapter.

1. Control procedures are typically inadequate to rule out the contributions of nonspecific changes in attitude and motivation. Adequate designs, such as the use of credible noncontingent feedback (Lubar, 1982), the comparison of biofeedback with other active treatments (Whitehead *et al.*, 1986), and the use of appropriate single-case experimental designs (Bird & Catalado, 1978) are still rarely employed.

2. Interpretation is often clouded by the mixing of biofeedback with other behavioral interventions including relaxation training, behavioral skills training, cognitive therapy, and behavior modification. This is a thorny issue in biofeedback studies as additional treatment approaches, such as relaxation training, are often used as home practice aids designed to help maintain symptom control in the home or school situation. Although there may be much clinical wisdom in applying a treatment package rather than an isolated biofeedback intervention, these confounds obviously make it impossible to determine which treatment should be credited for the obtained therapeutic gains.

3. Information concerning potentially important patient characteristics is usually not reported. For example, hyperactive children vary widely in their levels of cortical and autonomic arousal (Fin-

ley, 1983). Despite this, not one study considered measures of physiological arousal when selecting patients for biofeedback interventions and only one investigation (Denkowski *et al.*, 1984) correlated baseline measures of muscle tension with therapeutic gains. The implications of individual differences for the choice of a biofeedback intervention have been inadequately explored.

4. Follow-up data should be routinely collected. Erosions in therapeutic gains are the norm and this possibility must be assessed. When appropriate, treatments should be altered to include elements promoting the maintenance of symptom control (e.g., the gradual fading of biofeedback contingencies, providing feedback both during resting conditions and during situational challenges).

5. There is a tradition in behavioral medicine for the use of relaxation as an intervention with broad-spectrum healing powers. This has resulted in the prescription of relaxation even when no compelling rationale for its usage has been empirically documented. For example, the use of frontal region EMG biofeedback in the treatment of learning disabilities has as much justification as the use of increased exercise, adequate nutrition, or other formulas for improving general well-being. In addition, Burish has argued that frontal region EMG biofeedback provides only minimal benefit as a generalized relaxation procedure. Indeed, he and his colleagues have employed this form of biofeedback as a control intervention when evaluating the impact of other more potent relaxation procedures (Shirley, Burish, & Rowe, 1982). Taken as a whole, the data do not support the relatively widespread use of this intervention for the pediatric problems reviewed in this chapter.

6. Few researchers adopt a developmental perspective in the design of their studies (Marcon & Labbe, 1990). Similar interventions are offered to children who differ in their level of cognitive and emotional development. For example, Marcon and Labbe point out that a child's concept of self-regulation or locus of control shifts over time with an external locus of control typically emerging around age 9. They speculate that

> children who consistently understand that their actions could reduce the likelihood of [a symptom] may respond differently to treatments that incorporate self-regulation than [younger] children who place responsibility for their [symptom] on external factors such as chance or intervention by powerful others.

This sound advice is rarely reflected in the design or analyses of the studies reviewed in this chapter.

Patient–Treatment Interactions and the Art of Biofeedback

The successful application of appropriate biofeedback interventions with children and adolescents often requires modifications in the training procedures developed for adult clients. Experienced clinicians have long recognized this point and helpful guidelines are provided by Attanasio *et al.* (1985), Linkenhoker (1983), and Marcon and Labbe (1990). For example, whereas adults typically tolerate the procedures involved in electrode applications, young children may require greater reassurance about the safety of instrumentation. To date, most of the available advice is based on unsystematic observations of patients. However, some useful data are beginning to emerge.

Clinical researchers have commented on the challenges presented by the sometimes fragile motivation level and attention span of children referred for biofeedback training. Denkowski and Denkowski (1984) observed that across several research studies of EMG biofeedback with hyperactive children, a tendency emerged for physiological learning to plateau by the fourth session. They tentatively attributed any lack of further learning to boredom with the feedback task. One possible strategy for preventing boredom is to reduce the length of biofeedback sessions or to include a larger number of rest breaks (Attanasio *et al.*, 1985). Unfortunately, little is known about the impact of these procedural changes.

Others have attempted to maintain attention either by employing tangible reinforcers or by altering the nature of the feedback display. Finley *et al.* (1981) developed an automated reward system involving a universal feeder that presented children with reinforcers, such as candy or small toys, contingent on appropriate changes in physiology. The use of this system led to greater and more rapid reductions in EMG in a group of children with cerebral palsy than did the use of an audio feedback signal alone. Other recommended changes in reinforcement have included the use of music instead of a feedback tone (Walmsley, Crichton, & Droog, 1981) and the use of video game-like feedback displays. However, it will be important to determine if the enhanced stimulation provided by these changes leads to counterproductive increases in physiological arousal.

Many of the studies reviewed in this chapter combined biofeedback with medical interventions, most commonly medication. Despite this, interactions between behavioral and pharmacologic therapies have received little attention. Linkenhoker (1983) alerted clinicians to potential dangers caused by failures to alter the dosage of medications whose physiological effects parallel the physiological consequences of biofeedback. For example, Seeburg and DeBoer (1980) reported a case study where EMG biofeedback training in a diabetic patient reduced her need for insulin leading to harmful side effects until the medication regimen was adjusted. In a more positive vein, Surwit, Allen, Gilgor, and Duvic (1982) investigated the concurrent effects of autogenic training and sympathetic blocking agents on skin temperature changes in patients with Raynaud's disease. Statistically significant changes in skin temperature were only obtained when both interventions were applied simultaneously. On a related issue, Cleeland (1981) suggested that the addition of behavioral training methods to medical regimens might allow for a reduction of medications, such as anticonvulsants, which often suppress symptoms only at levels that are either toxic or produce unpleasant side effects.

Finally, researchers are beginning to identify patient variables that predict success or failure with biofeedback interventions. Denkowski et al. (1984) employed multiple regression analyses to relate patients' age, pretreatment EMG level, degree of hyperactivity, and locus of control to decreases in EMG levels following biofeedback training. The subjects were 59 hyperactive males aged 8–15. Only locus of control predicted posttreatment changes in EMG, with internal locus of control associated with better outcomes. Whitehead et al. (1986) also found that age did not predict response to biofeedback training in their patients with neurogenic incontinence. Children as young as 5 were able to successfully profit from biofeedback training as long as tangible reinforcers were used to maintain their attention. The authors did find, however, that physiological parameters were important in determining which patients benefit from biofeedback versus behavior modification approaches. Quite obviously, we are only beginning to understand the impact of demographic, cognitive, behavioral, and physiological characteristics of patients on the biofeedback learning experience. Much worthwhile research remains to be done.

References

Adams, R. D., & Victor, M. (1977). *Principles of neurology.* New York: McGraw–Hill.

Allen, K., & McKeen, L. (1991). Home-based multicomponent treatment of pediatric migraine. *Headache, 31,* 467–472.

American Psychiatric Association. (1994). *Diagnostic and statistical manual of mental disorders* (4th ed.). Washington, DC: Author.

Andrasik, F., & Attanasio, V. (1985). Biofeedback in pediatrics: Current status and appraisal. In M. C. Wolraith & D. K. Routh (Eds.), *Advances in developmental and behavioral pediatrics.* Greenwich, CT: JAI Press.

Andrasik, F., Blake, D. D., & McCarran, M. S. (1985). A biobehavioral analysis of pediatric headache. In N. A. Kasenegor, J. D. Arasteh, & M. S. Cataldo (Eds.), *Child health behavior: A behavioral pediatrics perspective.* New York: Wiley.

Attanasio, V., Andrasik, F., Burke, E. J., Blake, D. D., Kabela, E., & McCarran, M. S. (1985). Clinical issues in utilizing biofeedback with children. *Clinical Biofeedback and Health, 8,* 134–141.

Barkley, R. A. (1977). A review of stimulant drug research with hyperactive children. *Journal of Child Psychology and Psychiatry, 18,* 137–165.

Barkley, R. A. (1987). *Defiant children: A clinician's manual for parent training.* New York: Guilford Press.

Barkley, R. A. (1990). *Attention deficit hyperactivity disorder: A handbook for diagnosis and treatment.* New York: Guilford Press.

Barkley, R. A. (1993). Continuing concerns about EEG biofeedback/neurofeedback. *The ADHD Report, 1,* 1–3.

Bassotti, G., & Whitehead, W. E. (1994). Biofeedback as a treatment approach to gastrointestinal tract disorders. *The American Journal of Gastroenterology, 89,* 158–164.

Benson, H. (1975). *The relaxation response.* New York: Morrow.

Bhatara, V., Arnold, L. E., Lorance, T., & Gupta, D. (1979). Muscle relaxation therapy in hyperkinesis: Is it effective? *Journal of Learning Disabilities, 12,* 49–53.

Bird, B., & Cataldo, M. (1978). Experimental analysis of EMG feedback in treating dystonia. *Annals of Neurology, 3,* 310–315.

Blanchard, E. B., & Andrasik, F. (1987). Biofeedback treatment of vascular headache. In J. Hatch, J. Rugh, & J. Fisher (Eds.), *Biofeedback studies in clinical efficacy.* New York: Plenum Press.

Borkovec, T. D., & Nau, S. D. (1972). Credibility of analogue therapy rationales. *Journal of Behavior Therapy and Experimental Psychiatry, 3,* 257–260.

Borkovec, T. D., & Sides, J. K. (1979). Critical procedural variables related to the physiological effects of progressive relaxation: A review. *Behavior Research and Therapy, 17,* 119–126.

Braud, L. W. (1978). The effects of frontal EMG biofeedback and progressive relaxation upon hyperactivity and its behavioral concomitants. *Biofeedback and Self-Regulation, 3,* 69–89.

Braud, L. W., Lupin, M. N., & Braud, W. G. (1975). The use of electromyographic biofeedback in the control of hyperactivity. *Journal of Learning Disability, 7,* 420–425.

Burish, T. G. (1983). EMG biofeedback in the treatment of stress-related disorders. In C. Prokop & L. Bradley (Eds.), *Medical psychology: Contributions to behavioral medicine* (pp. 395–421). New York: Academic Press.

Burke, E., & Andrasik, F. (1989). Home- vs. clinic-based biofeedback treatment for pediatric migraine: Results of treatment through one-year follow-up. *Headache, 29,* 434–440.

Carter, J. L., & Russell, H. L. (1980). Biofeedback and academic attainment of LD children. *Academic Therapy, 15,* 483–486.

Carter, J. L., & Russell, H. L. (1981). Changes in verbal–performance IQ discrepancy scores after left hemisphere EEG frequency control training—A pilot report. *American Journal of Clinical Biofeedback, 4,* 66–67.

Carter, J. L., & Russell, H. L. (1985). Use of EMG biofeedback procedures with learning disabled children in a clinical and an educational setting. *Journal of Learning Disability, 18,* 214–216.

Cataldo, M. F., Bird, B. L., & Cunningham, C. E. (1978). Experimental analysis of EMG feedback in treating cerebral palsy. *Journal of Behavioral Medicine, 1,* 311–322.

Cerulli, M. A., Nikoomanesh, P., & Schuster, M. M. (1979). Progress in biofeedback conditioning for fecal incontinence. *Gastroenterology, 76,* 742–746.

Christie, D. J., DeWitt, R. A., Kaltenbach, P., & Reed, D. (1984). Using EMG biofeedback to signal hyperactive children when to relax. *Exceptional Children, 50,* 547–548.

Cleeland, C. S. (1981). Biofeedback as a clinical tool: Its use with the neurologically impaired patient. In S. B. Filskov & T. J. Boll (Eds.), *Handbook of clinical neuropsychology* (pp. 734–753). New York: Wiley.

Cobb, D. E., & Evans, J. R. (1981). The use of biofeedback techniques with school aged children exhibiting behavioral and/or learning problems. *Journal of Abnormal Child Psychology, 9,* 251–281.

Connoly, D. P., Besserman, R., & Kirschvink, J. (1974). Electromyography (EMG) biofeedback on hyperkinetic children. *Journal of Biofeedback, 2,* 24–30.

Cott, A., Pavloski, R. P., & Black, A. H. (1979). Reducing epileptic seizures through operant condition of central nervous system activity: Procedural variables. *Science, 203,* 73–75.

Cunningham, M. D., & Murphy, P. J. (1981). The effects of bilateral EEG biofeedback on verbal, visual–spatial, and creative skills in learning disabled male adolescents. *Journal of Learning Disabilities, 14,* 204–208.

DeBacher, G. (1983). Biofeedback in spasticity control. In J. V. Basmajian (Ed.), *Biofeedback: Principles and practice for clinicians* (2nd ed., pp. 111–129). Baltimore: Williams & Wilkins.

Denkowski, K. M., & Denkowski, G. C. (1984). Is group progressive relaxation training as effective with hyperactive children as individual EMG biofeedback treatment? *Biofeedback and Self-Regulation, 9,* 353–364.

Denkowski, K. M., Denkowski, G. C., & Omizo, M. M. (1983). The effects of EMG-assisted relaxation training on the academic performance, locus of control, and self-esteem of hyperactive boys. *Biofeedback and Self-Regulation, 8,* 363–375.

Denkowski, K. M., Denkowski, G. C., & Omizo, M. M. (1984). Predictors of success in the EMG biofeedback training of hyperactive male children. *Biofeedback and Self-Regulation, 9,* 253–264.

Doehring, D., Hoshko, J., & Bryans, B. (1979). Statistical classification of children with reading problems. *Journal of Clinical Neuropsychology, 1,* 5–16.

Donhoffer, H., & Lissak, K. (1962). EEG changes associated with the elaboration of conditioned reflexes. *Acta Physiologica Academy of Science, Hungary, 21,* 249–255.

Duckro, P., N., & Cantwell-Simmons, E. O. (1989). A review of studies evaluating biofeedback and relaxation training in the management of pediatric headache. *Headache, 29,* 428–433.

Dunn, F. M., & Howell, R. J. (1982). Relaxation training and its relationship to hyperactivity in boys. *Journal of Clinical Psychology, 38,* 92–100.

Engel, B. T., Nikoomanesh, P., & Schuster, M. M. (1974). Operant conditioning of rectosphincteric responses in the treatment of fecal incontinence. *New England Journal of Medicine, 290,* 646–649.

Fenichel, G. M. (1985). Migraine in children. *Neurology Clinics, 3,* 77–94.

Fentress, D., Masek, B., Mehegan, J., & Benson, H. (1986). Biofeedback and relaxation response training in the treatment of pediatric migraine. *Developmental Medicine & Child Neurology, 28,* 139–146.

Finley, W. W. (1976). Effects of sham feedback following successful SMR training in an epileptic: A follow-up study. *Biofeedback and Self-Regulation, 1,* 227–235.

Finley, W. W. (1983). Biofeedback with children. In C. E. Walker & M. C. Roberts (Eds.), *Handbook of clinical child psychology* (pp. 1050–1068). New York: Wiley.

Finley, W. W., Etherton, M. D., Dickmen, D., Karimian, D., & Simpson, R. W. (1981). A simple EMG-reward system for biofeedback training of children. *Biofeedback and Self-Regulation, 6,* 169–180.

Finley, W. W., Niman, C. A., Standley, J., & Wansley, R. A. (1977). Electrophysiologic behavior modification of frontal EMG in cerebral palsied children. *Biofeedback and Self-Regulation, 2,* 59–79.

Flemings, P. G. (1979). A study of electromyographic biofeedback as a method to teach hyperactive children how to relax within a public school setting. *Dissertation Abstracts International, 39,* 6693A.

Gargiulo, R. M., & Kuna, D. J. (1979). Arousal level and hyperkinesis: Implications for biofeedback. *Journal of Learning Disabilities, 12,* 4–5.

Gracenin, C. T., & Cook, J. E. (1977). Alpha biofeedback and LD children. *Academic Therapy, 12,* 275–279.

Green, E. E., Green, A. M., Walters, E. D., Sargent, J. D., & Meyer, R. G. (1975). Autogenic feedback training. *Psychotherapy and Psychosomatics, 25,* 88–98.

Guarnieri, P., & Blanchard, E. (1990). Evaluation of home-based thermal biofeedback treatment of pediatric migraine headache. *Biofeedback and Self-Regulation, 15,* 179–184.

Haight, M. J. (1976). The response of hyperkinesis to EMG biofeedback. (ERIC Document Reproduction Service No. ED. 125–169).

Hampstead, W. J. (1979). The effects of EMG-assisted relaxation training with hyperkinetic children. *Biofeedback and Self-Regulation, 4,* 113–125.

Hoelscher, T. J., & Lichstein, K. L. (1984). Behavioral assessment and treatment of child migraine: Implications for clinical research and practice. *Headache, 24,* 94–103.

Holroyd, K. A., Penzien, D. B., Hursey, K. G., Tobin, D. L., Rogers, L., Holm, J. E., Maralle, P. J., Hall, J. R., & Chila, A. G. (1984). Change mechanisms in EMG biofeedback training: Cognitive changes underlying improvements in tension headache. *Journal of Consulting & Clinical Psychology, 52*(6), 1039–1053.

Howe, R. C., & Sterman, M. B. (1972). Cortical–subcortical EEG correlates of suppressed motor behavior during sleep and waking in the cat. *Electroencephalography and Clinical Neurophysiology, 32,* 681–695.

Hughes, H., Henry, D., & Hughes, A. (1980). The effect of frontal EMG biofeedback training on the behavior of children with activity-level problems. *Biofeedback and Self-Regulation, 5,* 207–219.

Hunter, S. H., Russell, H. I, Russell, E. D., & Zimmerman, R. I. (1976). Control of fingertip temperature increases via biofeedback in learning disabled and normal children. *Perceptual and Motor Skills, 43,* 743–755.

Jeffrey, T. B. (1976). The effects of operant conditioning and electromyographic biofeedback on the relaxed behavior of hyperkinetic children. *Dissertation Abstracts International, 36,* 2510B.

Kewman, D. C., & Roberts, A. H. (1983). An alternative perspective on biofeedback efficacy studies: A reply to Steiner and Dince. *Biofeedback and Self-Regulation, 8,* 487–497.

Krause, T. R. (1978). Psychophysiological changes in hyperactive and normal children as a function of medication and biofeedback training. *Dissertation Abstracts International, 38,* 6219B.

Kuhlman, W. N. (1978). EEG feedback training of epileptic patients: Clinical and electroencephalographic analysis. *Electroencephalography and Clinical Neurophysiology, 45,* 699–710.

Labbe, E. L., & Williamson, D. A. (1984). Treatment of childhood migraine using autogenic feedback training. *Journal of Consulting and Clinical Psychology, 52,* 968–976.

Lee, S. W. (1991). Biofeedback as a treatment for childhood hyperactivity: A critical review of the literature. *Psychological Reports, 68,* 163–192.

Leslie, S. C., Davidson, R. J., & Batey, O. B. (1985). Purdue pegboard performance of disabled and normal readers: Unimanual versus bimanual differences. *Brain and Language, 24,* 359–369.

Linkenhoker, D. (1983). Tools of behavioral medicine: Applications of biofeedback treatment for children and adolescents. *Developmental and Behavioral Pediatrics, 4,* 16–20.

Linn, R. T., & Hodge, J. K. (1979). Use of EMG biofeedback training in increasing attention span and internalizing locus of control in hyperactive children. *Proceedings of the Biofeedback Society of America,* 11th Annual Meeting, pp. 81–84.

Loening-Baucke, V., Desch, L., & Wolraich, M. (1988). Biofeedback training for patients with myelomeningocele and fecal incontinence. *Developmental Medicine and Child Neurology, 30,* 781–790.

Loux, R. W., & Ascher, L. M. (1980). The effect of biofeedback-assisted relaxation upon the classroom behavior of hyperkinetic children. *Proceedings of the Biofeedback Society of America,* 11th Annual Meeting, pp. 85–86.

Lubar, J. F. (1982). EEG operant conditioning in severe epileptics: Controlled multidimensional studies. In L. White & B. Tursky (Eds.), *Clinical biofeedback: Efficacy and mechanisms* (pp. 288–310). New York: Guilford Press.

Lubar, J. F., & Bahler, W. W. (1976). Behavioral management of epileptic seizures following EEG biofeedback training of the sensorimotor rhythm. *Biofeedback and Self-Regulation, 1,* 77–104.

Lubar, J. F., Bianchini, K. J., Calhoun, W. H., Lambert, E. W., Brody, Z. H., & Shabsin, H. S. (1985). Spectral analysis of EEG differences between children with and without learning disabilities. *Journal of Learning Disabilities, 7,* 403–408.

Lubar, J. F., & Shouse, M. N. (1976). EEG and behavioral changes in a hyperkinetic child concurrent with training of the sensorimotor rhythm (SMR): A preliminary report. *Biofeedback and Self-Regulation, 1,* 293–306.

Lubar, J. O., & Lubar, J. F. (1984). Electroencephalographic biofeedback of SMR and beta for treatment of attention deficit disorders in a clinical setting. *Biofeedback and Self-Regulation, 9,* 1–23.

Marcon, R., & Labbe, E. (1990). Assessment and treatment of children's headaches from a developmental perspective. *Headache, 30,* 586–592.

Masterson, J. P., Jr., & Turley, W. B. (1980). Biofeedback training with children. *American Journal of Clinical Biofeedback, 3,* 137–143.

Miller, N. E. (1969). Learning of visceral and glandular responses. *Science, 163,* 434–445.

Moore, L. L. (1977). Behavior modification and electromyographic biofeedback as alternative to drugs for the treatment of hyperkinesis in children. *Dissertation Abstracts International, 38,* 77-27-560.

Murphy, P. J., Darwin, J., & Murphy, D. (1977). EEG feedback training for cerebral dysfunction: A research program with learning disabled adolescents. *Biofeedback and Self-Regulation, 2,* 288.

Nall, A. (1973). Alpha training and the hyperkinetic child: Is it effective? *Academic Therapy, 9,* 5–19.

Nash, J., & Holroyd, K. (1992). Home-based behavioral treatment for recurrent headache: A cost effective analysis? *APS Bulletin, 2,* 1–6.

Omizo, M. M. (1980a). The effects of biofeedback-induced relaxation training in hyperactive adolescent boys. *The Journal of Psychology, 105,* 131–138.

Omizo, M. M. (1980b). The effects of relaxation and biofeedback training on dimensions of self-concept (DOSC) among hyperactive male children. *Educational Research Quarterly, 5,* 22–30.

Omizo, M. M., Cubberly, W. E., Semands, S. G., & Omizo, S. A. (1986). The effects of biofeedback and relaxation training on memory tasks among hyperactive boys. *The Exceptional Child, 33,* 56–64.

Omizo, M. M., & Michael, W. B. (1982). Biofeedback-induced relaxation training and impulsivity, attention to task, and locus of control among hyperactive boys. *Journal of Learning Disabilities, 15,* 414–416.

Omizo, M. M., & Williams, R. E. (1982). Biofeedback-induced relaxation training as an alternative for the elementary school learning-disabled child. *Biofeedback and Self-Regulation, 7,* 139–148.

Pelham, W. E., & Murphy, H. A. (1986). Attention deficit and conduct disorders. In M. Hersen (Ed.), *Pharmacological and behavioral treatments: An integrative approach* (pp. 108–148). New York: Wiley.

Potashkin, B. D., & Beckles, N. (1990). Relative efficacy of Ritalin and biofeedback treatments in the management of hyperactivity. *Biofeedback and Self-Regulation, 15,* 305–315.

Rivera, E., & Omizo, M. M. (1980). An investigation of the effects of relaxation training and biofeedback on attention to task and impulsivity among hyperactive male children. *Exceptional Child, 27,* 41–51.

Roberts, A. C. (1966). *The aphasic child.* Springfield, IL: Thomas.

Roth, S. R., Sterman, M. B., & Clemente, C. D. (1967). Comparison of EEG correlates of reinforcement, internal inhibition and sleep. *Electroencephalography and Clinical Neurophysiology, 23,* 509–520.

Saper, J. R. (1983). *Headache disorders: Current concepts and treatment strategies.* Boston: John Wright.

Saper, J., Silberstein, S., Gordon, C., & Hamel, R. (1993). *Handbook of headache management: A practical guide to diagnosis and treatment of head, neck, and facial pain.* Baltimore: Williams & Wilkins.

Sargent, J. D., Green, E. E., & Walters, E. D. (1973). The use of autogenic feedback techniques in the treatment of migraine headaches. *Psychosomatic Medicine, 35,* 129–135.

Satterfield, J., & Dawson, M. (1971). Electrodermal correlates of hyperactivity in children. *Psychophysiology, 8,* 191–197.

Satz, P., Rardin, D., & Ross, J. (1971). An evaluation of a theory of specific developmental dyslexia. *Child Development, 42,* 2009–2021.

Schultz, J. H., & Luthe, W. (1969). *Autogenic therapy* (Vol. 1). New York: Grune & Stratton.

Seeburg, K. N., & DeBoer, K. F. (1980). Effects of EMG biofeedback in diabetes. *Biofeedback and Self-Regulation, 5,* 289–294.

Seeger, B. R., & Caudrey, D. J. (1983). Biofeedback therapy to achieve symmetrical gait in children with hemiplegic cerebral palsy: Long-term efficacy. *Archives of Physical Medicine and Rehabilitation, 64,* 160–162.

Seeger, B. R., Caudrey, D. J., & Scholes, J. R. (1981). Biofeedback therapy to achieve symmetrical gait in hemiplegic cerebral palsied children. *Archives of Physical Medicine and Rehabilitation, 62,* 364–368.

Seifert, A. R., & Lubar, J. F. (1975). Reduction of epileptic seizures through EEG biofeedback training. *Biological Psychology, 3,* 81–109.

Shepherd, K., Hickstein, R., & Shepherd, R. (1983). Neurogenic faecal incontinence in children with spina bifida: Rectosphincteric responses and evaluation of a physiological rationale for management, including biofeedback conditioning. *Australian Pediatric Journal, 19,* 97–99.

Shirley, M., Burish, T., & Rowe, C. (1982). Effectiveness of multiple-site EMG biofeedback in the reduction of arousal. *Biofeedback and Self-Regulation, 7,* 167–184.

Shouse, M. N., & Lubar, J. F. (1978). Physiological basis of hyperkinesis treated with methylphenidate. *Pediatrics, 62,* 343–351.

Shouse, M. N., & Lubar, J. F. (1979). Operant conditioning of EEG rhythms and Ritalin in the treatment of hyperkinesis. *Biofeedback and Self-Regulation, 4,* 299–312.

Silberstein, S. D. (1990). Twenty questions about headaches in children and adolescents [review]. *Headache, 30,*(11), 716–724.

Silberstein, S. D. (1992). Advances in understanding the pathophysiology of headache [review]. Neurology, *42,*(3) (suppl. 2), 6–10.

Silver, B. V., & Blanchard, E. B. (1978). Biofeedback and relaxation training in the treatment of psychophysiological disorders: Or are the machines really necessary? *Journal of Behavioral Medicine, 1,* 217–239.

Sterman, M. B. (1982). EEG biofeedback in the treatment of epilepsy: An overview circa 1980. In L. White & B. Tursky (Eds.), *Clinical biofeedback: Efficacy and mechanisms* (pp. 311–330). New York: Guilford Press.

Sterman, M. B., & Friar, L. (1972). Suppression of seizures in an epileptic following sensorimotor EEG feedback training. *Electroencephalography and Clinical Neurophysiology, 33,* 89–95.

Sterman, M. B., LoPresti, R. W., & Fairchild, M. D. (1969). *Electroencephalographic and behavioral studies of monomethylhydrazine toxicity in the cat* (Technical report, AMRL-TR-69-3). Ohio: Air Systems Command, Wright-Patterson Air Force Base.

Sterman, M. B., & Macdonald, L. R. (1978). Effects of central cortical EEG feedback training on the incidence of poorly controlled seizures. *Epilepsia, 19,* 207–222.

Sterman, M. B., & Macdonald, L. R., & Stone, R. V. (1974). Biofeedback training of the sensorimotor rhythm in man: Effects on epilepsy. *Epilepsia, 15,* 395–416.

Sterman, M. B., & Shouse, M. N. (1980). Quantitative analysis of training, sleep EEG and clinical response to EEG operant conditioning in epileptics. *Electroencephalography and Clinical Neurophysiology, 49,* 558–576.

Surwit, R., Allen, L., Gilgor, R., & Duvic, M. (1982). The combined effect of prazosin and autogenic training on cold reactivity in Raynaud's phenomenon. *Biofeedback and Self-Regulation,7,* 537–544.

Tansey, M. A. (1984). EEG sensorimotor rhythm biofeedback training: Some effects on the neurologic precursors of learning disabilities. *International Journal of Psychophysiology, 1,* 163–177.

Turk, D. C., Meichenbaum, D. H., & Berman, W. H. (1979). Application of biofeedback for the regulation of pain: A critical review. *Psychological Bulletin, 86,* 1322–1338.

Wald, A. (1981). Use of biofeedback in treatment of fecal incontinence in patients with meningomyelocele. *Pediatrics, 68,* 45–49.

Wald, A. (1983). Biofeedback for neurogenic fecal incontinence: Rectal sensation in a determinant of outcome.
Journal of Pediatric Gastroenterology and Nutrition, 2,
302–306.

Walmsley, R. P., Crichton, L., & Droog, D. (1981). Music as a
feedback mechanism for teaching head control to severely
handicapped children: A pilot study. *Developmental Medicine and Child Neurology, 23,* 739–746.

Whitehead, W. E., Parker, L. H., Bosmajian, L., Morrill-Corbin,
E. D., Middaugh, S., Garwood, M., Cataldo, M. F., & Freeman, J. (1986). Treatment of fecal incontinence in children
with spina bifida: Comparison of biofeedback and behavior modification. *Archives of Physical Medicine and Rehabilitation, 67,* 218–224.

Whitehead, W. E., Parker, L. H., Masek, B. J., Cataldo, M. F.,
& Freeman, J. M. (1981). Biofeedback treatment of
fecal incontinence in patients with myelomeningocele.
Developmental Medicine and Child Neurology, 23,
313–322.

Whitmer, P. O. (1977). EMG biofeedback manipulation of
arousal as a test of the overarousal and underarousal theories of childhood hyperactivity. *Dissertation Abstracts International, 38,* 3423B.

Wyler, A. R., Robbins, C. A., & Dodrill, C. B. (1979). EEG
operant conditioning for control of epilepsy. *Epilepsia,
20,* 279–286.

22

Approaches to the Cognitive Rehabilitation of Children with Neuropsychological Impairment

KENNETH D. McCOY, BARBARA C. GELDER, RENEE E. VanHORN, AND RAYMOND S. DEAN

From its beginning, clinical neuropsychology in North America has focused on the diagnosis and localization of cortical lesions (e.g., Boll, 1974; Dean, 1985a; Reitan, 1974). This has been the case because few other procedures existed to locate a soft tissue lesion. However, advances in radiologic techniques have provided structural (CT scan, MRI scan) and functional images (PET scans) of the brain not available 25 years ago (Bigler, 1988). This increased sophistication of imaging techniques has resulted in a deemphasis of neuropsychological assessment in diagnosis and localization in the neurologic setting. Recent data continue to stress the utility of a neuropsychological approach in the treatment planning of cognitive impairment (see Diller & Gordon, 1981; Uomoto, 1992). In fact, a number of authors have argued that the future of clinical neuropsychology lies in advances in our understanding of patients' functional deficits and planning rehabilitation approaches following cortical damage (Dean, 1982; 1985a; Diller & Gordon, 1981; Piasetsky, 1981). Indeed, Uomoto (1992) argued that clinical neuropsychology needs to assume the pivotal role in evaluation and rehabilitation of neurologic impairment.

Cortical damage generally results in some degree of impairment in sensory and/or motor functioning, attention, reasoning, judgment, and abstraction. Cognitive rehabilitation involves not only the relearning of cognitive skills, but also may include daily living impaired by brain damage. Consistent with these goals, cognitive rehabilitation involves the identification of neuropsychological deficits and the design of treatment strategies that retrain or compensate for impaired functions. These deficits are viewed on a continuum from basic living skills to more complex cognitive executive functions. Successful cognitive rehabilitation must have as its utmost goal the reintegration of patients into their premorbid social and vocational environment. For the child, this reintegration involves reentry into the academic setting.

This chapter examines the present status of cognitive rehabilitation with cortically impaired children. Theoretical approaches are examined, with emphasis on specific cognitive rehabilitation programs. The focus here is on the potential utility of these approaches in both clinical and school settings. Finally, current issues pertaining to the efficacy and availability of rehabilitation services will be considered.

History of Cognitive Rehabilitation

The effects of head injury on behavior have been observed since ancient times. Descriptions of

KENNETH D. McCOY, BARBARA C. GELDER, RENEE E. VanHORN, AND RAYMOND S. DEAN • Neuropsychology Lab, Ball State University, Muncie, Indiana 47306.

such cases date as early as 400 B.C. An enormous body of literature has accumulated concerning the language, perceptual, motoric, cognitive, and behavioral/emotional sequelae following cortical damage.

Reports of early 19th century investigators provide the foundation for our understanding of aphasia and language disorders (Bouillaud, 1825; Hughlings-Jackson, 1932; Wernicke, 1874). Functional impairment of brain-injured veterans allowed further insights into brain–behavior relationships. Although considerable documentation of deficits that result from acquired brain damage continued, strategies to assist with compensation and/or recovery of impaired functions were sorely lacking.

Early on, researchers reported data suggesting that the potential for recovery of higher cerebral functions was greater than many other functions mediated by the central nervous system. However, as early as 1911, Von Monakow argued that what appeared to be recovery following brain injury was, in fact, diaschisis—the process of uninjured brain systems resuming normal function. On the other hand, clinicians working with veterans who had sustained brain injuries (e.g., Goldstein, 1942) proposed that recovery of function could result only from restoration of an anatomical substrate. More recently, Pirozzolo and Papanicolaou (1986) discussed "plasticity" in terms of either or both neural and behavioral resilience. Neural plasticity refers to the brain's ability to regain function through neuron proliferation, migration, and synaptic interactions. Behaviorally, plasticity is seen as altered behavioral strategies. The patient's age at the time of injury is believed to be a factor in plasticity as well. Earlier research (Kennard, 1936; Teuber, 1974) suggested that greater recovery of function occurs in young children. However, other research suggested that insults in later life impair more specific functions than found in children, who present with more global or diffuse dysfunction. In general, recovery from brain damage is dependent on age, neural site, and behavioral function involved. So too, Luria (1963) argued that recovery of higher cerebral functions was the result of an emergence of interconnected and overlapping functional systems.

In the late 19th and early 20th century, children who exhibited patterns of deficits in language and perceptual motor functions similar to adults with acquired brain damage began to be studied. While specific traumas were not documented in these children, speculations were made regarding minimal brain damage. Strauss (1947) was among the early investigators who considered children's learning problems within the context of minimal brain dysfunction.

As increasing number of adults and children who exhibited patterns of deficits attributable to brain injury were identified, efforts were made to develop techniques that would aid functional recovery and/or teach compensatory strategies for daily living. Researchers working with brain-injured soldiers following WWI (e.g., Goldstein) and WWII (e.g., Wepman) began relating the findings of early attempts at rehabilitation based on both clinical assessment and research. The efforts of these early researchers laid the foundation for current neuropsychological rehabilitation approaches which incorporate both advances in assessment and past research into retraining.

Additionally, improvements attributed to rehabilitation must be separated from the progress in functioning that occurs spontaneously. For example, traumatic brain-injured patients experience the most rapid period of recovery in the first 6 months after the injury. These patients may continue to improve, albeit more slowly, up to 24 months postinjury (Bond, 1975). Improvements made beyond this time frame, without cognitive rehabilitation, have not yet been established in the literature.

Special Issues with Children

With over 1 million cases reported each year, traumatic brain injury (TBI) is the most prevalent of the childhood conditions with neuropsychological sequelae (Bigler, 1987; Nelson, 1992). According to Nelson (1992), the etiology of brain trauma varies with age, severity, geographic location, and season of the year. For infants and toddlers, brain trauma is usually a result of abuse (Raimondi & Hirschauer, 1984). The leading causes of brain injury among older children are vehicular accidents, assaults, firearms, and play activities (Kraus, Fife, Cox, Ramstein, & Conroy, 1986). Male children are twice as likely to suffer brain trauma, and the degree of severity of their injuries tends to be much greater than for females (Annegers, 1983; Kraus, 1980; Kraus et al., 1986). Overall incidence figures are believed to be gross underestimates, because the physical symptoms and neuropsychological impairments of milder cases often go undiagnosed (Evans, 1992). Of the injuries that are reported, approximately one-sixth are serious enough to require hospitalization (Eiben et al., 1984).

Subsequent to medical stabilization and hospital discharge, few options are available to treat residual neuropsychological deficits in these patients. Indeed, options are generally limited to inpatient rehabilitation facilities for those with severe deficits and outpatient physical, occupational, and speech therapy services for patients with mild to moderate deficits. While some children may be released to long-term residential facilities, many are not. In fact, Di Scala, Osberg, Gans, Chin, and Grant (1991) reported that 46.5% of more seriously affected children are discharged to the home from the hospital. On their return home, children are often expected to make a reentry into school with rehabilitation. Although some of these brain-injured children continue to receive rehabilitation services through outpatient community programs, often they are unrealistically expected to make relatively smooth transitions back into daily home and school life without such rehabilitation services.

The most common sequela of brain damage in children is generalized impairment in cognitive functions. This impairment typically involves deficits in memory, attention, and perception (Levin, Benton, & Grossman, 1982; Levin & Eisenberg, 1979a,b). Additionally, complaints often include fatigue, initiating and staying on task, organizing the environment, and academic performance. Furthermore, behavior and emotional problems are prominent complaints in this population (Nelson, 1992). With such neuropsychological symptoms, it is not surprising that a significant number of these children subsequently experience difficulties in school (e.g., Klonoff, Low, & Clark, 1977).

Children with TBI have special needs that are best addressed in a structured, stable, predictable, and unambiguous environment (Bigler, 1988). Given that school is the primary vocation for children, this institution is in a pivotal position to offer rehabilitation services. However, schools are often ill-equipped to handle the unique physical, cognitive, and behavioral challenges of this pediatric population. Moreover, school personnel do not understand and are inadequately trained to treat this population (Telzrow, 1987). Until recent legal mandates (i.e., Section 504, PL 94-142, PL 101-476), the needs of children with TBI either were ignored or were attempted within the context of traditional special education classifications. These traditional placement options are inappropriate because of qualitative differences between brain-injured children and those of the traditional special education categories such as learning disabled, emotionally handicapped, and mentally handicapped. These differences are perhaps best conceptualized within a dynamic–static framework.

As a result of both the spontaneous recovery of brain function and continuing developmental changes, children's clinical course is constantly changing, thus requiring the monitoring of academic progress, daily living skills, and emotional functioning on a regular basis. Such a dynamic nature of patient recovery requires more frequent review and modification of individual educational and treatment plans than required for adults. Clearly, these dynamic needs also differentiate the TBI patient from the traditional special education child who generally presents with more static needs that fluctuate less over time. As a result, reevaluations and updated educational plans are more urgent for TBI students.

Because the impairment associated with a brain injury is variable, each patient presents with a unique pattern of adequate and impaired functions requiring the design of an individualized rehabilitation program. Special concerns involve the child's premorbid functioning, developmental/maturational levels as well as family and social issues (McGuire & Sylvester, 1987). For example, in adults, the impairment of abstract thinking may be indicative of cortical impairment, whereas in children it may simply reflect the developmental age of the child. Therefore, the assessment of premorbid functioning must include consideration of the patient's developmental level.

Medication for the management of residual symptoms may serve either to retard or to facilitate cognitive rehabilitation (Prigatano, 1987). Categories of medications commonly used in the treatment of brain injuries include antidepressants, antipsychotics, anticonvulsants, antihistamines, and antianxiety agents. Sedation, confusion, dizziness, and impaired memory are some of the side effects of these drugs that may adversely affect neuropsychological evaluation and subsequent cognitive rehabilitation efforts. Thus, repeated assessment and constant monitoring of brain-injured patients undergoing drug treatment is essential (Prigatano, 1987). For example, the use of antipsychotics is discouraged in brain injury because of potential interference with cognitive recovery. However, positive effects such as reductions in aggression and stabilization of mood may outweigh the negative aspects (Prigatano, 1987).

Strategies of Cognitive Rehabilitation

Cognitive rehabilitation of neuropsychologically impaired children is in its infancy. Although relatively few empirically based programs of cognitive rehabilitation presently exist, a number of specific techniques have been studied in the treatment of attentional, perceptual, and memory deficits often associated with neurological impairment.

The frequency of attentional deficits in children and adults with TBI and neurologically based learning disabilities is well documented (Brown & Alford, 1984). Rehabilitation programs for the most part include some form of cognitive self-control or self-monitoring techniques. In general, research in this area has reported modest success in increasing attention (Brown & Alford, 1984; Hallahan & Sapona, 1983). One procedure involves teaching the patient to cognitively monitor the "on task" behavior via an array of learned self-messages (e.g., "Was I paying attention?").

Using a self-monitoring technique, Hallahan and Sapona (1983) reported significant improvement of the "on-task" behavior as well as the academic productivity of an 11-year-old male with attentional deficits. Importantly, the behavior effects of this strategy were found to maintain to a $2\frac{1}{2}$-month follow-up examination. Although the single subject design of this investigation limits the generalizability of the findings, it appears that a self-monitoring procedure may be effective in the remediation of some attentional deficits. The validity of the approach was further supported by Brown and Alford (1984), who used a self-instructional technique to remediate both attentional deficits and academic difficulties in 20 learning-disordered children. In this study, children receiving the cognitive training showed significant improvement on tests of learning aptitude, reading recognition, and the Matching Familiar Figures Test relative to the control group.

In a somewhat different approach to selective attention deficits, Ben-Yishay and his colleagues (e.g., Ben-Yishay, Diller, & Rattok, 1978; Ben-Yishay et al., 1980) developed a set of tasks that focus on systematic remediation. Organized in a hierarchy, these tasks require the patient to actively respond to stimulus lights, estimate time, consciously scan and identify various stimulus signals, and freely discriminate auditory and visual stimuli. The lack of a control group notwithstanding, Rattok et al. (1982) reported that these techniques improved the selective attention of brain-injured patients.

A number of rather innovative techniques have been proposed for use with cortically impaired patients with perceptual deficits. For example, Diller and his associates (e.g., Diller et al., 1974; Diller & Weinberg, 1977) reported the effective use of visual cancellation exercises in the remediation of visual scanning deficits. Initially the patient was taught to use a stimulus cue in the left/right visual field to compensate for visual neglect. After this anchoring procedure was learned, visual stimuli were presented in the neglected field until the patient was able to follow the stimuli to the outermost edges of that visual field. Weinberg et al. (1977) also reported data consistent with anchoring skill generalization to paper-and-pencil exercises as well as reading tasks.

It has been well established that brain-damaged patients often present with deficits in encoding, storage, and/or retrieval of information (e.g., Levin et al., 1982). Remediating memory impairment has occupied a good deal of research and clinical efforts. Memory impairment may relate to attention problems as well as actual dysfunction of regulation, storage, or retrieval of information. Consistent with the notion that children with neuropsychologically based learning disorders may fail to spontaneously utilize mnemonic strategies such as rehearsal (e.g., Bauer, 1977; Hallahan & Sapona, 1983; Tarver, Hallahan, Kaufman, & Ball, 1976), remedial efforts often focus on the systematic instruction of the child in the effective use of mnemonic strategies (Hallahan & Sapona, 1983). Similarly, various mnemonic techniques have been used with brain-damaged patients (e.g., Gianutsos & Gianutsos, 1979; Jones, 1974; Leftoff, 1981; Lewinsohn, Danaher, & Kikel, 1977). For instance, Leftoff (1981) reported that similar to normals, when verbal information (i.e., high-frequency nouns) was presented in the same serial order over repeated trials, patients with left hemisphere dysfunction recalled significantly more words than when the words were presented in a random fashion. Based on these data, Leftoff concluded that serial presentation of information may serve as a salient cuing device. In other words, patients were better able to retrieve verbal information if it was presented in an organized fashion. In another investigation of mnemonic devices, Jones

(1974) showed that visual imagery was effective in improving the paired-associative learning of patients with documented lesions of the left temporal lobe. In this study, patients were initially presented with word pairs accompanied by drawings depicting the two words interacting with one another (e.g., for the word pair elephant–bouquet, the picture depicted an elephant holding a bouquet of flowers). After a number of practice trials, the patient was required to develop his or her own unique images for each pair of words. Importantly, a follow-up of a number of the original patients indicated that they continued to use this technique on a daily basis (Jones, 1974). The success of this technique which involves linking verbal to visual information during the encoding process lends support to the dual encoding hypothesis proposed by Paivio (1971).

Cognitive Rehabilitation Programs

Cognitive rehabilitation has been broadly defined as a systematic effort to teach patients to overcome intellectual deficits arising from brain dysfunction (Task Force on Head Injury, 1984). This effort is seen to involve the reinforcement and strengthening of previously learned patterns of cognitive behavior, as well as the teaching of new patterns that allow the patient to compensate for neurological dysfunction that remains after recovery (Task Force on Head Injury, 1984). Consistent with this definition, Ben-Yishay (1981) argued that the objective of cognitive rehabilitation must be to "overcome, i.e., to correct (and if that is not feasible, then at the very least, to significantly ameliorate), the effects of generic cognitive deficits in such a way as to enable the individual patient to find alternative and adequate means of achieving specific functional goals" (p. 20).

As a prelude to cognitive rehabilitation, an assessment of the patient's overall neuropsychological functioning is necessary. Specifically, the patient's ability to formulate, plan, and implement goal-directed behaviors, selectively attend to a stimulus, process and retain various forms of information, grasp the essential nature of problem situations, and verbally interact must be evaluated. This information is needed to plan rehabilitation that integrates the patient's unique needs and takes advantage of specific strengths. The results of the neuropsychological examination are also of use in estimating the patient's readiness to benefit from different remedial strategies (Ben-Yishay, 1983). This patient-specific

regimen of rehabilitation is seen as appropriate with both adults and pediatric patients.

Orientations to Rehabilitation

A number of approaches to the rehabilitation of the neurologic impairment have been offered (e.g., Barth & Boll, 1981; Bolger, 1981; Diller & Gordon, 1981). Although related, each views neuropsychological impairment and treatment rather uniquely.

One basic approach to rehabilitation is the psychometric model. Impairment is conceptualized in terms of performance on measures of cognitive and neuropsychological functioning. As such, remedial strategies focus on ameliorating individual test-specific deficits. Generalized cognitive/neuropsychological improvement is hypothesized to occur even though it is the specific deficits that are targeted during therapy (e.g., Gudeman, Golden, & Craine, 1978).

Diller and Gordon (1981) described the psychometric model as using "saturation cuing" or "mastery learning" as the means to promote retraining (Diller & Gordon, 1981). Rehabilitation then relies on the analysis of task requirements and the systematic shaping and cuing of patient responses (Block, 1971). Initially the patient is provided with many cues which are gradually faded out as rehabilitation progresses. This approach virtually eliminates failure, which in turn reinforces learning. Ben-Yishay and his colleagues reported success in the rehabilitation of cognitive deficits using such a "saturated cuing" approach with brain-damaged adults (Ben-Yishay et al., 1979; Diller et al., 1974).

Ben-Yishay (1981) prioritized domains in cognitive rehabilitation as they related to: (1) self-help and daily living; (2) psychomotor, perceptual, and cognitive skills that underlie successful vocational or school functioning; and (3) socioemotional/interpersonal skills. Telzrow's (1985) rehabilitation priorities directed toward pediatric populations stressed independent eating, dressing, and toileting; adequate perceptual–motor skills; proficiency in reading, writing, and arithmetic; and interpersonal relationships at home and at school. Clearly, the goal of any rehabilitation program must be the reintegration of the patients into their premorbid environments.

Of particular interest to the present discussion, Ben-Yishay (1981) offered essential conditions for successful cognitive remediation. Perhaps most important, the patient must be aware of the potential benefits of the specific exercise and must be motivated to participate in the process. If one makes the assumption that repeated failure on a task may result in motivational deficits (e.g., see Dean & Rattan, 1986; Fowler & Peterson, 1981; Seligman, 1975), it follows that a cognitive rehabilitation program must be constructed to emphasize success and reduce error. As mentioned previously, Ben-Yishay (1981) espoused a remedial approach in which tasks are "orchestrated" in such a fashion that success is "guaranteed." Of course, errorless learning is not unique to Ben-Yishay's (1981) program. In fact, small incremental learning with minimal errors is the foundation of programmed instruction (see Anderson & Faust, 1967). It is clear that programming for success serves to elevate patient motivation and continued participation.

Psychometric Approach to Cognitive Rehabilitation

Reitan and Wolfson (1985) offered an approach to cognitive rehabilitation that is related to a hierarchical system of brain functioning (Reitan & Wolfson, 1985). The Reitan Evaluation of Hemispheric Abilities and Brain Improvement Training (REHABIT) program uses information obtained from the Halstead–Reitan Neuropsychological Battery (HRNB) as the basis of planning the rehabilitation program. The utility of the HRNB for developing specific programs of retraining has been documented (Reitan & Sena, 1983; Reitan & Wolfson, 1985; Sena, 1985, 1986; Sena & Sena, 1986). The HRNB is a comprehensive neuropsychological battery that is designed to measure the full range of functions. It is normed for both adults and children and the child versions do acknowledge the developmental aspects of pediatric patients (Reitan & Wolfson, 1988).

REHABIT's design is well suited for individualized educational planning for the brain-injured child. Many of the tasks are modeled from both conventional and special education curriculum plans. However, REHABIT extends traditional special education programming to incorporate higher-level neuropsychological functions. Although most preliminary research studies have included limited numbers of subjects, results have nonetheless demonstrated significant improvement in cognitive functioning above and beyond spontaneous recovery (Alfano & Meyerink, 1986).

REHABIT consists of five tracks of remediation. Patients are treated uniquely and special programs are designed specifically to meet the patient's needs or impairments based on patterns of deficits found in the HRNB assessment. Regardless of which track or plan is implemented, the rudimentary functions of attention, concentration, and memory are emphasized.

The first level of processing according to the REHABIT model includes the rudimentary functions of attention, concentration, and memory. These functions are critical for attending to incoming stimuli and are necessary to the general level of processing. At the second level of processing, information from level one is directed to either the left or right hemisphere. From a brain–behavior point of view, the left hemisphere is seen to mediate verbal information whereas the right hemisphere serves information of a visual/spatial nature. At the third and highest level, information is processed by abstraction, concept formation, and logical analysis.

In sum, REHABIT provides a comprehensive program for cognitive retraining. The strength of REHABIT lies in its integration of theory, assessment, and brain retraining. Thus, a program can be designed to remediate the specific deficits of the individual.

Stimulus-Based Approach

A second basic approach to cognitive rehabilitation is seen as a biologically based orientation. This approach focuses on groups or patterns of behaviors (e.g., Barth & Boll, 1981) and emphasizes elements of the stimulus itself (Diller & Gordon, 1981). The major task in cognitive rehabilitation is the identification of the specific components of a stimulus that contribute to the patient's impairment. From this perspective, treatment involves alteration of the stimulus in such a way as to offset the patient's behavioral deficits. Moreover, proponents of this approach to cognitive rehabilitation argue that these stimulus alterations promote patient awareness of the nature and extent of the impairment as well as potential compensatory strategies. It has been argued that such insight is important if rehabilitation is to generalize to other problem behaviors and settings (Diller & Gordon, 1981).

Perhaps the best example of this approach to cognitive rehabilitation can be found in attempts to remediate spatial neglect in brain-damaged patients (e.g., Diller, 1976; Diller et al., 1974; Diller & Weinberg, 1977; Weinberg & Diller, 1968; Weinberg et al., 1977). In accord with the "biological" model of rehabilitation, patients are initially trained to perform visual scanning tasks that focus the patient's awareness on visual field deficits. In one study by Diller and Weinberg (1977), patients who received scanning exercises after approximately 1 month were compared with groups of brain-damaged patients who received a standard occupational therapy regimen. With minor exceptions, those patients in the experimental treatment group showed significant improvement in attention to the complete visual field, relative to the control group. Of interest, the ability of patients to scan selectively all pertinent visual information was reported to generalize to other more complex tasks (e.g., reading, arithmetic, copying).

Developmental Approach to Cognitive Rehabilitation

Brain injury results in the loss of numerous behavioral sequences that, prior to the injury, had been habitual (Wood, 1988). Consistent with this notion, Bolger (1981) developed a comprehensive program of cognitive retraining. The underlying hypothesis is that efficient processing of information is dependent on the ability to execute cognitive operations automatically. Thus, remediation efforts must reestablish, and progressively build on automaticity of rudimentary functions. Underlying Bolger's (1981) approach to cognitive rehabilitation is the notion that rudimentary skills (e.g., attention, word recognition) must be made "automatic" before more higher-level cognitive skills can be addressed. Based on this reasoning, each task is repeatedly practiced beyond initial mastery. This technique assumes that "overlearning" facilitates the patient's ability to spontaneously perform a number of important cognitive functions. Indeed, such "automatic" processing is a prerequisite for successful educational or vocational generalization (Nelson, 1992).

If one subscribes to the idea that attentional capacity is limited at any given time, it would follow that many cognitive tasks place excessive demands on brain-damaged patients (Case, 1972; Case, Kurland, & Goldberg, 1982; Hasher & Zack, 1979). Evidence of difficulties related to limited attentional capacity may be demonstrated by deficits in both storage and retrieval of information for neuropsychologically impaired patients (e.g., Bolger, 1981). Based on this premise, remedial efforts are designed to improve the patient's execution of cognitive operations and provide processing strategies to reduce the cognitive demands. Bolger (1981) argued that the goal of cognitive remediation "is to increase the mental capacity of the individual to process larger amounts of stimuli with more accuracy and with greater attention to subtleties" (p. 67). Such an increase in the patient's ability to process information is viewed as a necessary component in the performance of complex cognitive tasks. For Bolger (1981), remedial tasks that focus on rudimentary (e.g., perceptual and attentional) processes as well as higher cortical functions are presented to the patient continuously throughout the rehabilitation program. The essential feature of the program is the emphasis on the patient's ability to integrate these higher-level cognitive functions.

Although this approach to cognitive training as described by Bolger (1981) has clinical appeal, data demonstrating its efficacy are lacking. Research with groups that differ on specific patterns of neurological deficits would allow examination of the utility of this approach.

Behavioral Engineering Approach

A third model of rehabilitation can best be characterized as behavioral engineering (Diller & Gordon, 1981). Behavioral engineering relies heavily on principles grounded in the behaviorism models of Skinner, Bandura, and others. The underlying premise holds that behavior is determined by its consequences; therefore, altering reinforcement contingencies alters behavior. From this viewpoint, the patient's impairments are operationalized as behavioral deficits. Inherent in this model is the assumption that behavioral deficits are maintained by environmental conditions. Therefore, the major objective in treatment is to identify and systematically modify the environmental antecedents that are assumed to underlie the problem behavior. To this end, rehabilitation therapists utilize a number of common behavioral analytic techniques (see Wilson & O'Leary, 1980, for a review).

Consistent with a behavioral orientation, the initial stages of treatment are marked by the identification of target behaviors amenable to therapy. Once behavioral deficits have been operationalized and their antecedents identified, the emphasis shifts to the establishment of a reliable baseline of behaviors against which to evaluate progress. The target behavior(s) is made contingent on a systematic program of reinforcement and is shaped in such small increments that failure is minimized. The ultimate goal is generalizing the response behavior from one set of stimuli to another appropriate set.

As part of a comprehensive rehabilitation program, Ben-Yishay and his colleagues (e.g.,

Ben-Yishay & Diller, 1981) have developed a systematic, hierarchical program of cognitive rehabilitation. Divided into five separate, yet interrelated modules, treatment emphasizes the remediation of both lower-level (e.g., attention) and more complex (e.g., verbal–abstract reasoning) cognitive deficits. Modules are organized such that patients initially receive tasks requiring more rudimentary cognitive skills (e.g., psychomotor manipulations), followed by more complicated exercises involving abstract reasoning and mental manipulation. The patient is presented with each module in such a fashion that failure is minimized. To this end, the remedial tasks are initially broken down into their smallest logical component parts. The patient is then guided through the tasks with the aid of prompts. The cues are made less explicit with each trial until the patient is able to perform tasks within the module without making errors or requiring prompting. In this way the patient proceeds in a sequential fashion until the final module is reached. Depending on the nature and degree of the neuropsychological impairment, this program is often highly redundant, which is believed to promote generalization (Silver *et al.*, 1983).

Horton (1979a,b; 1981) argued in favor of a behavioral approach with neuropsychologically impaired adults and children. Indeed, in support of this stance, a number of investigators have reported behavioral techniques to be effective in treating hyperactivity, impulsivity, and perseveration in brain-damaged children (e.g., Hall & Broden, 1967; Krop, 1971) and short-term memory loss in adult, brain-injured patients (e.g., Cooke, 1973). However, it is not clear how such an atomistic therapy generalizes to system deficits experienced by the neurologically impaired patient.

Computer Programs in Cognitive Rehabilitation

Advances in computer technology have produced a vast amount of software for use in cognitive rehabilitation. Some of these programs include THINKable (Giaquinto & Fiori, 1992), BFT (Buffery, 1987), and CIV (Speight, Laufer, & Mattes, 1993). A number of features make microcomputers attractive components of rehabilitation treatment. One of the most salient features of computer programs is the flexibility they provide when designing treatment programs that meet individualized needs (Lynch, 1981). Additionally, the computer is able to generate multiple exemplars of a targeted domain of impairment in a novel fashion. Moreover, as computer costs become more affordable, software is more accessible to wider populations and settings.

Generally speaking, these computer programs are organized such that patients can work at home. Similar to the programs previously discussed, this approach initially focuses on more rudimentary cognitive functions such as attention and stimulus discrimination and generalization. On mastery of these basic cognitive skills, the patient is administered programming that is seen to provide training in higher levels, such as memory and problem-solving. However, unlike the clinically based programs described above, little professional supervision or evaluation is involved.

Aside from the systematic repetition of rehabilitation routines, microcomputers hold potential for automating and individualizing cognitive rehabilitation in a cost-effective fashion. Indeed, the use of computers, programmed to automatically record data, would free the neuropsychologist from record keeping, allowing a focus on structuring cognitive therapy that meets the patient's assessed needs. Moreover, unlike most individual approaches to cognitive rehabilitation, the psychologist could monitor the performance for several patients simultaneously.

Presently, a number of microcomputer-based cognitive remediation programs have been developed for use with brain-damaged adults and children (e.g., Bracy, 1983; Buffery, 1987; Giaquinto & Fiori, 1992). These programs are clinically based and focus on improving the patient's functioning in the areas of selective and sustained attention, verbal and nonverbal auditory discrimination, visual discrimination, and stimulus differentiation and generalization. Over the past decade, case studies have been presented showing cognitive improvement for both children and adults involved with these programs (Bracy, 1983; Grishy & Schacter, 1988). While these claims appear promising, methodological problems continue to confound any generalization. Given the high variability inherent in TBI populations, the use of traditional research designs that involve comparison groups is not feasible. Therefore, as Wood (1988) points out, single-case design methods may be needed to evaluate these clinical procedures that have such variable criteria.

Although a number of authors have extolled the virtues of computer-based rehabilitation programs, few controlled studies exist that account for spontaneous recovery. To be sure, the majority of cited evidence has been based on case studies. Consequently, the generalizability of these results is highly questionable. Investigations using larger numbers of patients, adequate control groups, and standardized criterion measures would allow a test of the potential for many unsubstantiated claims.

A task force created by the Clinical Neuropsychology Division of the American Psychological Association has recently addressed the role and efficacy of computer technology in neuropsychological evaluation and rehabilitation. While encouraging further research, the task force report cautioned against the use of computers as the sole component of a cognitive rehabilitation treatment program. According to the report, computers should be used by trained and experienced professionals in a goal-directed manner to address specific rather than general cognitive functions (Matthews, Harley, & Malec, 1991).

Neurobehavioral Issues in Cognitive Rehabilitation

Few cognitive rehabilitation strategies consider the potential interaction between cognitive impairment and emotional functioning. Indeed, attempts that have focused on various underlying cognitive processes often do not consider the patient's behavior history and learned methods of coping with failure (e.g., Dean, 1978). This is a rather curious state of affairs when one considers the frequency with which patients having neurological disorders also present with maladaptive emotional patterns (see Boll, 1981; Dean, 1985b). These emotional factors would seem especially pertinent for children with cognitive deficits given the problems inherent in their return to the family, peer group, and school environment.

Emotional–cognitive dysfunction is portrayed quite clearly in children with long-standing learning disorders. Negative reactions to specific cognitive tasks and school in general exist in a large number of school-age children but may be masked by seemingly unrelated behaviors (e.g., withdrawal, lack of compliance). Moreover, research indicates that neurologically impaired children may develop maladaptive methods of coping with the stress of "cognitive failure" (Bender, 1985; Dean & Rattan, 1986). The emotional reaction to cognitive impair-

ment seen in children with congenital learning disorders is also evident in children with closed head injuries (Klonoff & Low, 1974).

In fact, children who experience repeated cognitive failure may develop what could be likened to a phobic reaction to the specific area of impairment. These phobias or aversive reactions are viewed to generalize beyond the immediate training session to produce an emotional reaction to any situation that involves the impaired cognitive skill. Unlike the adult who may avoid situations in which cognitive deficits are highlighted, the child who is expected to return to school does not have the same avoidance options. Thus, what begins as a neuropsychological dysfunction may lead to a response set of failure–aversion–failure, as the child attempts to cope with the stress of cognitive demands.

Systematic desensitization is a behavioral technique aimed at modifying phobic responses. This procedure includes the identification of an individual's hierarchy of aversive reactions to stimuli and then proceeds to pair positive (reinforcing) events with those that have produced negative reactions (see Land, 1964; Wolpe, 1969). This approach has been shown to be successful in desensitizing children's aversions and irrational emotional responses (see Wolpe, 1969). With such a perspective in mind, it would seem that this treatment would be of value in treating children's acquired aversive reactions to cognitive tasks. Specifically, this procedure may be applicable during the actual process of cognitive training. Suggested some years ago by Severson (1970) with learning-disabled children, this format allows both systematic desensitization of emotional aspects and cognitive rehabilitation simultaneously. However, few investigators have integrated this approach with more emotional-learning-based interventions. Dean (1982) argued that children with neuropsychological deficits cannot be treated simplistically from either a cognitive or a mental health point of view. It would seem that children with cognitive impairment would benefit from an approach that offers academic remediation while attempting to modify negative emotional responses.

Conclusion

While the field of cognitive rehabilitation/cognitive retraining has made modest progress in recent years, its application to children continues to be in its infancy. Indeed, as more children survive brain injury, they face a plethora of obstacles in the acquisition of skills that are vital to their daily living and vocational future. Increasingly, the public schools have been forced to assume much of the responsibility for TBI children's rehabilitation and reintegration into schools. However, traditional strategies used for children with chronic brain impairment (e.g., cerebral palsy) and learning disabilities do not adequately address the needs and challenges of this population. Similarly, rehabilitation priorities typically used with adult patients may not be viable with the child, who differs developmentally.

A number of cognitive rehabilitation programs presently exist. However, there is a general paucity of empirical support for these programs. Where data exist, there are inherent difficulties in drawing clear conclusions concerning the cognitive rehabilitation approaches most useful with a specific neuropsychologically impaired patient. Problems relating to the heterogeneity of samples, lack of control groups, and failure to control for spontaneous recovery combine to make the results of such investigations equivocal at best (Adamovich, Henderson, & Auerbach, 1985). Although many of the proposed rehabilitation programs have intuitive appeal for use with cognitively impaired children, little data support their use. Based on the accumulation of case studies, there does seem to be support for the expenditure of time, energy, and money required for cognitive rehabilitation research.

Clearly neuropsychology has the potential to continue making contributions to rehabilitation in general and cognitive retraining specifically. Indeed, the inertia of the field is moving toward a treatment emphasis (Dean, 1982, 1985a). Neuro-psychology with its empirical emphasis on brain–behavior relationships may be the most relevant of the healthcare professions to provide treatment for neurologically related cognitive deficits. Although such a trend in neuropsychology is clear (see Seretny, Dean, Gray, & Hartlage, 1986), we may be entering clinical practice without benefit of a firm empirical foundation.

References

Adamovich, B. B., Henderson, J., & Auerbach, S. (1985). *Cognitive rehabilitation of closed head injured patients.* San Diego: College-Hill Press.

Alfano, A. M., & Meyerink, L. H. (1986). Cognitive retraining with brain-injured adults. *VA Practitioner, 12,* 13.

Anderson, R. L., & Faust, G. F. (1967). The effects of strong formal prompts in programmed instruction. *American Educational Research Journal, 4,* 345–352.

Annegers, J. F. (1983). The epidemiology of head trauma in children. In K. Shapiro (Ed.), *Pediatric head trauma* (pp. 1–10). Mount Kisco, NY: Futura.

Barth, J. T., & Boll, T. J. (1981). Rehabilitation and treatment of central nervous system dysfunction: A behavioral medicine perspective. In *Medical psychology: Contributions to behavioral medicine* (pp. 241–266). New York: Academic Press.

Bauer, R. H. (1977). Memory processes in children with learning disabilities: Evidence for deficient rehearsal. *Journal of Experimental Child Psychology, 24,* 415–430.

Bender, W. N. (1985). Differences between learning disabled and non-learning disabled children in temperament and behavior. *Learning Disability Quarterly, 8,* 11–18.

Ben-Yishay, Y. (1981). Cognitive remediation after TBD: Toward a definition of its objectives, tasks, and conditions. In *Working approaches to remediation of cognitive deficits in brain damaged persons* (Rehabilitation Monograph No. 62). New York: New York University Medical Center, Institute of Rehabilitation Medicine.

Ben-Yishay, Y. (1983). Cognitive remediation viewed from the perspective of a systematic clinical research program in rehabilitation. *Cognitive Rehabilitation, 1,* 4–6.

Ben-Yishay, Y., & Diller, L. (1981). Rehabilitation of cognitive and perceptual defects in people with traumatic brain damage. *International Journal of Rehabilitation Research, 4,* 208–210.

Ben-Yishay, Y., Diller, L., & Rattok, J. (1978). A modular approach to optimizing orientation, psychomotor alertness, and purposive behavior in severe head trauma patients. In *Working approaches to cognitive deficits in brain damage* (Rehabilitation Monograph No. 59). New York: New York University Medical Center, Institute of Rehabilitation Medicine.

Ben-Yishay, Y., Diller, L., Rattok, J., Ross, B., Schaier, A., & Scherger, P. (1979, May). *Working approaches to remediation of cognitive deficits in brain damaged persons.* Supplement to the seventh annual workshop for rehabilitation professionals, New York.

Ben-Yishay, Y., Rattok, J., Ross, B., Lakin, P., Cohen, J., & Diller, L. (1980). A remedial module for the systematic amelioration of basic attentional disturbance in head trauma patients. In *Working approaches to cognitive deficits in brain damaged persons* (Rehabilitation Monograph No. 61). New York: New York University Medical Center, Institute of Rehabilitation Medicine.

Bigler, E. D. (1987). Acquired cerebral trauma: Behavioral, neuropsychiatric, psychoeducational assessment and cognitive retraining issues. *Journal of Learning Disabilities, 20,* 579–580.

Bigler, E. D. (1988). Acquired cerebral trauma: Attention, memory, and language disorders. *Journal of Learning Disabilities, 21,* 325–326.

Block, J. H. (Ed.). (1971). *Mastery learning: Theory and practice.* New York: Holt, Rinehart & Winston.

Bolger, J. P. (1981). Cognitive retraining: A developmental approach. *Clinical Neuropsychology, 4,* 66–70.

Boll, T. J. (1974). Behavioral correlates of cerebral damage in children nine through fourteen. In R. M. Reitan & L. A. Davison (Eds.), *Clinical neuropsychology: Current status and applications* (pp. 171–191). New York: Wiley.

Boll, T. J. (1981). The Halstead–Reitan neuropsychology battery. In S. B. Filskov & T. J. Boll (Eds.), *Handbook of clinical neuropsychology* (pp. 42–65). New York: Wiley.

Bond, M. R. (1975). Assessment of the psychosocial outcome after severe head injury. In R. Porter & D. W. Fitzsimons (Eds.), *Outcome of severe damage to the central nervous system* (Ciba Foundation Symposium 34) (pp. 141–157). Amsterdam: Elsevier.

Bouillaud, J. (1825). Recherches cliniques propre a demontrer que le perte de la parole correspond a la lesion de lobules anterieurs du cerveau et a confirmer l'opinion de M. Gall sur le siege de l'organe du language articule. *Archives of General Medicine, 8,* 25–45.

Bracy, O. (1983). Computer based cognitive rehabilitation. *Cognitive Rehabilitation, 1,* 7–8, 18.

Brown, R. T., & Alford, N. K. (1984). Ameliorating attentional deficits and concomitant academic deficiencies in learning disabled children through cognitive training. *Journal of Learning Disabilities, 17,* 20–26.

Buffery, A. W. (1987). Brain function therapy: Computerized neuropsychological rehabilitation. *Carrier Foundation Letter* (April, No.124), 1–3.

Case, R. (1972). Validation of a neo-Piagetian capacity construct. *Journal of Experimental Child Psychology, 14,* 45–49.

Case, R., Kurland, D. M., & Goldberg, J. (1982). Operational efficiency and the growth of short-term memory span. *Journal of Experimental Child Psychology, 33,* 386–403.

Cooke, N. (1973). Neuropsychology: From theory into practice. *Newsletter for Research in Mental Health and Behavioral Sciences, 15,* 43–46.

Dean, R. S. (1978). The use of the WISC-R in distinguishing learning disabled and emotionally disturbed children. *Journal of Consulting and Clinical Psychology, 46,* 381–382.

Dean, R. S. (1982). Neuropsychological assessment. In T. R. Kratochwill (Ed.), *Advances in school psychology* (Vol. 2, pp. 171–201). Hillsdale, NJ: Erlbaum.

Dean, R. S. (1985a). Perspectives on the future of neuropsychological assessment. In B. S. Plake & J. C. Witt (Eds.), *Buros–Nebraska series on measurement and testing: Future of testing and measurement* (pp. 203–244). Hillsdale, NJ: Erlbaum.

Dean, R. S. (1985b). Neuropsychological assessment. In J. D. Cavenar, R. Michels, H. K. Brodie, A. M. Cooper, S. B. Guze, L. L. Judd, G. L. Klerman, & A. J. Solnit (Eds.), *Psychiatry* (pp. 1–175). Philadelphia: Lippincott.

Dean, R. S., & Rattan, A. I. (1986). *Measuring the effects of failure with learning disabled children.* Paper presented at the annual convention of the National Academy of Neuropsychologists.

Diller, L. (1976). A model for cognitive retraining in rehabilitation. *The Clinical Psychologist, 29,* 13–15.

Diller, L., Ben-Yishay, Y., Gerstman, L. J., Gordon, W., Weinberg, J., Mandelberg, R., Schulman, P., & Shah, N. (1974). *Studies in cognition and rehabilitation in hemiplegia* (Rehabilitation Monograph No. 50). New York: New York University Medical Center, Institute of Rehabilitation Medicine.

Diller L., & Gordon, W. A. (1981). Rehabilitation and clinical neuropsychology. In S. B. Filskov & T. J. Boll (Eds.), *Handbook of clinical neurology* (pp. 702–733). New York: Wiley.

Diller, L. V., & Weinberg, J. (1977). Hemiinattention in rehabilitation: The evolution of a rational remediation program. *Advances in Neuropsychology, 18,* 63–82.

Di Scala, C., Osberg, J. S., Gans, B. M., Chins, L. J., & Grant, C. C. (1991). Children with traumatic head injury: Morbidity and post-acute treatment. *Archives of Physical Medicine and Rehabilitation, 7,* 662–666.

Eiben, C. F., Anderson, T. P., Lockman, L., Matthews, D. J., Dryja, R., Martin, J., Burrill, C., Cottesman, N., O'Brian, P., & Witte, L. (1984). Functional outcome of closed head injury in children and young adults. *Archives of Physical Medicine and Rehabilitation, 65,* 168–170.

Evans, R. W. (1992). Mild traumatic brain injury. *Traumatic Brain Injury, 3*(2), 427–439.

Fowler, J. W., & Peterson, P. L. (1981). Increasing reading persistence and altering attributional style of learned helpless children. *Journal of Educational Psychology, 73,* 251–260.

Gianutsos, R., & Gianutsos, J. (1979). Rehabilitating the verbal recall of brain-injured patients by mnemonic training: An experimental demonstration using single-case methodology. *Journal of Clinical Neuropsychology, 1,* 117–135.

Giaquinto, S., & Fiori, M. (1992). THINKable, a computerized cognitive remediation: First results. *Acta Neurologica, 14,* 546–560.

Goldstein, K. (1942). *Aftereffects of brain-injuries in war* (p. 204). New York: Grune & Stratton.

Grishy, E. L., & Schacter, D. L. (1988). Acquisition of domain-specific knowledge in patients with organic memory disorders. *Journal of Learning Disabilities, 21,* 333–339.

Gudeman, H., Golden, C., & Craine, J. (1978). The role of neuropsychological evaluation in rehabilitation of the brain injured patient: A program in neurotraining. *JSAS Catalog of Selected Documents in Psychology, 8,* 44 (MS No. 1693).

Hall, R., & Broden, M. (1967). Behavior changes in brain-injured children through social reinforcement. *Journal of Experimental Child Psychology, 5,* 463–479.

Hallahan, D. P., & Sapona, R. (1983). Self-monitoring of attention with learning disabled children: Past research and current issues. *Journal of Learning Disabilities. 16,* 616–620.

Hasher, L., & Zacks, R. T. (1979). Automatic and effortful processes in memory. *Journal of Experimental Psychology: General, 108,* 356–388.

Horton, A. M., Jr. (1979a). Behavioral neuropsychology: A clinical case study. *Clinical Neuropsychology, 1* (3), 44–47.

Horton, A. M., Jr. (1979b). Behavioral neuropsychology: Rationale and research. *Clinical Neuropsychology, 1*(2), 20–23.

Horton, A. M., Jr. (1981). Behavioral neuropsychology in the schools. *School Psychology Review, 10*(3), 367–372.

Hughlings-Jackson, J. (1932). Remarks of dissolution of the nervous system as exemplified by certain post-epileptic conditions. In J. Tayler (Ed.), *Selected writings of John*

Hughlings-Jackson (Vol. 2). London: Hodder & Stoughton.

Jones, M. K. (1974). Imagery as a mnemonic aid after left temporal lobectomy: Contrasts between material-specific and generalized memory disorders. *Neuropsychologia, 12,* 21–30.

Kennard, M. A. (1936). Age and other factors in motor recovery from precentral lesions in monkeys. *American Journal of Physiology, 115,* 138–146.

Klonoff, H., & Low, M. (1974). Disordered brain function in young children and early adolescents: Neuropsychological and electroencephalographic correlates. In R. M. Reitan & L. A. Davison (Eds.), *Clinical neuropsychology: Current status and applications* (pp. 121–165). New York: Wiley.

Klonoff, H., Low, M. D., & Clark, L. (1977). Head injuries in children: A prospective five year follow-up. *Journal of Neurology, Neurosurgery, and Psychiatry, 40,* 1211–1219.

Kraus, J. F. (1980). A comparison of recent studies on the extent of the head and spinal cord injury problem in the United States. *Journal of Neurosurgery, 53* (Suppl.), 35–43.

Kraus, J. F., Fife, D., Cox, P., Ramstein, K., & Conroy, C. (1986). Incidence, severity, and external causes of pediatric brain injury. *American Journal of Diseases of Children, 140,* 687–693.

Krop, H. (1971). Modification of hyperactive behavior of a brain-damaged, emotionally disturbed child. *Training School Bulletin (Vineland), 68,* 49–54.

Land, P. (1964). Experimental studies of desensitization psychotherapy. In J. Wolpe, A. Salter, & L. J. Peyna (Eds.). *The conditioning therapies* (pp. 260–291). New York: Holt, Rinehart & Winston.

Leftoff, S. (1981). Learning functions for unilaterally brain damaged patients for serially and randomly ordered stimulus material: Analysis of retrieval strategies and their relationship to rehabilitation. *Journal of Clinical Neuropsychology, 3,* 301–313.

Levin, H. S., Benton, A. L., & Grossman, R. G. (1982). *Neurobehavioral consequences of closed head injury.* London: Oxford University Press.

Levin, H. S., & Eisenberg, H. M. (1979a). Neuropsychological impairment after closed head injury in children and adolescents. *Journal of Pediatric Psychology, 4,* 389–402.

Levin, H. S., & Eisenberg, H. M. (1979b). Neuropsychological outcome of closed head injury in children and adolescents. *Child's Brain, 5,* 281–292.

Lewinsohn, P. M., Danaher, B. G., & Kikel, S. (1977). Visual imagery as a mnemonic aid for brain injured persons. *Journal of Consulting and Clinical Psychology, 45,* 717–723.

Luria, A. R. (1963). *Restoration of function after brain injury.* New York: Macmillan Co.

Lynch, W. J. (1981). The use of electronic games in cognitive rehabilitation. In L. E. Trexler (Ed.), *Cognitive rehabilitation: Conceptualization and intervention* (pp. 263–274). New York: Plenum Press.

McGuire, T. C., & Sylvester, C. E. (1987). Neuropsychiatric evaluation and treatment of children with head injuries. *Journal of Learning Disabilities, 20,* 590–595.

Matthews, C. G., Harley, J. P., & Malec, J. F. (1991). Guidelines for computer-assisted neuropsychological rehabilitation and cognitive remediation. *Clinical Neuropsychology, 5,* 3–19.

Nelson, V. S. (1992). Pediatric head injury. *Traumatic Brain Injury, 3*(2), 461–474.

Paivio, A. (1971). *Imagery and verbal processes.* New York: Holt, Rinehart & Winston.

Piasetsky, E. B. (1981). The relevance of brain–behavior relationships for rehabilitation. In L. E. Trexler (Ed.), *Cognitive rehabilitation: Conceptualization and intervention* (pp. 115–130). New York: Plenum Press.

Pirozzolo, F. J., & Papanicolaou, A. C. (1986). Plasticity and recovery of function in the central nervous system. In J. E. Obrzut & G. W. Hynd (Eds.), *Child neuropsychology* (Vol. 1). New York: Academic Press.

Prigatano, G. P. (1987). Recovery and cognitive retraining after craniocerebral trauma. *Journal of Learning Disabilities, 20,* 603–613.

Raimondi, A. J., & Hirschauer, J. (1984). Head injury in the infant and toddler. *Child's Brain, 11,* 12–35.

Rattok, J., Ben-Yishay, Y., Ross, B., Lakin, P., Silver, S., Thomas, L., & Diller, L. (1982). A diagnostic–remedial system for basic attentional disorders in head trauma patients undergoing rehabilitation: A preliminary report. In *Working approaches to remediation of cognitive deficits in brain damaged persons* (Rehabilitation Monograph No. 64). New York: New York University Medical Center, Institute of Rehabilitation Medicine.

Reitan, R. M. (1974). Methodological problems in clinical neuropsychology. In R. M. Reitan & L. A. Davison (Eds.), *Clinical neuropsychology: Current status and applications* (pp. 140–191). New York: Wiley.

Reitan, R. M., & Sena, D. A. (1983). *The efficacy of the REHABIT technique in remediation of brain-injured people.* Paper presented at the meeting of the American Psychological Association, Anaheim, CA.

Reitan, R. M., & Wolfson, D. (1985). The Halstead–Reitan Neuropsychological Test Battery and REHABIT: A model for integrating evaluation and remediation of cognitive impairment. *Cognitive Rehabilitation,* 10–17.

Reitan, R. M., & Wolfson, D. (1988). *Traumatic brain injury, Volume II: Recovery and rehabilitation.* Tucson, AZ: Neuropsychology Press.

Seligman, M. E. P. (1975). *Helplessness: On depression, development, and death.* San Francisco: Freeman.

Sena, D. A. (1985). The effectiveness of cognitive retraining for brain-impaired individuals. *The International Journal of Clinical Psychology, 7,* 62.

Sena, D. A. (1986). The effectiveness of cognitive rehabilitation for brain-impaired patients. *Journal of Clinical and Experimental Neuropsychology, 8,* 142.

Sena, H. M., & Sena, D. A. (1986). A quantitative validation of the effectiveness of cognitive retraining. *Archives of Clinical Neuropsychology, 1,* 74.

Seretny, M. L., Dean, R. S., Gray, J. W., & Hartlage, L. C. (1986). The practice of clinical neuropsychology in the United States. *Archives of Clinical Neuropsychology, 1,* 90–94.

Severson, R. A. (1970). *Behavior therapy with severe learning disabilities.* Unpublished manuscript, University of Wisconsin.

Silver, S., Ben-Yishay, Y., Rattok, J., Ross, B., Lakin, P., Piasetsky, E., Ezrachi, O., & Diller, L. (1983). Occupational outcomes in severe TBD's following intensive cognitive remediation: An interim report. In *Working approaches to remediation of cognitive deficits in brain damaged persons* (Rehabilitation Monograph No. 66). New York: New York University Medical Center, Institute of Rehabilitation Medicine.

Speight, I., Laufer, M. E., & Mattes, K. (1993). CIV (computer-aided interactive video): A novel application in neuropsychological rehabilitation. *Computers in Human Behavior, 9,* 95–104.

Strauss, A. A. (1947). Therapeutic pedagogy, a neuropsychiatric approach to special education. *American Journal of Psychiatry, 104,* 60–63.

Tarver, S. G., Hallahan, D. P., Kaufman, J. M., & Ball, D. W. (1976). Verbal rehearsal and selective attention in children with learning disabilities: A developmental lag. *Journal of Experimental Child Psychology, 22,* 375–385.

Task Force on Head Injury. (1984). *Standards for cognitive rehabilitation.* Erie, PA: American Congress of Rehabilitation Medicine.

Telzrow, C. F. (1985). The science and speculation of rehabilitation in developmental neuropsychological disorders. In L. C. Hartlage & C. F. Telzrow (Eds.), *The neuropsychology of individual differences* (pp. 271–304). Elmsford, NY: Pergamon Press.

Telzrow, C. F. (1987). Management of academic and educational problems in head injury. *Journal of Learning Disabilities, 20,* 536–545.

Teuber, H. L. (1974). Recovery of function after lesions of the central nervous system: History and prospects. *Neuroscience Research Progress Bulletin, 12,* 197.

Uomoto, J. M. (1992). Neuropsychological assessment and cognitive rehabilitation after brain injury. *Traumatic Brain Injury, 3*(2).

Weinberg, J., & Diller, L. (1968). *On reading newspapers by hemiplegic denial of visual disability.* Paper presented at the annual meeting of the American Psychological Association, New York.

Weinberg, J., Diller, L., Gordon, W. A., Gerstman, L. J., Lieberman, A., Lakin, P., Hodges, G., & Ezrachi, O. (1977). Visual scanning training effect on reading-related tasks in acquired right brain damage. *Archives of Physical Medicine and Rehabilitation, 58,* 479–486.

Wernicke, C. (1874). *Der aphasische Symptomenkomplex.* Breslau, Poland: M. Cohn & Weigert.

Wilson, G. T., & O'Leary, K. D. (1980). *Principles of behavior therapy.* Englewood Cliffs, NJ: Prentice–Hall.

Wolpe, J. (1969). *The practice of behavior therapy.* Elmsford, NY: Pergamon Press.

Wood, R. L. (1988). Attention disorders in brain injury rehabilitation. *Journal of Learning Disabilities, 21,* 327–332.

23

Pediatric Brain Injury Rehabilitation in a Neurodevelopmental Milieu

ELAINE FLETCHER-JANZEN AND H. DENNIS KADE

Introduction

Traumatic brain injury (TBI) has been coined the "silent epidemic" because its frequency and disabling effects have largely been unrecognized by the professional community and the public (Ylvisaker, 1985). TBI is the leading cause of death and disability in children and adolescents in the United States and it is the principal cause of brain damage in young adults (Miller, 1992). More than one million children sustain brain injuries annually, and approximately 165,000 require hospitalization (National Information Center for Children and Youth with Disabilities [NICCYD], 1993). Between 30 and 50% of injuries are moderate, severe, or fatal (Begali, 1992). In addition to the incidence of TBI, 5000 new cases of epilepsy caused by head trauma are reported each year (Miller, 1992). The incidence of TBI is not randomly distributed through the population. Males are about twice as likely as females to sustain a brain injury and their death rate from these injuries is four times that of females (Ball & Zinner, 1993). The most frequent causes of TBI are motor vehicle crashes (with alcohol involvement) (Ball & Zinner, 1993; Rusonis, 1990), falls, sports, and abuse/assault (Goldstein & Levin, 1990; NICCYD, 1993).

Recent advances in medical science and technology such as increased effectiveness of hospital trauma units, availability of neurosurgeons, and de-

velopments in critical and acute care management have all contributed to the increased survival rates of severely brain-injured individuals (Bigler, 1990; Levin, 1990; Uomoto, 1989). Trauma survival has required the development of programs to meet the long-term needs of these individuals. The demand for services by patients and their families has preceded the development of theoretical models, and therefore, research evidence of efficacy, which is a common phenomenon in medical care (Kreutzer, 1991). Indeed, it is estimated that between 5 and 10 billion dollars is spent each year to provide medical care and rehabilitation to TBI survivors (Bigler, 1990; Burke, 1988).

The responsibility for advances in treatment of the neurocognitive impairments, functional and behavioral disabilities, and the chronic handicapping condition has come to rest with professionals who understand brain–behavior relationships. Neuropsychologists have played a critical role in documenting and evaluating brain injury for patients whose deficits were formerly misunderstood (Ball & Zinner, 1993; Crokett, Clark, & Klonoff, 1981). Before our current knowledge base existed, professionals had to either infer the degree and amount of structural brain damage or wait until a postmortem examination could be performed. Current technology allows a more accurate means of assessing structural damage, which, in turn, permits better understanding of brain injury mechanisms and the correlation between area of brain damage and related changes in behavior (Bigler, 1990). However, it is only recently that patients with brain injury have received comprehensive treatment programs dealing with various cognitive and behav-

ELAINE FLETCHER-JANZEN • The Brown Schools of West Texas, Midland, Texas 79706. H. DENNIS KADE • Psychology Department, Cumberland Hospital for Children and Adolescents, New Kent, Virginia 23124.

ioral outcome deficits that accompany brain injury. Although there is a common scenario of frontal impact causing an acceleration/deceleration in closed head injury that produces associated posttraumatic deficits, each brain injury is unique. There is no single constellation of symptoms or unitary TBI syndrome for either children or adults. The recovery process also varies considerably. Therefore, reference to an average recovery curve would be of little use in predicting the course of a particular case in practice.

The focus of this chapter is the development of a pediatric brain injury rehabilitation program, based on a neurodevelopmental model and a neuropsychological paradigm of rehabilitation. The historical development of the treatment of brain injury will be reviewed and followed by an examination of the theoretical paradigms that have led to current models of service delivery in acute and inpatient facilities. In addition, differences between pediatric and adult programming and outcomes are addressed. The neurodevelopmental model of inpatient programming is based on the unique needs of the pediatric brain injury population and on holistic principles, and is dedicated to a continuum of service delivery from acute to reentry.

Historical Development of Clinical Neuropsychology and Brain Injury

The development of neuropsychological approaches to the rehabilitation of individuals with brain injury in the United States has been influenced by two main forces. The first is that of natural events in the world that have led to demands on the field of medicine to focus on the brain, such as World War I and the return of soldiers with severe brain injuries. Although in World War I, brain injury casualties promoted the study of the functional aspects of brain anatomy, the institutionalized care of brain-injured soldiers in the United States did not occur until World War II (Boake, 1989). At that time, the first speech disorders unit affiliated with a military neurosurgical center was formulated in Fort Sam Houston, Texas, and by 1945, 13 speech units were in operation. Also included in the units were other professionals such as physical therapists, occupational therapists, and psychotherapists (Boake, 1989). A long lapse in treatment development then followed and did not reemerge until the late 1960s and early 1970s when, undoubtedly, the effects of motor vehicle accidents prompted the need for treatment (Sohlberg & Mateer, 1989). It

was at this time that rehabilitation treatment units were developed that closely mirror those of today. Previously, the special team approach had primarily been used in spinal cord units. The first replications of this model were at Lowenstein Rehabilitation Hospital near Tel Aviv and the Rancho Los Amigos Hospital near Los Angeles where the guidelines for therapy with patients at different stages of recovery were established and the latter facilities' efforts brought forth the Rancho Los Amigos Cognitive Scale that is in use today (Boake, 1989, 1991).

The treatment protocols generated for the different levels of coma reflected by the Rancho Los Amigos scale began a field of cognitive rehabilitation, the efficacy of which is still questioned in the scientific literature (Rattok *et al.,* 1992). At the same time, in 1973, the Yom Kippur war in Israel produced a sharp increase in brain-injured soldiers. This led to the development of a day treatment program that was under the joint direction of the Rehabilitation Department of the Israeli Ministry of Defense and the New York University Institute of Rehabilitation Medicine under the direction of the neuropsychologists Yehuda Ben-Yishay and Leonard Diller (Ben-Yishay & Gold, 1990; Boake, 1991). In the late 1970s, day treatment centers were established in the United States and, simultaneously, residential treatment programs for post acute head injury patients in Illinois, Texas, and Toronto, Canada. Although many treatment programs have since been established all over the United States, most have been based on program models developed before 1980 (Boake, 1989, 1991). Much of these treatment models have the patient repeatedly attempt to do the things that are difficult to do in the hope that the patient and therapist will discover new ways to accomplish the same neurocognitive task using areas of functioning that are relatively spared (Gronwall, Wrightson, & Waddell, 1990).

The second force that shaped the development of the present-day treatment programs for individuals with brain injury is that of the theoretical and sociopolitical factors associated with Western psychology, and in particular, the individualist/reductionistic interplay with psychometrics inherent in the United States. Although some would argue that, in the United States, psychological study of the individual organism is treatment of the individual "*in vacuo,*" it may be viewed as a natural response to the sociopolitical emphasis on the study of the individual as opposed to the individual in a community or social context. This view was forwarded by such eminent Russian neuroscientists as L. S. Vygotsky,

A. N. Leontev, and, perhaps the best known, A. R. Luria. Luria's development of a functional system(s) model of the brain became very well known and is still in full force today both in Russia and in the United States (Luria, 1973, 1980; Obrzut & Hynd, 1990). Many rehabilitation programs for individuals with brain injury use this model as the basis of the organized understanding of a patient's deficits (Schara, 1991).

Historically, primary foci of U. S. neuropsychologists were the localization and documentation of structural damage and deficits associated with brain injury. There were no imaging machines to assist a physician's diagnosis and localization. The development of neuropsychological test batteries offering standardized and normative information was in response to a medical need. Not until the rapid advancement of diagnostic imaging technology did the entire field of neuropsychology in the United States shift from the assessment of brain structure to a combination of brain structure and brain function. It was realized by neuropsychologists that the goal was "to re-form the interrupted functional systems and those that have failed to develop" and efforts were made to "integrate the several facets of neurological, educational, and emotional functions" (Golden, 1979, p. 201). Thus, even neuropsychologists outside the field of TBI rehabilitation were increasingly called on to establish the existence and magnitude of any cognitive deficits related to the brain insult, estimate the patient's ability to return to her or his previous life-style, and suggest remediation programs (Trexler, 1987).

Neuropsychology and Rehabilitation

The primary focus of traditional clinical neuropsychology has been the diagnosis of generic cognitive deficits which are identified by responses to standardized tests (Ben-Yishay & Gold, 1990). The entrance of clinical neuropsychology into the rehabilitation arena has precipitated requests to translate test scores and statements about mild, moderate, or severe impairment into more functional terms and to describe disabilities in terms of daily living that can be used for therapeutic goals (Ylvisaker, 1985). There still remains, however, some fundamental differences between neuropsychology and rehabilitation that require recognition. Diller (1987) proposes that the main difference between disciplines is that neuropsychology conducts studies to help elucidate and clarify the nature of impairments. Rehabilitation, on the other hand, is concerned with the remediation of impairments and teaching patients to manage their disabilities.

The natural forces that are currently operating on the field of neuropsychological rehabilitation of children and adolescents with brain injury are dramatically different from those of the past three decades and are essentially fourfold: (1) the advances in neuroscience are changing our understanding of brain–behavior relationships almost exponentially (Bigler, 1990); (2) the expansion of knowledge in cognitive psychology and cognitive neuropsychology is just beginning to be integrated into clinical neuropsychology (Margolin, 1992); (3) the incidence of brain injury in this population is rapidly increasing despite preventative efforts of the government in the regulation of safety in motor vehicles and media education from organizations such as the National Head Injury Foundation; and (4) the pressures of cost containment for rehabilitation for individuals with brain injury are being controlled by the financial community rather than the clinical community. Indeed, the average length of stay for adults in inpatient rehabilitation facilities has shrunk from an average of 93 to 53 days in the past decade (Gerring & Carney, 1992). As the insurance industry is often only interested in managing costs, the "managed care" concept of the 1990s is, so far, something of a misnomer (Kade, 1994). Hospital management personnel's interest is in increased efficiency and outcomes arising from the Continuous Quality Improvement movement, and may be expanded when managed care evolves to a system of payment by capitation. But at present it is the neuropsychologist and clinical personnel delivering care to patients with brain injury who will be most interested in a model of care more likely to produce better efficiency and better outcomes than the pre-1980 models currently in use.

Biomedical versus Service Neuropsychological Delivery Paradigms

Stanczak and Hutcherson (1992) have examined the differences in the neuropsychological and rehabilitative approaches to the treatment of brain injury. Giles and Fussey (1988) and Ylvisaker *et al.* (1990) observe that it is this absence of a fundamental, shared philosophy between the two disciplines that results in fragmented and disjointed delivery of rehabilitative services. For many years, rehabilitation professionals have worked within a biomedical paradigm. The latter paradigm has a fundamental notion of disease, and patients can be understood from a reductionistic examination of their constituent physical parts (Howard, 1991). Patient deficits are considered a deviation from biological norms and the disease process lies within the patient. From this perspective, neuropsychologists are looked to for a more holistic representation of the functional aspects of the patient, e.g., how the patient's brain functioning relates to the patient's behavior. It is interesting how the reductionistic versus dynamic theoretical antagonism is present not only between specialties but within specialties as well. Stanczak and Hutcherson (1992) assert that:

> the linear notion of a disease, with its demand of diagnosis and treatment, is no longer a viable one. Instead, the neuropsychological paradigm emphasizes the nonlinear notions of assessment and adaptation. Assessment is the identification and measurement of variables that affect the patient's performance. Adaptation is the systematic control of those variables to maximize the patient's functional autonomy. But assessment and adaptation are continuous processes that, in practice, occur concomitantly and repetitively. Instead of searching for "treatment" which effects change just within the head injury victim, rehabilitation specialists seek to maximize adaptation in two ways: (1) by altering the manner in which the patient interacts with his/her environment, and (2) by altering the way the environment affects the patient. Thus, within the neuropsychological paradigm, the range of possible "treatment" is limited only by the number of relevant variables identified and by the training and creativity of the health care provider. (p. 127)

It is essential that the differences between the biomedical and neuropsychological theoretical positions are understood by those who develop programs for patients with TBI in inpatient settings. The theoretical bias will determine which patient outcomes are considered important for treatment and the approaches to therapy and treatment. The Stanczak and Hutcherson (1992) comparison of the biomedical and neuropsychological paradigms of rehabilitation service delivery reproduced in Table 1 clearly documents the linear versus holistic methods of treatment.

What is not mentioned in the Stanczak and Hutcherson (1992) comparison, however, is the probable need for different foci at different stages of treatment. In terms of a continuum of care, the biomedical emphasis for brain injury takes its place in the initial acute phase of treatment and slowly gives way to neuropsychological emphasis as the patient's locus of control (in a medical and psychological sense) emerges. In other words, the para-

digm should reflect the patient need. In the acute stages of treatment, service delivery is primarily focused on the biomedical needs of the patient such as stabilization and maintenance while the patient is comatose. However, as the patient emerges from coma, interaction with the environment becomes a factor within the patient's control. At this point, the neuropsychological paradigm begins a dynamic assessment process that should help the patient mediate his or her environment. The comatose patient is dependent on the biomedical response to his or her condition. As the patient's brain and body regain independent homeostasis, the acute period closes, the biomedical needs lessen, and the rehabilitative and neuropsychological needs increase (Grimm & Bleiberg, 1986). As the patient is discharged from a medical-surgical setting into a rehabilitation facility, the neuropsychological paradigm is in full force (except for those patients who continue to have major medical issues). Stanczak and Hutcherson (1992) state that programs that rely solely on one paradigm or the other probably do not exist. Most rehabilitative efforts are combinations of biomedical and neuropsychological interventions. However, it should be noted that unless a strong neuropsychology presence and a specific neuropsychological theoretical foundation exist in a brain injury rehabilitation program, that program is much more likely to reflect the supervision of the medical personnel involved. Reorientation of a biomedically managed program to a combination program that responds heavily to the neuropsychological needs of the patient is difficult and likely to deprive medical personnel of their considerable status and influence (Howard, 1991; Stanczak & Hutcherson, 1992). Therefore, the theoretical design of any brain injury rehabilitation program must be consciously held in the minds of the professionals involved and openly discussed and revised (Grimm & Bleiberg, 1986). A lack of theoretical perspective will reduce service delivery to reflecting the individual beliefs of the therapists or supervisors involved. The nature and complexity of brain injury rehabilitation demands cohesive and synergistic efforts from allied professionals and systems.

Models of Program Service Delivery

The neuropsychological rehabilitation programs that pioneered the methodology and designs of current programs were the Brain Injury Rehabilitation Unit of the Palo Alto Veteran's

TABLE 1. A Comparison of the Biomedical and Neuropsychological Paradigms of Rehabilitation Service Delivery[a]

	Biomedical paradigm	Neuropsychological paradigm
Philosophy	Materialistic, reductionistic	Emergent, holistic
Primary model	Disease model	Dysfunctional model
	Linear diagnosis and treatment	Nonlinear assessment and adaptation
Theories	Little heuristic value	Proven heuristic value
	Brain viewed as internal organ	Brain viewed as organ of interface
	Presumes plasticity of neural tissue	Presumes learning occurs
Locus of dysfunction	Organismic	Is the interface between the individual and the environment
Role of provider	Healer	Consultant
Locus of power	Provider	Patient and family
	Patient blamed for lack of success	Treatment blamed for lack of success
Intrapsychic pathologizing	Accepted	Eschewed
Premorbid factors	Secondary importance	Primary importance
Role of patient	Passive recipient of services	Equal and active participant
Treatment options	Nil set	Unlimited
Behavioral disturbances	Viewed negatively	Viewed positively
	Treated by chemical restraints and behavioral treatment plans	Treated by environment modification plans and operant learning
Staff	Passive	Active
Meaning	For provider	For patient
Service delivery	Traditional static pyramidal model	Flexible systems model
	Authoritarian leadership	Authoritative leadership
	Vertical communication	Horizontal communication
	Leader decision-making and conflict resolution	Team decision-making and conflict resolution
	Focuses on tertiary and secondary interventions	Focuses on primary and secondary interventions
	Narrow scope	Broad scope
	Inefficient	Efficient
	Relatively inexpensive	Relatively expensive
	Architectural isolation	Architecture promotes resocialization
	Multidisciplinary	Transdisciplinary
	Fragmented treatment plans	Integrated treatment plans
	Staff competition	Staff collaboration
	Professional frustration	Professional autonomy
	Deficit management model	Health promotion model

[a]From Stanczak & Hutcherson (1992).

Administration Medical Center, the Neuropsychological Rehabilitation Program at Presbyterian Hospital of Oklahoma City, and the Cognitive Rehabilitation Program at the Robert Wood Johnson Jr. Lifestyle Institute. These programs were begun in the 1970s and 1980s and led the way for practical activities of daily living, psychotherapeutic interventions, and interventive cognitive neuropsychology to be included in programming for adults with TBI (Trexler, 1987).

Within the brain injury rehabilitation program, the focus of neuropsychological assessment has changed. Ben-Yishay and Gold (1990) have suggested that assessment should reflect psychometric, neurological, remedial, and functional perspectives. This holistic approach has received support (Prigatano, 1988, 1990, 1991a), and is probably a marriage of earlier efforts that were reductionistic and dynamic. Reductionistic approaches in neuropsychology focused on the diagnostic validity and reliability of specific tests and test batteries. Accuracy and prediction were the tenets of assessment. Once a function was defined and measured, then restoration of the deficits to some specific predetermined criteria was the practice and the goal. On the other hand, the dynamic thinking in neuropsychological rehabilitation placed emphasis on the therapist/patient relationship and a larger perspective of general adaptation in a variety of contextual situations.

As with others, Trexler (1987) proposed a model of treatment that included the reductionistic and dynamic approaches and described three basic dimensions for rehabilitation programming. The dimensions included the promotion of the patient being aware of her or his neuropsychological deficits, the treatment of general and specific deficits, and the promotion of generalization to the home or outpatient setting. This model may reflect the different views of the goals of rehabilitation. Neuropsychologists tend to focus on impairments reflecting brain–behavior relationships, whereas other re-habilitation professionals center their efforts on disability through readaptation at a functional level.

Other models that are currently in the forefront of programming for individuals with brain injury use multimodal approaches to cognitive rehabilitation and holistic approaches to team intervention. Embodied in the holistic conception of rehabilitation is the premise that patients allow themselves to be guided by clinicians. Individuals who were autonomous before the trauma learn to accept direction for their relearning (Ben-Yishay & Gold,

1990). Outcome studies of young adults with brain injury show that the best predictors of postrehabilitation vocational attainments are improved self-awareness and acceptance. Ben-Yishay (1993) of the NYU brain injury program states:

> On one level the goal of neuropsychological rehabilitation is to ameliorate interferences with cognitive functions and aid in mastery of compensatory repertoires to improve functional competence. On another level the goal is to promote in TBI patients the necessary alteration of their sense of self or ego-identity so that in spite of the current limitations imposed by the brain injury they can reattain a minimum degree of self-esteem and self-worth. (p. 210)

The NYU group program is essentially a day treatment program for adults with brain injury. The program is divided into two main phases where the individual receives intensive assessment and remediation within a therapeutic community, and then treatment progresses to supervision of the patient in an *in vivo* occupation work trial. Outcome studies for the cognitive remediation portion of the program indicated significant but modest improvement on test scores. Small group therapy has been the more potent predictor of success in vocational attainment (Ben-Yishay & Gold, 1990).

This program has flourished for three decades, demonstrates clear outcomes such as returning patients to work, and continues essentially unchanged because of this success (Ben-Yishay & Gold, 1990; Ben-Yishay & Prigatano, 1990). Patients attend the Rusk Institute for 20-week cycles of treatment. The program provides day treatment for individuals between the ages of 18 and 55 who meet certain admission criteria (ability to tolerate extensive pretreatment neuropsychological testing, postinjury IQ above 80, a history of work or school attendance immediately before the brain injury, and lack of severe ambulatory and communication deficits, substance abuse, and physical aggression). After the initial assessment and evaluation period, remedial interventions begin within a small milieu including ten other patients. The day is organized around intensive group and individual activities with weekly counseling for the patient and family. Counseling sessions are often used to prepare the patient for an imminent group activity that is expected to be difficult for the patient. Periodically the patients prepare presentations that address the nature of the program and their individual problems and progress. The presentations sometimes resemble a 12-step program as the patient rises to address the assembly of peers (and sometimes family) and goes on to announce that she or he has a brain injury, and lists the impairments that result from the injury, and the challenges of the neuropsychological rehabilitation program. Occupational trials and *in vivo* training end the cycle of treatment. Systematic bridging techniques are included to help the application of skills to functional daily living.

Perhaps the best way to represent the overall objective of the holistic program model is to describe the clinical challenges that the patient with brain injury must face. The NYU group (Ben-Yishay & Gold, 1990; Ben-Yishay & Prigatano, 1990; Prigatano, 1990) developed a hierarchy of six stages of cognitive adjustment in the remedial program. The first is engagement, where the patient is encouraged to engage in the rehabilitation activities designed to optimize alertness, attention, and concentration. Awareness is the next stage. It is characterized by the patient beginning to focus on progressive awareness of his or her problems. The objective of this stage is to make sure that the patient has an understanding of the consequences of the brain injury and the commitment to undergo intensive rehabilitative efforts. The third and fourth stages of the program are the mastery and control, respectively, of compensatory strategies. These stages are also involved when the patient attempts to use compensatory techniques for daily problem-solving. The fifth stage, acceptance, is achieved when the patient attains a sense of realization that the limits of compensation for residual impairments have been met. According to Prigatano (1990), the latter is "never purely a cognitive act" (p. 297). The last stage concerns identity and refers to the culmination of the successful precedent stages. The patient established a new identity "hopefully with dignity and enthusiasm" (Prigatano, 1990, p. 287). At this point the patient achieves a perspective that the course of his or her life was permanently altered by the brain injury, but the new course is also a life worth living (Cossu, 1994).

Psychosocial Aspects of Holistic Programs

The outcome of brain injury is affected by neuropathological, physical, functional, familial, vocational, and neuropsychological factors (Trexler, 1987). However, there is increasing recognition of the importance of psychosocial aspects. Patients with TBI are much more seriously handicapped by emotional and personality disturbance than by their residual cognitive and physical disabilities (Divak, Herrle, & Scott, 1985; Lezak & O'Brien, 1990; McGuire &

Sylvester, 1990). Also, cognitive deficits significantly influence the degree of disability and handicap associated with a physical impairment (Kaplan & Corrigan, 1994). The level of stress experienced by the family, the ultimate caregivers after rehabilitation has ended, varies with cognitive impairment and psychological adjustment to the brain injury (Allen, Linn, Guiterrez, & Willer, 1994). With the publication of the DSM-IV (American Psychiatric Association, 1994) the category of Personality Change Due to a Medical Condition has emerged as a diagnosis. In children, a deviation in development or change in behavior lasting for more than a year is substituted for personality change. Subtypes include labile affect, disinhibition, aggression, apathy, paranoia, and personality change associated with a seizure disorder. This category provides the first formal opportunity for psychological aspect of brain injury to be recognized by diagnosis. Postconcussional Disorder is now listed in Appendix B of DSM-IV as worthy of further study and is more specific to brain injury. In the holistic genre, psychotherapy is an integral part of rehabilitation because the physical and mental domains are not artificially separated. Thus, the psychologist is viewed as a rehabilitation therapist on the same footing as the physical, occupational, and speech language therapists. Psychotherapy provides a key ingredient through the process of teaching the patient to operate in her or his own best interest. Prigatano (1991a) states:

> at its core, psychotherapy is a teaching experience in which a socially sanctioned healer uses whatever learning techniques are culturally acceptable to the individual and society. These teaching techniques must "make sense" to the patient and to the therapist. They must reflect a method of interaction that considers the cognitive and personality characteristics of the individual being served. In post acute neurorehabilitation, the psychotherapist of TBI patients must demonstrate that the teaching methods are appropriate for a given patient and measure, directly or indirectly, the outcome to these interventions. (p. 3)

Many have argued that "patients with a brain injury" are not "psychologically minded" and are therefore not candidates for psychotherapy. However, a neuropsychological model of rehabilitation simply takes the psychotherapeutic goals for a given patient and addresses them from multiple perspectives. The goal is to assist the patient with psychosocial adjustment (Prigatano, 1988). Others (Deaton, 1990; Jackson & Gouvier, 1992) use cognitive behavioral interventions to help the patient comply with psychotherapy instructions or to provide psychotherapy reminders when fluctuations in motivational or emotional state are likely to occur. Cognitive behavioral therapy teaches the patient to become aware of the need for self-regulation and/or link the executive-intentional control of behavior with the motivational/emotional states.

Pediatric versus Adult Programming for Individuals with Brain Injury

There is a significant lack of documentation of rehabilitation treatment with brain–injured children and adolescents in the research literature (Deaton, 1990; Ewing-Cobbs & Fletcher, 1990; Lehr, 1990; Rourke, Bakker, Fisk, & Strang, 1983). The data base that supports the Traumatic Brain Injury Model Systems Project funded by the National Institute on Disability and Rehabilitation Research includes only patients aged 16 or older (Dahmer, Shilling, Hamilton, Bontke, & Smith, 1993). Some research reports results with patients that include adolescents (and rarely children), but the pediatric cases are not analyzed separately. Reitan's REHABIT program for cognitive rehabilitation, described in Goldstein (1987), showed moderate to marked improvement in pre and post test scores for 23 of 26 patients aged 5 to 56 years with brain injuries (Brodsky, Brodsky, Lee, & Sever, 1986). However, they subsequently noted that the youngest patient, 7 years old at 25-month follow-up, had significant decline in verbal ability (Brodsky, 1988). The effectiveness of intervention for children with brain damage in general has been questioned, but the position of providers is that "the fields of rehabilitation medicine and developmental pediatrics are based on the principle that improving function, in spite of the permanence of handicap, is both desirable and possible" (Kaminer, 1986, p. 1101). Notwithstanding the staggering incidence of brain injury among the child and adolescent age group, and the demands of Public Law 101-476 mandating services for students with brain injury in the public schools (Gerring & Carney, 1992), little is written about the specialized training and inpatient programming needed for these individuals. Gans, Mann, and Ylvisaker (1990) suggest that the two most important aspects of difference between adults and children with TBI are that "the child is a growing organism, and that functioning development is incomplete" (p. 593). In terms of inpatient treatment, the following general areas should be considered when describing a pediatric population and brain injury.

Age of Injury

The primary consideration of pediatric brain injury and long-term outcome is the age at which the injury occurred. It has become apparent that the extent of recovery following TBI in children and youth is determined by a variety of factors such as etiology, length of recovery interval, size of lesion, and lesion site (Ewing-Cobbs, Fletcher, & Levin, 1985; Lehr, 1990). Much has been documented about the plasticity of the newly developing brain and will not be reiterated here. However, in general, it was thought for some time that "the earlier the insult the better the chance of functional reorganization of the brain, or that plasticity of the young brain provided some measure of protection from the effects of the injury" (Sohlberg & Mateer, 1989, p. 388). Lately, however, this assumption has been modified more to children over the age of 5, in that they may have substrates to provide the takeover of function. Younger children who sustain diffuse, widespread, or bilateral brain injury probably do not have the substrates necessary for domain specificity and may suffer serious compromises in the development of the basic cognitive structures that are necessary for psychoeducational and psychosocial functioning in later childhood and adolescence (Boll & Barth, 1981). More recent research (Lehr, 1990) suggests that short-term recovery from shifting functions to an area of the brain not yet specialized in function may result in compromise of later abilities to meet developmental milestones. The shift to new locations may make the child appear superficially intact but contribute to the slowing of reaction time, inefficient information processing, and ineffective memory for new learning that characterize much of postinjury functioning. Damage to immature areas of the brain may not have behavioral sequelae until neurodevelopment of functions associated with those structures fails to keep pace with environmental demands. Furthermore, there is an increased risk of hearing loss and seizure disorders that have extensive effects when combined with normal developmental demands (Sellers & Vegter, 1993). One possible pathway of the effects of a minor head trauma is subclinical posttraumatic seizures. Verduyn and colleagues studied 17 patients aged 11 to 56 who developed multiple, partial seizure-like symptoms after minor closed head trauma

(Verduyn, Hilt, Roberts, & Roberts, 1992). Neuropsychological assessment in this study often suggested static and episodic cognitive impairment and most of the subjects benefited from treatment with anticonvulsant medication without fully returning to premorbid levels of social and vocational functioning. If seizures are uncontrolled, they continue to provide insults to the brain. In general, therefore, research concurs that children suffer greater effects of TBI than adults, and younger children suffer greater deficits than older children and adolescents (Mira, Tucker, & Tyler, 1992). Indeed, Stein (1988) offers a particularly succinct viewpoint:

> after an injury, the remaining nervous system should be considered as a new, reorganized structure and not just as a structure minus one part. In my view, the symptoms that follow brain damage do not stem from the missing or damaged part, but rather from the organism's attempt to adapt, cope, and survive. (p. 34)

Assessment

The neuropsychological assessment of the child with brain injury goes far beyond the administration of a standardized set of test instruments (Ewing-Cobbs & Fletcher, 1990; Sohlberg & Mateer, 1989). Ylvisaker (1985) states that "traditional methods of assessment often require modification or flexibility in interpretation as a result of the particular combinations of cognitive, psychosocial, and motor problems that in many cases distinguish head injured children from those whose impairments are congenital" (p. 558). However, the procedure for assessment is similar for the pediatric and adult populations and, according to Sohlberg and Mateer (1989), includes: (1) examination of the premorbid history, (2) review of the medical history, (3) interview and behavioral observations, (4) administration and scoring of neuropsychological tests, (5) drawing of conclusions describing the cognitive/behavioral strengths and weaknesses, (6) formulation of recommendations for a remedial plan, and (7) attempts at prognosis for recovery.

In terms of assessment of consciousness in the acute phase of treatment, the depth of coma is tracked in a variety of ways, including the Glasgow Coma Scale, Coma Recovery Scale (CRS), Rancho Los Amigos (RLA) Level, and the Disability Rating Scale (DRS). The first two scales are based on a specific examination of the patient and the latter two scales are based on observations of what changes the patient has exhibited since the last rating. The Rancho Los Amigos Scales have been changed to fit pediatric assessment needs. Therefore, not only does the summary table of Levels of Consciousness reflect overall pediatric assessment, Records of Consciousness Levels focus on three separate pediatric groups: infant (6 months to 2 years), preschool (2 to 5 years), and school-age children (5 years and older) (Sellers & Vegter, 1993). Loss of consciousness (LOC) is tracked because the duration of unconsciousness is a gauge of the severity of the injury. However, as the coma gradually lightens, it can be difficult to agree on a precise time at which the coma ended because there is not consensual definition of coma boundaries. Posttraumatic amnesia (PTA) refers to how long the person remains confused, disoriented, and has trouble with memory. In a mild brain injury the person may not have been unconscious and patients can experience brain injury without head injury such as is seen in "occult brain injury" in spinal cord patients (see review by Hinnant & Kade, 1992). Thus, it is not surprising that PTA is a better general gauge of how seriously the brain was injured than LOC and the best predictor of neurobehavioral outcome in children 1 year postinjury (McDonald *et al.* 1994).

Telzrow (1990) has described and compared the different domains of assessment suggested by leading neuropsychologists in the field of pediatric neuropsychology. Most neuropsychological assessments address the following areas: intelligence, organizational skills, tactile perceptual, visual perceptual, auditory perceptual, memory, attention, problem-solving, abstract reasoning, manual dexterity, effects of feedback on performance, new learning ability, speech and language, personality, social skills, behavior, and family functioning. The domains are similar for adult and pediatric populations, but the latter group is more difficult to assess for a variety of reasons. The assessment is being conducted at a time when developmental processes are proceeding in the child. The processes vary from child to child and are subject to changes, spurts, and plateaus that complicate the establishment of valid measurements of neurocognitive function. Individuals at different ages may use different cognitive approaches to the same task (test) and possibly different areas of the brain as well (Hynd & Willis, 1988). The reliable and valid measurement of dynamic processes requires that tests reflect these developmental changes (see Franzen, 1989, for a review of specific tests). Like the Wechsler intelligence scales, neuropsychological tests for children are largely downward extensions of adult measures. They may be validated for brain-behavior relationships but have inadequate developmental norms (Hynd & Willis, 1988; Spreen & Strauss, 1991). Conversely, cognitive measures with better developmental norms are not validated for brain–behavior relationships (Reitan, 1993). One attempt used the Woodcock–Johnson-Revised Tests of Cognitive Ability (WJTCA) from the Woodcock–Johnson Psycho-Educational Battery-Revised with 39 patients aged 17 to 57 with closed head injury (Tupper, 1990). It found significant correlations between coma duration and performance on the Perceptual Speed and Memory clusters of the WJTCA, between Trail Making test performance and many WJTCA clusters, but no relationships with the Halstead Category test and any of the other Halstead–Reitan neuropsychological measures used. One attempt at the development of valid and functional assessment techniques that affects those reaching driving age involves fitness to drive. Galski and colleagues compared an off-road, predriving evaluation of skills regarded as important in driving and an on-road, behind-the-wheel evaluation of abilities needed to drive in actual traffic situations with patients who had a head injury or stroke. Only 4 out of 21 items on the predriving evaluation significantly predicted the outcome of the predriving evaluation and none predicted the outcome of the behind-the-wheel evaluation. Only 6 of the 26 tasks on the behind-the-wheel evaluation significantly predicted the outcome of the behind-the-wheel evaluation (Galski, Ehle, & Bruno, 1990, p. 709).

A subsequent study of 106 patients aged 16–87 showed residual deficits in cognition less related than behavior in determining fitness, and when behavioral measures were included, off-road and on-road evaluation reached sensitivities of 90 and 92% (Galski, Bruno, & Ehle, 1993).

Arguments against the validity of inferences from neuropsychological tests are well known (Reschly & Gresham, 1989); however, little else is offered as a guideline for assessing children and adolescents with brain injury. Consensus has been reached on measures that discriminate degree of brain injury and are sensitive to change over time (Kreutzer, Gordon, Rosenthal, & Marwitz, 1993), but most of these lack adequate norms and similar validity data for children. The process of assessment of younger patients with brain injury is further clouded by the difficulty that clinicians and parents have distinguishing between neurobehavioral prob-

lems caused by the injury versus the emotional reactions to the trauma surrounding the event itself (Waaland & Raines, 1991). Nonetheless, neuropsychological assessment is helpful in determining the individual patient's initial status, establishing a comprehensive baseline for future comparison, identifying strengths and weaknesses, developing prescriptions for treatment, and assisting with prediction and determination of outcomes (Lynch, 1990).

Developmental Stage

Notwithstanding the neurological aspects of brain development and brain injury, the developmental stage of psychosocial adjustment is also an important difference between pediatric and adult populations (Deaton, 1990). Preschool children have limited executive function. Traditional belief based on behavioral function was that supramodal or tertiary zones became functional between 5 and 8 years of age whereas prefrontal regions did not reach functional maturity until age 12 (Risser & Edgell, 1988). However, neuroscience research now suggests that prefrontal regions begin a process of maturation at 6 to 12 months of age and continue, perhaps in stages, to maturity (Pennington, 1991). In addition, there appears to be a correlation with neo-Piagetian stages of cognitive development. Thus, latency-aged children do not have the neuropsychological apparatus for the identity formation and executive functions that pubescent and adolescent individuals exhibit. Therefore, certain aspects of rehabilitation that would be addressed with adults would simply not be appropriate for adolescents and younger children. For example, the rehabilitation goal of acceptance and the formulation of a new identity that incorporates brain injury would not be a goal for an 8-year-old. The focus of acceptance of a new identity (or perhaps a different vision of the child as an adult) would be emphasized more with the family than with the patient in this case. With a patient who is 15 at time of injury, the developmental stage would be the emergence of identity. The latter would be incorporated into the therapeutic goals because psychosocial adjustment in rehabilitation incorporates realistic appraisal of abilities and expectations in life. Adolescent needs do not essentially have a long-established sense of self preinjury, as do those of adults (Lehr, 1990). Adolescents are in the process of individuation and emancipation from the family and brain injury interrupts the natural unfolding of these events. Therefore, the adolescent's "identity development and independence striving can be significantly threatened or interrupted by injury" (Lehr, 1990, p. 4).

Stage of Recovery

Many pediatric rehabilitative programs use a three-phase structure for rehabilitation with individualized plans based on the child's stage of recovery, developmental age, and specific impairments (Henry, 1983; Ylvisaker, 1986). Although the benefit of treatment beyond nursing and nutritional care of the comatose patient is controversial, studies have shown that patients in a coma can learn to do simple tasks such as removing a cloth from their face via backward chaining teaching technique (Sheil, Wilson, Horn, Watson, & Smith, 1993). Thus, a more reliable response to specific stimuli can be taught to a patient normally thought to be unresponsive. A study of 47 patients aged 14 to 55 with severe TBI has found a greater likelihood of functional change in those admitted to treatment less than 6 months postinjury. There was also a relationship between the amount of intervention provided and the level of functional change, suggesting some benefit to intervention even for those at a low level of functioning (Timmons, Gasquoine, & Scibak, 1987). The goals of rehabilitation shift over the course of recovery as the patient emerges from coma and can reliably communicate, and yet is still disoriented and experiencing PTA. Research suggests that in this second phase the patient can acquire skills (i.e., use procedural memory) during motor performance and pattern analyzing tasks, but cannot recognize words they learn to read in mirror orientation or recall recent events (i.e., use declarative memory) (Ewert, Levin, Watson, & Kalisky, 1989).

In the third phase of rehabilitation, the patient has become oriented and PTA has ended. Formal assessment makes possible a delineation of the specific impairments that will become the foci of treatment. In this phase metacognitive and executive functions have received increasing attention by therapists from a variety of disciplines. For example, it is felt that "awareness, goal setting, planning, self-initiation, self-inhibition, self-monitoring, ability to change set, and strategic behavior" are necessary for completion of rehabilitation, community reentry, and social independence (Pollens, McBratnie, & Burton, 1988, p. 26). Ylvisaker and Szerkeres (1989) state that "metacognitive dysfunction

involves deficits in both the knowledge base and executive system" with the latter involving "self-planning, self-directing, self-monitoring, and problem solving" (p. 34). Inclusion of these factors in treatment plans for speech–language therapy was seen as very important. Initial findings of limited functional improvements from interventions to improve memory resulted in additional interventions in executive functions to improve an adolescent patient's "ability" to identify a memory problem and to initiate a general plan for dealing with that problem (Lawson & Rice, 1989). Others have intervened in attentional processes with the logic that poor attention leads to poor encoding of information into memory (Mateer, 1993). However, studies of attentional deficits in 88 patients aged 16 to 45 with severe traumatic head injuries versus 59 age-matched, orthopedic rehabilitation patients provided no evidence of deficits of focused attention, sustained attention, or supervisory attentional control, but significant deficits in speed of information processing on tests such as the Symbol Digit Modalities Test, simple and choice reaction time tasks, and color naming and word reading scores on the Stroop (Ponsford & Kinsella, 1992). It has been suggested that treatment produces limited improvement in speed of information processing; therefore, patient and family education and supportive counseling are suggested (Lezak, 1994).

Psychosocial aspects are also dealt with in the third phase of rehabilitation. It is acknowledged that rehabilitation of a child with a condition such as cerebral palsy requires physical and occupational therapy, but a child with an acquired brain injury also requires psychological intervention and an intensive educational program (Russman, 1990). Self-esteem, self-image, and identity are key issues in brain injury rehabilitation. Garske and Thomas (1992) studied 47 individuals aged 16 to 35 with a history of severe closed head injury and found 55% mildly to severely depressed on the Beck Depression Inventory. Depression and lower self-esteem on the Rosenberg Self-Esteem Scale were significantly related to each other and to rehabilitation need satisfaction. McCabe and Green (1987) presented case reports of three 4- to 18-year-old boys who developed socially disinhibited behaviors following severe head injuries. Treatment helped them "to manage their maturational tasks of adolescence . . . including . . . identity issues" (p. 111). Secondary changes in self-image have been studied and found significant. A study of eight patients aged 16 to 57 with head injuries found that both patients and their close relatives saw "significant changes on a semantic differential rating scale of the patient's present, past, and future self . . . [Patients] tended to see themselves in a more positive light than relatives regarding a present self. Both . . . anticipate a return to past self within a year" (McWilliams, 1991, p. 246). The issues and interventions of this third phase of rehabilitation are the focus of this chapter, because the differences in pediatric programming are most apparent once the patient is oriented.

Modalities of Treatment

Rehabilitation can be viewed at the level of the program or at the level of the therapeutic dyad of therapist and patient. Both levels of intervention must provide structure in the form of alteration between activity and rest (Gronwall *et al.*, 1990). The comatose patient has difficulty regulating exposure to stimuli. The latter is usually evidenced in behaviors that represent frustration from overstimulation and fatigue. In addition, the level of regulation has an important influence on function and mood during the therapy sessions. Therefore, more (treatment) is not necessarily better (treatment). Later in the recovery process the patient's need for structure is balanced against an increasing need for self-control via shared decision-making. Of course, a child's ability to make decisions will vary by age and functioning level.

The obvious and well-established differences between child and adult therapies involve matching techniques to the developmental age of the child. These include such techniques as play therapy, the use of games and toys in speech, occupational, physical, and cognitive retraining therapies, and generally child-oriented materials and activities. The concept that play (and later school) is the work of the child takes on special meaning in rehabilitation because the traditional goal of adult rehabilitation is return to work: For the child it is return to play and to school. Play is intrinsically motivating to the child and an endeavor mediated by language with peers and more able models. Research studies have shown that "the proficiency of the therapist and his/her relationship with the patient proves to be the most significant variable related to the effectiveness of a therapy" (Rourke *et al.*, 1983, p. 156). This therapeutic relationship may be determined, in part, by the presentation and interaction style of the therapist matching the neuropsychological strengths or weaknesses of the patient. For example, a patient with auditory processing deficits may

have difficulty experiencing success with a therapist who favors highly verbal psychoeducational methods. A patient approaching a task greatly affected by her or his neuropsychological impairments and lacking in motivation and self-confidence may have limited success with a therapist providing emotional support but little structure. The amount of success patient and therapist experience together will probably greatly affect the therapeutic relationship. Therefore, the link between neuropsychological assessment and therapist flexibility in terms of treatment modality and style is imperative for successful outcomes.

Family Involvement

The obvious difference between family involvement with pediatric versus adult patients is that the family expectation on reentry for children is that the family will resume primary guidance and structure for the patient. In one way, this may reduce the amount of change for the family because they do not necessarily have to make the adjustment that a former autonomous adult is now a dependent adult, requiring a shift in family dynamics. The family of a pediatric patient expects to continue a guidance role when the child reenters. However, the adjustment for the idealized child to a child with special needs has its own set of emotional and psychosocial sequelae (Waaland & Raines, 1991). The adolescent patient may significantly interfere with the natural development of the family. The family may plunge from the developmental stage of family separation back into the school-aged developmental stage. Younger siblings at this time may resent the attention that the injured child receives. In addition, the greater need for supervision and structure sets the injured child apart from his or her siblings. The "birth order" among the siblings can be temporarily rearranged as an older child with an acute brain injury becomes more dependent on parents than younger siblings who may have to step into the "big brother or sister" role vacated by the patient. This can reverse with good recovery and then reverse again if the younger sibling later overtakes the patient whose development slows at later milestones. If the child is the survivor of an accident where other family members were killed, then special issues and difficulties may arise within the family (Mira *et al.*, 1992). Patients who were premorbidly difficult children may precipitate the family's anger by becoming even more difficult after emerging from an initially docile postinjury phase (Miller, 1993). The family with a child who is brain injured is placed in a special situation:

> Related to the issue of dependency is that of protection. The child who has become disinhibited and socially fearless is now at increased risk for social and sexual exploitation, as well as for harming others, and the parents face the challenging dilemma of fostering independence and recovery, while at the same time providing control and structure to maintain safety. (Miller, 1993, p. 214).

Any assessment of the family should include assessment of the patient as a member of that family system and acknowledge individual differences within the system. Willer and colleagues used structured small-group discussions with 13 young men aged 14 to 25 with TBI, their mothers, and their siblings to document problems from each perspective (Willer, Allen, Durnan, & Ferry, 1990). Patients saw problems with peer relations, autonomy, and success at school. Mothers focused on problems with the service system and its accessibility. Siblings saw family stress as the biggest problem. Patients coped through accepting personal responsibilities for progress. Mothers' acceptance of the patient was their most important means of coping. Siblings primarily coped by suppressing frustrations.

The stages in family adaptation when a child has sustained a TBI include shock, denial or disbelief, sorrow, anger, and adaptation (Martin, 1988). The "sudden and dramatic changes in the child's cognitive abilities and personality, ambiguity about recovery, . . . increased dependency and long term care needs" and the "lack of financial resources, lack of respite care, and lack of appropriate rehabilitation and educational programs in the community" are sources of family stress (Martin, 1988, p. 464). Clearly, the family must be prepared to accept the child's reentry into the home.

Reentry Issues

Adult patients are rehabilitated to achieve a return to capacity and children are trained to develop capacity (Rourke *et al.*, 1983). Adults and children relearn information in rehabilitation. However, children are in a constant state of maturation and new learning (Shapiro, 1987) and will return to an environment (i.e., school) where new learning is essential for success. Closed head in-

juries often involve the frontal and temporal lobes and therefore compromise problem-solving, higher-order processing, initiative, memory, and new learning (Levin, 1990). It is proposed (Lehr, 1990) that pediatric brain injury rehabilitation can be understood "as one process imposed on another" (p. 41).

Considering these specialized problems for children and adolescents reentering school, the lack of programming for youngsters with TBI in the public schools is surprising (Begali, 1992; Lash & Scarpino, 1993; Rourke *et al.*, 1983; Ylvisaker, 1985). It is unfortunately usual that a child or adolescent will reenter school and interact with personnel who have little or no training in the special needs of youngsters with TBI. Although an influx of publications about TBI is emerging because of federal legislation, overall staff development for a low-incidence population is not economical, and therefore staff training is and will probably be done on a case-by-case method. This will obviously hamper any given student's progress with new learning or psychosocial adjustment because the staff and student are learning about TBI reentry as they go along. This may also alter rehabilitation decisions as to reentry placement. If the pediatric patient is ready for community reentry and needs specific programming in the public schools, the rehabilitation team has the responsibility of making sure that the continuum of services available support the timing of reentry.

Savage and Carter (1988) present guidelines for rehabilitation professionals to use to contact school personnel, initiate school/hospital visits, conduct inservice training for educators, design appropriate education programming, and provide follow-up service. Although services are provided by public school systems, children with closed head injury differ from children traditionally served in special education programs and the burden is currently on rehabilitation professionals to facilitate reentry. Carney and Gerring (1990) present two cases that illustrate the necessity of cooperation between hospital and school to obtain the proper "assessment, environment, class size, teaching style, behavioral programs, instructional emphases, and integrated therapies" (p. 222). The informational needs of the school may dictate a different assessment. Specific elements of a functional assessment for adolescents who are reentering a classroom setting include visual processing, conversational processing, critical thinking, and skill integration (Milton, Scaglione, Flanagan, Cox, & Smith, 1991).

Program Evaluation

Practices in measuring outcome in rehabilitation in general, and in brain injury programs in particular, have become increasingly important (Johnston, Keith, & Hinderer, 1992; Malkmus & Evans, 1992). Program evaluation proposed specifically for adults with brain injuries focuses on questions of whether the patient is still living at the same place and employed 1 year postdischarge. These measures have little meaning in pediatric rehabilitation because most children with brain injuries will still be at home and, unlike jobs, opportunity to return to school is legally mandated and therefore may artificially inflate simply defined success rates. The following research helps illustrate this point. A study of 93 patients aged 12 to 65 with severe head injuries found that at 6 months, 18% of former workers had returned to gainful employment and 62% of former students had returned to school (Ruff, Marshall, Crouch, Klauber, & Smith, 1993). Of the remaining patients, 31% of the former workers and 66% of the former students had returned by 12 months. "Age, length of coma, speed for both attending and motor movements, spatial integration, and intact vocabulary were all significantly related to returning to work or school" (Ruff et al., 1993, p. 101). The best predictors of return to work or school were verbal ability, speed of information processing, and age.

In many rehabilitation families the program evaluation methodology is often based on subjective assessments by the therapists who treated the patient. The potential for bias toward positive outcome in such an approach is obvious (Barber, 1976; Neale & Liebert, 1973), but unstudied. Furthermore, the new pediatric measures such as the Functional Independence Measure for Children or WeeFIM (Uniform Data System for Medical Rehabilitation, 1994) are downward extensions of adult measures with no specific procedures to adjust each measure to the developmental age of the individual patient. The alternative approach of calculating "percent of therapists' goals met by discharge date" has the effect of encouraging therapists to set lower goals to make outcomes appear most positive. Program evaluation for children with brain injuries is just beginning to develop measures that are adjusted to the child's specific age and include the behavioral, emotional, and social sequelae of prime im-

portance to long-term outcome (Kade, 1993, 1994). In addition, many have documented the difficulty of determined outcomes with children because of the inherent problems that come with standardization of treatment in scientific investigations with children (Rourke et al., 1983).

Outcome Measurement

As the Glasgow Coma Scale predicts outcome, the Glasgow Outcome Scale measures outcome. The five areas of outcome are (1) death, (2) persistent vegetative state, (3) severe disability (conscious but disabled), (4) severe disability (disabled but independent), and (5) good recovery (Taylor, 1992). The latter category of the Glasgow Outcome Scale does not necessarily imply that there is an absence of persistent limitations for the patient. Only approximately one-third to one-half of all survivors of severe closed head injury can achieve good recovery (Begali, 1992). The Glasgow Outcome Scale may be popular because most patients have mild to moderate head injuries and these patients may simply be rated as "good recovery" at discharge from the acute medical-surgical hospital. The issue about the use of this scale with children, however, is that the term *good recovery* does not accurately reflect the academic and developmentally related criteria required for appropriate assessment of outcome. For example, good recovery of any injury sustained at age 4 may be the initial diagnostic impression until severe reading problems are discovered at age 8. Rourke et al. (1983) have stated that:

> In the case of brain injury, the first and most obvious initial symptom (e.g., attentional deficiencies and impairment of motor functions) may represent only the "tip of the iceberg" with respect to the problems that the child will face over the span of a lifetime. For example, in cases in which the parietal region of the right cerebral hemisphere has been damaged, the child's social skills and awareness of self, particularly in relation to others, may prove to be one of the most outstanding and difficult areas to remediate. Although this may not be a prominent feature of the child's adaptive deficiencies during the first weeks or months following brain injury, one of the most important targets of remediation is to teach such children those skills that would help to alleviate their immediate and eventual difficulties in social responsiveness. (p. 157)

Therefore, Begali (1992) suggests that outcome scales with children and adolescents should be supplemented with formal and objective measures of "cognitive functioning, behavior, motor function, achievement, social skills, personality, and neuropsychological functioning" (p. 58). Research focusing on congenital malformations of the brain and early hydrocephalus from congenital or perinatal causes, but including childhood-acquired left hemisphere stroke and traumatic head injury, shows that these children exhibit deficits in word-finding, anomia, and verbal fluency, with impairments persisting in some 7 years after injury (Dennis, 1992). Although gross linguistic impairments in children with severe head injury are typically transient, more subtle problems such as work retrieval, verbal organization, comprehension, verbal learning, and effective conversation are common (Ylvisaker, 1986). Indeed, it has been felt that deficits in "attention, perception, organizing processes, and functional integrative performance" can influence functioning in these areas (Ylvisaker, 1986, p. 112). Thus, a comprehensive approach to neuropsychological functioning is needed.

The neuropsychological approach must be comprehensive enough to include psychological functioning. A study of 32 patients aged 16 to 55 with severe TBI found that initial assessments of medical factors were related to adaptive physical functioning at discharge (Torkelson, Jellinek, Malec, & Harvey, 1983). However, those who were minimally aware of their physical abilities and limitations at admission improved in their adaptive physical functioning during treatment. The psychological factors were related to relative improvement in adaptive physical functioning when change occurred. Both physical and psychological functioning were related to length of rehabilitation stay.

Psychosocial outcome is equally important. The adult (defined as over 18 years old) outcome of severe closed head injury sustained by 12 adolescents discharged home and returned to school was dependence in many areas of adult functioning when assessed from the perspective of the patient and a primary caregiver (Bergland & Thomas, 1991). A recent review concluded that:

> Studies measuring psychosocial outcome in children and adolescents have shown that head injury leads to cognitive impairment that is directly related to the severity of injury in those with very severe head injury. Psychiatric disorders are also related to the severity of injury, but the relationship suggests that mediating factors are involved. No specific pattern of posttraumatic psychological/psychiatric dysfunction emerges from the studies, but it is clear that, as with adults, psychosocial recovery lags behind physical. Head injury affects the functioning of the young person in the family, at school, and within the wider community, often resulting in a secondary handicap of low self-esteem. (Livingston & McCabe, 1990, p. 255)

The Pediatric Rehabilitation Milieu

Diller and Gordon (1981) cite three types of environments that enter into rehabilitation: (a) physical (e.g., housing and transportation); (b) interpersonal (i.e., the immediate network of people around the patient); and (c) social (i.e., overt legal and covert norms and political/economic forces; for example, in a depressed economy, employment prospects for the disabled decline).

The interpersonal environment mentioned by Diller and Gordon could also be called the milieu. Much has been written about the social milieu of rehabilitation programs for individuals with TBI (Moore & Plovnik, 1991; Rattok et al., 1992). However, apart from the examination of the treatment team and its effectiveness within the social milieu with adult populations, formal manipulation of the sociotherapeutic environment for the pediatric populations has not been addressed. Prigatano and Ben-Yishay are probably credited with bringing milieu therapy per se into the neurorehabilitation arena with adults with brain injury, and it has long been recognized that an effective rehabilitation program should provide "individualized, round-the-clock service aimed at integrating therapeutic goals and objectives into day-to-day living so that the individual can achieve maximum independence" (Moore & Plovnik, 1991, p. 29).

Prigatano is perhaps the foremost proponent of using the psychotherapeutic milieu with individuals with brain injury. He extended the role of social work in rehabilitation from one of helping the patient and family adjust to brain injury and its sequelae to include an understanding of personality factors associated with successful outcomes. Prigatano (1988) also addressed the clinical understanding of the interplay between psychopathology and brain injury. In addition, small cohesive groups provide peer feedback about social skill deficits, a factor that provides therapeutic leverage (Grimm & Bleiberg, 1986; Rattok et al., 1992). Therefore, Prigatano's definition of the milieu (or holistic) approach to neurological rehabilitation is basically a program that "incorporates cognitive retraining activities with psychotherapy activities within the context of day treatment program" (Prigatano, 1990, p. 297).

The effectiveness of milieu therapy, especially with adolescents, has long been established by those who work in pediatric psychiatric setting (Abrahms, 1969; Bettleheim, 1969; Schwartz, Myers, & Astrachan, 1973). It is also well known to professionals in mental health rehabilitation who acknowledge that an appropriately structured rehabilitation milieu provides a nurturing, organizing, and generally helpful world for head-injured patients (Haarbauer-Krupa, Henry, Szekeres, & Ylvisaker, 1985; Rattok *et al.*, 1992). The growth in the last decade of pediatric rehabilitation settings that are designed for chronic and/or residential needs has prompted the establishment of planned therapeutic communities. The rehabilitation milieu provides a " . . . 'proving ground' gradually approximating a more naturalistic uncontrolled environment for patients to refine and experiment with their developing skills, hopefully without the tragic and negative consequences characteristic of highly demanding everyday life" (Grimm & Bleiberg, 1986, p. 526). Romano (1984) summarizes Kelman's three processes of influence at work in a rehabilitation milieu: (1) Compliance, when a patient is influenced to behave in a certain way in order to obtain rewards or punishments without regard to the content at hand; (2) identification, when the patient's behavior is influenced because he or she wants to establish or maintain a relationship with the group; and (3) internalization, when a patient accepts behavior because it is inherently rewarding and congruent with a value system.

In terms of structure, a milieu provides the patients with "stimulation, which can either confuse them further or contribute to cognitive recovery" (Haarbauer-Krupa, Moser, Smith, Sullivan, & Szekeres, 1985, p. 287). The rehabilitation team assists patients in making sense of the new environment and manipulates the programmatic structures within the milieu to reflect the patients' neuropsychological needs. Haarbauer-Krupa, Henry, Szekeres, and Ylvisaker (1985) propose seven principles of milieu treatment that describe the structure of rehabilitation milieu. The principles focus on the analysis of the complexity, relation, and duration of stimuli in the patient's external environment; coordination of family and staff approaches; predictability and familiarity of the physical setting; routines and repetition of events such as meals; use of a journal by the patient; and communication between the team members. A 6- to 39-month follow-up study of 24 patients with severe brain injury (aged 13 to 62 at admission) who had posttraumatic behavior disorders that had prevented rehabilitation in a more common setting showed lasting improvement from a token economy (Eames & Wood, 1985). It is impossible not to have

a milieu in a treatment program because an environment or milieu exists wherever individuals gather. On the other hand, it is a different question altogether as to whether the milieu is planned or unplanned. The proponents of interdisciplinary versus multidisciplinary teaming in rehabilitation settings have long considered the consequences of unplanned communities or milieu.

Interdisciplinary versus Multidisciplinary Rehabilitation Treatment Teams

Historically, the ideology of the team treating the individual with brain injury was aligned with the biomedical model. That team was made up of a neuropsychologist, clinical psychologist, medical social worker, dietitian, physical therapist, occupational therapist, speech–language pathologist, educational therapist, and other consultants as needed.

Cognitive rehabilitation was provided by the neuropsychologist, occupational therapist, or speech–language pathologist. The individual leading the team was the primary care physician or appropriate medical-surgical specialist in a model derived from medical-surgical care and codified in standards of the JCAHO (Joint Commission on Accreditation of Healthcare Organizations, 1993).

Essentially, the multidisciplinary model presupposes that the individual disciplines work on their separate treatment goals and report to the team leader (usually the attending physician) at regular intervals (Howard, 1991). In some models of rehabilitation treatment, the clinical psychologist and social work personnel are not included in the team. Sometimes the neuropsychologist is limited in role to that of consultant or diagnostician rather than rehabilitation therapist. Indeed, for many years rehabilitation has been viewed as the domain of physical, occupational, speech, recreation, and vocational therapists along with nursing staff. The multidisciplinary team is essentially a set of somewhat related disciplines brought together by one or two individuals. The patient's environment is essentially the living space that she or he shares with other patients interrupted by clinicians taking the patient from the unit to designated therapy rooms. This is not a milieu designed to view the patient as a whole. It is a planned milieu in that the program design reflects the needs of the biomedical model. However, the biomedical model does not plan a holistic view or treatment of the patient, and in this sense, it is a nontherapeutic milieu. Thus, it is not surprising that Ben-Yishay has suggested using such programs as the "control group" treatment to contrast with the results of a planned, holistic, neuropsychological milieu (Ben-Yishay, 1992).

The interdisciplinary team approach, although made up of the same disciplines, demands that team members work collaboratively on treatment goals, and the general themes of neuropsychological and functional rehabilitation are woven into all aspects of treatment (Campbell, 1981). This idea is not new to pediatric rehabilitation. Henry described an interdisciplinary cognitive rehabilitation therapy for school-age children with head injuries that emphasized strategies to compensate for deficits (Henry, 1983). In the current formulation of this model for rehabilitation, the physician and neuropsychologist work closely to facilitate the team's decisions about selection and assessment of treatment goals, but decisions are team centered rather than physician centered. The clinicians are a part of the patient's milieu at all times. Each clinician understands the individual goals of his or her discipline and the connection of each goal to the whole team and whole patient. The key premise behind the interdisciplinary process is that "the group produces a resultant quality of health care to patients that is greater than the sum of the care they would produce if working separately" (Schultz & Texidor, 1991, p. 2).

Interdisciplinary intervention has produced significant gains using a neurodevelopmental model with infants and children. It produced similar general progress and recovery patterns beyond maturation effects in infants and preschool children with acquired and congenital brain injuries (Bagnato & Mayes, 1986). Progress in this age group was measured in terms of developmental quotients, neurodevelopmental and neurobehavioral skills, and rhythmic behavior patterns (Bagnato & Neisworth, 1986). The measures used to set and prioritize goals, track progress, and assess outcome reflect the conceptual model of the therapists. Bagnato's group uses two levels of appraisal (administrative and clinical child) and three bases of assessment (normative, adaptive curriculum, and clinical judgment) (Bagnato, Mayes, Nichter, Domoto, & Smith, 1988). A 2-year follow-up of 14 of the 17 original cases was conducted (Bagnato & Neisworth, 1989). The average age at follow-up was 6 years 3 months. It was found that children with congenital impairments made better progress than those with acquired brain insult. Patient progress was related to number of days enrolled in early childhood education programming, frequency of therapy services, and parental involvement. The size of the study is very small. However, it is exemplary in being a rehabilitation treatment outcome study with children published in referred journals. In addition, the findings support the importance of rehabilitation rather than relying on the traditional belief in the power of spontaneous recovery in children.

The purpose of the model proposed in this chapter is to take the interdisciplinary, holistic, and neurodevelopmental program models and include inpatient psychotherapy with school-age populations into the design. If the milieu becomes the true focus of the program, then every clinician is working on the whole patient with good lateral communication between clinicians. Lateral communication with nursing staff extends the effects throughout the milieu, beyond the bounds of the therapy room. Thus, cost-effectiveness is achieved through replication of clinical effects throughout the milieu. This is a living and breathing program design that constantly fluctuates with the input of new learning and interchange between clinicians and the ever-changing nature of the patients involved.

The Neurodevelopmental Model of Pediatric Brain Injury Rehabilitation

The synthesis of successful elements of brain injury rehabilitation into a working paradigm is probably best illustrated by Ben-Yishay and the NYU group at the Rusk Institute in New York. A large part of the model presented in this chapter utilizes and adapts the clinical stages of the NYU program to a pediatric population that has an ongoing post-acute inpatient milieu. In addition, the model represents an interdisciplinary clinical paradigm for the treatment of children and adolescents with brain injury that lends itself to successful functional outcomes through the mechanism of holism and respect for the developmental autonomy of the patient; hence the term *neurodevelopmental rehabilitation model.*

The differences between the biomedical and neuropsychological paradigms of service delivery are clearly described in Table 1. Neither of these models, however, addresses the developmental concerns of the pediatric population. The neurodevelopmental model extends the elements of the neuropsychological paradigm by reflecting the status of the child within the environment, the fluid nature of pediatric development, and the responsibility of the team toward a minor individual. The specific extensions are outlined in Table 2.

The neurodevelopmental model was formulated to: (1) utilize the proven heuristic value of the clinical/cognitive stages originated by the NYU group, (2) extend the neuropsychological model to include pediatric concerns, (3) incorporate psychotherapeutic milieu elements into the rehabilitation treatment paradigm, and (4) sustain the interdisciplinary team as an effective component of rehabilitation treatment. The neurodevelopmental model is designed for the patient who has emerged from coma, become medically stable, and may or may not have returned home before admission to a post-acute rehabilitation setting. The program is characterized by the NYU cognitive adjustment stages that have been adapted to represent

TABLE 2. The Extension of the Neuropsychological Paradigm to the Neurodevelopmental Paradigm of Rehabilitation Service Delivery[a]

	Neuropsychological paradigm	Neurodevelopmental paradigm
Philosophy	Emergent, holistic	and, dynamic, adaptive
Primary mode.	Dysfunctional model	and functional/adaptive model
	Nonlinear assessment	and age-appropriate comparisons
Theories	Brain viewed as organ of interface presumes learning occurs	and, developmental level
Locus of dysfunction	In the interface between the individual and the environment	and as defined by authority figures
Role of provider	Consultant	and authority figure
	Treatment blamed for lack of success	and developmental level (ceiling)
Intrapsychic pathologizing	Eschewed	unless in familial framework
Premorbid factors	Primary importance	plus prediction of future performance
Role of patient	Equal and active participant	and subject to authority
Treatment options	Unlimited	and matched to developmental stage
Behavioral disturbances	Viewed positively	and developmentally with peer support
Staff	Active	and authority figures
Meaning	For patient	and family/peers
Service delivery	Flexible systems model	with family/peer/ milieu/direction
	Authoritative leadership	and consultants to family
	Team decision-making and conflict resolution	with family input and treatment continuation
	Staff collaboration	and family representation
	Health promotion model	and strength model of remediation
	Integrated treatment plans	tied to school reintegration and programming

[a]From Stanczak & Hutcherson (1992).

clinical stages of neurorehabilitation. Each stage marks the clinical task for the patient and team, allows for ongoing assessment of progress toward outcome, and is useful for program evaluation. The process of rehabilitation (as opposed to the content) is the central focus at all times.

In the neurodevelopmental model, the first meeting of the pediatric interdisciplinary team marks the beginning of the synthesis of treatment. Each discipline is aware of the stages of clinical adjustment and translates their assessment and treatment recommendations through the language of these stages. In order for a large team of professionals to understand each other and work on the same goals, there must be a common language and a consensus about treatment approach that speaks to all disciplines at once without compromising the integrity of those disciplines. Hence, a speech pathologist and social worker can be working with the same patient, with their respective discipline-specific goals and yet be synchronous. If the team is to work consistently within a given paradigm, the central principles of the paradigm must be ones that can be easily remembered, understood, and translated. These central principles must be stated in a common language that is efficient and elegant. The following stages of rehabilitation treatment are adapted from the cognitive adjustment stages devised by Ben-Yishay and his colleagues. They can provide a universal language for the interdisciplinary team that is concise and simple to remember. At the first treatment team meeting, the team will describe the patient's initial status in terms of the six stages of clinical adjustment.

Stage 1: Engagement

Engagement is the patient's minimum level of investment in the rehabilitation program. It is possible for a patient to be admitted into the hospital and for a variety of reasons refuse to mediate the environment. Many times, this entry for adolescents is not essentially voluntary. The patient has become medically stable but is far from functional independence, and the continuation of treatment is a disappointing and frustrating detour from the initial hopes of returning home. The adolescent does not essentially have a legal or medical say in the decision for inpatient rehabilitation, and the involuntary nature of admission may result in the patient denying any need for treatment, grieving the lack of ability to return home, and refusing to engage. Therefore, after perhaps months of challenging circumstances in the acute care hospital, the patient and family face a new set of rules, expectations, and information.

The team members assess the patient's level of cognitive and affective engagement in treatment. This can be done by answering an assortment of questions that translate directly to treatment goals. An example of questions used for assessment and documentation of progress through this process is shown in Table 3. The patient's adjustment is observed in the milieu. The questions that must be addressed include: "Does the patient acknowledge that he or she has a reason for being in the hospital?" "Does the patient acknowledge the therapist's expertise and authority?" "Does the patient attend therapies willingly?" "Does the patient understand the milieu/unit rules and expectations?" All disciplines may measure engagement by documenting such instances as number of therapies refused, frequency of agitation and oppositional behaviors at initiation of therapy times, and instances when the patient denies knowledge of milieu rules (not accounted for by memory impairment). Documenting observable instances of nonengagement and engagement will assist the team in (1) determining what level of engagement is necessary or acceptable for individual patients, and (2) developing specific treatment goals related to facilitating transition to the next step of adjustment.

The patient who is unengaged may be so for many reasons. This could simply be a time of orientation and initial adjustment. The patient may need some time to reserve judgment as to whether the program is an appropriate placement for her or him. Entry could also be hampered by typical neuropsychological deficits associated with brain injury such as memory difficulties, lack of impulse control, unawareness of prominent features of brain injury, separation from family, and general disruption in surroundings. The team must be wary of producing oppositional behavior by overcontrolling the patient under the guise of providing structure, or by using a schedule that perpetuates fatigue.

In most cases, if a patient is not engaged in therapy, it will be reported by most or all team members. This, then, becomes the focal point for the group and the point of treatment entry for the patient. The manner in which the team assists the patient with engagement is a key interdisciplinary goal for the whole team. Each discipline has specific goals to target engagement within a specific period of time (e.g., 2 weeks) until a reevaluation can be made by the team. For example, the team may decide that engagement is best facilitated by each therapist allowing the patient to choose a "fun" activity for therapy after they have engaged in "work" for a specified number of minutes. The "work" time can be extended as the patient achieves compliance and rapport with the therapists. In other cases of nonengagement the team may simply want to allow rapport to naturally build between the patient and the team. In some cases, peer modeling of engagement can be very powerful and is developed simply by observation of the milieu. The child who is able to acknowledge verbal communication may benefit from empathic statements by therapists about how hard it is for someone of the patient's age to accept help from adults outside the family (or if the patient is an adolescent, help from any adult) balanced by statements about how that help is necessary because of the brain injury. Any intervention is designed by the team after an extensive evaluation, and is tailored to each patient. If the patient does not have difficulties engaging in therapy and the treatment process, then this area is acknowledged but not addressed.

There may be instances where a patient in treatment is engaged and then becomes disengaged because of frustration, family issues, and the like. At this time, the team may wish to revisit this stage and problem-solve the cause of the disengagement and strategies for reengagement. In the event that some team members report engagement and other team members do not, then this is an ideal time for the team to problem-solve the strong and weak areas of both programming and individual therapist and strategies for assisting individual therapist and strategies for assisting individual team members or disciplines. From a psychosocial viewpoint, nonengagement could be a simple lack of adjustment to a new and highly structured environment. A psychotherapeutic view of nonengagement may be that rapport has not been established with the patient. Physical therapists may interpret a lack of engagement as avoidance of physical pain. Each discipline can tap into the issue of nonengagement and develop discipline-specific and team goals to solve the problem. It should be stressed that engagement, regardless of discipline interpretation, is fundamental to the course of rehabilitation treatment. If engagement is not established with the team, then successes in different therapies will appear seldom and random. The superficially compliant but unengaged patient may demonstrate more functional behavior in the context of the therapy room, but fail to later show change in other environments. The latter is symptomatic of fragmented services that service discipline-specific goals at the expense of therapeutic movement for the patient as a whole. It is all too easy for multidisciplinary therapists to proceed with discipline-specific goals for an unengaged patient and then attempt to explain the predictable lack of progress with labels such as "unmotivated" or references to the patient's premorbid personality characteristics. Much of the psychological and psychiatric consultation in a multidisciplinary model is for teams trying to treat an unengaged patient as if the patient were engaged in therapy. A conscious and planned system of interdisciplinary intervention should produce general therapeutic movement.

Stage 2: Awareness

Anosognosia (a lack of knowledge about a recognition deficit) was formally recognized as long ago as 1914 by Babinski (Kilstrom & Tobias, 1991; Prigatano & Schacter, 1991). According to Kilstrom and Tobias, Babinski defined unawareness as the patient being unaware of any problems in memory, language, perception, or voluntary movement. Unawareness could be evidenced by: (1) the patient not acknowledging that there is anything wrong, (2) the patient acknowledging difficulty but attributing it to some source other than the known cause, or (3) the patient actively denying any difficulty at all. In addition, Prigatano and Klonoff (1991) argue that a deficit in self-awareness is the most limiting factor in the psychotherapeutic treatment of individuals with TBI and therefore results in a negative impact on long-term outcome. Schacter and Prigatano (1991) believe that "describing patients as 'aware' or 'unaware' of their deficits does not do full justice to the subtleties of awareness disturbances" (p. 261). They make distinctions between defensive denial of deficits versus neural bases of unawareness and note a lack of formal or objective measures of unawareness in brain-injured individuals. Prigatano (1991b) states that an understanding of individual awareness deficits is important not only to assist the patient in the process of self-appraisal but because:

> self awareness emerges primarily in the areas of the brain deemed heteromodal cortex. This region is important for integrating what might broadly be called "cognitive" and "affective" components of experience. Learning any new behavior, as well as attempts at relearning "old" behaviors, might well require involvement from these structures. That is, awareness of various components of the self (or higher cerebral mediated activities) is by definition important for relearning necessary in neurorehabilitation. (p. 123)

It is important for the team treating pediatric patients to distinguish yet a third possible factor associated with unawareness and that is the cognitive and/or developmental level of the patient. Is it reasonable to expect a 12-year-old with severe TBI to ever be aware of his or her specific cognitive and psychosocial deficits and the long-term impact of those deficits? If so, to what extent? Would the impact of brain injury at latency age permanently alter a child's ability to develop awareness? Is it developmentally appropriate for adolescents with brain injury to exhibit moderate amounts of defensive denial/unawareness? All of these questions must be posed with each pediatric patient. The developmental expectations for the patient will determine awareness goals, and in some cases the reverse may be true.

Awareness, then, is a process for the pediatric patient with brain injury. It is a progression of understanding about her or his residual or anticipatory neurobehavioral deficits that result from the injury. The patient is aware that there are specific sequelae from the brain injury that affect everyday functioning. In addition, this awareness includes "optimum responsiveness to treatments and the ability and willingness to modify one's maladaptive behaviors" (Ben-Yishay & Gold, 1990, p. 197). The compensatory strategies that are patient specific are usually domain specific and are introduced to the patient by the individual therapist. The unaware patient is introduced to assessments made about his or her psychosocial and neuropsychological strengths and weaknesses. In addition, assessment results are tied to interventions and specific therapy goals. Many times in rehabilitation, the introduction of compensatory strategies and techniques for the adolescent with brain injury occurs via the rules of the program. The patients "learn by doing in the clinical environment" (Moore & Plovnik, 1991, p. 501). For example, all patients may use a memory notebook or journal. It is expected of all patients, and therefore the individual becomes aware of a milieu-based strategy simply because it is the rule. Staff members are knowledgeable of the benefits of memory books and reiterate the usage and benefits on a daily basis in the milieu. In this way, many patients become aware of one of the common sequelae to brain injury.

Awareness is the conscious extension of the engagement stage. The patient is cooperative in therapies for the most part, and exhibits membership in the milieu. The team evaluates awareness by addressing obvious questions about patient performance. "How does the patient respond to assessment results given by the team?" "Does the patient express interest in his or her individual progress?" "Does the patient exhibit community awareness in the milieu?" "Does the patient participate in the milieu and therapies?" "Does the patient acknowledge that she or he has deficits associated with her or his medical condition and/or brain injury?" "Does the patient understand the consequences of the deficits?" "Does the patient understand specific treatment goals targeted in the treatment plan?" "Does the patient accept/agree with treatment goals?" (See Table 3.)

The awareness stage of treatment may be very difficult for adolescents because emotional lability and behavior problems are inherently severe for this age group (McGuire & Sylvester, 1990). Becoming aware of severe and long-term sequelae is not a pleasant process and many adolescents will typically resist limits and authority (Barin, Hanchett, Jacob, & Scott, 1985). The usual education that assists normalization with regard to adjustment to injury for adults is not as reassuring for adolescents. The life experience for adolescents is short, and they have fewer overlearned coping skills premorbidly on which to draw for assistance (Haarbauer-Krupa, Moser, Smith, Sullivan, & Szekeres, 1985). It is difficult to normalize experiences that have to be synchronized with the separation and individuation tasks of the adolescent. Hence, the team must satisfy the need of the adolescent patient to feel that his or her adjustment to the brain injury is appropriate and yet he or she can remain or become an independent entity. Although an adult's self-confidence can be bolstered by accessing memories of previous success at becoming independent after passing through adolescence, the adolescent has nothing to access other than the normal facade or feigning of not needing help from an adult. The milieu must make up for this by providing more support and structure to the adolescent than the adult patient would need.

Stage 3: Mastery

This is the stage where the patient is in the process of mastering compensatory techniques for the deficits identified by the interdisciplinary team. For most patients, a repertoire of skills must be learned that focus on functional or cognitive deficits. Haarbauer-Krupa, Henry, Szekeres, and Ylvisaker (1985) provide a detailed list of variables to consider in the selection and training of compensatory strategies. The variables range from the consideration of developmental factors to type and extent of brain injury. The list provides a comprehensive framework for the team when the mastery stage is negotiated. This stage is, perhaps, the easiest to assess because treatment goals are distinct and measurable. For example, the patient learning a selection of cognitive behavioral techniques to reduce physical aggression is a common task set for an adolescent. The techniques can be taught in the milieu, community groups, individual and group therapies, or essentially anywhere in the rehabilitation setting. The individual counselor or psychotherapist may be the person responsible for the direct teaching of the strategies but the team is responsible for incorporating and/or facilitating generalization of training.

In terms of assessment, the patient receives the information and demonstrates retention of the information. Questions that would be appropriate for this stage may be: "Does the patient exhibit understanding of the concept of the compensatory strategies?" "Does the patient exhibit engagement in learning compensatory strategies?" "Does the patient exhibit consistent advancement in content knowledge of strategies?" "Does the patient effectively use compensatory strategies when prompted?" "Does the patient exhibit at least 90% mastery of strategies?" For each brain injury patient, the team develops a list of specific goals that are presented to the patient for mastery. Knowledge of a compensatory strategy and spontaneous use of a strategy, however, are two different things.

Stage 4: Control

Control is represented by the patient demonstrating mastery of a compensatory strategy and also demonstrating spontaneous employment of that strategy in the milieu. In the case of the first example above, a patient would demonstrate understanding and knowledge of compensatory strategies to extinguish physical aggression and then would demonstrate use of one or more of the strategies to extinguish physical aggression and then would demonstrate use of one or more of the strategies when confronted with a situation that would normally evoke physical aggression. The patient may, for example, start a verbal altercation with a peer in the milieu and instead of escalating to aggression, the patient requests staff to assist him or her in a self-imposed time-out to cool down. The strategy is initiated spontaneously by the patient and the results or consequences of the employment of the strategy are immediate (i.e., the patient is positively reinforced for choosing the strategy).

The team assesses this stage by observing the patient spontaneously using compensatory strategies in the milieu. It may be the observation that the patient is using a memory notebook on a consistent basis, is refraining from entering the personal space of peers, or is utilizing social skills (e.g., introductions, eye contact, nonverbal cues). The latter examples are measurable and dependent on the clinicians being aware of the patient not only in specific therapies but in the general milieu as well. Questions that the team may ask at this stage could be: "Does the patient spontaneously demonstrate compensatory strategies in the milieu?" "Does the patient demonstrate compensatory strategies in different environments? "Does the patient remark on inappropriate behaviors of peers?" "Does the patient need significantly less cues to use compensatory techniques?"

This completion of the control stage is critical if the patient is able to live outside an institution or at least a constantly supervised setting. If the patient cannot control the compensatory strategies in the inpatient milieu, then the chances for generalization on reentry are slim. Laments of patients being successful in the rehabilitation setting and failures in real life are replete in the rehabilitation literature (Ben-Yishay & Prigatano, 1990; Bruce, 1990; Cicerone & Tupper, 1991; Grimm & Bleiberg, 1986). The essence of control, therefore, is the emergence of generalization.

With regard to the patient who does not demonstrate control of any compensatory strategies, the team must revisit the initial goals for mastery and assess if the level of mastery is sufficient for generalization. It may be that in some cases the nature (deficits in executive functioning or metacognition) or severity of the brain injury may preclude a desirable level of control. For the "patient with a brain injury," it is a difficult process to recognize when a problem is developing or exists, inhibit an initial and perhaps "emotional" response, imagine a desired outcome, consider multiple possible responses based on matching previous experiences with the present problem in context, and then choose a response based on predictions of the likelihood of success. Yet to be efficient, the patient must also sometimes allow the quick overlearned response to occur without conscious, verbal mediation. For the team, it is easy to have assumed that the patient needed a program of instruction in coping skills when more careful assessment may reveal the patient has more coping skills than are used because of metacognitive and executive deficits. Brain injury rehabilitation borrowed self-instructional training (literally teaching the patient how to think himself or herself through solving a problem) from clinical psychology where it became popular in the treatment of impulsive children with attention deficit hyperactivity disorder (ADHD) (Haarbauer-Krupa, Henry, Szekeres, & Ylvisaker, 1985; Szerkeres, Ylvisaker, & Holland, 1985). Unfortunately, after 20 years of research there is still a lack of scientific evidence that this approach leads to mastery outside the therapy room for impulsive children (Abikoff, 1985, 1991). Without scientific evidence, there is no reason to persist in using the same techniques for brain-injured children in the hope that they will somehow achieve generalization and mastery through that approach.

If the patient with brain injury does not master use of compensatory strategies, then discharge planning is facilitated by the fact that the patient has reached a level of independence and will require a given level of structure in the next placement. For example, a patient may be able to master the memory notebook in the milieu with staff assistance and cues. Whether the patient moves to self-sufficiency regarding the memory notebook or remains dependent on external cues to use the book is the fundamental difference between mastery and control. The difference will have far-reaching effects for independent living on patient reentry.

Stage 5: Acceptance

Acceptance is related to control in that now the patient incorporates the changes in her or his life while consciously accepting personal deficits. The patient and team have an ongoing verbal discourse at this time that has been predicated on the patient learning new aspects of the self that have been transformed into measurable and successful tasks. This stage is characterized by the patient taking pride in her or his accomplishments and demonstrating generalization of training. In addition, many times the patient becomes a role model for other patients and is an active member of the milieu. For adolescents, membership in the milieu includes an acceptance of the authority and expertise of staff as well as acceptance from peers as an experienced patient. In terms of the example given above, a patient would spontaneously use compensatory strategies to solve problems on a regular basis. In terms of team assessment, the frequency of use of compensatory strategies would be higher than in the mastery and/or control

stages. In addition, the team would observe the patient identifying deficits in peers and offering advice to those peers as to how to use compensatory strategies to avoid physical aggression, for example. Peer-to-peer redirection is a powerful intervention in the adolescent milieu (Grimm & Bleiberg, 1986) and is only evidenced when more experienced and successful patients achieve acceptance and serve as guides to patients who have not yet achieved control of compensatory strategies. Therefore, assessment of this stage would be characterized by questions such as: "Does the patient consistently use compensatory strategies in therapy?" "Does the patient consistently use compensatory strategies across environments?" "Does the patient refer to himself or herself as a patient retrospectively?" "Does the patient consistently take on role model status in groups and milieu?" "Does the patient incorporate compensatory strategies into reentry planning?" (See Table 3.)

Stage 6: Identity

Identity is the last stage of clinical adjustment in the neurodevelopmental model. It consists of the patient becoming temporarily aware of his or her progress through the former stages. This stage, as with the others, is interpreted within a developmental context. It is not appropriate for a 13-year-old to exhibit the formulation of identity that we would expect with an 18-year-old. The latter has a component of emancipation from the family that is developmentally desirable and predictable. The 13-year-old, on the other hand, is not ready for emancipation and identity formation. Indeed, the goal for this age group is to exhibit age-appropriate movement *toward* identity formation. The successful patient, in the identity stage, exhibits developmentally appropriate understanding of the events surrounding the injury, the residual deficits, and the mastery and control of compensatory strategies. Developmental issues are critical in assessing the identity stage. It is the reintegration of the patient at an age-specific period and is assessed with questions such as: "Does the patient initiate changes in design/content of compensatory strategies?" "Does the patient take an active part in discharge planning?" "Does the patient exhibit realistic goals for reentry?" "Does the patient refer to himself or herself as a person who has worked through trauma?"

The patient is consciously aware of the progress made in treatment and is cognizant of the realistic implications of the brain injury. The patient also exhibits

TABLE 3. Example of Patient Progress Summary of the Milestones in Cognitive Adjustment to Brain Injury

I	I	I	I	I	I
Engagement	Awareness	Mastery	Control	Acceptance	Identity

Stage 1: Engagement   Date demonstrated

   Acknowledges at least one sequela as a reason for being in the hospital

   Separates from his/her family to attend therapy

   Understands the milieu/unit rules and expectations (May be shown by trying to find "loopholes")

   Understands the rules and expectations of individual and group therapies

   Attends a majority of therapies willingly

   Cooperates with a majority of therapist requests

Stage 2: Awareness   Date demonstrated

   Acknowledges sequelae beyond concrete (such as inability to walk or speak clearly) symptoms

   Attributes impairments to brain injury and functional disabilities that result from impairments

   Can discuss his/her brain injury directly rather than use terms such as "the accident" or "my head injury"

   Accepts/agrees with at least some treatment goals beyond concrete symptoms

Stage 3: Mastery   Date demonstrated

   Exhibits understanding of concept of the compensatory strategies

   Exhibits engagement in learning compensatory strategies

   Contributes suggestions (by work or deed) as to how to compensate for disabilities

   Exhibits consistent advancement in content knowledge of strategies

Stage 4: Control   Date demonstrated

   Spontaneously demonstrates compensatory strategies for therapists

   Uses compensatory strategies in the milieu when coached through the process

   Uses compensatory strategies in the milieu when told which strategy to use

   Uses compensatory strategies in the milieu when simply cued to "stop and think"

   Spontaneously demonstrates compensatory strategies in the milieu

   Demonstrates compensatory strategies in different environments

   Remarks on inappropriate behaviors of peers

Stage 5: Acceptance   Date demonstrated

   Acknowledges present and future need for compensatory strategies

   Refers to his/her rehabilitation as a necessary process that is nearing completion

   Takes on role model status in groups and milieu (for example, recommends same compensatory strategies to peers)

   Incorporates compensatory strategies into planning for future events such as reentry

Stage 6: Identity   Date demonstrated

   Initiates changes in design/content of compensatory strategies (within his/her ability)

   Takes an active part in discharge planning

   Exhibits goals for reentry as realistic as expected for age

   Refers to him/herself as a person who has worked through trauma or risen to the challenge of the injury

   Possesses a sense of personal dignity and positive self-worth and sees the course of his/her life as altered but worth living

age-appropriate levels of identity formation. At all times, the emphasis is on the patient making choices for the future that are as realistic as would be expected for his or her age. The team's focus is on the appropri-ateness of placement at discharge and an accumulation of *in vivo* experiences that assist the maintenance of skills developed in treatment at this stage. Hence, discharge planning and reentry issues are the focus of treatment. Many times, the level of synthesis needed for this stage may be precluded by the severity of brain injury and/or level of maturity. In addition, the duration of stay in many facilities does not allow patients the time necessary to accomplish the goals of the identity stage or even earlier stages with patients who are unengaged in the rehabilitation process at admission. This places additional pressure on reentry into school or the services that bridge the gap between the rehabilitation hospital and the school.

Summary and Conclusions

This chapter has focused on the history of brain injury treatment as it pertains to the development and gradual definition of the role of neuropsychology in rehabilitation. Neuropsychology has played an important part in assisting the medical profession in the diagnosis and localization of brain damage. With the increase in objective medical technology and the advancement of the field of rehabilitation, neuropsychology has come to serve in the areas of assessment and treatment of cognitive and neurobehavioral strengths and weaknesses associated with brain injury. The shift from localization to function has been reflected in the development of theoretical paradigms that are holistic versus reductionistic. Holistic programs represent neuropsychological principles whereas reductionistic programs serve the biomedical position.

While the biomedical and neuropsychological paradigms have a large research base with adult populations, little has been written about pediatric groups. The differences between adult and pediatric programming are substantial and essentially entail the problem of assessing and predicting outcomes for individuals who are in the process of developing. Issues surrounding family involvement must be handled differently within the educational and inclusion approach of interdisciplinary rehabilitation. Determining appropriate school placement is difficult, given that most teacher training in TBI is sparse and brief (Sohlberg & Mateer, 1989). Reentry is challenging for children and it is compounded by decreasing lengths of stay which are financially rather than clinically determined.

The neurodevelopmental model was formulated to: (1) utilize the proven heuristic value of the clinical/cognitive stages originated by the NYU group, (2) extend the neuropsychological model to include pediatric concerns, (3) incorporate psychotherapeutic milieu elements into the rehabilita-

tion treatment paradigm, and (4) sustain the interdisciplinary team as an effective component of rehabilitation treatment. The neurodevelopmental model aligns the interdisciplinary team with a framework of assisting the patient through six clinical stages of rehabilitation. The first two stages, engagement and awareness, seek to orient the patient to the difficult task at hand, set limits and expectations, and mark the beginning of a partnership between the patient and team. The next two stages, mastery and control, involve the learning of compensatory strategies that are individualized for each patient and the beginning of generalization of those strategies in the milieu. The last two stages, acceptance and identity, focus on patients incorporating their experiences (both positive and negative) into their self-concept and rehearsing reentry and discharge decisions and actions. The clinical stages are the unifying elements that allow different disciplines to communicate and accurately assess patient progress at any time. At any given stage, the team can assess patient progress and task analyze problems in progression. In essence, most patients will enter treatment unengaged and leave treatment with a synthesis of what and how treatment has affected them. In addition, the team may predict the stage at discharge that is appropriate for the patient and recommend placements that are commensurate with mastery and control. Program evaluation is essential and must include this six-step linear model of patient progress.

The neurodevelopmental model is concrete and therefore provides a means for quantifiable evaluation of its effectiveness and basis for further empirical studies that are important in the development of effective pediatric rehabilitation programs. In addition, the model becomes an effective teaching tool for patients, families, and staff. The framework allows for anyone in the milieu to be aware of the patient's immediate rehabilitation and milieu needs, and it allows those individuals to have a basic means of assessment of patient progress. Families are much more likely to participate in treatment and feel a part of the team if they understand and use the same language to describe their experience. The families, after all, are the individuals who carry the pediatric patient from one setting to another. Most often, the patient makes the transition from facility to home and, notwithstanding the best of discharge planning, the family members shoulder much (or all) of the responsibility for supporting the continuum of care and ultimately are the caregivers after formal rehabilitation is finished. It is up to the rehabilitation treatment team, then, to support the pediatric patient and family with treatment that transcends discipline and setting.

References

Abikoff, H. (1985). Efficacy of cognitive training interventions in hyperactive children: A critical review. Special Issue: Attention deficit disorder: Issues in assessment and intervention. *Clinical Psychology Review, 5* (5), 479–512.

Abikoff, H. (1991). Cognitive training in ADHD children: Less to it than meets the eye. *Journal of Learning Disabilities, 24* (4), 205–209.

Abrahms, G. M. (1969). Milieu therapy. *Archives of General Psychiatry, 21,* 259– 286.

Allen, K., Linn, R. T., Guiterrez, H., & Willer, B. S. (1994). Family burden following traumatic brain injury. *Rehabilitation Psychology, 39* (1), 29–48.

American Psychiatric Association. (1994). *Diagnostic and statistical manual of mental disorders* (4th ed.). Washington, DC: Author.

Bagnato, S. J., & Mayes, S. D. (1986). Pattern of developmental and behavioral progress for young brain-injured children during interdisciplinary intervention. *Developmental Neuropsychology, 2* (3), 213–240.

Bagnato, S. J., Mayes, S. D., Nichter, C., Domoto, V., & Smith, E. A. (1988). An interdisciplinary neurodevelopmental assessment model for brain-injured infants and preschool children. *Journal of Head Trauma Rehabilitation, 3* (2), 75–86.

Bagnato, S. J., & Neisworth, J. T. (1986). Tracing developmental recovery from early brain injury. *Remedial and Special Education, 7* (5), 31–36.

Bagnato, S. J., & Neisworth, J. T. (1989). Neurodevelopmental outcomes of early brain injury: A follow-up of fourteen case studies. *Topics in Early Childhood Special Education, 9* (1), 72–89.

Ball, J. D., & Zinner, E. S. (1993). Pediatric traumatic brain injury: Psychoeducation for parents and teachers. *Advances in Medical Psychotherapy, 7,* 39–50.

Barber, T. X. (1976). *Pitfalls in human research: Ten pivotal points.* New York: Pergamon Press.

Barin, J. J., Hanchett, J. M., Jacob, W. L., & Scott, M. B. (1985). Counseling the head injured patient. In M. Ylvisaker (Ed.), *Head injury rehabilitation: Children and adolescents* (pp. 361–382). Boston: College-Hill.

Begali, V. (1992). *Head injury in children and adolescents.* Brandon, VT: Clinical Psychology Publishing Company.

Ben-Yishay, Y. (1992, August). *Psychotherapeutic intervention following head injury.* Seminary presented at the Albert Einstein College of Medicine's Cape Cod Institute, North Eastham, MA.

Ben-Yishay, Y. (1993). Cognitive remediation in traumatic brain injury. *Archives of Physical Medicine and Rehabilitation. 74,* 205–213.

Ben-Yishay, Y., & Gold, J. (1990). Therapeutic milieu approach to neuropsychological rehabilitation. In R. L. Wood (Ed.),

Neuro-behavioral sequelae of traumatic brain injury (pp. 194–215). Hillsdale, NJ: Erlbaum.

Ben-Yishay, Y., & Prigatano, G. P. (1990). Cognitive remediation. In M. Rosenthal, E. R. Griffith, M. R. Bond, & J. D. Miller (Eds.), *Rehabilitation of the adult and child with traumatic brain injury* (2nd ed., pp. 393–409). Philadelphia: Davis.

Bergland, M. M., & Thomas, K. R. (1991). Psychosocial issues following severe head injury in adolescence: Individual and family perceptions. *Rehabilitation Counseling Bulletin, 35* (1), 5–22.

Bettleheim, B. (1969). *Children of the dream.* New York: Macmillan Co.

Bigler, E. (1990). *Traumatic brain injury.* Austin, TX: PRO-ED.

Boake, C. (1989). A history of cognitive rehabilitation of head-injured patient, 1915 to 1980. *Journal of Head Trauma Rehabilitation, 4* (3), 1–8.

Boake, C. (1991). History of cognitive rehabilitation following head injury. In J. Kreutzer & P. H. Wehman (Eds.), *Cognitive rehabilitation for persons with traumatic brain injury* (pp. 3–12). Baltimore: Brookes.

Boll, T. J., & Barth, J. T. (1981). Neuropsychology of brain damage in children. In T. J. Boll & S. B. Filsov (Eds.), *Handbook of clinical neuropsychology* (pp. 418–452). New York: Wiley

Brodsky, P. (1988). Follow-up on youngest REHABIT client: Importance of caution. *Perceptual and Motor Skills, 66* (2), 383–386.

Brodsky, P., Brodsky, M., Lee, H., & Sever, J. (1986). Two evaluation studies of Reitan's REHABIT program for the retraining of brain dysfunctions. *Perceptual and Motor Skills, 63* (2, Pt. 1), 501–502.

Bruce, D. A. (1990). Scope of the problem—Early assessment and management. In M. Rosenthal, E. R. Griffith, M. R. Bond, & J. D. Miller (Eds.), *Rehabilitation of the adult and child with traumatic brain injury* (2nd ed., pp. 521–537). Philadelphia: Davis.

Burke, W. (1988). *Head injury rehabilitation: An overview.* Houston: HDI.

Campbell, R. J. (1981). *Psychiatric dictionary* (5th ed.). London: Oxford University Press.

Carney, J., & Gerring, J. (1990). Return to school following severe closed head injury: A critical phase in pediatric rehabilitation. *Pediatrician, 17* (4), 222–229.

Cicerone, K. D., & Tupper, D. E. (1991). Neuropsychological rehabilitation: Treatment of errors in everyday functioning. In K. D. Cicerone & D. E. Tupper (Eds.), *The neuropsychology of everyday life: Issues in development and rehabilitation* (pp. 271–292). Boston: Kluwer.

Cossu, S. (1994, April). Invited lunch speaker at the Carolinas Brain Injury Symposium, Columbia, SC.

Crokett, D., Clark, C., & Klonoff, H. (1981). Introduction—An overview of neuropsychology. In S. B. Filsov & T. J. Boll (Eds.), *Handbook of clinical neuropsychology* (pp. 1–37). New York: Wiley.

Dahmer, E. R., Shilling, M. A., Hamilton, B. B., Bontke, C. F., & Smith, E. A. (1993). A model systems database for traumatic brain injury. *Journal of Head Trauma Rehabilitation, 8* (2), 12–25.

Deaton, A. (1990). Behavioral change strategies for children and adolescents with traumatic brain injury. In E. Bigler (Ed.), *Traumatic brain injury* (pp. 231–250). Austin, TX: PRO-ED.

Dennis, M. (1992). Word finding in children and adolescents with a history of brain injury. *Topics in Language Disorders, 13* (1), 66–82.

Diller, L. (1987). Neuropsychological rehabilitation. In M. Meier, A. Benton, & L. Diller (Eds.), *Neuropsychological rehabilitation* (pp. 1–3). New York: Guilford Press.

Diller, L., & Gordon, W. A. (1981). Rehabilitation and clinical neuropsychology. In T. J. Boll & S. B. Filsov (Eds.), *Handbook of clinical neuropsychology* (pp. 702–733). New York: Wiley.

Divak, J. A., Herrle, J., & Scott, M. B. (1985). Behavior management. In M. Ylvisaker (Ed.), *Head injury rehabilitation* (pp. 347–360). Boston: College-Hill.

Eames, P., & Wood, R. (1985). Rehabilitation after severe brain injury: A follow-up of a behavior modification approach. *Journal of Neurology, Neurosurgery and Psychiatry, 48* (7), 613–619.

Ewert, J., Levin, H. S., Watson, M. G., & Kalisky, Z. (1989). Procedural memory during posttraumatic amnesia in survivors of severe closed head injury: Implications for rehabilitation. *Archives of Neurology, 46* (8), 911–916.

Ewing-Cobbs, L., & Fletcher, J. M. (1990). Neuropsychological assessment of traumatic brain injury in children. In E. D. Bigler (Ed.), *Traumatic brain injury* (pp. 107–128). Austin, TX: PRO-ED.

Ewing-Cobbs, L., Fletcher, J. M., & Levin, H. S. (1985). Neuropsychological sequela following pediatric head injury. In M. Ylvisaker (Ed.), *Head injury rehabilitation: Children and adolescents* (pp. 71–89). Boston: College Hill.

Franzen, M. D. (1989). *Reliability and validity in neuropsychological assessment.* New York: Plenum Press.

Galski, T., Bruno, R. L., & Ehle, H. T. (1993). Prediction of behind-the-wheel driving performance in patients with cerebral brain damage: A discriminant function analysis. *American Journal of Occupational Therapy, 47* (5), 391–396.

Galski, T., Ehle, H. T., & Bruno, R. L. (1990). An assessment of measures to predict the outcome of driving evaluations in patients with cerebral damage. *American Journal of Occupational Therapy, 44* (8), 709–713.

Gans, B. M., Mann, N. R., & Ylvisaker, M. (1990). Rehabilitation management approaches. In M. Rosenthal, E. R. Griffith, M. R. Bond, & J. D. Miller (Eds.), *Rehabilitation of the adult and child with traumatic brain injury* (2nd ed., pp. 593–614). Philadelphia: Davis.

Garske, G. G., & Thomas, K. R. (1992). Self-reported self-esteem and depression: Indexes of psychosocial adjustment following severe traumatic brain injury. *Rehabilitation Counseling Bulletin, 36* (1), 44–52.

Gerring, J. P., & Carney, J. M. (1992). *Head trauma* (2nd ed.). San Diego: Singular.

Giles, G. M., & Fussey, I. (1988). Models of brain injury rehabilitation: From theory to practice. In I. Fussey & G. M. Giles

(Eds.), *Rehabilitation of the severely brain injured adult: A practical approach* (p. 1029). London: Croom-Helm.

Golden, C. J. (1979). Neurotherapy for the brain injured child. *Academic Therapy, 15* (2), 201–207.

Goldstein, F. C., & Levin, H. S. (1990). Epidemiology of traumatic brain injury: Incidence, clinical characteristics and risk factors. In E. Bigler (Ed.), *Traumatic brain injury* (pp. 51–67). Austin, TX: PRO-ED.

Goldstein, G. (1987). Neuropsychological assessment for rehabilitation: Fixed batteries, automated systems and non-psychometric methods, In M. J. Meier, A. L. Benton, & L. Diller (Eds.), *Neuropsychological rehabilitation* (pp. 18–40). New York: Guilford Press.

Grimm, B. H., & Bleiberg, J. (1986). Psychological rehabilitation in traumatic brain injury. In T. J. Boll & S. B. Filsov (Eds.), *Handbook of clinical neuropsychology* (Vol. 2, pp. 495–560). New York: Wiley.

Gronwall, D., Wrightson, P., & Waddell, P. (1990). *Head injury: the facts: A guide for families and care-givers.* London: Oxford University Press.

Haarbauer-Krupa, J., Henry, K., Szekeres, S. F., & Ylvisaker, M. (1985). Cognitive rehabilitation therapy: Late stages of recovery. In M. Ylvisaker (Ed.), *Head injury rehabilitation: Children and adolescents* (pp. 311–346). Boston: College-Hill.

Haarbauer-Krupa, J., Moser, L., Smith, G., Sullivan, D. M., & Szekeres, S. F. (1985). Cognitive rehabilitation therapy: Middle stages of recovery. In M. Ylvisaker (Ed.), *Head injury rehabilitation: Children and adolescents* (pp. 287–310). Boston: College-Hill.

Henry, K. (1983). Cognitive rehabilitation and the head-injured child. *Journal of Children in Contemporary Society, 16* (1–2), 189–205.

Hinnant, D. W., & Kade, H. D. (1992). Cognitive deficits following cervical trauma. In D. D. Tollison & J. R. Satterthwaite (Eds.), *Painful cervical trauma: Diagnosis and rehabilitative treatment of neuromusculoskeletal injuries* (pp. 395–413). Baltimore: Williams & Wilkins.

Howard, M. E. (1991). Interdisciplinary team treatment in acute care. In P. M. Deutsch & K. B. Fralish (Eds.), *Innovations in head injury rehabilitation* (pp. 3.01–3.05). New York: Matthew Bender.

Hynd, G. W., & Willis, W. G. (1988). *Pediatric neuropsychology.* New York: Grune & Stratton.

Jackson, W. T., & Gouvier, W. D. (1992). Group psychotherapy with brain-damaged adults and their families. In C. J. Long & J. K. Ross (Eds.), *Handbook of head trauma* (pp. 309–328). New York: Plenum Press.

Johnston, M. V., Keith, R. A., & Hinderer, S. R. (1992). Measurement standards for interdisciplinary medical rehabilitation. *Archives of Physical Medicine and Rehabilitation, 73* (12-S), S3–S23.

Joint Commission on Accreditation of Healthcare Organizations. (1993). *The Joint Commission 1994 Accreditation Manual for Hospitals.* Oakbrook Terrace, IL: Author.

Kade, H. D. (1993, April). *Maximizing outcome for brain injury survivors through behavior change.* Paper presented at the Carolina Brain Injury Symposium, Charlotte, NC.

Kade, H. D. (1994, April). *Behavior change after brain injury: Setting priorities and measuring change.* Paper presented at the Carolinas Brain Injury Symposium, Columbia, SC.

Kaminer, R. K. (1986). Infant stimulation programs. *Archives of Neurology, 43* (11), 1101.

Kaplan, C. P., & Corrigan, J. D. (1994). The relationship between cognition and functional independence in adults with traumatic brain injury. *Archives of Physical Medicine and Rehabilitation, 75,* 643–647.

Kilstrom, J. F., & Tobias, B. A. (1991). Anosognosia, consciousness, and the self. In G. P. Prigatano & D. L. Schacter (Eds.), *Awareness of deficit after brain injury* (pp. 198–222). London: Oxford University Press.

Kreutzer, J. (1991, May). *Issues in brain injury rehabilitation research.* Symposium presented by the Research, Resource & Training Center of the Medical College of Virginia, Tysons Corner.

Kreutzer, J., Gordon, W., Rosenthal, M., & Marwitz, J. (1993). Neuropsychological characteristics of patients with brain injury: Preliminary findings from a multi-center investigation. *Journal of Head Trauma Rehabilitation, 2,* 47–59.

Lash, M., & Scarpino, C. (1993). School reintegration for children with traumatic brain injuries: Conflicts between medical and educational systems. *Neurorehabilitation, 3,* (3), 13–25.

Lawson, M. J., & Rice, D. N. (1989). Effects of training in use of executive strategies on verbal memory problem resulting from closed head injury. *Journal of Clinical and Experimental Neuropsychology, 11* (6), 842–854.

Lehr, E. (1990). *Psychological management of traumatic brain injuries in children and adolescents.* Rockville, MD: Aspen.

Levin, H. S. (1990). Predicting the neurobehavioral sequelae of closed head injury. In R. L. Wood (Ed.), *Neurobehavioral sequelae of traumatic brain injury* (pp. 70–88). Hillsdale, NJ: Erlbaum.

Lezak, M. D. (1994, November). *Neurobehavioral characteristics of diffuse damage in brain disease (multiple sclerosis, traumatic brain injury, HIV+).* Workshop presented at the 14th annual conference of the National Academy of Neuropsychology, Orlando, FL.

Lezak, M. D., & O'Brien, K. P. (1990). Chronic emotional, social, and physical changes after traumatic brain injury. In E. Bigler (Ed.), *Traumatic brain injury* (pp. 365–380). Austin, TX: PRO-ED.

Livingston, M. G., & McCabe, R. J. (1990). Psychosocial consequences of head injury in children and adolescents: Implications for rehabilitation. *Pediatrician, 17* (4), 255–261.

Luria, A. R. (1973). *The working brain: An introduction to neuropsychology.* New York: Basic Books.

Luria, A. R. (1980). *Higher cortical functions in man* (2nd ed.). New York: Basic Books.

Lynch, W. J. (1990). Neuropsychological assessment. In M. Rosenthal, E. R. Griffith, M. R. Bond, & J. D. Miller (Eds.), *Rehabilitation of the adult and child with traumatic brain injury* (pp. 310–327). Philadelphia: Davis.

McCabe, R. J., & Green, D. (1987). Rehabilitating severely head-injured adolescents: Three case reports. *Journal of Child Psychology and Psychiatry and Allied Disciplines, 28* (1), 111–126.

McDonald, C. M., Jaffe, K. M., Fay, G. C., Polissar, N. L., Martin, K. M., Liao, S., & Rivara, J. B. (1994). Comparison of indices of traumatic brain injury severity as predictors of neurobehavioral outcome in children. *Archives of Physical Medicine and Rehabilitation, 75,* 328–337.

McGuire, T. L., & Sylvester, C. E. (1990). Neuropsychiatric evaluation and treatment of traumatic brain injury. In E. Bigler (Ed.), *Traumatic brain injury* (pp. 209–229). Austin, TX: PRO-ED.

McWilliams, S. (1991). Affective changes following severe head injury as perceived by patients and relatives. *British Journal of Occupational Therapy, 54* (7), 246–248.

Malkmus, D. D., & Evans, R. W. (Eds.). (1992). Special issue on quality, outcome, and value. *Journal of Head Trauma Rehabilitation, 7.*

Margolin, D. I. (Ed.). (1992). *Cognitive neuropsychology in clinical practice.* London: Oxford University Press.

Martin, D. A. (1988). Children and adolescents with traumatic brain injury: Impact on the family. *Journal of Learning Disabilities, 21* (8), 464–470.

Mateer, C. A. (1993, October). *Cognitive rehabilitation: Treating acquired disorders of memory and attention.* Workshop presented at the 13th annual conference of the National Academy of Neuropsychology, Phoenix, AZ.

Meier, M., Benton, A., & Diller, L. (Eds.). (1987). *Neuropsychological rehabilitation.* New York: Guilford Press.

Miller, J. H. (1992). Management and evaluation of head trauma. In C. J. Long & L. K. Ross (Eds.), *Handbook of head trauma* (pp. 3–18). New York: Plenum Press.

Miller, L. (1993). *Psychotherapy of the brain-injured patient: Reclaiming the shattered self.* New York: Norton.

Milton, S. B., Scaglione, C., Flanagan, T., Cox, J. L., & Smith, E. A. (1991). Functional evaluation of adolescent students with traumatic brain injury. *Journal of Head Trauma Rehabilitation, 6* (1), 35–46.

Mira, M. P., Tucker, B. F., & Tyler, J. S. (1992). *Traumatic brain injury in children and adolescents.* Austin, TX: PRO-ED.

Moore, M. K., & Plovnik, N. (1991). Post-acute programs. In P. M. Deutsch, & K. B. Fralish (Eds.), *Innovations in head injury rehabilitation* (pp. 5.01–5.202). New York: Matthew Bender.

National Information Center for Children and Youth with Disabilities. (1993). *Traumatic brain injury.* Fact sheet number 18 (FS18). Washington, DC: NICCYD.

Neale, J. M., & Liebert, R. M. (1973). *Science and behavior.* Englewood Cliffs, NJ: Prentice–Hall.

Obrzut, J. E., & Hynd, G. W. (1990). Cognitive dysfunction and psychoeducational assessment in traumatic brain injury. In E. Bigler (Ed.), *Traumatic brain injury* (pp. 165–179). Austin, TX: PRO-ED.

Pennington, B. F. (1991). *Diagnosing learning disorders: A neuropsychological framework.* New York: Guilford Press.

Pollens, R. D., McBratnie, B. P., & Burton, P. L. (1988). Beyond cognition: Executive functions in closed head injury. *Cognitive Rehabilitation, 6* (5), 26–32.

Ponsford, J., & Kinsella, G. (1992). Attentional deficits following closed-head injury. *Journal of Clinical and Experimental Neuropsychology, 14* (5), 822–838.

Prigatano, G. P. (1988). Bringing it up in milieu: Toward effective TBI rehabilitation: *Journal of Rehabilitation Psychology, 34* (2), 135–144.

Prigatano, G. P. (1990). Effective traumatic brain injury rehabilitation: Team/patient interaction. In E. Bigler (Ed.), *Traumatic brain injury* (pp. 297–312). Austin, TX: PRO-ED.

Prigatano, G. P. (1991a). Disordered mind, wounded soul: The emerging role of psychotherapy in rehabilitation after brain injury. *Journal of Head Trauma Rehabilitation, 6*(4), 1–10.

Prigatano, G. P. (1991b). Disturbances of self-awareness of deficit after traumatic brain injury. In G. P. Prigatano & D. L. Schacter (Eds.), *Awareness of deficit after brain injury* (pp. 111–126). London: Oxford University Press.

Prigatano, G. P., & Klonoff, P. S. (1991). Psychotherapy and neuropsychological assessment after brain injury. In E. Bigler (Ed.), *Traumatic brain injury* (pp. 313–330). Austin, TX: PRO-ED.

Prigatano, G. P. & Schacter, D. L. (1991). *Awareness of deficit after brain injury.* London: Oxford University Press.

Rattok, J., Ben-Yishay, Y., Ezrachi, O., Lakin, P., Piasetsky, E., Ross, B., Silver, S., Vakil, E., Zide, E., & Diller, L. (1992). Outcome of different treatment mixed in a multidimensional neuropsychological rehabilitation program. *Neuropsychology, 6* (4), 395–415.

Reitan, R. M. (1993). RE: Development of a "nationally normed" neuropsychological test battery. *Bulletin of the National Academy of Neuropsychology, 10* (2), 1–2.

Reschly, D. J., & Gresham, F. M. (1989). Current neuropsychological diagnosis of learning problems: A leap of faith. In C. R. Reynolds & E. Fletcher-Janzen (Eds.), *Handbook of clinical child neuropsychology* (pp. 503–519). New York: Plenum Press.

Risser, A. H., & Edgell, D. (1988). Neuropsychology of the developing brain. In M. G. Tramontana & S. R. Hooper (Eds.), *Assessment issues in child neuropsychology* (pp. 41–65). New York: Plenum Press.

Romano, M. D. (1984). The therapeutic milieu in the rehabilitation process. In D. W. Krueger (Ed.), *Rehabilitation psychology* (pp. 43–50). Rockville, MD: Aspen.

Rourke, B. P., Bakker, D. J., Fisk, J. L., & Strang, J. D. (1983). *Child neuropsychology.* New York: Guilford Press.

Ruff, R. M., Marshall, L. F., Crouch, J., Klauber, M. R., & Smith, E. A. (1993). Predictors of outcome following severe head trauma: Follow-up data from the Traumatic Coma Data Bank. *Brain Injury, 7* (2), 101–111.

Rusonis, E. S. (1990). Adolescents with closed head injury. *Adolescent Medicine, 3,* 1311–1319.

Russman, B. S. (1990). Rehabilitation of the pediatric patient with a neuromuscular disease. *Neurologic Clinics, 8* (3), 727–740.

Savage, R., & Carter, R. (1988). Transitioning pediatric patients into educational systems: Guidelines for rehabilitation professionals. *Cognitive Rehabilitation, 6* (4), 10–14.

Schacter, D. L., & Prigatano, G. P. (1991). Forms of unawareness. In G. P. Prigatano, & D. L. Schacter (Eds.), *Awareness of deficit after brain injury* (pp. 258–262). London: Oxford University Press.

Schara, J. (1991). Evaluation. In P. M. Deutsch & K. B. Fralish (Eds.), *Innovations in head injury rehabilitation* (pp. 6.01–6.100). New York: Matthew Bender.

Schultz, I. L., & Texidor, M. S. (1991). The interdisciplinary approach: An exercise in futility or a song of praise? *Medical Psychotherapy, 4,* 1–8.

Schwartz, C., Myers, J. K., & Astrachan, B. M. (1973). The outcome study in psychiatric evaluation research. *Archives of General Psychiatry, 29,* 98–102.

Sellers, C. W., & Vegter, C. H. (1993). *Pediatric brain injury.* Tucson, AZ: Communication Skill Builders.

Shapiro, K. (1987). Special considerations for the pediatric age group. In P. R. Cooper (Ed.), *Head injury* (2nd ed., pp. 367–389). Baltimore: Williams & Wilkins.

Sheil, A., Wilson, B., Horn, S., Watson, M., & Smith, E. A. (1993). Can patients in coma following traumatic head injury learn simple tasks? Special Issue: Coma and the persistent vegetative state. *Neuropsychological Rehabilitation, 3* (2), 161–175.

Sohlberg, M. M., & Mateer, C. A. (1989). *Introduction to cognitive rehabilitation.* New York: Guilford Press.

Spreen, O., & Strauss, E. (1991). *A compendium of neuropsychological tests: Administration, norms, and commentary.* London: Oxford University Press.

Stanczak, D. E., & Hutcherson, W. L. (1992). Acute rehabilitation of the head-injured individual: Toward a neuropsychological paradigm of treatment. In C. J. Long & L. K. Ross (Eds.), *Handbook of head trauma* (pp. 225–236). New York: Plenum Press.

Stein, D. (1988). In pursuit of new strategies for understanding recovery from brain damage: Problems and perspectives. In T. J. Boll & B. K. Bryant (Eds.), *Clinical neuropsychology and brain function: Research, measurement and practice* (pp. 13–51). Washington, DC: APA.

Szerkeres, S. F., Ylvisaker, M., & Holland, A. L. (1985). Cognitive rehabilitation therapy: A framework for intervention. In M. Ylvisaker (Ed.), *Head injury rehabilitation: Children and adolescents* (pp. 361–382). Boston: College-Hill.

Taylor, D. A. (1992). Traumatic brain injury: Outcome and predictors of outcome. In C. J. Long & L. K. Ross (Eds.), *Handbook of head trauma* (pp. 125–136). New York: Plenum Press.

Telzrow, K. (1990). Management of academic and educational problems in traumatic brain injury. In E. Bigler (Ed.), *Traumatic brain injury* (pp. 251–272). Austin, TX: PRO-ED.

Timmons, M., Gasquoine, L., & Scibak, J. W. (1987). Functional changes with rehabilitation of very severe traumatic brain injury survivors. *Journal of Head Trauma Rehabilitation, 2* (3), 64–73.

Torkelson, R. M., Jellinek, H. M., Malec, J. F., & Harvey, R. F. (1983). Traumatic brain injury: Psychological and medical factors related to rehabilitation outcome. *Rehabilitation Psychology, 28* (3), 169–176.

Trexler, L. E. (1987). Neuropsychological rehabilitation in the United States. In M. Meier, A. Benton, & L. Diller (Eds.), *Neuropsychological rehabilitation* (pp. 430–436). New York: Guilford Press.

Tupper, D. E. (1990). Some observations on the use of the Woodcock–Johnson Tests of Cognitive Ability in adults with head injury. *Journal of Learning Disabilities, 23* (5), 306–310.

Uniform Data System for Medical Rehabilitation. (1994). *Guide for the uniform data set for medical rehabilitation for children (WeeFIM).* Buffalo: State University of New York at Buffalo.

Uomoto, J. M. (1989). Care continuum in traumatic brain injury rehabilitation. *Rehabilitation Psychology, 34* (2), 71–79.

Verduyn, W. H., Hilt, J., Roberts, M. A., & Roberts, R. J. (1992). Multiple partial seizure-like symptoms following "minor" closed head injury. *Brain Injury, 6* (3), 245–260.

Waaland, P., & Raines, S. R. (1991). Families coping with childhood neurological disability. *Neurorehabilitation, 1* (2), 19–27.

Willer, B., Allen, K., Durnan, M. C., & Ferry, A. (1990). Problems and coping strategies of mothers, siblings and young adult males with traumatic brain injury. *Canadian Journal of Rehabilitation, 3* (3), 167–173.

Ylvisaker, M. (1985). *Head injury rehabilitation: Children and adolescents.* Boston: College-Hill.

Ylvisaker, M. (1986). Language and communication disorders following pediatric head injury. *Journal of Head Trauma Rehabilitation, 1* (4), 48–56.

Ylvisaker, M., Chorazy, A. J., Cohen, S. B., Mastrilli, J. P., Molitor, C. B., Nelson, J., Szekeres, S. F., Valko, A. S., & Jaffe, K. M. (1990). Rehabilitative assessment following head injury in children. In M. Rosenthal, E. R. Griffith, M. R. Bond, & J. D. Miller (Eds.), *Rehabilitation of the adult and child with traumatic brain injury* (pp. 558–583). Philadelphia: Davis.

Ylvisaker, M., & Szekeres, S. F. (1989). Metacognitive and executive impairments in head-injured children and adults. *Topics in Language Disorders, 9* (2), 34–49.

24

Treating Traumatic Brain Injury in the School

Mandates and Methods

RUTH ADLOF HAAK AND RONALD B. LIVINGSTON

In the last few years, a proliferation of information has become available to the professionals who serve children with traumatic brain injury (TBI). The scientific community, government-sponsored research and development centers, new professional activities, and new professional societies dealing with the education and credentialing of workers in these activities have all contributed a wealth of information. Numerous medical facilities have also sprung up to treat children with TBI and to offer their expertise to the growing field. Rarely has a field of endeavor in the human services grown so quickly as has the recent effort to deal more effectively with our brain-injured population.

This chapter will attempt to present a comprehensive overview of current information considered to be essential to the proper educational programming of students with TBI.

The Mandate for Education of Students with TBI

Annually in the United States, there are approximately 1 million cases of head trauma severe enough to require hospitalization. An estimated 40% of these patients are below the age of 18 (Bigler, 1990), and TBI is listed as one of the top three medical problems causing disability in children (Goldstein & Levin, 1990; Lehr & Savage, 1990; Russell & Sharratt, 1992). The majority of these injuries are relatively mild, with fatal and severe head injuries comprising approximately 10% of the cases (Fletcher & Levin, 1988). Although the majority of these children and adolescents appear to recover fully (Rosman, 1986), many return to the public school system with special needs. The 1990 Individuals with Disabilities Education Act (IDEA) (Public Law 101-476, a revision and reenactment of former Public Law 94-142) designated TBI as a new disability category for students requiring special education services. Under this law, TBI is defined as

> an acquired injury to the brain caused by an external physical force, resulting in total or partial functional disability or psychosocial impairment, or both, that adversely affects a child's educational performance. The term applies to open or closed head injuries resulting in impairment in one or more areas such as cognition; language; memory; attention; reasoning; abstract thinking; problem solving; sensory, perceptual, and motor abilities; psychosocial behavior; physical functions; information processing; and speech. The term does not apply to brain injuries that are congenital or degenerative, or brain injuries induced by birth trauma. (*Federal Register,* 1992, p. 44802)

Public Law 101-476 mandates that individual states must provide an appropriate individualized educa-

RUTH ADLOF HAAK • Eanes Independent School District, Austin, Texas 78746. RONALD B. LIVINGSTON • Department of Psychology, University of Texas at Tyler, Tyler, Texas 75701.

tional program for children who have identified disabilities. TBI now specifically constitutes such a disability.

Although the mandate to provide services for students with TBI is a federal requirement, individual states must write guidelines for providing services. To date, not all states have completed this process. States that have completed the process have approached it differently. An example of a comprehensive set of guidelines is that developed by the Virginia Department of Education (Virginia Department of Education and the Rehabilitation Research Center on Severe Traumatic Brain Injury, 1992). These guidelines address family needs, the training of school personnel, program planning, and implementation. Another approach is that of the North Carolina Department of Public Instruction, which produced a directive formalizing criteria for qualified providers of services to students with TBI (North Carolina Department of Public Instruction, 1994).

The Basics of Brain Injury and Its Functional Effects on Educability

Educators vary in the level of information they need to have regarding brain functioning, depending on their individual responsibilities. The information reviewed in this section is intended to be basic, relating to the mechanisms of brain injury and its functional effects on the ability of the student with TBI to learn. Such basic information also includes much of the fundamental terminology that educators will encounter in dealing with TBI cases.

Epidemiology of TBI Incidence

Epidemiological studies suggest that approximately 200 per 100,000 individuals in the United States experience TBI annually (e.g., Naugle, 1990). This rate varies considerably across the life span. For example, some studies reveal a high incidence of TBI during the first 5 years of life (Naugle, 1990; Parente, 1994). These young children are chiefly at risk for head injuries from falls, but are also vulnerable to head injuries resulting from motor vehicle accidents and physical abuse (Parente, 1994). Relative to younger children and adolescents, children in elementary and middle school are at slightly lower risk for head injury. Most head injuries during these early grades are the result of motor vehicle accidents, bicycle accidents, or sports-related head trauma (Parente, 1994).

Epidemiological studies have consistently found a pronounced increase in TBI incidence between the ages of 15 and 24 (Goldstein & Levin, 1990; McAllister, 1992; Naugle, 1990; Parente, 1994). The primary cause of brain injury in these adolescents and young adults is motor vehicle accidents (Naugle, 1990). There is a final increase in TBI incidence that begins at approximately age 70. This third peak is largely the result of an increased vulnerability to falls (Naugle, 1990).

Epidemiological studies have consistently shown that males are more likely than females to sustain a head injury, with an average reported ratio of 2:1 (Goldstein & Levin, 1990; McAllister, 1992; Naugle, 1990; Savage & Wolcott, 1994). Additionally, males experience more severe cerebral trauma, with a mortality ratio as high as 4:1 over females (Goldstein & Levin, 1990; Naugle, 1990). Rutter, Chadwick, and Shaffer (1983) emphasized that children experiencing brain trauma are not a random sample of the general population, and reported characteristics, individual (e.g., impulsiveness and aggressiveness) and family (e.g., parental illness and level of supervision), that contribute to a child's risk of sustaining TBI.

Survey of Neurobehavioral Sequelae

The effects of TBI in children are complex, multiply determined, and unique to the individual patient (Deaton, 1990). As a result, children and adolescents with brain injuries represent a heterogeneous population with regard to neurobehavioral characteristics and outcome. Nevertheless, it is possible to describe broad categories of residual deficits that may influence the educational adjustment and performance of children following TBI (Telzrow, 1990). As closed head injuries (as opposed to open injuries) are most common, the majority of the research has addressed these injuries.

Effects of Brain Injury on Mental Functioning

General Cognitive/Intellectual Abilities

The literature provides considerable evidence of intellectual decline in children with severe brain injuries (Ewing-Cobbs & Fletcher, 1990; Goldstein &

Levin, 1985; Klonoff, Crockett, & Clark, 1984; Obrzut & Hynd, 1990; Rutter *et al.*, 1983; Telzrow, 1990; Wilkening, 1989). There is also considerable evidence suggesting a direct relationship between the severity of the brain injury and the degree of cognitive/intellectual impairment (Bawden, Knights, & Winogron, 1985; Oddy, 1993; Rutter *et al.*, 1983; Winogron, Knights, & Bawden, 1984). Generally, intellectual impairment is greatest immediately following the injury, with patients displaying improvement during the first 1–2 years postinjury (Klonoff, Low, & Clark, 1977; Rutter *et al.*, 1983). Although recovery of intellectual functioning can be significant, evidence suggests that many severely injured children achieve only a partial recovery of intellectual abilities (Ewing-Cobbs & Fletcher, 1990; Levin & Eisenberg, 1979).

In adults, the pattern of cognitive deficits following unilateral brain injury generally differs according to which hemisphere (lateral half of the brain) is damaged. That is, verbal skill deficits are commonly associated with damage to the left hemisphere whereas visuospatial deficits are generally related to right hemisphere damage. In pediatric populations, however, the cognitive deficits associated with unilateral (one hemisphere) brain lesions tend to be less specific and less differentiated than in adults (Obrzut & Hynd, 1990). Although there is a tendency for verbal and academic skills to be more impaired following left hemisphere damage and visuospatial skills to be more impaired following right hemisphere lesions, the differences are relatively small (Rutter *et al.*, 1983; Wilkening, 1989).

Although formal measures of intelligence are sensitive to the effects of cerebral damage, they only assess a limited number of neuropsychologial (more brain-based) abilities (Fletcher & Levin, 1988). As a result, a student may perform within normal limits on intellectual tests and still demonstrate significant impairments in other areas (Bawden *et al.*, 1985; Telzrow, 1990). Additionally, Telzrow (1990) notes that intellectual tests are administered in a highly structured environment, and therefore may overestimate the ability of the student with TBI to function in the less controlled school environment.

Language Functions

Language function is a salient factor influencing academic performance, but relatively few studies have focused on residual speech–language deficits in children with TBI (Ewing-Cobbs & Fletcher, 1990). Although language abilities often show significant recovery following TBI in children, children returning to school may continue to display language processing deficits (Fletcher & Levin, 1988; Goethe & Levin, 1986; Telzrow, 1990). The specificity of the language disabilities associated with TBI varies as a function of age and localization of damage (Wilkening, 1989). For example, written language skills appear to be more impaired in children than in adolescents following closed-head injuries (Ewing-Cobbs & Fletcher, 1990; Ewing-Cobbs, Levin, Eisenberg, & Fletcher, 1987). With regard to localization, Aram, Ekelman, Rose, and Whitaker (1985) found that left hemisphere lesions interfere with syntactic development to a greater extent than right hemisphere lesions.

Regardless of age or site of damage, expressive language abilities are generally more impaired than receptive language abilities (Goethe & Levin, 1986; Wilkening, 1989). Also, pragmatic or conversational language skills, which require an interplay of cognitive, linguistic, and social skills, are particularly susceptible to disruption following TBI in children (Russell, 1993). In summary, residual language deficits are frequently associated with TBI in children and adolescents, and these deficits may interfere with academic performance and social interactions.

Memory

Despite the extensive literature addressing memory deficits in adults following TBI, relatively few studies have specifically examined posttraumatic memory functions in children (Ewing-Cobbs & Fletcher, 1990). Similar to adult populations, evidence suggests that memory deficits are among the most common and enduring neuropsychological deficits of brain-injured children (Fletcher & Levin, 1988; Goethe & Levin, 1986; Levin, Benton, & Grossman, 1982; Telzrow, 1985). For example, Levin and Eisenberg (1979) reported that nearly half of their patients (aged 6–18) exhibited verbal memory deficits with a median injury-to-test interval of 19 days. The occurrence of memory deficits in this study was strongly related to severity of injury (i.e., as measured by the Glasgow Coma Score). Evidence suggests that improvement in memory following TBI may be slower and less complete than other abilities (e.g., motor and language skills) (Farr, Greene,

& Meyers, 1983; Fuld & Fisher, 1977; Goethe & Levin, 1986). Although most patients demonstrate complete recovery of memory abilities, data suggest that in some cases verbal memory deficits may continue for up to 10 years postinjury (Gaidolfi & Vignolo, 1980).

Attention and Concentration

Deficits in attention/concentration are extremely common following TBI in both adults (e.g., Cullum, Kuck, & Ruff, 1990) and children (Ylvisaker, Szekeres, Hartwick, & Tworek, 1994). Studies of adults have found a significant relationship between severity of injury and attentional impairments, and it has been postulated that attentional problems are related to a slowed rate of information processing (van Zomeren & Brouwer, 1994). Less is known about attentional impairments following TBI in children, but the available evidence suggests similar patterns to adults. For example, consistent with the report of increased reaction times following closed-head injuries in adults, children with severe brain injury exhibit similar deficits on reaction time tasks (e.g., Bawden et al., 1985). In the context of pediatric TBI, Ylvisaker et al. (1994) reported that patients returning to school often display difficulties with sustained attention, selective attention, switching attention, and divided attention. The authors postulate that these attentional difficulties contribute to a variety of problems involving memory, learning, language, and social interactions.

Visuospatial, Visuoconstructive, and Visuoperceptive Skills

A wide variety of nonverbal abilities may be affected in TBI (Cullum et al., 1990). As previously noted, performance on nonverbal tasks such as those represented on the Performance subtests of the WISC-R (or WISC-III) tend to be disrupted by TBI more than performance on the Verbal subtests (Ewing-Cobbs & Fletcher, 1990; Rutter, et al., 1983; Telzrow, 1990). Bawden et al. (1985) found that children with severe head injury demonstrated more impairment on tasks emphasizing motor speed and visuospatial skills than children with mild or moderate head injury. The authors reported that tests of speeded motor or visuospatial functioning were able to detect

subtle cognitive deficits not apparent on intelligence tests.

Motor/Sensory/Physical Functioning

Brain injury may impact a variety of motor abilities (Cullum et al., 1990; Telzrow, 1991). Although motor skills frequently demonstrate good recovery, some children will continue to display significant motor sequelae (e.g., ataxia, irregular muscular activity; tremor, shaking; or spasticity, involuntary muscular contractions; Telzrow, 1990). As a result, measures of fine motor speed, dexterity, and strength should be included in the comprehensive assessment of functioning following TBI. Commonly occurring sensory problems following TBI include hearing and vision deficits, and such patients should undergo complete audiological and ophthalmological examinations (Mira, Tucker, & Tyler, 1992). Other physical effects may include reduced stamina, posttraumatic seizures, and headaches (Mira et al., 1992).

Behavioral and Emotional Changes

Behavioral disturbances are common following TBI in children and adolescents, and these behavioral changes may be the most prominent features of the injury (Goethe & Levin, 1986; Hartlage, 1990; Oddy, 1993; Telzrow, 1990). Behavioral disturbances often reflect an exacerbation of premorbid behavioral tendencies and often persist in spite of significant improvement in cognitive functioning (Brown, Chadwick, Shaffer, Rutter, & Traub, 1981; Rutter et al., 1983). There is no well-defined pattern of behavioral problems following TBI in children, although there are constellations of problems that occur more often. Hartlage (1990) and Dilks and Hartlage (1990) found statistically significant increases in children's behaviors after TBI in absentmindedness, agitation, complaining, confusion, being cross, depression, disagreeableness, distractibility, forgetfulness, short-temperedness, slowness, and being easily upset. Socially uninhibited behavior following severe TBI is prevalent (Rutter et al., 1983). As noted, there is a fairly direct relationship between the severity of TBI and residual cognitive impairments, but the relationship between severity of injury and behavioral adjustment is more complex (Ewing-Cobbs & Fletcher, 1990). Injury severity is an important variable influencing behavioral outcome, and other factors such as premorbid characteristics and the postinjury environment are also influential (Fletcher & Levin, 1988; Rutter *et al.*, 1983).

Academic Sequelae

Although the acquisition of academic skills is a critical developmental task for children and adolescents, few studies have systematically examined the types or severity of academic problems associated with TBI (Fletcher & Levin, 1988). Nevertheless, the existing evidence indicates that academic achievement is often significantly impacted by TBI (Fletcher & Levin, 1988; Telzrow, 1990). Certainly, many of the cognitive and behavioral sequelae of TBI can directly impact academic learning. Based on her review, Telzrow (1990) concluded that many children and adolescents with TBI require some form of instructional modification (e.g., special education services or adjusted school programs). She noted that even children returning to a regular classroom setting often experience significant academic problems, including grade repetition. The detrimental effects of TBI on academic achievement may be most apparent in younger children who have not previously acquired basic reading, writing, and arithmetic skills (Lehr & Savage, 1990).

Course of Recovery

Methodological differences in outcome studies make it difficult to make broad statements regarding the course of recovery for children sustaining TBI. For example, studies use different criteria to grade the severity of brain injury. Similarly, studies frequently vary in the techniques used to assess neurobehavioral functioning or outcome. To compound the methodological problems, there is considerable individual variability in recovery. Some children demonstrate rapid and impressive "spontaneous" recoveries from TBI, and others demonstrate substantial long-term impairments. The factors contributing to good versus poor recovery are not clearly understood, but injury severity is a primary determinant of recovery (Fletcher & Levin, 1988; Oddy, 1993; Warzak, Ford, & Evans, 1992). In general, children with severe TBI often display a variety of the neurobehavioral problems previously discussed. Nevertheless, one should not assume that all mild brain injuries are of little or no consequence. For example, Boll (1983) provided evidence suggesting that even mild TBI can result in neurobehavioral sequelae that interfere with school achievement.

Recent efforts to delineate other factors influencing recovery have met with some success. For example, the presence of brain stem abnormalities (e.g., oculomotor and oculocephalic signs) has been associated with poor outcome on global measures of recovery (Fletcher & Levin, 1988). Additionally, long-term outcome appears to reflect the influence of diverse factors such as the child's reaction to the injury, the rehabilitation options available, and family factors (Ewing-Cobbs & Fletcher, 1990).

As a general rule, cognitive recovery from TBI is most obvious immediately after the injury, with substantial improvement continuing throughout the first year posttrauma (Rutter *et al.*, 1983). However, some studies have demonstrated progressive intellectual improvements up to 5 years following the injury (Fletcher & Levin, 1988). Whereas cognitive deficits following TBI show considerable recovery during the first years after the injury, behavioral and academic problems appear to be more enduring (Rutter *et al.*, 1983).

Influence of Age at Injury

The "Kennard principle" suggests that brain injury sustained in childhood is less deleterious than a comparable injury sustained in adults (Bolter & Long, 1985). Although this principle has received considerable acceptance, mounting evidence argues against preferential recovery in juvenile brains (e.g., Levin *et al.*, 1994; Thompson *et al.*, 1994). In fact, there is evidence that an immature nervous system is more susceptible to injury than a mature system (Goethe & Levin, 1986; Hynd & Willis, 1988; Nice & Logue, 1984; Obrzut & Hynd, 1990). Additionally, as brain damage may predominantly affect the acquisition of new skills (Hebb, 1942), early insult could be particularly detrimental, for children have more new learning to accomplish and fewer well-consolidated skills and knowledge to rely on (Rutter *et al.*, 1983). Assessment of recovery in children is complicated by the fact that neurobehavioral deficits may not emerge until a later development period (Horton, 1994). Fletcher and Levin (1988) concluded that

> comparative psychometric studies of adults and children show relatively similar patterns of recovery and provide little support for the view that recovery is better after diffuse CNS insult in children. Indeed, younger children seem more vulnerable to the effects of head injury than adults. (p. 290)

In summary, although it is clear that age influences the expression of cerebral injury (Kolb &

Fantie, 1989), results regarding age effects are inconsistent and prevent the development of definitive statements projecting the final outcomes of TBI (Oddy, 1993; Rutter *et al.,* 1983). For comprehensive references that can lead one into greater detail in the study of brain injuries and their effects, see Begali (1987), Bigler (1990), Lehr (1990), National Head Injury Foundation Task Force on Special Education (1989), Rourke, Bakker, Fisk, and Strang (1983), Savage and Wolcott (1994), and Ylvisaker (1985).

The Critical Issues in Appropriate Programming for the Student with TBI

There are a number of issues of importance to be addressed if an appropriate educational program is to be offered to students with TBI:

1. Issues of coordination of information and services between the medical facility and the school
2. Issues of assessment
3. Issues of programming
4. Issues of school reentry
5. Issues of family support
6. Issues of transition from school to community reintegration

Each of these rather broad issues will now be reviewed and addressed.

Issues of Coordination between the Medical Facility and the School

In the past it was too often the case that a child with brain injury simply appeared back in school one day without any preliminary notice and with no information in hand. Indeed, what information was available indicated the student was "ready to return to school." Unless the student was so obviously physically injured as to visually remind family and school personnel daily of the disability, normal expectations were immediately placed on the student, who then frustrated others and self by floundering and failing (Hartlage, 1990).

School reentry has generally improved from the scenario above. Nevertheless, it is still often far from optimal. Responsibilities remain in question. For example, Mira *et al.* (1992) advise that it is the school that should take the initiative in contacting the medical professionals when a child is injured. Their advice seems face valid that the school that

makes itself more visible and active while the child is in the hospital will receive much better information and cooperation. On the other hand, Savage (1994) states that "hospitals and/or rehabilitation professionals need to immediately inform the school that they are presently caring for one of their students" (p. 6). Some health professionals may feel that such voluntary informing violates rules of confidentiality.

In practice, schools know when a student is absent. Also, because the population that incurs head injuries is not a random one, many times students who suffer brain injuries are already receiving some special services that involve closer monitoring of attendance and progress. Therefore, it seems that in the interest of assuring that the student is properly served, the school should take the responsibility for knowing the student's status. This, however, is still not simple. State laws may automatically consider a student no longer a school district resident if he or she is in a nondistrict hospital. Parents and students have confidentiality rights and sometimes reject the school's efforts to contact them and/or their medical attenders, perhaps not wishing others to know the circumstances of the head injury. In these cases, the school may be stymied in its best efforts to keep informed of the student's needs. In most cases, however, it is thankfully so that parents appreciate and expect the school to contact them when a student is so seriously hurt as to have a brain injury. The classes of the student usually will be sending cards, visiting, and the like, and some school personnel normally will be personally involved. The school can thus contact the medical providers involved with the parents' permission.

Once parentally approved contact has been established between the parties, it will prove efficient to appoint a contact person on "both ends," so that communications do not get hopelessly confused (Mira *et al.,* 1992). Such contact persons will exchange information: The hospital will inform the school of the student's progress and expected dismissal and school reentry dates, providing assessments, and making recommendations; the school will keep the hospital up-to-date on its progress in preparing for the return of the student, its needs from the hospital in doing so, and the legal requirements it must fulfill for services to be provided.

Especially productive are visits and observations in the hospital by the school contact person and/or other educational personnel critically involved in the student's reentry. Optimal cooperation between the two institutions is attained by a case conference involving all important players considerably ahead of time for hospital dismissal.

Issues of Assessment

The school and the medical facility each have their own particular assessment needs and utilize their own types of assessments. Some medical assessments will be critical for educational planning and some less so; likewise, the school's assessment may include areas important to the hospital's rehabilitation program.

The school needs information from the hospital: How is the student injured and what can be expected to be the effects of these injuries on the student's ability to attend school and to learn? This information should be provided by both the student's medical report and, optimally, the results of a neuropsychological examination that offers practical implications of its findings. The school should expect to receive at least the former report and usually both reports, and if they are not voluntarily provided by the parents, the parents should be pressed to provide them with the explanation that a special education program cannot be properly planned without such information. If the hospital does not provide a neuropsychological assessment, the school will need to obtain one if at all possible (see below). The major responsibility for the comprehensive type of assessment needed for the education of a student with TBI, however, falls on the school.

The School's Assessment

The first assessment the school needs is the simple one of a reasonably practical test of whether the child is able to sustain instruction in any classroom setting. The commonly accepted standard suggested by Cohen, Joyce, Rhoades, and Welks (1985) asks these questions: (1) Can the child attend to a task 10–15 minutes at a time? (2) Can the child tolerate 20–30 minutes of general classroom stimulation? (3) Can the child function as a member of a group of two or more? (4) Can the child follow simple directions? (5) Can the child engage in any meaningful form of communication? (6) Does the child give evidence of learning potential? If most of these answers are negative, the school will need to make arrangements for other than classroom instruction at first, i.e., homebound teaching or day treatment programs.

When school reentry is entertained, another alternative that is used as a beginning for classroom instruction is the legal option of a shortened school day. One needs to take into consideration in developing schedules for students with TBI those amounts of time needed by related services offered at the school, such as occupational therapy and physical therapy. A very minimal amount of academic instruction together with the necessary related services time can amount to a considerable time period for a newly returning student with TBI. The total "day" that the returning student can tolerate needs to be divided as appropriately as possible into its needful components.

After the initial issue of school reentry is assessed, the school needs to assume a mind-set regarding assessment of the particular student that is somewhat different from its usual assessment course (Begali, 1987; Rourke, Fisk, & Strang, 1986; Telzrow, 1991). Two questions especially pertain:

1. Is an assessment supposed to predict eventual capacity or current readiness? Although actually this is always a pertinent question in assessing individuals with handicapping conditions, it is especially important in TBI assessments because such students may change rapidly (Rosen & Gerrig, 1986; Telzrow, 1991). Tests given under optimum conditions of one-to-one attention, a quiet atmosphere, pleasant and nonvarying encouragement, and short subtesting may produce scores that are little predictive of current abilities (but more of future capacity) (Telzrow, 1991).

2. Will changes in testing keep up with changes in the student? Telzrow (1991) points out that most experts in the field agree that periodic, ongoing reassessments, particularly within the educational context, are necessary so as to keep appropriately modifying programs for students with TBI. Once the mind-set is accepted that assessment of the student with TBI within the school will not be a simple every-3-year reevaluation, the questions of capacity versus readiness and appropriate times to reevaluate can be answered within *each discipline.*

The disciplines within the school that will need to conduct their assessments of the student include the special education assessment component, the neuropsychological testing component (if none, this test will need to be obtained; see below), the occupational therapy component, the physical therapy component, and the speech and language component, at a minimum. The student may return from the hospital with many of these testing needs met. Even in that case, however, it is necessary for the on-site school personnel to review these assessments carefully and to fill in any elements uniquely required by school practice or law.

Medical facilities and schools operate under different legal requirements. The medical facility often does not realize that a written report is not enough to make a child eligible for special education services. In special education, there is a special eligibility report to be completed that indicates specific criteria for classification have been met in the case of each disability. This is just one of many illustrations of how the pre-reentry coordination of hospital and home, referred to earlier in this chapter, can be helpful. The school can inform the hospital of the eligibility requirements, explain the criteria, supply the appropriate form(s), and often obtain the eligibility statement(s) along with the written report(s) from the hospital. This will save both institutions time and frustration and smooth the way for the student to obtain more timely services.

When the educational testing component of the school begins to conduct its assessment of the student with TBI, its mind-set will be mostly on tests that tap current functioning and can translate into immediate recommendations for educational interventions. Rapid changes are anticipated in such an approach, and Baxter, Cohen, and Ylvisaker (1985) indicate that brief screening measures (and less comprehensive measures than a tester might normally choose) are thus acceptable for setting short-term goals. Nevertheless, it is not acceptable to utilize tests of low quality in any situation: It is better to have no tests than misleading ones. Naturally, tests that are as close as possible to the actual activities one wishes to predict can be assumed to predict best.

Another general necessity of comprehensive educational assessment of students with TBI is the special need for the educational assessor to be the organizer of the total array of assessments that are going to be obtained from the various sources, namely, medical facilities and professional disciplines in and out of school. (The assessment information will be presented to a special education committee, which then must develop an individualized educational plan for the student; see PL 101-476.)

The greatest service the educational assessor can perform is to appear at the special education committee meeting with a comprehensive assessment that is an *organized* product, composed of the assessor's own testing and the various other assessments that are attached. This cannot be overempha-

sized. A special education committee is by intention a multidisciplinary group. The responsibility for guidance of the committee in making fitting recommendations for the student rests first on the person providing information on the student's status, i.e., the educational assessor. At times, with complicated cases such as TBI, this person may appear at the meeting with a huge pile of test results that are briefly discussed and then largely ignored. They are ignored because they are unusable, and when this happens the whole logical process set out in law for developing a handicapped student's individual educational plan (IEP) is derailed at the start. An IEP not firmly rooted in current assessment results is appropriate only by accident.

Mira *et al.* (1992) have a suggested list of questions that need answering before an IEP for a student can be developed (p. 53). Using some of their suggestions, the following list is proposed as a guideline to the educational assessor in pulling together information from his or her own testing and that of others into a unified report for presentation to the committee:

Elements of the Student's Status That Modify Goals and Instruction for the Student as of
Date: __ Student:__

Contextual Issues: Include any needs for control of noise level, time in school, room placement, class size, instructional intensity, special equipment, medical processes at school, toileting, special transportation, respite care, or other contextual needs of this student.

Behavioral Issues: Include behavioral issues that at the present time are going to impact instruction: try to account for which of these behaviors are recent and appear to originate with the brain injury, which may be historical, and which historical behaviors are aggravated by the brain injury so that a more logical behavioral plan can be developed, if needed. Such a plan will select first for modification, of course, those behaviors least related to the injury.

Cognitive Issues: Include historical information on the student's premorbid cognitive status in the best form obtainable for this information; present current ability and achievement test results, recognizing they may be inflated by ideal test conditions as far as current functioning goes; and particularly, present cognitive processing type information primarily derived from the neuropsychological testing, which deals with issues central to brain damage: for example, attentional behavior, speed at which the student can work, frustration tolerance, impulsivity, social controls, memory problems, abstraction difficulties, language problems, perceptual problems, self-awareness, emotional lability and others relevant to this student (see Ylvisaker & Szekeres, 1989, for example). Present as a separate listing those cognitive behaviors of greatest strength at the present time.

Physical Issues: Include as pertinent physical limitations, endurance, physical and/or occupational therapy needs, speech needs, needs for adaptive physical education (if appropriate), diets, and any other physical needs peculiar to this student.

Psychosocial Issues: Include emotional reaction to the injury, social needs, psychotherapeutic needs, and whether the student is able to profit from any psychotherapeutic or social intervention now and, if so, in what format.

Instructional Issues: Include areas of instruction and levels of performance of the student prior to the injury; areas of instruction to accent and avoid at the present time; and levels at which the student can perform at the present time in proposed subjects.

If the school in which the educational assessor works utilizes a standardized type of report format (see Appendix for an example), the educational assessor may prepare the above-outlined information in a separate handout to be provided each committee member at the beginning of (or before) the meeting. As subsequent discussion develops in the committee meeting, the separate assessments from the various disciplines can be referred to as needed.

Parents are often more concerned with eventual recovery of capacity than the immediate educational concerns listed above that are needed by educators. It is best to try to resist such pressures for long-term prediction. This is already an unsafe area when dealing with children, for developmental changes make such predictions notoriously shaky, and they are even more so with TBI (Baxter *et al.*, 1985). Another pressure that may arise in discussing TBI assessment results occurs when someone realizes that part of the child's current behavior is historical. A child who has had a disability previous to the brain injury will now have the same and additional disabilities. It is common for educational personnel or parents to say, "Aha, see here, this behavior went on before. It isn't caused by the injury." The assessor needs to explain that even though the behavior occurred previously, the level of the behavior may indeed be raised or lowered by the addition of the brain injury. Knowledge that certain behaviors preexisted is important (Bigler, 1990) and such information is liable to be contributed by family members and teachers, but realization that an insult to the brain makes it even more difficult for the student to deal with these prior behaviors is useful to these parents and teachers, who may otherwise view these behaviors as volitional (Hartlage, 1990).

The educational assessor's organized report is critical to the development of a proper IEP for the child with brain injury. He or she needs to be given the time necessary to pursue such an involved duty requiring so much coordination, judgment, and organization.

The Neuropsychological Evaluation

As stated above, if the hospital does not supply a neuropsychological evaluation when the student returns to school, it is critical for the school to perform this evaluation itself (if it has that capacity) or to obtain this evaluation (if it does not). Neuropsychological evaluation specializes in measuring behaviors thought to be directly affected by brain functioning. It is thus the most appropriate form of testing for a student with TBI.

A number of systems exist for the actual conducting of neuropsychological assessments with these students (references cited below). Neuropsychologists select from some of these systems to determine appropriate batteries for their situations. The educational assessor (and the special education committee), however, needs to have some idea of what domains they can expect to see addressed in an adequate neuropsychological examination and what elements should be covered in an adequate neuropsychological report.

In her article on the school psychologist's perspective in testing students with TBI, Telzrow (1991) organized a table of the major domains considered by seven experts or groups of experts to be essential for proper neuropsychological assessment (Telzrow, 1991, Table 1, p. 31). A reanalysis of that table (by the first author), which organized the domains by category, found the elements considered most essential to be, in order: first, perceptual and language testing; second, executive functioning processes; third, motor, sensory, and intelligence testing; fourth, memory and learning functions; fifth, attentional variables; sixth, academic functioning; and lastly, various others preferred by individual assessors. The educational assessor in the school can supply many of these assessments to the neuropsychologist: the language testing, intelligence testing, and academic testing at the least, with contributions toward some of the other areas (such as the basic sensory function testing the school performs, sensory motor testing by the occupational and/or physical therapists, memory and learning functions the educational assessor may do him- or herself, and other contributions such as observations within settings and behavioral observations). The neuropsychologist should request, expect to receive, and incorporate into his or her report these various contributions if properly current and thus avoid duplication in testing.

When the neuropsychological report is received, the adequacy and usefulness of this report may be judged by guidelines presented by a number of workers, one useful system being the outline of Kreutzer, Devany, Myers, and Harris-Marwitz (1991) for a neuropsychological report: The report should contain (1) demographic data and injury data, (2) referral questions, (3) the basis of evaluation (e.g., previous tests, reports), (4) behavioral observations, (5) interview with informants, (6) records review, (7) test results, (8) impressions, (9) diagnoses, and (10) recommendations. One standard is almost always (and most beneficially) observed: specifying direct referral questions that the assessment gears itself to answer (No. 2 above). The school should be prepared to pose those questions for which it desires serious, working answers. The neuropsychological examination is thus not the esoteric type of assessment some would consider it but a focused examination and report: It tries to answer the practical questions put to it, citing both strengths and deficits of the brain–behavior relationships in question.

Neuropsychologists interested in the various systems of neuropsychological assessment proposed for the student with TBI may wish to consult Bigler (1990), Kreutzer and Marwitz (1991), and Waaland (1992) as examples. In addition, the assessor is referred to the entire second part of this volume for a discussion of current issues within the field of neuropsychological assessment.

Other Specialized Assessments

Included among the specialized assessments needed for a student with TBI, to be incorporated in the overall comprehensive assessment assembled by the educational assessor, are reports from an occupational therapist, a physical therapist, and a speech and language therapist, in many cases. The school nurse may contribute information. Additionally, there may be a report from a psychologist or behavioral specialist. The intervention of the latter may not be so necessary at the point of school reentry as it will be after the staff has had some time to get acquainted with the student. At reentry, it is probably productive to begin any behavioral management with whatever system the medical facility was using, if one was necessary. Later, the staff may be bewildered at some of the student's behavior, finding it difficult to separate TBI behavior from other nonfunctional behavior originating from non-TBI sources. The parents and the home may also be experiencing different types or degrees of behavioral problems, and one or the other may need assistance. The mind-set cited previously, i.e., that there will need to be ongoing assessment activity with the student with TBI, will have prepared all staff for such developing assessment needs. Nevertheless, there will be times when the psychologist or behavioral specialist is needed to generate a behavioral management plan before the student reenters.

Programming for TBI

Ideally, programming for TBI begins before the child has reentered school, not after; then it continues as changes in the child's functioning take place. Programming for a student with TBI is a matter for the special education committee of the school (called various names in various states, but whose composition is prescribed by PL 101-476). No other body or single person in the school, regardless of level of authority, has the right to create a school program for a student with TBI.

Again ideally, the school and the medical facility that served the student with TBI will have been in contact and cooperating with each other for some time. They will have discussed through their agents or through a staffing the proposed needs of the student on reentry. The school will have been preparing for these needs. (For example, if this is the school's first student with TBI, actual physical additions or changes to some of the school's facilities may be required.) When the time for reentry is near, the special education committee will meet to create the educational plan to be followed for the student, namely, the IEP. Hospital representatives may be invited to that meeting. The necessary comprehensive assessment, with attached specialized assessments (discussed above) to support reentry planning, will be ready to present. And the school will have present as a member of the committee an administrator who has the authority to commit the resources of the district.

The IEP is a lengthy, sequential, and comprehensive process, all the details of which are not pertinent here. The heart of the matter is programming: What is going to be done to educate the student, and what does it take to accomplish this? The IEP is supposed to be individualized to the particular student. Each student with TBI will differ, many being only mildly affected or affected only in certain areas; others will be severely affected, in certain areas or grossly. Ylvisaker, Hartwick, and Stevens (1991) feel that it is generally advisable to create a package of services that includes as much regular education as possible (with adaptations as needed), supported by some combination of resource room assistance, remedial programs, tutoring, consultants, ancillary services, and outpatient therapy. "The two primary—and sometimes competing—goals," they say, are "(1) a return to the child's pretrauma setting and (2) academic and social success" (p. 15). Thus, the traditional options already existing in special education (e.g., resource rooms, tutorial centers, team teaching in the regular room) may be completely adequate for a certain student with TBI or for certain activities of another student with TBI. Unfortunately, the majority of TBI cases will need additional programmatic options.

Very recently, many approaches and programs have been developed to address the remedial needs of these patients, some of them controversial. As the special education committee addresses the issues outlined above in the educational assessor's report to the committee, they will be developing the IEP. Adjustments in context, place, and time; specialized equipment; specialized therapies; and the other noninstructional needs listed are all necessities to be provided for the education of the student with TBI. However, when the committee gets to instruction, the core issue from an educational point of view is being attacked. Are there specialized instructional programs that should be used with students? Two that have been developed in recent years are often proposed: cognitive rehabilitation and neuropsychological programming.

Cognitive rehabilitation is now a formalized, credentialed field of practice that existed less than a decade ago as a fledgling endeavor (Boake, 1988). It bears some kinship to the earlier processing remediation efforts of special education inspired by works such as Bateman (1965), Cruikshank, Bentzen, Ratzburg, and Tannhauser (1961), Frostig (1975), Kirk (1967), Strauss and Lehtinen (1947), and others, now generally in disfavor following critical reviews (e.g., Kavale & Mattson, 1983; Mann, 1979). As Boake points out, cognitive rehabilitation actually traces back to head injury rehabilitation efforts in both Germany and the United States following World War I.

It is often proposed that cognitive rehabilitation attempts to teach or reteach specific mental processes; however, Boake gives a much broader role to cognitive rehabilitation: "Cognitive rehabilitation is a constellation of procedures that provide the patients with skills and strategies needed for the performance of tasks that are difficult or impossible for them to do due to cognitive deficits." Cognitive rehabilitationists try to achieve goals through the use of specific exercises, routines, and compensatory strategies and materials, much of it now computerized. Cognitive rehabilitation is a common aspect nowadays of a medical rehabilitation program for a patient with TBI. Many professionals are basically prepared to deliver cognitive rehabilitation from the point of view of their own disciplines (e.g., speech therapists, psychologists); cognitive rehabilitation is a multidisciplinary field of endeavor.

As with the older process of remediation, the newer cognitive rehabilitation is objected to by many educationists (and quite a few neuropsychologists). The issues are too complex to be discussed here but include, at the least, how exactly either is practiced, the accuracy of the neuropsychological or cognitive evaluations that establish the deficits being targeted, the appropriateness of remediation materials to the goals anticipated, rates of recovery in the individual, and the extreme reluctance of many educators to feel comfortable in teaching anything other than subject matter. Some studies (e.g., Schachter & Glisky, 1986; Singley & Anderson, 1989) question the ability of cognitive rehabilitation to restore cognitive processes *per se*. They do feel it is possible to improve cognitive outcomes by teaching such matters as organizational strategy, rather than by attempting to reteach components like sequencing and categorizing, for example. Others (e.g., Miller, 1984; Newcombe, 1985) provide reviews that suggest that residual skills are improved and mild improvement results from cognitive or neuropsychological retraining practices. Also to be considered is the very active state of cognitive rehabilitation practice and literature, and the fact that a young discipline has not had sufficient time to both set up practice and completely research itself. Taking a middle ground, Prigatano (1990) provides some guidelines for those who wish to pursue cognitive retraining. As Bigler indicates (1990, p. 413), the jury on cognitive rehabilitation is clearly still out.

Neuropsychological programming, or neuroeducation, builds on neuropsychological assessment capabilities. It is a model that supports brain-based teaching and learning for all students, especially those with neurologic (brain-based) problems (Savage & Mishkin, 1994). To help children with brain injuries succeed, Savage and Mishkin state that educators in the neuroeducational model need to consider four factors: (1) the environmental changes needed to help these students, (2) the critical transition issues in school reentry for such students, (3) developmental factors impacting on these students, and (4) a teaching–learning framework that utilizes current knowledge of the brain and brain injury (p. 395). Although it does not appear that the fourth component, the teaching–learning framework of neuroeducation, is a completely developed part of the model at this stage, Blosser and DePompei (1994) explicate many practical features of this approach. It should be noted also that the systematic way to build the IEP noted in this chapter already fulfills a large part of the requirements for a neuroeducational model (see previous section on the comprehensive assessment). Anyone following this assessment model is following a neuroeducational model.

When no existing option is in place for meeting the student's needs related to his or her TBI, then more specialized instructional situations must be created. These still may not call for formally different curricula, however. Cognitive rehabilitative strategies can be (in fact are averred to be) successfully taught within the context of traditional subject matter, according to most special education practice today (Ylvisaker, Szekeres, & Hartwick, 1991; Ylvisaker *et al.,* 1994). If the child is disorganized, for example, the language teacher or special education teacher who is teaching language can focus on organizing a theme or journal entry as easily as trying to teach organizational strategies and language content separately. What is critical is that all members of the special education committee come away from the committee meeting with a clear idea of the cognitive processing needs of the child so that each instructor may incorporate practice of these processes within the content of her or his instruction. The instructors need to have an equally clear idea of the student's strengths and to utilize them just as conscientiously.

Although the above discussion is supported by the weight of present knowledge regarding instruction for students with TBI, it is sometimes altogether a different matter to be sitting in an actual committee meeting with a set of parents who feel that a more formally designed cognitive rehabili-

tation program (or any other new therapeutic approach that holds out hope for their child) is something they are absolutely entitled to. Solutions to this problem are not easy. A productive solution, though one involving quite a team effort, is to remain open-minded on an issue of this nature: Organize a local team to investigate the new approach, in this case cognitive rehabilitation; organize a local curriculum of cognitive rehabilitation techniques, incorporating into this format the practices and strategies each discipline within the school already uses to attain cognitive rehabilitation goals; investigate materials from other sources, including cognitive rehabilitation and catalog sources; and include purchases of appropriate materials and software. In short, the best response to any challenge for services in special education is usually to investigate those services and to prepare to offer the applicable methods oneself if possible. For those who feel such continual growth and development is expensive and taxing, the answer is that this is the way a profession grows and serves children.

Issues of Family Support

The family has long been recognized as an important factor in the overall rehabilitation of a student with TBI (e.g., Berroll & Rosenthal, 1989; Kreutzer, Marwitz, & Kepler, 1992; Waaland, 1990; Williams & Kay, 1991; Ylvisaker, 1991). The injury to the child is, in fact, an injury to the family system. Whole lives may have to be rearranged to take into account the awesome new responsibilities of caring for a child with brain injury. It is reasonable to suspect that families will vary greatly, based on their own characteristics and functionality, in their ability to care. A review of investigations of the impact of TBI on the family is presented by Florian, Katz, and Lahav (1989), and the needs of the family members are pinpointed by a very recent quantitative analysis of caregiver needs (Kreutzer, Serio, & Bergquist, 1994).

Blosser and DePompei have outlined a comprehensive set of factors in their chapter in Savage and Wolcott (1994) that require attention from the school in dealing with the family. They discuss effects on the family, how expectations may vary between family and professionals, empowering the family, and counseling and teaching with the family. Above all, the school needs to guard against assuming a possessive, all-knowing stance with the family. School personnel, as dedicated as they may be, are relieved after 8 hours; the family is not. Stress on the family can be severe (Martin, 1990).

When parents do not agree with school professionals, they often earn the judgment that they are in "denial." Sometimes they are. Sometimes the school is in denial of the total set of factors important to the family. The allegations of denial are often associated with Blosser and DePompei's factor of "expectations." Expectations can rarely be changed by one successful coup. Instead, changing expectations in a more realistic direction usually requires a number of (some say endless) IEPs, committee meetings, and years of time—not to mention patience and experience. It is the expectation of changing expectations that educators need to truly accept as a long-term proposition.

Empowering the family involves multiple instances of helping to increase the functionality of the family. Counseling and support group opportunities are productive methods for doing this, including support for the siblings of students with TBI.

Virtually nothing can recharge the family more concretely, however, than the school's guidance and help in obtaining respite care. States vary as to their resources in this regard, but typically there are funds available for respite care from the local or regional mental health authority and the state educational agency (as part of their effort to prevent the need for residential placement). Respite care is true help and as such may be the most useful help available for the families of certain seriously impaired students. Although funds for respite care are notoriously limited, and obtaining them is a frustrating experience, the school that helps the family in this regard is often viewed more positively in all of the other school and family interactions that take place between them.

Community Reintegration

In 1985, Hazaki, Gordon, and Roe found the unemployment rate for special education graduates to be 50%. Condeluci (1994) feels that much of the difficulty with transitioning special students into the adult mainstream relates to the way that services to students are presently structured, i.e., learning is teacher centered, students are approached from their deficits, and social roles are constricted. The latter point of view is developed extensively in the work of Wolfensberger (1972, 1983). Condeluci states that "without question . . . with passage of the Americans with Disabilities

Act . . . , a fundamental shift in the position of people with disabilities will occur in the United States" (p. 541). To help bring about this needed change, IDEA (PL 101-476) now requires for the first time that transitional services be provided by the school.

Although each state must abide by the requirements of IDEA, the state is allowed to write its own procedures for doing so. Therefore, the procedures for providing transitioning services for special education students may vary from state to state, but they should already exist in each state and need to be referred to and followed (for further assistance, refer to your state plan for special education or your state educational agency).

In general, the procedure will include points such as: (1) beginning the transition process at some point, (2) requiring an assessment of vocational potential from the points of view of student, parents, and teachers, (3) vocational testing, (4) updating the transition plan at regular intervals, (5) involving other, i.e., adult, service providers to be participants in the plan, such as state employment commission or state rehabilitation commission representatives, and (6) definite activities and responsibilities that will be assumed by the various participants at school completion. It needs to be remembered also that many students with TBI will be capable of continuing their educations postsecondary (Cook, 1991). More and more colleges and universities are providing modifications and support for students with disabilities.

The goal of transitional planning is to provide meaningful employment and independent living opportunities for young adults with severe disabilities on graduation from school (e.g., Wilcox & Bellamy, 1982; Will, 1984). Some current methods of effecting readiness for such independence while the student is still in school include, in addition to the many varieties of vocational education classes, the supported employment models (Kreutzer & Wehman, 1991) and the life coach model (Jones, Patrick, Evans, & Wulff, 1991). Life care planning (Riddick & Kitchen, 1992; Waaland & Riddick, 1992) can also be an important activity necessary in the case of some students with brain injury. No longer is it acceptable to leave employability as a postschool concern; students with severe handicaps should be receiving a secondary program that prepares them as much as is reasonable for independent or assisted living. Reintegration into the community is a very robust area of research and development at the present time.

Appendix: Traumatic Brain Injury Screening Measure

Please rate the student's behavior (in comparison to same-age classmates) using the following rating scale:

Not at All
Occasionally
Often
Very Severe and Frequent Problem

Not at All	Occasionally	Often	Very Severe and Frequent Problem	
				Confused with time (day, date), place (classroom, bathroom, schedule changes), and personal information (birth date, address, phone, schedule)
				Appears sleepy or fatigues easily
				Inattentive, easily distracted, cannot sustain concentration
				Confused or requires prompts about where, how, or when to begin assignment
				Gives up quickly on challenging tasks
				Forgets things that happened even the same day
				Problems learning new concepts, facts, or information
				Forgets information learned from day to day (does well on quizzes, but fails tests covering several weeks of learning)
				Unable to comprehend or break down instructions and requests
				Processes information at a slow pace
				Difficulty fluently expressing ideas (speech disjointed or slurred; stops midsentence)
				Cannot track when reading, skips problems, or neglects a portion of a page of written material
				Gets lost in halls and cannot follow maps or graphs
				Slow, inefficient motor output (drawing, notetaking, boardwalk)
				Poor motor dexterity (cutting, drawing)

Not at All	Occasionally	Often	Very Severe and Frequent Problem	
				Difficulty with sequential steps of task (getting out materials, turning to page, starting an assignment)
				Confuses the sequence of events or other time-related concepts
				Unable to categorize (size, species), understand abstract concepts, or make cause–effect inferences
				Difficulty applying what they know in different or new situations
				Difficulty breaking down complex tasks (term papers, projects)
				Sets unrealistic goals
				Makes unrelated statements or responses
				Acts without thinking (leaves class, throws things, sets off alarms)
				Extremes in activity level (lethargic or underaroused to hyperactivity)
				Peculiar manners and mannerisms (stands too close, interrupts, unusually loud, poor hygiene)
				Becomes argumentative, aggressive, or destructive with little provocation
				Apathetic and disinterested in friends or activities
				Appears depressed, anxious, or self-conscious
				Identified problems with sensory (hearing, vision) or motor (fine motor or gross motor)
				Problems with visual acuity, blurring, or tracking
				Poor sense of body in space (loses balance, negotiating obstacles)
				A. Orientation and Attention to Activity
				Confused with time (day, date), place (classroom, bathroom, schedule changes), and personal information (birth date, address, phone, schedule)
				Seems "in a fog" or confused
				Stares blankly
				Appears sleepy or to fatigue easily

Not at All	Occasionally	Often	Very Severe and Frequent Problem	
				Fails to finish things started
				Cannot concentrate or pay attention
				Daydreams or gets lost in thoughts
				Inattentive, easily distracted
				B. Starting, Changing, and Maintaining Activities
				Confused or requires prompts about where, how, or when to begin assignment
				Does not know how to initiate or maintain conversation (walks away, etc.)
				Confused or agitated when moving from one activity, place, or group to another
				Stops midtask (math problem, worksheets, story, or conversation)
				Unable to stop (perseverates on) inappropriate strategies, topics, or behaviors
				Gives up quickly on challenging tasks
				C. Taking in and Retaining Information
				Forgets things that happened even the same day
				Problems learning new concepts, facts, or information
				Cannot remember simple instructions or rules
				Forgets classroom materials, assignments, and deadlines
				Forgets information learned from day to day (does well on quizzes, but fails tests covering several weeks of learning)
				D. Language Comprehension and Expression
				Confused with idioms ("climbing the walls") or slang
				Unable to recall word meaning or altered meaning (homonym or homographs)
				Unable to comprehend or break down instructions and requests
				Difficulty understanding "Wh" questions

Not at All	Occasionally	Often	Very Severe and Frequent Problem	
				Difficulty understanding complex or lengthy discussion
				Processes information at a slow pace
				Difficulty finding specific words (may describe but not label)
				Stammers or slurs words
				Difficulty fluently expressing ideas (speech disjointed, stops mid-sentence)
				E. Visual–Perceptual Processing
				Cannot track when reading, skips problems, or neglects a portion of a page of written material
				Orients body or materials in unusual positions when reading or writing
				Gets lost in halls and cannot follow maps or graphs
				Shows left–right confusion
				F. Visual–Motor Skills
				Difficulty copying information from board
				Difficulty with notetaking
				Difficulty with letter formation or spacing
				Slow, inefficient motor output
				Poor motor dexterity (cutting, drawing)
				G. Sequential Processing
				Difficulty with sequential steps of task (getting out materials, turning to page, starting an assignment)
				Confuses the sequence of events or other time-related concepts
				H. Problem-Solving, Reasoning, and Generalization
				Fails to consider alternatives when first attempt fails
				Does not use compensatory strategies (outlining or underlining)
				Problems understanding abstract concepts (color, emotions, math and science)

Not at All	Occasionally	Often	Very Severe and Frequent Problem	
				Confusion with cause–effect relationships
				Unable to categorize (size, species)
				Problems making inferences or drawing conclusions
				Can state facts, but cannot integrate or synthesize information
				Difficulty applying what they know in different or new situations
				I. Organization and Planning Skills
				Difficulty breaking down complex tasks (term papers, projects)
				Problems organizing materials
				Problems distinguishing between important and unimportant information
				Difficulty making plans and setting goals
				Difficulty following through with and monitoring plans
				Sets unrealistic goals
				J. Impulse or Self-Control
				Blurts out in class
				Makes unrelated statements or responses
				Acts without thinking (leaves class, throws things, sets off alarms)
				Displays dangerous behavior (runs into street, plays with fire, drives unsafely)
				Disturbs other pupils
				Makes inappropriate or offensive remarks
				Shows compulsive habits (masturbation, nail biting, tapping)
				Hyperactive, out-of-seat behavior
				K. Social Adjustment and Awareness
				Acts immature for age
				Too dependent on adults

Not at All	Occasionally	Often	Very Severe and Frequent Problem	
				Too bossy or submissive with peers
				Peculiar manners and mannerisms (stands too close, interrupts, unusually loud, poor hygiene)
				Fails to understand social humor
				Fails to correctly interpret nonverbal social cues
				Difficulty understanding the feelings and perspective of others
				Does not understand strengths, weaknesses, and self-presentation
				Does not know when help is required or how to get assistance
				Denies any problem or changes resulting from injury
				L. Emotional Adjustment
				Easily frustrated by tasks or if demands not immediately met
				Becomes argumentative, aggressive, or destructive with little provocation
				Cries or laughs too easily
				Feels worthless or inferior
				Withdrawn, does not get involved with others
				Becomes angry or defensive when confronted with changes resulting from injury
				Apathetic and disinterested in friends or activities
				Makes constant inappropriate sexual comments and gestures
				Unhappy or depressed affect
				Nervous, self-conscious, or anxious behavior
				M. Sensorimotor Skills
				Identified problems with smell, taste, touch, hearing, or vision
				Problems discriminating sound or hearing against background noise
				Problems with visual acuity, blurring, or tracking

Not at All	Occasionally	Often	Very Severe and Frequent Problem	
				Problems with tactile sensitivity (e.g., cannot type or play an instrument without watching hands)
				Identified problems with oromotor (e.g., swallowing), fine motor, or gross motor skills
				Poor sense of body in space (loses balance, negotiating obstacles)
				Motor paralysis or weakness of one or both sides
				Motor rigidity (limited range of motion), spasticity (contractions), and ataxia (erratic movements) (circle one)
				Impaired dexterity (cutting, writing) or hand tremors
				Difficulty with skilled motor activities (dressing, eating)
				/24 A. Orientation/Attention
				/18 B. Task Initiation, Transition, Maintenance
				/15 C. Information Encoding and Retention
				/27 D. Language Comprehension and Expression
				/12 E. Visual–Perceptual Processing
				/15 F. Visual–Motor Skills
				/6 G. Sequential Processing
				/24 H. Problem-Solving, Reasoning, & Generalizing
				/18 I. Organization and Planning Skills
				/24 J. Impulse or Self-Control
				/27 K. Social Adjustment and Awareness
				/30 L. Emotional Adjustment
				/30 M. Sensorimotor Skills

This chapter has attempted to offer a comprehensive but fundamental framework for persons who have the responsibility of administrating, monitoring, and providing appropriate education for students with TBI. Like any map, this chapter outlines current conditions. As such, it is hoped that the chapter is useful to those who face this serious challenge.

Note: The Rehabilitation Research and Training Center on Severe Traumatic Brain Injury (RRTCSTBI) provides a wide range of materials on most subjects covered in this chapter. Request their document, "Materials Available through the National Information Clearinghouse," for a complete listing of resources they provide. RRTCSTBI, Medical College of Virginia, Virginia Commonwealth University, MCV Box 434, Richmond, VA 23298-0434 (804-786-7290).

References

Aram, D., Ekelman, B., Rose, D., & Whitaker, H. (1985). Verbal and cognitive sequelae following unilateral lesions acquired in early childhood. *Journal of Clinical and Experimental Neuropsychology, 7,* 55–78.

Bateman, B. (1965). An educator's view of a diagnostic approach to learning disabilities. In J. Hellmuth (Ed.), *Learning disorders* (Vol. I). Seattle, WA: Special Child Publications.

Bawden, H. N., Knights, R. M., & Winogron, H. W. (1985). Speeded performance following head injury in children. *Journal of Clinical and Experimental Neuropsychology, 7,* 39–54.

Baxter, R., Cohen, S. B., & Ylvisaker, M. (1985). Comprehensive cognitive assessment. In M. Ylvisaker (Ed.), *Head injury rehabilitation: Children and adolescents.* San Diego, CA: College-Hill Press.

Begali, V. (1987). *Head injury in children and adolescents: A resource and review for school and allied professionals.* Brandon, VT: Clinical Psychology Publishing.

Berroll, S., & Rosenthal, M. (1989). Families of the brain injured [Special issue]. *Journal of Head Trauma Rehabilitation, 3*(4).

Bigler, E. (1990). Neuropathology of traumatic brain injury. In E. Bigler (Ed.) *Traumatic brain injury* (pp. 13–14). Austin, TX: PRO-ED.

Blosser, L., & DePompei, R. (1994). Creating an effective classroom environment. In R. C. Savage & G. F. Wolcott (Eds.), *Educational dimensions of acquired brain injury* (pp. 393–411). Austin, TX: PRO-ED.

Boake, C. (1988). *A history of cognitive rehabilitation: Where have we come from?* [Lecture: available as a tape]. Richmond: Rehabilitation Research and Training Center on Severe Traumatic Brain Injury, Medical College of Virginia.

Boll, T. J. (1983). Minor head injuries in children: Out of sight, but not out of mind. *Journal of Clinical Child Psychology, 12,* 74–80.

Bolter, J. F., & Long, C. J. (1985). Methodological issues in research in developmental neuropsychology. In L. Hartlage & C. Telzrow (Eds.), *The neuropsychology of individual differences* (pp. 42–60). New York: Plenum Press.

Brown, G., Chadwick, O., Shaffer, D., Rutter, M., & Traub, M. (1981). A prospective study of children with head injuries: III. Psychiatric sequelae. *Psychological Medicine, 11,* 49–61.

Cohen, S., Joyce, C., Rhoades, K., & Welks, D. (1985). Educational programming for head injured students. In M. Ylvisaker (Ed.) *Head injury rehabilitation: Children and adolescents* (pp. 384–385). Austin, TX: PRO-ED.

Condeluci, A. (1994). Transition to employment. In R. C. Savage & G. F. Wolcott (Eds.), *Educational dimensions of acquired brain damage* (pp. 519–542). Austin, TX: PRO-ED.

Cook, J. (1991). Higher education: An attainable goal for students who have sustained head injuries. *Journal of Head Trauma Rehabilitation, 6*(1), 64–72.

Cruikshank, W. M., Bentzen, A., Ratzburg, F. H., & Tannhauser, M. T. (1961). *A teaching method for brain-injured and hyperactive children, Syracuse University Special Education and Rehabilitation Monograph Series 6.* Syracuse, NY: Syracuse University Press.

Cullum, C. M., Kuck, J., & Ruff, R. M. (1990). Neuropsychological assessment of traumatic brain injury in adults. In E. Bigler (Ed.), *Traumatic brain injury* (pp. 129–164). Austin, TX: PRO-ED.

Deaton, A. V. (1990). Behavioral change strategies for children and adolescents with traumatic brain injury. In E. Bigler (Ed.), *Traumatic brain injury* (pp. 231–250). Austin, TX: PRO-ED.

Dilks, J. D., & Hartlage, L. C. (1990). *Common behavior problems following head injury in children.* Paper presented at the Annual Conference on Traumatic Head Injury, Williamsburg, VA.

Ewing-Cobbs, L., & Fletcher, J. M. (1990). Neuropsychological assessment of traumatic brain injury in children. In E. Bigler (Ed.), *Traumatic brain injury* (pp. 107–128). Austin, TX: PRO-ED.

Ewing-Cobbs, L., Levin, H. S., Eisenberg, H. M., & Fletcher, J. M. (1987). Language function following closed head injury in children and adolescents. *Journal of Clinical and Experimental Neuropsychology, 9,* 575–592.

Farr, S. P., Greene, R. L., & Meyers, P. G. (1983). Changes in neuropsychological functioning in patients recovering from closed head injury. *Clinical Neuropsychology, 5,* 44–55.

Fletcher, J. M., & Levin, H. S. (1988). Neurobehavioral effects of brain injury in children. In D. Routh (Ed.), *Handbook of pediatric psychology.* New York: Guilford Press.

Florian, F., Katz, S., & Lahav, V. (1989). Impact of traumatic brain damage on family dynamics and functioning. *Brain Injury, 3,* 219–234.

Frostig, M. (1975). The role of perception in the integration of psychological functions. In W. M. Cruikshank & D. P. Hallahan (Eds.), *Perceptual and learning disabilities in children* (Vol. I.) Syracuse, NY: Syracuse University Press.

Fuld, P. A., & Fisher, P. (1977). Recovery of intellectual ability after closed head injury. *Developmental Medicine and Child Neurology, 19,* 495–502.

Gaidolfi, E., & Vignolo, L. A. (1980). Closed head injuries of school-age children: Neuropsychological sequelae in early adulthood. *International Journal of Neuroscience, 19,* 495–502.

Goethe, K. E., & Levin, H. S. (1986). Neuropsychological consequences of head injury in children. In G. Goldstein & R. Tarter (Eds.), *Advances in clinical neuropsychology* (pp. 213–241). New York: Plenum Press.

Goldstein, F. C., & Levin, H. S. (1985). Intellectual and academic outcome following closed head injury in children and adolescents: Research strategies and empirical findings. *Developmental Neuropsychology, 1,* 195–214.

Goldstein, F. C., & Levin, H. S. (1990). Epidemiology of traumatic brain injury: Incidence, clinical characteristics and risk factors. In E. Bigler (Ed.), *Traumatic brain injury* (pp. 51–68). Austin, TX: PRO-ED.

Hartlage, L. (1990). Behavior and emotional changes after head injury. *Journal of Head Injury, II*(1), 17–19.

Hazaki, S. B., Gordon, L. R., & Roe, C. A. (1985). Factors associated with the employment status of handicapped youth exiting high school from 1979–1983. *Exceptional Children, 51*(6), 455–469.

Hebb, D. O. (1942). The effect of early and late brain injury upon test scores and the nature of normal adult intelligence. *Proceedings of the American Philosophical Society, 1,* 265–292.

Horton, A. M. (1994). *Behavioral interventions with brain-injured children.* New York: Plenum Press.

Hynd, G. W., & Willis, W. G. (1988). *Pediatric neuropsychology.* New York: Grune & Stratton.

Jones, M. L., Patrick, P. D., Evans, R. W., & Wulff, J. J. (1991). The life coach model of community re-entry. In B. T. McMahon & L. R. Shaw (Eds.), *Work worth doing: Advances in brain injury rehabilitation.* Orlando, FL: Paul M. Deutsch.

Kavale, K., & Mattson, P. (1983). One jumped off the balance beam: Meta-analysis of perceptual–motor training. *Journal of Learning Disabilities, 16,* 165–173.

Kirk, S. A. (1967). The ITPA: Its origins and implications. In J. Hellmuth (Ed.), *Learning disorders. Special Child Publications, 3.* Seattle, WA: Bernie Straub.

Klonoff, H., Crockett, D., & Clark, C. (1984). Head injuries in children: A model for predicting course of recovery and prognosis. In R. Tarter & G. Goldstein (Eds.), *Advances in clinical neuropsychology* (pp. 139–157). New York: Plenum Press.

Klonoff, H., Low, M., & Clark, C. (1977). Head injuries in children: A prospective five-year follow-up. *Journal of Neurology, Neurosurgery and Psychiatry, 40,* 1121–1219.

Kolb, B., & Fantie, B. (1989). Development of the child's brain and behavior. In C. R. Reynolds & E. Fletcher-Janzen (Eds.), *Handbook of clinical child neuropsychology* (pp. 17–39). New York: Plenum Press.

Kreutzer, J. S., Devany, C., Myers, S., & Harris-Marwitz, J. (1991). Neurobehavioral outcomes following traumatic brain injury: Review, methodology and implications for cognitive rehabilitation. In J. S. Kreutzer & P. H. Wehman (Eds.), *Cognitive rehabilitation for persons with traumatic brain injury* (pp. 55–73). Baltimore: Paul H. Brookes.

Kreutzer, J. S., & Marwitz, J. H. (1991). Neuropsychological evaluation for persons with traumatic brain injury. In *Practical strategies for scientifically-based rehabilitation* (pp. 168–202). Richmond: Rehabilitation Research and Training Center on Severe Traumatic Brain Injury, Medical College of Virginia.

Kreutzer, J. S., Marwitz, J. H., & Kepler, K. (1992). Traumatic brain injury: Family response and outcome. *Archives of Physical Medicine and Rehabilitation, 73,* 771–778.

Kreutzer, J. S., Serio, C. D., & Bergquist, S. (1994). Family needs following brain injury. *Journal of Head Trauma Rehabilitation, 9*(3).

Kreutzer, J. S., & Wehman, P. H. (Eds.). (1991). *Cognitive rehabilitation for persons with traumatic brain injury: A functional approach.* Baltimore: Paul H. Brookes.

Kreutzer, J. S., Zasler, N. D., Wehman, P. H., & Devany, C. W. (1992). Neuromedical and psychosocial aspects of rehabilitation after traumatic brain injury. In G. F. Fletcher, B. B. Jann, S. L. Wolf, & J. D. Banja (Eds.), *Rehabilitation medicine: Contemporary clinical perspectives* (pp. 63–102). Philadelphia: Lea & Febiger.

Lehr, E. (1990). *Psychological management of traumatic brain injuries in children and adolescents.* Rockville, MD: Aspen.

Lehr, E., & Savage, R. (1990). Community and school integration from a developmental perspective. In J. S. Kreutzer & P. H. Wehman (Eds.), *Community integration after traumatic brain injury* (pp. 301–309). Baltimore: Paul H. Brookes.

Levin, H. S., Benton, A. L., & Grossman, R. G. (1982). *Neurobehavioral consequences of closed head injury.* New York: Oxford University Press.

Levin, H. S., & Eisenberg, H. M. (1979). Neuropsychological impairment after closed head injury in children and adolescents. *Journal of Pediatric Psychology, 4,* 389–402.

Levin, H. S., Mendelsohn, D., Lilly, M. A., Fletcher, J. M., Culhane, K. A., Chapman, S. B., Harward, H., Kusnerik, L., Bruce, D., & Eisenberg, H. M. (1994). Tower of London performance in relation to magnetic resonance imaging following closed head injury in children. *Neuropsychology,* 171–179.

McAllister, T. W. (1992). Neuropsychiatric sequelae of head injuries. *Psychiatric Clinics of North America, 15,* 395–413.

Mann, L. (1979). *On the trail of process: A historical perspective on cognitive processes and their training.* New York: Grune & Stratton.

Martin, D. A. (1990). Family issues in traumatic brain injury. In E. Bigler (Ed.), *Traumatic brain injury* (pp. 381–394). Austin, TX: PRO-ED.

Miller, E. (1984). *Recovery and management of neuropsychological impairment.* New York: Wiley.

Mira, M. P., Tucker, B. F., & Tyler, J. S. (1992). *Traumatic brain injury in children and adolescents.* Austin, TX: PRO-ED.

National Head Injury Foundation Task Force on Special Education. (1989). *An educator's manual: What educators need to know about students with traumatic brain injury.* Southborough, MA: NHIF.

Naugle, R. I. (1990). Epidemiology of traumatic brain injury in adults. In E. Bigler (Ed.), *Traumatic brain injury* (pp. 69–106). Austin, TX: PRO-ED.

Newcombe, F. (1985). Rehabilitation in clinical neurology: Neuropsychological aspects. In P. J. Vinken, G. W. Bruyn, H. L. Klawans, & J. A. M. Frederiks (Eds.), *Handbook of clinical neurology* (Vol. 46). Amsterdam: Elsevier/North-Holland.

Nice, J., & Logue, P. (1984). Neuropsychological consequences of head injuries. In R. A. Hock (Ed.), *The rehabilitation of a child with a traumatic brain injury* (pp. 177–207). Springfield, IL: Thomas.

North Carolina Department of Public Instruction. (1994). Registry of Approved Providers for Traumatic Brain Injury. Raleigh, NC: Author.

Obrzut, J. E., & Hynd, G. W. (1990). Cognitive dysfunction and psychological assessment in traumatic brain injury. In E. Bigler (Ed.), *Traumatic brain injury* (pp. 165–181). Austin, TX: PRO-ED.

Oddy, M. (1993). Head injury during childhood. *Neuropsychological Rehabilitation, 3,* 301–320.

Parente, R. (1994). Academic re-entry after traumatic brain injury. In S. Menaldino (Ed.), *Newsletter of the society for cognitive rehabilitation.* (Available from the Society for Cognitive Rehabilitation, P.O. Box 53067, Albuquerque, NM 87153-3067)

Prigatano, G. P. (1990). Recovery and cognitive retraining after cognitive brain injury. In E. Bigler (Ed.), *Traumatic brain injury* (pp. 283–284). Austin, TX: PRO-ED.

Riddick, S., & Kitchen, J. (1992). *Life care planning in adult TBI.* Lecture (available as a tape) presented at the Case Management Training Conference. Richmond: RRTCSTBI, Medical College of Virginia.

Rosen, C. D., & Gerrig, J. P. (1986). *Head trauma: Educational reintegration.* San Diego, CA: College-Hill Press.

Rosman, N. P. (1986). Acute head injuries in children. In M. A. Fisman (Ed.), *Pediatric neurology* (pp. 275–306). New York: Grune & Stratton.

Rourke, B. P., Bakker, D. J., Fisk, J. L., & Strang, J. D. (1983). *Child neuropsychology: An introduction to theory, research and clinical practice.* New York: Guilford Press.

Rourke, B., Fisk, J. L., & Strang, J. D. (1986). *Neuropsychological assessment of children: A treatment-oriented approach.* New York: Guilford Press.

Russell, D., & Sharratt, A. (1992). *Academic recovery after head injury.* Springfield, IL: Thomas.

Russell, N. K. (1993). Educational considerations in traumatic brain injury: The role of the speech–language pathologist. *Language, Speech, and Hearing Services in the Schools, 24,* 267–275.

Rutter, M., Chadwick, O., & Shaffer, D. (1983). Head injury. In M. Rutter (Ed.), *Developmental neuropsychiatry* (pp. 83–111). New York: Guilford Press.

Savage, R.C. (1994). Educational issues for students with traumatic brain injury (TBI). In S. Menaldino (Ed.), *Newsletter of the Society for Cognitive Rehabilitation.* (Available from the Society for Cognitive Rehabilitation, P.O. Box 53067, Albuquerque, NM 87153-3067)

Savage, R. C., & Mishkin, L. (1994). A neurobehavioral model for teaching students with acquired brain injury. In R. C. Savage and G. F. Wollcott (Eds.), *Educational dimensions of acquired brain injury* (pp. 393–412). Austin, TX: PRO-ED.

Savage, R. C., & Wolcott, G. F. (Eds.). (1994). *Educational dimensions of acquired brain injury.* Austin, TX: PRO-ED.

Schachter, D. L., & Glisky, E. L. (1986). Memory remediation: Restoration, alleviation, and the acquisition of domain-specific knowledge. In B. P. Uzzell & Y. Gross (Eds.), *Clinical neuropsychology of intervention* (pp. 257–282). The Hague: Nijhoff.

Singley, M. K., & Anderson, J. R. (1989). *Transfer of cognitive skills.* Cambridge, MA: Harvard University Press.

Strauss, A. A., & Lehtinen, L. (1947). *Psychopathology and education of the brain-injured child* (Vol. 1). New York: Grune & Stratton.

Telzrow, C. (1985). The science and speculation of rehabilitation in developmental neuropsychological disorders. In L. C. Hartlage & C. Telzrow (Eds.), *The neuropsychology of individual differences* (pp. 271–308). New York: Plenum Press.

Telzrow, C. (1990). Management of academic and educational problems in traumatic brain injury. In E. Bigler (Ed.), *Traumatic brain injury* (pp. 251–272). Austin, TX: PRO-ED.

Telzrow, C. F. (1991). The school psychologist's perspective on testing students with traumatic brain injury. *Journal of Head Trauma Rehabilitation, 6,* 23–34.

Thompson, N. M., Francis, D. J., Stuebing, K. K., Fletcher, J. M., Ewing-Cobbs, L., Miner, M. E., Levin, H. S., & Eisenberg, H. M. (1994). Motor, visual–spatial, and somatosensory skills after closed head injury in children and adolescents: A study of change. *Neuropsychology, 8,* 333–342.

van Zomeren, A. H., & Brouwer, W. H. (1994). *Clinical neuropsychology of attention.* London: Oxford University Press.

Virginia Department of Education and Rehabilitation Research Center on Severe Traumatic Brain Injury. (1992). *Guidelines for educational services for students with traumatic brain injury.* Richmond, VA: Department of Education.

Waaland, P. K. (1990). Family response to childhood traumatic brain injury. In J. S. Kreutzer & P. H. Wehman (Eds.), *Community integration following traumatic brain injury* (pp. 225–247). Baltimore: Paul H. Brookes.

Waaland, P. K. (1992). Neuropsychological assessment of children and youth with TBI. Case Management Training Program in Traumatic Brain Injury. Richmond: Rehabilitation Research and Training Center on Severe Traumatic Brain Injury, Medical College of Virginia.

Waaland, P. K., & Riddick, S. (1992). *Life care planning in pediatric TBI.* Lecture (available as a tape) presented at the Case Management Training Program in TBI. Richmond, VA: RRTCSTBI, Medical College of Virginia.

Warzak, W. J., Ford, L., & Evans, J. (1992). Working with the traumatically brain-injured patient: Implications for rehabilitation. *Comprehensive Mental Health Care, 2,* 115–130.

Wilcox, B., & Bellamy, G. T. (1982). *Design of high school programs for severely handicapped students.* Baltimore: Paul H. Brookes.

Wilkening, G. N. (1989). Techniques of localization in child neuropsychology. In C. R. Reynolds & E. Fletcher-Janzen (Eds.), *Handbook of clinical child neuropsychology* (pp. 291–309). New York: Plenum Press.

Will, M. C. (1984). *OSERS programming for the transition of youth with disabilities: Bridges from school to working life.* Washington, DC: Office of Special Education and Rehabilitative Services, U.S. Department of Education.

Williams, J. M., & Kay, T. (Eds.). (1991). *Head injury: A family matter.* Baltimore: Paul H. Brookes.

Winogron, H. W., Knights, R. M., & Bawden, H. N. (1984). Neuropsychological deficits following head injury in children. *Journal of Clinical Neuropsychology, 6,* 269–286.

Wolfensberger, W. (1972). *Normalization.* Toronto: National Institute on Mental Retardation.

Wolfensberger, W. (1983). *PASSING.* Toronto: National Institute on Mental Retardation.

Ylvisaker, M. (1985). *Head injury rehabilitations: children and adolescents.* San Diego: College Hill Press.

Ylvisaker, M. (1991). What families can expect from schools after TBI. Neuro-Developments Newsletter of the Pediatric Brain Injury Resource Center, *1,* (3)1.

Ylvisaker, M., Hartwick, P., & Stevens, M. (1991). School reentry following head injury: Managing the transition from hospital to school. *Journal of Head Trauma Rehabilitation, 6*(1).

Ylvisaker, M., & Szekeres, S. F. (1989). Metacognitive and executive impairment in head-injured children and adults. *Topics in Language Disorders, 9,* 34–39.

Ylvisaker, M., Szekeres, S. F., & Hartwick, P. (1991). Cognitive rehabilitation following traumatic brain injury in children. In M. Tramontana & S. Hooper (Eds.), *Advances in child neuropsychology* (Vol. 1). Berlin: Springer-Verlag.

Ylvisaker, M., Szekeres, S., Hartwick, P., & Tworek, P. (1994). Cognitive intervention. In R. C. Savage & G. F. Wolcott (Eds.), *Educational dimensions of acquired brain injury* (pp. 121–173). Austin, TX: PRO-ED.

25

The Neuropsychology of Epilepsy
Overview and Psychosocial Aspects

PATRICIA L. HARTLAGE and LAWRENCE C. HARTLAGE

Although estimates of the prevalence of childhood epilepsy in the United States vary, review of a number of epidemiological studies suggests that this condition may affect up to one million children (Hartlage & Telzrow, 1984). Children with epilepsy (recurrent seizures), like all children, differ from one another on a variety of dimensions; however, children with epilepsy are subject to three conditions that contribute to increased variability. Two of these conditions are primarily neuropsychological in nature. One involves the fact that epilepsy may be symptomatic of some type of brain dysfunction, and such factors as locus, extent, type, age of acquisition, and resultant seizure manifestations may each or in combination have implications for how the child's adaptive behavior may be affected. Another neuropsychological condition involves the effects of anticonvulsant drug therapy on the child's development or manifestation of adaptive behavior. The third condition represents an interaction between such social factors as the reactions of the child's parents, peers, and teachers; the neuropsychological substrates of appropriate adaptation to the requirements of given ages; and the effects of anticonvulsant medication on both peer response and the child's potential for utilization of underlying neuropsychological assets. Although for a given child with epilepsy these three conditions are likely to be interactive, it may be helpful to overview each

condition as a separate entity before attempting to address the more complex issues involved in the interactions of these conditions.

Neuropsychological Substrates of Childhood Epilepsy

Not all children with epilepsy have intellectual deficits, but for many years it has been reported that unselected populations of children with epilepsy were likely to have mean IQs ranging up to a standard deviation lower than average (Henderson, 1953; Holmes, 1987; Somerfield-Ziskind & Ziskind, 1940; Sullivan & Gahagan, 1935; Whitehouse, 1971). More recent research has identified factors that contribute to our understanding of correlations of depressed IQ in children with epilepsy. Frequency of seizures is associated with mental deficit, greater frequency being correlated with more severe intellectual deficit in most (Chaudhry & Pond, 1961; Farwell, Dodrill, & Batzel, 1985; Keith, Evert, Green, & Gage, 1955) but not all series (Bourgeois, Prensky, Palkes, Talent, & Busch, 1983).

Type of seizure appears to be an important correlate of intellectual ability in that intellectual levels within a given seizure classification are much more homogeneous than those found among the spectrum of childhood epilepsy. Typical childhood or juvenile absence seizures, despite occurring many times per day, are unlikely to show intellectual deficit (Collins & Lennox, 1946; O'Leary, Seidenberg, Berent, & Boll, 1981; Zimmerman, Burgemeister, & Putnam, 1948). Generalized tonic–clonic seizures are most

PATRICIA L. HARTLAGE • Section of Child Neurology, Medical College of Georgia, Augusta, Georgia 30912. LAWRENCE C. HARTLAGE • Augusta Neuropsychology Center, Evans, Georgia 30809.

506

likely to show greatest intellectual deficit, with partial complex seizures resulting in intermediate levels of intellectual impairment (Tarter, 1972). Although these findings are likely fairly compatible with impressions of clinicians who work with unselected populations of children with epilepsy, a screened sample of tertiary center childhood epilepsy patients shows Full Scale IQ levels of 70 for minor motor; 74 for atypical absence; 96 for partial plus generalized; 98 for partial; 99 for generalized tonic–clonic; and 106 for classic absence (Farwell et al., 1985). In this sample, the lower Full Scale IQ scores were found to differ ($p < 0.05$) only between the minor motor and atypical absence children and all other types. The finding of highest IQ scores in the children with only classic absence type of seizures is similar to the average IQ levels of 106 and 113 reported, respectively, by Zimmerman et al. (1948) and Collins and Lennox (1946) for samples of children with classic absence seizures. Specific childhood epilepsy syndromes are even more predictive of cognitive impairment. Like children with typical absence, those with the syndromes of benign rolandic epilepsy and juvenile myoclonic epilepsy rarely decline intellectually regardless of number of seizures (Holmes, 1991), while progressive mental retardation is observed in 75–95% of children with Lennox Gastaut syndrome (Chevrie & Aicardi, 1972) and over 70% of those with infantile spasms syndrome (Bellman, 1983).

Another important correlate of cognitive or intellectual deficit in childhood epilepsy relates to age of onset, an important factor because the highest incidence of seizure onset is in the first year of life (Hauser, 1994). Many years ago, research indicated that IQ scores were lower among children with epilepsy whose seizures began before age 5 (Sullivan & Gahagan, 1935). More recent studies (Chevrie & Aicardi, 1978; O'Leary et al., 1981; Scarpa & Carassini, 1982) find the greatest intellectual impairment associated with seizure onset in the first year of life although others (Bourgeois et al., 1983; Ellenberg, Hirtz, & Nelson, 1984) failed to confirm this finding. An important component of age of onset of seizures is that of duration of seizures, in that earlier onset typically is related to duration. Recent computations show that overlap (r^2) between intelligence and age of onset accounts for 9% of variance, with duration accounting for 16% and number of years with seizures accounting for most (38%) variance (Farwell et al., 1985).

Holmes (1991) reviewed the evidence for whether or not seizures cause brain damage and concluded that the most important factors responsible for a child's eventual IQ were intelligence before the onset of seizures and etiology of the seizures. He states that for most children seizures are benign and not responsible for subsequent damage and cites recent clinical and animal data suggesting that the immature brain is less likely to suffer sequelae of seizures than the mature brain.

It is likely that studies of intellectual findings among children with epilepsy will not show a great deal of uniformity across settings because the types of children with epilepsy who are evaluated at different types of referral centers may differ on variables related to intellectual abilities. In tertiary centers, such as major medical center epilepsy programs, there is a likelihood that the more difficult cases will be studied because the relatively uncomplicated cases are less likely to be referred there. In a large series of epileptic children, Gregoriades (1972) found that 11% had classic absence seizures, whereas a report from a major teritiary care epilepsy program found only 6% of children with this problem (Farwell et al., 1985). Similarly, Gregoriades found that 50% of children in his sample had only generalized tonic–clonic seizures, whereas Farwell and colleagues' sample had only 25% of this seizure type. In light of findings concerning intellectual correlates of seizure types, it is obvious that conclusions concerning intellectual levels among children with epilepsy may be expected to vary as a function of the types of children seen in a given setting. Although there are no specific data relating to this phenomenon, it seems likely that the extent of intellectual deficit in childhood epilepsy may be somewhat exaggerated by the fact that careful psychometric studies of children with epilepsy are somewhat more likely to be reported from large epilepsy programs, to which the more complicated and difficult-to-manage seizure cases may be referred.

Formal neuropsychological studies involving assessment of children with epilepsy typically have not found a specific profile or pattern of impairment. In terms of seizure types, one study of children tested with the age-appropriate Reitan Neuropsychological Battery (Reitan & Davison, 1974) found no significant impairment among children with only classic absence seizures; and only very mild or mild impairments in children with minor motor, atypical absence, and classical absence plus generalized tonic–clonic seizures (Farwell et al., 1985). These researchers also found differences among seizure types on a screen for aphasia, with the aphasia screening scale differentiating between children with minor motor and atypical absence seizures compared with other seizure types, significance being more pronounced ($p < 0.05$) for younger children. Somewhat similar findings were reported by Matthews and Kløve (1967) who found that children with various types of epilepsy performed poorer than controls on neuropsychological measures. Somewhat more specific findings were reported by Epir, Renda, and Baser (1984) in a study of Turkish children, wherein receptive language and drawing ability were more impaired in children with epilepsy. The children in the Epir *et al.* study were somewhat atypical from those usually studied in that 80% were not receiving seizure medication. With respect to reliability, one of the few such studies was by Dodrill and Troupin (1975), who found that the majority of neuropsychological measures used for evaluation of patients with epilepsy did not demonstrate significant practice effects. However, they concluded that performance on Wechsler scales may be more affected by anticonvulsant medication than many other neuropsychological measures, thus raising the possibility that specific tests used for assessment in epilepsy may have reliability differentially affected by anticonvulsant drug therapy.

Medication–Performance Interactions

The possible influence of anticonvulsant medication on the mental performance of children with epilepsy is of obvious relevance to neuropsychological study, in that the vast majority of children with epilepsy who receive neuropsychological evaluation will likely be taking one or more anticonvulsant medications at the time of testing. This factor has, however, tended to be ignored in much neuropsychological research in childhood epilepsy.

Perhaps the first long-range approach to studying anticonvulsant medication effects on mental test performance was reported by Lennox (1942), who studied more than 1000 patients of varying ages who had received anticonvulsant medications for seizure control. He concluded that there was no relationship between anticonvulsant medications and psychological function. Similar conclusions were reached by other early investigators, who studied such anticonvulsant medications as phenobarbital (Somerfield-Ziskind & Ziskind, 1940), diphenylhydantoin (Loveland, Smith, & Forster, 1957), and primidone (Chaudhry & Pond, 1961; Loveland *et al.*, 1957; Roye & Martin, 1959). Thus, for ap-

proximately three decades there was both belief, and research evidence in support of this belief, that any behavioral impairment in children with epilepsy was not related to their anticonvulsant medication.

A problem in the investigation of possible relationships between anticonvulsant medication and mental function in children involved the individual variability in drug metabolism and the considerable variability in size found in children at different ages. At a given dosage level of anticonvulsant medication, for example, a child weighing 20 pounds would show a different response than a child weighing 80 pounds. Such fourfold variability in body weight is relatively uncommon in adults, so that the technical considerations involved in studying drug–behavior interactions in children posed a considerably greater challenge. Increased pharmacokinetic variability is also seen in children as various enzyme systems mature at different rates.

With the advent of gas–liquid chromatography (Woodbury, Penry, & Schmidt, 1972), it became possible to assess the amount of anticonvulsant medication in the child's serum at the time of mental testing. Approximately corresponding to the increased availability of gas–liquid chromatography to investigators in epilepsy was the recognition of relationships between the medications used for seizure control and mental test performance in both children and adults (Idestrom, Schalling, Carlquist, & Sjöquist, 1972; Reynolds & Travers, 1974; Trimble & Reynolds, 1976). Although the reported spectrum of psychotropic action of anticonvulsant medications in general is expected to produce psychomotor improvement (diminished retardation), cognitive improvement (especially concentration and attention), and affective improvement (diminished irritability, anxiety, and depression) (Parnas, Gram, & Flachs, 1980), it is interesting to note that apparently the opposite effect appears to represent the rule rather than the exception. Bourgeois *et al.* (1983) in a prospective study of the stability of IQ in children with seizure disorders and sibling controls found that children who had a greater number of toxic drug levels and whose epilepsy began at a younger age were more likely to show a persistent decrease in IQ. Specific relationships between given anticonvulsant medications and performance on given psychological tests were studied in a series of investigations wherein serum anticonvulsant levels were determined on serial visits with psychological testing done at the time serum levels were collected (Hartlage, 1984; Hartlage, Hynd, & Telzrow, 1981; Hartlage & Linz, 1984;

Hartlage, McCuiston, & Noonan, 1982; Hartlage, Nance, Noonan, & Shaw, 1983; Hartlage, Noonan, & Prim, 1983). For the major types of anticonvulsant medications studied (phenobarbital, primidone, carbamazepine, diphenylhydantoin, and valproic acid), most striking relationships were found between phenobarbital and primidone and neuropsychological measures. The neuropsychological measures most sensitive to serum anticonvulsant levels were coding, digit symbol, and symbol digit tests, all of which correlated ($p < 0.05$) with phenobarbital level. Two of these measures (symbol digit and digit symbol) correlated ($p < 0.05$) with primidone serum levels. Neuropsychological measures that correlated with phenobarbital serum levels ($p < 0.05$) were finger oscillation (bilateral), digit span forward and total, and a subscale involving a rapid symbol marking from the General Aptitude Test Battery. Primidone correlated ($p < 0.05$) with nondominant hand finger oscillation and Minnesota Rate of Manipulation Test, bilateral Minnesota Rate of Manipulation Test, digit span forward, and the General Aptitude Test Battery subscale. With respect to actual levels of performance, high serum barbiturate levels were associated with raw scores of 15.2, 15.5, and 11.6, compared with low serum barbiturate level scores of 27.2, 27.9, and 31.1, respectively, for performance on digit symbol, coding, and symbol digit measures (Hartlage, 1981). Relationships between neuropsychological measures and other types of anticonvulsant medications (carbamazepine, diphenylhydantoin, and valproic acid) did not exceed chance levels, and there were no significant relationships between either phenobarbital or primidone and measures of word knowledge, concept formation, or dominant hand performance on the Minnesota Rate of Manipulation Test. Dodrill (1975) reported that diphenylhydantoin depressed performance on a variety of motor tasks, but not with tasks emphasizing higher motor function, and MacLeod, Dekaban, and Hunt (1978) found relationships between phenobarbital concentration and short-term but not long-term memory. Skilbeck (1984) found memory impairment on reaction time for memory scanning affected by diphenylhydantoin, with slower reaction times related to higher dosage levels. Trimble and Cull (1989) reviewed the effects of antiepileptic drugs on children's cognition and behavior and concluded that phenobarbital was most and valproate and carbamazepine least likely to impair function. Meador et al. (1991) found that carbamazepine and phenytoin have comparable cognitive effects in adults and phenobarbital is more likely to have an adverse effect. Although there have been fewer studies of the effects of phenytoin on children, Aman, Werry, Paxton, and Turbott (1994) recorded little or no cognitive or motor effects at fluctuations in levels of the order of 50% in children with well-controlled seizures receiving moderate doses of phenytoin. These and other findings suggest that the relationship between anticonvulsant medications and neuropsychological test performance may be fairly specific, both with respect to anticonvulsant medication and the abilities affected (MacLeod et al., 1978). In any case, however, there appear to be relationships between some medications used for seizure control and performance on special mental ability measures, to an extent that merits consideration in the evaluation of the performance of a given child with epilepsy.

Social and Emotional Correlates of Childhood Epilepsy

Although there has always been fairly consistent agreement that children with epilepsy differ from their nonepileptic peers on a number of social and emotional variables (Bagley, 1971; Livingston, 1972), there is no good agreement concerning either the nature or the possible causes of these differences. Early work implicated psychopathology related to temporal lobe dysfunction (Gibbs, Gibbs, & Furster, 1948) as etiologic, although a more recent review (Dodrill & Batzell, 1986) has indicated that the incidence of emotional and psychiatric problems in persons with epilepsy is similar to that in persons with other neurological disorders, with persons having temporal lobe onset seizures showing an incidence no higher than found for those with other seizure types. Whitman, Hermann, and Gordon (1980) found that, as a group, individuals with epilepsy do not manifest behavior disturbances at a level different from that found in groups with chronic illness or nonepileptic neurological disorder. However, these same investigators found that when psychopathology was present in individuals in each of the three groups, the possibility of a more serious psychopathology was greatest in persons with epilepsy. This raises the possibility that, although epilepsy may not necessarily be etiologic in social–emotional problems, it may be a condition that exacerbates such problems. Such a possibility does not necessarily preclude the potential for specific types or causes of epilepsy to be associated with increased likelihood of social–emotional problems, and there is speculation that temporal lobe epilepsy may have different social–emotional correlates than other types because both the seizures and the behavioral disturbances may reflect dysfunctions in the limbic system. Aggressive behavior during or between seizures has been the subject of many studies. Ounsted (1969) found that children who experienced only temporal lobe epilepsy were unlikely to have social–emotional pathology although catastrophic rages occurred in those with concomitant low intelligence and hyperkinetic behavior; however, others have reported contradictory findings (Bear, 1979; Blumer, 1975; Glass & Mattson, 1973; Waxman & Geschwind, 1975). Hermann (1982) compared children with epilepsy who had impaired or unimpaired neuropsychological function. Presence of impairments demonstrated on the Luria–Nebraska battery children's version was associated with aggressive behavior and psychosocial dysfunction. At the end of a seizure the person may resist being restrained, but violence during a seizure is an extremely rare event. Only 7 of 54,000 patients with videotapes of the events had directed ictal aggression, all occurring during partial complex seizures. These were of sudden onset, brief (<30 s) duration, and consisted of stereotyped simple acts not supported by a consecutive series of purposeful movements (Delgado-Escueta *et al.,* 1981). Hermann, Dikmen, and Wilensky (1982) found that combined seizure types are most likely associated with emotional pathology, whereas no relationships between seizure types and emotional pathology have been found by other researchers (Hermann & Stevens, 1980; Lacher, Lewis, & Kupke, 1979; Matthews & Kløve, 1967; Standage & Fenton, 1975).

Although there is no common agreement concerning relationships between seizure types and behavioral pathology, there is agreement that emotional adjustment among individuals with epilepsy may be impaired. In a study of epilepsy in four countries (Canada, Finland, German Democratic Republic, and the United States), Dodrill *et al.* (1984) found a number of common problems, with emotional adjustment always representing the major area of concern. Although these findings were limited to adults, they are compatible with those of Bagley (1971) with children. Austin, Smith, Risinger, and McNelis (1994) compared quality of life in 136 children with epilepsy to 134 with asthma and found that although the asthmatics had a more compromised quality of life in the physical domain, children with epilepsy were more compromised in psychological, social, and academic domains. A feature of social–emotional problems in childhood epilepsy, when compared with healthy nonepileptic

and chronically ill diabetic children, has been found to involve the attribution of control over their lives to external sources (Matthews, Barabas, & Ferrari, 1982), with a secondary feature involving lower self-concept. This feeling of external control over their lives may be related to a finding of increased dependency in epileptic children who were matched with (otherwise healthy) tonsillectomy patients (Hartlage, Green, & Offutt, 1972). Other investigators have hypothesized that dependency in epileptic children may be related to parental attitudes (Bayley & Schaefer, 1960; Heathers, 1953), and this hypothesized relationship has received some support from Hartlage and Green (1972), who also found parental attitudes to be related to academic and social achievement in children with epilepsy. When compared with matched controls, children with epilepsy tended to perform less well academically than their ability levels would suggest, as well as tending to have poorer language usage than what would be suggested by their measured communication abilities (Green & Hartlage, 1971). Although no causal relationships between epilepsy and academic underachievement have been identified, there are a number of factors that may be involved. One involves the possibility of some depressing effect of anticonvulsant medication on academic performance. Another factor may relate to dependency, whatever origin it may have. Yet another possible factor suggested by Dodrill (1980) involves some interrelationship between neuropsychological substrates of learning. Although presumably impaired neuropsychological functioning might also be expected to depress intellectual level, Matthews, Barabas, and Ferrari (1983) reported the incidence of specific learning disorder to range from 15 to 30% among children with epilepsy, and Breger (1975) also identified learning impairments in children with epilepsy. Aldenkamp, Alperts, Dekker, and Overweg (1990) propose three major types of learning problems in children with epilepsy: memory and attention deficits and a speed of processing factor which might be affected by anticonvulsant drugs. Camfield, Camfield, Smith, Gordon, and Dooley (1993), looking at predictors of social outcome in over 300 intellectually normal schoolchildren with epilepsy, found that the presence of a learning disability was the strongest predictor of social outcome and that 35% of the children experienced school failure or needed special education. Academic underachievement corrected for intelligence in children with epilepsy has been found to be increasingly depressed with advancing age (Mitchell, Chavez, Lee, & Guzman, 1991; Seidenberg *et al.,* 1986) similar to children with specific learning disabilities (Satz, Taylor, Fried, & Fletcher, 1978), which adds another factor compounding social function.

Thus, there is agreement that problems in social–emotional spheres are not uncommon among children with epilepsy, although the causes or at least correlates of such problems, the interpretation of findings, and implementation of intervention approaches for a given child still must depend heavily on the skills and insights of the clinician working with the child.

Diagnostic and Classificatory Issues

A unique feature of epilepsy, when compared with most other chronic diseases, is that most of the time the symptoms (seizures) are not present. Further, it is relatively uncommon for the child with convulsive seizures to demonstrate them on examination, so that the diagnosis is not as straightforward as it might be with many other childhood disorders. The primary laboratory diagnostic tool, the EEG, may well not be definitive because estimates of normal (i.e., nonepileptic) individuals with abnormal EEGs are approximately 25% (Kaufman, 1981), and nearly that percentage of individuals with recurrent seizures do not have abnormal EEGs (Harris, 1976). Standard electroencephalographic recordings are more useful in children than adults with epilepsy. Below age 10, 80% will have positive findings; the yield declines with age to less than 40% after age 40 (Ajmone Marsan & Zivin, 1970). Nevertheless, the normal EEG cannot exclude seizures. Analysis of paroxysmal events by prolonged video EEG monitoring helps clarify seizure type and site of onset, and may uncover alternative diagnoses such as cardiac arrhythmias or psychogenic seizures (Kaplan & Lesser, 1990).

Seizures can be classified in a number of ways. The most widely used current classification (Commission on Classification and Terminology of the International League Against Epilepsy, 1989) involves two types, partial and generalized. In the latter, clinical and electrographic abnormalities involve the entire brain and consciousness is interrupted, briefly in absence or petit mal, and more obviously in generalized tonic–clonic or grand mal convulsions. In simple partial seizures with unilateral hemispheric involvement, consciousness is preserved, whereas in complex partial seizures, consciousness is impaired or altered. Seizures that begin locally may become secondarily generalized. Also included in the latest revision of classification are epilepsy syndromes, clusters of signs and symptoms occurring together, most with onset in childhood. The etiologies and incidence of various types of seizures differ between children and adults and the impact of seizures may vary in the different stages of development so that in a number of respects childhood epilepsy represents a somewhat different phenomenon than adult epilepsy. Complicating classification is the fact that a given child with epilepsy, whether symptomatic or idiopathic, may demonstrate different seizure types at different stages of life.

The usual system of classifying epilepsy is by seizure types but it may be helpful to keep in mind that epilepsy represents a symptom rather than a specific disease entity; in addition to multiple manifestations, there may be multiple causes. Epilepsy may represent evidence of an irritative reaction to some type of brain injury. If the nature of the brain injury is known, such as might result in the case of an identified neoplasm, the resultant epilepsy is referred to as symptomatic. In the more common cases where no specific cause is identified, epilepsy is referred to as idiopathic. Some of the idiopathic seizures with no identifiable brain lesion or history of brain injury are clearly genetic. Simple febrile convulsions, the most prevalent form of seizures in early life, clearly represent an inherited response to fever, and other age-limited epilepsy syndromes such as childhood absence and benign rolandic epilepsy are often familial. Specific chromosomal loci have been identified for seven epilepsy genes. A gene for juvenile myoclonic epilepsy and two for benign neonatal convulsions have been identified but there is genetic heterogeneity, i.e., not all affected families have these genetic loci. Genes for various forms of progressive myoclonic epilepsy have been mapped to four autosomal chromosome sites and to genetic material contained in mitochondria (Delgado-Escueta *et al.,* 1994).

Although issues involving classification are important for epileptologists, and for researchers who wish to define patient populations, the complexity of criteria for classification of seizures tends to preclude understanding by professionals from other specialties. As a result, the symptoms (epilepsy) of a variety of central nervous system disorders may be treated as if they represented a meaningful unitary classification in neuropsychological research or clinical practice. Given the heterogeneity of epilepsy, it is often difficult to generalize across studies, even involving children who have seizures within a given class, in such a way as to generate hypotheses with implications for neuropsychological assessment or intervention for a given child with epilepsy.

Treatment and Rehabilitation

Most children with epilepsy can have their seizures controlled by medication. There are more than a dozen currently used antiepilepsy drugs (NINCDS, 1980) with an equal number in development (Leppik, 1994). Four new drugs have had trials in children: felbamate, gabapentin, lamotrigine, and vigabatrin. Most are reported to be less sedating and may offer a better quality of life than "old" drugs all in use for over two decades, but no large-scale comparative studies have been done (Pellock, 1994). Felbamate, the first of the drugs to be marketed in the United States in September 1993, after several years in clinical trials with adults and children, was found after less than a year of general use to cause fetal bone marrow and liver failure, making it unsuitable for routine use in treatment of seizures. Like all new medications, antiepilepsy drugs are generally developed first for use in adults; smaller studies are then performed in children with specific types of epilepsy to investigate efficacy and age-related pharmacokinetic and safety factors. Guidelines for new drug trials in children now include careful monitoring of cognition and behavior (Commission on Antiepileptic Drugs of the International League Against Epilepsy, 1994).

The surgical treatment of epilepsy has been in use for many years (Penfield & Flanigin, 1950) and continues to be better established as an effective treatment in children and adults. Children who do not respond to medical therapy and have definable lesions like tumors or clearly focal onset seizures, especially in the anterior temporal lobe, are candidates for focal resections. In hemiplegic children with seizures arising from the damaged hemisphere, a functional hemispherectomy may control their seizures. Sectioning the corpus callosum, which connects the two hemispheres, may result in significant improvements in children with akinetic (drop) attacks or focal secondarily generalized seizures (Engel, 1993). The growth of epilepsy centers, most of which include surgery in their treatment armamentarium, has led to a number of technological advances in understanding the pathophysiology and neuropsychology of epilepsy. Supplementing video EEG monitoring and neuroimaging techniques such

as computerized axial tomography (CAT) and magnetic resonance imaging (MRI) are functional imaging studies. Studies of metabolism by positron emission tomography (PET) and circulation by single photon emission computerized tomography (SPECT) can detect epileptic foci which may not have been visualized by the morphological neuro-images (Chugani *et al.,* 1990). Neuropsychological testing has remained the gold standard of function and has contributed much to improving the efficacy and safety of epilepsy surgery, and neuropsychologists have, in turn, profited from these unique opportunities to study brain–behavior relationships.

Factors such as level of mental function, psychosocial and interpersonal adjustment, and seizure type and frequency are variables with important implication for rehabilitative prognosis. These variables, in turn, may interact with treatment variables; for example, seizure type and frequency may influence the regimen of drug or surgical therapy, which in turn may influence level of mental function and psychosocial adjustment and how teachers, parents, and peers react to the child; how well the child may perform academically with respect to his or her level of mental abilities; and so on. Prognosis for rehabilitative outcome of the child with epilepsy thus represents a multifaceted issue, with so many potentially pertinent variables as to suggest that specific prognostic statements for a given child may need to be done on an individualized, case-by-case basis.

The adjustment requirements for a child with epilepsy, as for any other child, change with age. The child with epilepsy who has been overprotected by solicitous parents may have special difficulty in separating from this protective environment to enter school and make adjustments to teachers and peers who may be much less protective or supportive.

In middle school years the child with epilepsy may encounter problems with self-esteem and peer acceptance as a result of being "different," especially if seizures occurring during school attendance are remarkable and violent. Further adjustment difficulties during this age span may relate to learning problems, whether the result of neuropsychological impairment or medication effects. Participation in some playground activities or contact sports may be prohibited, and represent yet another indication of being different. Even out-of-school activities, such as swimming or bicycle riding, can be limited, providing additional limitations to normal peer interactions or skill development.

Adolescence represents a time of special adjustment difficulty for the child with epilepsy. Successful treatment of the symptom is not enough. Adolescents with well-controlled grand mal epilepsy have been found to have poorer self-image, lower achievement, and lower expectations for their future than those with uncontrolled epilepsy (Hodgman *et al.,* 1979). Driving a car, an important adolescent milestone, may be precluded, or may be the major motivator for an adolescent with epilepsy in assuming control of her or his own health habits. Adolescence is a challenge for every individual and the individual's family and these challenges are magnified for the adolescent with epilepsy. The emerging need for independence may be clouded by accumulative academic deficiencies, limited vocational or educational options, and rejecting social attitudes (Hartlage, 1974; Hartlage & Roland, 1971; Hartlage, Roland, & Taraba, 1971; Hartlage & Taraba, 1971).

Summary

Children with epilepsy are a high-risk group for neuropsychological dysfunction. Prevention of cognitive and psychosocial problems or at least amelioration of these problems involves knowledge about the individual child's particular seizure disorder and treatment options, involvement of the child in the treatment process, early identification of academic emotional problems, minimizing restrictions in activities, and encouraging age-appropriate independence. At the first sign of academic difficulty the child with epilepsy should have a comprehensive psychological assessment to help plan appropriate educational strategies. The psychologist must be aware of the potential side effects of antiepileptic medications and the unique vulnerability of children with this unpredictable disorder to feelings of loss of control and low self-esteem. Children and adolescents with epilepsy offer to the psychologist many opportunities for fruitful research and offer great rewards from clinical service in helping these young people succeed in living with and growing up with epilepsy.

References

Ajmone Marsan, C., & Zivin, L. S. (1970). Factors related to the occurrence of typical paroxysmal abnormalities in the EEG records of epileptic patients. *Epilepsia, 11,* 361–381.

Aldenkamp, A. P., Alpherts, W. C. J., Dekker, M. J. A., & Overweg, J. (1990). Neuropsychological aspects of learning disabilities in epilepsy. *Epilepsia, 31*(4), 9–20.

Aman, M. G., Werry, J. S., Paxton, J. W., & Turbott, S. H. (1994). Effects of phenytoin on cognitive–motor performance in children as a function of drug concentration, seizure type, and time of medication. *Epilepsia, 35*(1), 172–180.

Austin, J. K., Smith, M. S., Risinger, M. W., & McNelis, A. M. (1994). Childhood epilepsy and asthma: Comparison of quality of life. *Epilepsia, 35*(3), 608–615.

Bagley, C. (1971). *The social psychology of the epileptic child.* Coral Gables, FL: University of Miami Press.

Bayley, N., & Schaefer, E. (1960). Maternal behavior and personality development data from the Berkeley growth study. *Psychiatric Research Reports of the American Psychiatric Association, 13,* 155–173.

Bear, D. M. (1979). Temporal lobe epilepsy: A syndrome of sensory–limbic hyperconnection. *Cortex, 15,* 357–384.

Bellman, M. (1983). Infantile spasms. In T. A. Pedley & B. S. Meldrum (Eds.), *Recent advances in epileptology* (pp. 1031–1034). Edinburgh: Churchill Livingstone

Blumer, D. (1975). Temporal lobe epilepsy and its psychiatric significance. In D. F. Benson & D. Blumer (Eds.), *Psychiatric aspects of neurologic disease* (pp. 171–198). New York: Grune & Stratton.

Bourgeois, B. F. D., Prensky, A. L., Palkes, H. S., Talent, B. K., & Busch, S. G. (1983). Intelligence in epilepsy: A prospective study in children. *Annals of Neurology, 14,* 438–444.

Breger, E. (1975). Psychiatric consultation to the epileptic child and his family: A study of 60 cases—Part 3: Follow-up study. *Maryland State Medical Journal,* 47–50.

Camfield, C., Camfield, P., Smith, B., Gordon, K., & Dooley, J. (1993). Biological factors as predictors of social outcome of epilepsy in intellectually normal children: A population-based study. *Journal of Pediatrics, 122,* 869–873.

Chaudhry, M. R., & Pond, D. A. (1961). Mental deterioration in epileptic children. *Journal of Neurology, Neurosurgery & Psychiatry, 24,* 213–219.

Chevrie, J. J., & Aicardi, J. (1972). Childhood epileptic encephalopathy with slow spike-wave: A statistical study of 80 cases. *Epilepsia, 13,* 259–271.

Chevrie, J. J., & Aicardi, J. (1978). Convulsive disorders in the first year of life: Neurological and mental outcome and mortality. *Epilepsia, 19,* 67–74.

Chugani, H. T., Shields, W. D., Shewmon, D. A., Olson, D. M., Phelps, M. E., & Peacock, W. J. (1990). Infantile spasms: I. PET identifies focal cortical dysgenesis in cryptogenic cases for surgical treatment. *Annals of Neurology, 27,* 406–413.

Collins, L. A., & Lennox, W. G. (1946). Intelligence of 300 private epileptic patients. *Research Publication of the Association for Nervous and Mental Disorder, 26,* 586–597.

Commission on Antiepileptic Drugs of the International League Against Epilepsy. (1994). Guidelines for antiepileptic drug trials in children. *Epilepsia, 35*(1), 94–100.

Commission on Classification and Terminology of the International League Against Epilepsy. (1989). Proposal for revised classification and terminology of the International League Against Epilepsy. Proposal for the revised classification of epilepsies and epileptic syndromes. *Epilepsia, 30*(4), 389–399.

Delgado-Escueta, A. V., Mattson, R. H., King, L., Goldensohn, E. S., Speigel, H., Madsen, T., Crandall, P., Dreifuss, F., &

Porter, R. J. (1981). Special report. The nature of aggression during epileptic seizures. *New England Journal of Medicine, 305,* 711–716.

Delgado-Escueta, A. V., Serratosa, J. M., Liu, A., Weissbecker, K., Medina, M. T., Gee, M., Treiman, L. J., & Sparkes, R. S. (1994). Progress in mapping human epilepsy genes. *Epilepsia, 35*(1), S29–S40.

Dodrill, C. B. (1975). Diphenylhydantoin serum levels, toxicity, and neuropsychological performance in patients with epilepsy. *Epilepsia, 16,* 593–600.

Dodrill, C. B. (1980). Interrelationships between neuropsychological data and social problems in epilepsy. In R. Canger, F. Angeleri, & J. Penry (Eds.), *Advances in epileptology* (pp. 191–197). New York: Raven Press.

Dodrill, C. B., & Batzell, L. W. (1986). Interictal behavioral features of patients with epilepsy. *Epilepsia, 27*(2), S64–74.

Dodrill, C. B., Beir, R., Kasparik, M., Tacke, I., Tacke, U., & Tan, S. (1984). Psychosocial problems in adults with epilepsy: Comparison of findings from four countries. *Epilepsia, 25,* 176–183.

Dodrill, C. B., & Troupin, A. S. (1975). Effects of repeated administration of a comprehensive neuropsychological battery among chronic epileptics. *Journal of Nervous and Mental Disease, 161,* 185–190.

Ellenberg, T. H., Hirtz, D. G., & Nelson, K. B. (1984). Age of onset of seizures of young children. *Annals of Neurology, 15,* 127–134.

Engel, J. (Ed.). (1993). *Surgical treatment of the epilepsies.* New York: Raven Press.

Epir, S., Renda, R., & Baser, N. (1984). Cognitive and behavioral characteristics of children with idiopathic epilepsy in a low-income area of Ankara, Turkey. *Developmental Medicine and Child Neurology, 28,* 200–207.

Farwell, J. R., Dodrill, C. B., & Batzel, L. W. (1985). Neuropsychological abilities of children with epilepsy. *Epilepsia, 26,* 395–400.

Gibbs, F. A., Gibbs, E. R., & Furster, B. (1948). Psychomotor epilepsy. *Archives of Neurology, 60,* 331–340.

Glass, D. W., & Mattson, R. (1973). Psychopathology and emotional precipitation of seizures in temporal lobe and nontemporal lobe epileptics. *Proceedings, American Psychological Association Convention,* p. 427.

Green, J. B., & Hartlage, L. C. (1971). Comparative performance of epileptic and non-epileptic children and adolescents. *Diseases of the Nervous System, 32,* 418–421.

Gregoriades, A. D. (1972). A medical and social survey of 231 children with seizures. *Epilepsia, 13,* 13–20.

Harris, H. (1976). Clinical and biochemical aspects of epilepsy. In H. F. Bradford & C. D. Marsden (Eds.), *Biochemistry and neurology* (pp. 213–240). New York: Academic Press.

Hartlage, L. C. (1974). Ten year changes in attitudes toward different types of handicaps. *Interamerican Journal of Psychology, 8,* 1–2.

Hartlage, L. C. (1981). Neuropsychological assessment of anticonvulsant drug toxicity. *Clinical Neuropsychology, 3,* 20–22.

Hartlage, L. C. (1984, August). *False positive lateralizing signs related to anticonvulsant medications.* Paper presented at the American Psychological Association, Toronto.

Hartlage, L. C., & Green, J. B. (1972). The relation of parental attitudes to academic and social achievement in epileptic children. *Epilepsia, 13,* 21–26.

Hartlage, L. C., Green, J. B., & Offutt, L. (1972). Dependency in epileptic children. *Epilepsia, 13,* 27–30.

Hartlage, L. C., Hynd, G., & Telzrow, C. (1981, October). *Canonical variate analysis of anticonvulsant medication effects in neurological measures.* Paper presented at the National Academy of Neuropsychologists, Orlando.

Hartlage, L. C., & Linz, T. (1984, October). *Differential stability of neuropsychological tests with epileptic patients.* Paper presented at the National Academy of Neuropsychologists, San Diego.

Hartlage, L. C., McCuiston, M., & Noonan, M. (1982, October). *Stability of correlations between serum phenobarbital levels and neuropsychological test performance.* Paper presented at the National Academy of Neuropsychologists, Atlanta.

Hartlage, L. C., Nance, L., Noonan, M., & Shaw, J. (1983, February). *A neuropsychological screening battery for drug toxicity.* Paper presented at the International Neuropsychological Society, Mexico City.

Hartlage, L. C., Noonan, M., & Prim, J. (1983, October). *Anticonvulsant serum level vs. dosage correlated with neuropsychological test performance.* Paper presented at the National Academy of Neuropsychologists, Houston.

Hartlage, L. C., & Roland, P. E. (1971). Attitudes toward different types of handicapped workers. *Journal of Applied Rehabilitation Counseling, 2,* 155–161.

Hartlage, L. C., Roland, P. E., & Taraba, D. (1971). Perceptions of various types of disabilities by employers. *Psychological Aspects of Disability, 18,* 122–124.

Hartlage, L. C., & Taraba, D. (1971). Implications of differential employer acceptance of individuals with physical, mental and social handicaps. *Rehabilitation Research and Practice Review, 2,* 45–48.

Hartlage, L. C., & Telzrow, C. F. (1984). Neuropsychological aspects of childhood epilepsy. In R. Tarter & G. Goldstein (Eds.), *Advances in clinical neuropsychology* (pp. 159–179). New York: Plenum Press.

Hauser, W. A. (1994). The prevalence and incidence of convulsive disorders in childhood. *Epilepsia, 35*(2), S2–S26.

Hauser, W. A., & Hessdorffer, D. H. (1990). *Epilepsy: Frequency, causes and consequences.* New York: Demons Press.

Heathers, G. (1953). Acquiring dependence and independence: A theoretical orientation. *Journal of Genetic Psychology, 87,* 277–291.

Henderson, P. (1953). Epilepsy in school children. *British Journal of the Preventive Society of Medicine, 7,* 9–13.

Hermann, B. P. (1982). Neuropsychosocial functioning and psychopathology in children with epilepsy. *Epilepsia, 23,* 545–554.

Hermann, B. P., Dikmen, S., & Wilensky, A. (1982). Increased psychopathology associated with multiple seizure types: Fact or artifact? *Epilepsia, 23,* 587–595.

Hermann, B. P., & Stevens, J. R. (1980). Interictal behavioral correlates of the epilepsies. In B. P. Hermann (Ed.), *A Multidisciplinary handbook of epilepsy* (pp. 272–307). Springfield, IL: Thomas.

Hodgman, C. H., McAnarney, E. R., Myers, G. T., Iker, H. I., McKinney, R., Parmalee, D., Schuster, B., & Tutihasi, M. (1979). Emotional complications of adolescent grand mal epilepsy. *Journal of Pediatrics, 95,* 309–312.

Holmes, G. L. (1987). *Diagnosis and management of seizures in children.* Philadelphia: Saunders.

Holmes, G. L. (1991). Do seizures cause brain damage? *Epilepsia, 32* (Suppl. 5), 14–28.

Idestrom, C. M., Schalling, D., Carlquist, U., & Sjöquist, F. (1972). Behavioral and psychophysiological studies: Acute effects of diphenylhydantoin in relation to plasma level. *Psychological Medicine, 2,* 111–120.

Kaplan, P. W., & Lesser, R. P. (1990). Long-term monitoring. In D. D. Daly & T. A. Pedley (Eds.), *Current practice of clinical electroencephalography* (pp. 513–534). New York: Raven Press.

Kaufman, D. H. (1981). *Clinical neurology for psychiatrists.* New York: Grune & Stratton.

Keith, H. M., Evert, J. C., Green, M. W., & Gage, R. P. (1955). Mental status of children with convulsive disorders. *Neurology, 5,* 419–425.

Lacher, D., Lewis, R., & Kupke, T. (1979). MMPI in differentiation of temporal lobe and nontemporal lobe epilepsy: Investigation of three levels of test performance. *Journal of Clinical and Consulting Psychology, 47,* 186–188.

Lennox, W. G. (1942). Brain injury, drugs and environment as causes of mental decay in epilepsy. *American Journal of Psychiatry, 99,* 174–180.

Leppik, I. E. (1994). Antiepileptic drugs in development: Prospects for the near future. *Epilepsia, 35*(4), S29–S40.

Livingston, S. (1972). *Comprehensive management of epilepsy in infancy, childhood, and adolescence.* Springfield, IL: Thomas.

Loveland, N., Smith, B., & Forster, F. (1957). Mental and emotional changes in epileptic patients on continuous anticonvulsant medication. *Neurology, 7,* 856–865.

MacLeod, C. M., Dekaban, A., & Hunt, L. (1978). Memory impairment in epileptic patients: Selective effects of phenobarbital concentration. *Science, 202,* 1102–1104.

Matthews, C. G., & Kløve, H. (1967). Differential psychological performances in major motor, psychomotor, and mixed seizure classifications of known and unknown etiology. *Epilepsia, 8,* 117–128.

Matthews, W., Barabas, G., & Ferrari, M. (1982). Emotional concomitants of childhood epilepsy. *Epilepsia, 23,* 671–684.

Matthews, W., Barabas, G., & Ferrari, M. (1983). Achievement and school behavior among children with epilepsy. *Psychology in the Schools, 26,* 10–13.

Meador, K. J., Loring, D. W., Allen, M. E., Zambrini, E. Y., Moore, E. E., Abney, O. L., & King, D. W. (1991). Comparative cognitive effects of carbamazepine and phenytoin in healthy adults. *Neurology, 41,* 1537–1540.

Mitchell, W. G., Chavez, J. M., Lee, H., & Guzman, B. L. (1991). Academic underachievement in children with epilepsy. *Journal of Child Neurology, 6,* 65–72.

NINCDS. (1980). *Epilepsy, the NINCDS Research Program.* Bethesda, MD: National Institutes of Health.

O'Leary, D. S., Seidenberg, M., Berent, S., & Boll, T. J. (1981). Effects of age of onset of tonic–clonic seizures on neuropsychological performance in children. *Epilepsia, 22,* 197–204.

Ounsted, C. (1969). Aggression and epilepsy: Rage in children with temporal lobe epilepsy. *Journal of Psychosomatic Research, 13,* 237–242.

Parnas, J., Gram, L., & Flachs, H. (1980). Psychopharmacological aspects of antiepileptic treatment. *Progress in Neurobiology, 15,* 119–138.

Pellock, J. M. (1994). Role of new medications in the treatment of childhood epilepsy. *International Pediatrics, 9,* 100–108.

Penfield, W., & Flanigin, H. (1950). Surgical therapy of temporal lobe seizures. *Archives of Neurology and Psychiatry, 64,* 491–500.

Reitan, R. M., & Davison, L. A. (Eds.). (1974). *Clinical neuropsychology: Current status and applications.* Washington, DC: Winston.

Reynolds, E. M., & Travers, D. (1974). Serum anticonvulsant concentrations in epileptic patients with mental symptoms. *British Journal of Psychiatry, 124,* 440–445.

Roye, D., & Martin, F. (1959). Standardized psychometrical test applied to the analysis of effect of anticonvulsant medication on the intellectual proficiency of young epileptics. *Epilepsia, 1,* 189–207.

Satz, P., Taylor, H. G., Fried, J., & Fletcher, J. (1978). Some developmental and predictive precursors of reading disability. In A. L. Benton & D. Pearl (Eds.), *Dyslexia: An appraisal of current knowledge* (pp. 313–348). London: Oxford University Press.

Scarpa, P., & Carassini, B. (1982). Partial epilepsy in childhood: Clinical and EEG study of 261 cases. *Epilepsia, 23,* 333–341.

Seidenberg, M., Beck, N., Geisser, M., Giordani, B., Sackellaris, J. C., Berent, S., Dreifuss, F. E., & Boll, T. J. (1986). Academic achievement in children with epilepsy. *Epilepsia, 27,* 753–759.

Skilbeck, C. (1984). Computer assistance in the management of memory and cognitive impairment. In B. Wilson & N. Moffat (Eds.), *Clinical management of memory problems* (pp. 112–131). New York: Aspen.

Somerfield-Ziskind, E., & Ziskind, E. (1940). Effect of phenobarbital on the mentality of epileptic patients. *Archives of Neurology and Psychiatry, 125,* 678–685.

Standage, K. F., & Fenton, G. W. (1975). Psychiatric symptom profiles of patients with epilepsy: A controlled investigation. *Psychological Medicine, 5,* 152–160.

Sullivan, E. B., & Gahagan, L. (1935). On intelligence of epileptic children. *Genetic Psychology Monography, 17,* 309–375.

Tarter, R. E. (1972). Intellectual and adaptive functioning in epilepsy: A review of fifty years of research. *Diseases of the Nervous System, 33,* 763–770.

Trimble, M. R., & Cull, C. A. (1989). Antiepileptic drugs, cognitive function, and behavior in children. *Cleveland Clinic Journal of Medicine, 56,* S140–S146.

Trimble, M. R., & Reynolds, E. M. (1976). Anticonvulsant drugs and mental symptoms: A review. *Psychological Medicine, 6,* 169–178.

Waxman, S. G., & Geschwind, N. (1975). The interictal behavior syndrome of temporal lobe epilepsy. *Archives of General Psychiatry, 32,* 1580–1588.

Whitehouse, D. (1971). Psychological and neurological correlates of seizure disorders. *Johns Hopkins Medical Journal, 129,* 36–42.

Whitman, S., Hermann, B. P., & Gordon, A. (1980, December). *Psychopathology in epilepsy: How great is the risk?* Paper presented at the annual meeting of the American Epilepsy Society, San Diego.

Woodbury, D. M., Penry, J. K., & Schmidt, R. P. (Eds.). (1972). *Antiepileptic drugs.* New York: Raven Press.

Zimmerman, F. T., Burgemeister, B., & Putnam, T. (1948). The ceiling effect of glutamic acid upon intelligence in children and adolescents. *American Journal of Psychiatry, 104,* 593.

26

The Neuropsychology of Pediatric Epilepsy and Antiepileptic Drugs

THOMAS L. BENNETT AND MAILE R. HO

Epilepsy is a nervous system disturbance that abruptly interferes with ongoing behavior, perception, movement, consciousness, or other brain functions. Individual attacks are called seizures, and when the problem is consistent it is called either a seizure disorder or epilepsy. Seizures are relatively common among infants, children, and adolescents with Hauser (1994) estimating 30,000 newly diagnosed cases of epilepsy in children in the United States for 1990 alone. Probably 8 of every 1000 children experience some sort of seizure activity, even if it is only a single occurrence of a febrile seizure (Lechtenberg, 1984). Occasionally, a seizure disorder will disappear as a child matures, but in a majority of cases, epilepsy persists into adulthood, and in 80% of adults with epilepsy, this condition developed when they were children. The purpose of this chapter is to describe the neuropsychology of pediatric epilepsy, and the emphasis will be to discuss the emotional/behavioral and cognitive concomitants of epilepsy and antiepileptic drugs (AEDs). We use the term *concomitants* to underscore the fact that epilepsy is a complex phenomenon, and the behavioral and cognitive events associated with it are the product of a complex interaction among neurological, medication, and psychosocial variables (Hermann & Whitman, 1986).

The apparent association between cognitive impairment and epilepsy has been observed for at least several centuries. For example, in his 17th century Oxford Lectures, Thomas Willis remarked: "It often happens that epileptic patients, during their paroxysm and afterwards, suffer a severe loss of memory, intellect, and phantasy" (Dewhurst, 1980). This view of epilepsy pervaded the thinking of physicians through the 19th century as clinicians continued to note a high frequency of cognitive impairment in patients with epilepsy (e.g., Turner, 1907).

A significant limitation of the early observations was that they were typically confined to investigating patients in institutions. Thus, even when IQ began to be used as an index of intellectual ability (e.g., Fox, 1924), the results were biased by sampling error. Since the 1950s, the trend has been to sample the population more generally and to investigate intellectual functions in noninstitutionalized individuals. As these latter studies were published, it soon became quite evident that epilepsy and cognitive impairment were not highly correlated. Lack of cognitive impairment began to be stressed (e.g., Keating, 1960; Lennox & Lennox, 1960). In a study of 1905 individuals with epilepsy, Lennox and Lennox concluded that fully two-thirds of their patients were intellectually normal, and only one-seventh were clearly impaired.

Many problems were encountered in the early studies of cognitive impairment in epilepsy. Major factors known to affect cognitive processes in patients with epilepsy were not controlled, and indeed, this remains a major problem for research conducted on this topic today. These factors include age at onset and duration of the seizure disorder, seizure type, seizure frequency, medication variables, and whether the seizures are idiopathic or symptomatic. These variables are discussed later in this chapter.

THOMAS L. BENNETT AND MAILE R. HO • Department of Psychology, Colorado State University, Ft. Collins, Colorado 80523.

A second major problem deals with the assessment of epilepsy. Early studies that employed objective measures used IQ testing. However, although IQ testing is in general a good measure of a person's biological level of adaptive functioning, it is nevertheless highly dependent on achievement. Furthermore, having not been developed originally to evaluate cerebral dysfunction, IQ tests are not particularly sensitive to the types of cognitive problems that people with brain injury experience. Neuropsychologists use IQ scores along with other information to estimate premorbid functioning in brain-injured individuals because of the IQ's resistance to brain injury.

Rather than using IQ as a measure of cognitive functions, recent research has used a cognitive process approach in evaluating cognitive abilities in epileptic populations. The cognitive processes investigated have included sensory processes, attention and sustained concentration, learning and memory, language skills, perceptual abilities, conceptualization and reasoning, and motor abilities. The majority of studies do not investigate all of these processes, and within a given process such as attention, one is struck by the fact that few investigators use the same task. Another problem is that a test may not evaluate what it purports to evaluate. Thus, a test of memory may actually be a test of attention, or it might be failed because of impaired attention, language, or conceptualization processes.

This latter difficulty can potentially be circumvented by utilizing a battery approach in assessment, an example of which is the Halstead–Reitan Neuropsychological Test Battery (Reitan & Wolfson, 1993). Reitan (1974) believed that this approach would be sensitive to the aggregate of cognitive impairments that might characterize a particular type of epilepsy under investigation.

Although generally in agreement with Reitan's view, Carl Dodrill has further refined the battery approach in the assessment of individuals with epilepsy (e.g., Dodrill, 1978, 1981). He has modified and/or extended the Halstead–Reitan Battery to optimally assess cognitive deficits associated with epilepsy. His battery uses 16 measures of performance. Eleven of these are from the Halstead–Reitan Battery [Category Test, Tactual Performance Test, total time, memory, and localization scores; Seashore Rhythm Test; Finger Tapping, total; Trails B; Aphasia Screening Test errors; Constructional Dyspraxia; Sensory/Perceptual exam; and Name Writing, total (letter/second)]. To this core, he added the following: Seashore Tonal Memory; Stroop Test, and the logical and visual reproduction portions of the Wechsler Memory Scale. Norms that reliably distinguished performance of patients with epilepsy from that of closely matched control subjects were established. The two groups were matched according to sex, age, education, occupational status, and race.

The sensitivity to cognitive deficits associated with epilepsy that Dodrill attempted to achieve was apparently realized as illustrated in a study by Dodrill and Troupin (1977). This study investigated the effects of phenytoin and carbamazepine on cognitive function. Use of the standardized Halstead–Reitan Battery yielded no statistically significant findings. However, several important differences emerged when Dodrill's Epilepsy Battery was employed. The application of neuropsychological test batteries to evaluate the cognitive effects of epilepsy and Dodrill's development of a battery specific to epilepsy represent advances. Unfortunately, the most common approach still remains narrow, and the majority of inquiries on this topic have continued to focus on a single, or only a few, cognitive abilities.

Four major topics are discussed in this chapter. First to be considered are the effects of epilepsy on cognitive processes such as attention, memory, and reasoning ability. That section is introduced by a model of the brain's functions in neuropsychological processes. Neural factors underlying cognitive deficits are discussed next. These include such factors as the age of onset and duration of the seizure disorder, seizure type, seizure frequency, and whether the seizures are idiopathic or symptomatic. Third, the influence of AEDs on cognitive processes is considered. Finally, alternative treatment options (nonmedication) are considered.

Epilepsy and Cognitive Processes

Because patients with epilepsy frequently present with a variety of cognitive and psychomotor deficits, as will be described in this chapter, neuropsychological assessment can be a valuable aid in establishing the severity of these impairments and monitoring the effects of treatments on these deficits. Specifically, neuropsychological evaluation before and after treatment is begun, and before and after major medication changes, should be used to determine if such changes produced positive effects for the patient; the evaluations could help determine an AED regimen that would strike an optimal balance between seizure control and adverse cognitive effects (Trimble & Thompson, 1986). Finally, knowledge of the nature and extent of neuropsychological deficits may be of help in devising remedial programs or compensatory strategies to alleviate these deficits.

The neuropsychologist can provide a direct role in treatment through traditional group and individual psychotherapy. The neuropsychologist can be an educational source for the child and his or her family about the nature of epilepsy, can help the child deal with psychosocial stressors associated with the disorder, and can help the family or teachers of the child to devise methods to manage objectionable behavior. As indicated, remedial or compensatory strategies can be devised to alleviate cognitive deficits. The neuropsychologist may also be involved in stress management and/or biofeedback training whose goal it is to reduce seizure frequency. Behavioral approaches to the treatment of epilepsy will be described later in this chapter.

This section of the chapter discusses the effects of epilepsy on cognitive processes. We discuss this against a model of neuropsychological function, which is described following a brief discussion of the effects of epilepsy on general intelligence.

Epilepsy and General Intelligence

While the vast majority of children with epilepsy fall within the normal limits of intelligence, the distribution for children with epilepsy is skewed toward the low-normal range of scores because of the underlying mechanisms/pathophysiology of the epilepsy, and not the epilepsy itself. Intelligence and the difficulties that will be discussed apply to all children, regardless of whether or not they have epilepsy, but are more frequently seen in children with epilepsy.

The importance of understanding a child's intelligence capabilities is key to being able to decipher underlying causes of poor academic performance. Material beyond a child's difficulty level or boredom with material beneath his or her level can both lead to poor academic performance. Frustration with these academic difficulties and misplaced parental and teacher expectations can lead the child to behave in improper manners during school and thus to be classified as a behaviorally problematic child. Pressures to perform at unrealistic levels by parents and teachers may be alleviated early in the child's academic career by recognizing the contributions and appropriateness of intelligence testing to academic

placement and performance. Learning problems caused by interrupted auditory or visual information processing secondary to the seizure activity are common. Lack of concentration and distractibility are also more common to children with epilepsy than children without such conditions. Particular care must be taken to evaluate the possible influences of AEDs on learning and attentional deficiencies as they all can cause problems (Freeman, Vining, & Pillas, 1990). Such sequelae are common causes of academic difficulties in children with epilepsy and careful evaluation of the causes of academic problems must be made.

Neuropsychological Model of Brain Functioning

To appreciate fully the effects of epilepsy on cognitive processes, it is helpful to consider these processes within a theoretical or conceptual model of the behavioral correlates of brain functioning. In our own conceptualizations, we have found it helpful to expand on and modify the model presented by Reitan and Wolfson (1993), which denotes six categories of brain–behavior relationships. Bennett (1988) has expanded the number of categories to seven to separate attention from memory and to emphasize the dependence of memory on attention and concentration. He expanded on their level of logical analysis and renamed it "executive functions." Note that this is a process model and not an anatomical model. With the exceptions of language skills and visuospatial, visuoconstructive, and manipulospatial skills, which are more represented, respectively, in the left and right hemispheres, these processes are bilaterally represented. This model is diagrammed in Figure 1 (from Bennett, 1988).

According to this model, the first level of neuropsychological processing is input to the brain via one of the sensory systems. It should be remembered that input could also arise endogenously from within the brain. The input must be attended to or concentrated on for information processing to occur and for the significance of the input to be ascertained (second level). Determining the significance of the stimulus or remembering it for later reference requires involvement of the memory system (third level).

The interdependence of attention and memory illustrates the fact that this neural system is dynamic, with activity flowing in both directions. In general, if information is to be remembered, it must be attended to, although, on the other hand, attention is

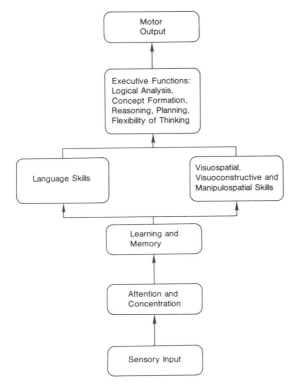

FIGURE 1. Conceptual model of the behavioral correlates of brain functioning (after Reitan & Wolfson, 1993; modified by Bennett, 1988).

no guarantee for memory. Similarly, attention is dependent on memory in terms of attentional processes being involved in such activities as habituation and filtering of gated-out nonrelevant information.

Input material that is verbal in nature requires the processing activities of a fourth neuropsychological category, language skills. Nonverbal material similarly requires processing mechanisms of a fifth category, visuospatial, visuoconstructive, and manipulospatial skills.

Executive functions represent the highest level of information processing. These activities are involved in logical analysis, conceptualization, planning, self-monitoring, and flexibility of thinking. Poor performance on tests of executive functions can result from a primary deficit to those functions themselves, or it can result from a primary deficit to one of the lower levels of processing on which executive functions depend. Executive functions quickly become quite impaired in the person who is distractible, forgetful, language impaired, or who cannot perform higher-level perceptual processes.

Motor functions are the basis for responding and represent the final common path of the neuropsychological processes. They reflect the output capabilities of the system. This is the rationale for placing motor output at the top of Figure 1. With this neuropsychological model as a backdrop, the effects of epilepsy on specific cognitive processes can be discussed.

Effects of Epilepsy on Specific Cognitive Processes

Sensory Input

Both impairment and exaggeration of sensory input can be said to result from seizures. Absence or petit mal attacks are generalized nonconvulsive seizures that occur particularly in children. They are characterized by brief episodes of loss of consciousness lasting approximately 5 to 15 seconds. During these episodes, the child seems to be unaware of his or her surroundings and stares with a vacant expression. Sensory input occurring during these periods is neither attended to nor registered.

Complex partial seizures, on the other hand, may be manifested as sensory misperceptions and/or hallucinations. Misperceptions are often visual and complex. They typically involve distortions in depth perception or size. Size misperceptions can result in objects being perceived as much smaller (micropsia) or larger (macropsia) than they are. Visual misperceptions reflect a posterior temporal lobe seizure focus. For example, they were observed to occur in a patient of ours prior to discovery of a right temporal lobe astrocytoma, and they diminished following its removal.

Misperception of voices results from a focal discharge of the anterior temporal lobe neocortex, especially from the left hemisphere. Voices will be perceived as too high or too low in pitch or as being too loud or too soft. The patient might complain that the voices around him or her sound like they are coming out of a tunnel.

Hallucinations or auras that are experienced by patients with complex partial seizures are typically simple. In general, olfactory–gustatory sensations, which are often quite displeasing, result from a focal discharge in the uncus of the hippocampus. Our patients who experience these auras most typically report salty or bitter taste sensations and/or olfactory sensations best described as burning flesh or putrid. One patient, whose seizures were particularly refractory to anticonvulsant therapy, and who experienced secondary generalized seizures correlated with menstruation, was anosmic except when she experienced olfactory auras just prior to and during menstruation each month.

Abdominal and epigastric sensations typically arise from an amygdala focus. Simple auditory phenomena, such as buzzing, ringing, and hissing sounds, are produced by focal activity on the surface of the temporal lobe, especially the primary auditory reception area. Complex visual hallucinations, although uncommon, arise from the temporo-parieto-occipital junction (Rodin, 1984).

Cephalgic auras reflect discharge originating in the central regions of the temporal lobes. They consist of severe, sharp, stabbing knifelike head pains that are often associated with the head feeling too big, too small, or off the body. Cephalgic auras will occasionally be misdiagnosed as migraine headaches and subsequently incorrectly medicated.

An important feature of auras is that they are passive experiences. The patient feels like an observer to these ictal (seizure) events, dissociated from the actual experience. This is different from the schizophrenic who firmly believes his or her hallucinations are "real" experiences. The ictal events are unrelated to the environment, except for rare seizures triggered by specific stimuli (e.g., musicogenic seizures, sexual seizures). We once had a patient whose seizures were reliably triggered whenever he played the arcade game Foosball! More typically for the complex partial seizure patient, the ictal events begin spontaneously with an arrest of all activity, and the aura and/or psychomotor responses follow. Finally, while attention is usually paid to the most salient attribute of the epileptic patient's aura, the dreamlike quality of the epileptic aura will often encompass many experiences. For example, a patient of ours regularly experienced a series of events including epigastric sensations, time distortion, detachment from her surroundings, and olfactory sensations as components of her seizure episodes.

Attention and Concentration

Impairment of attention and concentration, in the absence of overt clinical seizures, has been documented by several writers. For example, Holdsworth and Whitmore (1974) reported that 42% of their population of children with epilepsy were rated by their teachers as being markedly inattentive, and other writers have noted the detrimental effects of epilepsy-associated inattention on school success (e.g., Stores, 1973). In adults, Mirsky and Van Buren (1965) noted that the presence of epileptic spike waves was associated with decreased attention and concentration that was particularly apparent just prior to onset and following spike wave activity.

Attention difficulties in epilepsy are related to seizure type. Patients with generalized seizures are more impaired on measures of sustained attention than are patients with focal seizures (Lansdell & Mirsky, 1964; Mirsky, Primoc, Ajmone-Marsan, Rosvold, & Stevens, 1960). Mirsky and his colleagues argue that this occurs because generalized seizures are more likely than focal seizures to affect central subcortical structures that are responsible for maintaining attention.

In contrast, it appears that patients with focal seizures are more impaired on selective attention than are patients with generalized seizures (Loiseau, Signoret, & Strube, 1984; Stores, 1973). Louiseau et al. (1984) demonstrated that individuals with focal seizures and those with generalized seizures performed significantly worse on a test of selective attention than nonepileptic individuals. The worst performance was seen in the group with focal seizures. Stores interpreted this phenomenon as indicating that subcortical structures are important in determining what to pay attention to (selective attention). Focal seizures in the cortex thus produce inattentiveness by disrupting selective attention.

Learning and Memory

Memory deficits in association with epilepsy have been documented for over 100 years. Evidence has accumulated associating these deficits with temporal lobe epilepsy foci. In an early study that compared cognitive abilities in patients with generalized seizures versus those with focal complex partial seizures of temporal lobe origin, Quadfasel and Pruyser (1955) found that memory impairment was significant only in the focal group.

It should be noted, however, that most studies have been based on investigations of patients who were surgical candidates for intractable epilepsy. Little attention has been directed toward patients with complex partial seizures who were not candidates for surgical intervention. In addition, the findings from existing studies have not been entirely consistent.

When present, the memory deficit seen in individuals with complex partial seizures can exist in isolation. For example, when a complex partial seizure patient was initially evaluated using the Halstead–Reitan Battery, he showed a severe memory deficit that was more pronounced when he attempted to learn verbal material than when he attempted to learn nonverbal material (patterns). His Full-Scale WAIS-RIQ score was in the high average range, and his performance on all of the tests of the Halstead–Reitan Battery was within the normal range. Unfortunately, he showed a more global disruption of cognitive ability when tested a year later. Although his overall intellectual ability, as evaluated by the WAIS-R, had not significantly changed, he showed, in addition to his memory deficits, impairments in word-finding (dysnomia), psychomotor speed, and attention and sustained concentration. His conceptualization and logical analysis abilities remained unimpaired, but his memory deficits were even more pronounced than they had been in the initial evaluation.

The pattern of the neuropsychological deficits may prove to be an aid in determining the laterality of a temporal lobe focus, just as it is in determining the laterality of dysfunction after brain damage. One discrepancy worth noting is a difference in the severity of a deficit in processing, consolidating, and recalling verbal versus nonverbal information. It is well established that left temporal lobe dysfunction yields greater verbal than nonverbal deficit, and the opposite pattern is obtained with right temporal lobe dysfunction (Jarvis & Barth, 1984; Milner, 1975). An analogous phenomenon occurs in patients with left versus right temporal lobe foci. For example, the patient we described who had a greater deficit in verbal memory than in nonverbal memory apparently had a left temporal lobe focus, as indicated by his EEG evaluations.

Although clinical evidence that memory disorders exist in complex partial seizures is longstanding, few carefully designed experiments on this topic have been carried out, and verbal memory has been studied more often than nonverbal memory. Studies of verbal memory in complex partial seizure patients indicate that those individuals with a left temporal lobe focus perform worse on tests of verbal memory than those with a right temporal lobe focus (Masui et al., 1984; Mayeux, Brandt, Rosen, & Benson, 1980).

Fedio and Mirsky (1969) studied verbal and nonverbal memory in children with right versus left seizure foci. Although no differences on short-term memory were found, recall of verbal material after a 5-minute delay was significantly poorer in the left-focus group. In contrast, delayed recall of nonverbal material was significantly poorer in the right-focus children. Glowinski (1973) confirmed the direction of these laterality differences in adults, but the magnitude of these differences was not significant.

Since these initial studies were conducted, methodology for categorizing and matching patients has improved, and the basic findings have been confirmed, with long-term memory more significantly affected than short-term memory. For example, Lavadas, Umitta, and Provinciali (1979) investigated patients with epileptic foci in either the left or right temporal lobe who had no evidence of structural lesion on their CT scans. Short- and long-term memory were assessed. No difference in short-term memory was observed. On the other hand, patients with a left temporal lobe focus were more impaired on verbal long-term memory tasks. Delaney, Rosen, Mattson, and Novelly (1980) reported similar findings in right- and left-temporal-lobe-focus patients matched for age of onset, duration of epilepsy, and seizure frequency.

Taken together, these studies suggest a significant impairment of memory functions in patients with complex partial seizures of temporal lobe origin. A word of caution comes from Mayeux et al. (1980), who reported findings indicating that dysnomia contributes greatly to the interictal memory impairment seen in patients with complex partial seizures. Impairment on memory testing was highly correlated with deficits on the Boston Naming Test. They wrote that "the relative anomia demonstrated in temporal lobe epilepsy patients may have been interpreted by these patients and their relatives as poor memory" (p. 123). The authors further suggested that the verbosity and circumstantiality observed in some patients with complex partial seizures (e.g., Bear & Fedio, 1977; Bennett, 1987) may be the expression of a compensatory mechanism for dysnomia. This research points to the difficulty in attempting to evaluate deficits in specific cognitive processes for patients with epilepsy.

Language Skills

Both experimental inquiry and clinical observation indicate that epilepsy may adversely affect language skills. As indicated earlier, Mayeux et al. (1980) demonstrated that dysnomia was prominent in their complex partial seizure patients who had a left temporal lobe focus as indexed by scores on the Boston Naming Test. They also suggested that dysnomia contributed to the verbosity and circumstantial speech that are often observed in these individuals.

Circumstantiality is seen in both their spoken and written communication. Their communications are often overinclusive and include excessive background detailing, precise times, clarifications, and other nonessentials (Bear, Freeman, & Greenberg, 1984) and can prevent conversations from reaching a normal end. This interpersonal communication style can lead to such patients being shunned.

Hypergraphia is also often seen in patients with complex partial seizures. Hypergraphia refers to a tendency toward excessive and compulsive writing, and it was first well documented in these patients by Waxman and Geschwind (1984). It is often characterized by verbosity and circumstantiality, but it facilitated the writing of complex partial seizure victim and legendary author Fyodor Dostoyievski (Geschwind, 1984).

Impaired language skills as a consequence of epilepsy are also suggested by studies indicating that children with epilepsy have difficulty learning to read. Tizard, Rutter, and Whitmore (1969), for example, reported that 25% of their sample of children with epilepsy who were 9 to 12 years old were more than 28 months behind in reading and comprehension versus only 4% of the general population. In their Isle of Wight study, Rutter and his colleagues found that children with epilepsy showed a 12-month lag in reading ability compared with their chronological age (Rutter, Graham, & Yule, 1970). Bagley (1971) and Long and Moore (1979) have reported similar findings.

Perceptual–Motor Skills

There has not been a great deal of research investigating the effects of epilepsy on perceptual–motor skills, but the following has been reported. As was noted earlier, Dodrill (1978, 1981) found that total time, memory, and localization scores from the Tactual Performance Test were sensitive measures of the effects of epilepsy on cognitive processes. The total time score is a measure of perceptual–motor (manipulospatial) ability. A deficit in spatial memory can be evaluated via the localization score if a significant discrepancy exists between the localization score and the memory score from this task.

Several studies using the Bender–Gestalt test have indicated that children with epilepsy perform more poorly than control subjects (e.g., Schwartz & Dennerll, 1970; Tymchuk, 1974). Tymchuk found that a score that combined errors with reproduction time reliably distinguished between children with epilepsy and children with school/behavioral problems and borderline to mildly retarded children without epilepsy. No attempt was made to distinguish differential effects according to seizure type in these studies. Regarding this last factor, Morgan and Groh (1980) reported greater impairment on the Frostig Test of Developmental Visual Perception in children with focal seizures than in those with generalized seizures.

Executive Functions

Because of their dependence on lower-level neuropsychological functions, executive functions of the brain involved in such processes as conceptualization, logical analysis, reasoning, planning, sequential thinking, flexibility of thinking, and self-monitoring are especially sensitive to dysfunction, including that associated with epilepsy. As indicated earlier in this chapter, executive functions will typically be impaired in the person who is distractible, has a poor memory, is language impaired, or who has difficulty with perceptual–motor skills. In a general sense, executive functions are the basis for a person's ability to effectively meet the demands of his or her environment. Although these impairments may be easily overlooked, they are commonly seen in individuals with epilepsy as indicated by performance on such tests as the Trail Making Tests, the Wisconsin Card Sorting Test, and the Category Test. Trails B and the Category Test from the Halstead–Reitan Battery are components of Dodrill's Epilepsy Battery, and both Reitan (1974) and Dodrill (1981) stress the use of tests of executive functions in evaluating cognitive function in patients with epilepsy.

An interesting study by Hermann, Wyler, and Richey (1988) investigated Wisconsin Card Sorting Test performance (a test of frontal lobe functions) in patients with complex partial seizures of temporal lobe origin. Performance was studied in individuals whose seizures arose from the dominant versus nondominant temporal lobe as well as in an epilepsy control group composed mainly of patients with primarily generalized seizures. Thirty-seven percent of the dominant hemisphere-focus group and 79% of nondominant-temporal-lobe groups were impaired on this task, suggesting frontal lobe involvement. Only 17% of the epilepsy controls were impaired. It was suggested that these findings reflected dysfunction of the frontal lobes because of epileptic discharge ("neural noise") being propagated from a temporal lobe/hippocampal epileptic focus. Pathways that could transmit such temporal–frontal discharges are well known. After partial resection of the epileptogenic temporal lobe, Wisconsin Card Sorting Test performance improved, presumably because of a significant diminution of neural noise. A similar explanation was used to account for the finding by Novelly *et al.* (1984) that patients who underwent unilateral temporal lobectomy experienced a postoperative improvement in material-specific memory mediated by the hemisphere contralateral to the resection.

Motor Output

Decreased reaction time and psychomotor speed are common difficulties for individuals with epilepsy. Thus, McGuckin (1980) proposed that lack of speed is one of four main barriers to competitive employment faced by individuals with epilepsy. Using subjects with absence seizures, Goode, Penry, and Dreifuss (1970) reported that the presence of spike-wave activity was accompanied by disruption of attention, increased reaction time, and impaired movement on tasks of motor performance, thereby producing more errors. Errors further increased when spike waves were present for more than 3 seconds. Bruhm and Parsons (1977) also showed that slowed reaction time was common in patients with epilepsy.

Neural Factors Underlying Cognitive Deficits

Cognitive and behavioral changes associated with epilepsy are commonly attributed to neurophysiological dysfunction associated with ictal (seizure) events or long-term alterations in the central nervous system associated with repeated discharge. An example of the latter would be the kindling phenomena (e.g., see Post, 1983) or Bear's (1979) hypothesis that personality changes associated with complex partial seizures reflect a hyperconnectivity or a hyperexcitability of the limbic system. A number of variables, as reviewed by Hermann and Whitman (1986), have been posited as determining the magnitude of behavioral changes. In general, more significant effects are thought to result if the seizure disorder starts at an early age, in

patients with poor seizure control, in individuals who have had the disorder for a relatively long period of time, and if the person exhibits multiple seizure types. Complex partial seizures, particularly those of temporal lobe origin, are typically believed to produce more obvious cognitive and behavioral changes than most seizure types.

This section of the chapter briefly considers some of the neural variables that must be considered in evaluating the effects of epilepsy on cognitive processes. The following factors are discussed: etiology of the seizure disorder, seizure type and frequency, and age at onset and duration of the seizure disorder.

Etiology of the Seizure Disorder

Of the intellectual correlates associated with epilepsy and the variables that alter them, the most predictable is that of etiology and its relationship to IQ. In his review of research concerned with intellectual and adaptive functioning in epilepsy, Tarter (1972) summarized studies in which etiological factors were considered. IQ scores of individuals whose seizures were idiopathic ranged from 4 to 11 points higher than scores attained by patients whose seizures were secondary to other etiology in both institutionalized and noninstitutionalized children and adults.

Etiology can significantly confound attempts to study neuropsychological processes in persons with epilepsy. For example, Fowler, Richards, Berent, and Boll (1987) conducted a study, utilizing a modified Halstead–Reitan Neuropsychological Test Battery, to assess cognitive impairments in persons with epilepsy and to investigate correlations between deficits on these tests and EEG indices of focus localization. They were able to demonstrate cognitive impairments on most of the measures employed and, where applicable, correlate these findings with EEG localization. For example, persons scoring low on tests of verbal comprehension usually had a left temporal lobe focus. However, approximately half of the subjects in this study knew the origin of their seizure disorder. Etiologies included head injury, infectious disease (e.g., encephalitis), intracranial tumors, and cerebrovascular disease (e.g., stroke). Given that brain damage alone can severely impair cognitive functioning and that the Halstead–Reitan Neuropsychological Test Battery is highly sensitive to the effects of these conditions, it would seem impossible to sort out the cognitive impairments related to epilepsy from those related to the disorder underlying the epilepsy in this inquiry.

Dikmen and Reitan's (1978) results would support this view. They have demonstrated that, when coupled with head injury with or without persistent focal cortical signs, persons with post-traumatic epilepsy demonstrate impaired performance on the Halstead–Reitan Neuropsychological Test Battery. It is not surprising that such impairments are seen in persons with persistent focal cortical signs since there are obvious signs of brain pathology. It is their contention that it is not possible to tell if the impairments seen in persons without persistent cortical signs are related to the epilepsy or to the effects of the head injury. They argue, however, that they are most likely the result of the residual effects of the head injury picked up by a neuropsychological test sensitive to these effects.

Recent research in our laboratory by Sandra Haynes took great care to rule out prior history of head injury or neurological disease in her study of the cognitive effects of epilepsy in adults with clear evidence of focal left versus right temporal lobe seizures (Haynes & Bennett, 1991). Subjects with epilepsy were closely matched to a normal group on sex, age, IQ, and education. The test battery administered included the WAIS-R, Lateral Dominance Exam, Seashore Rhythm Test, Speech Sounds Perception Test, Seashore Tonal Memory Test, Rey–Osterreith Figure Memory Test, Story Memory Test, Boston Naming Test, Trail Making Tests, Category Test, Finger Oscillation Test, and the Grooved Pegboard Test.

The number of experimental subjects was small (four in each group), but in the absence of prior head injury or neurological disease, there were no lateralized deficits observed. The only trend found was that the subjects with epilepsy as a group exhibited generalized deficits in the areas of psychomotor speed, selective attention, and reasoning ability. This study emphasizes the importance of ruling out underlying cerebral pathology related to head injury or other neurological disease in studying cognitive processes in persons with epilepsy *per se*.

Seizure Type and Frequency

In addition to etiological factors, type and frequency of seizures constitute important variables influencing the nature and extent of intellectual and cognitive dysfunction. A number of studies have shown generalized tonic–clonic seizures to be asso-

ciated with greater intellectual and cognitive impairment than other types of seizures. An early study by Zimmerman, Burgemeister, and Putnam (1951) investigated intellectual ability in children and adults using the Stanford Binet, Wechsler–Bellevue, and Merrill–Palmer Performance Tests. Mean IQ measured in children and adults with idiopathic absence seizures ranged from 10 to 14 points higher than in patients with tonic–clonic seizures. Using the WAIS and the Halstead–Reitan battery, Matthews and Kløve (1967) found that adult patients who experienced generalized seizures demonstrated greater overall intellectual–cognitive impairment than patients with other types of seizures regardless of whether the seizures were idiopathic or symptomatic. Wilkus and Dodrill (1976) also observed poorer performance by adults with EEG evidence of generalized discharged versus a focal seizure group. In addition, they noted that more frequent seizures were associated with greater deficits. This negative correlation between cognitive ability and frequency of seizures was also reported by Dikmen and Matthews (1977) in a study of 72 adults with tonic–clonic seizures of known and unknown etiology.

A similar relationship between seizure frequency and intellectual–cognitive impairment has been reported in children. In an early study, Keith, Ewert, Green, and Gage (1955) reviewed medical records of 296 children and found a regular increasing progression in percentage of retarded children as frequency of seizures increased. This relationship was consistent across all seizure types considered. Also, cases on which the seizures were symptomatic showed a greater incidence of retardation (73%) than those on which the cause of seizures could not be attributed to organic abnormality (22.2%).

Farwell, Dodrill, and Batzel (1985) evaluated a large group of children whose ages ranged from 6 to 15 years. Within each seizure type studied, lower seizure frequency was associated with higher scores on the WICS-R. In addition, seizure type was found to be a discriminating factor when both IQ and neuropsychological functions were evaluated. The minor motor and atypical absence groups showed statistically significant lower IQ scores than all other groups. However, children with partial or generalized tonic–clonic seizures demonstrated proportions of Full-Scale IQ scores comparable to those observed in the control group. When considered together, children with epilepsy showed significantly greater neuropsychological impairment than controls as measured by the age-appropriate

Halstead–Reitan battery. Overall, neuropsychological impairment was found to differentiate between seizure types with greater sensitivity than did Full-Scale IQ (WISC-R). Children with minor motor or atypical absence seizures demonstrated no detectable neuropsychological impairment, but when seizure types were mixed (classical absence plus generalized tonic–clonic), impairment was again evident.

Seizure type has been found to affect selected cognitive functions differentially. Quadfasel and Pruyser (1955) compared cognitive abilities in adult male patients with generalized seizures versus complex partial seizures and found that memory was impaired only in the partial seizure group. Fedio and Mirsky (1969) assessed the performance of outpatient groups of children (6 to 14 years old) who had left temporal lobe epileptic focus, right temporal focus, or centrencephalic epilepsy (generalized seizures). Children were evaluated using measures of attention, verbal and nonverbal learning and memory, and IQ. Regardless of seizure type, the performance of children with epilepsy was below that of the epileptic control group. Of greater interest, however, was the pattern of deficits observed between seizure types and within the temporal lobe seizures groups. Children with left temporal lobe focus showed learning and memory deficits on measures that required delayed recall of verbal material whereas children with right temporal lobe focus had greater difficulty with recall tasks involving visuospatial abilities. Significant differences between performance on measures of short-term memory were not evident between groups. Further, children whose seizures were centrencephalic in nature performed at a significantly lower level on tasks of sustained attention than did the temporal lobe groups, but they did not demonstrate either short- or long-term memory impairment.

Patterns of intellectual performance on the Wechsler Intelligence Scales (WAIS or WISC-R) that varied with seizure type were observed by Giordani et al. (1985). Adults and children with partial seizures performed better on Digit Span, Digit Symbol (or Coding), Block Design, and Object Assembly than did patients with either generalized or partial secondarily generalized seizures although significant differences between groups on Full-Scale IQ scores were not present.

In contrast, some studies have not shown a clear relationship between seizure type and cognitive impairment (Arieff & Yacorzynski, 1942; Scott, Moffett, Matthews, & Ettlinger, 1967) or frequency of seizures and greater intellectual impairment (Delaney et al., 1980; Loiseau et al., 1980; Scott et al., 1967). O'Leary et al. (1983) found only one variable that showed a significant difference in performance between groups of children with differing seizure disorders. Children with partial seizures performed significantly better on the Tactual Performance Test (TPT-total time) than children with generalized seizures. The partial seizure group in this study, however, was composed of simple partial, complex partial, and partially secondarily generalized seizure types, and this wide variation of seizure types within one group may have accounted for the limited differences seen when groups were compared.

Because seizure classifications and their inclusion criteria have not been consistent, particularly in the earlier studies, and populations tested have not been uniform across investigations (institutionalized versus noninstitutionalized), direct comparisons between studies are not always possible. The study of seizure type and frequency and its effect on intellectual and cognitive function is further complicated by the severity of seizures and the levels of antiepileptic medications necessary to achieve adequate seizure control. It is also possible that in some cases, the association between observed cognitive deficits and frequency of seizures is related to the extent of cerebral damage which is responsible for both. When considered as a whole, however, current studies suggest that the extent of intellectual and cognitive dysfunction in epilepsy varies with type of seizure and increases with greater seizure frequency.

Age at Onset and Duration of Disorder

More than a century ago, Gowers recognized the relationship between early onset of seizure disorder and poor prognosis for mental functioning (Browne & Reynolds, 1981). In general, current research supports this observation. Studies of intellectual and neuropsychological functions in children with epilepsy, regardless of seizure type, indicate that onset of seizures early in life and a consequently long duration of seizure disorder places children at higher risk for cognitive dysfunction. It should be noted that in studies of children, long duration of seizure disorder is necessarily associated with early onset. Many studies of the effect of age of onset in the past have considered only major motor (generalized tonic–clonic seizures). Dikmen, Matthews, and Harley (1977) found that adult patients with early onset of major motor seizures (0 to 5 years of age) achieved significantly lower Verbal, Performance, and Full-Scale IQ scores (WAIS) than a group of patients with later onset of seizures (10–15 years of age). Both seizure groups showed impaired neuropsychological functions (Halstead–Reitan) relative to a nonepileptic control group. However, differences in performance between the early and late-onset epileptic groups were not significant. On the other hand, Matthews and Kløve (1967) found that early onset of generalized tonic–clonic seizures resulted in greater impairment of both intellectual and neuropsychological abilities. This difference was observed in both idiopathic seizures and seizures secondary to known pathology (symptomatic seizures).

O'Leary et al. (1983) studied the effects of early onset of epilepsy in children 9 to 15 years of age with partial versus generalized seizures. Results indicated that both groups of children with early seizure onset performed more poorly on measures of neuropsychological abilities than children whose seizures began at a later age. These findings remain consistent with observations of the effect of seizure onset by Farwell et al. (1985), who studied a variety of seizure types, and Scarpa and Carassini (1982) in their study of children with partial seizures.

As in studies of seizure frequency, investigation of the effects of age at onset is complicated by AEDs. These have been found to affect cognitive performance in both children and adults (Browne & Reynolds, 1981; Trimble, 1981). In cases of early seizure onset, the effects of AEDs on the developing brain become an important consideration as does the subsequent long-term drug therapy that must follow.

Intellectual and Cognitive Effects of AEDs

AEDs or anticonvulsant medications have been implicated in producing negative cognitive and emotional effects in patients with seizure disorders. As a general rule, toxic blood serum levels of all AEDs adversely affect behavior and cognition (Reynolds, 1983; Wyllie, 1993), but adverse behavioral effects are sometimes associated with serum levels of AEDs that are within the therapeutic range (Thompson, Huppert, & Trimble, 1981). Polypharmacy increases the risk of epilepsy patients developing cognitive and emotional disorders with reductions in polytherapy resulting in improved cognition (Duncan, Shorvon, & Trimble, 1990;

Thompson & Trimble, 1982). Generally, phenobarbital and primidone (20% of which is metabolized into phenobarbital) are thought to produce the most significant effects, but phenytoin has also been implicated. In a double-blind study of polytherapy reduction, removal of phenytoin from drug therapy resulted in significant improvements in motor speed and in attention and concentration. Discontinuation of sodium valproate and carbamazepine in polytherapy have also resulted in increases in motor speed but no improvement in attention and concentration (Duncan et al., 1990). Generally, AEDs can magnify behavioral and cognitive changes produced by the seizure disorder itself, but in contrast, carbamazepine and sodium valproate have been argued to produce positive psychotropic effects.

Intellectual and cognitive impairments in people with epilepsy, especially memory deficits, were observed and noted in the literature over 100 years ago, long before current AEDs were utilized (Trimble & Thompson, 1981). Unfortunately, there is increasing evidence not only that cognitive deficits occur as a direct result of seizures themselves but also that many, if not most, AEDs affect cognitive abilities. As a result, AEDs may thereby compound the cognitive difficulties and behavioral problem seen in persons with epilepsy (American Academy of Pediatrics, 1985; Bellur & Hermann, 1984; Blumer & Benson, 1982; Committee on Drugs, 1985; Corbett, Trimble, & Nichol, 1985; Himmelhock, 1984; Reynolds & Trimble, 1985; Walker & Blumer, 1984; Wilson, Petty, Perry, & Rose, 1983). Therefore, the disentangling of medication effects from seizure effects represents a formidable challenge to researchers.

For most AEDs, favorable reports, usually based on subjective impressions, have been noted immediately after the drugs have been introduced for general use. With widespread use and experimental inquiry into their neuropsychological influence, adverse effects soon have emerged for most AEDs. Toxic doses of virtually all AEDs can affect mental functioning. It is, however, the possibility of cognitive impairment resulting from serum concentrations of AEDs within therapeutic ranges that is of most concern in the long-term treatment of epilepsy.

For example, Reynolds and Travers (1974) studied a group of 57 outpatients some of whom were experiencing intellectual deterioration, psychiatric illness, personality change, or psychomotor slowing. Those who were experiencing these difficulties had significantly higher blood levels of phenytoin or phenobarbital than those without such changes even though these individuals all had blood levels of these drugs that were within the optimum or therapeutic range. Patients with overt drug toxicity, detectable cerebral lesions, or psychiatric illness that preceded the onset of epilepsy had been excluded from the study. These observations were also not simply related to seizure frequency. Similar findings were reported by Trimble and Corbett (1980) in a study of 312 children in a residential hospital school. Children who experienced a decline in IQ of between 10 and 40 points over a 1-year interval had significantly higher levels of phenytoin and primidone, with a similar trend for phenobarbital, than those who did not. Farwell *et al.* (1990) found that children receiving phenobarbital after at least once febrile seizure and who were at risk for further seizures scored an average of 8.4 IQ points lower than those receiving placebos. Again, blood levels of these AEDs were within the therapeutic range for both studies.

The nature and extent of these deficits vary with the drug or combination of drugs administered, as well as the serum concentration of the drug. As would be expected, polytherapy (administration of more than one AED) has been found to result in greater deficits than monotherapy (MacLeod, Dekaban, & Hunt, 1978; Shorvon & Reynolds, 1979; Thompson & Trimble, 1982). Shorvon and Reynolds (1979) were able to reduce polytherapy to monotherapy in 29 of 40 outpatients studied. In over half of the patients reduced to monotherapy, improvements in alertness, concentration, drive, mood, and sociability were observed. This was especially noted in association with withdrawal of phenobarbital or primidone. Similarly, Fischbacher (1982) reported that reduction of at least one AED in institutionalized patients improved alertness, psychomotor performance, and behavior. Most investigations of AEDs have been conducted with adults. However, there is no evidence suggesting that the pathophysiological mechanisms or properties of anticonvulsant medications in childhood (partial) epilepsy differ from adult partial epilepsy (Pellock, 1994). The body of a child, however, utilizes the medications quite differently than adults and, further, each child will metabolize and eliminate the AED differently (Dodson & Pellock, 1993). While the cognitive effects of the older AEDs on children have been investigated quite extensively, the cognitive effects of the newer AEDs on children remain to be established. Many reports of the mechanisms of action of the new AEDs have been published (e.g., Fisher, 1993; Kalviainen, Keranen, & Riekkinen, 1993; Vajda, 1992) and more specific information in children will follow suit

as was the case with previous AEDs. To date, the known cognitive effects produced by commonly prescribed AEDs include the following.

Phenobarbital

Early studies investigating the cognitive effects of phenobarbital led to the conclusion that, despite its sedative properties, the drug had no adverse effects on cognitive ability (Grinker, 1929; Lennox, 1942; Somerfield-Ziskind & Ziskind, 1940). However, with the development of more sensitive neuropsychological tests and the medical technology necessary to accurately monitor serum anticonvulsant levels, intellectual and cognitive dysfunction associated with phenobarbital soon became apparent. For example, Hutt, Jackson, Belsham, and Higgins (1968) tested phenobarbital on nonepileptic volunteers and found that it impaired sustained attention and psychomotor performance.

Hyperactivity is often a paradoxical side effect of phenobarbital therapy (McGowan, Neville, & Reynolds, 1983; Painter & Gaus, 1993; Wolf & Forsythe, 1978). In a comparative study of monotherapy with four major anticonvulsants in previously untreated children with epilepsy, McGowan *et al.* (1983) found that five of the ten children assigned to the phenobarbital group developed hyperactivity or aggressive behavior or difficulty coping with schoolwork. This necessitated withdrawal of the drug from the patients and discontinuing its use in the study.

Primidone

Primidone (Mysoline) is a barbiturate analogue that is metabolized to phenobarbital and phenylethylmalonamide (PEMA) whose actions may be synergistic. There is little direct experimental evidence with respect to the effects of primidone on cognitive ability in children, but it is generally believed that the effects closely parallel those produced by phenobarbital.

Phenytoin

When phenytoin (Dilantin) was initially introduced as an AED, it was thought to improve alertness (Trimble, 1981). Past research has indicated that phenytoin has adverse effects on psychomotor performance (Idestrom, Schelling, Carlquist, & Sjoquist, 1972; Thompson & Trimble, 1982), concentration (Andrewes, Tomlinson, Elwes, & Reynolds, 1984; Dodrill & Troupin, 1977), memory (Andrewes *et al.,* 1984; Thompson & Trimble, 1982), and problem-solving (Dodrill & Troupin, 1977). However, the most recent indications are that the negative cognitive effects associated with phenytoin (and phenobarbital) were not large in psychometric magnitude and that conflicting results in previous studies may be related to problems in patient selection, study design, and serum concentration levels (Dodrill & Troupin, 1991; Duncan *et al.,* 1990; Meador, Loring, Huh, Gallagher, & King, 1990). Meador *et al.* (1990) found no evidence of adverse cognitive effects of phenytoin at moderate doses.

A reversible phenytoin-induced encephalopathy, observed without other clear neurological evidence of toxicity such as nystagmus or ataxia and characterized by intellectual and memory impairment, has been reported (Trimble & Reynolds, 1976). This encephalopathy can occur in adults, but is most often seen in children and especially those with preexisting mental retardation or brain damage. The deterioration of intellectual functioning in the absence of classical signs of toxicity may result in a misinterpretation of the reversible encephalopathy as a progressive neurological disease.

Ethosuximide

Browne *et al.* (1975) studied the effects of ethosuximide on psychometric performance and noted an improvement in 17 of 37 children. Blood levels of ethosuximide were monitored and remained within therapeutic ranges over the 8-week duration of the study. These findings were inconsistent with earlier reports (Guey, Charles, Coquery, Roger, & Soulayrol, 1967). However, 15 of 25 children studied by Guey *et al.* (1967) were mentally retarded and taking other drugs in addition to ethosuximide. Nevertheless, there have been additional reports of psychosis or encephalopathy resulting from ethosuximide administration (Roger, Grangeon, Guey, & Lob, 1968).

Valproic Acid (Sodium Valproate)

Trimble and Thompson (1984) reported minimal adverse side effects associated with the administration of valproic acid on neuropsychological test performance. Barnes and Bower (1975) had previously suggested that sodium valproate improved alertness and school performance. On the negative side, there have been several reports of sodium valproate-induced encephalopathy, similar to that described for phenytoin (Davidson, 1983;

Reynolds, 1985). Dean (1993) suggests that when at-risk populations are correctly identified, sodium valproate clearly remains the drug of choice for most forms of generalized epilepsy because of its effectiveness, broad spectrum of activity, and relative lack of CNS side effects. Dean (1993) further points out that sodium valproate exhibits lower cognitive dulling and behavioral disturbances when compared to phenytoin, phenobarbital, primidone, and the benzodiazepines.

Carbamazepine

Carbamazepine (Tegretol), like sodium valproate, appears to produce minimal adverse side effects on cognitive processes. Dalby (1975) reported the occurrence of behavioral alterations associated with complex partial seizures of temporal lobe origin. Specifically, decreases in speed of information processing, interpersonal viscosity, emotional lability, and increased aggressivity all improved with carbamazepine in approximately 50% of his patients.

An interesting study by Schain, Ward, and Guthrie (1977) evaluated the cognitive consequences of replacing phenobarbital and primidone with carbamazepine in the treatment of children with tonic–clonic and complex partial seizure disorders. A battery of neuropsychological tests intended to assess general intelligence, problem-solving ability, and inattentiveness was administered. Substantial improvement in problem-solving measures were noted with carbamazepine drug therapy. In addition, the children appeared to be more alert and attentive than when they were treated with phenobarbital or primidone. Carbamazepine control of seizures remained adequate. Thompson and Trimble (1982), using adults, also found carbamazepine to have a less detrimental effect on cognitive functioning than did phenobarbital or primidone.

Overall, carbamazepine appears to be a promising AED that is most effective as monotherapy but also effective as polytherapy, with seizure reduction shown for focal, generalized tonic–clonic (primary and secondary), and some types of symptomatic generalized seizures. Its efficacy appears to be comparable to phenytoin, phenobarbital, primidone, and valproate with some positive psychotropic effects observed with a controlled release (Sillanpää, 1993).

Felbamate

Of the current and new antiepileptic medications, initial investigation indicated that felbamate

(Felbatol) was effective both in monotherapy and in polytherapy treatment of complex partial seizures with the added benefit of low toxicity. The speculated mechanism of action is that felbamate appears to prevent the spread of seizures by increasing the seizure threshold (Graves & Leppick, 1991; Wagner, 1994) but its specific mechanism of action remains unclear (Ramsay & Slater, 1993).

However, felbamate can and does have complex interactions with other AEDs (see Ramsay & Slater, 1993, for a complete reporting). A double-blind safety and efficacy trial of felbamate in polytherapy, sponsored by the National Institutes of Health (NIH), indicated significant changes in serum levels of phenytoin and carbamazepine. These pharmacokinetic changes necessitated a redistribution of relative doses of phenytoin and carbamazepine to alleviate toxicity (Graves & Leppick, 1991). It is suggested that polytherapy with felbamate be carefully titrated and that doses of felbamate and concurrent AEDs be adjusted accordingly. Most adverse effects associated with felbamate are observed in polytherapy (Wagner, 1994). Initial clinical trials indicate that phenytoin and valproic acid doses were routinely reduced by 20% following administration of felbamate. It should be noted that while felbamate has been found to significantly alter serum levels of phenytoin and carbamazepine, the latter have likewise been found to alter serum levels of felbamate. Additionally, felbamate has not been linked to any neurotoxic effects independent of phenytoin and carbamazepine (Graves & Leppick, 1991).

During the summer of 1994, the manufacturers of felbamate recommended discontinuation of therapy utilizing felbamate due to reports of its adverse effects on the liver and incidents of aplastic anemia (Trimble, 1994). Felbamate usage was resumed shortly thereafter, but it continues to be underutilized because of the 1 in 10,000 incidence rate of aplastic anemia. Frequent monitoring of complete blood counts is recommended with current felbamate usage.

Gabapentin

Early studies of gabapentin indicate that it is moderately to highly effective in the treatment of partial and tonic–clonic seizures (Crawford, Ghadiel, Lane, Blumhardt, & Chadwick, 1987). A double-blind, add-on study by Sivenius, Kalviainen, Ylinken, and Riekkinen (1991) showed that patients who received 1200 mg/day gabapentin for 3 months reduced their partial seizure frequency by 57% whereas patients receiving 900 mg/day and patients in the placebo group experienced no significant reduction in seizure frequency. Transient mild to moderate somnolence was the only consistent adverse effect reported in gabapentin add-on use. Despite the encouraging early figures touting gabapentin as an interaction-free AED (Schmidt, 1989), more recent polytherapy efficacy reports for gabapentin doses have been conflicting. As of 1993, nearly 800 patients with refractory partial seizures have been followed by Browne. Of these, 15% of the patients administered 900 mg/day and 19% of the patients administered 1200 mg/day dropped out of the study because they had no decreases in seizure frequency by 12 and 18 months. The remaining patients experienced decreases in seizure frequencies of 45 and 46% at 12 and 18 months, respectively, after beginning polytreatment with gabapentin. Some patients with generalized tonic–clonic and absence seizures have shown some benefit from gabapentin (Abou-Khalil, Shellenberger, & Anhut, 1992; Bauer, Bechinger, Castell, Deisenhammer, & Egli, 1989). Clinical safety and efficacy trials continue to show support for gabapentin's utility as an AED (see Graves & Leppick, 1991; Ramsay & Slater, 1993) and variations reported should take into account the lack of well-defined therapeutic range of gabapentin dosage.

Monotherapy utilizing 1200 mg/day of gabapentin reduced seizures in 50% of the test population but was less effective than the same dose of carbamazepine or polytherapy with gabapentin and carbamazepine (Wilensky, Temkin, Ojeman, Rischer, & Holubkov, 1992). Of 127 patients with refractory partial epilepsy administered either 1.2 g/day gabapentin or a placebo in a double-blind parallel design, 26% of the patients exhibited a greater than 50% reduction in seizure frequency versus 10% of those receiving the placebo (Graves & Leppick, 1991). A similar study by Schmidt (1989) produced like findings for patients receiving comparable doses of gabapentin and additionally reported best responses by generalized tonic–clonic and absence seizure types.

Dodrill, Wilensky, Ojeman, Temkin, and Shellenberger (1992) compared monotherapy gabapentin and carbamazepine patients' neuropsychological performances after treatment for 4 to 8 months. Results indicate no significant performance differences between the two groups. Interestingly, after patient reports of a general improvement in feelings of well-being, a 1986 study of ten healthy volunteers by Saletu, Grunberger, and Linzmayer showed that improvements in concentration, alphabetical reaction tests, and numerical memory were observed after 200-mg and again after 400-mg doses of gabapentin (in Ramsay & Slater, 1993).

Lamotrigine

Lamotrigine was recently developed as an AED whose mechanism of action is postsynaptic and has a profile similar to phenytoin. Lamotrigine's efficacy has been extensively studied with an exhaustive overview by Richens and Yuen (1991) reporting 27 to 30% of subjects from various studies and populations achieving at least 50% reduction in total seizures (Vajda, 1992).

Although studies of lamotrigine safety are ongoing, initial results from an adult population of over 1000 subjects indicate a low incidence of adverse reactions. This double-blind design with lamotrigine as an add-on to existing antiepileptic medications resulted in no higher than 14% of the population reporting mild adverse experiences including dizziness, diplopia, somnolence, headache, ataxia, and asthenia (Betts, Goodwin, Withers, & Yuen, 1991). Similar rates of adverse effects were reported by Gram (1989). See Ramsay and Slater (1993) for a comprehensive report of seven efficacy trials that suggest an overall result profile of lamotrigine as an effective AED in add-on polytherapy in partial seizure disorders and possibly in primary generalized seizures with relatively minor adverse effects.

Of 36 pediatric subjects exposed to lamotrigine for over 12 weeks, add-on results indicate similar results with up to 50% reductions in seizures previously resistant to AEDs. Myoclonic jerks, myoclonic absences, and tonic and atonic seizures responded best to lamotrigine (Dulac, Withers, & Yuen, 1991). Recent studies in pediatric epilepsy have indicated that lamotrigine is well tolerated and exhibits best results in absence epilepsy, Lennox–Gastaut syndrome, and other symptomatic generalized epilepsy (Schlumberger et al., 1994; Wallace, 1990).

While lamotrigine appears to operate without altering serum levels of concurrently administered AEDs, the reverse is not true. Lamotrigine pharmacokinetics are significantly altered by valproic acid (Gram, 1989) and may have significant interactions with other AEDs (Graves & Leppick, 1991).

Vigabatrin

The study of the role of GABA inhibition in the reduction of seizure activity has led to the development of vigabatrin (Sabril), whose mechanism of antiepileptic action is tied to its ability to increase GABA levels in the brain (Beyers, 1993). Patients with chronic refractory epilepsy receiving predominately polytherapy, showed significant reductions in seizure activity. Ring, Heller, Farr, and Reynolds (1990) found that the addition of vigabatrin was associated with a 48% reduction in seizure frequency. Adverse side effects including headache, depression, increased lability of mood, dizziness, and confusion led to the withdrawal of 7 of the original 51 subjects. Six other subjects were withdrawn because they failed to achieve a 50% reduction in seizures. A 1991 study by Reynolds, Ring, Farr, Heller, and Elwes showed even greater promise for the utility of vigabatrin with a third of their sample showing greater than 75% reductions in seizures. Two of their subjects became seizure free and adverse side effects were similar to other AEDs in nature and frequency. Such results have led to vigabatrin's consideration as one of the most promising new AEDs available. Despite the fact that vigabatrin is well documented to significantly reduce serum levels of phenytoin as well as primidone and phenobarbital concentrations, the number of efficacy and safety studies in support of it have not been surpassed. Ben-Menachem et al. (1989) report favorable and comparable efficacy between adults and children treated with vigabatrin. In children, both controlled and open clinical efficacy studies indicate that vigabatrin is a safe and effective AED in the treatment of partial seizures (Gillham, Blacklaw, McKee, & Brodie, 1993; Grant & Heel, 1991; Herranz et al., 1991; Livingston, Beaumont, Arzimanoglou, & Aicardi, 1989; McGuire, Duncan, & Trimble, 1992; Mumford, Beaumont, & Gisselbrecht, 1990). Adding to vigabatrin's appeal is the apparent lack of tolerance to the medication following long-term use (Browne et al., 1989; Tartara et al., 1989).

When collectively considered, these studies indicate that some AEDs can have negative effects on cognitive functions. These findings allow us to conclude that some of the neuropsychological changes that are observed in children with epilepsy occur as a result of anticonvulsant therapy rather than a consequence of the many variables, reviewed earlier, that can themselves alter cognitive ability in these individuals. This is an important consideration in prescribing these agents. Although these subtle, yet significant, cognitive effects may easily be overlooked without careful neuropsychological monitoring, they may be a large price to pay for seizure control, or quite commonly, inadequate seizure control. This is especially true for children and others in academic pursuits (Stores, 1981) and for adults whose occupations require psychomotor speed, sustained concentration, and high levels of information processing. Studies of the efficacy and cognitive effects of the newer AEDs continue, however, and show promise in the treatment of certain refractory childhood epilepsy syndromes.

In addition to the specific effects of AEDs on cognitive functioning, one should also take into account the 1994 study by Austin, Smith, Risinger, and McNelis examining the quality of life for children with epilepsy versus those with asthma. While a reduction in seizure activity is certainly an improvement in one's quality of life, their results indicate that children with epilepsy still have a greater degree of compromised quality of life in terms of psychological, social, and school domains than children with a comparable chronic illness. The role of psychosocial problems in the lives of adolescents with epilepsy has been recognized by the development of the Adolescent Psychosocial Seizure Inventory (APSI). The APSI is an objective assessment tool covering eight areas of psychosocial adjustment (Batzel et al., 1991).

Nonmedication Alternative Treatments

Surgical Treatment

Ten to twenty percent of the 150,000 people who develop epilepsy each year are deemed to have intractable seizure disorders that fail to be controlled by AEDs (NIH, 1990). Advances in neuro-imaging technique have improved the accuracy of locating epileptogeneses, thus minimizing the possible adverse effects of surgical intervention. With these advances in surgical management and localization of seizures, investigators estimate that "2000 to 5000 new patients in the United States might be suitable for operations each year, compared with the present annual rate of about 500" (NIH, 1990). Surgical success rates of up to 75% have been reported with patients remaining seizure free for 5 years postoperatively. When deemed appropriate, surgical therapy may prevent the development of long-term AED-related toxicity, psychosocial, educational, and vocational problems (Graves & Leppick, 1993).

Guldvog, Løyning, Hauglie-Hanssen, Flood, and Bjørnaes (1991) compared surgical and med-ical treatment outcomes in a retrospective parallel longitudinal cohort study in Norway that spanned the years 1949 to 1988. Subjects were closely matched on appropriate demographics. Results indicated that partial seizure frequency is better controlled by surgical treatment but that neurologic deficits may be more frequent in surgically treated than in medically treated patients. Recent advances have been made in the definitive diagnosis and identification of potential surgical candidates most likely to benefit from epilepsy surgery. However, careful consideration of the trade-off between seizure frequency reduction and neurologic deficit must be made.

Surgical therapy is not without its risks and precise and exhaustive evaluation of candidates is necessary. The NIH Consensus Development Conference on Surgery for Epilepsy (1990) has recommended that a specialized epilepsy center with comprehensive evaluation and treatment services for intractable epilepsy lead the surgical candidacy evaluation. They further espouse that such a center should include epilepsy-specific trained neurologists, neurosurgeons, neuropsychologists, and neurodiagnostic personnel. Personnel trained to deal with social, psychological, and psychiatric problems as well as educational and vocational rehabilitation should also participate in the holistic evaluation and ensuing treatment. A minimum of electroencephalographic (EEG), magnetic resonance imaging (MRI), and neuropsychological testing facilities should also be available in an effective and comprehensive epilepsy center.

Behavioral Treatment

Following an initially serendipitous discovery, Sterman and his colleagues have found consistently over the past 20 years, a reliable correspondence between 12- and 15-Hz activity and resistance to seizure activity (see Sterman, 1993). In his initial findings, cats trained to maintain the 12- to 14-Hz frequency were more resistant to drug-induced seizures than when the 12- to 14-Hz frequency range was not maintained (Wyrwicka & Sterman, 1968). He has termed this frequency of activity the *sensorimotor rhythm* (SMR) and since his first case study described in 1972 (Sterman & Friar, 1972), has found success in training epileptic patients in maintaining the frequency and thus enhancing normal thalamocortical regulation which, Sterman proposes, acts to increase seizure thresholds. The scalp-recorded SMR has been shown to correlate quite well with subcortical thalamocortical firing (Sterman & Bloomfield, 1987), whose abnormality in firing has been established as a factor in epileptogenesis.

In his most recent work, Sterman (1993) reported two cases in which successful SMR training has enabled reductions in both monotherapy and polytherapy antiepileptic medication regimens in high-functioning females. Lantz and Sterman (1992) demonstrated that subjects who were most successful in acquiring the SMR response exhibited greater improvements on neuropsychological test performance than did less successful subjects. Sterman warns, however, that SMR training is not effective in all individuals and that factors such as education and motivation play integral roles in successful training.

Dietary Treatment

Prior to the 1920's development and widespread use of AEDs, a common technique in the treatment of epilepsy was nutritionally based mimicking, originally based on the observation of a faith healer who successfully demonstrated that fasting and prayer reduced seizures. Further medical investigation revealed that when one fasts, the body first uses glucose in the bloodstream for energy but that when glucose is depleted, the body switches to burning fat deposits. This is the ketogenic state in which there results the release of ketone bodies. The presence of ketone bodies in urinary sampling has been shown to be very important in indicating the physiological state of fasting. The onset of ketosis, clinical improvement, and prognosis have been correlated with the normalization of EEG for more than 20 years (Nellhaus, 1971). Obviously, fasting indefinitely may reduce seizures indefinitely, but is inherently dangerous and impractical.

The ketogenic diet is based on mimicking of the fasting state through the massive intake of fats in proportion to daily caloric intake (80 to 90%). Minimal intake of proteins and carbohydrates are allowed—just exactly enough to maintain the child's weight. Virtually no glucose is allowed. Extra carbohydrates, protein, and all forms of glucose become primary energy sources (versus the stored energy in fat) and would take the body out of the ketogenic state. The diet must be followed exactly as prescribed, with absolutely no deviation, and monitored continually to ensure maintenance of the ketogenic state. Even slight deviations in the diet (e.g., 2 g of extra protein or a child not finishing her

or his meal completely) can result in the child leaving the ketogenic state and have been accompanied by the reoccurrence of seizure activity (Schwartz, Boyes, & Aynsley-Green, 1989; Schwartz, Eaton, Bower, & Aynsley-Green, 1989). If the child remains seizure free for 2 years, the diet is usually discontinued and deemed a success (Hendricks, 1995). With renewed public interest in the ketogenic diet, Kinsman, Vining, Quaskey, Mellits, and Freeman (1992) reported the actuarial results of 58 children started on the diet between 1980 and 1985. These were among the most refractory pediatric epilepsy cases and all children were having a minimum of three seizures a day despite proper maintenance of multiple medications. Of the 58 children, 88% were in polytherapy and 80% had multiple seizure types. Improvement in seizure control was generally noted within the first 2 weeks of being on the diet. Improvement was defined as a 50% or more reduction in seizure frequency for a minimum of 4 weeks. Of the 67% of the children who exhibited improved seizure control, 28% exhibited *complete* seizure control. That is, 16 of the 58 children had complete cessation of seizures while on and after completion of the strict dietary regimen. Of the 58 children, 64% were able to reduce one or more AEDs while 28% were able to reduce two or more AEDs and 10% were able to completely discontinue use of AEDs. Note again that these results are particularly striking when one considers that this population consisted of the most resistant cases of pediatric epilepsy seen at Johns Hopkins. Additional benefits of the diet noted in the Kinsman *et al.* (1992) study included improvements in alertness, behavior, and cognition. These effects can most likely be attributed to the benefits in reducing AEDs, whose cognitive effects have been discussed throughout this chapter.

Schwartz, Eaton, *et al.* (1989) suspect the beneficial effect of the ketogenic state to be a decreased neuronal excitation due to an alteration in nerve-cell lipid membranes. However, despite 70 years of study and use, the specific mechanisms of action that make the classical ketogenic diet (and other modified versions) so successful remain unclear (Hendricks, 1995; Schwartz, Boyes, & Aynsley-Green, 1989). Its absolute strict guidelines and 2-year length of adherence for long-term benefit make it impractical for controlled experimental study. The classical diet's efficacy, however, remains clearly demonstrated (Kinsman *et al.,* 1992; Schwartz, Eaton, *et al.,* 1989) and as its reputation spreads, increasing numbers of patients as well as less severe cases continue to consider the diet, and the waiting lists for the dozen centers that administer the diet grow (Hendricks, 1995).

References

Abou-Khalil, B., Shellenberger, M. K., & Anhut, H. (1992). Two open-label, multicenter studies of the safety and efficacy of gabapentin in patients with refractory epilepsy. *Epilepsia, 33,* 77.

American Academy of Pediatrics. (1985). Behavioral and cognitive effects of anticonvulsant therapy. *Pediatrics, 76*(4), 644–647.

Andrewes, D. G., Tomlinson, L., Elwes, R. D., & Reynolds, E. H. (1984). The influence of carbamazepine and phenytoin on memory and other aspects of cognitive function in new referrals with epilepsy. *Acta Neurologica Scandinavica, 69*(Suppl. 99), 23–30.

Arieff, A. J., & Yacorzynski, G. K. (1942). Deterioration of patients with organic epilepsy. *Journal of Nervous and Mental Disease, 96,* 49–55.

Austin, J. K., Smith, M. S., Risinger, M. W., & McNelis, A. M. (1994). Childhood epilepsy and asthma: Comparison of quality of life. *Epilepsia, 35*(3), 608–615.

Bagley, C. (1971). *The social psychology of the child with epilepsy.* London: Routledge & Kegan Paul.

Barnes, S. E., & Bower, B. D. (1975). Sodium valproate in the treatment of intractable childhood epilepsy. *Developmental Medicine and Child Neurology, 17,* 175–181.

Batzel, L. W., Dodrill, C. B., Dubinsky, B. L., Ziegler, R. G., Connolly, J. E., Freeman, R. D., Farwell, J. R., & Vining, E. P. G. (1991). An objective method for the assessment of psychosocial problems in adolescents with epilepsy. *Epilepsia, 32*(2), 202–211.

Bauer, G., Bechinger, D., Castell, M., Deisenhammer, E., & Egli, M. (1989). Gabapentin in the treatment of drug-resistant epileptic patients. *Advances in Epileptology, 17,* 219–221.

Bear, D. M. (1979). Temporal lobe epilepsy: A syndrome of sensory–limbic hyperconnection. *Cortex, 15,* 357–384.

Bear, D. M., & Fedio, P. (1977). Quantitative analysis of interictal behavior in temporal lobe epilepsy. *Archives of Neurology, 34,* 454–467.

Bear, D. M., Freeman, R., & Greenberg, M. (1984). Behavioral alterations in patients with temporal lobe epilepsy. In D. Blumer (Ed.), *Psychiatric aspects of epilepsy* (pp. 197–227). Washington, DC: American Psychiatric Press.

Bellur, S., & Hermann, B. P. (1984). Emotional and cognitive effects of anticonvulsant medications. *The International Journal of Clinical Neuropsychology, 6,* 21–23.

Ben-Menachem, E., Persson, L. I., Schechter, P. J., Haegele, K. D., Huebert, N., Hardenberg, J., Dahlgren, L., & Mumford, J. P. (1989). The effect of different vigabatrin treatment regimens on CSF biochemistry and seizure control in epileptic patients. *British Journal of Clinical Pharmacy, 27,* 79S–85S.

Bennett, T. L. (1987). Neuropsychological aspects of complex partial seizures: Diagnostic and treatment issues. *The International Journal of Clinical Neuropsychology, 9*(1), 37–45.

Bennett, T. L. (1988). Use of the Halstead–Reitan Neuropsychological Test Battery in the assessment of head injury. *Cognitive Rehabilitation, May/June,* 18–24.

Betts, T., Goodwin, G., Withers, R. M., & Yuen, A. W. C. (1991). Human safety of lamotrigine. Human safety of lamotrigine. *Epilepsia, 32*(Suppl. 2), S17–S19.

Beyers, V. L. (1993). Novel antiepileptic drugs: Nursing implications. *Journal of Neuroscience Nursing, 25*(6), 375–379.

Blumer, D., & Benson, D. F. (1982). Psychiatric manifestations of epilepsy. In D. F. Benson & D. Blumer (Eds.), *Psychiatric aspects of neurological disease* (Vol. 2, pp. 25–48). New York: Grune & Stratton.

Browne, S. W., & Reynolds, E. H. (1981). Cognitive impairment in epileptic patients. In E. H. Reynolds & M. R. Trimble (Eds.), *Epilepsy and psychiatry* (pp. 147–164). London: Churchill Livingstone.

Browne, T. (1993). Long-term efficacy and toxicity of gabapentin. *Neurology, 43,* A307.

Browne, T. R., Dreifuss, F. E., Dyken, P. R., Goode, D. J., Penry, J. K., Porter, R. J., White, B. J., & White, P. T. (1975). Ethosuccimide in the treatment of absences (petit mal) seizures. *Neurology, 25,* 515–525.

Browne, T. R., Mattson, P. H., Penry, J. K., Smith, D. B., Treiman, D. M., Wilder, B. J., Ben-Menachem, E., Miketta, R. M., Sherry, K. M., & Szabo, G. K. (1989). A multicentre study of vigabatrin for drug-resistant epilepsy. *British Journal of Clinical Pharmacy, 27,* 95S–100S.

Bruhm, P., & Parsons, O. A. (1977). Reaction time variability in epileptic and brain-damaged patients. *Cortex, 13,* 373–384.

Committee on Drugs. (1985). Behavioral and cognitive effects of anticonvulsant therapy. *Pediatrics, 76,* 644–647.

Corbett, J. A., Trimble, M. R., & Nichol, T. C. (1985). Behavioral and cognitive impairments in children with epilepsy: The long-term effects of anticonvulsant therapy. *Journal of the American Academy of Child Psychiatry, 24,* 17–23.

Crawford, P., Ghadiel, E., Lane, R., Blumhardt, L., & Chadwick, D. (1987). Gabapentin as an antiepileptic drug in man. *Journal of Neurology, Neurosurgery, and Psychiatry, 49,* 1251–1257.

Dalby, M. A. (1975). Behavioral effects of carbamazepine. In J. K. Penry & D. D. Daly (Eds.), *Advances in Neurology* (Vol. 11, pp. 331–343). New York: Raven Press.

Davidson, D. L. W. (1983). A review of the side effects of sodium valproate. *British Journal of Clinical Practice, 27*(Suppl.), 79–85.

Dean, J. C. (1993). Valproate. In E. Wyllie (Ed.), *The treatment of epilepsy: Principles and practices* (pp. 915–923). Philadelphia: Lea & Febiger.

Delaney, R. C., Rosen, A. J., Mattson, R. H., & Novelly, R. A. (1980). Memory function in focal epilepsy: A comparison of non-surgical, unilateral temporal lobe and frontal lobe samples. *Cortex, 16,* 103–117.

Dewhurst, K. (1980). *Thomas Willis' Oxford Lectures.* Oxford: Sanford.

Dikmen, S., & Matthews, C. G. (1977). Effect of major motor seizure frequency upon cognitive–intellectual function in adults. *Epilepsia, 18,* 21–29.

Dikmen, S., Matthews, C. G., & Harley, J. P. (1977). Effect of early versus late onset of major motor epilepsy upon cognitive-intellectual function in adults. *Epilepsia, 16,* 73–81.

Dikmen, S., & Reitan, R. (1978). Neuropsychological performance in posttraumatic epilepsy. *Epilepsia, 18,* 31–36.

Dodrill, C. B. (1978). A neuropsychological battery for epilepsy. *Epilepsia, 19,* 611–623.

Dodrill, C. B. (1981). Neuropsychology of epilepsy. In S. B. Filskov & T. J. Boll (Eds.), *Handbook of clinical neuropsychology* (pp. 366–395). New York: Wiley.

Dodrill, C. B., & Troupin, A. S. (1977). Psychotropic effects of carbamazepine in epilepsy: A double-blind comparison with phenytoin. *Neurology, 27,* 1023–1028.

Dodrill, C. B., & Troupin, A. S. (1991). Neuropsychological effects of carbamazepine and phenytoin: A reanalysis. *Neurology, 41,* 141–143.

Dodrill, C. B., Wilensky, A. J., Ojeman, L., Temkin, N., & Shellenberger, K. (1992). Neuropsychological, mood, and psychosocial effects of gabapentin. *Epilepsia, 33,* 117–118.

Dodson, W. E., & Pellock, J. M. (Eds.). (1993). *Pediatric epilepsy: Diagnosis and therapy.* New York: Demos.

Dulac, O., Withers, R. M., & Yuen, A. W. C. (1991). Add-on lamotrigine in pediatric patients with resistant epilepsy (Abstract). *Epilepsia, 32*(Suppl. 3), 10.

Duncan, J. S., Shorvon, S. D., & Trimble, M. R. (1990). Effects of removal of phenytoin, carbamazepine, and valproate on cognitive function. *Epilepsia, 31*(5), 584–591.

Farwell, J. R., Dodrill, C. B., & Batzel, L. W. (1985). Neuropsychological abilities in children with epilepsy. *Epilepsia, 26*(5), 395–400.

Farwell, J. R., Lee, Y. J., Hirtz, D. G., Sulzbacher, S. I., Ellenberg, J. H., & Nelson, K. B. (1990). Phenobarbital for febrile seizures: Effects on intelligence and on seizure recurrence. *New England Journal of Medicine, 322,* 364–369.

Fedio, P., & Mirsky, A. F. (1969). Selective intellectual deficits in children with temporal lobe or centrencephalic epilepsy. *Neuropsychologia, 7,* 287–300.

Fischbacher, E. (1982). Effect of reduction of anticonvulsants on wellbeing. *British Medical Journal, 285,* 425–427.

Fisher, R. S. (1993). Emerging antiepileptic drugs. *Neurology, 43*(Suppl. 5), S12–S20.

Fowler, P. C., Richards, H. C., Berent, S., & Boll, T. J. (1987). Epilepsy, neuropsychological deficits, and EEG lateralization. *Archives of Clinical Neuropsychology, 2,* 81–92.

Fox, J. T. (1924). Response of epileptic children to mental and educational tests. *British Journal of Medical Psychology, 4,* 235–248.

Freeman, J. M., Vining, E. P. G., & Pillas, D. J. (1990). *Seizures and epilepsy in childhood: A guide for parents.* Baltimore: Johns Hopkins University Press.

Geschwind, N. (1984). Dostoievsky's epilepsy. In D. Blumer (Ed.), *Psychiatric aspects of epilepsy* (pp. 325–334). Washington, DC: American Psychiatric Press.

Gillham, R. A., Blacklaw, J., McKee, P. J. W., & Brodie, M. J. (1993). Effect of vigabatrin on sedation and cognition function in patients with refractory epilepsy. *Journal of Neurology, Neurosurgery, and Psychiatry, 56,* 1271–1275.

Giordani, B., Berent, S., Sackellares, J. C., Rourke, D., Seidenberg, M., O'Leary, D. S., Dreifuss, F. E., & Boll, T. J. (1985). Intelligence test performance of patients with partial and generalized seizures. *Epilepsia, 26*(1), 37–42.

Glowinski, H. (1973). Cognitive deficits in temporal lobe epilepsy. *The Journal of Nervous and Mental Disorders, 157,* 129–137.

Goode, D. J., Penry, J. J., & Dreifuss, F. E. (1970). Effects of paroxysmal spike wave on continuous visuo-motor performance. *Epilepsia, 11,* 241–254.

Gram, L. (1989). Potential antiepileptic drugs: Lamotrigine. In R. Levy, F. E. Dreifuss, R. Mattson, B. S. Dreifuss, & J. K. Penry (Eds.), *Antiepileptic drugs* (3rd ed., pp. 947–953). New York: Raven Press.

Grant, S. M., & Heel, R. C. (1991). Vigabatrin. A review of its pharmodynamics and pharmacokinetic properties, and therapeutic potential in epilepsy and disorders of motor control. *Drug, 41,* 889–926.

Graves, N. M., & Leppick, I. E. (1991). Antiepileptic medications in development. *DICP Annals of Pharmacotherapy, 25,* 978–986.

Graves, N. M., & Leppick, I. E. (1993). Advances in pharmacotherapy: Recent developments in the treatment of epilepsy. *Journal of Clinical Pharmacy and Therapeutics, 18,* 227–242.

Grinker, R. R. (1929). The proper use of phenobarbital in the treatment of the epilepsies. *Journal of the American Medical Association, 93,* 1218–1219.

Guey, J., Charles, C., Coquery, C., Roger, J., & Soulayrol, R. (1967). Study of psychological effects of ethosuximide (Zaraontin) on 25 children suffering from petit mal epilepsy. *Epilepsia, 8,* 129–141.

Guldvog, B., Løyning, Y., Hauglie-Hanssen, E., Flood, S., & Bjørnaes, H. (1991). Surgical versus medical treatment for epilepsy. I. Outcome related to survival, seizures, and neurologic deficit. *Epilepsia, 32*(3), 375–388.

Hauser, W. A. (1994). The prevalence and incidence of convulsive disorders in children. *Epilepsia, 35*(Suppl. 2), s1–s6.

Haynes, S. D., & Bennett, T. L. (1991). Cognitive impairment in adults with complex partial seizures. *International Journal of Clinical Neuropsychology, 12,* 74–81.

Hendricks, M. (1995, April). High fat and seizure free. *Johns Hopkins Magazine,* 14–20.

Hermann, B. P., & Whitman, S. (1986). Psychopathology in epilepsy: A multi-etiological model. In S. Whitman & B. P. Hermann (Eds.), *Psychopathology in epilepsy: Social dimensions* (pp. 5–37). London: Oxford University Press.

Hermann, B. P., Wyler, A. R., & Richey, E. T. (1988). Wisconsin Card Sorting Test performance in patients with complex partial seizures of temporal lobe origin. *Journal of Clinical and Experimental Neuropsychology, 10*(4), 467–476.

Herranz, J. L., Arteaga, R., Farr, I. N., Valdizan, E., Beaumont, D., & Armijo, J. A. (1991). Dose–response study of vigabatrin in children with refractory epilepsy. *Journal of Child Neurology, 6*(Suppl.), 2S25–2S51.

Himmelhock, J. M. (1984). Major mood disorders related to epileptic changes. In D. Blumer (Ed.), *Psychiatric aspects of epilepsy* (pp. 271–294). Washington,DC: American Psychiatric Press.

Holdsworth, L., & Whitmore, K. (1974). A study of children with epilepsy attending ordinary schools, I: Their seizure patterns, progress, and behavior in school. *Developmental Medicine and Child Neurology, 16,* 746–758.

Hutt, S. J., Jackson, P. M., Belsham, A. B., & Higgins, G. (1968). Perceptual–motor behavior in relation to blood phenobarbitone level. *Developmental Medicine and Child Neurology, 10,* 626–632.

Idestrom, C. M., Schelling, D., Carlquist, V., & Sjoquist, F. (1972). Behavioral and psychophysiological studies: Acute effects of diphenylhydantoin in relation to plasma levels. *Psychological Medicine, 2,* 111–120.

Jarvis, P. E., & Barth, J. T. (1984). *Halstead–Reitan Test Battery: An interpretative guide.* Odessa, FL: Psychological Assessment Resources.

Kalviainen, R., Keranen, T., & Riekkinen, P. J. (1993). Place of newer antiepileptic drugs in the treatment of epilepsy. *Drugs, 46*(6), 1009–1024.

Keating, L. E. (1960). A review of the literature on the relationship of epilepsy and intelligence in school children. *Journal of Mental Science, 106,* 1042–1059.

Keith, H. M., Ewert, J. C., Green, M. W., & Gage, R. P. (1955). Mental status of children with convulsive disorders. *Neurology, 5,* 419–425.

Kinsman, S. L., Vining, E. P. G., Quaskey, S. A., Mellits, D., & Freeman, J. M. (1992). Efficacy of the ketogenic diet for intractable seizure disorders: Review of 58 cases. *Epilepsia, 33*(6), 1132–1136.

Lansdell, H., & Mirsky, A. F. (1964). Attention in focal and centrencephalic epilepsy. *Experimental Neurology, 9,* 463–469.

Lantz, D., & Sterman, M. B. (1992). Neuropsychological prediction and outcome measures in relation to EEG feedback training for the treatment of epilepsy. In T. L. Bennett (Ed.), *The neuropsychology of epilepsy* (pp. 213–222). New York: Plenum Press.

Lavadas, E., Umitta, C., & Provinciali, L. (1979). Hemisphere dependent cognitive performances in epileptic patients. *Epilepsia, 20,* 493–502.

Lechtenberg, R. (1984). *Epilepsy and the family.* Cambridge, MA: Harvard University Press.

Lennox, W. G. (1942). Brain injury, drugs, and environment as causes of mental decay in epileptics. *American Journal of Psychiatry, 99,* 174–180.

Lennox, W. G., & Lennox, M. A. (1960). *Epilepsy and related disorders.* Boston: Little, Brown.

Livingston, J. H., Beaumont, D., Arzimanoglou, A., & Aicardi, J. (1989). Vigabatrin in the treatment of epilepsy in children. *British Journal of Clinical Pharmacology, 27*(Suppl. 1), 109S–112S.

Loiseau, P., Signoret, J. L., & Strube, E. (1984). Attention problems in adult epileptic patients. *Acta Neurologica Scandinavia, 69*(Suppl. 99), 31–34.

Loiseau, P., Strube, E., Brouslet, D., Battellochi, S., Gomeni, C., & Morselli, P. L. (1980). Evaluation of memory function in a population of epileptic patients and matched controls. *Acta Neurologica Scandinavia, 62*(Suppl. 80), 58–61.

Long, C. G., & Moore, J. T. (1979). Parental expectations for their epileptic children. *Journal of Child Psychology and Psychiatry, 20,* 313–324.

McGowan, M. E. L., Neville, B. G. R., & Reynolds, E. H. (1983). Comparative monotherapy trial in children with epilepsy. *British Journal of Clinical Practice, 27*(Symp. Suppl.), 115–118.

McGuckin, H. M. (1980). Changing the world view of those with epilepsy. In R. Canger, F. Angeleri, & J. K. Penry (Eds.), *Advances in epileptology: Eleventh epilepsy international symposium* (pp. 205–208). New York: Raven Press.

McGuire, A. M., Duncan, J. S., & Trimble, M. R. (1992). Effects of vigabatrin on cognitive function and mood, when used as add-on therapy in patients with intractable epilepsy. *Epilepsia, 33,* 128–134.

MacLeod, C. M., Dekaban, A., & Hunt, E. (1978). Memory impairment in epileptic patients: Selective effects of phenobarbital concentration. *Science, 202,* 1102–1104.

Masui, K., Niwa, S., Anzai, N., Kameyama, T., Saitoh, O., & Rymar, K. (1984). Verbal memory disturbances in left temporal lobe epileptics. *Cortex, 20,* 361–368.

Matthews, C. G., & Kløve, H. (1967). Differential psychological performances in motor, psychomotor, and mixed seizure classification of known and unknown etiology. *Epilepsia, 8,* 117–128.

Mayeux, R., Brandt, J., Rosen, J., & Benson, F. (1980). Interictal memory and language impairment in temporal lobe epilepsy. *Neurology, 30,* 120–125.

Meador, K. J., Loring, D. W., Huh, K., Gallagher, B. B., & King, D. W. (1990). Comparative cognitive effects of anticonvulsants. *Neurology, 40,* 391–394.

Milner, B. (1975). Hemispheric specialization: Scope and limits. In B. Milner (Ed.), *Hemispheric specialization and interaction* (pp. 75–89). Cambridge, MA: MIT Press.

Mirsky, A. F., Primoc, D. W., Ajmone-Marsan, C. A., Rosvold, H. E., & Stevens, J. R. (1960). A comparison of the psychological test performance of patients with focal and nonfocal epilepsy. *Experimental Neurology, 2,* 75–89.

Mirsky, A. F., & Van Buren, J. M. (1965). On the nature of the "absence" in centrencephalic epilepsy: A study of some behavioral, electroencephalographic, and autonomic factors. *Electroencephalography and Clinical Neurophysiology, 18,* 334–348.

Morgan, A., & Groh, C. (1980). Changes in visual perception in children with epilepsy. In B. Kulig, H. Meinardi, & G. Stores (Eds.), *Epilepsy and behavior '79.* Lisse: Swets & Zeitlinger.

Mumford, J. P., Beaumont, D., & Gisselbrecht, D. (1990). Cognitive function, mood, and behaviour in vigabatrin treated patients. *Acta Neurologica Scandinavica, 82*(Suppl. 133), 15.

National Institutes of Health. (1990). *Consensus development conference on surgery for epilepsy* (NIH Publication No. HE20.3615/2:90-1). Washington, DC: U.S. Department of Health and Human Services.

Nellhaus, G. (1971). The ketogenic diet reconsidered (abstract). *Neurology, 21,* 424.

Novelly, R. A., Augustine, E. A., Mattson, R. H., Glaser, G. H., Williamson, P. D., Spencer, D. D., & Spencer, S. S. (1984). Selective memory improvement and impairment in temporal lobectomy for epilepsy. *Annals of Neurology, 15,* 64–67.

O'Leary, D. S., Lovell, M. R., Sackellares, J. C., Berent, S., Giordani, B., Seidenberg, M., & Boll, J. T. (1983). Effects of age of onset of partial and generalized seizures on neuropsychological performance in children. *Journal of Nervous and Mental Disease, 171*(10), 624–629.

Painter, M. J., & Gaus, L. M. (1993). Phenobarbital in seizure disorders. In E. Wyllie (Ed.), *The treatment of epilepsy: Principles and practices* (pp. 900–908). Philadelphia: Lea & Febiger.

Pellock, J. M. (1994). The use of new anticonvulsant drugs in children. In M. R. Trimble (Ed.), *New anticonvulsants: Advances in the treatment of epilepsy.* (pp. 127–143). New York: Wiley.

Post, R. M. (1983). Behavioral effects of kindling. In M. Parsonage (Ed.), *Advances in epileptology: XIVth international symposium* (pp. 173–180). New York: Raven Press.

Quadfasel, A. F., & Pruyser, P. W. (1955). Cognitive deficits in patients with psychomotor epilepsy. *Epilepsia, 4,* 80–90.

Ramsay, R. E., & Slater, J. D. (1993). Antiepileptic drugs in clinical development. In J. A. French, M. A. Dichter, & I. E. Leppick (Eds.), *New antiepileptic drug development: Preclinical and clinical aspects* (Epilepsy research suppl. 10, pp. 45–67). Amsterdam: Elsevier.

Reitan, R. M. (1974). Psychological testing of epileptic patients. In O. Magnus & L. de Hass (Eds.), *The handbook of clinical neurology: Vol. 15. The epilepsies* (pp. 559–575). Amsterdam: Elsevier.

Reitan, R. M., & Wolfson, D. (1993). *The Halstead–Reitan Neuropsychological Test Battery: Theory and clinical interpretation* (2nd ed.) Tucson, AZ: Neuropsychology Press.

Reynolds, E. H. (1983). Mental effects of antiepileptic medication: A review. *Epilepsia, 24*(Suppl. 2), 85–96.

Reynolds, E. H. (1985). Antiepileptic drugs and psychopathology. In M. R. Trimble (Ed.), *The psychopharmacology of epilepsy* (pp. 49–63). New York: Wiley.

Reynolds, E. H., Ring, H. A., Farr, I. N., Heller, A. J., & Elwes, R. D. (1991). Open, double-blind, and long-term study of vigabatrin in chronic epilepsy. *Epilepsia, 32*(4), 530–538.

Reynolds, E. H., & Travers, R. D. (1974). Serum anticonvulsant concentrations in epileptic patients with mental symptoms. *British Journal of Psychiatry, 124,* 440–445.

Reynolds, E. H., & Trimble, M. R. (1985). Adverse neuropsychiatric effects of anticonvulsant drugs. *Drugs, 29,* 570–581.

Richens, A., & Yuen, A. W. C. (1991). Overview of the clinical efficacy of lamotrigine. *Epilepsia, 32*(Suppl. 2), S13–S16.

Ring, H. A., Heller, A. J., Farr, I. N., & Reynolds, E. H. (1990). Vigabatrin: Rational treatment for chronic epilepsy. *Journal of Neurology, Neurosurgery, and Psychiatry, 53*(12), 1051–1055.

Rodin, E. (1984). Epileptic and pseudoepileptic seizures: Differential diagnostic considerations. In D. Blumer (Ed.), *Psychiatric aspects of epilepsy* (pp. 179–195). Washington, DC: American Psychiatric Press.

Roger, J., Grangeon, H., Guey, J., & Lob, H. (1968). Psychiatric and psychological effects of ethosuximide treatment in epileptics. *Encephale, 57,* 407–438.

Rutter, M., Graham, P., & Yule, W. (1970). A neuropsychological study in childhood. *Clinics in Developmental Medicine, 35/36.* London: S. I. M. P. & Heinemann.

Saletu, B., Grunberger, J., & Linzmayer, L. (1986). Evaluation of encephalotropic and psychotropic properties of gabapentin in man by pharmaco-EEG and psychometry. *International Journal of Clinical Pharmacology and Toxicology, 24,* 362–373.

Scarpa, P., & Carassini, B. (1982). Partial epilepsy in childhood: Clinical and EEG study in 261 cases. *Epilepsia, 23,* 333–341.

Schain, R. J., Ward, J. W., & Guthrie, D. (1977). Carbamazepine as an anticonvulsant in children. *Neurology, 27,* 476–480.

Schlumberger, E., Chavez, F., Palacios, L., Rey, E., Pajot, N., & Dulac, O. (1994). Lamotrigine in treatment of 120 children with epilepsy. *Epilepsia, 35*(2), 359–367.

Schmidt, B. (1989). Potential antiepileptic drugs. I. Gabapentin. In R. Levy, R. Mattson, B. Meldrum, J. K. Penry, & F. E. Dreifuss (Eds.), *Antiepileptic drugs* (3rd ed., pp. 925–935). New York: Raven Press.

Schwartz, M. L., & Dennerll, R. D. (1970). Neuropsychological assessment of children with and without questionable epileptogenic dysfunction. *Perceptual and Motor Skills, 30,* 111–121.

Schwartz, R. H., Boyes, S., & Aynsley-Green, A. (1989). Metabolic effects of three ketogenic diets in the treatment of severe epilepsy. *Developmental Medicine and Child Neurology, 31,* 152–160.

Schwartz, R. H., Eaton, J., Bower, B. D., & Aynsley-Green, A. (1989). Ketogenic diets in the treatment of epilepsy: Short-term clinical effects. *Developmental Medicine and Child Neurology, 31,* 145–151.

Scott, D., Moffett, A., Matthews, A., & Ettlinger, G. (1967). Effects of epileptic discharges on learning and memory in patients. *Epilepsia, 8,* 188–194.

Shorvon, S. D., & Reynolds, E. H. (1979). Reduction of polypharmacy for epilepsy. *British Medical Journal, 2,* 1023–1025.

Sillanpää, M. (1993). Carbamazepine. In E. Wyllie (Ed.), *The treatment of epilepsy: Principles and practices* (pp. 867–886). Philadelphia: Lea & Febiger.

Sivenius, J., Kalviainen, R., Ylinen, A., & Riekkinen, R. (1991). Double-blind study of gabapentin in the treatment of partial seizures. *Epilepsia, 32,* 539–542.

Somerfield-Ziskind, E., & Ziskind, E. (1940). Effect of phenobarbital on the mentality of epileptic patients. *Archives of Neurology and Psychiatry, 43,* 70–79.

Sterman, M. B. (1993). Sensorimotor EEG feedback training in the study and treatment of epilepsy. In D. I. Mostofsky & Y. Løyning (Eds.), *The neurobehavioral treatment of epilepsy* (pp. 1–18). Hillsdale, NJ: Erlbaum.

Sterman, M. B., & Bloomfield, S. (1987). Limbic neuronal discharge correlates of sensorimotor EEG feedback training in presurgical patients with intractable epilepsy. In D. I. Mostofsky & Y. Løyning (Eds.), *The neurobehavioral treatment of epilepsy* (pp. 1–18). Hillsdale, NJ: Erlbaum.

Sterman, M. B., & Friar, L. R. (1972). Suppression of seizures in an epileptic following sensorimotor EEG feedback training. *Electroencephalography and Clinical Neurophysiology, 33,* 89–95.

Stores, G. (1973). Studies of attention and seizure disorders. *Developmental Medicine and Child Neurology, 15,* 376–382.

Stores, G. (1981). Problems of learning and behavior in children with epilepsy. In E. H. Reynolds & M. R. Trimble (Eds.), *Epilepsy and psychiatry* (pp. 33–48). Edinburgh: Churchill Livingstone.

Tartara, A., Manni, R., Galimberti, C. A., Mumford, J. P., Iudice, A. S., & Perucca, E., (1989). Vigabatrin in the treatment of epilepsy: A long-term follow-up study. *Journal of Neurology, Neurosurgery, and Psychiatry, 52,* 467–471.

Tarter, R. E. (1972). Intellectual and adaptive functioning in epilepsy: A review of 50 years of research. *Diseases of the Nervous System, 33,* 763–770.

Thompson, P. J., Huppert, F. A., & Trimble, M. R. (1981). Phenytoin and cognitive function: Effects on normal volunteers and implication for epilepsy. *British Journal of Clinical Psychology, 20,* 155–162.

Thompson, P. J., & Trimble, M. R. (1982). Anticonvulsant drugs and cognitive functions. *Epilepsia, 23,* 531–544.

Tizard, J., Rutter, M., & Whitmore, K. (1969). *Education, health, and behavior.* London: Longsmans.

Trimble, M. (1981). Anticonvulsant drugs, behavior, and cognitive abilities. *Current Developments in Psychopharmacology, 6,* 65–91.

Trimble, M. R. (Ed.). (1994). *New anticonvulsants: Advances in the treatment of epilepsy.* New York: Wiley.

Trimble, M. R., & Corbett, J. A. (1980). Behavioral and cognitive disturbances in epileptic children. *Irish Medical Journal, 73,* 21–28.

Trimble, M. R., & Reynolds, E. H. (1976). Anticonvulsant drugs and mental symptoms. *Psychological Medicine, 6,* 169–178.

Trimble, M. R., & Thompson, P. J. (1981). Memory, anticonvulsant drugs, and seizures. *Acta Neurologica Scandinavica, 89,* 31–41.

Trimble, M. R., & Thompson, P. J. (1984). Sodium valproate and cognitive function. *Epilepsia, 25*(Suppl. 1), 560–564.

Trimble, M. R., & Thompson, P. J. (1986). Neuropsychological aspects of epilepsy. In I. Grant & K. M. Adams (Eds.), *Neuropsychological assessment of neuropsychiatric disorders* (pp. 321–346). London: Oxford University Press.

Turner, W. A. (1907). *Epilepsy.* London: Macmillan & Co.

Tymchuk, A. J. (1974). Comparison of Bander error and time scores for groups of epileptic, retarded, and behavior-problem children. *Perceptual and Motor Skills, 38,* 71–74.

Vajda, F. J. E. (1992). New anticonvulsants. *Current Opinions in Neurology and Neurosurgery, 5,* 519–525.

Wagner, M. L. (1994). Felbamate: A new antiepileptic drug. *American Journal of Hospital Pharmacy, 51*(13), 1657–1666.

Walker, A. E., & Blumer, D. (1984). Behavioral effects of temporal lobectomy for temporal lobe epilepsy. In D. Blumer (Ed.), *Psychiatric aspects of epilepsy* (pp. 295–323). Washington, DC: American Psychiatric Press.

Wallace, S. J. (1990). *Add-on open trial of lamotrigine on resistant childhood seizures.* Eighteenth ICNA meeting, Tokyo, p. 734.

Waxman, S. A., & Geschwind, N. (1984). Hypergraphia in temporal lobe epilepsy. *Neurology, 30,* 314–317.

Wilensky, A. J., Temkin, N. R., Ojeman, L. M., Rischer, B., & Holubkov, A. (1992). Gabapentin and carbamazepine as monotherapy and combined: A pilot study (Abstract). *Epilepsia, 33,* 77.

Wilkus, R. J., & Dodrill, C. B. (1976). Neuropsychological correlates of the EEG in epileptics. I. Topographic distribution and average rate of epileptiform activity. *Epilepsia, 17,* 89–100.

Wilson, A., Petty, R., Perry, A., & Rose, R. C. (1983). Paroxysmal language disturbance in an epileptic treated with clobazam. *Neurology, 33,* 652–654.

Wolf, S. M., & Forsythe, A. (1978). Behavior disturbance, phenobarbital, and febrile seizures. *Pediatrics, 61,* 728–731.

Wyllie, E. (Ed.). (1993). *The treatment of epilepsy: Principles and practices.* Philadelphia: Lea & Febiger.

Wyrwicka, W., & Sterman, M. B. (1968). Instrumental conditioning of sensorimotor cortex EEG spindles in the waking cat. *Physiology and Behavior, 3,* 703–707.

Zimmerman, F. T., Burgemeister, B. B., & Putnam, T. J. (1951). Intellectual and emotional makeup of the epileptic. *Archives of Neurology and Psychiatry, 65,* 545–556.

27

Neuropsychological Effects of Stimulant Medication on Children's Learning and Behavior

RONALD T. BROWN, ELIZABETH DREELIN, AND ARDEN D. DINGLE

Introduction

Historical Overview and Evolving Research

Stimulants refer to a class of drugs that produce excitation of the central nervous system (CNS) and have been used in the treatment of children and adolescents since the 1930s (Bradley, 1937). Since then, there has been consistent interest in the clinical application of stimulant medication; however, systematic research efforts did not begin until the 1960s (Brown & Borden, 1989), when more rigorous methodology was employed. The focus of this research was on the identification and assessment of target behaviors and side effects in controlled clinical trials. These investigations emphasize several different areas: short-term efficacy, atypical drug response, organic etiologies, predictors of drug response, long-term outcome of treatment, negative consequences, and the use of additional therapeutic modalities in conjunction with stimulants (Jacobvitz, Sroufe, Stewart, & Leffert, 1990). The short-term efficacy studies include carefully controlled drug placebo trials, use in various settings, effects on learning and achievement, dose–response curves, and impact on socialization (Jacobvitz et al., 1990). Atypical drug effects have focused on the examination of stimulant response in symptomatic and nonsymptomatic samples. Extensive investigation has focused on determining the etiology of symptoms as well as the mechanisms underlying drug response. Considerable empirical efforts have concentrated on the identification of factors predicting positive drug response. Additionally, numerous studies have been devoted to tracing the long-term outcome of academic performance, peer relations, and delinquent behaviors of children treated with stimulants over the course of several years. Attention also has focused on the iatrogenic and physical side effects of stimulants. Finally, recent research has focused on the integration of stimulant drug therapy with nonsomatic therapies.

Because of the interdisciplinary efforts of clinical child psychologists, neuropsychologists, neurologists, pediatricians, and child psychiatrists, much progress has been made over the past several years in the understanding of the actions of stimulants on children's learning and behavior. Distinct bodies of knowledge are available from both laboratory and clinical settings that have significantly influenced treatment of children and adolescents in behavioral pediatrics and child psychiatry. Promising areas await investigation, the most exciting of which are the effects of stimulants on neurological functioning as evidenced by more recent technologies in assessing brain functioning.

RONALD T. BROWN AND ARDEN D. DINGLE • Departments of Psychiatry and Behavioral Sciences and Pediatrics, Emory University, Atlanta, Georgia 30322. ELIZABETH DREELIN • Department of Psychiatry and Behavioral Sciences, Emory University, Atlanta, Georgia 30322.

TABLE 1. Commonly Used Stimulants in Children: Indications, Adverse Effects, and Medical Management

	Dextroamphetamine (Dexedrine)	Methylphenidate (Ritalin)	Pemoline (Cylert)
Indications	Overactivity, impulsivity, inattention		
Work-up	Physical and neurological examination (height, weight, blood pressure, pulse, and dyskinetic movements), routine laboratory tests (CBC with differential, blood chemistry profile, urinalysis		Physical and neurological examination (height, weight, blood pressure, pulse and dyskinetic movements), routine laboratory tests (CBC with differential, blood chemistry profile, urinalysis), liver function tests
Pharmacology			
How supplied (mg)	5, 10, 15	5, 10, 20, SR-20	18.75, 37.5, 75
Single-dose range	0.15 to 0.5	0.3 to 0.7	0.5 to 2.5
Daily dose range			
mg/kg/day	0.3 to 1.25	0.6 to 2.0	0.5 to 3.0
mg/day	5 to 40	10 to 70	18.75 to 112.5
Initial dosage	2.5 mg 2 to 3 times/day	5 mg 2 to 3 times/day	18.75 mg each morning
Peak plasma level	2 to 3 hr	1.5 to 2.5 hr	2 to 4 hr
Plasma half-life	4 to 6 hr	2 to 3 hr	7 to 8 hr (children)
Peak clinical effect	1 to 2 hr	1 to 3 hr	If prescribed as indicated, several weeks after treatment begins therapeutic effect is generally sustained over several hours
Onset of behavioral effect	30 to 60 min	30 to 60 min	Variable
Duration of behavioral effect	4 to 6 hr	3 to 5 hr	6 to 8 hr
Side effects			
Common adverse reactions	Difficulty in falling asleep, mild elevation of pulse and blood pressure		
Less frequent adverse reactions	Decreased appetite (temporary), crying and dysphoria, growth retardation (height and weight, mild), drowsiness, anxiety, and irritability		
Serious but unusual adverse reactions	Psychotic thoughts, lowering seizure threshold, worsening of tic disorder or dyskinesia, potential for medication abuse, hypertension		Psychotic thoughts, lowering seizure threshold, worsening of tic disorder or dyskinesia, potential for medication abuse, hypertension, hepatocellular injury, elevated serum glutamic pyruvic transaminase
Special considerations			
Relative contraindications	Marked anxiety, agitation or psychosis, glaucoma, verbal–motor tic (Tourette's syndrome)		
Toxicity/overdose	Irritability, restlessness, agitation, nausea, diarrhea, high fever, sweating, pallor, flushing, arrhythmias, tachycardia, significant hypertension, delirium, tremor, convulsions, coma		High fever, sweating, pallor, flushing, arrhythmias, tachycardia, significant hypertension, delirium, tremor, convulsions, coma
Drug interactions	Increased blood level of tricyclic antidepressants, increased metabolism of phenytoin, opposes effect of antihypertensives, acetazolamide increases renal absorption of amphetamines		
Follow-up	Follow height, weight, and blood pressure and pulse on a regular basis; observe for dyskinetic movements; perform yearly physical examination and routine laboratory tests		

Prevalence

Stimulants in children have been the most widely used and meticulously studied psychotropic medication. Evidence indicates that management of children with stimulants has increased steadily over the past two decades (Wilens & Biederman, 1992). From a survey of Baltimore County schools, Safer and Krager (1988) have provided evidence to indicate that the rate of prescribing stimulants has doubled every 4 to 7 years since 1971. Further, of prescribed psychotropic medication for attention deficit hyperactivity disorder (ADHD) over the past several years, stimulants increased from 76% to 99%. Thus, stimulants are the primary medications prescribed by primary care physicians for ADHD (Wolraich *et al.*, 1990). Although stimulant medication continues to be prescribed and studied extensively, misconceptions persist about its effects and appropriate application. In fact, the disparity is striking between the empirical evidence and some commonly held views regarding treatment with stimulants. Thus, to effectively assess and treat children, it is important for the child psychologist to have a clear understanding of the empirical literature about stimulants as well as the application of stimulants.

Pharmacology

Mechanism of Action

This discussion will be limited to the most commonly prescribed stimulant medications in the United States, namely, dextroamphetamine (Dexedrine), methylphenidate (Ritalin), and pemoline (Cylert). Dextroamphetamine and methylphenidate have been reported to alter the availability of neurotransmitters, primarily dopamine and norepinephrine, by stimulating the release of newly synthesized dopamine into the synaptic cleft, preventing presynaptic reuptake of these neurotransmitters, and inhibiting monoamine oxidase activity (Wilens & Biederman, 1992). Evidence supporting the idea that stimulants affect the dopaminergic system has been presented by Levy and Hobbes (1988) who found that haloperidol, a commonly used antipsychotic drug (which primarily affects the dopamine system), blocked the effect of methylphenidate in children with attention problems. The effects of stimulants on the serotonergic system appear to be minimally related to its clinical actions (Zametkin & Rapoport, 1987). Pemoline is structurally dissimilar from methylphenidate or dextroamphetamine; it has only mild or no sympathomimetic activity and primarily influences dopamine neurotransmission (Barkley, DuPaul, & Costello, 1993). Lou, Henrikson, Bruhn, Borner, and Nielsen (1989) have found methylphenidate to partially correct cerebral blood flow abnormalities in individuals with ADHD visualized by means of positron emission tomography (PET), indicating an increase in dopamine use.

Although this research has been of significant interest, other studies have focused on the physiological mechanisms of stimulants and their connections to behavior. Specifically, this body of research posits that stimulants influence the regulation of arousal, attention, and reactivity (Douglas & Peters, 1979). Much of the work has come from the literature that indicates children with ADHD have abnormalities in their levels of arousal and activity.

Despite considerable exploration into the effects of stimulants on the CNS, there is no definitive conceptualization of their mechanism of action (Pelham, 1993). As Pelham observed, an understanding of the neurophysiological effects of stimulants is not necessary for effective clinical application. Actually, the most illuminating information about stimulant drug effects has come from the behavioral pharmacology literature that has examined learning, cognition, and behavior.

Types of Stimulants

As noted previously, the most commonly used stimulants are dextroamphetamine (Dexedrine), methylphenidate (Ritalin), and pemoline (Cylert). Their basic effects are presented in Table 1. There are other stimulants including caffeine and deanol that will not be discussed because they are not used clinically and are not as effective as the CNS stimulants. Dextroamphetamine and methylphenidate, which are sympathomimetic amines, are structurally similar; methylphenidate is a piperidine derivative. Pemoline is structurally dissimilar from amphetamines.

These medications are administered orally several times a day and are quickly absorbed from the gastrointestinal tract. Moreover, they easily cross the blood–brain barrier and are rapidly eliminated from the body within 24 hours (Barkley *et al.*, 1993). There is considerable variation among individuals in terms of optimal dosage, duration, and efficacy. Plasma level has been demonstrated to be dose related with increasing plasma level being related to higher doses (Dulcan, 1990). However, blood levels are not predictive of behavioral response to stimulants (Swanson, 1988). Both dextroamphetamine and methylphenidate are available in regular and long-acting forms (Dexedrine Spansules and Ritalin-SR). Recent empirical evidence attests to the equivalent efficacy and minimal side effects of both the sustained release (SR) and standard forms of stimulants (Fitzpatrick, Klorman, Brumaghim, & Borgstedt, 1992; Pelham *et al.*, 1990). A possible advantage of the long-acting forms is that administration may not be required during the school day, thus eliminating the possible problematic school issues.

Dextroamphetamine

The oldest of the stimulants, dextroamphetamine (the long-acting form) reaches peak plasma level within 2 to 3 hr with a plasma half-life between 4 and 6 hr. It is metabolized primarily by the liver, even though a significant amount of the drug is excreted in the urine. Behavioral effects are often observable within 30 to 60 min, appear to peak within 1 to 2 hr following administration, and typically dissipate within 4 to 6 hr (Barkley *et al.*, 1993).

Methylphenidate

The most commonly prescribed stimulant, methylphenidate, achieves its peak in the plasma within 1.5 to 2.5 hr after ingestion. The plasma half-life is usually within 2 to 3 hr and the drug is entirely metabolized within 12 to 24 hr (Barkley *et al.*, 1993). Swanson, Sandman, Deutsch, and Baren (1983) have concluded that the medication may be administered either during or after meals, although plasma concentration peaks sooner after a meal. The behavioral effects of the drug typically occur 30 to 60 min after administration and peak within 1 to 3 hr and dissipate within 3 to 5 hr. It is primarily converted to various inactive compounds and little of the drug is available in the urine. SR methylphenidate has a plasma half-life between 2 and 6 hr with a peak level occurring within 1 to 4 hr. Behavioral effects typically occur within 1 to 2 hr and peak within 3 to 5 hr and slowly diminish until approximately 8 hr postingestion (Barkley *et al.*, 1993).

Some well-controlled clinical trials have examined the comparative efficacy of dextroamphetamine and methylphenidate and have demonstrated similar benefits as well as side effects. However, clinical experience clearly suggests response is idiosyncratic and that failure to respond to one of these medications warrants a trial of the other (Barkley *et al.*, 1993).

Pemoline

Finally, a third stimulant medication, pemoline, has a plasma half-life of 7 to 8 hr in children, which is shorter than the half-life in adults. Peak plasma levels are reached 2 to 4 hr following ingestion. Within 24 hr 50 to 75% of the dose is excreted in the urine (Barkley *et al.*, 1993). The duration of efficacy and behavioral response patterns have not been documented as well as have the other stimulants. The half-life of pemoline may increase with duration of use, thereby resulting in a higher plasma level, which may explain the considerably delayed behavioral effects of the drug; the beneficial clinical effects of the medication may not be observed until after several weeks of consecutive administration. However, one recent study has suggested that pemoline may be effective for the classroom behavior of ADHD children within 2 hr of ingestion on the second consecutive day of administration (Pelham *et al.*, 1990). The long-term efficacy of pemoline has been questioned in the literature (Brown & Borden, 1989); and, coupled with the need to carefully monitor liver functioning (Goodman & Gilman, 1980), this has resulted in less frequent use of pemoline relative to the other stimulants. Unfortunately, pemoline has not received as widespread attention in the empirical literature as dextroamphetamine and methylphenidate, and further research is necessary to guide its clinical application.

Administration and Dose Response

Schedule

The dosing schedules of dextroamphetamine and methylphenidate vary depending on which form of the drug is used and the child's daily activities. Typically these stimulants are administered on a twice-daily schedule, with a third late afternoon dose if necessary. Pemoline is administered once a day because of its longer half-life.

Dose Response

There has been considerable interest in determining optimal dose response. Previously, there was some evidence to suggest that cognition was best enhanced by lower doses of stimulants (Brown & Sleator, 1979; Sprague & Sleator, 1977), whereas behavior was most improved on higher doses (Sprague & Sleator, 1977). However, although theoretically interesting, these findings have not been supported by additional research and have not been useful clinically. Rapport and Kelly (1991) have challenged the notion of specific dose–response relationships. The original dose–response studies were analyzed for groups of children and do not consider each child's dose response. Rather, stimulant effects are interactive with and interdependent on a variety of variables including dose of medication, duration of the drug effect, individual differences, task and performance characteristics, and prevailing social and environmental conditions. In essence, response will vary according to the structure of the environment, the activity with which the child is involved, and the individual metabolism and temperament of the child. Group effects do not necessarily translate to individual dose response and every patient's dose must be considered individually.

Therapeutic Application

Stimulants are primarily indicated for the clinical management of ADHD, although within the past decade additional research has examined the effectiveness of stimulants for other disorders, both psychiatric and physical. There is increasing recognition that stimulants are effective for a particular constellation of symptoms (inattention, impulsivity, and overactivity) and may be helpful in the treatment of a variety of disorders. Literature on the effects of stimulants for each diagnostic category will be reviewed.

Attention Deficit Hyperactivity Disorder

ADHD is a syndrome characterized by inattention, impulsivity, and difficulty focusing, which may be accompanied by physical overactivity (American Psychiatric Association, 1994). ADHD has had a checkered and somewhat confusing history and the diagnostic criteria have undergone numerous revisions. Studies have employed different criteria depending on the current nomenclature; to understand this literature, it is necessary to be familiar with the criteria for sample selection. The literature reviewed here is based primarily on the *Diagnostic and Statistical Manual*, versions *III* (American Psychiatric Association, 1980) and *III-R* (American Psychiatric Association, 1987). In the most current edition of the *Diagnostic and Statistical Manual-IV* (American Psychiatric Association, 1994), it is recognized that there are two diagnostic entities: attention deficits with and without hyperactivity.

Mechanisms of Action

Several interesting theories exist regarding the mode of action of stimulants in children with ADHD. Gittelman-Klein and Klein (1973) hypothesized that stimulants enhance processes related to attention, resulting in an improved ability to focus and sustain attention. Other researchers have provided data indicating that stimulants are effective in a subgroup of children who experience underarousal of the CNS and poor inhibitory control (Satterfield, Cantwell, & Satterfield, 1974). Brown and Borden (1989) have reviewed the popular clinical lore that the actions of stimulants are paradoxical. However, it has been found that normally developing children and adults have similar cognitive and behavioral responses to stimulants as do children with ADHD. In a seminal study, Rapoport and associates (Rapoport, 1983; Rapoport *et al.,* 1980) examined the effects of dextroamphetamine in both hyperactive and normally developing boys as well as normal male college students. In a crossover design, under placebo-controlled, double-blind procedures, Rapoport *et al.* (1980) found all groups to show a decrease in motoric activity and demonstrate improved attention in response to dextroamphetamine. Further, as Brown and Borden (1989) have observed, normally developing and ADHD children have similar physiological responses (e.g., slowing of heart rate before a reaction time task), which suggests that the actions of stimulants are not specific to children with ADHD. Rapport and Kelly (1991) have recommended that greater research efforts be undertaken to systematically study the effects of stimulants with normally developing children before making any definitive conclusions regarding the actions of these drugs.

Treatment Prevalence

Although investigators have reported various rates of prevalence, it has been estimated that up to

6% of all elementary-school-age children are receiving stimulant medication for overactivity and inattention (Jacobvitz *et al.*, 1990). In fact, Safer and Krager (1988) have demonstrated that prescribing practices for stimulant medication have increased dramatically over the past two decades. As Henker and Whalen (1989) have observed, stimulants continue to be the most pervasive therapy for ADHD. Many practicing clinicians as well as the lay press have implied that stimulant medication may be overused by professionals. This opinion is partly responsible for an intense research effort to determine the advantages and disadvantages of treatment with these medications. In fact, an overwhelming amount of literature has resulted, leading Henker and Whalen to conclude that stimulant drug therapy is the most thoroughly researched and meticulously studied therapeutic modality in child and adolescent psychiatry and pediatric psychopharmacology. Thus, its clinical use rests on a firm foundation of empirical rigor.

Cognitive Effects

There has been a plethora of studies that have consistently demonstrated the ability of stimulant drugs to enhance performance on laboratory tasks of cognitive performance (Rapport & Kelly, 1991). For example, Rapport and Kelly reviewed 84 studies that examine a wide array of cognitive tasks and found stimulant medication to exert effects on tasks tapping vigilance and sustained attention (Klorman, Brumaghim, Fitzpatrick, & Borgstedt, 1991; Rapport, Carlson, Kelly, & Petaki, 1993; Rapport & Kelly, 1991), matching to sample tasks or measures of inhibitory control (Brown & Sleator, 1979; Douglas, 1988; Douglas, Barr, Amin, O'Neill, & Britton, 1988; Malone & Swanson, 1993; Rapport *et al.*, 1993; Rapport & Kelly, 1991; Tannock, Schachar, Carr, Chajczyk, & Logan, 1989; Vyse & Rapport, 1989), more efficient search strategies (Klorman *et al.*, 1991), stimulus–reaction time tasks (Douglas *et al.*, 1988; Tannock, Schachar, Carr, Chajczk, & Logan, 1989), enhanced performance on long- and short-term recall tasks (Dalby, Kinsbourne, & Swanson, 1989; Douglas *et al.*, 1988; Evans, Gualtieri, & Amara, 1986; Rapport, Quinn, DuPaul, Quinn, & Kelly, 1989), paired associate learning (Dalby *et al.*, 1989; Douglas *et al.*, 1988; Rapport *et al.*, 1989), picture recognition tasks (Kupietz, Winsberg, Richardson, Maitinsky, & Mendell, 1988; Peloquin & Klorman, 1986; Reid & Borkowski, 1984; Sprague & Sleator, 1977), stimulus identification tasks with

and without distraction (Reid & Borkowski, 1984; Sebrechts *et al.*, 1986), and improvement on tasks related to perceptual and motoric functioning (Douglas *et al.*, 1988; Gittelman, Klein, & Feingold, 1983).

As the data support the efficacy of stimulants on basic cognition, there has been a burgeoning of research to examine their actions on higher-order cognitive tasks. Keith and Engineer (1991) found methylphenidate to improve receptive language capacity and auditory processing in children with ADHD. Although these findings are encouraging, in the absence of a double-blind trial, replication is needed before definitive conclusions are made regarding the effects of stimulants on language. In another investigation of language processing, Malone, Kershner, and Seigel (1988) conclude that methylphenidate selectively improves the phonological level of word processing and that its therapeutic effects are produced through inhibition of excessive right-hemisphere activity in response to task demands that engage the left hemisphere. Additionally, Balthazor, Wagner, and Pelham (1991) found methylphenidate to improve nonspecific aspects of information processing.

Many investigators have employed the Paired Associates Learning task, in which the child is presented with word pairs and subsequently requested to respond with the initial stimulus. In their use of this task, Rapport *et al.* (1989) demonstrated that methylphenidate facilitated the acquisition and accuracy on paired associate learning. Differential rates of acquisition and accuracy were found to vary with dose of medication and exposure to the learned material. Specifically, accuracy was enhanced with methylphenidate and speed of acquisition improved with prior experience to the task. This study is important as it suggests that medication influences specific cognitive processes while other cognitions may be unaffected.

Previously it was believed that stimulants exert their influence only on rote cognitive tasks and that higher-order information processing was minimally affected (Brown & Borden, 1989; Douglas & Peters, 1979). However, the current research that we reviewed has provided some preliminary data to suggest that stimulants exert some action, albeit specific, on some higher-order cognitive skills.

Academic Achievement

A major unresolved issue is whether stimulant treatment exerts a positive influence on academic achievement and learning. Classroom behavior of children with ADHD has been demonstrated to benefit from stimulants, and many parents and teachers report that children show marked improvement in their schoolwork in response to stimulants (DuPaul & Rapport, 1993; Gadow, 1993). However, a number of investigations have been unable to detect these improvements on standardized academic achievement tests (for review see Brown & Borden, 1989). Several hypotheses have been posited to explain this discrepancy including variability of dose response on learning, inadequate duration of psychopharmacology, insensitive assessment tools, and state-dependent learning (Brown & Borden, 1989). Recent studies have continued to address this issue. Vyse and Rapport (1989) studied the effect of methylphenidate on the acquisition of trained and untrained complex visual relationships in children with ADHD. Methylphenidate promoted children's learning of both taught and untaught visual relations and these improvements were similar to the changes observed in the children's attention and classroom work efficiency.

Another investigation (Tannock, Schachar, Carr, & Logan, 1989) examined the impact of methylphenidate on the academic functioning and overt behavior of children with ADHD and found that methylphenidate improved both academic efficiency and behavior in these children. In the Pelham laboratory (Balthazor et al., 1991), methylphenidate was found to affect nonspecific aspects of information processing on a classroom reading comprehension measure. These investigators conclude that methylphenidate exerts its beneficial effects on academic processing through general rather than specific aspects of information processing.

Although the results of these studies are suggestive, they are limited because they did not employ standardized assessments of academic achievement. In contrast, Elia, Welsh, Gullotta, and Rapoport (1993) studied the effects of both dextroamphetamine and methylphenidate on ADHD children's performance on standardized reading and mathematics. On both medications, children attempted more reading and mathematics tasks with an increased number of percent correct on the reading series. An increased percent correct for the mathematics series occurred only for dextroamphetamine.

Forness and associates (Forness, Cantwell, Swanson, Hanna, & Youpa, 1991) evaluated the effects of methylphenidate on standardized academic achievement in children with ADHD, some of whom also had conduct disorder. There were no significant findings except that medication enhanced reading comprehension only in the group with conduct disorder. In a follow-up investigation, findings were similar in a longer-term (6 weeks) medication trial (Forness, Swanson, Cantwell, Youpa, & Hanna, 1992).

What few studies are available regarding this issue suggest that stimulant medications exert their effects primarily on academic efficiency, rather than achievement as measured by standardized assessment instruments. As Henker and Whalen (1989) have observed, a major unresolved controversy is the mechanism by which stimulants exert their influence. Whether or not stimulants directly enhance learning and academic achievement or produce alterations in attitude, motivation, and possibly self-regulatory strategies remains equivocal. Finally, Forness et al. (1992) have recommended that future research efforts in this area also should focus on subgroups of children with ADHD since differential responses to stimulants seem to occur with specific samples.

Behavioral and Motoric Effects

There is voluminous literature on the effects of stimulant medication on the behaviors of ADHD children that parallels the cognition literature. It has been demonstrated that stimulant drugs have beneficial influences on rule-governed behavior and compliance with commands (Pelham, 1993), parent–child interactions (Barkley, Karlsson, Strzelecki, & Murphy, 1984), and physical and verbal aggression (Hinshaw, 1991). Most of this work either has employed teacher and parent ratings of behavior (DuPaul & Rapport, 1993; Gadow, Nolan, Sverd, Sprafkin, & Paolicelli, 1990; Klorman et al., 1989) to assess these behaviors or has actually made use of direct observations of children's behavior in a classroom or laboratory-type classroom setting (Pelham, 1993). Typically, these studies have been conducted under double-blind controlled trials. The results of these studies have unequivocally demonstrated the efficacy of stimulants in decreasing classroom disruption, increasing time on task in completing assignments, and following classroom rules (Pelham & Hoza, 1987; Pelham, Vallano, Hoza, Greiner, & Gnagy, 1992). In fact, DuPaul and Rapport (1993) have provided data to indicate that methylphenidate exerted a significant effect on classroom measures of attention and academic efficiency for children with ADHD to the point that, as a group, the children received scores that no longer deviated from those obtained by normal control children.

Pelham, Vallano, *et al.* (1992) have extended these techniques of behavioral observations and controlled trials of stimulant medication in a summer camp, classroom-type program at the University of Pittsburgh. In one very interesting study, Pelham and colleagues (Pelham *et al.,* 1990) evaluated the efficacy of methylphenidate on children's attention while playing baseball. Dependent measures included on-task behavior, ability to answer questions correctly regarding the status of the game, judgment during batting, batting skill, and performance on skill drills. Findings were that children were on task twice as often when medicated, although it did not improve their baseball skills.

Because hyperactivity may be a core symptom of ADHD, some researchers have investigated the effects of stimulants on motor functioning. The results have shown generally decreased activity in structured settings with variable results in unstructured settings (Brown & Borden, 1989; Porrino, Rapoport, Behar, Ismond, & Bunney, 1983). Effects on fine motor skills have been more equivocal. Gittelman *et al.* (1983) reported significant placebo and stimulant drug effects on the Purdue Pegboard, Raven's Matrices, and Draw-a-Person test for children with reading disorders, whereas Douglas (1988) has found little or no differences on a maze tracking Etch-a-Sketch task. Finally, Whalen, Henker, and Finch (1981) found that methylphenidate improved handwriting. It is likely that the effect of stimulants on inhibitory control (Malone & Swanson, 1993; Rapport *et al.,* 1988; Tannock, Schachar, Carr, Chajczyk, & Logan, 1989) increases the capacity of children to delay responding, thereby producing greater control over their actions and improving general motor skills.

Aggression

Given that violence and delinquent behavior have increased in this country over the past several years (Kazdin, 1987), there has been considerable interest in psychopharmacological interventions for aggressive behaviors. Hinshaw (1991) recently reviewed the empirical evidence regarding the efficacy of stimulants in treating aggressive and antisocial behaviors in children with ADHD. These studies have been conducted primarily in both laboratory and large-group natural settings. This analysis points out a clear discrepancy between the effects of stimulants in the laboratory, which have been small and typically nonsignificant, and the rather large effects obtained when naturalistic observations of aggression are made in either the classroom or outdoor play setting.

Murphy, Pelham, and Lange (1992), who found minimal effects of methylphenidate on aggression on a laboratory provocation task, have attributed the differences in findings of laboratory versus naturalistic setting to the type of aggression sampled in each of the settings. For example, laboratory settings typically include primarily planned and retaliatory aggression whereas naturalistic environments typically elicit a mixture of proactive and reactive peer- and adult-directed intentional and accidental aggressive acts. Hinshaw, Buhrmester, and Heller (1989) have provided evidence to indicate that larger doses of stimulants reduce aggressive behaviors in a laboratory and relatively lower doses diminish aggressive behavior in a naturalistic setting. Pelham, Vallano, *et al.* (1992) did not find methylphenidate to produce any effect on anger or provocation in a laboratory setting for aggressive children diagnosed with ADHD, thus lending further support to the observations of Murphy *et al.* (1992) that aggression in laboratory settings is minimally affected by stimulants.

Generally, both aggressive and nonaggressive subtypes of children with ADHD show positive responses to stimulant medication as indicated by ratings by teachers (Klorman *et al.,* 1988; Klorman, Brumaghim, Fitzpatrick, Borgstedt, & Strauss, 1994), parents (Barkley, McMurray, Edelbrock, & Robbins, 1989), and program staff in a summer camp (Hinshaw, Henker, Whalen, Erhardt, & Dunnington, 1989). Gadow and associates (Gadow *et al.,* 1990) have provided further evidence to suggest that methylphenidate reduces nonphysical, physical, and verbal aggression in the classroom, and some preliminary support has been provided for a contagion effect. Having a less aggressive child with ADHD resulted in decreased nonphysical aggression by peers who did not receive stimulants (Gadow, Paolicelli, *et al.,* 1992).

Some researchers have explored the possibility of a differential cognitive response in aggressive and nonaggressive children with ADHD. Matier, Halperin, Sharma, Newcorn, and Sathaye (1992) found both aggressive and nonaggressive groups of children to exhibit similar responses to methylphenidate on measures of attention, whereas activity decreased only in the nonaggressive group. These investigators interpreted their findings to indicate that the various symptom dimensions influenced by stimulants, including aggressive behaviors, are mediated by differential neurotransmitters (Miczek, 1987).

In conclusion, the initial studies conducted with aggressive youngsters, particularly laboratory based, suggested that aggressive behaviors are little affected by stimulants; however, later naturalistic investigations provided greater support for the efficacy of methylphenidate on aggressive behaviors. In part, these differences have been attributable to different assessment strategies and doses of stimulants given in each type of setting. Although correlates of stimulant drug effects in animal studies have raised several interesting hypotheses for studies with humans, much more research is needed. Further investigation is also needed to understand the effects of stimulants on specific types of aggression.

Social Relations and Peer Status

It is well known that children with ADHD experience significant problems in their relationships with others (Henker & Whalen, 1989; Whalen & Henker, 1991). These children have been found to have an impulsive, immature, and disruptive manner of interacting with others (Pelham & Bender, 1982). Because of the efficacy and widespread use of stimulants for ADHD, a natural direction for investigation has been the effects of stimulants on social behavior. Research that has examined this issue with both peers (Pelham, 1993) and adults (Granger, Whalen, & Henker, 1993a; Milich & Landau, 1982; Pelham & Bender, 1982; Whalen, 1989) has come primarily from two laboratories (Henker & Whalen, 1989; Pelham, 1993; Whalen & Henker, 1991). Whalen *et al.* (1989) examined the effects of methylphenidate on peer relationships and discovered that peers rated medicated hyperactive boys higher on social standing (e.g., increased peer nominations as best friend, cooperative, and fun to be with), but these improvements did not normalize peer appraisals.

When children with ADHD were observed interacting with younger children, stimulant medication generally muted social behavior, decreasing social engagement and increasing dysphoria relative to the placebo condition (Buhrmester, Whalen, Henker, McDonald, & Hinshaw, 1992). Compared with the normals, the placebo group was more socially engaged, employed more aversive leadership techniques, and was rated less likable by the younger children. No differences were found between comparison and unmedicated hyperactive boys for any aspect of prosocial behavior.

Similarly, adult observers rated medicated and placebo control ADHD children during an interactional task with several peers (Granger *et al.*, 1993a). All of the children received more negative behavioral descriptions than positive. Placebo controls received negative evaluations for noncompliance, aggression, and disruption, whereas children on active medication were negatively assessed for passive and submissive behaviors.

In another investigation, Granger, Whalen, and Henker (1993b) examined the malleability of adults' social impressions of children with ADHD. Undergraduate students were requested to observe two videotaped scenarios of a boy with symptoms of ADHD. The targets were receiving either methylphenidate or placebo for the two sessions. The students' cumulative social evaluations of the children were assessed following their viewing of both videotaped segments. Findings were that the undergraduates combined their perceptions of the two behavior samples into a composite impression. Even when children's behavior improved in response to methylphenidate, the undergraduates' ratings of the children's undercontrolled behavior were quite high. The findings are important as they suggest that the overall behavior of children with ADHD plays a rather influential role in shaping adults' impressions regardless of whether the children are receiving active stimulant medication.

Although these studies indicate that stimulants do not appear to increase prosocial behaviors, they do influence compliance and level of intrusiveness. Pelham (1993) has suggested that to use stimulants effectively for the purpose of increasing prosocial behaviors may require the simultaneous use of additional therapies such as behavioral interventions. Pelham provided data to indicate the beneficial effects of methylphenidate and behavioral therapy in the social domain. However, these dependent measures of socialization appeared to assess aggression (i.e., stealing, lying, and negative verbalizations) rather than prosocial behaviors as assessed in the Whalen and Henker laboratory. In short, the research is not definitive regarding the effects of stimulant medication on social behaviors. Clearly, greater research efforts are needed in this area, particularly studies that compare the effects of stimulants with nonsomatic therapies for increasing prosocial behaviors.

Learning Disabilities

Learning disabilities is a general category used to describe a heterogeneous group of children with deficits in a variety of abilities such as reading, arithmetic, language, writing, and motor skills (American Psychiatric Association, 1994). Attention disturbances and problems with distractibility have been observed in this population (Douglas & Peters, 1979). Further, a significant number of children with ADHD also have learning disabilities (Barkley, 1990). The few studies investigating the use of stimulants on basic learning disabilities were conducted primarily with children who evidenced reading disabilities; the stimulants demonstrated little or no effects on reading performance (for review see Brown & Borden, 1989). There is clear evidence that stimulants are not an effective treatment modality for basic learning disabilities.

Most of the literature focusing on the effects of stimulants on learning disabilities typically has emphasized ADHD children with learning disabilities. Because all of the stimulant and learning disabilities literature is not within the scope of this chapter, we will review only those major studies published within the last 10 years. Kupietz and associates (Kupietz et al., 1988; Richardson, Kupietz, Winsberg, Maitinsky, & Mendell, 1988) examined the effects of methylphenidate on children diagnosed with ADHD and developmental reading disorders. Placebo and three doses of methylphenidate were compared over a 6-month period employing measures of associative learning and academic achievement scores. Although improvement in academic performance was noted, it could not be directly attributed to methylphenidate. Similarly, Forness et al. (1991) found methylphenidate to exert little effect on reading performance in children with ADHD and learning disabilities. Another investigation of the effect of stimulants on academic achievement, in a subset of children with ADHD and learning disabilities, found that a diagnosis of learning disabilities is not related to drug-induced improvements on academic measures (Elia et al., 1993).

Thus, consistent with previous observations (Brown & Borden, 1989), the literature clearly suggests that stimulants exert little specific influence on learning disabilities. The majority of the research has examined children with both ADHD and learning disabilities, and the benefits of stimulants in this group appear to be specific to enhanced attention rather than improved academic processing. In conclusion, stimulants may have an adjunct role in the treatment of learning-disabled children who also have attentional problems; however, nothing can substitute for educational remediation.

Conduct Disorders

Conduct disorder is characterized by persistent patterns of aggression, oppositional behavior, and behaviors that violate the norms of society (Gadow, 1992). Few studies have examined the effects of stimulants for children with conduct disorders. There is encouraging support for the effects of stimulants on disruptive and aggressive behaviors (Pelham & Murphy, 1986), the core symptoms found in youth with conduct disorders. Further, as Rapoport (1983) has pointed out, many of the subjects in the earlier successful stimulant drug trials were delinquent populations (Eisenberg et al., 1963), lending some evidence to the hypothesis that conduct-disordered youth would respond to these agents.

In a placebo-controlled, double-blind investigation of the effect of methylphenidate on aggression in hospitalized adolescents diagnosed with both conduct disorder and ADHD, Kaplan, Busner, Kupietz, Wassermann, and Segal (1990) found a significant reduction in aggression as rated by ward staff, but no significant differences were found for teacher ratings of overactivity and aggression. Although this study was a valuable first step, it has some limitations. It is important both theoretically and clinically to examine the effects of stimulants on conduct-disordered youth without a diagnosis of ADHD.

To address the effects of stimulants on conduct-disordered youth, Brown and associates (Brown, Jaffe, Silverstein, & Magee, 1991) examined the efficacy of methylphenidate on hospitalized conduct-disordered youth on teacher ratings of behavior, a measure of classroom learning, and a laboratory measure of impulsivity. Twenty-two male adolescents with conduct disorder, 12 to 18 years of age, participated in a double-blind, placebo-controlled, crossover study in which each youth received three doses of methylphenidate (10, 15, and 20 mg) and a placebo in a randomly assigned, counterbalanced order. Seven of the subjects had a comorbid diagnosis of ADHD. Significant overall medication effects were shown on teacher ratings of conduct, on number of arithmetic questions correctly completed, and on time spent on task. In addition, an interaction was found between diagnosis and dose, with the conduct-disordered adolescents requiring higher doses to increase arithmetic accuracy and inhibitory control, whereas lower doses were found to enhance academic proficiency in the comorbid ADHD and conduct-disordered group. Brown *et al.* (1991) postulate that having ADHD may produce a greater sensitivity to stimulant response. It should be noted that this investigation was an acute clinical trial, evaluating the children on each medication dose for only 2 weeks. Thus, the effects of medication on aggression in conduct disorder were unclear as aggressive acts tend to occur at a lower frequency than ADHD symptoms (e.g., overactivity, distractibility, and emotional lability).

It should be noted that stimulants in the two studies reviewed employed controlled trials in an inpatient psychiatric setting in which any potential risks could be tightly controlled by medical staff; subjects also received adjunctive treatments such as behavior modification and psychotherapy. Given the social ramifications of aggression, the aforementioned studies are of theoretical importance. Current research suggests the potential efficacy of stimulants for conduct-disordered adolescents with or without ADHD. Clearly further research in this area is warranted. Despite the tentative empirical support of the use of stimulants for conduct-disordered youth, we advise caution in using these findings for clinical practice, particularly in an outpatient setting. Conduct-disordered youth have many problems and their potential for drug abuse is quite high (Elliott, 1988) resulting in a substantial risk that stimulants could be misused. There is some evidence that stimulant treatment in ADHD is related to a decrease in abuse of drugs (Loney, Kramer, & Milich, 1981), although no studies can be found that have examined this issue for conduct-disordered adolescents. In the absence of additional trials, the careful and systematic monitoring of stimulant drug effects for this population seems most prudent, and the clinical use of these stimulants seems best confined to a controlled inpatient facility.

Mental Retardation

Frequently, children who are mentally retarded also have symptoms consistent with ADHD; stimulants have been commonly prescribed for those children with both conditions (Gadow, 1985). However, the efficacy of stimulants for behavior disorders in the mentally retarded has been questioned (Aman, 1982). In studies of the use of stimulants in the mentally retarded, the drugs produced therapeutic benefits comparable to those observed in children who are not mentally retarded. It was suggested that the degree of improvement is related directly to the severity of retardation with the more

severely mentally retarded children benefiting the least (Gadow, 1985).

A single-case study was conducted with three mildly mentally retarded children with ADHD to assess the effectiveness of methylphenidate and dextroamphetamine, and findings demonstrated a reduction in excessive movement and an increase in task behavior in response to these medications (Payton, Burkhart, Hersen, & Helsel, 1989). In another study of 12 children whose IQs ranged from 50 to 74 and who met rigorous diagnostic criteria for ADHD, Handen, Breaux, Gosling, Ploof, and Feldman (1990) examined the efficacy of methylphenidate versus placebo. Improvement with medication was found in 75% of the patients. Significant improvements in work output, on-task behavior, and attentional skills were noted. Consistent with the ADHD literature, improvements in attention were not associated with concomitant gains in learning and social interaction with peers. Findings were interpreted to support the notion that stimulant medication produces similar effects across similar domains in ADHD children, both retarded and nonretarded.

In a controlled trial of methylphenidate, thioridazine (a widely used neuroleptic), and placebos in children identified as mentally retarded with ADHD and/or conduct disorder (IQs ranged from profound retardation to low average) (Aman, Marks, Turbott, Wilsher, & Merry, 1991a), methylphenidate consistently and highly significantly reduced teacher ratings of problem behavior. Parental ratings showed no behavioral effects as a whole. When the children were categorized by attention span, mental age, and IQ level, higher-functioning subjects were found to show a generally favorable response to methylphenidate on both parent and teacher behavioral scales. Lower-functioning children showed an adverse or indifferent response to stimulants. The authors conclude that IQ and mental age may in fact be important determinants of response to stimulants. However, thioridazine produced less absolute change than methylphenidate and was worse than methylphenidate on teacher ratings of inattention and global ratings of behavior. Additionally, methylphenidate improved accuracy on a memory task, reduced omission errors on an attention task, and reduced seat movements (Aman, Marks, Turbott, Wilsher, & Merry, 1991b). In a related investigation, Aman, Kern, McGhee, and Arnold (1993) discovered that children with higher IQs responded more favorably to methylphenidate than did children with IQs less than 45.

Another double-blind investigation of methylphenidate versus placebo examined 14 children with ADHD whose IQs ranged from 48 to 74 (Handen et al., 1992). Nine children (64%) responded positively to methylphenidate with significant enhancement of on-task behavior and attention skills. Consistent with previous studies, no improvement on measures of learning or social interactions was observed. Handen and associates (Handen, Feldman, Gosling, Breaux, & McAuliffe, 1991) reviewed the incidence of side effects in their cohort and conclude that the mentally retarded may be at greater risk for developing motor tics and social withdrawal. For this reason, their use with the mentally retarded should be monitored carefully.

This literature indicates similar efficacy of stimulants with retarded and nonretarded children with ADHD. There appears to be a significant relationship between IQ score and positive response with higher-functioning children evidencing better response. Additional studies are necessary with larger cohorts of children with various intellectual abilities to clarify the association between stimulant response, intellectual functioning, and side effects.

Acquired Neurological Conditions

There has been burgeoning literature about the neuropsychological, social, and emotional sequelae of acquired brain injuries in pediatric populations. This research has meticulously documented characteristic deficits that include cognitive, academic, and behavioral disturbances using numerous measures (Fletcher & Levin, 1988; Levin, Eisenberg, Wigg, & Kabayashi, 1982). The neurocognitive functions most vulnerable to acquired brain injuries appear to be attention, memory, and problem-solving abilities. Deficits in these areas may persist many years after the original insult (Evans, Gualtieri, & Patterson, 1987). Evidence has accumulated to suggest that these attentional deficits and related neurocognitive disorders (Levin & Eisenberg, 1979a,b; Levin & Grossman, 1976) significantly impede cognition, achievement, and social development in children with acquired brain injuries (Eiben et al., 1984; Ewing-Cobbs, Fletcher, & Levin, 1985; Levin et al., 1982). Fletcher and Levin (1988) carefully reviewed the studies concerning pediatric closed head injuries and concluded that these children demonstrate a chronic pattern of poor inhibitory control and sustained attention. Moreover, this high frequency of attention deficits has been found to be pervasive and chronic

in children with other acquired brain injuries such as brain tumors (Fletcher, Levin, & Landry, 1984) and sustained hypoxic–ischemic events (Morris, Krawiecki, Wright, & Walters, 1993).

As Fletcher and Levin (1988) have suggested, the attentional, memory, and problem-solving deficits displayed by children with acquired brain injuries crucially affect the recovery–rehabilitation process. It has been well documented that these children have "impressive" academic difficulties (Goldstein & Levin, 1985) and a significant proportion of them require special education placement (Shaffer, Bijur, Chadwick, & Rutter, 1980).

Although serious attention, cognitive, and academic deficits in children with acquired brain injuries have been substantiated, the best-documented sequelae for these children have been behavioral and psychosocial difficulties (Fletcher & Levin, 1988; Noll, LeRoy, Bukowski, Rugosch, & Kulkarni, 1991). Problems include poor impulse control, overactivity, aggression, emotional lability, and difficulties with self-monitoring (Klonoff, Crockett, & Clark, 1984).

Unfortunately, cognitive and behavioral rehabilitation programs with these children have met limited success (Prigatano, 1987; Telzrow, 1985). Many clinicians have used stimulant medication as a treatment component because inattention, emotional lability, aggression, impulsivity, distractibility, and overactivity commonly occur in these children. The stimulants seem to be an appropriate match to the essential cognitive and behavioral sequelae of children with acquired brain injuries. And it seems that the neurobiological basis for this response is similar for ADHD children and those with acquired brain injuries.

The late 1970s and 1980s were a very important tertiary stage in the refinement of drug trials and systematic study of stimulants for ADHD children's learning and behavioral problems (Rapport & Kelly, 1991). The studies reviewed in this chapter support the potential efficacy of stimulant medication as a viable pharmacotherapy for the treatment of children with acquired brain injuries who have attentional and overactivity difficulties. Those symptoms in both ADHD and normally developing children that have demonstrated the most improvement with stimulants include impaired capacity to sustain attention and effort, impulsivity, emotional lability, overactivity, communication competence, and aggression (Rapport & Kelly, 1991), deficits that are well documented for children with acquired brain injuries. Because normal and ADHD children have comparable physiological responses to stimulant medication (Rapoport *et al.,* 1980), it is likely that stimulants in children with acquired brain injuries work similarly. The effects of stimulants in this population are theoretically important to examine as this research may shed additional light on the actions of the drug.

Gualtieri (1991) has delineated specific reasons why stimulants should prove efficacious in the clinical management of children with acquired head injuries. First, as previously noted, stimulants have been demonstrated to improve symptoms of inattention, distractibility, disorganization, overactivity, impulsivity, and emotional lability in children with ADHD (Barkley, 1990; Rapport & Kelly, 1991). Many children with acquired brain injuries and with similar symptoms should respond well to sympathomimetic medications. Second, stimulants have been found to improve symptoms of hypersomnia, apathy, energia, and hypoarousal in narcoleptic patients (Orlosky, 1982). Thus, children with acquired brain injuries who are afflicted with these symptoms may respond favorably to stimulant medication. Third, stimulants have been found to improve long-term memory in ADHD children through a direct mechanism, dissociated from medication effects on attention and fatigue (Evans *et al.,* 1986). It is plausible that they would have similar effects in children with acquired head injuries. Fourth, there is some evidence to suggest that stimulants improve perceptual functioning in ADHD children (Rapport & Kelly, 1991) as well as enhance fine motor speed, accuracy, and steadiness (Gualtieri, Hicks, Levitt, Conley, & Schroeder, 1986). Because these deficits frequently have been characteristic of children with acquired head injuries, it is reasonable to hypothesize that stimulants would have comparable therapeutic effects for them. Gualtieri and Evans (1988) have suggested that stimulants exert their effects by enhancing dopaminergic neurotransmission to rostral brain structures, particularly in the frontal cortex. Thus, the stimulants may be particularly useful for those patients with acquired brain injury whose deficits are attributable to frontal lobe or frontal–subcortical system injuries (more typical of closed head injuries).

Although there have been some anecdotal reports of stimulant effects throughout the neuropsychiatric literature in patients with acquired brain injuries (Weinstein & Wells, 1981), only two double-blind trials have been found that employed stimulant medication in adolescents and adults (Evans *et al.,* 1987; Gualtieri & Evans, 1988). No published studies have examined the efficacy of stimulant therapy for children with acquired brain injuries.

Evans *et al.* (1987), in the first double-blind, placebo-controlled, dose–response study, separately examined the effects of methylphenidate and dextroamphetamine in a young male with a closed head injury. Memory and attention were found to be significantly improved as a function of both stimulants. In a follow-up of this case study, Gualtieri and Evans (1988) conducted double-blind trials of methylphenidate in 15 adolescent and adult patients with brain trauma. There was some improvement in the areas of attention, memory, verbal fluency, and emotional lability with specific behaviors responding differentially to high and low doses of methylphenidate.

Although these findings are promising, they raise more questions than answers. In the Evans *et al.* (1987) case study, the patient evidenced the most optimal response to the higher of the two doses studied (0.3 versus 0.15 mg/kg b.i.d.), whereas in the second group trial, some variability was noted across tasks with the majority of patients evidencing improvement on the low dose of methylphenidate.

Gualtieri and Evans (1988), in their work with adolescents and young adults, have reported carryover effects from one drug condition to another, including crossover from active medication to placebo. These carryover effects have not been observed in ADHD children or other adolescent patient groups (Brown *et al.,* 1991); and the investigators suggest that methylphenidate may change neuronal responsiveness, which enhances the recovery process. This hypothesis also has been espoused by Feeny, Gonzalez, and Law (1982) in a clinical trial with adults that demonstrated improved acute postinjury learning as a function of stimulant medication. The underlying suggested mechanism is that dopamine agonists will enhance the cortical recovery process. For children, it is unclear whether such carryover effects occur and if stimulants hasten the rehabilitation process following their acute recovery. Thus, although these data are encouraging in supporting the use of stimulants for children with acquired brain injuries, much more research is needed before endorsing their efficacy for this population.

Tourette's Syndrome

Tourette's syndrome is a hereditary neurobehavioral disorder characterized by multiple motor and verbal tics. Behavioral and attentional problems frequently are concomitant with Tourette's syndrome; some research had suggested that ADHD is often a core symptom of Tourette's syndrome and that Tourette's constitutes a major etiological subgroup of ADHD (Gadow & Sverd, 1990). In fact, prevalence rates of ADHD in Tourette's patients exceeded 70%.

Over the years, there has been some clinical evidence to suggest that stimulant medication can precipitate motor tics, stereotypies, or exacerbate symptoms associated with Tourette's syndrome. In fact, a small percentage of ADHD children who receive methylphenidate have been found to develop tics, although they typically have been reversible on cessation of medication. More recently, there have been greater systematic efforts to study the effects of stimulant medication in ADHD children with comorbid tic disorders.

One earlier single-blind, placebo-controlled study examined the effects of methylphenidate on teacher ratings and observed playroom behavior in four boys diagnosed with ADHD and Tourette's syndrome (Sverd, Gadow, & Paolicelli, 1989). Results indicated that methylphenidate produced no more tics than did the placebo. In fact, for each of the children, the highest dose of methylphenidate improved classroom ratings of the tics compared with the placebo, even though some mild tic exacerbation was noted on the lower dose of medication. Sverd and colleagues interpret their findings to suggest that methylphenidate alone may prove to be both safe and effective for the treatment of attention problems and behavior difficulties in children with Tourette's.

Sprafkin and Gadow (1993) present case studies in which methylphenidate appears to have induced tic exacerbation. However, on careful analyses of the course of stimulant therapy, data were not convincing regarding the role of stimulants in exacerbating Tourette's disorder. Although one patient's tic disorder seemed to become more severe with methylphenidate, the child was found to have less severe tic symptoms with higher doses of methylphenidate. Another patient appeared to develop Tourette's syndrome while receiving methylphenidate but subsequently was determined to have a preexisting undiagnosed tic disorder. Sprafkin and Gadow (1993) emphasize the importance of careful and unbiased assessment regarding pretreatment symptoms, variability in symptomatology over time, and careful assessment of any possible link between stimulant medication and tic exacerbation.

Finally, in a controlled clinical trial investigating the effects of methylphenidate in boys diagnosed with both ADHD and Tourette's, Gadow and associates (Gadow, Nolan, & Sverd, 1992) observed these children in a classroom setting for 6 weeks. Methylphenidate suppressed overactive and disruptive behavior in the classroom and physical aggression on the playground. Similar findings were reported by parents on behavioral ratings of the same children (Sverd, Gadow, Nolan, Sprafkin, & Ezor, 1992). Most importantly, methylphenidate was found to reduce the occurrence of vocal tics at school; however, no differences were found during routine assessments. Of the 11 children studied, only 1 boy experienced motor tic exacerbation.

Finally, Borcherding, Keysor, Rapoport, Elia, and Amass (1990) studied the effects of methylphenidate and dextroamphetamine and found that abnormal movements and perseverative compulsive behaviors occurred with both medications. These abnormalities frequently were subtle, transient, and usually occurred on one drug. Only one patient had to discontinue medication because of tic severity. Based on their findings, Borcherding and colleagues conclude that monitoring of stimulants is important. It may not be necessary to discontinue medication because of these symptoms, but adjusting the dose or selecting another stimulant may ameliorate these manifestations.

Although the recent studies are encouraging and suggest that stimulants are an effective and safe intervention for ADHD children with tic disorders, more clinical trials are needed to definitively determine the safety and efficacy in this population. Families of ADHD children, particularly those with Tourette's, must be apprised of the potential risks of stimulants; and, if a trial of stimulants is elected, careful monitoring should always be the rule.

Depression in Medically Ill Groups

Although stimulants primarily have been used to treat problems of inattention and impulsivity, a significant body of literature exists describing the use of stimulants to treat depression in medically ill adults for whom traditional antidepressant therapy was contraindicated (Stoudemire, Morau, & Fogel, 1991). Based on these data, there has been considerable interest in using stimulants for a similar population of children and adolescents. However, a careful examination of the literature reveals only one case report using methylphenidate in a depressed adolescent with AIDS. This 15-year-old with hemophilia, AIDS, and major depressive disorder, who manifested numerous side effects on a traditional antidepressant, showed marked improvement in mood, energy level, and appetite on methylphenidate (Walling & Pfefferbaum, 1990). Although these findings are suggestive, additional research must be conducted to empirically validate the benefits of stimulants for this population.

Developmental Issues

Although stimulants have been used primarily in the elementary-school-age population, there has been an increasing recognition that attention difficulties span the entire developmental life span and that stimulants are an appropriate treatment modality for many age groups.

Preschoolers

Response to stimulants in preschoolers with ADHD has been found to be quite variable (Brown & Borden, 1989). Unfortunately, only a few studies have investigated the efficacy of stimulants for this group (Barkley, DuPaul, et al., 1993; Speltz, Varley, Peterson, & Beilke, 1988). Generally, these data have suggested minimal effect of stimulants on preschool children. Some investigators have suggested that older preschoolers may benefit from these drugs (Pelham, 1993), but the clinical literature has sounded caution regarding the potential of untoward side effects (Dulcan, 1990). Alessandri and Schramm (1991), in a single-subject study, investigated the effects of dextroamphetamine in a preschooler with ADHD. On stimulants, improvements were noted in sustained attention and play behavior. Given the limited research data in this area, coupled with the potential for problematic side effects and the unknown impact of stimulants on critical aspects of growth and development, stimulants should be used judiciously only after other therapies and adjunctive treatments have been employed.

Adolescents

In the past, ADHD was conceptualized as a disorder of childhood. It has become increasingly clear that as children grow older they continue to have significant problems with attention and impulsivity but may become less physically overactive (Klorman, 1986). As a result, there has been a paucity of information pertaining to the pharmacology of stimulants in adolescents.

Now there is burgeoning literature attesting to the efficacy of stimulants in ADHD adolescents. Coons and associates (Coons, Klorman, & Borgstedt, 1987), in a double-blind trial of methylphenidate, found superior behavioral ratings, as rated by parents, and increased accuracy on a task of sustained attention. In a similar investigation, Klorman, Brumaghim, Fitzpatrick, and Borgstedt (1990) examined the effects of methylphenidate in a double-blind trial with previously undiagnosed and untreated ADHD adolescents. On medication, teacher and parent ratings of hyperactivity, inattention, and oppositional behavior were significantly decreased. The adolescents rated themselves as clinically improved and reported an improvement in mood. Treatment benefits were comparable for adolescents regardless of the presence or absence of a comorbid disorder (i.e., conduct, oppositional, or depressive disorder). In an investigation of methylphenidate in adolescents diagnosed with ADHD and conduct disorder, Kaplan et al. (1990) found a significant reduction of aggression as rated by ward staff, yet no significant differences were found for teacher ratings.

In our laboratory (Brown et al., 1991), conduct-disordered adolescents were compared on various doses of methylphenidate on measures of behavior, classroom learning, and impulsivity. Significant overall medication effects were demonstrated on teacher ratings of conduct and on arithmetic accuracy and academic performance. Similar effects were noted for younger black adolescents diagnosed with ADHD (Brown & Sexson, 1988); significant increases in blood pressure were noted for this group of adolescents, already at risk for hypertension (Brown & Sexson, 1989), suggesting that these youth be carefully monitored while receiving stimulants.

Other investigators have confirmed the beneficial effects of stimulants with ADHD adolescents but have documented a lower medication response rate relative to prepubertal boys (Pelham, Vodde-Hamilton, Murphy, Greenstein, & Vallano, 1991). Additionally, Evans and Pelham (1991) conducted a controlled trial of pemoline and methylphenidate in young adolescents ranging in age from 11 to 15 and found a 66% response rate.

In summary, the literature with ADHD adolescents has paralleled the data obtained from their school-age counterparts. The data have generally suggested improved cognitive performance, impulse control, academic efficiency, and diminished aggression. However, more work needs to be conducted to determine optimal dosing, side effects, and the long-term effects of stimulants in this population, as many of these individuals will continue to be symptomatic in adulthood.

Adults

The recognition that ADHD persists throughout adulthood has stimulated immense interest in the diagnosis, treatment, and outcome of this disorder. Thus, a logical extension of research with stimulants has been to study their effects in adults with ADHD. Although a discussion of the spectrum of stimulant effects in adults is not within the scope of this chapter, data from preliminary investigations are consistent with the pediatric literature and are encouraging regarding clinical efficacy (Wender, Reimherr, Wood, & Ward, 1985).

Issues of Assessment

Physiological Correlates

There has been an increasing interest in the anatomical, biochemical, and physiological processes of the brain in children with various types of psychopathology including ADHD (Hynd *et al.*, 1991; Zametkin *et al.*, 1993). Although not yet conclusive, these studies have generally suggested that differences in structure, metabolism, and activity occur as a function of psychopathology. One aspect of this line of investigation is determining the effects of stimulants on the central and autonomic nervous system.

Central and Autonomic Nervous System Variables

Although a number of promising studies investigating the effects of stimulants on the brain are under way, few reports have been published in this area. The studies generally suggest that the effects of stimulants are associated with a normalizing of several nervous system variables (Brown & Borden, 1989). However, the specific actions of stimulants on central and autonomic nervous system variables are not well understood.

Zahn, Rapoport, and Thompson (1980) compared the psychostimulant effects on autonomic nervous system responses in normal and ADHD boys. The autonomic responses included heart rate, cardiac regulation, and skin temperature. The in-

vestigators concluded that stimulants have similar behavioral and autonomic nervous system effects in ADHD and normally developing children, although the magnitude of the effects may differ.

Several studies have found various abnormalities in the electroencephalograms (EEGs) of ADHD children (Yellin, 1986). Surwillo (1980) observed that the EEGs of ADHD children are immature in relation to their chronological age and that stimulants have a maturing effect on the EEGs.

The best-researched brain measure is the event-related potential (ERP), which is the electrical change in the brain in response to specific stimuli, either internal or external (Klorman, 1991; Yellin, 1986). Abnormalities have been found in ADHD children relative to their normal peers, especially during tasks requiring sustained attention (Brown & Borden, 1989). The P_{300} component of the ERP was noted to be smaller in amplitude in ADHD children than in normal controls (Klorman, 1991). Methylphenidate has been demonstrated to increase the amplitude of the P_{300} in both ADHD and normal children (Klorman, 1991). These findings were interpreted to indicate reduced capacity allocation for ADHD children, which is enhanced by methylphenidate.

Although not well understood, these processes clearly underlie the physiological mechanism by which the stimulants exert their influence. The majority of this work has been done with ERPs; however, other biochemical and physiological processes show the potential to be good barometers of CNS responses to stimulants. As the development of new technology continues, exciting avenues of research are likely to emerge.

Learning

Although stimulants have not been found to demonstrate strong positive influences on basic learning processes by stimulants, academic efficiency has been found to be enhanced. One major issue has been whether or not stimulants exert their effects on learning through the development of dependent states. State-dependent learning is characterized by the failure to transfer learning in a medicated state to an unmedicated state (i.e., information learned while the child is medicated is not easily retrieved while the child is not medicated). Most of the studies examining this issue have not found evidence for state-dependent learning for placebo and active stimulant drug conditions (for review see Brown & Borden, 1989). Nonetheless, practitioners need to be concerned about how stimulants affect learning and need to monitor the academic performance of their patients carefully.

Behavioral Correlates

Currently, behavioral assessment is the major means by which children are evaluated for stimulant medication and by which they are monitored. A variety of techniques exist for assessing behavior and these include the use of direct observation, rating scales, and sociometric ratings. Direct observations provide clearly delineated measures that minimize inference on the part of observers (Atkins & Pelham, 1991), thus decreasing the subjectivity of the responses. Typically, direct observations are conducted in a classroom or playroom situation, ideally where observers are blind to either the diagnostic or medication status of the subjects. The use of this technique has been effective in documenting stimulant drug effects and distinguishing stimulant drug from placebo effects (Gadow, 1993).

Rating scales provide a summary of behavior and, over the years, have played an essential role in evaluating response to stimulants. They have several advantages including simplicity, cost-effectiveness, and reduced subjectivity. Typically, rating scales, whether completed by teachers or parents, tap similar domains of children's behavior (Atkins & Pelham, 1991; Gadow, 1993). Multiple rating scales exist; the most commonly used for stimulant drug evaluation to assess ADHD children have included the Conner's Teacher Rating Scale (Trites, Blouin, & LaPrade, 1982), the Iowa Conners Rating Scale (Loney & Milich, 1982), and the Swanson Nolan and Pelham Rating Scale (Pelham, Atkins, Murphy, & Swanson, 1984). Teacher rating scales are particularly useful for assessing stimulant response during the day, and parent ratings may be useful for other time periods.

Atkins and Pelham (1991) have recommended the use of a multivariate approach as a means of assessing drug response. Thus, obtaining ratings from sources that include teachers, parents, peers, and the children themselves across a variety of situations will yield the most comprehensive assessment as each group has a different perspective and provides independent information.

Psychological Testing

Over the years, delineating and refining the appropriate psychological measures for the assessment of stimulant drug effects has been a prolific and marketable enterprise. Although a discussion of each of these measures is not possible within the space constraints of this chapter, those instruments that have been found to differentiate stimulant drug effects from placebo are primarily related to attention and concentration (Rapport & Kelly, 1991). Psychological testing is merely one facet of a comprehensive battery used to evaluate a child for a possible stimulant drug trial (Fischer & Newby, 1991). Psychological testing may identify deficits in attention and concentration, but its primary function is to identify basic learning disabilities and concomitant emotional and behavioral problems. More recently, the trend has been to utilize direct observations, rating scales, computerized tasks of vigilance, and sustained attention to evaluate drug response. Typically, the computer tasks involve the repetitious presentation of specific stimuli over time. Data have demonstrated repeatedly that results on such tasks are sensitive to placebo and active doses of stimulant medication (Brown & Borden, 1989).

Neuropsychological Evaluation

There has been consistent enthusiasm for developing a package of neuropsychological instruments designed to identify children with attention difficulties and for monitoring their drug responses. A variety of measures are available and have demonstrated good psychometric properties (Lezak, 1983). The majority of these tools have been found to assess frontal lobe functioning. In a very recent investigation, Barkley and Grodinsky (1994) evaluated the predictive power of a group of frontal lobe measures commonly employed to assess children with ADHD. The measures included the Continuous Performance Task (Gordon, 1983), the Controlled Word Association Test (Benton & Hamsher, 1978), the Hand Movement Scale (Kaufman & Kaufman, 1983), the Porteus Mazes (Porteus, 1965), the Rey–Osterrieth Complex Figure Test (Lezak, 1983), the Stroop Color-Word Association Test (Stroop, 1935), the Trail Making Test (Parts A and B) (Reitan & Wolfson, 1985), the Wisconsin Card Sorting Task (Heaton, 1981), and the Grooved Pegboard Test (Reitan & Wolfson, 1985). The measures were administered to attention-deficit-disordered children with and without hyperactivity, learning-disabled children, and normally developing children. The level of sensitivity for the ADHD group was low, i.e., the measures did not adequately discriminate the ADHD children from the other diagnostic groups. Some positive prediction was found on the Continuous Performance Task for the ADHD subgroup. These investigators conclude that abnormal scores on the Continuous Performance Task are predictive of attention problems, but are not very useful in designating subtypes of the disorder. More importantly, having a score that falls within the normal range does not necessarily indicate the absence of attention abnormalities. Thus, their usefulness in monitoring drug effects for these children also would be questionable. As these tests are labor intensive and costly to administer, their clinical appropriateness for evaluating drug response must be judiciously evaluated.

Clinical Evaluation

Despite extensive exploration of a variety of diagnostic instruments, attention problems and stimulant response are best assessed clinically. Of primary importance is the gathering of historical data and the collection of behavioral observations from multiple sources including the classroom (Atkins & Pelham, 1991; Fischer & Newby, 1991; Gadow, 1993; Gadow, Nolan, Paolicelli, & Sprafkin, 1991a,b; Nolan & Gadow, 1994), the home environment (Barkley, DuPaul, & McMurray, 1991; Fischer & Newby, 1991; McBride, 1988), peer interaction (Pelham & Hoza, 1987), and the clinical setting (McBride, 1988). For the consideration of a trial of stimulants, specific symptoms (e.g., inattention, impulsivity, and overactivity) should be present across the assessed domains (i.e., at home, at school, and possibly in the clinic).

After obtaining baseline data and making a careful diagnosis, a trial of stimulants may be warranted. Some have suggested that double-blind procedures be followed even in the clinical setting (Fischer & Newby, 1991; Gadow *et al.,* 1991a,b; Varley & Trupin, 1982), which allows for an objective evaluation of stimulant drug effects across both the home and school situation as well as systematic documentation of side effects (Barkley *et al.,* 1993). This approach also should be applied in the titration of dose (Barkley *et al.,* 1991). Consistent data-based procedures have been demonstrated to be the most appropriate techniques for the assessment and treatment of children on stimulants.

Predicting Responses

A common question that arises is whether or not a positive response to stimulants may be predicted by test data. Not only would this be of theoretical interest, it also would be invaluable clinically. Previously, the data have been equivocal with some suggesting that response to stimulants could be predicted by measures of attention and concentration (Barkley, 1976), whereas other investigators have insisted that no single variable is useful for predicting stimulant drug response (Loney, 1986). DuPaul and associates (DuPaul, Barkley, & McMurray, 1994) studied a sample of ADHD children and found that children with ADHD and comorbid internalizing symptoms were less likely to respond positively to methylphenidate than were their noninternalizing counterparts. Similarly, Handen, Janosky, McAuliffe, Breaux, and Feldman (1994) found, in mentally retarded ADHD youth, that more elevated parent ratings of activity and impulsivity and higher teacher ratings of activity, impulsivity, inattention, and conduct problems were associated with the best response to stimulants. In addition, subjects who were male, white, and from families of higher socioeconomic status were more likely to evidence positive response to stimulants. Finally, some investigations have centered around documenting the optimal measure for predicting drug response, and generally this has proved unproductive. At this point, a systematic drug trial is most appropriate for assessing response.

Limitations of Stimulants

Iatrogenic and Emanative Effects

Physical

As with any medication, stimulants have both positive and negative effects, and the practitioner must carefully weigh the benefits of the medication against the side effects. Stimulants have been used for nearly 60 years and consistently have been found to be one of the safest psychotropic drugs available. An extensive literature is available regarding the side effects of stimulants in pediatric populations. The most common side effects reported are insomnia and decreased appetite. Irritability and weight loss also have been reported frequently, as well as headaches and abdominal pain. Other less common side effects include negative mood changes, tics and other nervous movements, dizziness, drowsiness, nail biting, anxiety, social withdrawal, euphoria, nightmares, and staring (DuPaul & Barkley, 1990). In an investigation of the side effects of methylphenidate, Barkley and his group (Barkley, McMurray, Edelbrock, & Robbins, 1990) found that over one-half of the sample demonstrated decreased appetite, insomnia, anxiousness, irritability, or proneness to crying. Many of these side effects also were apparent during the placebo condition. The investigators suggest that these symptoms may represent characteristics associated with ADHD rather than side effects of stimulants. It also should be noted that the side effects tended to be mild. Finally, they demonstrated that side effects were related to dose with greater side effects occurring at higher doses.

One untoward effect, particularly noted with methylphenidate, has been the behavioral rebound phenomenon, which typically is described as a deterioration in behavior (worse than baseline) that occurs in the late afternoon or evening following daytime drug therapy (Johnston, Pelham, Hoza, & Sturges, 1988). Johnston *et al.* (1988) found limited evidence for behavioral rebound effects for children receiving methylphenidate during the day. They note, however, that there is considerable variability both across subjects and within each particular child. They conclude that rebound effects were not large and for the great majority of the children, these effects were not significant. Typically if rebound is a problem, alterations in dosing and scheduling can be helpful (DuPaul & Barkley, 1990).

One potentially serious side effect with the use of stimulants is the development of abnormal motor movements (i.e., tics). It has been estimated that fewer than 1% of stimulant-treated children develop a tic disorder. When pharmacotherapy is discontinued, these tics often remit. However, a small percentage of children will continue to have tics and may develop Tourette's disorder. Currently, it is not clear whether stimulants can induce Tourette's or other tic disorders in previously normal children or if stimulants trigger symptoms in children having an underlying, previously unexpressed tic disorder (DuPaul & Barkley, 1990). Screening for personal or family history of tics or Tourette's before prescribing stimulants is of utmost importance and decisions to use stimulants for children with tic disorders must be considered carefully.

It also should be noted that each of the stimulants has unique side effects (DuPaul & Barkley, 1990). Children receiving pemoline have developed allergic skin reactions, lip licking and biting, and light picking of the fingertips. These problems resolve by decreasing the dose or stopping medication. Finally, an uncommon but serious side effect of all of the stimulants is psychosis. Tactile and visual hallucinations have been most commonly reported, although there have been instances of abnormalities in thought processing (Barkley, 1981). A case study describes a 6-year-old male with ADHD who developed a florid psychotic disturbance (primarily delusional thinking) while receiving methylphenidate which resolved when medication was discontinued (Bloom, Russell, Weisskopf, & Blackerby, 1988). There have been some isolated cases in the clinical literature to suggest that children's social interaction may decrease in response to stimulants. Additional clinical observations of stimulant-treated children include increased dysphoria, lack of spontaneity, and overcontrol (DuPaul & Barkley, 1990).

Some research has suggested that side effects are dose related (Brown & Sexson, 1988) and transitory. It is important to keep in mind that side effects encountered with one stimulant may not be produced by another stimulant (Barkley *et al.*, 1993). Stimulants work well in the majority of children when prescribed for appropriate symptoms and for the most part are tolerated fairly well. Nonetheless, the physician must carefully monitor children receiving these medications and balance associated benefits with potential untoward side effects.

Psychosocial Attitudes and Beliefs about Medication

A vital aspect of evaluating the merit of stimulant drug treatment for children is a consideration of treatment acceptability and satisfaction by the child, family, and other involved individuals (teachers, physician, and peers). As described by Kazdin (1980), this concept suggests that consumer attitudes about the appropriateness of prescribed treatments may influence their willingness to accept and comply with treatment requirements. Thus, the probability that an intervention will successfully ameliorate a child's difficulties may be constrained by various factors such as popular beliefs about the severity of the child's problems, the availability of alternative treatments, the time and effort required to institute the treatment, the reported efficacy of the therapy, potential untoward side effects, and previous medication experience (Cross-Calvert & Johnston, 1990; Elliott, 1988). Most of this research has been conducted for children with ADHD with emphasis on the attitudes of the children being treated, parents, teachers, physicians, and peers.

Child and Peer Attitudes

There has been a burgeoning interest in children's attitudes and expectations toward medication. Considering that most stimulants require multiple doses during the day, children frequently receive their medication while at school surrounded by peers. Other children's knowledge of stimulant use may intrude on the social relations of ADHD children (Whalen & Henker, 1991). Sigelman and Shorokey (1986) investigated children's attributions and the relative likeability of a hypothetical hyperactive child receiving medication or exerting personal effort to control problem classroom behavior. Findings indicated that the boy was perceived as more likeable in the effort situation and suggest that children's knowledge of an ADHD child's medication status may ultimately mediate social status.

Another concern has been that pharmacological treatment may have cognitive and affective consequences for the child (Whalen & Henker, 1976). Specifically, these investigators have argued that stimulant treatment for ADHD may convey an undesirable message to the child about personal control and competence (Henker & Whalen, 1989). Children may ascribe the benefits of the medication to external causes and consider their efforts and capabilities irrelevant; this attribution then could impede further learning. Milich and colleagues (Carlson, Pelham, Milich, & Hoza, 1993; Milich, Carlson, Pelham, & Licht, 1991; Pelham, Murphy, et al., 1992) have meticulously addressed this issue in several definitive studies. In a series of investigations, ADHD boys were exposed to success and failure conditions in a counterbalanced methylphenidate trial. Medication appeared to exert a differential effect on performance; medication enhanced persistence, but only in the face of failure. When attributions for success and failure were examined, boys did not differ in their attributions when exposed to solvable tasks. However, following failure, boys made significantly more external (i.e., task difficulty) and significantly fewer internal (i.e., effort) attributions on medication versus placebo. These results were replicated with an additional no-pill condition, where on medication, children attributed success to ability or effort and failure to medication or program staff (Pelham, Murphy, et al., 1992). Thus, the medication diminished the boys' sense of personal responsibility following failure, a pattern consistent with a more adaptive and healthy response style (Taylor & Brown, 1988). These results contradicted the earlier work of Whalen and Henker (1991). Recently, Ialongo and associates (Ialongo, Lopez, Horn, Pascoe, & Greenberg, 1994) investigated the effects of methylphenidate and found no decrease in self-perceptions of competence, control, and mood for ADHD children. Additionally, a study reported by Milich, Licht, Murphy, and Pelham (1989) found that ADHD boys were significantly more accurate in assessing the quality of their vigilance performance on a task of sustained attention when receiving medication. Children on medication behaved in a mastery-oriented fashion, whereas their unmedicated ADHD peers tended to display helplessness (Milich, 1994). Finally, Cohen and Thompson (1982), in their sample, found that most ADHD children believed that they have greater internal control while on medication and two-thirds indicated their desire to remain on stimulant medication. This point is corroborated further by Bowen, Fenton, and Rappaport (1991) who found that the majority of children who were being treated with a stimulant found it to be helpful, and parents corroborated this.

Parental Attitudes

For many years, the use of stimulants for children with ADHD has generated considerable controversy among parents, which has been elaborated in the lay press. Both clinical and research reports have documented considerable discrepancies between the recommendations regarding stimulant drug treatment and the actual practice. Significant interest has developed in examining the influence of parental attitudes on treatment compliance. Liu and associates (Liu, Robin, Brenner, & Eastman, 1991) surveyed mothers of ADHD children and mothers of normally developing children regarding the acceptability of methylphenidate, behavior modification, and their combination in the treatment of ADHD. Both groups rated behavior modification as the most acceptable treatment and methylphenidate as the least acceptable. Mothers' knowledge of ADHD was related to greater acceptability of medication.

To address known parental concerns about the use of stimulant medication for the treatment of ADHD, Slimmer and Brown (1985) investigated the effects of a decision-making conference on the treatment acceptance process. Findings indicated that a mother's decision to elect a trial of medication was more likely when mothers were encouraged to express their feelings of guilt about the disorder, to consider other treatment alternatives, and to rank treatment options.

Borden and Brown (1989) examined the attributional effects of combining medication with cognitive therapy in the treatment of children with ADHD. All of the children received an intensive program in cognitive therapy focusing on self-control. Children also were randomly assigned to a methylphenidate, placebo, and a no-pill condition. Parents in the no-pill group believed most strongly that their children were capable of solving their own presenting problems. The placebo group most strongly believed that solutions would result from external and uncontrollable factors.

Teacher Attitudes

Most children receiving stimulants require a dose during the school day so that the knowledge and beliefs of educators about stimulant use can have a significant impact on treatment for children. Epstein and associates (Epstein, Matson, Repp, & Helsel, 1986) surveyed regular and special education student teachers to rate the acceptability of various treatments for a first-grade boy with ADHD described in a case vignette. Treatment choices included medication, behavior modification, counseling, and special education. Both groups reported that special education was the most appropriate intervention and that medication was the least acceptable. Similarly, Kasten, Coury, and Heron (1992) discovered that 41% of special educators believe that too many students receive stimulant medication and 35% stated that stimulants are provided too frequently for ADHD.

The literature also indicates that teachers are concerned by the lack of communication between physicians and teachers regarding the medication status of children (Gadow, 1982). Other studies have supported this conclusion with special education teachers complaining that school personnel have little influence on medication decisions (Epstein, Singh, Luebke, & Stout, 1991; Singh, Epstein, Luebke, & Singh, 1990). The opinions of teachers also are vital in making medication decisions, as the most prevalent method to assess treatment efficacy involves obtaining the teacher's ratings and impressions of the child's behavior in response to stimulants. Unfortunately, 86% of the teachers of learning-disabled pupils and 95% of the teachers of seriously emotionally disturbed (Ep-

stein *et al.*, 1991) indicated that they needed more training in issues related to drug therapy in children.

Finally, Malyn, Jensen, and Clark (1993) recently compared medication beliefs among teachers and school psychologists based on a survey of their knowledge of the efficacy and side effects of stimulants in the treatment of ADHD. Additionally, teachers were asked if they would recommend stimulant medication to a parent of an ADHD child. The majority reported that methylphenidate would be beneficial for most ADHD children. However, only one-third of the school psychologists and one-half of the teachers indicated that they would inform parents regarding the option of stimulant medication even though 82% of the psychologists believed that stimulants benefited most ADHD children.

Societal Attitudes

In today's society, there is considerable concern about the inappropriate use of drugs (both illegal and prescribed). These attitudes may have significant impact on the parent decision-making process. Summers and Caplan (1987) surveyed lay people about the relative merits of stimulant treatment for a boy with ADHD and in a second case anticonvulsant medication for a seizure disorder. In each vignette the boy was described as walking around the classroom and disrupting the class during academic activities. Subjects indicated that the use of medication would be more justified for the epileptic child whose disorder they considered to be of organic etiology. In contrast, subjects believed that ADHD was more likely of a psychosocial origin, that the child was able but not willing to control his behavior, and had a more negative attitude toward using medication. In fact, those participants who considered ADHD to be a psychosocial problem thought that medication would exacerbate the child's symptoms.

In summary, the literature pertaining to attitudes and expectations about stimulants indicates that these cognitions have important implications for clinical practice and underscores the importance of carefully talking to children, parents, and teachers about their expectations regarding medication effects as well as considering the attitudes of peers.

Long-Term Outcome of Children Treated with Stimulants

Despite the impressive short-term track record of stimulants, much is unknown about their long-term effects. Few studies employing rigorous methodology have addressed this issue (DuPaul & Barkley, 1990; Rapport & Kelly, 1991) because of the difficulties of systematically examining the long-term effects of stimulants and the ethical limitations of placing children in no-medication or placebo-control groups for extensive periods. Those studies that have attempted to investigate the effects of stimulants with ADHD children over the course of several years have not yielded very encouraging results (Barkley, 1990). Generally, the findings of these studies have indicated that ADHD children who were treated with stimulants during the course of at least 5 years did not differ in any meaningful way from children who had never received pharmacotherapy for their ADHD disorder (Hechtman, Weiss, & Perlman, 1984). It should be noted that the children participating in these investigations were off medication at the time of follow-up, which may in part have contributed to the negative results (Brown, Borden, Wynne, Schleser, & Clingerman, 1986). Continued rigorous evaluation of the long-term effects of stimulants remains essential because of the increasing use of these medications for longer periods of time through adolescence and possibly adulthood. The long-term effects of these drugs on behavior and learning need clarification. The most informative follow-up studies available regarding the long-term effects of stimulants have focused on possible deleterious side effects.

Growth Suppression

Growth suppression and weight loss were reported in the earlier literature, particularly with dextroamphetamine and methylphenidate (Safer & Allen, 1973). Moreover, evidence has suggested that stimulants may have some direct effects on growth hormone levels in the blood (Barkley, 1990). However, more recent studies have found height and weight suppression to be dose related and to occur more frequently during the first year of therapy. Gittelman-Klein and associates (Gittelman-Klein, Landa, Mattes, & Klein, 1988) have carefully addressed the effects of methylphenidate and growth in ADHD children. They measured the effects of methylphenidate withdrawal on the growth of ADHD children randomly assigned to be taken off, or remain on, their medication regimen over two consecutive summers. After one summer, no group difference in height was found, but children taken off methylphenidate therapy

weighed more. Being off medication for two summers resulted in a positive effect on height but not weight. However, this study did not address the continued long-term impact of methylphenidate on eventual height and weight. In a follow-up investigation, Gittelman-Klein and Mannuzza (1988) examined the height of young adults (off medication) who had been treated with methylphenidate for ADHD and compared them to nonmedicated controls with a history of behavior problems. No differences were found between treated patients and controls; both groups were at the national norm for stature. Based on their studies, the authors conclude that methylphenidate therapy does not compromise final height, even when it compromises a child's growth during the active treatment phase. Gittelman-Klein and Mannuzza (1988) conclude that a compensatory growth rate, or growth rebound, occurs following discontinuation of stimulant therapy. These results seem promising, yet stimulants are increasingly being used for longer periods, well into adolescence and young adulthood without significant intervals off medication. Thus, although growth suppression seems to be a transitory phenomenon and appears to have a minor influence on adult height or weight, further investigation is needed and the clinician should carefully monitor growth in children receiving stimulants.

Cardiac System

Although limited empirical data exist, questions have been raised regarding the effects of stimulant drugs on the cardiovascular system. Stimulants increase heart rate, respiration, and blood pressure (Barkley *et al.*, 1993). These effects have been found to be transitory and tend to dissipate with the metabolism and elimination of the medication from the body. Brown and Sexson (1988, 1989) found that young black males show significantly increased blood pressure following methylphenidate administration, although it was still within the normal range. One concern has been that children treated with stimulants for several years may be at increased risk for cardiovascular problems during middle adulthood or later in life. Unfortunately, the follow-up studies examining the functioning of ADHD children who were treated with stimulants for several years have not addressed this issue. This remains a ripe area for future research.

Addiction

Parents, in particular, are frequently quite concerned about their children's possible addiction to these drugs or their increased risk of abusing other drugs as teenagers. To date, there are no reports in the literature of addiction or serious drug dependence with stimulants when it is prescribed to treat symptoms for which the medication is indicated. Although much more research is needed to address this issue, the evidence from the few available studies has failed to confirm the notion that children medicated with stimulants are more at risk for drug and alcohol abuse than unmedicated children (Gadow, 1981; Henker, Whalen, Bugenthal, & Barker, 1981) or their normal peers (Gadow & Sprague, 1980). In fact, according to some empirical data, a positive clinical response to stimulants may be associated with a lower probability of drug and alcohol abuse later in life than found in the general population (Blouin, Bornstein, & Trites, 1978; Loney *et al.*, 1981). Also, it has been reported that many older children frequently dislike taking medication and wish to discontinue its use prematurely (Brown, Borden, Wynne, Clingerman, & Spunt, 1987). It appears that the risk of addiction is fairly low. Nonetheless, this area is another one that has received too little attention in the literature. Given that there are many ADHD children treated with stimulants who also have aggressive behavior and may be at particular risk for problems associated with addiction as a result of family history and peer pressure, the potential for addiction must be carefully monitored. This is an important area that merits more systematic study.

Multimodal Therapies

In this time of budgetary constraints, biological psychiatry, and healthcare reform, employing medication alone has been hailed as a cost-effective strategy for managing children with chronic behavioral disorders. However, there are decided limitations of stimulant therapies. First, not all children who receive stimulant medication evidence a positive response. Stimulants have a short half-life; so, although a large majority of children demonstrate positive changes, their reduction in symptoms seems to be short-lived or may last only as long as the medication regimen continues (Whalen & Henker, 1991). Further, unlike antibiotic therapy, stimulants are not curative; rather, they manage symptoms. As Brown, Dingle, and Landau (1994) have observed, no psychotropic medications "normalize" a child's functioning; in fact, symptoms frequently may reappear following cessation of medication. Although positive changes may be observed, these effects typically are circumscribed in duration and in extent of response and rarely influence actual learning. Finally, these medications are not without potential side effects and there is concern about the subtle messages associated with medications used to alter behavior (Borden & Brown, 1989; Whalen & Henker, 1991).

In ADHD children for whom stimulants are employed most frequently, there is increasing recognition that the disorder is lifelong, with a guarded prognosis (Weiss & Hechtman, 1986) and affects many areas of functioning. For this reason, experts in the field have concluded that "appropriate psychosocial and psychoeducational interventions should form a component of treatment for most children . . . even where pharmacotherapy is helpful" (Pelham, 1993, p. 219). Thus, there has been an increasing emphasis on identifying adjunctive nonpharmacological treatments to be used either alone or together with stimulants to effect a broader scope of behavioral change perhaps over a longer period of time than has been demonstrated with stimulants used alone. Moreover, there has been some hope that a combination of psychotherapy and pharmacotherapy would produce effects superior to either therapy employed alone. Based on this rationale, a number of studies over the past decade have systematically investigated the effects of stimulants alone and in combination with cognitive and behavioral therapies.

Cognitive behavioral therapy has been hailed as a natural fit between the essential deficits in self-control characteristic of ADHD children and the regulation of self-control, which is a prime focus of cognitive therapy. Those outcome studies that have examined the effects of cognitive therapy, either alone or in combination with stimulant treatments, have been decidedly disappointing (Abikoff *et al.*, 1988; Abikoff & Gittelman, 1985; Brown, 1980; Brown *et al.*, 1986; Brown, Wynne, & Medenis, 1985). The results have been less than expected even when performance on specific cognitive tasks was examined (Abikoff *et al.*, 1988; Brown *et al.*,

1985, 1986). In each of these studies, medication alone produced superior effects than cognitive therapy alone, and the addition of cognitive therapy to medication did not yield any stronger effect than medication alone.

Another line of research has investigated the effect of stimulant medication versus behavior therapy or the therapies combined on the classroom performance of ADHD children. The majority of these studies have been conducted in the Pelham laboratory (Carlson, Pelham, Milich, & Dixon, 1992; Pelham *et al.*, 1988, 1993). Specifically, methylphenidate has been found to be superior to behavior modification alone and the combination of the two therapies was only slightly better than medication alone (Pelham *et al.*, 1993).

Similar findings have been reported by other research groups in examining the additive effects of stimulants, parent training, and self-control training with ADHD children (Horn *et al.*, 1991). Horn and colleagues found no evidence of the superiority of combined medication and parent training to medication used alone. Although some limited initial support was found for the combination of a low dose of methylphenidate (0.4 mg/kg) and parent training versus a higher dose (0.8 mg/kg) of medication used alone, these findings were not supported when the children were evaluated 9 months later (Ialongo *et al.*, 1993). In fact, at follow-up, no support was found for the hypothesis that the combined therapies would produce greater maintenance of treatment gains than medication alone.

In addition, for classroom performance and academic achievement, Carlson *et al.* (1992) found significantly improved classroom behavior when stimulant therapy and behavior management each was employed alone. Only methylphenidate was found to improve academic productivity and accuracy. Of particular interest was the finding that the combination of behavior therapy and a relatively low dose of methylphenidate (0.3 mg/kg) produced superior classroom behavior, which was nearly identical to the improvements produced by a relatively higher dose of methylphenidate (0.6 mg/kg). These results are striking and lend the most support to the use of combined treatment modalities and suggest that behavioral therapies may have an augmenting effect on medication.

Although clinical experience would suggest that children fare better with adjunctive therapies and stimulants, the data have not necessarily borne this out. More research efforts are needed with larger numbers of children over longer periods of time. However, there is a critical investigation of multimodal therapies on the empirical horizon. This large-scale, federally supported study offers much promise in clarifying the efficacy of combined treatments, particularly the mediation of stimulant effects by behavioral therapies.

Treatment Acceptability, Satisfaction, and Compliance

Despite the extensive literature documenting the beneficial effects of stimulant treatment for ADHD, many parents remain hesitant about this treatment (Liu *et al.*, 1991) and generally perceive medication as less acceptable than behavioral approaches for the management of their children's behavior (Kazdin, 1984; Summers & Caplan, 1987). Interestingly, these observations are consistent with the pediatric psychology literature, where parents generally view pharmacological means of managing pain as less acceptable than nonpharmacological approaches (Tarnowski, Gavaghan, & Wisniewski, 1989).

When particular interventions are not entirely acceptable to parents, satisfaction and compliance with treatment are at significant risk (Cross-Calvert & Johnston, 1990; Tarnowski, Kelly, & Mendlowitz, 1987). Parental concerns may mean that stimulants may be underutilized for children who might benefit from their use. Additionally, children and their parents may fail to adhere to the prescribed regimen of the medication or may prematurely discontinue treatment. Both alteration of drug administration procedures and premature discontinuation of treatment have been well documented for children treated with stimulants (Brown *et al.*, 1987; Firestone, 1982; Kauffman, Smith-Wright, Reese, Simpson, & Fowler, 1981).

Firestone (1982) reported that one-fifth of families whose children began methylphenidate treatment discontinued treatment by the fourth month, and this figure increased to nearly one-half by the end of the tenth month. Fewer than 10% of these families consulted project staff prior to stopping the medication. Firestone indicated that parents cited discomfort with the medication as their primary reason for noncompliance. In a similar investigation, Brown *et al.* (1987) found that even in short-term clinical trials of methylphenidate, 25% of the methylphenidate doses were missed as verified by pharmacist counts. Finally, Kauffman *et al.* (1981), from their analyses of urine samples, found that one-third of their ADHD sample did not adhere to prescribed methylphenidate regimens in any given week.

Johnston and Fine (1993) have noted that the problems of acceptability, satisfaction, and compliance with methylphenidate treatment are intricately related. As Brown and Borden (1989) have observed, these difficulties may be attributed to numerous factors including the need for long-term treatment, negative publicity in the lay press, and fears regarding negative side effects. Brown and Borden described the long-course treatment of ADHD with stimulants as being analogous to a learned-helplessness situation whereby the family is unable to envision meeting hoped-for goals within a reasonable amount of time and experiences a lack of a sense of control over symptoms. These phenomena may act synergistically, resulting in families being too discouraged to follow through on treatment plans.

In an effort to address typical noncompliance with stimulant medication, Johnston and Fine (1993) compared two methods of evaluating the efficacy of methylphenidate on measures of parental acceptance, satisfaction, and compliance. ADHD children were assigned randomly either to a controlled double-blind medication trial or to a typical clinical evaluation that was nonblind and without placebo controls. Although all parents became more accepting of the stimulant medication after participating in each of the evaluations, ratings of satisfaction with treatment were higher in the controlled trial condition. Consistent with previous studies of adherence (Brown *et al.*, 1987; Firestone, 1982; Kauffman *et al.*, 1981), approximately 20% of the sample was not compliant with treatment at both the 6-week and 3-month follow-up. Although no differences were found for rates of adherence between the two treatment groups, this investigation does support the use of systematic clinical drug trial evaluations in enhancing consumer satisfaction among parents.

The study by Johnston and Fine (1993) clearly suggests that attending to parents as well as children in developing therapeutic rapport and providing support to parents and children will assist with patient satisfaction and hopefully enhance adherence. In addition, parents and children must be given adequate information about stimulants and be provided with appropriate strategies for overcoming any obstacles that may impede compliance with the medication. Finally, adherence must be carefully assessed before drawing any definitive conclusions regarding either the short- or long-term efficacy of any treatment with stimulants.

Training Issues

A number of reasons exist for the active participation of clinical neuropsychologists in the management of children receiving stimulants. Clinical psychologists are proficient in evaluation and assessment procedures, particularly those that use behavioral rating scales, observational techniques, and psychometric testing, all of which can be helpful in monitoring drug responses as well as determining those behaviors that require nonpharmacological treatment (DuPaul & Barkley, 1990). Moreover, clinical psychologists have sound training in research methodology, enabling them to empirically evaluate the effects of stimulants on children's cognition and behavior. In fact, clinical psychologists have directed the major laboratories producing the seminal work with stimulants (Barkley, 1990; Pelham, 1993; Rapport & Kelly, 1991; Whalen & Henker, 1991).

Because most clinical neuropsychologists undoubtedly will have contact with children receiving stimulants, a question arises as to what training is necessary to work effectively with these children. Clearly, clinical neuropsychologists need graduate course work in neuroanatomy, physiology, and principles of basic psychopharmacology. As most clinical child neuropsychology training occurs at the internship and postdoctoral level, it is recommended that training programs include didactic seminars in pediatric psychopharmacology, that trainees receive supervised experiences in working with medicated children, and that they have ongoing communication with physicians regarding drug response and evaluation of side effects. Additionally, because the stimulants have a significant impact on school performance, it also is recommended that school psychologists receive specialized course work and supervised experiences in assessment of children for stimulants and in monitoring the effects of medication on cognition and learning (Brown *et al.*, 1994).

Concluding Comments

There is a plethora of research attesting to the efficacy of stimulants for behaviors such as inattention, impulsivity, physical overactivity, and difficulty focusing. The research literature is conclusive that the stimulants are an effective and appropriate treatment modality for various disorders that share these symptoms. In fact, the number of studies supporting this conclusion is overwhelming. Despite the unequivocal evidence for its appropriateness, stimulants still receive less than favorable endorsements, particularly in the lay press. Perhaps children and their parents' feelings and beliefs about the medication are as important as the effects of the medication on cognition and behavior. Often it appears that the expectations regarding stimulant efficacy are inappropriate and unrealistic. For example, like many other pharmacotherapies, stimulants only exhibit their effects within a time-limited period. Thus, to expect generalization from the stimulants would be unreasonable and inconsistent. Given their benefits and continued documented safety, they are an appropriate adjunctive therapy for the symptoms discussed in this chapter.

Despite the vast knowledge about the behavioral effects of stimulants, little is known about their biological actions. Although considerable efforts have been made to delineate the biological model of stimulant effects, as of yet there are no definitive data to support any existing theory. An understanding of brain physiology and its interaction with stimulants is an exciting ongoing area of investigation. With significant advancements in magnetic resonance imaging, PET, and research on neurotransmitters, more conclusive explanations are likely to emerge over the next decade.

Although multimodal therapies have shown significant theoretical promise, the data thus far have been decidedly disappointing. This is counter to clinical experience, although the effects of stimulants are fairly striking and it is difficult to surpass their effectiveness with other nonsomatic therapies. As environments appear to mediate the effects of stimulants, the results of the federally supported multimodal therapies, which correct previous methodological weaknesses characteristic in a new program of research, provide hope for empirically validating these techniques.

In our review of this voluminous literature, what has been striking is the meticulousness with which the stimulants have been investigated. Of all of the therapies discussed in the childhood psychopathology literature, the stimulants are the most carefully and extensively documented. Its approach in examining effects across situations, informants, and time is an ideal model from which to study therapeutic outcome and would be valuable for evaluating other modalities of treatment for children and adolescents.

References

Abikoff, H., Ganeles, D., Reiter, G., Blum, C., Foley, C., & Klein, R. G. (1988). Cognitive training in academically deficient ADHD boys receiving stimulant medication. *Journal of Abnormal Child Psychology, 16*, 411–432.

Abikoff, H., & Gittelman, R. (1985). Hyperactive children treated with stimulants: Is cognitive training a useful adjunct? *Archives of General Psychiatry, 42*, 953–961.

Alessandri, S. M., & Schramm, K. (1991). Effects of dextroamphetamine on the cognitive and social play of a preschooler with ADHD. *Journal of the American Academy of Child and Adolescent Psychiatry, 30*, 768–772.

Aman, M. G. (1982). Stimulant drug effects in developmental disorders and hyperactivity—Toward a resolution of disparate findings. *Journal of Autism and Developmental Disorders, 12*, 385–398.

Aman, M. G., Kern, R. A., McGhee, D. E., & Arnold, L. E. (1993). Fenfluramine and methylphenidate in children with mental retardation and ADHD: Clinical and side effects. *Journal of the American Academy of Child and Adolescent Psychiatry, 32*, 851–859.

Aman, M. G., Marks, R. E., Turbott, S. H., Wilsher, C. P., & Merry, S. N. (1991a). Clinical effects of methylphenidate and thioridazine in intellectually subaverage children. *Journal of the American Academy of Child and Adolescent Psychiatry, 30*, 246–256.

Aman, M. G., Marks, R. E., Turbott, S. H., Wilsher, C. P., & Merry, S. N. (1991b). Methylphenidate and thioridazine in the treatment of intellectually subaverage children: Effects on cognitive–motor performance. *Journal of the American Academy of Child and Adolescent Psychiatry, 30*, 816–824.

American Psychiatric Association. (1980). *Diagnostic and statistical manual of mental disorders* (DSM-III) (3rd ed.). Washington, DC: Author.

American Psychiatric Association. (1987). *Diagnostic and statistical manual of mental disorders* (DSM-III-R) (3rd. ed. rev.). Washington, DC: Author.

American Psychiatric Association. (1994). *Diagnostic and statistical manual of mental disorders* (DSM-IV) (4th ed.). Washington, DC: Author.

Atkins, M. S., & Pelham, W. E. (1991). School-based assessment of attention deficit-hyperactivity disorder. *Journal of Learning Disabilities, 24*, 197–204.

Balthazor, M. J., Wagner, R. K., & Pelham, W. E. (1991). The specificity of the effects of stimulant medication on classroom learning-related measures of cognitive processing for attention deficit disorder children. *Journal of Abnormal Child Psychology, 19*, 35–52.

Barkley, R. A. (1976). Predicting the response of hyperkinetic children to stimulant drugs: A review. *Journal of Abnormal Child Psychology, 4*, 327–348.

Barkley, R. A. (1981). *Hyperactive children: A handbook for diagnosis and treatment.* New York: Guilford Press.

Barkley, R. A. (1990). *Attention deficit hyperactivity disorder: A handbook for diagnosis and treatment.* New York: Guilford Press.

Barkley, R. A., DuPaul, G. J., & Costello, A. (1993). Stimulants. In J. S. Werry & M. G. Aman (Eds.), *Practitioners' guide to psychoactive drugs for children and adolescents* (pp. 205–237). New York: Plenum Press.

Barkley, R. A., DuPaul, G. J., & McMurray, M. B. (1991). Attention deficit disorder with and without hyperactivity: Clinical response to three dose levels of methylphenidate. *Pediatrics, 88,* 519–531.

Barkley, R. A., & Grodinsky, G. M. (1994). Are tests of frontal lobe functions used in the diagnosis of attention deficit disorders? *The Clinical Neuropsychologist, 8,* 121–139.

Barkley, R. A., Karlsson, J., Strzelecki, E., & Murphy, J. V. (1984). Effects of age and Ritalin dosage on the mother–child interactions of hyperactive children. *Journal of Consulting and Clinical Psychology, 52,* 739–749.

Barkley, R. A., McMurray, M., Edelbrock, C. S., & Robbins, K. (1989). The response of aggressive and nonaggressive ADHD children to two doses of methylphenidate. *Journal of the American Academy of Child and Adolescent Psychiatry, 28,* 873–881.

Barkley, R. A., McMurray, M., Edelbrock, C. S., & Robbins, K. (1990). Side effects of methylphenidate in children with attention deficit hyperactivity disorder: A systemic, placebo-controlled evaluation. *Pediatrics, 86,* 184–192.

Benton, A. L., & Hamsher, K. deS. (1978). *Multilingual Aphasia Examination* (manual, revised). Iowa City: University of Iowa.

Bloom, A. S., Russell, L. J., Weisskopf, B., & Blackerby, J. L. (1988). Methylphenidate-induced delusional disorder in a child with attention deficit disorder with hyperactivity. *Journal of the American Academy of Child and Adolescent Psychiatry, 27,* 88–89.

Blouin, A. G. A., Bornstein, R. A., & Trites, R. L. (1978). Teenage alcohol use among hyperactive children: A five-year follow-up study. *Journal of Pediatric Psychology, 3,* 188–194.

Borcherding, B. G., Keysor, C. S., Rapoport, J. L., Elia, J., & Amass, J. (1990). Motor/vocal tics and compulsive behaviors on stimulant drugs: Is there a common vulnerability? *Psychiatry Research, 33,* 83–94.

Borden, K. A., & Brown, R. T. (1989). Attributional outcomes: The subtle messages of treatments for attention deficit disorder. *Cognitive Therapy and Research, 13,* 147–160.

Bowen, J., Fenton, T., & Rappaport, L. (1991). Stimulant medication and attention deficit-hyperactivity disorder: The child's perspective. *American Journal of Diseases of Children, 145,* 291–295.

Bradley, C. (1937). The behavior of children receiving Benzedrine. *American Journal of Psychiatry, 94,* 577–585.

Brown, R. T. (1980). Impulsivity and psycho-educational intervention in hyperactive children. *Journal of Learning Disabilities, 13,* 249–254.

Brown, R. T., & Borden, K. A. (1989). Neuropsychological effects of stimulant medication on children's learning and behavior. In C. R. Reynolds & E. Fletcher-Janzen (Eds.), *Handbook of clinical child neuropsychology* (pp. 443–474). New York: Plenum Press.

Brown, R. T., Borden, K. A., Wynne, M. E., Clingerman, S. R., & Spunt, A. L. (1987). Compliance with pharmacological and cognitive treatments for attention deficit disorder. *Journal of the American Adacemy of Child and Adolescent Psychiatry, 26,* 521–526.

Brown, R. T., Borden, K. A., Wynne, M. E., Schleser, R., & Clingerman, S. R. (1986). Methylphenidate and cognitive therapy with ADD children: A methodological reconsideration. *Journal of Abnormal Child Psychology, 14,* 481–497.

Brown, R. T., Dingle, A., & Landau, S. (1994). Overview of psychopharmacology in children and adolescents. *School Psychology Review, 9,* 4–25.

Brown, R. T., Jaffe, S., Silverstein, J., & Magee, H. (1991). Methylphenidate and adolescents hospitalized with conduct disorder: Dose effects on classroom behavior, academic performance, and impulsivity. *Journal of Clinical Child Psychology, 20,* 282–292.

Brown, R. T., & Sexson, S. B. (1988). A controlled trial of methylphenidate in black adolescents: Attentional, behavioral, and physiological effects. *Clinical Pediatrics, 27,* 74–81.

Brown, R. T., & Sexson, S. B. (1989). Effects of methylphenidate on cardiovascular responses in attention deficit hyperactivity disordered adolescents. *Journal of Adolescent Health Care, 10,* 179–183.

Brown, R. T., & Sleator, E. K. (1979). Methylphenidate in hyperkinetic children: Differences in dose effects on impulsive behavior. *Pediatrics, 64,* 408–411.

Brown, R. T., Wynne, M. E., & Medenis, R. (1985). Methylphenidate and cognitive therapy: A comparison of treatment approaches with hyperactive boys. *Journal of Abnormal Child Psychology, 13,* 69–87.

Buhrmester, D., Whalen, C. K., Henker, B., McDonald, V., & Hinshaw, S. P. (1992). Prosocial behavior in hyperactive boys: Effects of stimulant medication and comparison with normal boys. *Journal of Abnormal Child Psychology, 20,* 103–121.

Carlson, C. L., Pelham, W. E., Milich, R., & Dixon, J. (1992). Single and combined effects of methylphenidate and behavior therapy on the classroom performance of children with attention-deficit hyperactivity disorder. *Journal of Abnormal Child Psychology, 20,* 213–232.

Carlson, C. L., Pelham, W. E., Milich, R., & Hoza, B. (1993). ADHD boys' performance and attributions following success and failure: Drug effects and individual differences. *Cognitive Therapy and Research, 17,* 269–287.

Cohen, N. J., & Thompson, L. (1982). Perceptions and attitudes of hyperactive children and their mothers regarding treatment with methylphenidate. *Canadian Journal of Psychiatry, 27,* 40–42,

Coons, H. W., Klorman, R., & Borgstedt, A. D. (1987). Effects of methylphenidate on adolescents with a childhood history of attention deficit disorder. II. Information processing. *Journal of the American Academy of Child and Adolescent Psychiatry, 26,* 368–374.

Cross-Calvert, S., & Johnston, C. (1990). Acceptability of treatments for child behavior problems: Issues and implications for future research. *Journal of Clinical Child Psychology, 19,* 61–74.

Dalby, J. T., Kinsbourne, M., & Swanson, J. M. (1989). Self-paced learning in children with attention deficit disorder with hyperactivity. *Journal of Abnormal Child Psychology, 17,* 269–275.

Douglas, V. I. (1988). Cognitive deficits in children with attention deficit disorder with hyperactivity. In L. M. Bloomingdale & J. Sergeant (Eds.), *Attention deficit disorder: Criteria, cognition, intervention* (pp. 65–81). New York: Pergamon Press.

Douglas, V. I., Barr, R. G., Amin, K., O'Neill, M. E., & Britton, B. G. (1988). Dosage effects and individual responsivity to methylphenidate in attention deficit disorder. *Journal of Child Psychology and Psychiatry, 29,* 453–475.

Douglas, V. I., & Peters, K. (1979). Toward a clearer definition of the attention deficit of hyperactive children. In G. A. Hale, & M. Lewis (Eds.), *Attentional and cognitive development* (pp. 173–247). New York: Plenum Press.

Dulcan, M. K. (1990). Using psychostimulants to treat behavioral disorders of children and adolescents. *Journal of Child and Adolescent Psychopharmacology, 1,* 7–20.

DuPaul, G. J., & Barkley, R. A. (1990). Medication therapy. In R. A. Barkley (Ed.), *Attention deficit hyperactivity disorder: A handbook for diagnosis and treatment* (pp. 573–612). New York: Guilford Press.

DuPaul, G. J., Barkley, R. A., & McMurray, M. B. (1994). Response of children with ADHD to methylphenidate: Interaction with internalizing symptoms. *Journal of the American Academy of Child and Adolescent Psychiatry, 33,* 894–903.

DuPaul, G. J., & Rapport, M. D. (1993). Does methylphenidate normalize the classroom performance of children with attention deficit disorder? *Journal of the American Academy of Child and Adolescent Psychiatry, 32,* 190–198.

Eiben, C. G., Anderson, T. P., Lockman, L., Matthews, D. J., Dryja, R., Burrill, D., Gottesman, N., O'Brien, P., & Witte, L. (1984). Functional outcome of closed head injury in children and young adults. *Archives of Physical Medicine and Rehabilitation, 65,* 168–170.

Eisenberg, L., Lachman, R., Molling, P. A., Lockner, A., Mizelle, J. D., & Conners, C. K. (1963). A psychopharmacological experiment in a training school for delinquent boys: Methods, problems, findings. *American Journal of Orthopsychiatry, 33,* 431–447.

Elia, J., Welsh, P. A., Gullotta, C. S., & Rapoport, J. L. (1993). Classroom academic performance: Improvement with both methylphenidate and dextroamphetamine in ADHD boys. *Journal of Child Psychology and Psychiatry, 34,* 785–804.

Elliott, S. N. (1988). Acceptability of behavioral treatments in educational settings. In J. C. Witt, S. W. Elliott, & F. M. Gresham (Eds.), *Handbook of behavior therapy in education* (pp. 121–150). New York: Plenum Press.

Epstein, L., Singh, N. N., Luebke, J., & Stout, C. E. (1991). Psychopharmacological intervention. II. Teacher perceptions of psychotropic medication for students with learning disabilities. *Journal of Learning Disabilities, 24,* 477–483.

Epstein, M. H., Matson, J. L., Repp, A., & Helsel, W. J. (1986). Acceptability of treatment alternatives as a function of teacher status and student level. *School Psychology Review, 15,* 84–90.

Evans, R. W., Gualtieri, C. T., & Amara, I. (1986). Methylphenidate and memory: Dissociated effects on hyperactive children. *Psychopharmacology, 90,* 211–216.

Evans, R. W., Gualtieri, C. T., & Patterson, D. (1987). Treatment of chronic CHI with psychostimulant drugs: A controlled case study and an appropriate evaluation procedure. *Journal of Nervous and Mental Disease, 165,* 106–110.

Evans, S. W., & Pelham, W. E. (1991). Psychostimulant effects on academic and behavioral measures for ADHD junior high school students in a lecture format classroom. *Journal of Abnormal Child Psychology, 19,* 537–552.

Ewing-Cobbs, L., Fletcher, J. M., & Levin, H. S. (1985). Neuropsychological sequelae following pediatric head injury. In M. Ylvisaker (Ed.), *Head injury rehabilitation: Children and adolescents* (pp. 71–89). San Diego: College Hill Press.

Feeny, D. M., Gonzalez, A., & Law, W. A. (1982). Amphetamine, haloperidol, and experience interact to affect rate of recovery after motor cortex injury. *Science, 217,* 855–857.

Firestone, P. (1982). Factors associated with children's adherence to stimulant medication. *American Journal of Orthopsychiatry, 52,* 447–457.

Fischer, M., & Newby, R. F. (1991). Assessment of stimulant response in ADHD children using a refined multimethod clinical protocol. *Journal of Clinical Child Psychology, 20,* 232–244.

Fitzpatrick, P. A., Klorman, R., Brumaghim, J. T., & Borgstedt, A. D. (1992). Effects of sustained-release and standard preparations of methylphenidate on attention deficit disorder. *Journal of the American Academy of Child and Adolescent Psychiatry, 31,* 226–234.

Fletcher, J. M., & Levin, H. (1988). Neurobehavioral effects of brain injury in children. In D. K. Routh (Ed.), *Handbook of pediatric psychology* (pp. 258–295). New York: Guilford Press.

Fletcher, J. M., Levin, H. S., & Landry, S. H. (1984). Behavioral consequences of cerebral insult in children, In C. R. Amli & S. Finger (Eds.), *Early brain damage* (Vol. 1, pp. 189–213). New York: Academic Press.

Forness, S. R., Cantwell, D. P., Swanson, J. M., Hanna, G. L., & Youpa, D. (1991). Differential effects of stimulant medication on reading performance of boys with hyperactivity with and without conduct disorder. *Journal of Learning Disabilities, 24,* 304–310.

Forness, S. R., Swanson, J. M., Cantwell, D. P., Youpa, D., & Hanna, G. L. (1992). Stimulant medication and reading performance: Follow-up on sustained dose in ADHD boys with and without conduct disorders. *Journal of Learning Disabilities, 25,* 115–123.

Gadow, K. D. (1981). Drug therapy for hyperactivity: Treatment procedures in actual settings. In K. D. Gadow & J. Loney

(Eds.), *Psychosocial aspects of drug treatment for hyperactivity* (pp. 325–378). Boulder, CO: Westview Press.

Gadow, K. D. (1982). School involvement in pharmacotherapy for behavior disorders. *Journal of Special Education, 16,* 385–399.

Gadow, K. D. (1985). Prevalence and efficacy of stimulant drug use with mentally retarded children and youth. *Psychopharmacology Bulletin, 21,* 291–303.

Gadow, K. D. (1992). Pediatric psychopharmacotherapy: A review of recent research. *Journal of Child Psychology and Psychiatry, 33,* 153–195.

Gadow, K. D. (1993). A school-based medication evaluation program. In J. L. Matson (Ed.), *Handbook of hyperactivity in children* (pp. 186–219). Boston: Allyn & Bacon.

Gadow, K. D., Nolan, E. E., Paolicelli, L. M., & Sprafkin, J. (1991a). A procedure for assessing the effects of methylphenidate on hyperactive children in public school settings. *Journal of Clinical Child Psychology, 20,* 268–276.

Gadow, K. D., Nolan, E. E., Sprafkin, J., & Paolicelli, L. (1991b). A procedure for assessing the effects of methylphenidate on hyperactive children in public school settings. *Journal of Clinical Child Psychology, 20,* 268–276.

Gadow, K. D., Nolan, E. E., & Sverd, J. (1992). Methylphenidate in hyperactive boys with comorbid tic disorder: II. Short-term behavioral effects in school settings. *Journal of the American Academy of Child and Adolescent Psychiatry, 41,* 462–471.

Gadow, K. D., Nolan, E. E., Sverd, J., Sprafkin, J., & Paolicelli, L. (1990). Methylphenidate in aggressive–hyperactive boys: I. Effects on peer aggression in public school settings. *Journal of the American Academy of Child and Adolescent Psychiatry, 29,* 710–718.

Gadow, K. D., Paolicelli, L. M., Nolan, E. E., Schwartz, J., Sprafkin, J., & Sverd, J. (1992). Methylphenidate in aggressive hyperactive boys: II. Indirect effects of medication treatment on peer behavior. *Journal of Child and Adolescent Psychopharmacology, 2,* 49–61.

Gadow, K., & Sprague, R. L. (1980). *An anterospective follow-up of hyperactive children into adolescence: Licit and illicit drug use.* Paper presented at the annual meeting of the American Psychological Association, Montreal.

Gadow, K. D., & Sverd, J. (1990). Stimulants for ADHD in child patients with Tourette's syndrome: The issue of relative risk. *Developmental and Behavioral Pediatrics, 11,* 269–271.

Gittelman, R., Klein, D. F., & Feingold, I. (1983). Children with reading disorders: II. Effects of methylphenidate in combination with reading remediation. *Journal of Child Psychology and Psychiatry, 24,* 193–212.

Gittelman-Klein, R., & Klein, D. F. (1973). *The relationship between behavioral and psychological test changes in hyperkinetic children.* Paper presented at the 12th Annual Meeting of the American College of Neuropsychopharmacology, Palm Springs, CA.

Gittelman-Klein, R., Landa, B., Mattes, J. A., & Klein, D. F. (1988). Methylphenidate and growth in hyperactive children: A controlled withdrawal study. *Archives of General Psychiatry, 45,* 1127–1130.

Gittelman-Klein, R., & Mannuzza, S. (1988). Hyperactive boys almost grown up: III. Methylphenidate effects on ultimate height. *Archives of General Psychiatry, 45,* 1131–1134.

Goldstein, F. C., & Levin, H. S. (1985). Intellectual and academic outcome following closed head injury in children and adolescents: Research strategies and empirical findings. *Developmental Neuropsychology, 1,* 195–241.

Goodman, A., & Gilman, L. S. (1980). *The pharmacological basis of therapeutics.* New York: Macmillan Co.

Gordon, M. (1983). *The Gordon Diagnostic System.* DeWitt, NY: Gordon Systems.

Granger, D. A., Whalen, C. K., & Henker, B. (1993a). Malleability of social impressions of hyperactive children. *Journal of Abnormal Child Psychology, 21,* 631–647.

Granger, D. A., Whalen, C., & Henker, B. (1993b). Perceptions of methylphenidate effects on hyperactive children's peer interactions. *Journal of Abnormal Child Psychology, 21,* 535–549.

Gualtieri, C. T. (1991). *Pharmacotherapy and the neurobehavioral sequelae of traumatic brain injury.* Unpublished manuscript, University of North Carolina, Chapel Hill.

Gualtieri, C. T., & Evans, R. W. (1988). Stimulant treatment for the neurobehavioral sequelae of traumatic brain injury. *Brain Injury, 2,* 273–290.

Gualtieri, C. T., Hicks, R. E., Levitt, J., Conley, R., & Schroeder, S. R. (1986). Methylphenidate and exercise: Additive effects on motor performance. *Neuropsychobiology, 15,* 84–88.

Handen, B., Breaux, A. M., Gosling, A., Ploof, D. L., & Feldman, H. (1990). Efficacy of methylphenidate among mentally retarded children with attention deficit hyperactivity disorder. *Pediatrics, 86,* 922–930.

Handen, B., Breaux, A. M., Janosky, J., McAuliffe, S., Feldman, H., & Gosling, A., (1992). Effects and noneffects of methylphenidate in children with mental retardation and ADHD. *Journal of the American Academy of Child and Adolescent Psychiatry, 31,* 455–461.

Handen, B., Feldman, H., Gosling, A., Breaux, A. M., & McAuliffe, S. (1991). Adverse side effects of methylphenidate among mentally retarded children with ADHD. *Journal of the American Academy of Child and Adolescent Psychiatry, 30,* 241–245.

Handen, B., Janosky, J., McAuliffe, S., Breaux, A. M., & Feldman, H. (1994). Prediction of response to methylphenidate among children with ADHD and mental retardation. *Journal of the American Academy of Child and Adolescent Psychiatry, 33,* 1185–1193.

Heaton, R. K. (1981). *A manual for the Wisconsin Card Sorting Test.* Odessa, TX: Psychological Assessment Resources.

Hechtman, L., Weiss, G., & Perlman, T. (1984). Young adult outcome of hyperactive children who received long-term stimulant treatment. *Journal of the American Academy of Child Psychiatry, 23,* 261–269.

Henker, B., & Whalen, C. K. (1989). Hyperactivity and attention deficits. *American Psychologist, 44,* 216–223.

Henker, B., Whalen, C., Bugenthal, D. B., & Barker, C. (1981). Licit and illicit drug patterns in stimulant treated children and their peers. In K. D. Gadow & J. Loney (Eds.), *Psy-*

chosocial aspects of drug treatment for hyperactivity (pp. 443–462). Boulder, CO: Westview Press.

Hinshaw, S. P. (1991). Stimulant medication and the treatment of aggression in children with attentional deficits. *Journal of Clinical Child Psychology, 20,* 301–312.

Hinshaw, S. P., Buhrmester, D., & Heller, T. (1989). Anger control in response to verbal provocation: Effects of stimulant medication for boys with ADHD. *Journal of Abnormal Child Psychology, 17,* 393–407.

Hinshaw, S. P., Henker, B., Whalen, C. K., Erhardt, D., & Dunnington, R. E., Jr. (1989). Aggressive, prosocial, and nonsocial behavior in hyperactive boys: Dose effects of methylphenidate in naturalistic settings. *Journal of Consulting and Clinical Psychology, 57,* 636–643.

Horn, W. F., Ialongo, N. S., Pascoe, J. M., Greenberg, G., Packard, T., Lopez, M., Wagner, A., & Puttler, L. (1991). Additive effects of psychostimulants, parent training, and self-control therapy with ADHD children. *Journal of the American Academy of Child and Adolescent Psychiatry, 30,* 233–240.

Hynd, G. W., Semrud-Clikeman, M., Lorys, A. R., Novey, E. S., Eliopulos, D., & Lyytinen, H. (1991). Corpus callosum morphology in attention deficit-hyperactivity disorder: Morphometric analysis of MRI. *Journal of Learning Disabilities, 24,* 141–146.

Ialongo, N. S., Horn, W. F., Pascoe, J. M., Greenberg, G., Packard, T., Lopez, M., Wagner, A., & Pyttler, L. (1993). The effects of a multimodal intervention with attention deficit hyperactivity disorder children: A 9-month follow-up. *Journal of the American Academy of Child and Adolescent Psychiatry, 32,* 182–189.

Ialongo, N. S., Lopez, M., Horn, W. F., Pascoe, J. M., & Greenberg, G. (1994). Effects of psychostimulant medication on self-perceptions of competence, control, and mood in children with attention deficit hyperactivity disorder. *Journal of Clinical Child Psychology, 23,* 161–173.

Jacobvitz, D., Sroufe, A., Stewart, M., & Leffert, N. (1990). Treatment of attentional and hyperactivity problems in children with sympathomimetic drugs: A comprehensive review. *Journal of the American Academy of Child and Adolescent Psychiatry, 29,* 677–688.

Johnston, C., & Fine, S. (1993). Methods of evaluating methylphenidate in children with attention deficit hyperactivity disorder: Acceptability, satisfaction, and compliance. *Journal of Pediatric Psychology, 18,* 717–730.

Johnston, C., Pelham, W. E., Hoza, J., & Sturges, J. (1988). Psychostimulant rebound in attention deficit disordered boys. *Journal of the American Academy of Child and Adolescent Psychiatry, 27,* 806–810.

Kaplan, S. L., Busner, J., Kupietz, S., Wassermann, E., & Segal, B. (1990). Effects of methylphenidate on adolescents with aggressive conduct disorder and ADHD: A preliminary report. *Journal of the American Academy of Child and Adolescent Psychiatry, 29,* 719–723.

Kasten, E. F., Coury, D. L., & Heron, T. E. (1992). Educators' knowledge and attitudes regarding stimulants in the treatment of attention deficit hyperactivity disorder. *Journal of Developmental and Behavioral Pediatrics, 13,* 215–219.

Kauffman, R. E., Smith-Wright, D., Reese, C. A., Simpson, R., & Fowler, J. (1981). Medication compliance in hyperactive children. *Pediatric Psychopharmacology, 1,* 231–237.

Kaufman, A. S., & Kaufman, N. L. (1983). *Kaufman Assessment Battery for Children—Interpretive manual.* Circle Pines, MN: American Guidance Service.

Kazdin, A. E. (1980). Acceptability of alternative treatment for deviant behavior. *Journal of Applied Behavior Analysis, 13,* 259–273.

Kazdin, A. E. (1984). Acceptability of aversive procedures and medication as treatment alternatives for deviant child behavior. *Journal of Abnormal Child Psychology, 12,* 289–302.

Kazdin, A. E. (1987). Treatment of antisocial behavior in children: Current status and future directions. *Psychological Bulletin, 102,* 187–203.

Keith, R. W., & Engineer, P. (1991). Effects of methylphenidate on the auditory processing abilities of children with attention deficit-hyperactivity disorder. *Journal of Learning Disabilities, 24,* 630–636.

Klonoff, H., Crockett, D. D., & Clark, C. (1984). Closed head injuries in children: A model for predicting course of recovery and prognosis. In R. E. Tarter & G. Goldstein (Eds.), *Advances in clinical neuropsychology* (Vol. 2, pp. 139–157). New York: Plenum Press.

Klorman, R. (1986). Attention deficit disorder in adolescence. In R. A. Feldman & A. R. Stiffman (Eds.), *Advances in adolescent mental health* (Vol. 1, pp. 19–62). Greenwich, CT: JAI Press.

Klorman, R. (1991). Cognitive event-related potentials in attention deficit disorder. *Journal of Learning Disabilities, 24,* 130–140.

Klorman, R., Brumaghim, J. T., Fitzpatrick, P. A., & Borgstedt, A. D. (1990). Clinical effects of a controlled trial of methylphenidate on adolescents with attention deficit disorder. *Journal of the American Academy of Child and Adolescent Psychiatry, 29,* 702–709.

Klorman, R., Brumaghim, J. T., Fitzpatrick, P. A., & Borgstedt, A. D. (1991). Methylphenidate speeds evaluation processes of attention deficit disorder adolescents during a continuous performance test. *Journal of Abnormal Child Psychology, 19,* 263–283.

Klorman, R., Brumaghim, J. T., Fitzpatrick, P. A., Borgstedt, A. D., & Strauss, J. (1994). Clinical and cognitive effects of methylphenidate on children with attention deficit disorder as a function of aggression/oppositionality and age. *Journal of Abnormal Psychology, 103,* 206–221.

Klorman, R., Brumaghim, J. T., Salzman, L. F., Strauss, J., Borgstedt, A. D., McBride, M., & Loeb, S. (1988). Effects of methylphenidate on attention-deficit hyperactivity disorder with and without aggressive/noncompliant features. *Journal of Abnormal Psychology, 97,* 413–422.

Klorman, R., Brumaghim, J. T., Salzman, L. F., Strauss, J., Borgstedt, A. D., McBride, M. C., & Loeb, S. (1989). Comparative features of methylphenidate on attention-deficit hyperactivity disorder with and without aggressive/noncompliant features. *Psychopharmacology Bulletin, 25,* 109–113.

Kupietz, S. S., Winsberg, B. G., Richardson, E., Maitinsky, S., & Mendell, N. (1988). Effects of methylphenidate dosage in hyperactive reading-disabled children: I. Behavior and cognitive performance effects. *Journal of the American Academy of Child and Adolescent Psychiatry, 27,* 70–77.

Levin, H. S., & Eisenberg, H. M. (1979a). Neuropsychological outcome of closed head injury in children and adolescents. *Children's Brain, 5,* 281–292.

Levin, H. S., & Eisenberg, H. M. (1979b). Neuropsychological impairment after closed head injury in children and adolescents. *Journal of Pediatric Psychology, 4,* 389–402.

Levin, H. S., Eisenberg, H. M., Wigg, N. R., & Kabayashi, K. (1982). Memory and intellectual ability after head injury in children and adolescents. *Neurosurgery, 11,* 668–673.

Levin, H. S., & Grossman, R. G. (1976). Effects of closed head injury on storage and retrieval in memory and learning of adolescents. *Journal of Pediatric Psychology, 1,* 38–42.

Levy, F., & Hobbes, G. (1988). The action of stimulant medication in attention deficit disorder with hyperactivity: Dopaminergic, noradrenergic, or both. *Journal of the American Academy of Child and Adolescent Psychiatry, 27,* 802–805.

Lezak, M. D. (1983). *Neuropsychological assessment.* London: Oxford University Press.

Liu, C., Robin, A. L., Brenner, S., & Eastman, J. (1991). Social acceptability of methylphenidate and behavior modification for treating attention deficit hyperactivity disorder. *Pediatrics, 88,* 506–565.

Loney, J. (1986). Predicting stimulant drug response among hyperactive children. *Psychiatric Annals, 16,* 16–19.

Loney, J., Kramer, J., & Milich, R. (1981). The hyperactive child grows up: Predictors of symptoms, delinquency and achievement at follow-up. In K. D. Gadow & J. Loney (Eds.), *Psychosocial aspects of drug treatment for hyperactivity* (pp. 381–415). Boulder, CO: Westview Press.

Loney, J., & Milich, R. (1982). Hyperactivity, inattention and aggression in clinical practice. In M. Wolraich & D. K. Routh (Eds.), *Advances in developmental and behavioral pediatrics* (3rd ed., pp. 113–147). Greenwich, CT: JAI Press.

Lou, H. C., Henrikson, L., Bruhn, P., Borner, H., & Nielsen, J. B. (1989). Striatal dysfunction in attention deficit and hyperkinetic disorder. *Archives of Neurology, 46,* 48–52.

McBride, M. C. (1988). An individual double-blind crossover trial for assessing methylphenidate response in children with attention deficit disorder. *Journal of Pediatrics, 113,* 137–145.

Malone, M. A., Kershner, J. R., & Seigel, L. (1988). The effects of methylphenidate on levels of processing and laterality in children with attention deficit disorder. *Journal of Abnormal Child Psychology, 16,* 379–395.

Malone, M. A., & Swanson, J. M. (1993). Effects of methylphenidate on impulsive responding in children with attention deficit hyperactivity disorder. *Journal of Child Neurology, 8,* 157–163.

Malyn, D., Jensen, W. R., & Clark, E. (1993). *Myths and realities about ADHD: A comprehensive survey of school psychologists and teachers about causes and treatments.* Paper presented at the annual convention of the National Association of School Psychologists, Washington, DC.

Matier, K., Halperin, J. M., Sharma, V., Newcorn, J. H., & Sathaye, N. (1992). Methylphenidate response in aggressive and nonaggressive DHD children: Distinctions on laboratory measures of symptoms. *Journal of the American Academy of Child and Adolescent Psychiatry, 31,* 219–225.

Miczek, K. A. (1987). The psychopharmacology of aggression. In L. L. Iversen, S. D. Iversen, & S. H. Snyder (Eds.), *Handbook of psychopharmacology: New directions in behavioral pharmacology* (pp. 183–328). New York: Plenum Press.

Milich, R. (1994). ADHD children's response to failure: If at first you don't succeed, do you try, try, again? *School Psychology Review, 23,* 11–18.

Milich, R., Carlson, C. L., Pelham, W. E., & Licht, B. G. (1991). Effects of methylphenidate on the persistence of ADHD boys following failure experiences. *Journal of Abnormal Child Psychology, 19,* 519–536.

Milich, R., & Landau, S. (1982). Socialization and peer relations in hyperactive children. In K. D. Gadow & I. Bialer (Eds.), *Advances in learning and behavioral disabilities: A recent annual* (Vol. 1, pp. 283–339). Greenwich, CT: JAI Press.

Milich, R., Licht, B., Murphy, D. A., & Pelham, W. E. (1989). Attention-deficit hyperactivity disordered boys' evaluations of attributions for task performance on medication versus placebo. *Journal of Abnormal Child Psychology, 98,* 280–284.

Morris, R., Krawiecki, N., Wright, J., & Walters, W. (1993). Neuropsychological, academic, and adaptive functioning in children who survive in-hospital cardiac arrest and resuscitation. *Journal of Learning Disabilities, 26,* 46–51.

Murphy, D. A., Pelham, W. E., & Lange, A. (1992). Aggression in boys with attention deficit-hyperactivity disorder: Methylphenidate effects on naturalistically observed aggression, response to provocation, and social information processing. *Journal of Abnormal Child Psychology, 20,* 451–466.

Nolan, E. E., & Gadow, K. D. (1994). Relation between ratings and observations of stimulant drug response in hyperactive children. *Journal of Clinical Child Psychology, 23,* 78–90.

Noll, R., LeRoy, S., Bukowski, W. M., Rugosch, F. A., & Kulkarni, R. (1991). Peer relationships and adjustment in children with cancer. *Journal of Pediatric Psychology, 16,* 307–326.

Orlosky, M. J. (1982). The Klein–Levin syndrome: A review. *Psychosomatics, 23,* 609–617.

Payton, J. B., Burkhart, J. E., Hersen, M., & Helsel, W. J. (1989). Treatment of ADHD in mentally retarded children: A preliminary study. *Journal of the American Academy of Child and Adolescent Psychiatry, 28,* 761–767.

Pelham, W. E. (1993). Pharmacotherapy for children with attention-deficit hyperactivity disorder. *School Psychology Review, 22,* 199–227.

Pelham, W. E., Atkins, M. S., Murphy, D. A., & Swanson, J. (1984). *A teacher rating scale for the diagnosis of attention deficit disorder: Teacher norms, factor analyses, and reliability.* Unpublished manuscript, University of Pittsburgh.

Pelham, W. E., & Bender, M. E. (1982). Peer relationships in hyperactive children: Description and treatment. In K. D. Gadow & I. Bialer (Eds.), *Advances in learning and behavioral disabilities: A research annual* (Vol. 1, pp. 365–436). Greenwich, CT: JAI Press.

Pelham, W. E., Carlson, C., Sams, S. E., Vallano, G., Dixon, M. J., & Hoza, B. (1993). Separate and combined effects of methylphenidate and behavior modification on boys with attention deficit hyperactivity disorder in the classroom. *Journal of Consulting and Clinical Psychology, 61,* 506–515.

Pelham, W. E., Greenslade, K. E., Vodde-Hamilton, M., Murphy, D., Greenstein, J. J., Gnagy, E. M., Guthrie, K. J., Hoover, M. D., & Dahl, R. E. (1990). Relative efficacy of long-acting stimulants on children with attention deficit-hyperactivity disorder: A comparison of standard methylphenidate, sustained-release methylphenidate, sustained-release dextroamphetamine, and pemoline. *Pediatrics, 86,* 226–237.

Pelham, W. E., & Hoza, J. (1987). Behavioral assessment of psychostimulant effects on ADD children in a summer day treatment program. In R. Prinz (Ed.), *Advances in behavioral assessment of children and families* (Vol. 3, pp. 3–34). Greenwich, CT: JAI Press.

Pelham, W. E., & Murphy, D. A. (1986). Attention deficit and conduct disorders: In M. Hersen (Ed.), *Pharmacological and behavioral treatments: An integrative approach* (pp. 108–148). New York: Wiley.

Pelham, W. E., Murphy, D. A., Vannatta, K., Milich, R., Licht, B. G., Gnagy, E. M., Greenslade, K. E., Greiner, A. R., & Vodde-Hamilton, M. (1992). Methylphenidate and attributions in boys with attention-deficit hyperactivity disorder. *Journal of Consulting and Clinical Psychology, 60,* 282–292.

Pelham, W. E., Schnedler, R. W., Bender, M. E., Miller, J., Nilsson, D., Budlow, M., Ronnei, M., Paluchowski, C., & Marks, D. (1988). The combination of behavior therapy and methylphenidate in the treatment of hyperactivity: A therapy outcome study. In L. Bloomingdale (Ed.), *Attention deficit disorders* (pp. 29–48). Elmsford, NY: Pergamon Press.

Pelham, W. E., Vallano, G., Hoza, B., Greiner, A. R., & Gnagy, E. M. (1992). *Methylphenidate dose effects on ADHD children: Individual differences across children and domains.* Unpublished manuscript, University of Pittsburgh.

Pelham, W. E., Vodde-Hamilton, M., Murphy, D. A., Greenstein, J., & Vallano, G. (1991). The effects of methylphenidate on ADHD adolescents in recreational, peer group, and classroom settings. *Journal of Clinical Child Psychology, 20,* 293–300.

Peloquin, L. J., & Klorman, R. (1986). Effects of methylphenidate on normal children's mood, event related potentials, and performance in memory scanning and vigilance. *Journal of Abnormal Psychology, 95,* 88–98.

Porrino, L. J., Rapoport, J. L., Behar, D., Ismond, D., & Bunney, W. E. (1983). A naturalistic assessment of the motor activity of hyperactive boys: II. Stimulant drug effects. *Archives of General Psychiatry, 40,* 688–693.

Porteus, S. D. (1965). *Porteus Maze Test: Fifty years application.* New York: Psychological Corporation.

Prigattano, G. P. (1987). Recovery and cognitive training after craniocerebral trauma. *Journal of Learning Disabilities, 20,* 603–613.

Rapoport, J. L. (1983). The use of drugs: Trends in research. In M. Rutter (Ed.), *Developmental neuropsychiatry* (pp. 385–403). New York: Guilford Press.

Rapoport, J. L., Buchsbaum, M. S., Weingartner, H., Zahn, T., Ludlow, C., & Mikkelsen, E. J. (1980). Dextroamphetamine: Its cognitive and behavioral effects in normal and hyperactive boys and normal men. *Archives of General Psychiatry, 37,* 933–943.

Rapport, M. D., Carlson, G. A., Kelly, K. L., & Petaki, C. (1993). Methylphenidate and desipramine in hospitalized children: I. Separate and combined effects on cognitive function. *Journal of the American Academy of Child and Adolescent Psychiatry, 32,* 333–342.

Rapport, M. D., & Kelly, K. L. (1991). Psychostimulant effects on learning and cognitive function: Findings and implications for children with attention deficit hyperactivity disorder. *Clinical Psychology Review, 11,* 61–92.

Rapport, M. D., Quinn, S. O., DuPaul, G. J., Quinn, E. P., & Kelly, K. (1989). Attention deficit disorder with hyperactivity and methylphenidate: The effects of dose and mastery level on children's learning performance. *Journal of Abnormal Child Psychology, 17,* 669–689.

Rapport, M. D., Stoner, G., DuPaul, G. J., Kelly, K. L., Tucker, S. B., & Schoeller, T. (1988). Attention deficit disorder and methylphenidate: A multilevel analysis of dose response effects on children's impulsivity across settings. *Journal of the American Academy of Child and Adolescent Psychiatry, 27,* 60–69.

Reid, M. K., & Borkowski, J. G. (1984). Effects of methylphenidate (Ritalin) on information processing in hyperactive children. *Journal of Abnormal Child Psychology, 12,* 169–186.

Reitan, R. M., & Wolfson, D. (1985). *The Halstead–Reitan Neuropsychological Battery.* Tucson: Neuropsychological Press.

Richardson, E., Kupietz, S. A., Winsberg, B. G., Maitinsky, S., & Mendell, N. (1988). Effects of methylphenidate dosage in hyperactive reading-disabled children. II. Reading achievement. *Journal of the American Academy of Child and Adolescent Psychiatry, 27,* 78–87.

Safer, D. J., & Allen, R. P. (1973). Factors influencing the suppressant effects of two stimulant drugs on the growth of hyperactive children. *Pediatrics, 51,* 660–667.

Safer, D. J., & Krager, J. M. (1988). A survey of medication treatment for hyperactive/inattentive students. *Journal of the American Medical Association, 260,* 2256–2258.

Satterfield, J. H., Cantwell, D. P., & Satterfield, B. P. (1974). Pathophysiology of the hyperactive child syndrome. *Archives of General Psychiatry, 31,* 839–844.

Sebrechts, M. M., Shaywitz, S. E., Shaywitz, B. A., Jatlow, P., Anderson, G. M., & Cohen, D. J. (1986). Components of attention, methylphenidate dosage, and blood levels in children with attention deficit disorder. *Pediatrics, 77,* 222–228.

Shaffer, D., Bijur, P., Chadwick, O. F. D., & Rutter, M. (1980). Head injury and later reading disabilities. *Journal of the American Academy of Child Psychiatry, 18,* 592–610.

Sigelman, C. K., & Shorokey, J. J. (1986). Effects of treatments and their outcomes on peer perceptions of a hyperactive child. *Journal of Abnormal Child Psychology, 14,* 397–410.

Singh, N. N., Epstein, M. H., Luebke, J., & Singh, Y. N. (1990). Psychopharmacological intervention. I: Teacher perceptions of psychotropic medication for students with serious emotional disturbance. *The Journal of Special Education, 24,* 283–295.

Slimmer, L. W., & Brown, R. T. (1985). Parents' decision-making process in medication administration for control of hyperactivity. *Journal of School Health, 55,* 221–225.

Speltz, M. L., Varley, C. K., Peterson, K., & Beilke, R. L. (1988). Effects of dextroamphetamine and contingency management on a preschooler with ADHD and oppositional defiant disorder. *Journal of the American Academy of Child and Adolescent Psychiatry, 27,* 175–178.

Sprakfin, J., & Gadow, K. D. (1993). Four purported cases of methylphenidate-induced tic exacerbation: Methodological and clinical doubts. *Journal of Child and Adolescent Psychopharmacology, 3,* 231–244.

Sprague, R. L., & Sleator, E. K. (1977). Methylphenidate in hyperkinetic children: Differences in dose effects on learning and social behavior. *Science, 198,* 1274–1276.

Stoudemire, A., Morau, M. G., & Fogel, B. S. (1991). Psychotropic drug use in the medically ill: Part II. *Psychosomatics, 32,* 34–36.

Stroop, J. R. (1935). Studies of interference in serial verbal reactions. *Journal of Experimental Psychology, 18,* 643–662.

Summers, J. A., & Caplan, P. J. (1987). Lay people's attitudes toward drug treatment for behavioral control depend on which disorder and which drug. *Clinical Pediatrics, 26,* 258–263.

Surwillo, W. W. (1980). Changes in the electroencephalogram accompanying the use of stimulant drugs (methylphenidate and dextroamphetamine) in hyperactive children. *Biological Psychiatry, 12,* 787–799.

Sverd, J., Gadow, K. D., Nolan, E. E., Sprafkin, J., & Ezor, S. N. (1992). Methylphenidate in hyperactive boys with comorbid tic disorder. *Advances in Neurology, 58,* 271–281.

Sverd, J., Gadow, K. D., & Paolicelli, L. M. (1989). Methylphenidate treatment of attention-deficit hyperactivity disorder in boys with Tourette syndrome. *Journal of the American Academy of Child and Adolescent Psychiatry, 28,* 574–579.

Swanson, J. M. (1988). Measurement of serum concentrations and behavioral response of ADHD children to acute doses of methylphenidate. In L. M. Bloomingdale (Ed.), *Attention deficit disorder: New research in attention, treatment, and psychopharmacology* (pp. 107–126). New York: Pergamon Press.

Swanson, J. M., Sandman, C. A., Deutsch, C., & Baren, M. (1983). Methylphenidate hydrochloride given with or before breakfast. I. Behavioral, cognitive, and electrophysiological effects. *Pediatrics, 72,* 49–55.

Tannock, R., Schachar, R., Carr, R. P., Chajczyk, D., & Logan, G. D. (1989). Effects of methylphenidate on inhibitory control in hyperactive children. *Journal of Abnormal Child Psychology, 17,* 473–491.

Tannock, R., Schachar, R., Carr, R. P., & Logan, G. D. (1989). Dose–response effects of methylphenidate on academic performance and overt behavior in hyperactive children. *Pediatrics, 84,* 648–657.

Tarnowski, K. J., Gavaghan, M. P., & Wisniewski, J. J. (1989). Acceptability of interventions for pediatric pain management. *Journal of Pediatric Psychology, 14,* 463–472.

Tarnowski, K. J., Kelly, P. A., & Mendlowitz, D. R. (1987). Acceptability of behavioral pediatric interventions. *Journal of Consulting and Clinical Psychology, 55,* 435–436.

Taylor, S. E., & Brown, J. D. (1988). Illusion and well-being: A social-psychological perspective on mental health. *Psychological Bulletin, 103,* 193–210.

Telzrow, C. F. (1985). The science and speculation of rehabilitation in developmental neuropsychological disorders. In L. C. Hartlage & C. F. Telzrow (Eds.), *Neuropsychological aspects of individual differences: A developmental perspective* (pp. 271–307). New York: Plenum Press.

Trites, R. L., Blouin, A. G., & LaPrade, K. (1982). Factor analysis of the Conners' Teacher Rating Scale based on a large normative sample. *Journal of Consulting and Clinical Psychology, 50,* 615–623.

Varley, C. K., & Trupin, E. (1982). Double-blind administration of methylphenidate to mentally retarded children with attention deficit disorder: A preliminary study. *American Journal of Mental Deficiency, 86,* 560–566.

Vyse, S. A., & Rapport, M. D. (1989). The effects of methylphenidate on learning in children with ADHD: The stimulus equivalence paradigm. *Journal of Consulting and Clinical Psychology, 57,* 425–435.

Walling, V. R., & Pfefferbaum, B. (1990). The use of methylphenidate in a depressed adolescent with AIDS. *Developmental and Behavioral Pediatrics, 11,* 195–197.

Weinstein, G. S., & Wells, C. E. (1981). Case studies in neuropsychiatry: Post-traumatic psychiatric dysfunction—Diagnosis and treatment. *Journal of Clinical Psychiatry, 42,* 120–122.

Weiss, G., & Hechtman, L. T. (1986). *Hyperactive children grown up.* New York: Guilford Press.

Wender, P. H., Reimherr, F. W., Wood, D., & Ward, M. (1985). A controlled study of methylphenidate in the treatment of attention deficit disorder, residual type, in adults. *American Journal of Psychiatry, 142,* 547–552.

Whalen, C. K. (1989). Attention deficit-hyperactivity disorder. In T. H. Okendick & M. Hersen (Eds.), *Handbook of child psychopathology* (2nd ed., pp. 131–159). New York: Plenum Press.

Whalen, C. K., & Henker, B. (1976). Psychostimulants and children: A review and analysis. *Psychological Bulletin, 83,* 1113–1130.

Whalen, C. K., & Henker, B. (1991). Therapies for hyperactive children: Comparisons, combinations, and compromises. *Journal of Consulting and Clinical Psychology, 59,* 126–137.

Whalen, C. K., Henker, B., Buhrmester, B., Hinshaw, S. P., Huber, A., & Laski, K. (1989). Does stimulant medication improve the peer status of hyperactive children? *Journal of Consulting and Clinical Psychology, 57,* 545–549.

Whalen, C. K., Henker, B., & Finch, D. (1981). Medication effects in the classroom: Three naturalistic indicators. *Journal of Abnormal Child Psychology, 9,* 419–433.

Wilens, T. E., & Biederman, J. (1992). The stimulants. *Pediatric Psychopharmacology, 15,* 191–222.

Wolraich, M. L., Lindgren, S., Stromquist, A., Milich, R., Davis, C., & Watson, D. (1990). Stimulant medication use by primary care physicians in the treatment of attention deficit hyperactivity disorder. *Pediatrics, 86,* 95–101.

Yellin, A. M. (1986). Psychophysiological correlates of attention deficit disorder. *Psychiatric Annals, 16,* 29–34.

Zahn, T. P., Rapoport, J. L., & Thompson, C. L. (1980). Autonomic and behavioral effects of dextroamphetamine and placebo in normal and hyperactive prepubertal boys. *Journal of Abnormal Child Psychology, 8,* 145–148.

Zametkin, A. J., Leibenauer, L. L., Fitzgerald, G. A., King, A., Minkunas, D. V., Herscovitch, P., Yomada, E. M., & Cohen, R. M. (1993). Brain metabolism in teenagers with attention-deficit hyperactivity disorder. *Archives of General Psychiatry, 50,* 333–340.

Zametkin, A. J., & Rapoport, J. L. (1987). Neurobiology of attention deficit disorder with hyperactivity: Where have we come in 50 years? *Journal of the American Academy of Child and Adolescent Psychiatry, 26,* 676–686.

28

Nonstimulant Psychotropic Medication

Desired Effects and Cognitive/Behavioral Adverse Effects

MANUEL L. CEPEDA

Most behavioral adverse effects of medications do not differ in quality from similar behaviors that may be present when a child is free of medication. Cognitive adverse effects that are demonstrated with specialized testing may not be apparent in the classroom or when testing with routine educational batteries. Some impairments demonstrated in the laboratory cannot be corroborated during real-life activities, such as operating a motor vehicle. The literature may report adverse events that occur following the administration of a single dose of medication to a healthy volunteer during a drug trial study. The same adverse event may not occur during long-term administration of the same drug to a patient. The medical literature does not always clarify whether problems are life-threatening major medical events, transient effects that will dissipate rather quickly, or "nuisance" effects limited to subjective somatic complaints that are of no demonstrable consequence.

This chapter reviews the literature and presents guidelines for understanding medication adverse events that may influence behavior and cognition in an educational setting and during counseling and testing. Target behaviors (symptoms) that do respond to medications are also described.

Adverse Effects

Adverse effects are somatic, psychological, and behavioral responses to medication that are not pertinent to the desired therapeutic response. They are also known as side effects. Sometimes the term "adverse event" is used. Adverse effects are not necessarily undesirable. Sedation, a common initial side effect of some antidepressants, may be undesirable when medication is taken during the workday. The same side effect is beneficial when the depressed patient, with sleep onset disturbance as one of the symptoms, takes the medication at bedtime. When discussing the frequency of adverse effects, the following nomenclature is often used. Common adverse events occur one or more times in more than 5% of patients using a given medication. Frequent adverse events occur in at least 1% and less than 5% of patients. Infrequent refers to the range from 1 in 1000 and up to but not including 1 in 100. Rare events occur in less than 1 in 1000 patients while using the drug. An adverse event must occur about twice as often in patients using active drug as it does in control subjects using a placebo for the event to be clearly an adverse event caused by medication.

Two different dropout rates (percentage of patients who discontinue medication) are reported in the medical literature. One is the overall dropout rate. The other is the adverse event dropout rate. The former is the number of patients who discontinue medication for any reason. The latter is the number discontinuing because of adverse events. Both are important. The adverse event dropout rate

MANUEL L. CEPEDA • Department of Psychiatry, College of Medicine, University of South Alabama, Mobile, Alabama 36693-3327.

reflects not only serious medical risk, but also the physician's tolerance of potentially dangerous side effects and the patient's or responsible adult's concurrence with continuing a medication after balancing risks and benefits. Some patients are quicker than others to discontinue after experiencing nuisance side effect. The overall dropout rate is always higher than the adverse event dropout rate. Expenses, lack of support from the family to take medication, and the propensity to discontinue any treatment that is not of immediate benefit contribute to the higher overall dropout rate. Annoying or subjective complaints attributed to medication may be present prior to starting medication. Depressed or anxious patients may become more attentive to these same complaints once medication is started. Encouragement by parents, teachers, and therapists to continue medication or to talk further with the prescribing physician prior to discontinuing medication can be critical to reducing the overall dropout rate.

For drugs newly marketed in the last 5 to 10 years, information from the medication package inserts (official package circulars) is available in the *Physicians' Desk Reference* (Medical Economics, 1995). This information is prepared by each drug manufacturer and contains data approved by the Food and Drug Administration (FDA) for use by drug manufacturers in labeling and advertising. The information may reflect only the data from the investigational new drug clinical trials prior to initial approval for marketing the drug. Once approved, the manufacturer is not required to update the package insert to reflect new medical literature. When new indications and dosing practices appear in the medical literature, the drug manufacturer cannot use the material without updating the clinical trials and again requesting FDA approval. It is important to understand that restraints placed by the FDA on what the drug manufacturer places in the package inserts is not synonymous with placing restraints on physicians' prescribing practices. Physicians prescribe within guidelines suggested by the current medical literature and common practice. Prescribing practices of physicians can differ significantly from the FDA constraints placed on medication package inserts and reprinted in the *Physicians' Desk Reference*. The FDA has made clear to physicians that the current medical literature is to be used for those guidelines and for the indications for new uses of drugs (Department of Health and Human Services, 1982).

Medication package inserts always address the adverse effects profile. This includes profiles for both healthy volunteers versus placebo and mental disorder versus placebo adverse events. Usually, the adverse effects reported for healthy volunteers are those that result from a single-dose administration of the drug. The data from patients with a mental disorder are usually from a drug trial that has extended over several weeks to several months. The original medical literature must be reviewed since details of the studies are not given in the medication package inserts supplied by manufacturers. Sources of the data are rarely cited. During drug trials, over 50 common treatment emergent somatic complaints are monitored. Items include skin rashes, flulike complaints, respiratory complaints, palpitations, musculoskeletal aches, sexual dysfunction, neuropsychiatric problems, and weight change. Some of these complaints are reported by up to 20 to 25% of subjects using a placebo. Blood chemistries to assess for possible hematologic or hepatic damage and electrocardiograms are a standard part of drug trials. The clinician must consider any medical reports about adverse events against a knowledge of the placebo response rate for the same event.

Psychopharmacology with Children

The use of psychotropic medications in the treatment of childhood psychopathology began in the late 1930s with the stimulant medication Benzedrine. It was almost 15 years later, following the introduction of the antipsychotics such as chlorpromazine (Thorazine) and thioridazine (Mellaril), that additional drugs were administered for the treatment of childhood mental disorders. Most of the early target behaviors involved psychomotor excitement, restless behavior, anxiety, and hyperactivity. Many of the initial drug trials involved children with a diagnosis of delinquent behavior, brain damage, cerebral palsy, or mental retardation. Quickly, antianxiety (anxiolytic) medications such as hydroxyzine (Atarax) and later, the tricyclic antidepressants such as imipramine (Tofranil) were added. These have been followed more recently by a newer generation of antidepressants, the selective serotonin reuptake inhibitors (SSRI). Now the antimania drug lithium and several anticonvulsants are being used by child psychiatrists, child neurologists, and other physicians who treat the medication-responsive aspects of childhood psychopathology. The field of childhood psychopharmacology has always been one of symptom treatment. Although many behavioral concomitants of specific diagnoses are medication responsive, the underlying disease process has yet to be treated directly.

Overview of Nonstimulant Psychotropic Drugs

Six general groups of psychotropic medications are given to children: antipsychotic, antidepressant, antianxiety, antimania, anticonvulsive, and stimulant medications. The first five are discussed in this chapter. The antiparkinsonian drugs are also reviewed. Stimulant medications are reviewed elsewhere in this book.

Representative antipsychotic medications (also called neuroleptics or major tranquilizers) prescribed for children and adolescents include chlorpromazine (Thorazine), thioridazine (Mellaril), haloperidol (Haldol), thiothixene (Navane), and fluphenazine (Prolixin). Clozapine (Clozaril) is of a different class (dibenzodiazepine) and has a quite different adverse effects profile. The latter drug is the only one in the psychopharmacology armamentarium that requires weekly laboratory monitoring. Blood must be drawn for white blood cell counts for as long as the drug is administered because of the risk of agranulocytosis (failure of the body to produce white blood cells). If the latter occurs, life-threatening infections may quickly develop. There is no clinical evidence that the antipsychotic efficacy of any one is clearly superior to the others. They do differ with respect to the degree of anticholinergic effect and because of this (and for other pharmacological reasons), the adverse effects profiles differ.

The antidepressant drugs have four major subclasses (tricyclics, aminobetones, monoamine oxidase inhibitors, and selective serotonin reuptake inhibitors). Representative tricyclic antidepressants include imipramine (Tofranil), amitriptyline (Elavil), desipramine (Norpramine), and clomipramine (Anafranil). The latter is actually a selective serotonin reuptake inhibitor that belongs to the tricyclic antidepressant class. The only example from the aminobetone subclass is bupropion (Wellbutrin). The monoamine oxidase inhibitors include tranylcypromine (Parnate) and phenelzine (Nardil). The selective serotonin reuptake inhibitors include fluoxetine (Prozac) and sertraline (Zoloft).

As with the antipsychotics, there is little difference in clinical efficacy between antidepressants. There are differences in the side effects profiles. The selective serotonin reuptake inhibitors have a far safer adverse event profile when taken in amounts that exceed normal therapeutic levels (e.g., drug overdose). Overdoses with tricyclic antidepressants are significantly more life threatening.

Most of the antianxiety drugs are of the benzodiazepine class. Commonly prescribed are chlordiazepoxide (Librium), diazepam (Valium), and alprazolam (Xanax). A relatively new antianxiety agent is from the azaspirodecanedione class. This is buspirone (Buspar). It is not related to the benzodiazepines and does not cause psychological or physical dependence as do the benzodiazepines. It is also less sedating. It may take several weeks of continuous treatment for anxiety symptoms to respond to buspirone. The benzodiazepines produce immediate relief of anxiety. Buspirone is also less efficacious overall than the benzodiazepines. The antihistamine hydroxyzine (Atarax or Vistaril) is used as an antianxiety agent. A drawback is that patients report that it loses efficacy during long-term use. It does not have the abuse or dependence profile of the benzodiazepines. It may be administered (intramuscular) on an as-needed basis to children or adolescents hospitalized on a psychiatric inpatient unit for attenuation of nonpsychotic rage behavior.

Lithium carbonate is a salt. It has a life-threatening adverse effects profile that closely parallels the level of drug in the blood. Initially, frequent monitoring of blood levels is necessary. Later, monitoring of serum blood levels can be done every 3 to 6 months. Patients are warned to avoid sodium chloride (table salt)-free diets, which might increase the serum levels of lithium carbonate. Adverse effects may appear quickly when serum blood levels exceed the upper therapeutic range.

Representative anticonvulsant drugs include carbamazepine (Tegretol) and clonazepam (Klonopine). Clonazepam has many properties characteristic of the benzodiazepine class of anxiolytics. This includes withdrawal symptoms similar to those seen with alcohol withdrawal and the risk of abuse and dependence. Carbamazepine does not have the same abuse or dependence potential. The antiparkinsonian agents include benztropine (Cogentin) and amantadine (Symmetrel). They are important because they are often prescribed at the same time as the antipsychotic drugs to treat musculoskeletal system side effects that might occur. Benztropine can contribute to an anticholinergic delirium when used in conjunction with the more anticholinergic antipsychotic medications.

The following sections first address the common diagnoses (psychopathology) treated with each medication. Next, the specific target symptoms that respond to medications are listed. A discussion of representative adverse effects and guidelines for testing while on medication follows.

Antipsychotic Medications

The antipsychotic drugs are of well-established benefit in the treatment of schizophrenia, schizophreniform disorder, schizoaffective disorder, and delusional disorder. They are also useful in the treatment of major depression with psychosis and the manic phase of the bipolar disorder. The psychotic symptoms responsive to medication include rapid-onset delusions and hallucinations, incoherent or disorganized speech, agitated behavior, and catatonic excitement or stupor. Additional target symptoms include the press of speech, flight of ideas, and motoric hyperactivity of mania. A significant response may be seen during the first few days of treatment. To prevent relapse, the antipsychotic drugs are continued even when the psychosis is in remission.

Patients with pervasive developmental disorders or significant mental retardation who have symptoms of agitation, physical aggression, or self-mutilatory behavior are also prescribed antipsychotic drugs. Significant attenuation of these behaviors over several months is the goal. Seldom is a total remission achieved. Hyperactive behaviors are quicker to respond. Medication may need to be continued for several years. Antipsychotic drugs are used to treat the multiple tic disorders (Tourette's disorder). They are prescribed for the occasional psychotic symptoms and frequent irritability seen early in the course of Huntington's disease. None treat the underlying disease or alter the ultimate course.

Agitation, aggression, and rage that is not a part of a psychotic or dementing disorder may also be treated with neuroleptics. The indications for this use are not as well established. Examples include the aggressive component of a conduct disorder, aggression as a part of an intermittent explosive disorder, and low frustration tolerance, rages, and hostility in conjunction with several of the Cluster B personality disorders (antisocial, borderline, and narcissistic disorders). Medical literature to support neuroleptic use for target symptoms not associated with a psychotic disorder is limited and only marginally supportive.

The common behavioral adverse effects of the antipsychotic drugs involve central nervous system-mediated pathways. An acute dystonic reaction with the sudden onset of muscle spasms may be seen. Although a dystonic reaction may look frightening to an observer, it usually causes little physical discomfort. Spasm of the masseter muscles may cause the jaw to pull over to one side and look as if it is dislocated. The head and neck may twist back and to one side because of sternocleido-mastoid muscle spasm. This is called torticollis. The child may complain that the tongue is being pulled into the back of the mouth, or that there is a feeling of swallowing the tongue or that he or she cannot swallow. Both eyes may roll up (oculogyric crisis) leaving only the bottom part of each pupil and iris showing. Rarely, the truncal muscles may be involved. The child may twist into an opisthotonos position with the head pulled backwards in extension and back arched with arms drawn up and legs extended. With the exception of the tongue complaint, the presence of acute dystonic reactions should be easily identified by an observer.

Akathesia is easily recognized. It is an apparent inability to sit still. Both legs may behave as if they are pacing while the individual is sitting or "standing" in place. It is sometimes called "walking in place." In children, the "fidgetiness" of the hyperactive child may be mistaken for akathesia. Identification is less a problem in adolescents.

A parkinsonian picture may be seen. There may be muscular rigidity, a pill-rolling hand tremor, drooling, and masklike facies. The reduced movement may be confused with catatonia or with the appearance of a retarded depression.

Dyskinesias should also be easily recognized. These include facial tics and blinking (blepharospasm). These symptoms may occur in children independent of any medication use.

Tardive dyskinesia can be a troubling adverse effect. Symptoms include abnormal mouth movements that look like persistent chewing, lip-smacking, or repetitive tongue protrusions (fly catchers tongue). Another name for this is buccolingual–masticatory (BLM) movements. The movements may abate if neuroleptic medication is lowered or discontinued and may be temporarily hidden or masked if medication is increased. BLM movements can intensify and cause physical derangement. The clinical picture is difficult to assess because withdrawal dyskinesias which may occur when a neuroleptic dose is decreased are indistinguishable in appearance from early tardive dyskinesia. Those at greatest risk for tardive dyskinesia are elderly females. Although reported in children, it is not common.

Acute dystonic reactions and akathesias should clear within an hour or less when antiparkinsonian drugs such as benztropine (Cogentin) or diphenhydramine (Benadryl) are administered. Parkinsonian symptoms may take longer to clear. Seldom is it necessary to decrease or discontinue the antipsychotic medication because of these effects. The BLM movements may be attenuated over the short term with the daily use of antiparkinsonian drugs. The recommended management is to lower or if necessary discontinue the antipsychotic medication. Because BLM movements may become chronic and continue even after medication is discontinued, physicians may screen high-risk patients on antipsychotic medications for early signs as often as every 1 or 2 months.

Most of the antipsychotic medications cause sedation when first given or whenever high doses are first prescribed. This effect should abate over several days, or possibly weeks for the very high doses. Usually the physician decreases the medication from the initial treatment dose to lower maintenance levels after a few weeks as a normal course of treatment. This also will help alleviate any sedation that is occurring. Instead of sedation, patients may report they feel "drugged up."

It is the anticholinergic component of a neuroleptic's pharmacological effect that causes the initial confusion, memory problems, and disorganization when medication is first prescribed. This is a dose-related effect. In combination with a highly anticholinergic antiparkinsonian drug such as benztropine (Cogentin), delirium may occur. It may take a week or more for a serious anticholinergic delirium to clear once medication is stopped. Generally, those drugs with a greater risk for anticholinergic-mediated adverse effects have a lesser risk for causing dystonic reactions. However, there is a greater risk for dystonic reactions from those drugs with a less pronounced anticholinergic profile.

If antipsychotic medication is discontinued, clinically significant pharmacologic effects persist for about 24 to 36 hours. Almost all of the drug will be metabolized and cleared from the body within 3 or 4 days following cessation. At that point, there is no longer any noticeable clinical effect. With prolonged administration, metabolites may persist in the urine for several months to over a year. This latter finding is not of importance because there is no clinical effect.

Most research into the effects of antipsychotic medications on cognition has studied children with mental retardation or with autism. Some 70% of this latter group have an IQ in the range for mental retardation. When patients are symptomatic with medication-responsive target behaviors, it is not possible to design studies that assess the effects of antipsychotic medications on cognition or learning alone. Several studies emphasize that as the symptoms of aggression, restlessness, and poor concentration improve, tasks such as learning and school achievement improve (Anderson *et al.,* 1984; Campbell *et al.,* 1982; Helper, Wilcott, & Garfield, 1963; Sprague, Barnes, & Werry, 1970; Weise, O'Reilly, & Hesbacher, 1972; Werry, Weiss, Douglas, & Martin, 1966). None of the studies suggest that medication directly improves learning ability. Improvement in learning is a consequence of treating symptoms of the mental disorder. Most of the improvement follows the first month or two of medication treatment.

When antipsychotic medications were given to children with a spectrum of nonpsychotic disorders (adjustment reaction, hyperactivity, psychoneurotic reaction, conduct disorder, and personality disturbance), the results more often were inconclusive or actually suggested a deterioration in test performance. For subjects with these diagnoses, it was concluded that any untoward effects on testing or learning were related to the sedation seen on initial administration. Higher doses also affected test scores.

Studies with adults yield similar findings (Braff & Saccuzzo, 1982; Spiegel & Keith-Spiegel, 1967; Weiss, Robinson, & Dasberg, 1973). Those symptomatic with schizophrenia showed improved intelligence test scores following the administration of antipsychotics. Other aspects of cognitive function, including attention, improved with the use of medications (King, 1990; Strauss & Kleiser, 1990; Strauss, Kleiser, & Leuthcke, 1988). Again, the improvement came following a reduction in the severity of symptoms of the illness and was not attributed to a direct effect of antipsychotic drug on learning. Any decrement in performance caused by medication was masked by the improved performance as target symptoms abated.

In nonpsychotic subjects, higher doses of antipsychotics are associated with poorer performances on psychomotor speed and attention tasks, independent of clinical diagnosis and level of intelligence (Sweeney, Keilp, Haas, Hill, & Weiden, 1991). The data suggest that for the drugs with a more prominent anticholinergic side effect profile, the impairment is more severe. The addition of selected antiparkinsonian medications intensifies the impairment (Cleghorn, Kaplan, Szechtman, Szechtman, & Brown, 1990; Eitan, Levin, Ben-Artzi, Levy, & Neumann, 1992).

Thioridazine is associated with inhibition of ejaculation during masturbation and sexual intercourse (Greenberg & Carrillo, 1968). This is a less frequent problem with the other neuroleptics. It should be anticipated and discussed along with other risks and benefits prior to prescribing thioridazine. Should this problem occur, a change of medication may be necessary.

In children with autism, it is difficult to distinguish stereotypies (repetitive senseless movements or verbalizations) which can be characteristic of autism from the neuroleptic-mediated dyskinesias (Shay et al., 1993). As with adults who gain weight when taking neuroleptics, weight gain greater than expected for age has been reported in children and adolescents (Silva, Malone, Anderson, Shay, & Campbell, 1993). Neuroleptics may induce tics in children with attention deficit hyperactivity disorder (Guatrieri & Patterson, 1986).

Drug-induced dysphagia (difficulty swallowing) can occur with neuroleptic use. Choking on food and possible aspiration (food enters trachea and lungs) may occur. This may lead to pneumonitis (inflammation of the lungs) or asphyxia (literally a "stopping of the pulse" resulting from lack of oxygen). This is a critical problem for patients with brain injuries who receive neuroleptics for control of psychomotor agitation. Some 25 to 30% of these patients already have dysphagia as a consequence of the brain injury (Silwa & Lis, 1993).

The following are clinical guidelines for psychological or educational testing of children prescribed antipsychotic medication. For children with nonpsychotic disorders receiving antipsychotics, adverse effects of medication on test results may be seen during the initial days to a week or two after the medication is started. At reasonable clinical doses, any adverse effect on testing should be negligible after the child has been on medication for at least 2 weeks. A different guideline applies for patients with psychotic disorders. If testing is to be used for educational placement, it should be delayed for at least 4 to 8 weeks after medication is started. At this point, the adolescent should be relatively free of symptoms and on a stable maintenance dose. Avoid testing whenever obvious sedation is present. If the child or adolescent must be tested free of antipsychotic medication, a 2- to 4-day delay following cessation of drug should be sufficient.

Antidepressants

The antidepressants are prescribed to treat major depressive disorder, dysthymia, and the depressive phase of a bipolar disorder. The target symptoms most clearly responding to antidepressants include spontaneous crying spells, decreased appetite, weight loss, diurnal mood variation (less energy on arising than later in the day), difficulty in falling asleep, middle of the night awakening, early morning awakening, decreased libido, and impairment of concentration. Less responsive to medications are sustained feelings of depression (mood) and anhedonia. Antidepressants do not alleviate ongoing depressed mood if it is unaccompanied by the specific biological symptoms associated with clinical depression.

Some attenuation of anxiety symptoms accompanying a depressive illness may be seen as quickly as 2 or 3 days after starting an antidepressant. It takes between 3 and 8 weeks for the core clinical symptoms of depression that are going to respond to medication to do so. Because of the length of time necessary for response, antidepressants are not used to treat stress symptoms that might be expected to remit over a week or two without treatment. Likewise, during a brief hospitalization for crisis stabilization, antidepressants are not started immediately.

In the early 1970s, the tricyclic antidepressant imipramine (Tofranil) was used to treat hyperactive children. Most of the target clinical improvements included improved conduct in general, improved attention span, and reduced motor activity. Most studies concluded that the antidepressant was effective and also that the degree of improvement was the same as with stimulant medication (Quinn & Rapoport, 1975; Rapoport, Quinn, Bradbard, Riddle, & Brooks, 1974; Werry, Aman, & Diamond, 1979). This course of treatment did not gain popularity, however, and now the stimulant medications are used almost exclusively.

The selective serotonin reuptake inhibitor antidepressants such as clomipramine, fluoxetine, and sertraline are used to treat symptoms of obsessive–compulsive disorder. The compulsions or repetitive behaviors such as checking, touching, or hand washing respond better to medication than does obsessional thinking alone.

Enuresis may be treated with the tricyclic antidepressant imipramine. Although imipramine is the prototype antidepressant for use with this problem, any tricyclic antidepressant should help equally as well. The most optimistic reports come in the treatment of secondary nocturnal enuresis. It is called secondary because the child has periods of days or weeks free of enuresis. Primary enuresis (no significant period free of symptoms) is less responsive to medication. Half or more of those with secondary enuresis become asymptomatic with medication use. Antidepressant treatment of enuresis is superior to placebo treatment, but has not been demonstrated to be superior to the many other alternative treatments [bell and pad, token economy, desmopressin nasal spray (DDAVP), brief family or individual psychotherapy]. There is literature on this topic (Behrle, Elkin, & Laybourne, 1956; Kardash, Hillman, & Werry, 1968; Stenberg & Lackgren, 1994).

Some children with severe symptoms of separation anxiety disorder are treated with high doses of antidepressants. Most medication treatment for this disorder comes only after psychotherapeutic and psychosocial/educational therapies have failed. This is not a well-documented treatment and the more recent literature does not support earlier reports of usefulness (Gittelman-Klein & Klein, 1971, 1973).

Antidepressants have none of the dramatic musculoskeletal side effects described for the antipsychotics. Children are more comfortable if the dose is increased by increments every 2 or 3 days so that the therapeutic dose is reached after a week or two, but this is not an absolute necessity. If the dose is increased too rapidly, the child may complain of sleepiness, tiredness, or drowsiness. These effects are transient and should abate over a week or two. Mild fine hand tremors may be seen. There may be complaints about a dry mouth or blurred vision while reading. The latter symptoms are anticholinergic-mediated adverse effects, and should abate also. This may take a couple of months if the child is unduly sensitive or the dose must remain high. Rarely, a child will complain of difficulty paying attention even on a reasonable dose. A different class of antidepressant may need to be prescribed.

Both cognitive and behavioral effects of a single-dose administration or antidepressants have been studied (DiMascio, Heninger, & Klerman, 1964; Ross, Smallberg, & Weingartner, 1984; Thompson & Trimble, 1982). Some antidepressants are more sedating than others. For these, reports of feeling sleepy peak between 2 and 3 hours after administration and are gone by 7 hours after the drug is ingested. The same problems have not been reported during long-term administration. The more sedating tricyclics do impair performance on serial addition and digit substitution tasks when the drug is first administered.

The cognitive effects of antidepressants during long-term administration have been studied in children being treated for enuresis, hyperactivity, childhood depression, and aggression (Brumback & Staton, 1980; Campbell et al., 1982; Kupietz & Balka, 1976; Rapoport, 1965; Staton, Wilson, & Brumback, 1981; Werry, Dowrick, Lampen, & Vamos, 1975). The results may vary by diagnostic category. Scores on such measures as the Wechsler Intelligence Scale for Children improved as melancholic symptoms of depression lifted. Improvements came following 2 to 3 months of drug therapy. Performance on the Continuous Performance Test, a measure of sustained attention or vigilance, improved during administration of amitriptyline (Elavil). Several studies concluded that children using an antidepressant concentrated better. Studies of children with conduct disorder and enuresis that compared IQ scores before and after antidepressant treatment found no significant differences.

The memory and attention changes during ongoing tricyclic antidepressant treatment of adults with depression have received more attention (Glass, Uhlenhuth, & Weinreb, 1978; Glass, Uhlenhuth, Hartel, Matuzas, & Fischman, 1981; Henry, Weingartner, & Murphy, 1973; Keeler, Prange, & Reifler, 1966; Lamping, Spring, & Gelenberg, 1984; Legg & Stiff, 1976; Sternberg & Jarvik, 1976). Impairment in short-term memory is a clinical characteristic of depression. The greater the clinical improvement with antidepressant medications, the greater is the short-term memory improvement. Imipramine probably facilitates psychomotor tasks such as tapping or reaction time. Although the depressed patient is symptomatic, possible adverse medication effects on test scores cannot be separated from the significant improvement that is seen as a result of alleviation of the symptoms of depression. Clinical measures such as the Wechsler Adult Intelligence Scale are not sensitive enough to reflect adverse medication effect while a patient is asymptomatic and on a maintenance dose of tricyclic antidepressant. Although not as extensively studied, many of these findings are also true of the monoamine oxidase inhibitor class of antidepressants (Murphy, 1977).

When drug treatment is initiated, the tricyclic antidepressants with greater anticholinergic potential can cause memory disturbances. The same effects are less evident or not evident during chronic administration (Thompson, 1991).

Sexual dysfunction has been associated with the use of the tricyclic and monoamine oxidase inhibitor classes of antidepressants. This includes inhibition of ejaculation in males and anorgasmia in females (Jani & Wise, 1988; Rosenbaum & Pollack, 1988; Segraves, 1988; Shen & Lindbergh, 1990). Although the literature addresses adult dysfunction (young adult through geriatric ages) and does not report the problem in adolescents, there is no reason why the adolescent would not be at equal risk. A decreased libido (sex drive), rather than inhibition of ejaculation and anorgasmia, is associated with clinical depression. Even with a careful sexual function screen prior to starting antidepressants, it is difficult to differentiate dysfunction related to antidepressants from the sexual dysfunction so often associated with depression (Petrie, 1980).

Doses of tricyclics well above the usual treatment doses (drug overdose) have been associated with deaths resulting from cardiac arrhythmias. Sudden death (unexplained) has been reported in four children using a tricyclic antidepressant. None of the children were receiving unusually high treatment doses. Postmortem blood levels were not above the therapeutic range (Riddle et al., 1991; Tingelstad, 1991). Sudden deaths in general are associated with cardiac arrhythmias as the mechanism of death. Although three of the deaths occurred with desipramine, data suggest that electrocardiogram effects for desipramine are similar to those for other tricyclic antidepressants (Wilens, Biederman, Spencer, & Geist, 1993). At present, the conclusion is that if desipramine is linked to sudden death (because of an adverse cardiovascular event), the occurrence is rare (Biederman et al., 1993). It is not clear why desipramine would have a greater risk than other tricyclics. It is not certain at this time that the risk associated with the tricyclics is greater than the risk for sudden death in those free of medication.

The delirium caused by tricyclics is related to high blood levels of the drug (Meador-Woodruff,

Akil, Wisner-Carlson, & Grunhaus, 1988). The incidence of delirium is also related to increasing age (Livingston, Zucker, Isenberg, & Wetzel, 1983). None of the studies in the medical literature report the incidence of delirium in children and adolescents.

One study has concluded that depressed patients using antidepressant medication should be capable of driving (Hobi et al., 1982). The subjects were all patients using established clinical doses of antidepressant.

The following clinical guidelines apply for routine psychological and psychoeducational testing. If the child is receiving tricyclic antidepressants to treat a depression with melancholic symptoms, testing should be delayed until clinical improvement is seen if the results are to be used for long-term educational placement. This means delay should be at least 3 weeks and perhaps as long as 6 to 8 weeks after the correct therapeutic dose is initiated. Testing earlier than this (while the patient is still symptomatic) will reflect current function highly influenced by symptoms of depression. For the child receiving antidepressants for problems other than depression, the initial sedative and/or anticholinergic effect that may be seen in the first week or two of administration may influence the test results. It would be best to delay testing until the child has been on medication a couple of weeks. If the child must be tested free of antidepressant medication, only a 3- or 4-day delay following discontinuation is suggested. There are insufficient research data to conclude that long-term administration of tricyclic antidepressants impairs performance on any routine psychological or psychoeducational batteries.

Antimanic Drugs

Lithium carbonate is used for the treatment of the manic phase of bipolar disorders. Because clinical improvement of manic symptoms takes 7 to 10 days with lithium alone, an antipsychotic medication (which can reduce symptomatology over 3 or 4 days) is often prescribed at the same time lithium is started and discontinued once lithium reaches therapeutic levels. If the manic phase of a bipolar disorder does occur in young children, it is uncommon. It is more frequently seen in the adolescent. Lithium is of unclear benefit in the treatment of the depressive phase of a bipolar disorder. For many patients, it does not offer prophylaxis against reoccurring depression.

Lithium has been used to treat target symptoms of aggression, hostility, rage, and behavioral impulsivity in children and adolescents. These symptoms are seen in conduct disorders and intermittent explosive disorders. Lithium use for the latter problems is not as well established (Platt, Campbell, Green, & Grega, 1984).

At the usual therapeutic doses, as monitored via serum blood levels, lithium does not produce CNS-mediated behavioral side effects. One study (Judd, Hubbard, Janowsky, Huey, & Takahashi, 1977) reported that in normal volunteers, therapeutic levels of lithium did impair performance on the Digit Symbol subtest of the WAIS and the Trail Making A test. Another study concluded that lithium caused a decrement in WAIS IQ scores (Aminoff, Marshall, Smith, & Wyke, 1974) in patients being treated for Huntington's chorea, a neurological disorder associated with dementia.

Other studies have specifically studied memory tasks (Bonnel, Etevenon, Benyacoub, & Slowen, 1981; Christodoulous, Kokkevi, Lykouras, Stefanis, & Papadimitriou, 1981; Huey *et al.,* 1981; Kusumo & Vaughan, 1977; Marusarz, Wolpert, & Koh, 1981; Squire, Judd, Janowsky, & Huey, 1980). All of the studies used either specialized scales or selected parts of more common tests. Patients with a comorbid dementia and the elderly are at more risk for memory dysfunction when lithium is used. Some studies suggest that those with more severe psychiatric illness show more impairment. There is some evidence that lithium does not affect the more global measures on the WAIS or the Wechsler Memory Scale in nondemented patients. In contrast with the other drugs covered, studies with lithium did not show a clear improvement in cognitive function paralleling clinical improvement.

There is limited data from which to generalize concerning the testing of children using lithium. Because lithium is so short acting, one to two days after the last dose is a sufficient delay if the child must be drug free when tested.

Antianxiety Drugs

Antianxiety medications see widespread use for the symptomatic relief of anxiety in adults. They are less often prescribed for similar target symptoms in children and adolescents. The literature does not advocate the use of antianxiety medication to treat the common childhood diagnoses that include anxiety as a prominent symptom. Occasionally physicians do prescribe anxiolytics for brief symptomatic treatment of overwhelming stress in children as a part of crisis stabilization. Anxiolytics are also used to attenuate alcohol withdrawal symptoms (tremor, insomnia, psychomotor agitation, anxiety). They are used to treat pavor nocturnes (night terrors) and somnambulism (sleepwalking). Some anxiolytics are used to treat panic disorder.

Anxiety can be a prominent symptom during an acute psychosis. Hospitalized adolescents with these problems may receive anxiolytics until they respond to neuroleptics. Then the anxiolytic will be discontinued. Depressed patients may receive anxiolytics until sleep improves with concomitant antidepressant treatment.

There is a paucity of literature on the cognitive and behavioral adverse effects of anxiolytics in children. One study that did specifically evaluate anxiolytic drug effects on the cognitive function of children concluded that at therapeutic doses there is no adverse effect on cognition (Ferguson & Simeon, 1984). Most studies with adult subjects conclude that at common therapeutic doses, little if any difference between placebo and drug groups can be demonstrated (Healey, Pickens, Meisch, & McKenna, 1983; Pishkin, Fishkin, Shurley, Lawrence, & Lovallo, 1978; Zimmermann-Tansella, 1984). Single-dose administration of the drug may produce a reduced speed of performance on some items. At high doses, the sedative effect will impair cognitive performance.

For the benzodiazepine class, several reviews are available that summarize the effects (Cole, 1986; DiMascio, Giller, & Shader, 1968; Ghoneim & Mewaldt, 1990; Kornetsky, Williams, & Bird, 1990; Lister, 1985; Wittenborn, 1988). While using benzodiazepines, more problems occur with the acquisition of new information than the retrieval of previously learned material. If sedation is present, the impairment is more pronounced. The impairment is more pronounced for tasks that require more effort (e.g., learning new material) than for automatic processes requiring minimal attention. At nonsedating doses, short-term or working memory remains intact.

A decrease in vigilance may occur with single-dose administration (Gotestam & Anderson, 1978). Experienced drivers receiving diazepam for relief of anxiety had more difficulty with normal perception and anticipation of events. This may be more of a problem during less interesting, low-attention-level driving on highways than in dense city traffic where a high attention level is constantly required (deGier, 't Hart, Nelemans, & Bergman, 1981).

The addiction potential of the benzodiazepines is of concern during long-term administration. Possibly one patient in five using benzodiazepines over an extended period of time increases the dose surreptitiously. This suggests the development of tolerance and/or abuse. Even low doses are associated with withdrawal symptoms after about 4 months of use. Clinical evidence for dependence may appear after 4 to 6 weeks of daily use (Miller & Gold, 1990; Zisook & DeVaul, 1977).

Paradoxical rage reactions (aggressive dyscontrol) have been reported during benzodiazepine use. There is far more literature suggesting that antianxiety medications are helpful in reducing irritability and aggression. There is no clear conclusion that aggressive dyscontrol is a specific side effect of the antianxiety medications (Dietch & Jennings, 1988; Gardos, 1980).

Both the ability to sustain attention during a repetitive task under time pressure and visual–spatial ability may be impaired in those using benzodiazepines in normal therapeutic doses for 1 year or longer (Golombok, Moodley, & Ladner, 1988). Buspirone, a newer non-benzodiazepine class antianxiety agent, does not affect memory as adversely (Lucki, Rickels, Giesecke, & Geller, 1987). It is easier to show memory effects in the elderly. Less or no impairment is seen in young adults (Block, DeVoe, Stanley, Stanley, & Pomara, 1985). Analogous studies are not available for children and adolescents. Although the greatest effect may be on the acquisition of new material (episodic memory), tolerance to these problems does develop (Koelega, 1989).

As with the antimanic drugs, there are insufficient research data regarding the use of anxiolytic drugs in children to comment on the cognitive effects in relationship to routine psychological testing. The clinical effect for single-dose administration of most anxiolytics is about 4 to 6 hours. The half-life for most is much longer and drugs may be detected through routine blood and urine assays for 1 to 2 days following administration of a single dose. If the child must be free of anxiolytic medication effect at the time of testing, a delay of 1 day following the last dose should be sufficient.

Anticonvulsants

The use of anticonvulsants in the treatment of seizure disorders is well established. Less well established is their use for the treatment of episodic dyscontrol, aggression, and repetitive self-injury behavior (Israel & Beaudry, 1988). Carbamazepine has an additional established role in the treatment of the lithium-resistant bipolar disorders. Adverse effects such as mania, hypomania, increased irritability, impulsivity, hyperactivity, and aggression have been reported during clinical trials with carbamazepine (Pleak, Birmaher, Gavrilescu, Abichandani, & Williams, 1988). There is insufficient literature from which to base an opinion about the effects of the anticonvulsants on common psychoeducational testing batteries.

Antiparkinsonian Agents

Antiparkinsonian agents are used to treat acute dystonic reactions, parkinsonian symptoms, and akathesia associated with neuroleptic use. The antiparkinsonian drugs may temporarily suppress buccolingual or masticatory movements. The withdrawal dyskinesias associated with a relative reduction in dose of neuroleptic may also be subdued with antiparkinsonian drugs. They are usually prescribed only after a patient develops parkinsonian or dystonic symptoms. Most patients only need coverage for a few weeks, although for some patients daily use for months is necessary.

Brain-damaged patients of any age and the elderly are more sensitive to the anticholinergic effects of antiparkinsonian agents on memory (Fayen, Goldman, Moulthrop, & Luchins, 1988). The problem is not seen with amantadine (Symmetrel). It does not have the same anticholinergic profile and may be used in place of benztropine (Cogentin). Nondemented patients are far less sensitive to anticholinergic effects on cognitive performance (Thienhaus, Allen, Bennett, Chopra, & Zemlan, 1990). Some patients come to appreciate the stimulant-euphoric effect associated with high doses of antiparkinsonian medication and become skilled at self-inducing a mild anticholinergic delirium by using extra medication. This can develop into drug abuse (Dugas, 1977).

Summary

Childhood psychopharmacology began in the late 1930s with the use of Benzedrine, an amphetamine to treat "motorically driven" children. From there the search for behavior-modifying drugs expanded. Today it includes the use of antipsychotic, antidepressant, anxiolytic, anticonvulsant, and antimania drugs. For some of the drugs, serum blood levels help the physician adjust the dose quickly into the therapeutic range and also warn of levels that might be associated with adverse effects.

All medications have desired effects and adverse effects. The latter range from nuisance to life threatening and from transient to long term. For most side effects that occur early, such as sedation or confusion, adaptation occurs over days or weeks as the initially high treatment dose is lowered to a maintenance therapeutic dose or the child adapts to the ongoing dose. Other adverse effects occur independent of dose and at any time during the course of treatment. Some adverse effects are more frequent with prolonged therapy than early in the course of treatment. Some adverse effects are idiosyncratic to a single drug. Although generalizations can be made for classes of drugs, the medical literature must be reviewed for each individual drug since adverse effects do vary within each class.

Recommendations concerning educational testing while the patient is using psychotropic medication vary by class of drug, illness, dose, and length of treatment. Testing may be possible as early as several days after starting medication or may need to be delayed as long as 6 to 8 weeks after medication has begun.

The literature supports the conclusion that for the psychotropic medications in use today, common educational batteries are not affected once symptoms of psychosis or depression have remitted and the child is clinically stable on a maintenance dose. For disorders without symptoms of psychosis or depression, the delay must be long enough for any initial adverse medication effects to abate.

References

Aminoff, M. J., Marshall, J., Smith, E., & Wyke, M. (1974). Cognitive function in patients on lithium therapy. *British Journal of Psychiatry, 125,* 109–112.

Anderson, L. T., Campbell, M., Grega, D. M., Perry, R., Small, A. M., & Green, W. H. (1984). Haloperidol in the treatment of infantile autism: Effects upon learning and behavioral symptoms. *American Journal of Psychiatry, 141,* 1195–1202.

Behrle, F. C., Elkin, M. T., & Laybourne, P. C. (1956). Evaluation of a conditioning device in the treatment of nocturnal enuresis. *Pediatrics, 17,* 849–856.

Biederman, J., Baldessarini, R. J., Goldblatt, A., Lapey, K. A., Doyle, A., & Hesslein, P. (1993). A naturalistic study of 24-hour electrocardiographic recordings and echocardio-graphic findings in children and adolescents treated with desipramine. *Journal of the American Academy of Child and Adolescent Psychiatry, 32,* 805–813.

Block, R. I., DeVoe, M., Stanley, B., Stanley, M., & Pomara, N. (1985). Memory performance in individuals with primary degenerative dementia: Its similarity to diazepam-induced impairments. *Experimental Aging Research, 11,* 151–155.

Bonnel, H. L., Etevenon, P., Benyacoub, J., & Slowen, P. (1981). Intellectual efficiency in manic–depressive patients treated with lithium. *Acta Psychiatrica Scandinavica, 64,* 423–430.

Braff, D. L., & Saccuzzo, D. P. (1982). Effect of antipsychotic medication on speed of information processing in schizophrenic patients. *American Journal of Psychiatry, 139,* 1127–1130.

Brumback, R. A., & Staton, R. D. (1980). Neuropsychological study of children during and after remission and endogenous depressive episodes. *Perceptual and Motor Skills, 50,* 1163–1167.

Campbell, M., Small, A. M., Green, W. H., Jennings, M. A., Perry, R., Bennett, W. G., Pedron-Gayol, M., & Anderson, L. (1982). Lithium and haloperidol in hospitalized aggressive children. *Psychopharmacology Bulletin, 18,* 126–130.

Christodoulous, G. N., Kokkevi, A., Lykouras, E. P., Stefanis, C. N., & Papadimitriou, G. N. (1981). Effects of lithium on memory. *American Journal of Psychiatry, 18,* 847–848.

Cleghorn, J. M., Kaplan, R. D., Szechtman, B., Szechtman, H., & Brown, G. M. (1990). Neuroleptic drug effects on cognitive function in schizophrenia. *Schizophrenia Research, 3,* 211–219.

Cole, S. O. (1986). Effects of benzodiazepines on acquisition and performance: A critical assessment. *Neuroscience and Biobehavioral Reviews, 10,* 265–272.

deGier, J. J., 't Hart, B. J., Nelemans, F. A., & Bergman, H. (1981). Psychomotor performance and real driving performance of outpatients receiving diazepam. *Psychopharmacology, 73,* 340–344.

Department of Health and Human Services, United States Government. (1982). Use of approved drugs for unlabeled indications. *FDA Drug Bulletin, 12,* 4–5.

Dietch, J. T., & Jennings, R. K. (1988). Aggressive dyscontrol in patients treated with benzodiazepines. *Journal of Clinical Psychiatry, 49,* 184–188.

DiMascio, A., Giller, D. R., & Shader, R. I. (1968). Behavioral toxicity of psychotropic drugs: III. Effects on perceptual and cognitive functions. *Connecticut Medicine, 32,* 771–775.

DiMascio, A., Heninger, G., & Klerman, G. L. (1964). Psychopharmacology of imipramine and desipramine: A comparative study of their effects in normal males. *Psychopharmacologia, 5,* 361–371.

Dugas, J. E. (1977). Mood elevation and medication. *Diseases of the Nervous System, 38,* 958.

Eitan, N., Levin, Y., Ben-Artzi, E., Levy, A., & Neumann, M. (1992). Effects of antipsychotic drugs on memory functions of schizophrenic patients. *Acta Psychiatrica Scandinavica, 85,* 74–76.

Fayen, M., Goldman, M. B., Moulthrop, M. A., & Luchins, D. J. (1988). Differential memory function with dopaminergic versus anticholinergic treatment of drug-induced extrapyramidal symptoms. *American Journal of Psychiatry, 145,* 483–486.

Ferguson, H. B., & Simeon, J. G. (1984). Evaluating drug effects on children's cognitive functioning. *Progress in Neuropsychopharmacology and Biological Psychiatry, 8,* 683–686.

Gardos, G. (1980). Disinhibition of behavior by antianxiety drugs. *Psychosomatics, 21,* 1025–1026.

Ghoneim, M. M., & Mewaldt, S. P. (1990). Benzodiazepines and human memory: A review. *Anesthesiology, 72,* 926–938.

Gittelman-Klein, R., & Klein, D. F. (1971). Controlled imipramine treatment of school phobia. *Archives of General Psychiatry, 25,* 204–207.

Gittelman-Klein, R., & Klein, D. F. (1973). School phobia: Diagnostic considerations in the light of imipramine effect. *Journal of Nervous and Mental Disease, 156,* 199–215.

Glass, R. M., Uhlenhuth, E. H., Hartel, F. W., Matuzas, W., & Fischman, M. W. (1981). Cognitive dysfunction and imipramine in outpatient depressives. *Archives of General Psychiatry, 38,* 1048–1051.

Glass, R. M., Uhlenhuth, E. H., & Weinreb, H. (1978). Imipramine-reversible cognitive deficit in outpatient depressives. *Psychopharmacology Bulletin, 14,* 10–11.

Golombok, S., Moodley, P., & Ladner, M. (1988). Cognitive impairment in long term benzodiazepine users. *Psychological Medicine, 18,* 365–374.

Gotestam, K. G., & Anderson, B. E. (1978). Subjective effects and vigilance after diazepam and oxazepam in normal subjects. *Acta Psychiatrica Scandinavica, 274* (Suppl.), 117–128.

Greenberg, H. R., & Carrillo, C. (1968). Thioridazine-induced inhibition of masturbatory ejaculation in an adolescent. *American Journal of Psychiatry, 124,* 151–153.

Guatrieri, C. T., & Patterson, D. R. (1986). Neuroleptic-induced tics in two hyperactive children. *American Journal of Psychiatry, 143,* 1176–1177.

Healey, M., Pickens, R., Meisch, R., & McKenna, T. (1983). Effects of clorazepate, diazepam, lorazepam and placebo on human memory. *Journal of Clinical Psychiatry, 44,* 436–439.

Helper, M. M., Wilcott, R. C., & Garfield, S. L. (1963). Effects of chlorpromazine on learning and related processes in emotionally disturbed children. *Journal of Consulting Psychology, 27,* 1–9.

Henry, G. M., Weingartner, H., & Murphy, D. L. (1973). Influence of affective states and psychoactive drugs on verbal learning and memory. *American Journal of Psychiatry, 130,* 966–971.

Hobi, V., Gastpar, M., Gastpar, G., Gilsdorf, U., Kielholz, P., & Schwarz, E. (1982). Driving ability of depressive patients under antidepressants. *Journal of International Medical Research, 10,* 65–81.

Huey, L. Y., Janowsky, D. S., Judd, L. L., Abrams, A., Parker, D., & Clopton, P. (1981). Effects of lithium carbonate on methylphenidate-induced mood, behavior and cognitive process. *Psychopharmacology, 73,* 161–164.

Israel, M., & Beaudry, P. (1988). Carbamazepine in psychiatry: A review. *Canadian Journal of Psychiatry, 33,* 577–584.

Jani, N. N., & Wise, T. N. (1988). Antidepressants and inhibited female orgasm: A literature review. *Journal of Sex and Marital Therapy, 14,* 279–284.

Judd, L. L., Hubbard, B., Janowsky, D. S., Huey, L. Y., & Takahashi, K. I. (1977). The effect of lithium carbonate on the cognitive functions of normal subjects. *Archives of General Psychiatry, 34,* 355–357.

Kardash, S., Hillman, E. S., & Werry, J. (1968). Efficacy of imipramine in childhood enuresis: A double-blind control study with placebo. *Journal of the Canadian Medical Association, 99,* 263–266.

Keeler, M. H., Prange, A. J., & Reifler, C. B. (1966). Effects of imipramine and thioridazine on set and action. *Diseases of the Nervous System, 27,* 798–802.

King, D. J. (1990). The effect of neuroleptics on cognitive and psychomotor function. *British Journal of Psychiatry, 157,* 799–811.

Koelega, H. S. (1989). Benzodiazepine and vigilance performance: A review. *Psychopharmacology, 98,* 145–156.

Kornetsky, C., Williams, J. E. G., & Bird, M. (1990). Attentional and motivational effects of psychoactive drugs. *NIDA Research Monograph, 97,* 177–192.

Kupietz, S. S., & Balka, E. B. (1976). Alterations in the vigilance performance of children receiving amitriptyline and methylphenidate pharmacotherapy. *Psychopharmacology, 50,* 29–33.

Kusumo, K. S., & Vaughn, M. (1977). Effects of lithium salts on memory. *British Journal of Psychiatry, 131,* 453–457.

Lamping, D. L., Spring, B., & Gelenberg, A. J. (1984). Effects of two antidepressants on memory performance in depressed outpatients: A double blind study. *Psychopharmacology, 84,* 254–261.

Legg, J. F., & Stiff, M. P. (1976). Drug-related test patterns of depressed patients. *Psychopharmacology, 50,* 205–210.

Lister, R. G. (1985). The amnestic actions of benzodiazepines in man. *Neuroscience & Biobehavioral Reviews, 9,* 87–94.

Livingston, R. L., Zucker, D. K., Isenberg, K., & Wetzel, R. D. (1983). Tricyclic antidepressants and delirium. *Journal of Clinical Psychiatry, 44,* 173–176.

Lucki, I., Rickels, K., Giesecke, M. A., & Geller, A. (1987). Differential effects of the anxiolytic drugs, diazepam and buspirone, on memory function. *British Journal of Clinical Pharmacology, 23,* 207–211.

Marusarz, T. Z., Wolpert, E. A., & Koh, S. D. (1981). Memory processing with lithium carbonate. *Journal of Clinical Psychiatry, 42,* 190–192.

Meador-Woodruff, J. H., Akil, M., Wisner-Carlson, R., & Grunhaus, L. (1988). Behavioral, and cognitive toxicity related to elevated plasma tricyclic antidepressant levels. *Journal of Clinical Psychopharmacology, 8,* 28–32.

Medical Economics. (1995). *Physicians' desk reference.* Montvale, NJ: Author.

Miller, N. S., & Gold, M. S. (1990). Benzodiazepine tolerance, dependence, abuse and addiction. *Journal of Psychoactive Drugs, 22,* 23–33.

Murphy, D. L. (1977). The behavioral toxicity of monoamine oxidase-inhibiting antidepressants. *Advances in Pharmacology and Chemotherapy, 14,* 71–105.

Petrie, W. M. (1980). Sexual effects of antidepressants and psychomotor stimulant drugs. *Modern Problems of Pharmacopsychiatry, 15,* 77–90.

Pishkin, V., Fishkin, S. M., Shurley, J. T., Lawrence, B. E., & Lovallo, W. R. (1978). Cognitive and psychophysiologic response to doxepin and chlordiazepoxide. *Comprehensive Psychiatry, 19,* 171–178.

Platt, J. E., Campbell, M., Green, W. H., & Grega, D. M. (1984). Cognitive effects of lithium carbonate and haloperidol in treatment-resistant aggressive children. *Archives of General Psychiatry, 41,* 657–662.

Pleak, R. R., Birmaher, B., Gavrilescu, A., Abichandani, C., & Williams, D. T. (1988). Mania and neuropsychiatric excitation following carbamazepine. *Journal of the American Academy of Child and Adolescent Psychiatry, 27,* 500–503.

Quinn, P. O., & Rapoport, J. L. (1975). One year follow-up of hyperactive boys treated with imipramine or methylphenidate. *American Journal of Psychiatry, 132,* 241–245.

Rapoport, J. (1965). Childhood behavior and learning problems treated with imipramine. *International Journal of Psychiatry, 1,* 635–642.

Rapoport, J. L., Quinn, P. O., Bradbard, G., Riddle, K. D., & Brooks, E. (1974). Imipramine and methylphenidate treatments of hyperactive boys. *Archives of General Psychiatry, 30,* 789–793.

Riddle, M. A., Nelson, J. C., Kleinman, C. S., Rasmusson, A., Leckman, J. F., King, R. A., & Cohen, D. J. (1991). Sudden death in children receiving norpramin: A review of three reported cases and commentary. *Journal of the American Academy of Child and Adolescent Psychiatry, 30,* 845–846.

Rosenbaum, J. F., & Pollack, M. H. (1988). Anhedonic ejaculation with desipramine. *International Journal of Psychiatry in Medicine, 18,* 85–88.

Ross, R. J., Smallberg, S., & Weingartner, H. (1984). The effects of desmethylimipramine on cognitive function in healthy subjects. *Psychiatry Research, 12,* 89–97.

Segraves, R. T. (1988). Psychiatric drugs and inhibited female orgasm. *Journal of Sex and Marital Therapy, 14,* 202–207.

Shay, J., Sanchez, L. E., Cueva, J. E., Armenteros, J. L., Overall, J. E., & Campbell, M. (1993). Neuroleptic-related dyskinesias and stereotypies in autistic children: Videotaped ratings. *Psychopharmacology Bulletin, 29,* 359–363.

Shen, W. W., & Lindbergh, S. S. (1990). Inhibited female orgasm resulting from psychotropic drugs: A five year updated clinical review. *Journal of Reproductive Medicine, 37,* 11–14.

Silva, R. R., Malone, R. P., Anderson, L. T., Shay, J., & Campbell, M. (1993). Haloperidol withdrawal and weight changes in autistic children. *Psychopharmacology Bulletin, 29,* 287–291.

Sliwa, J. A., & Lis, S. (1993). Drug-induced dysphagia. *Archives of Physical Medicine and Rehabilitation, 74,* 445–447.

Spiegel, D. E., & Keith-Spiegel, P. (1967). The effects of carphenazine, trifluoperazine and chlorpromazine on ward behavior, physiological functioning and psychological test scores in chronic schizophrenic patients. *The Journal of Nervous and Mental Disease, 144,* 111–116.

Sprague, R. L., Barnes, K. R., & Werry, J. S. (1970). Methylphenidate and thioridazine: Learning, reaction time, activity and classroom behavior in disturbed children. *American Journal of Orthopsychiatry, 40,* 615–628.

Squire, L. R., Judd, L. L., Janowsky, D. S., & Huey, L. Y. (1980). Effects of lithium carbonate on memory and other cognitive functions. *American Journal of Psychiatry, 137,* 1042–1046.

Staton, R. D., Wilson, H., & Brumback, R. A. (1981). Cognitive improvement associated with tricyclic antidepressant treatment of childhood major depressive illness. *Perceptual and Motor Skills, 53,* 219–234.

Stenberg, A., & Lackgren, G. (1994). Desmopressin tablets in the treatment of severe nocturnal enuresis in adolescents. *Pediatrics, 94,* 841–846.

Sternberg, D. E., & Jarvik, M. E. (1976). Memory functions in depression. *Archives of General Psychiatry, 33,* 219–224.

Strauss, W. H., & Kleiser, E. (1990). Cognitive disturbances in neuroleptic therapy. *Acta Psychiatrica Scandinavica, 82*(Suppl. 358), 56–57.

Strauss, W. H., Kleiser, E., & Leuthcke, H. (1988). Dyscognitive syndromes in neuroleptic therapy. *Pharmacopsychiatry, 21,* 298–299.

Sweeney, J. A., Keilp, J. G., Haas, G. L., Hill, J., & Weiden, P. J. (1991). Relationships between medication treatments and neuropsychological test performance in schizophrenia. *Psychiatry Research, 37,* 297–308.

Thienhaus, O. J., Allen, A., Bennett, J. A., Chopra, Y. M., & Zemlan, F. P. (1990). Anticholinergic serum levels and cognitive performance. *European Archives of Psychiatry and Clinical Neuroscience, 240,* 28–33.

Thompson, P. J. (1991). Antidepressants and memory: A review. *Human Psychopharmacology, 6,* 79–90.

Thompson, P. J., & Trimble, M. R. (1982). Non-MAOI antidepressant drugs and cognitive functions: A review. *Psychological Medicine, 12,* 539–548.

Tingelstad, J. B. (1991). The cardiotoxicity of the tricyclics. *Journal of the American Academy of Child and Adolescent Psychiatry, 30,* 845–846.

Weise, C. C., O'Reilly, P. P., & Hesbacher, P. (1972). Perphenazine–amitriptyline in neurotic underachieving students: A controlled study. *Diseases of the Nervous System, 33,* 318–325.

Weiss, A. A., Robinson, S., & Dasberg, H. (1973). Changes in mental functioning accompanying antipsychotic drug therapy. *Annals of Psychiatry and Related Disciplines, 11,* 134–140.

Werry, J. S., Aman, M. G., & Diamond, E. (1979). Imipramine and methylphenidate in hyperactive children. *Journal of Child Psychology and Psychiatry, 21,* 27–35.

Werry, J. S., Dowrick, P. W., Lampen, E. L., & Vamos, M. J. (1975). Imipramine in enuresis—Psychological and physiological effect. *Journal of Child Psychology and Psychiatry, 16,* 289–299.

Werry, J. S., Weiss, G., Douglas, V., & Martin, M. A. (1966). Studies on the hyperactive child: The effect of chlorpromazine upon behavior and learning ability. *Journal of the American Academy of Child Psychiatry, 5,* 292–312.

Wilens, T. E., Biederman, J., Spencer, T., & Geist, D. E. (1993). A retrospective study of serum level and electrocardiographic effects of nortriptyline in children and adolescents. *Journal of the American Academy of Child and Adolescent Psychiatry, 32,* 270–277.

Wittenborn, J. R. (1988). Assessment of the effect of drugs on memory. *Psychopharmacology Series, 6,* 67–78.

Zimmermann-Tansella, C. (1984). Psychological performance of normal subjects on tasks commonly used in evaluation of anxiolytic drugs. *Perceptual and Motor Skills, 58,* 803–810.

Zisook, S., & DeVaul, R. (1977). Adverse behavioral effects of benzodiazepines. *The Journal of Family Practice, 5,* 963–966.

29

Neuropsychological Sequelae of Substance Abuse by Children and Youth

ROBERT WILLIAM ELLIOTT

Substance abuse by children and youths continues to be a problem of international scope. In comparison with a number of years ago, the drugs available for illicit use have become more potent, more addictive, and, as a consequence, perhaps more damaging to the central nervous system (CNS). Although not all illicit drugs are chronically damaging, all drugs produce acute neurological and neuropsychological impairment (Hartman, 1995). Youth, as a group, throughout history have used alcohol and other psychoactive substances to affect their sensory system, creating acute and sometimes permanent problems (Bukstein, 1995).

Incidence

In 1975, University of Michigan researchers initiated a longitudinal group of studies to investigate the prevalence of drug use by high school students (Johnston, O'Malley, & Bachman, 1993). Drug use increased until 1985 when a reverse trend became apparent. Their 1993 survey (Forrest, 1994; Quintanilla, 1994) revealed that high school seniors in the United States significantly increased their drug use in 1993 for the first time in more than a decade. The University of Michigan 1993 survey found that 42.9% of high school seniors had used an illicit drug at least once in their lives, up from 40.7% in 1992. This finding reported the first in-

crease of use of illicit drugs since 1981 when lifetime use by seniors reached a peak of 65.6%. The NIDA 1993 Monitoring the Future survey of adolescent drug use and related attitudes (Forrest, 1994) reported upswings in drug use among eighth, ninth, and tenth graders. In this survey, for the third year in a row, there was a significant increase in marijuana use by eighth-grade students. Among this group, 25.7% acknowledged that they had used illicit drugs in the past. The figure rose to 35.1% when inhalants such as glue or gasoline fumes were included. Cocaine use had also increased among eighth, tenth, and twelfth graders for the third year in a row (Swan, 1995). This survey found an increase in use of crack cocaine, heroin, and LSD among eighth graders.

The majority of adolescents experiment with substances, especially alcohol. Youth between the ages of 18 and 25 are still the most likely to use illicit drugs. Although there is evidence of a decline in illicit drug use thereafter (Yamaguchi & Kandel, 1994), the age at which an adolescent begins using illicit drugs is a powerful predictor of later alcohol and drug problems, especially if use begins before age 15 (Institute for Health Policy, 1993).

Developmental Issues

Because of the developing nervous system, children represent a particularly vulnerable population (Schroeder, 1995), yet children and young adults are populations rarely studied in drug abuse research (Grant & Reed, 1985; Ivnik, 1986). During adolescence, the higher-level cognitive attributes of

ROBERT WILLIAM ELLIOTT • Department of Student Services, Redondo Beach Unified School District, Redondo Beach, California 90277.

planning, evaluation, flexibility, internalized behavioral controls, higher-level abstracting skills, and ethical awareness are developing (Golden, 1985). The use of drugs during this period could interfere with development of one or more of these attributes and could adversely affect cognitive functions mediated by frontal and prefrontal regions of the neocortex (Elliott, 1989).

Newcomb and Bentler (1991) designed an 8-year prospective study that examined how patterns and types of adolescent drug use impacted physical health and use of health services in adulthood. The researchers discovered that increased quantity and frequency of alcohol, cannabis, cocaine, cigarettes, and hard drugs as a teenager increased the likelihood that various health problems would become apparent in adulthood. Increases in drug involvement beginning in adolescence through young adulthood had an adverse effect on health and increased the use of all health services in adulthood.

Assessment of Youth

The general purpose of a neuropsychological assessment is to evaluate brain–behavior relationships. This is accomplished by measuring behavior sensitive to CNS integrity. The assessment process evaluates abilities such as intellect, memory, speech and linguistic skills, perception, attention and concentration, problem-solving, decision-making, and planning. Impairment in any of these areas suggests either permanent or temporary dysfunction in those regions of the brain that subserve these abilities. During the last 5 years, neuropsychologists have become increasingly sensitive to issues regarding specificity and sensitivity of neuropsychological evaluation methods. As technology has advanced, computerized assessment batteries have become valuable tools for investigating gross as well as subtle behavior changes associated with neuropathology (Kay, 1995; The Risk Management Foundation of the Harvard Medical Institutions, 1993). Although many individuals typically will show no obvious evidence of brain damage during standard clinical interviews or neurological examinations, they do manifest cognitive deficits on sensitive neuropsychological measures (Fals-Stewart, Schafer, Lucente, Rustine, & Brown, 1994). Lezak (1995) has reviewed the most widely used noncomputerized measures.

Assessing youth is more complicated than assessing adults because of differences in emotional development and brain development and a need to recognize different stages of development at different ages. During adolescence and childhood there are spurts and plateaus in cognitive development creating a dynamic and unstable system. This dynamic system requires the use of different procedures and methodology for investigation than those designed for adults. Schroeder (1995) notes that even with environmental toxins, children show clinical effects at lower levels of exposure than adults. Children present different toxicokinetic response profiles than do adults because of their developing status. For instance, a low-level neurotoxic exposure may affect both the peripheral nervous system and the central nervous system in children. The same dose level in adults may only affect the peripheral nervous system. There are also differences in metabolic rate between adults and children and differences in reversibility of neurotoxic effects. In addition, the behavioral plasticity and capacity for reorganization of the immature brain, the different diagnostic considerations in adult and child neurology, variability in test-taking behavior at younger ages, and the dramatic impact of environmental and social factors on the developing organism ensure both a qualitative and a quantitative difference between the child and the adult (Baron, Fennell, & Voeller, 1995).

Definitions

This chapter will focus primarily on the chronic effects of alcohol abuse and illicit drug use. Chronic use implies the possibility of long-term consequences after ingestion of the drug has ceased (Ware, 1979). Acute effects are mentioned only when very few or no chronic effect studies have been reported. "Drug dependence," "substance dependence," and "substance abuse" are terms used synonymously in this chapter. DSM-IV (American Psychiatric Association, 1994) differentiates between substance-related disorders. Substance dependence lists tolerance, withdrawal, and compulsive drug-taking behavior occurring any time in the same 12-month period. Intoxication is defined as a reversible substance-specific syndrome with maladaptive behavior or psychological changes developing during or shortly after use.

The content in this chapter and the majority of research studies reviewed has been limited to those studies investigating children, adolescents, and young adults through the age of 25. The focus of the chapter is on drugs that are taken deliberately for abuse.

Drug Classification

There are a variety of classification systems available that categorize drugs based on differential criteria. Kissin's (1977) system is one of only a few that are based on behavioral and CNS consequences. He divides psychoactive drugs into depressants, stimulants, and hallucinogens. Parsons and Adams (1983) add inhalants to Kissin's classification system. Johnston *et al.* (1993) developed the most widely recognized drug survey nationally and identify the most popular drugs of abuse. Their classification scheme includes designer drugs. The order of discussion of each drug is based on the addictive potential inherent in the drug (Hastings, 1991). Polydrug abuse and research on steroids, because of the complexity of these chemicals, are discussed at the end of the chapter.

Cocaine

Cocaine has become one of the most widely abused, illicit drugs in the United States (Johnston *et al.*, 1993) and one of the most widely investigated drugs in the last several years (Harris, 1994). Cocaine is a stimulant of natural origin that shares many of the behavioral and biochemical properties found in psychomotor stimulants, amphetamines, and methylphenidate (Post, Weiss, Pert, & Uhde, 1987). Thus, cocaine's powerful combination as a local anesthetic and psychomotor stimulant makes its CNS effects difficult to interpret. Cocaine can be diluted or mixed with other inert substances, such as lactose, or mixed with other psychoactive substances, such as PCP or heroin. This mixture can produce a rapid and intense but brief experience. Cocaine can be converted to "crack," a form of cocaine converted to a free base form, by mixing it with ammonia or baking soda. Crack results in an immediate and intense euphoria that is of shorter duration than cocaine taken intranasally (Bukstein, 1995).

Kaplan, Freedman, and Sadock (1980) noted that if "used no more than two or three times a week, cocaine creates no serious problems" (p. 1621). The American Psychiatric Association's diagnostic manual (DSM-III; APA, 1980) listed a category for cocaine abuse but not for cocaine dependence (p. 173). The DSM-III advisory committee on substance abuse disorders concluded there was no evidence of withdrawal or tolerance and no evidence of physiologic addiction (Spitzer, Williams, & Skodal, 1980). The American Psychiatric Association, in their most recent diagnostic manual (DSM-IV, 1994), listed cocaine abuse as well as cocaine dependence. The authors noted that dependence could develop from short periods of use, tolerance occurred with repeated use, and discontinuance of use could cause withdrawal symptoms (p. 222).

Cocaine use is highly reinforcing and high doses can create rapid motor activity, rambling speech, impaired judgment, paranoid and psychotic behavior, irritability, and anxiety. Chronic effects on the CNS have been demonstrated with electrophysiologic and imaging techniques. EEGs have shown markedly reduced alpha power in frontal and temporal regions (Pascual-Leone, Dhuna, & Anderson, 1991a). Imaging studies by the same researchers indicated CNS abnormalities associated with chronic cocaine abuse. CT studies found evidence of cerebral atrophy in chronic cocaine abusers (Pascual-Leone, Dhuna, & Anderson, 1991b).

Johnston *et al.* (1993) indicated that cocaine use by adolescents appears to be declining from its peak use in the 1980s. Lifetime prevalence peaked at 17.3% of seniors in 1985 and then declined to 6.1% of high school seniors reporting using cocaine at least once during their lifetime in 1993. Daily use of cocaine by high school seniors has remained at a low level starting with 0.1% in 1975, 0.4% in 1985, and 2.3% in 1993 (University of Michigan, 1994).

Much of the research on cocaine affecting youth has focused on prenatal exposure. It is well recognized that such exposure can result in a broad range of deficits depending on the chronicity, severity, and timing of the exposure. Longitudinal studies with toddlers and preschoolers suffering from such exposure suggest that the majority of exposed children have low average to normal cognitive abilities but tend to be highly distractible and have significant difficulties with speech and language development, peer interactions, and fine motor control (Phelps & Cox, 1993). Addiction with cocaine develops much more rapidly than with other drugs. Addiction can develop in a few weeks or months, especially when smoked as free base (crack) (Washton & Stone-Washton, 1993).

In one of the few longitudinal studies that have evaluated the chronic effects of cocaine abuse on neuropsychological findings, Berry *et al.* (1993) administered a battery of neuropsychological tests to a group of 16 young adult subjects within 72 hours of their last cocaine use and again 2 weeks later. All subjects were hospitalized for treatment of cocaine dependence. They were matched with 21 non-cocaine-using control subjects. All of the cocaine-abusing subjects had used the drug for a minimum of 6 months prior to their admission. Both groups underwent neuropsychological testing with the Trail Making Test, Rey–Osterrieth Complex Figure, FAS, Block Design, Digit Symbol, Rey Auditory-Verbal Learning Test, PASAT, and Stroop to evaluate cognitive functioning. The results suggested that recent cocaine use resulted in specific neuropsychological impairment during the acute phase. Memory, visuospatial abilities, and concentration were affected during the acute phase. After 2 weeks of abstinence, the cocaine-dependent group continued to manifest deficits on measures of psychomotor speed, memory, and concentration. The authors concluded that these deficits were consistent with the neuropsychological deficits seen in dopamine depletion disorders, such as Parkinson's disease and progressive supranuclear palsy.

In a similar study (van Gorp *et al.,* 1995), 33 cocaine-dependent subjects were neuropsychologically assessed and compared with 22 nonabusing control subjects. The authors found that with a similar battery of tests there was no evidence of significant neuropsychological deficits in the cocaine-abusing groups after 3 weeks of abstinence. Assessments were performed at the time of admission and 14 and 21 days later. The deficits noted in the 1993 study were confirmed in this study after 2 weeks of abstinence. Although the authors found no deficits after 3 weeks, it is unknown whether the second group used cocaine to the same extent as the first group. In fact, the extent of cocaine use was not disclosed in the research reports for either study. During the acute phase, the performance of the subjects in the second group did not fall within the impaired range on any of the measures administered. Although the first group was impaired on selected measures on initial testing, they also were the group that failed to show any evidence of recovery on selected measures at 2 weeks. Thus, the differences between the two groups may have more to do with the degree of cocaine abuse than length of time.

These results are consistent with other test results suggesting deficits in planning and impulsivity even with sober, cocaine-addicted adults. Such evidence has been forthcoming from neuroimaging studies suggesting frontotemporal hypoperfusion on SPECT and frontal hypometabolism on PET (Ranlett, Gansler, & Kodituwakku, 1995).

Mittenberg and Motta (1993), in evaluating the effects of chronic cocaine abuse on memory and learning, found that users who were 10 days abstinent, compared with controls matched on age, education, race, and gender, showed evidence of significant residual impairment in verbal learning efficiency as a result of memory storage difficulty. A dose–response relationship was suggested.

In some of the most extensive follow-up evaluations on cocaine abusers, Strickland (Strickland, Mena, Villanueva-Meyer, & Miller, 1993; Strickland & Stein, 1995) found that with a group of subjects who had regularly used from 1.5 to 7 years in comparison with the reference groups, cocaine abusers demonstrated poor performance on measures of learning and memory, visuospatial skills, and executive functioning. These individuals had verifiable abstinence from their current sober living environment of between 5 and 12 months. With another group of subjects, Strickland *et al.* (1993) utilized CT and MRI brain scans as well as selected neuropsychological measures to study cerebral perfusion, brain morphology, and cognitive functioning. All subjects were drug free for 6 months, and showed significant cerebral hypoperfusion in the frontal, periventricular, and/or temporal–parietal areas. Neuropsychological testing revealed deficits in attention, concentration, new learning, visual and verbal memory, word production, and visual motor integration.

Elliott noted all of these effects as well as convulsions in his clinical work with recovering adolescent cocaine abusers (Elliott, 1987). Myers and Earnest (1984) noted that after three young adults, aged 20 to 25, injected 140–160 mg of cocaine, each sustained a generalized convulsion. A neurological examination completed shortly thereafter, which included EEG and CT evaluations, yielded normal results.

It is well accepted that cocaine is addictive and that tolerance does exist. Withdrawal signals are detectable on the EEG, neuropathological evidence is detected in the brain scans, and cognitive deficits are evident from the neuropsychological assessment test results. A preponderance of evidence indicates that there is a dose relationship with high use associated with long-term neuropsychological deficits. Nevertheless, the studies that have been presented have focused generally on young adults and not on children or adolescents. Careful, controlled, long-term studies of cocaine's effects on the neuropsychological performance of youth with at least 6 months of sobriety need to be performed. Researchers need to utilize brain imaging techniques and to correlate such information with neuropsychological findings.

The majority of recent research results suggest a positive correlation between use of cocaine and CNS damage. Because SPECT and other imaging techniques have indicated CNS damage, it is possible that the damage may be related to multiple microinfarctions resulting from vascular spasm or hypertensive crises (Ardila, Rosselli, & Strumwasser, 1990). As Stuss and Cummings (1990) have indicated, small vessel infarctions are associated with the development of subcortical vascular dementia. Lastly, it is known that hypoperfusion of subcortical, temporal, and frontal lobe areas can be associated with deficits in neuropsychological functioning (Strickland *et al.*, 1991).

Stimulants

After marijuana and inhalants, stimulants as a group of illicit drugs are the next most widely used drug by teenagers (University of Michigan, 1994). The University of Michigan survey found a lifetime use rate of 11.8% by eighth graders and 14.9% by tenth graders. Daily use of stimulants by high school seniors has remained at 0.2% since 1990 and is down from the years prior to 1990.

Stimulants can be grouped into three categories: amphetamines, dextroamphetamines, and methamphetamines. Although the structure of each of these synthetic drugs is different, each can produce similar long-lasting effects, similar to the effects reported with cocaine use. Stimulants differ primarily in their strength and duration of effect. Stimulants act on the CNS by potentiating the effects of norepinephrine and activating areas of the sympathetic nervous system (Young, Young, Klein, Klein, & Beyer, 1977).

Tolerance develops rapidly to the euphoric effects of stimulants and the large doses necessary to reproduce the original effect may produce adverse mental status changes. Stimulant toxicity may include repetitive teeth grinding, touching, picking of the face or extremities, perseveration of speech or

behavior, preoccupation with one's own behavior and mental activity, suspiciousness, paranoia with auditory and visual hallucinations, hyperactivity, confusion, hypertension, tachypnea, convulsions, cardiovascular collapse, and high fever progressing to death (Bukstein, 1995; Ricaurte & Langston, 1995). Withdrawal from stimulant use can produce extreme depression, fatigue somnolence up to 20 hours a day, and apathy. Persistent mood anxiety and minor perceptual changes may last up to several months (Bukstein, 1995; Cho, 1990).

In recent years a new illicit dosage form of methamphetamine has been introduced into the drug market. One form referred to as "ice" consists of pure dextro-methamphetamine which is crystallized and then usually inhaled or smoked. The potential toxic reactions from prolonged use are similar to other amphetamines. Despite these dangers, users often perceive smoking ice as easier to use and even safer than other drugs (Bukstein, 1995).

Some teenagers in search of a new high are snorting or injecting Ritalin, a prescriptive drug designed to treat attention deficit disorder. Although Ritalin was abused by teens in the 1970s, its use decreased in the 1980s. Ritalin has recently begun to reemerge. It shares the same properties as other stimulants and can cause heart attacks and strokes (Manning, 1995).

Trites, Suh, Offord, Neiman, and Preston (1974) evaluated the neuropsychological functioning of a group of adolescents of average IQ who were amphetamine users. Results of the Halstead–Reitan Neuropsychological Battery failed to indicate brain dysfunction. In another well-controlled study of chronic stimulant users, Grant, Adams, Carlin, and Rennick (1977) were uanble to find evidence of neuropsychological impairment. A few researchers (Rylander, 1972; Schuckit, 1994; Young *et al.*, 1977) have suggested that the use of stimulants may damage the CNS and disrupt memory, concentration, and abstract reasoning skills. None of the researchers presented collaborating evidence.

There is very little literature on the neuropsychological effects of amphetamine use with adults or with children. There are no data addressing the issue of the long-term effects of amphetamines (Hartman, 1995). There has been research investigating the exposure of infants to methamphetamine prenatally. The effects that have been documented are similar to those discovered in so-called "cocaine babies" including lethargy, tremor, increased intra-ventricular hemorrhage, and other CNS structural damage (Voorhees, 1994).

Alcohol

Alcohol is the most misused drug by children and adolescents in the United States. There has been a very modest decrease in lifetime prevalence of alcohol use among high school seniors from a peak of 93.2% in 1980 to 87% in 1993. The lifetime prevalence of alcohol use has not shown the same dramatic declines noted in the past decade with illegal substances such as marijuana and cocaine (University of Michigan, 1994). The latter survey found that over 50% of senior students reported consuming alcohol during a preceding 30-day period. It is noteworthy that for 12- to 17-year-olds, 25.2% of the students reported experiencing blackouts (U. S. DHHS, 1991). Ethyl alcohol, or ethanol, the same active ingredient used in beer, wine, and distillates, is classified as a CNS depressant. At modest blood levels below 100 mg/ml, there may be a few psychoactive effects. As the blood alcohol level passes 100 mg/ml, mild sedation, decreased anxiety, and increases in social disinhibition may take place. Impairment in visual motor skills and coordination, integration of sensory stimulation and information processing becomes apparent. Higher blood levels of alcohol eventually result in sedation, CNS depression, stupor, and coma (Bukstein, 1995). Tolerance and physical and psychological dependence develop over time with diagnosable alcoholism becoming established after 3 to 15 years of prolonged use (Young et al., 1977). Rarely do children or adolescents experience seizures, hallucinations, or DTs, which are frequently reported in heavy adult users who have used alcohol for a prolonged period of time. Because of its common use, alcohol may be taken with other psychoactive substances to potentiate or to soften the effects of the other substances (Bukstein, 1995). Frequent heavy drinking in adolescence appears to be self-limiting and does not appear to be predictive of alcoholism in adults (Blane, 1976).

In regard to reversibility of alcohol deficits, subjects under age 35 to 40 generally return to normal performance levels within 3 months after they have stopped drinking. Older subjects showed improvement but remain in the impaired range on neurocognitive tasks (Goldman, 1982). Parsons (1993) noted that there was sufficient biomedical evidence indicating that detoxified, sober alcoholics had altered brain structures and that even when sober had detriments on measures of intellectual functions involving cognitive, perceptual, and perceptual–motor skills. After reviewing a number of studies on recovery, Parsons (1993) concluded that improvement did occur but extended over a 5-year period for many alcoholics.

The area of the cerebral cortex that appears to be uniquely sensitive to alcohol abuse is the frontal lobes, although MRI scans and postmortem studies have implicated the temporal and parietal lobes as well (Jernigan, Butters, DiTraglia, & Cemark, 1991). Clinical signs associated with damage to the frontal cortex include emotional apathy, disinhibition, poor attention, and abnormal perseverative responding (Oscar-Berman & Hutner, 1993).

Although the study of the social and personality effects of alcohol on children, adolescents, and adults has received considerable attention in recent years, there have been very few studies of the neuropsychological effects of alcohol abuse on children and teens (Tarter & Edwards, 1985). Defining and differentiating alcohol abuse and alcohol dependence in these studies of youthful drinkers has been difficult because many of the characteristic medical problems, such as cirrhosis and pancreatitis associated with alcohol abuse, have not had enough time to develop in younger individuals.

Aasly, Storsaeter, Nilsen, and Smevik (1993) investigated the structural brain changes evident in twenty-three 20- to 29-year-old drug abusers and seventeen 21- to 30-year-old male controls. Each of the subjects underwent clinical and neurological examinations and MRI of the brain. The drug-abusing group used cannabis, inhalants, opiates, psychedelics, hallucinogens, amphetamines, and cocaine. The drug abuse was always combined with heavy alcohol consumption. One drug abuser had abnormal neurological findings and three others had mild imbalance. MRI examinations showed that drug abusers had significantly smaller vermes cerebelli compared with controls and there were significant white matter changes more often in the drug-abusing group. The researchers concluded that the results were probably related to high alcohol consumption in combination with drug abuse. They suggested that alcohol was a more potent brain toxic agent than the most commonly abused narcotic drugs.

Eckhardt, Stapleton, Rawlings, Davis, and Grodin (1995) investigated the cognitive functioning of detoxified alcoholics who had alcohol-related problems for a relatively brief period of time. The subjects were 101 detoxified, drug-free alcoholics between the ages of 18 and 35 (mean age 26 with 13 years of education) who had consumed an average of 114 g four to five times a week for an average of 6 years. An extensive battery of neuropsychological tests including measures of language skills, attention, motor skills, intelligence, memory, and cognitive functioning related to frontal lobe functioning were administered an average of 39 days after their last drink. All subjects were inpatients in a military recovery program who had been admitted with a diagnosis of alcohol dependence. The major finding of this study was that measures of language skills, attention, motor skills, intelligence, memory, and cognitive functioning related to frontal regions of the brain and cognitive style were all within normal limits. Only 4 of the 101 individuals performed at levels indicative of mild cognitive dysfunction. The researchers concluded that an average of 6 years of excessive alcohol consumption was not associated with clinically significant cognitive impairment in a group of relatively young alcoholics after an average of 39 days of abstinence.

A number of studies have identified neuropsychological deficits associated with adolescent alcohol abuse. Krull, Tivis, Blanco, Hames, and Smith (1994) compared a group of alcohol-abusing, conduct-disordered, and normal control adolescents on a battery of neuropsychological tests and electrophysiological measures. They utilized tests that were sensitive to frontal lobe functions and auditory and visual event-related potentials (ERPs). They found that alcohol abuse as well as familial history of alcoholism were associated with impaired performance on neuropsychological and electrophysiological measures. The effect of alcohol abuse was particularly noted on frontal lobe measures. The neurotoxic effects of alcohol during periods of cortical maturation adversely affected abstract reasoning and flexibility. The authors did not address the issue of length of sobriety and, therefore, may have been addressing issues related to acute alcohol abuse rather than chronic effects.

Pogge (1994) studied 11 adolescents admitted for alcohol abuse alone and 38 admitted for cannabis abuse with or without alcohol or other substance abuse problems. These two groups were compared with a group of adolescents with no history of substance abuse. The differences between the two groups were relatively small although the alcohol-abusing group manifested more cognitive and attentional abnormalities than the other sub-

stance abusers. Specifically, there was evidence of deficits in working memory on a serial addition test. The substance abusers made more errors of omission than control subjects on continuous performance tests, suggesting differences in sustained attention (Pogge, Stokes, & Harvey, 1992). Again, in this study there was a minimal period of time that had passed between last use of alcohol or other drugs and the assessment process. What may have been measured were acute rather than long-term or chronic effects.

The cognitive performance of young social drinkers was investigated by Hannon, Day, Butler, Larson, and Casey (1983). The Shipley, Wisconsin Card Sorting Test, Digit Symbol Test, Trail Making Test, and TPT were administered to a group of 52 female and 40 male college students (mean age 20.3 years). The subjects were asked to refrain from taking any drugs or consuming alcohol for 24 hours prior to testing. The results indicated decreased neuropsychological performance with increased quantity of alcohol per occasion and total lifetime consumption by both sexes. Women appeared to be more adversely affected neuropsychologically by social drinking than men.

Hannon et al. (1985) replicated their 1983 study with a larger sample, a longer period of no alcohol use, and made a few changes in the tests administered to the subjects. The 103 female and 67 male college students (mean age 20.8 years) were administered the Raven's Advanced Progressive Matrices, Shipley, Wisconsin Card Sorting Test, and Digit Symbol Test. The Trail Making Test and TPT were dropped from the test battery. The subjects were asked to refrain from consumption of any alcohol for 2 weeks prior to testing. With the 1-week added period of sobriety, there was a predicted negative relationship between quantity and cognitive variables for women, and three unpredicted relationships for men. The correlations were weak and conclusions speculative.

In one of the few studies that investigated the role of age of drinking onset on neuropsychological functioning, Portnoff (1982) administered the WAIS, Shipley, Wechsler Memory Scale, and an abbreviated version of the Halstead–Reitan Neuropsychological Battery to two groups of ten chronic alcoholics dichotomized by age of drinking onset. The early onset group had started drinking steadily at 14.1 years of age (range 12–18) and drank for an average of 19.4 years. The later-onset group started drinking steadily at 23.4 years (range 20–30) and drank for an average of 16.5 years. Prior to testing, all of the subjects discontinued taking all medication and had been alcohol free for an average of 3.8 weeks. The groups were matched for sex, education, race, and handedness. Significant differences on the Shipley, Wechsler Memory Scale, Category Test, Trails B, and Rhythm Test suggested that early onset alcoholics developed more impairment on measures of abstraction, rhythm perception, visuospatial sequencing, verbal memory, and figural memory. It appeared that individuals who started drinking at an early age may have been more vulnerable to the adverse neuropsychological effects of alcohol than individuals who started drinking at a later age. The researchers did not review early school or medical records to control for premorbid developmental differences between the two groups, the early onset drinkers had been drinking 3 years longer than the later-onset drinkers, and the sample sizes were very small. As a result, the findings of this study, although strongly suggestive, were not conclusive.

The few studies focusing on the neuropsychological effects of alcohol abuse on children and adolescents have suggested deficits in abstracting, attention, and problem-solving skills. Memory deficits have been implicated although very few child studies have adequately assessed memory functions. Complicating research conclusions with adolescents and children is the fact that adults suffer from alcohol-related and chronic medical problems and psychological withdrawal symptoms at a much greater rate than children and adolescents. This may be a result of children's relatively short drinking history. It is possible that related health problems compromise neuropsychological functioning but take a longer period of time to develop (Bukstein, 1994). Neuroimaging studies have demonstrated that chronic alcoholism produces widespread brain damage in older adults but such evidence has not been apparent with children and adults. In child and adolescent alcohol use studies, longitudinal investigations are needed to pinpoint specific neuropsychological functions affected by alcohol use correlated with chronological age. From the research reviewed, it is likely that neuropsychological impairment caused by alcohol abuse is more likely to become evident from neuropsychological assessments than from neuroimaging or standard physiologic investigative techniques.

Phencyclidine (PCP)

PCP was developed by pharmacological researchers as an animal anesthetic in 1956. In 1957 human clinical trials were initiated, but the discovery of adverse side effects forced discontinuation of all human research by 1965. PCP became available as a "street drug" in 1966 in San Francisco (Elliott, 1989). Although PCP is generally identified by users as a hallucinogen, it cannot be accurately placed in any single drug category. Among drug experts, PCP is identified as a tranquilizer/anesthetic with hallucinogenic properties (Young *et al.,* 1977). The effects can vary, depending on the dosage, other drug involvement, age of the user, personality traits, route of administration, and physical setting. PCP increases the activity of the brain dopamine system and interferes with the synaptic transmission between cells (Institute of Medicine, National Academy of Sciences, 1985). Since 1972, abuse of PCP has increased dramatically and episodically in several ways. In 1993, 1.4% of high school seniors reported using PCP during the past year, most within the preceding month (*Health and Human Services News,* January 31, 1994). PCP is most commonly used by persons between 12 and 25 years old.

Little is known about the neuropsychological effects of PCP, although clinical observations have indicated a progression from irritability to violence as PCP use is continued (Fauman & Fauman, 1979). One of the problems with evaluating the effects of PCP is that PCP-abusing populations are generally polydrug abusers, which makes the unique contributions of PCP to cognitive impairment difficult to establish. A further difficulty is that a sizable proportion of PCP sold on the streets contains other chemical agents with dissimilar pharmacological structure but similar behavioral effects (Lewis & Hordan, 1986). PCP produces dramatic changes in behavior, memory, perception, and orientation. Because of these effects, researchers have been concerned that PCP abuse may result in permanent damage to the CNS, yet there has been very little formalized research completed on neuropsychological sequelae of PCP abuse (Grant & Reed, 1985).

Ware (1979) studied the cognitive performance of eight chronic PCP users and that of a group of eight polydrug, non-PCP users. The subjects (mean age 19 to 20 years) were inpatients at a state hospital matched for age, education, sex, race, current medication and dosage level, and handedness. Testing was not initiated until all subjects had been free of any drug use for a minimum of 3 weeks. The Halstead–Reitan Neuropsychological Battery and the WAIS were administered to all subjects. The researchers found that PCP users performed worse than the polydrug users on WAIS IQ measures. They also performed worse on selected subtests of the WAIS and on the Speech Sounds Perception Test of the Halstead–Reitan Neuropsychological Battery. The PCP group was more neuropsychologically impaired than the polydrug group but the differences did not reach a level of statistical significance. Complicating the study findings were a failure to employ a non-drug-using control group, use of small sample sizes, and a recognition that half of the patients were on some type of psychotropic medication. The two groups also differed in IQ, history of alcohol consumption, and psychiatric disorders.

Carlin, Grant, Adams, and Reed (1979) investigated the chronic effects of PCP with chronic PCP users versus normal controls and polydrug abusers who did not use PCP. The three groups (average age 25.9 years) were matched for age, education, sex, and race. Both drug-using groups displayed deficits in abstracting abilities and complex perceptual–motor skills, but these groups could not be distinguished on the basis of the test results. Weaknesses in this study included use of a small sample size, reliance on self-reports for medical and drug use history, lack of external neurological criteria, higher IQ for the control than for the polydrug group, and failure to control for use of ethanol by both drug groups.

Crane (1984) evaluated the effects of chronic long-term PCP ingestion on cognitive functioning in adolescents. Three groups of individuals were selected from a residential treatment program and matched for age (average age 16 years, range 15–20), sex, ethnicity, and education. Group one included ten subjects with a history of polydrug and PCP use, group two included ten polydrug users who had not used PCP, and group three included ten non-drug-using controls. The drug-using groups had used drugs at least twice a week for 6 consecutive months but had not used any drug during the 3-month period prior to testing. A standard neurological examination, EEG, the WAIS, and the Halstead–Reitan Neuropsychological Battery were administered. The only significant difference between the groups was that the PCP/polydrug group displayed more abnormal findings on cranial nerve VIII measures. Crane concluded that PCP's long-term effects may not impair cortical but may impair subcortical functions regulated by the brain stem.

Lewis and Hordan (1986) studied 30 adolescents and young adults who were referred to drug abuse counseling (presumably PCP from the context of the article). Tests most sensitive to impairment in this population included Trails B, where 30% showed scores above the brain damage cutoff, and the Category Test, where more than 70% of the sample were in the mild, moderate, or severely impaired range. About 60% of the sample also performed "below normal" on the Finger Tapping Test, suggesting impaired fine motor performance or a motivational deficit. Baldridge and Bessen (1990) found that children under the age of 5 who become intoxicated on PCP show lethargy, staring, or depression of consciousness. Aggression or violence was unusual.

In a five-part study of the effects of PCP on adolescent cognitive functioning, Light (1984) reviewed medical records and test results to determine whether polydrug/non-PCP, moderate PCP, and heavy PCP use correlated with neuropsychological test results. In Study I, Light reviewed the medical records of one hundred sixteen 17-year-olds who had been assessed approximately 12 days after admission to a drug treatment facility. The Shipley, Wide Range Achievement Test, Benton Visual Retention Test, and MMPI were administered to each subject. Heavy PCP users scored lower than the other groups on the Shipley but there was a question whether the heavy PCP group had fully recovered from the acute effects of PCP at the time they were tested.

In Study II, Light (1984) administered a neuropsychological battery to fifty-two 18- to 21-year-olds who were classified as polydrug/non-PCP users, moderate PCP users, or heavy PCP users. The drug-using groups were assessed 4 to 6 days and the heavy PCP users were assessed 149 days after their last drug use. The Halstead–Reitan Neuropsychological Battery, two memory items from the Luria–Nebraska, Wide Range Achievement Test, WAIS, and Trail Making Test were administered. Only the Trails A time was significantly different across the three groups. Light was unable to match the subjects on a number of demographic variables, length of sobriety was much longer for the heavy PCP users, and the non-PCP group may have been more impaired because of problems associated with use of other drugs.

All researchers acknowledge that PCP has dramatic acute effects on the CNS but the effects vary greatly between individuals. Dosage level appears to be a critical element. Heavy users develop more pathology than light users. Because of the lingering acute effects of PCP, the study of chronic effects has been difficult. Whether chronic PCP abuse leads to long-lasting neuropsychological complications remains unclear. The confounds of high rates of head trauma, seizure, and childhood chronic otitis media, attention and learning disorder, together with the questionable nature of the substances sold as PCP, make these studies difficult to interpret (Lewis & Hordan, 1986). Still, most of the available research with adolescents and young adults does indicate neuropsychological impairment with chronic, long-term use. Motor performance skills appear to be more adversely affected than verbal skills. Memory and language disturbances have been reported but are not well documented (Aniline & Pitts, 1982).

Inhalants

Inhalant abuse involves the voluntary inhalation of the fumes from aerosols, anesthetics, or other substances, in an effort to achieve an intoxicated state. The "high" is dose related, cumulative over a short period of time, and may persist for periods ranging from a few minutes to a few hours. Most abusers began sniffing in their preteen or early adolescent years. Addictive behavior patterns associated with abuse of inhalants are common. The abuse of these substances can result in what has been called sudden sniffing death syndrome (SSDS) (Greer, 1984). All solvents depress CNS activity by an anesthetic action. Individuals who abuse solvents become progressively less sensitive to the solvent as a function of solvent concentration and exposure duration until unconsciousness, coma, or death occurs.

Inhalation of solvents has become a problem of international scope. Montoya-Cabrera (1990) estimated that in Mexico City there were about 500,000 children addicted to various substances, more commonly to organic solvents, because of their low cost and euphoriant effect. Children as young as 4 to 7 have been reported with "marked addiction" to organic solvent inhalation. The typical solvent abuser in the United States is a young male between 7 and 17 years old. Inhalants are one of the few illicit substances that have failed to show significant declines in use by adolescents during the past two decades. In fact, among high school seniors there has been a gradual increase over the past 16 years. Lifetime prevalence in 1990 was 18.0% and in 1993 17.4% for high school seniors (Bukstein, 1995).

Inhalants are diverse in their physiological, pharmacological, and behavioral effects, yet most researchers tend to treat inhalants as a single class of drugs. Toluene, contained in glues, solvents, and paint sprays (Callen, 1984), does not target a single organ system. Comstock and Comstock (1977) reported that nervous system and liver and kidney problems have been associated with toluene use. n-Hexane use has been clearly associated with polyneuropathy (Grant & Reed, 1985). Gasoline vapor inhalation can cause motor-neuronal degeneration, disorders of the hematopoietic system, and encephalopathy because of the various additives (i.e., TCP, lead, and benzene) found in gasoline. Aerosols containing Freon can cause hypercapnia, cardiac arrhythmia, renal tubular necrosis, uremia, and sudden death (Wilde, 1975). Inhalation of propane gas can cause vision and hearing problems as well as chronic memory problems (Stepp, 1994). Typewriter correction fluids have been associated with visual disturbances, multiple nerve palsies, and peripheral neuropathy (Greer, 1984).

Inhalants that have been identified as possible abusive substances include the medical anesthetic gases (ether, chloroform, halothane, nitrous oxide); industrial or household solvents (paint thinner, degreasers, solvents in glue); art and office-supply solvents (correction fluid and solvents in marker pens); gases used in household or commercial products (butane lighters, gasoline, whipped cream dispensers, electronic equipment dusters and cleaners, refrigerant replenishers); household aerosol propellants (as in paint, hair spray, and fabric protector spray); and aliphatic nitrates ("poppers").

Glue Sniffing

Hormes, Filley, and Rosenberg (1986) evaluated 20 subjects with a history of chronic solvent vapor abuse who were participants in a rehabilitation program. Most of the subjects were in high school when they began sniffing. The mean age was 27.4 years with 9.2 mean years of education. All subjects were evaluated with a detailed neurological and substance abuse history, a standard neurological examination, a standardized neurobehavioral examination, and lab evaluations including DDRL. Some of the subjects were also given EMG, EEG, CSF, and evoked potentials. All subjects had used one or two products that contained toluene for a mean duration of 145.1 months. Over half of the subjects also admitted to use of other substances including amphetamines, marijuana, and alcohol. All subjects were evaluated after an abstinence period of at least 4 weeks to reduce acute intoxication findings. Neurological impairment indicators were evident in 65% of the subjects. Sixty percent of the subjects had cognitive dysfunction with abnormalities in attention, memory, visuospatial functions, complex cognition, naming, and reading or writing. Diffuse atrophy of cerebral hemispheres, cerebellum, and, in severe cases, brain stem were evident in 88.8% of the subjects. Three of seven EEGs revealed diffuse continuous slowing. Four individuals revealed abnormalities of brain stem auditory evoked potentials. The researchers concluded that there was evidence of cognitive dysfunction and cerebellar, corticospinal, and brain stem signs suggesting diffuse CNS effects. There was continued improvement in five patients who had been abstinent for 6 or more months, suggesting that recovery may proceed after solvent use is discontinued.

Malm and Lying-Tunell (1980) evaluated an 18-year-old female who had inhaled pure toluene beginning at the age of 12 years. Development of neurological symptoms, including ataxic gait, incoordination of arms and legs, unsteadiness, dysarthria, poor coordination, and reduced abstracting ability, were evident. During a 5-week period of hospitalization during which time she did not inhale toluene, her symptoms persisted but decreased. After 8 months her symptoms had disappeared. Although the researchers indicated that her symptoms had disappeared, the only examination that was conducted at that time was a physical examination that included a measure of visual acuity. It is likely that the physical examination and test of visual acuity were not methods that would be sensitive to brain stem involvement or to other less obvious neuropsychological indices.

Foo, Jeyaratnam, and Koh (1990) assessed the neurobehavioral performance of a group of 30 female assembly workers who had been exposed to toluene. The toluene emanated from resinous glue used to cement component parts. A control group of 30 workers from a different part of the factory (mean age 25 years) were matched for age, sex, and ethnicity. A neurobehavioral test battery that included the Benton Visual Retention Test, Visual Reproduction Test, Trail Making Test, Grooved Pegboard, Digit Span and Digit Symbol subtests, Finger Tapping, and simple reaction time were administered to each of the subjects and controls. Test performance by the exposed subjects was weaker on most of the other measures compared with the control group. There was no difference on the Finger Tapping. A dose–effect relationship was noted on six of the eight neurobehavioral tests. Although

motor speed was not affected by exposure to toluene, manual dexterity, visual scanning, and verbal memory were adversely affected with exposure to toluene ranging from 49 to 130 ppm.

Allison and Jerrom (1984) compared the psychological test performance of ten Scottish adolescents (mean age 15 years) who had inhaled solvents for an average of 4½ years against ten matched control subjects who had never inhaled solvents. The primary toxic component in the glue was toluene/acetone. Using a number of measures of intelligence, memory, and attention, the researchers concluded that long-term abusers of toluene/acetone demonstrated weaker attention, verbal and visual memory, and visuospatial problem-solving skills compared with a control group. Verbal abilities remained intact. The conclusions of this study were tentative because the study was not blind, the test administrator being aware of the group assignment of each subject. Also, the assessment process may have been assessing acute rather than chronic residual effects of solvent abuse as the subjects had last used 10 days to 6 weeks prior to testing.

Channer and Stanley (1983) assessed a 16-year-old male who had begun to experience visual hallucinations after inhaling a toluene/acetone-based glue for 3 months. Four months after he stopped sniffing glue a normal CT scan was recorded with diffusely abnormal EEG and delayed visual evoked responses (VERs). Even after a period of 8 months of sobriety, the hallucinations continued. The EEG remained unchanged and the VERs only minimally improved.

Tsushima and Towne (1977) evaluated a group of 20 toluene-sniffing subjects (mean age 18.5 years) from low-income housing projects. Although other drugs had been used, paint fume inhalation was primary. The researchers reported the subjects inhaled an average of 2.3 cans of paint per day for periods ranging from 2 to 13 years. A matched control group of 20 non-paint-sniffing individuals, matched for age, education, and sex, was utilized. The Finger Tapping Test, Seashore Rhythm Test, Trail Making Test, Grooved Pegboard, WISC-R coding subtest, Stroop Color and Word Test, Memory for Designs, and Peabody Picture Vocabulary Test were administered. Significant differences (≥ 0.05) were evident between the sniffers and the controls on 11 of the 13 measured variables. Sniffers exhibited weaker performances on measures of motor speed, auditory discrimination, visual–motor function, and memory. Limitations of the study included a lack of information about the chemical elements in the paint and the possibility that there were preexisting deficits in the sniffers. In addition, the sniffers admitted to inhaling paint the day before the assessment.

In one of the earliest studies of glue sniffing, Massengale, Glaser, LeLievre, Dodds, and Klock (1963) assessed 12 boys (age 6 to 16 years with a mean age of 13) for cognitive functioning 12 hours to 7 days after their last contact with glue (toluene). Five tests assessing attention, fine motor performance, detection of changes, design integration, and design recall were administered. Despite inhalation of glue for periods ranging from 1 to 42 months, there were no significant differences between the performance or physical characteristics of glue sniffers and a matched control group.

Gasoline Inhalation

Prejean and Gouvier (1994) described the neuropsychological deficits experienced by two subjects (aged 19 and 20 years) who inhaled gasoline fumes, one leaded and the other unleaded. A number of sensory, motor function, language, sensorimotor integration, and language tests as well as the WAIS-R and Wechsler Memory Scale were administered to both subjects. The results of this assessment demonstrated residual left hemisphere deficits including weaker verbal IQ and verbal memory, fine sensory and motor dysfunction, and tactile memory deficits. The test results suggested that the deficits were related to factors other than the presence of lead additives. However, the study was compromised by a lack of awareness by the researchers of the subjects' premorbid IQ levels, and the subjects' use of other illicit drugs during the period of the assessment.

The inhalation of gasoline fumes for the purpose of intoxication became a widespread problem following World War I (Lewis & Patterson, 1974). This fad faded until the 1950s when literature on the effects of gas sniffing began to reappear (Faucett & Jensen, 1952), but the focus had changed from the effects on adults to the effects on children. Researchers began to express concern about the effects of leaded gasoline because lead, as a causative agent, had been implicated in irreversible changes in cognitive functioning (Ross, 1982).

Seshia, Rajani, Boeckx, and Chow (1978) completed standard neurological evaluations (EEG, nerve conduction study, ECG, blood profile, X ray, and urine assay) on 50 Native American subjects aged 4 to 20 who were being treated for inhalation of leaded gasoline. Inhalation of gas vapors occurred for 6 months in the youngest child to over 5 years in those older than 12. Acute, but abnormal, neurological signs were apparent in 92% of the subjects at day one. At 8 weeks, only one patient manifested residual neurological signs. This study suggested that although the acute neurological effects of gasoline vapor inhalation are acutely significant, over time the adverse effects dissipate.

These studies suggest that results of neurological examinations are usually normal except in the most severe cases. More subtle and subclinical psychological effects tend to be seen earlier in abusers' history of exposure. When neuropsychological symptoms are apparent, they tend to suggest diffuse cortical and subcortical damage.

Multisolvent Inhalation

Comstock (1977) evaluated twenty-two 17-year-olds (range 13 to 26) who were in treatment for solvent (toluene primarily) abuse. The patients had inhaled solvents for an average of 4 years (range 1 to 11). Twenty of the patients reported abuse of other drugs as well as inhalants. The evaluation process included EEG, EMG, nerve–muscle biopsy, and a general medical lab examination. The Halstead–Reitan Neuropsychological Battery was administered to two subjects. Despite heavy exposure to volatile solvents, the medical examination did not identify CNS abnormalities. The mental status examination identified "mental-grasp deficiencies" in 55% of the patients soon after their admission. Two weeks later there was a clearing of these deficiencies. Of the two patients administered the Halstead–Reitan Battery, one scored in the pathological range on a number of the subtests. The authors hinted at the possibility of residual impairment adversely affecting the ability of the patient to benefit from "talking psychotherapy." Limitations to this study included lack of a control group and a failure to report on preexisting or contributing conditions.

In one of the better, well-controlled studies of the effects of chronic inhalant abuse, Bigler (1979) completed extensive neuropsychological evaluations on 16- to 19-year-olds (mean age 17.8) with a history of chronic inhalant abuse (range 2 to 6 years). The same testing was performed on control groups matched for age, sex, and education. The control groups of ten patients each were: (a) brain damaged, (b) psychotic non-brain-damaged, and (c) non-brain-damaged/nonpsychotic. Neuropsychological evaluations were initiated about 48 days after admission and included administration of the WAIS, Category Test, TPT, Rhythm Test, Speech-Sounds Perception Test, Finger Tapping Test, and Trail Making Test. The inhalant abuse group scored within the impaired range on most measures and was similar to the brain-damaged group on neuropsychological measures. The deficits suggested diffuse cerebral dysfunction. The findings were compromised because seven of the ten inhalant abusers were on neuroleptic medication such as Thorazine, Haldol, Cogentin, Mellaril, or Navane at the time of testing.

Berry, Heaton, and Kirby (1978) evaluated 37 inhalant-abusing youths (average age 18 years, range 14 to 29) who were in treatment for drug abuse. The inhalant-abusing group snorted an average of more than three times a day for periods ranging from 1½ to 17 years (average 5.5). The control group consisted of 11 subjects matched for age, sex, ethnicity, education background, and use of substances other than inhalants. A complete neuropsychological evaluation revealed weaker neuropsychological test results with the inhalant group than with the control group. The researchers concluded that inhalant abuse caused impairment.

Korman, Matthews, and Lovitt (1981) tested 109 volunteer teenage subjects who had used drugs. The range of use was unreported but 68 reported inhalants to be their major drug of abuse. The Wechsler, Halstead–Reitan Neuropsychological Battery, grip strength, motor speed, and academic achievement measures were administered to all subjects. The researchers concluded that inhalant abusers developed deficits in a wider range of cognitive areas than was previously known. The integrity of these test findings was compromised because there was no drug-using control group and all of the abusers were multidrug users. The performances of both groups were weak and there was no mention of the time elapsed since last use of the drug.

Other Inhalants

Nitrous oxide, or laughing gas, has been abused in the past 100 years. Perhaps 5% of the population has inhaled laughing gas to achieve a high. Nitrous oxide is classified as an anesthetic characterized by sedation and decreased memory. Although intoxication with nitrous oxide is achieved very rapidly and dissipates within 5 minutes or so after stopping inhalation, there is evidence of impairments in memory and psychomotor performance (Schuckit, 1995a). Parry (1995) noted that

chronic intoxication with nitrous oxide produced a myeloneuropathy that was clinically identical to subacute degeneration of the spinal cord resulting from vitamin B_{12} deficiency.

The evidence is clear that inhalation of most, if not all, solvent fumes produces acute CNS effects, including peripheral neuropathy. The issue is much less clear about the long-term chronic effects of inhalants on cognitive functioning. The evidence is much more suggestive of permanent CNS impairment when multiple solvents are inhaled. Such impairment is apt to be general and most likely will affect complex and higher-order neuropsychological processes.

Methodological problems and experimental artifacts complicate any conclusions. Very few studies are longitudinal and rarely are presniffing differences reported in the research or addressed. Although radiologic investigations could add valuable diagnostic information, such techniques were generally not used. There are even fewer neuropsychological investigative reports to confirm or refute the presence of organic changes.

Marijuana/Hashish

Marijuana today is about ten times more potent than the marijuana available in the 1970s. Hashish is a refined form of marijuana containing about 8% marijuana and about eight times the amount of Δ-9-tetrahydrocannabinol (THC) found in most marijuana (Bell, 1985). Marijuana acts on the CNS as a depressant, although some researchers (Kissin, 1977) treat it as a hallucinogen. University of Michigan (1994) researchers, in an annual survey of 51,000 high school and eighth-grade youth, discovered that drug use by teenagers is on the rise again. They found that 9% of eighth graders, 19% of tenth graders, and 26% of twelfth graders reported using marijuana in the past year. This is an increase of 2 to 4% from the year earlier.

Marijuana users report euphoria, a relaxed state, sleepiness, heightened sexual arousal, hunger, decreased social interaction, short-term memory deficits, and difficulty completing multiple-step tasks (Schuckit, 1984). A large proportion of the animal and human research studies support the finding that at least mild levels of tolerance can be observed with repeated use. There are sufficient data to conclude that under some circumstances marijuana can produce a withdrawal syndrome. Such a syndrome is likely to be seen only after exceptionally high doses of marijuana or, perhaps, observed in a few highly vulnerable individuals responding to lower marijuana doses (Schuckit, 1995b). Addictive behavior patterns occur rarely.

Although Ricaurte and Langston (1995) indicated there was no evidence that chronic marijuana use produces long-term deleterious effects on the CNS, positive research findings have been published. Many of these studies included young abusers. Block and Ghoneim (1993) compared the performance of 23-year-old marijuana users with nonusers matched on intellectual functioning before the onset of drug use. The performance of chronic marijuana users and nonusers on the Iowa Test of Basic Skills taken during the fourth grade of grammar school was compared. The subjects were then given the twelfth grade versions of these tests and other computerized cognitive tests in successive test sessions. Marijuana users were identified as those individuals who had used marijuana at least weekly for a minimum of 2 years. The marijuana users promised to abstain from alcohol, marijuana, and other drugs for 24 hours before each testing session. Marijuana was smoked seven or more times weekly for 52 users, five or six times weekly for 28 users, and one to four times weekly for 64 users. The complication to the research study was that 90% of the heavy marijuana users had used cocaine, 8% had used psychedelics, 79% had used LSD, 79% had used amphetamines, 54% had used heroin, and 52% had used tranquilizers. Other drugs were also reported. The researchers found deficits in subjects who used marijuana seven or more times weekly in memory for high imaginary words. They also found deficits in mathematic skills and verbal expression on the Iowa Test of Educational Development in subjects who were previously matched by fourth grade test scores. Complicating their results was the fact that some of the marijuana users had used illicit drugs in the previous 30 days, which might have affected their performance. They relied on subjects to admit that they had not used marijuana and only had them commit to no use for 24 hours. Therefore, the effects may have been related to more acute factors than long-lasting factors. Yesavage, Leirer, Denari, and Hollister (1985) demonstrated that the flying performance of pilots was poor 24 hours after smoking marijuana.

Schwartz, Gruenewald, Klitzner, and Fedio (1989) evaluated the auditory–verbal and visual–spatial memory of 10 cannabis-dependent adolescents and compared the results with the performance of 17 subjects in two control groups. All three groups (median age 16 years) were matched for age, IQ, and absence of learning disability. A battery of seven neuropsychological tests was administered initially to all subjects and a parallel test battery was administered 6 weeks later. The study subjects were in an outpatient therapeutic community drug treatment program where the average duration of stay was 14 to 15 months. The 27 participants represented three groups of adolescents: cannabis-dependent (Group A), drug-free adolescents (Group B), and adolescent patients who had abused drugs but who had not been cannabis-dependent (Group C). To ensure that the study subjects remained drug free during the 6-week period, urine samples were taken. This study provided evidence of the lingering impact of marijuana use on selected short-term auditory and visual memory processes. Memory deficits persisted at the 6-week retest period. Limitations to the research findings were the small sample sizes and no differences between Groups A and C.

Fletcher (1987) studied the performance of 27 marijuana users and 30 nonusers in Costa Rica on sophisticated mental tests. Users in the all-male group averaged 6.4 marijuana cigarettes a day for an average of more than 30 years. This was a follow-up study to a 1973 study in Costa Rica. The researchers were successful in obtaining data on 61 of the 82 1973 subjects and conducted psychological tests on 57. Most of the users had continued smoking at the same level so they had been smoking heavily for more than 30 years. Subjects in the nonuser group were matched for age, education, IQ, and alcohol and tobacco consumption. The 1973 research had failed to find any impairment associated with even high levels of marijuana use. The follow-up study included several different psychological tests capable of detecting subtle changes in learning, memory, and concentration. Three of these tests indicated significant differences. The researchers found that on selected cognitive tests there were significant results. Users were slower in responding on a continuous performance test that required sustained attention and processing effort. Researchers tried to reduce the possibility that they were assessing acute, rather than chronic, effects of marijuana by asking the subjects to refrain from smoking the previous day and then testing early in the morning. The marijuana users had greater difficulties with sustained attention and short-term memory but the effects were very subtle and "subclinical." Limitations to the study included use of a small sample size, and not allowing a reasonable amount of time to pass to ensure that they were not assessing the user's last marijuana dose rather than any chronic effects.

Evidence of cerebral atrophy, including large left lateral ventricles, temporal lobe dilations, and damage to the region of the caudate nuclei and basal ganglia was found by air encephalography in ten male patients (average age 22 years) who had smoked marijuana over a period of 3 to 11 years (Campbell, Evans, Thompson, & Williams, 1971). Memory and concentration problems were evident in most of the subjects. A serious flaw to this research was introduced when the researchers failed to control for use of other drugs. Most of the subjects admitted to using other drugs. There was no indication as to when each subject had last used what drug.

Grant, Rochford, Fleming, and Stunkard (1973) evaluated 29 male medical students who had smoked marijuana an average of three times a month for 3 years and a non-drug-using control group. The median age of both users and controls was 23 years. The significant difference found between users and nonusers from a battery of tests was on the TPT Localization score. The sample was limited to bright, light to moderate users who may have been well compensated neurologically.

Carlin and Trupin (1977) evaluated a group of ten well-educated subjects (average age 24). The subjects were asked to abstain from marijuana use for 24 hours prior to administration of the Halstead Neuropsychological Battery. The only significant ($p < 0.05$) score difference between the users and nonusers was on the Trail Making Test, Part B. The researchers did find, surprisingly, that the user group performed better than the nonuser group.

Culver and King (1974) administered the Halstead Neuropsychological Battery, WAIS, Trail Making Test, Laterality Discrimination Test, and selected tests from the Kit of Factor-Referenced Cognitive Tests. The 84 subjects were 20 to 25 years of age. Three groups were created. Group 1 were LSD/mescaline users, Group 2 were marijuana/hashish users, and the third group served as controls. The marijuana/hashish users had used marijuana and/or hashish at least twice a month for at least 12 months. They could be classified as light to moderate users. The drug users agreed to abstain from all drug use for the 7 days preceding testing. There were no significant differences between the marijuana and hashish users and controls.

Millsaps, Azrin, Schneider, Burns, and Mittenberg (1995) compared 30 chronic marijuana users with 30 age-, education-, race-, occupation-, and sex-matched (average age 21 years) non-substance-using controls on the Wechsler Memory Scale-Revised and WAIS-R. Marijuana subjects had been abstinent for varying lengths of time (mean 29.1 days). Logical memory and visual reproduction retention results revealed no significant differences. The results suggested that marijuana use does not compromise memory or intelligence. The marijuana users met DSM-III-R criteria for marijuana dependence and had no significant history of alcohol or other substance abuse problems. Memory and intelligence did not appear to be adversely affected by marijuana use.

Conclusions cannot be drawn because most of the research generated to date on marijuana has been compromised by methodological problems and bias sampling. Nevertheless, with high use of marijuana there may be long-term effects. There is increasing research showing there may be subtle chronic effects even with adolescent users. There also may be a dose relationship. Memory test data appear to be the most significant generally showing reduced memory efficiency, at least during marijuana use.

Designer Drugs

Designer drugs are a group of substances that were created in an attempt to circumvent existing laws against production and distribution of certain controlled drugs. These drugs are similar in either structure or effect to substances already regulated by the Controlled Substances Act. The chemical variation is achieved by changing a few molecules of an existing illicit drug so that the newly created drug is modified enough molecularly to fall outside of existing regulations. Generally, designer drugs are hallucinogens or opiates. Because quality controls in the labs that create designer drugs are highly variable, the end product may be ten times weaker or ten times stronger than the drug being copied.

One designer drug that has become popular with adolescents is the consciousness-enhancing drug MDMA (3,4-methylenedioxymethamphetamine). MDMA, now a controlled substance, was recently banned because it was similar to a compound that had been shown to cause brain damage in animals. It is sold as Ecstasy, XTC, E, Adam, Eve, and

MDM. MDMA is a stimulating hallucinogen that has a number of characteristics in common with mescaline and LSD. There are data indicating possible chemical alterations in the brain that can last 6 months or longer after repeated use. Animal data demonstrate that relatively moderate doses of MDMA can cause potentially significant depletion of the brain chemical serotonin. Researchers studying MDMA have indicated there is no proof that it causes brain damage in humans (National Institute on Drug Abuse, 1994). Animal lab studies suggest that even after a single dose of MDMA, serotonin cells in the brain may be harmed (Turkington, 1986).

Another designer drug, the synthetic heroin substitute MPPP (methyl-4-phenyl-4-propionoxypiperidine), or when distilled at the wrong temperature or pH, the compound MPTP (1-methyl-4-phenyl-1,2,4,5-tetrahydropyridine) is created. This designer drug grew out of a chemist's attempt to elaborate an uncontrolled analogue of meperedine (Ricaurte & Langston, 1995). MPTP selectively destroys dopamine-producing neurons in the substantia nigra. The victims of this drug, most of whom are under 35 (Hartman, 1995), developed a syndrome that had all of the elemental features of Parkinson's disease including rigidity, stooped posture, tremor at rest, and difficulty speaking. There is no research on neurological evaluations of individuals who have taken MPTP or MPPP.

Recently, new synthetic analogues have appeared in the illicit drug market including 4-methyl-aminorex (Euphoria), *para*-methoxymethamphetamine (PMMA), and methcathinone (Cat), and there is preclinical evidence that at least PMMA and Cat are toxic to serotonin and dopamine neurons in rodents. The neurotoxic potential of these drugs in humans is unknown. Although no neuropsychological studies of designer drug effects have been published, the available information from emergency room visits and from animal research strongly indicates that the dangerous and toxic effects of these substances on the CNS may be substantial.

Lysergic Acid Diethylamide (LSD)

Although LSD is classified as a hallucinogen, it does not cause the user to hallucinate *per se*. The user of LSD views the world in a distorted fashion or misinterprets sensory experiences. LSD's acute effects are variable and unpredictable. Flashbacks can occur days or months after the initial dose; they are rare with the occasional user but are common with the frequent and repetitive user (Bukstein, 1995). LSD alters sensations, reasoning, mood states, and perception. The drug primarily acts on the visual cortex, limbic system, and reticular formation (Holbrook, 1983). Frequent and/or recurrent use of LSD may produce tolerance but there is no evidence of physical dependence or a withdrawal syndrome. As a hallucinogen there are other substances that, even though constructed with different synthetic compounds, produce many of the same effects. The group includes PCP, mescaline, psilocybin/psilocin, DOM, and DOB. Of all of the hallucinogens, LSD has the most neuropsychological research. Because of LSD's extreme psychopharmacological potency, various researchers have speculated that CNS damage might be a consequence of repeated exposure.

The National Senior or Monitoring the Future survey reports lifetime prevalence of total hallucinogen use at 10.9% of surveyed high school seniors. LSD makes up a majority of hallucinogen use with a lifetime prevalence of 10.3% in 1993. In 1993 eighth graders reported a lifetime prevalence of 3.9% for hallucinogens and a monthly prevalence of 1.2%. Generally, LSD use has been increasing gradually at the high school level during the last several years according to the Monitoring the Future survey. This increase follows a history of declines which came about after recognition of the dangers and risks attributed to LSD use (University of Michigan, 1994).

Cohen and Edwards (1969) completed one of the first studies of the effects of LSD on neuropsychological functioning. The Halstead–Reitan Neuropsychological Battery, Raven's Progressive Matrices, and a spatial orientation test were administered to two groups of 21-year-old volunteers matched for age, sex, and education. The LSD user group had an average of 70 LSD experiences but were known to also have used other drugs. The control group included inexperienced LSD users. It is not known if the control group used other drugs. Of the 15 scores obtained, the LSD user group displayed impaired functioning on the visual–spatial orientation and Trails A test. There appeared to be a positive correlation between frequency of use of LSD and performance on Trails A and Raven's Matrices. There was no evidence of generalized neuropsychological deficits. Confounds in this study that may have distorted the findings included a lack of knowledge of the premorbid levels of functioning of the subjects and lack of awareness of the use of alcohol and other drugs.

Wright and Hogan (1972) replicated the Cohen and Edwards (1969) study with 40 LSD users ranging in age from 17 to 24. The subjects had used LSD an average of 29 times during a period of 4½ to 27 months. At the time of testing it was determined that none of the LSD users were acutely toxic although four had used LSD the previous day. The Halstead–Reitan Neuropsychological Battery, Trail Making Test, WAIS, and an aphasia test were administered. No significant differences were found between the two groups but these findings may reflect the fact that the Wright and Hogan subjects used LSD, on average, less than half as many times as the Cohen and Edwards LSD users. It has been established in the literature that there is a dose-related effect.

Culver and King (1974) compared LSD/mescaline users and marijuana users with a control group who had no history of marijuana or LSD use. The Halstead–Reitan Neuropsychological Battery, WAIS, Laterality Discrimination Test, and three spatial–perceptual tests from the Kit of Factor-Referenced Cognitive Tests were administered to matched triads of 28 subjects each selected from a group of bright 20- to 25-year-old college seniors. The drug users were asked to stop using any drugs at least 7 days before testing. LSD users scored significantly lower than the marijuana and control groups on the WAIS performance and full scale IQ, Picture Completion subtest, cube comparison test, and the Trails A and B time scores. Culver and King repeated the same testing with new subjects who were similar to those in the first study. The second group of triads were more closely matched on the WAIS. In this study they found that the LSD user group was significantly weaker than the marijuana and control groups on the Trail Making Test. The only measure that reached a level of statistical significance on both studies for the LSD user group was the Trail Making Test. Although the LSD users' Trail Making Test times were slower than those of the marijuana and control groups, their performances were within the normal range.

Investigations of the effects of LSD on adolescent and young adult development have revealed very little new information during the last decade as evident by the paucity of new investigations on the effects of the drug. On those studies that have been reported, the researchers have generally used the same instrumentation. Although most studies reported impaired neuropsychological performance with chronic use of LSD, findings have been inconsistent from study to study. Some of these differences have resulted because of preexisting premorbid differences among the population studies, length of LSD use, and the time since last use of LSD. When significant findings have been evident, they have implicated abstract reasoning and speeded sequencing tasks, with overall levels of functioning remaining intact. Generally, the evidence suggests that LSD has subtle, dose-dependent effects on the CNS when used chronically.

Heroin and Other Opiates

Opiate analgesics include heroin, opium, codeine, hydromorphone (Dilaudid), oxycodone (Percodan), propoxyphene (Darvon), meperidine (Demerol), diphenoxylate (Lomotil), and pentazocine (Talwin) (Schuckit, 1984). The action of these drugs on the nervous system is homogeneous, tolerance develops rapidly, and all are extremely addictive. Heroin is a narcotic analgesic of the opiate class. It is a semisynthetic derivative of morphine that can be three times as potent as morphine (Young et al., 1977).

The Monitoring the Future survey revealed that only a small proportion of high school seniors report heroin or other opiate use. The peak of use was 2.2% of seniors in 1995. In 1991 the lifetime prevalence rate declined to 0.9%. The lifetime rate increased to 1.1% in 1993. The daily use of both heroin and other opiates is reported at almost insignificant levels in 1993, i.e., less than 0.1% of high school seniors (University of Michigan, 1994).

The physiologic effects of opium use include drowsiness, pinpoint pupils, reduced cough reflex, reduced vision, and constipation. Nausea, vomiting, and respiratory depression may result from large doses. In more severe states of intoxication, motor incoordination and slurred speech may be evident (Bukstein, 1995). Besides producing physiologic dependence, there is cross-tolerance between opiates.

Heroin is generally injected into the body but can also be taken orally, snorted, or smoked. Some addicts mix cocaine or amphetamines with heroin, producing a mixture called "speed ball." Parsons and Adams (1983) reported that 60% of persons who died of heroin overdose showed significant cerebral edema. Hill and Mikhad (1979) found significantly smaller sulci and ventricle–brain indexes in their study of adult heroin users.

The study of the neuropsychological effects of opiates began in 1974 when Fields and Fullerton reported an absence of performance differences on the Halstead–Reitan Neuropsychological Battery between a group of heroin addicts and medical controls. A third group included in the study had brain damage. The three groups of 25 subjects were matched for age, sex, and education. The heroin and control groups were also matched on IQ. The heroin addicts had used heroin an average of almost 5 years (range 1–10). The brain-damaged group performed significantly worse on the Halstead–Reitan Neuropsychological Battery than the heroin and control group, whose scores were equivalent. Information regarding premorbid history, use of alcohol, and extent of use of heroin was not provided.

Because of the absence of research on the chronic effects of heroin addiction on brain–behavior relationships, it is not clear what effects, if any, chronic heroin use has on long-term neuropsychological functions. Further study is required, particularly with youthful abusers and with heroin-using individuals who are not using other drugs.

Sedatives/Barbiturates

Barbiturates are CNS depressants that vary in duration of action. Barbiturates depress the CNS and interfere with synaptic functioning. Dosage, type of barbiturate, metabolism, use of other drugs, and environmental elements all affect the individual's reaction to the drug. Tolerance can quickly develop, thus making barbiturates highly dangerous. Most surveys separate sedatives and tranquilizers but both classes of agents are CNS depressants.

Although there is a great deal of research about cognitive impairment and affective consequences associated with alcohol abuse, there is a less extensive but nonetheless substantial literature on impairments produced by sedative hypnotics. A number of studies of long-term sedative abuse and dependence indicate that sedative hypnotics can cause depression, anxiety, and cognitive impairment (McLellan, Woody, & O'Brien, 1979). Most of these effects diminish with prolonged abstinence (Woody, McLellan, & O'Brien, 1990). The University of Michigan (1994) annual survey indicates that among high school seniors the lifetime use of sedatives has declined since the 1970s. In 1993 the use was 6.4% of surveyed seniors. Barbiturate use accounted for most of the sedative use by seniors with a similar pattern of decline reported over a lifetime. Lifetime tranquilizer use increased from a low of 6.0% in 1992 to 6.4% in 1993.

Bergman, Borg, Engelbrecktson, and Vikander (1989), in a follow-up to their 1980 study of 30 hypnotic–sedative abuse subjects, found a slight but significant improvement in neuropsychological functioning 4 to 6 years later. Although both subgroups improved significantly on seven of nine measures at the second evaluation, relapsed sedative–hypnotic abusers performed more poorly on a block design measure, the Trail Making Test, and on a measure of field dependence, compared with the abstinent subgroup. Confounds to the research findings included possible impairment of the drug-using group prior to the onset of drug use, and the very poor scores obtained at baseline by the relapsers posed the possibility that they had more room for improvement at second testing.

Judd and Grant (1975) administered the Halstead–Reitan Neuropsychological Battery, WAIS, and MMPI to a group of 18 polydrug users who were heavy users of depressants, 19 neurologically intact medical patients, and 19 brain-damaged patients (average ages 25, 24, and 22 years, respectively). After 2 to 3 weeks of sobriety, the drug users performed significantly worse than the medical patients on 13 of 29 measures. The drug-using group showed deficits in abstracting quality, accuracy of perception, motor speed, and nonverbal learning. A factor that compromised their findings was the age range of the drug-using group (14 to 54 years). With such a wide variation in age, it is possible that more significant results would become less apparent as it is known that there is considerably more variability in performance demonstrations with older adults than with younger subjects (Elliott, 1985).

A new street drug that breaks down inhibitions and can boost the high of alcohol, cocaine, and heroin has recently been introduced in the United States. Known by the street name "Roofie" or the "Forget Pill," it is an addictive sedative ten times stronger than Valium. Rohypnol has been used in Europe and elsewhere as a sleeping pill but is not legal in the United States. There are indications that users of the drug lose their inhibitions and forget what they have done. No information in the research literature is available about this new sedative (Levy, 1995).

In summary, it appears that for some young people, use of sedatives and barbiturates over a long period can lead to impaired neuropsychological functioning. The available research is not conclusive because research methods have been compromised by small sample sizes, a failure to control in research design for use of multiple drugs, and failure of researchers to control for acute effects, for differences between groups, and premorbid abilities.

Multiple Substance Abuse

Most individuals who misuse one drug tend to misuse at least one other drug as well (Mehrabian & Straubinger, 1989; Rainone, Deren, Kleinman, & Wish, 1987). As a result, in order to understand neurobehavioral consequences of any drug or combination of drugs, researchers must be prepared to deal with the additive or interactive effects of a multitude of substances. Maddux, Hoppe, and Costello (1986) surveyed 133 senior medical students and discovered that most had abused some type of psychoactive substance before entering medical school. Of those who admitted to using a drug, most reported use of more than one drug.

When two or more drugs are introduced into the body, the potential for an interactive effect exists. This interactive effect may be additive, potentiated, or inhibiting. An additive effect occurs when the effect of two or more drugs is greater than could be achieved by any single drug, but no greater than addition of the drug responses. Potentiation occurs when one drug enhances the effect of another drug when the two are taken together. The combination of the drugs may result in an effect that is greater than could be achieved by the simple addition of the drugs. Inhibition occurs when one drug diminishes or reverses the effect of another drug when the two drugs are taken together (Woolf, 1983). Multiple drug abuse is more common among adolescents than adults (Morrison, 1990).

Grant, Adams, Carlin, Rennick, Judd, and Schott (1978) completed an extensive study of polydrug abuse by investigating the neuropsychological functioning of a group of one hundred fifty-one 25-year-old multidrug users, sixty-six 28-year-old psychiatric patients, and fifty-nine 26-year-old non-drug-using, nonpatient volunteers. Each of the subjects was administered the Halstead–Reitan Neuropsychological Battery, WAIS, Grooved Pegboard Test, and MMPI. The polydrug users were evaluated between 21 and 30 days after enrollment in a treatment program. Test data indicated that 37% of the polydrug users, 26% of the psychiatric patients, and 8% of the nonpatient group scored within the neuropsychologically impaired range. The researchers indicated that age, ed-

ucation, premorbid medical factors, and extensive use of depressants and opiates in polydrug users, and extensive use of antipsychotic medications in the psychiatric group appeared to be related to impaired neuropsychological functioning. A factor analysis of the data revealed significantly weaker performance by the polydrug users on general verbal intelligence, visual–motor, tactile–motor, and perceptual skills.

Three months after the initial evaluation, 61% of the polydrug users, 77% of the psychiatric patients, and 86% of the nonpatient group were reevaluated. Mild improvement was noted in the polydrug group. Neuropsychological impairment was identified in 34% of the polydrug users, 27% of the psychiatric group, and 4% of the nonpatient group. Again, heavier use of depressants and opiates, premorbid illness history, and drug taking were related to neuropsychological impairment. The researchers speculated that impairment associated with abuse of depressants and opiates may be enduring and polydrug users might be deficient in verbally mediated problem-solving skills.

Ivnik (personal communication, February 1986) administered the WAIS-R or WISC-R, Arithmetic subtest of the WRAT, Reading section of the Woodcock–Johnson Psychoeducational Test Battery, Auditory Verbal Learning Test, and MMPI to 110 middle-class 13- to 19-year-olds (average age 15.9) who were admitted to treatment for drug abuse. The primary drugs of abuse were marijuana and alcohol. Polydrug abuse ranged from 1 to 4 years with wide variations in individual use. Testing was completed within 10 days after initial presentation. Test results failed to show significant cognitive dysfunction. Factors in the study that may have compromised the conclusions included an absence of a control group and wide variation between subjects in the extent of drug use.

Crane (1984) investigated the neurological and neuropsychological consequences of PCP use by adolescents; he compared 20 PCP/polydrug (except inhalant) users, 10 polydrug users who had not used PCP, and 10 nondrug users. The residential treatment facility subjects were between 15 and 20 years old and were matched for age, sex, and education. A neurological examination, neuropsychological examination, and EEG were administered to each subject. The subjects had been free of drugs for about 3 months at the time of testing. Although the author was unable to identify deficits in the polydrug user group, that group differed from the other two groups with respect to ethnicity and may have experienced a greater degree of social, psychological, and intellectual development differences.

Grant, Mohns, Miller, and Reitan (1976) found neuropsychological impairment in a group of 22 young, polydrug users who had been free of drugs an average of 2 months. They compared the performance levels of the polydrug users in a residential drug treatment program with those of a group of 19 medical and 19 neurological patients matched for age, education, and sex. At the time of testing, most subjects had been drug free for 2 months. Evaluation instruments included the Halstead–Reitan Neuropsychological Battery, WAIS, and MMPI. One-half of the polydrug users showed mild, generalized neuropsychological impairment. Impairment was judged to be evident in 11 to 26% of the medical patients and 84 to 89% of the neurological patients. There appeared to be no association between impairment and the use of any specific drug.

In contrast to these findings, Bruhn and Maage (1975) were unable to identify neuropsychological deficits associated with heavy use of combinations of marijuana, amphetamines, and opiates. A group of 87 Danish male prisoners (average age 23.1 years) matched for age and education were divided into four groups. The four groups ranged from no drug use to heavy use of four or more drug categories. Each subject was given the WAIS, Category Test, Learning and Memory Test, Seashore Rhythm Test, Hidden Pattern Test, and a reaction time test. There were no apparent differences between the groups in abstract reasoning, concentration, perception, learning capability, or any other area of cognitive functioning. Researchers assumed the subjects were not using drugs during testing because they were prisoners. With our current knowledge of the extent and use of drugs in the prison system, such an assumption seems naive.

Parsons and Farr (1981) found that polydrug abusers may show depressed performance on the Finger Tapping, Seashore Rhythm, Category, and Trail Making B Test. In contrast, Bruhn and Maage (1975) were unable to identify neuropsychological deficits associated with heavy use of combinations of marijuana, hallucinogens, amphetamines, and opiates.

Research findings on the effects of polydrug abuse in adolescents are mixed. A common finding of studies of drug use in adolescent delinquents is deficient verbal IQ on the Wechsler scales and a higher frequency of polydrug use compared with nondelinquent drug users. The studies that have failed to find neuropsychological deficits have focused on younger subjects. These studies have tended to lack a control group, or if there was a control group, the control group was poorly matched with the experimental group. Studies that have found a positive relationship between polydrug use and neuropsychological impairment have tended to associate the impairment with abuse of one of the depressants and opiates.

Steroids

Individuals who consume anabolic-androgenic steroids (AASs) experience changes in outward appearance, physical capabilities, and possible mood and social behavior and possible CNS damage. Although the emphasis and research on steroids has been focused on moods and behaviors, some data suggest that there may be a relationship between use of steroids and CNS functioning. As yet, the nature of the relationship is unclear.

Monitoring the Future first surveyed high school seniors on use of steroids in 1989. At that time, 3.0% of seniors reported lifetime use. In the 1993 survey, 2.0% of seniors reported use. Eighth graders reported a lifetime prevalence of 1.6% and tenth graders reported a lifetime prevalence of 1.7% (University of Michigan, 1994).

Attention to steroids increased during the late 1980s when the use of AASs by youth became prevalent for enhancement of athletic skills. Anabolic steroids are synthetic analogues of the male sex hormone testosterone which can be used legitimately to treat a variety of diseases and conditions in both adults and children. There are a number of steroids approved for clinical use but there are also numerous black market preparations that have no approved therapeutic use in humans (Bukstein, 1995). Although for decades scientists and athletes have felt that anabolic steroids could enhance physical performance and increase muscle mass, muscle strength, and aggressiveness, their use has also been associated with various harmful effects including liver abnormalities, changes in cardiovascular risk, endocrine effects, and psychological effects including severe mood changes and aggressive behavior (Hallagan, Hallagan, & Snyder, 1989).

Steroid abuse is common among athletes in a variety of sports such as weight lifting, body building, cycling, football, and track and field. Its use has also been prevalent among lower-level amateur and recreational athletes (Yesalis, Kennedy, Kopstein,

& Bahrke, 1993). Anabolic steroids are likely to have addictive potential. Some adolescents who abuse anabolic steroids will display indications of psychoactive substance abuse including continuous use despite adverse consequences, tolerance, and even withdrawal (Bower, 1992).

Steroids may affect the nervous system directly and indirectly. Ingestion of steroids can be a treatment modality and also a cause for dementia. Corticosteroid receptors are located in the hypothalamus, pituitary, hippocampus, septum, and amygdala. The set of interactions between the corticosteroids and the body systems is unknown at this time (Hartman, 1995). Varney, Alexander, and MacIndoe (1984) evaluated six patients who received 60–125 mg/day of prednisone for steroid-treatable diseases. Two of the six patients had contracted long-lasting cognitive sequelae subsequent to a resolving steroid psychosis. The four remaining patients showed global, but reversible, deficits in an 80-day to 2-year follow-up study. The patients were assessed with a neuropsychological battery that included the WAIS, Wechsler Memory Scale, Benton Visual Retention Test, Spatial Recognition Test, 3D Constructional Praxis Scale, as well as other measures. Deficits in "memory retention, attention, concentration, mental speed and efficiency in occupational performance" were noted. Each of the patients became impaired relative to his own prior and subsequent functioning (Varney et al., 1984, p. 372).

Impairment of both behavior and cognitive functioning as a result of steroid administration is dose related. Wolkowitz, Reus, Weingartner, and Thompson (1990) found increased intrusion (commission) errors in recall and diminished corrected free recall. The researchers felt that the steroids suppressed the brain's ability to filter out extraneous information (Wolkowitz et al., 1993). Because of the potential for AASs to create dependency in users, they were placed in Schedule III of the Controlled Substances Act in 1990. Schedule III is reserved for substances that are addictive (Nightingale, 1991).

Recent studies of active AAS users have indicated that there may be frequent use of addictive substances such as cocaine, alcohol, and marijuana (Perry, Yates, & Andersen, 1990; Pope & Katz, 1988). No studies have looked at the relationship between AAS use and use of other addictive drugs and neurological or neuropsychological functioning although it is recognized that steroids can act on CNS structures that are responsible for perception and interpretation of sensory information as well as for modulation of affect.

The first research studies on AASs have focused primarily on social, clinical, and physical effects. Although a few studies have examined the potential effect of AASs on the CNS, little is known about the potential long-term effects of AASs on any body system. No research studies have addressed the impact of AASs on the CNS of youthful illicit users. It has been suggested that anabolic steroids are similar to other common drugs of abuse but this issue has not been explored scientifically. Studies examining indications of physical and psychological dependence, as well as the rewarding value of steroids, have not been conducted. Such an area of inquiry would be productive and would allow researchers and treatment professionals to understand the nature of this drug as a drug of abuse.

Methodological Issues in Substance Abuse Research

There are several methodological considerations and pitfalls that should be addressed when conducting research in the field of alcoholism and drug abuse. One critical element deals with selection of subjects. Individuals who abuse alcohol and drugs are apt to differ from the general population in ways that may have implications for neuropsychological functioning. Some of the differences that abusers manifest may predate their use of illicit substances. Conclusions based on research results in such cases may have little to do with the adverse effects of any substance (Grant & Reed, 1985). Differences between drug abusers and the general population might involve education, sociocultural and ethnic influences, nutrition, personality differences, and history of medically related neurological damage. A large proportion of research studies that have focused on substance abuse failed to match subjects along these lines. Such a failure can compromise the interpretation of findings.

Other methodological flaws evident in drug and alcohol research involve a reliance on retrospective studies, use of inappropriate and unmatched control groups, use of small experimental and control groups, and reliance on neurological or neuropsychological data-gathering methods that have not yet been proven to be reliable or valid. Use of measures of central tendency, which assume a uniformity of impairment that may not exist, can cloud or distort test findings by averaging extremes (Carlin, 1986).

Two critical features in substance abuse research, when ignored, can invalidate findings. First, a number of research reports do not take into account periods of sobriety or how much time has elapsed since the last use of drugs before tests were administered. In some studies, subjects were tested days after they last used drugs, yet the researcher implies that chronic use issues were assessed and addressed. The second issue deals with the use of self-reported drug use surveys. Individuals who abuse drugs tend to use more than one drug (Parsons & Adams, 1983) and many of the drugs purchased on the streets by adolescents are often contaminated or contain ingredients other than the presumed drug. Many researchers rely exclusively on the drug users' self-reported drug use history. Self-reports by drug users, as to type and frequency of use, although convenient for researchers, make interpretation of results difficult and suspect. Such information may be partly responsible for the many seemingly contradictory findings in the field of substance abuse research.

The quantity of drug use, the specific drug used, and the duration of drug usage need to be documented. Research findings have indicated that type of drug, quantity, and duration of use are important elements when conducting research on drug effects (Korman, 1977). In solvent research, the type of solvent involved, the host agent for the drug, and the presence of toxic impurities may contaminate research. Alternative explanations for significant research findings need to be offered. It is not usual for what appears to be CNS neuropathology to actually be a consequence of peripheral nerve damage. Peripheral nerve damage is frequently recognized in research with solvents. Yet, few researchers perform nerve conduction studies, which could differentiate peripheral neuropathy from CNS impairment.

Research findings may be significant but conclusions may be obscured because the researcher combined all drug-using group information under one category. Researchers who inquire about drug use history most of the time find that drug users will admit to taking two or more drugs. Although these researchers assign a specific subject to a primary drug category, they fail to acknowledge the secondary drug use history or to identify the secondary drug and possible interactive effects.

During a research project, if residual drug effects exist, the researcher should describe and attempt to separate transient from the long-term effects. Such knowledge has implications not only for determination of CNS effects, but also for providing treatment and for predicting the clinical course of recovery (Spencer, 1990).

A final issue that has become increasingly recognized as a critical element in research is ecological validity (C. Long, personal communication, 1995). There needs to be a clear relationship between the degree of impairment associated with drug abuse and test performance and impairment in day-to-day life. Aitken, Chase, McCue, and Ratcliff (1993) demonstrated a substantial relationship between test performance and everyday capabilities in a brain-injured population. As a form of compromise to neuropsychological integrity, exposure to drugs should likewise be expected to be related to everyday capabilities.

Summary

The National Senior Survey (University of Michigan, 1994) found that over 50% of senior students reported consuming alcohol and 18% admit to using an illicit drug during the preceding 30-day period. Although this is a decline of the peak alcohol and drug use documented in 1980, the trend during the last 3 years indicates an increase in some drugs and a decrease in others. Specifically, between 1990 and 1993, seniors reported a slight increase in use of any illicit drug with a significant increase in marijuana, hallucinogens, including LSD, and sedatives. During the same period of time there was a corresponding decline in alcohol, cocaine, opiates other than heroin, inhalants, and steroids. The use of crack cocaine, heroin, and stimulants has remained unchanged between 1990 and 1993. Johnston et al. (1993) reported that 42.9% of adolescents in the United States have used an illicit drug before leaving high school and 2.5% of seniors report consuming alcohol on a daily basis. Almost 30% have had five or more drinks on one occasion during the preceding 2 weeks.

Although the trend in adolescent use of drugs, including alcohol, has been generally in decline during the last few years, the level of substance abuse remains disturbingly high and has implications for drug education, research, and rehabilitation programs. Relevant to rehabilitation, if research is able to demonstrate that abuse of a drug by youth adversely affects abstracting and conceptualization capabilities, then verbal, highly cognitively oriented therapeutic techniques may be useless or less appropriate than behavioral conditioning techniques. During the early phase of treatment, substance abusers may be cognitively impaired to the extent that information processing will be seriously compromised (Spencer, 1990). If perceptual motor, spatial, and sequencing skills are compromised, then a didactic and more verbally mediated therapeutic approach may be appropriate. Knowledge of the specific effects of certain drugs will allow those who provide rehabilitation services to intercede in family and environmental issues in a knowledgeable manner.

Definitive statements, offered by different researchers, about the effects of different drugs or combinations of drugs on the CNS of children, adolescents, and young adults are difficult to summarize as there are substantial differences in outcomes, methodology, and implications from study to study (Elliott, 1989). In every researcher's mind, the one question should be, "Did the drug cause the effect or did existence of the effect cause use of the drug?" Because the majority of drug users use more than one drug (especially alcohol), researching the effects of a specific drug on the CNS will be very difficult.

A large percentage of neuropsychological studies that have investigated drug effects have methodological or statistical design flaws that have compromised conclusions and made the information provided difficult to interpret. Although some of these flaws are within the control of the researcher, such as using a small number of subjects, failure to use a control group, and failure to control for premorbid abilities, other conditions are beyond the control of the researcher. For example, many drug abusers use a multitude of other drugs and practice poor nutrition. A number of them have histories of other complicating psychiatric conditions or conditions that would compromise the CNS such as head injuries, multiple sclerosis, or ADHD.

Many times researchers fail to investigate the subcomponents of behavior. If residual drug effects are to be identified, it will be useful for researchers to evaluate the components of certain cognitive skills. Examples include specific types of memory deficits (i.e., declarative versus procedural) that might provide important information on differences between drug-abstinent and non-drug-abusing children. Comprehensive descriptions of specific performance areas and descriptions of specific learning deficits need to be identified in evaluating children. It remains to be clarified whether drug-abstinent

children make the same types of errors that are apparent in generalized brain dysfunction in adults (Spencer, 1990). In research with adult drug abusers, polydrug studies have indicated that up to half of all drug users exhibit neuropsychological deficits during the first few weeks after discontinuance of drug taking. Although many drug abusers demonstrate signs of recovery 3 to 6 months after discontinuance, residual impairment remains (Grant & Reed, 1985).

Much of the drug research with adults and children relies on drug users' self-reports of their drug use. When severe use has been documented, even with young individuals (Grant *et al.*, 1976, 1977), some CNS impairment is apparent. The younger brain appears to be more resilient to the adverse effects of mild to moderate drug use, even over a period of years. As the brain matures and ages, it becomes increasingly sensitive to drugs, especially depressants (Greenblatt, Sellers, & Shader, 1982).

Although a large body of research data has been collected during the past three decades, reporting on the relationship between drug abuse and CNS deficits, relatively little is known about the long-term neuropsychological effects of most drugs. A great deal is known about acute intoxication and withdrawal features. In the field of toxicology, it is recognized that neurotoxic exposure can produce a syndrome characterized by subclinical neuropsychological injury. Injury to the nervous system may accumulate for months, or even years. The implications of the injury may not become apparent, except in the context of neuropsychological or neurological examinations, until the condition manifests itself in a clinical syndrome months, or even years, later (Calne, 1991). Research with animals has indicated that lesions produced during early development may not become apparent until the animal ages at which time cell reductions may deplete neuronal reserves below needed capacity. This phenomenon has been termed "the event threshold concept" (Reuhl, 1991, p. 343). It has become increasingly clear to neurotoxicology researchers that adverse effects of toxicants may not become clinically evident for months or years after exposure. This "grace" period reflects a period of time when the individual manifests no evidence of toxicity. It is also referred to as a "silent" period (Reuhl, 1991). This may explain why there are not the significant findings with children and adolescents that are seen with adults. Even when a youth discontinues using a drug, the toxic elements of the drug may not emerge for years. Damage to the structures during early development may not be evident as a deficit until there is a functional demand on the system. As pubertal changes develop, somatic or behavioral alterations may become apparent or exacerbate subtle, preexisting abnormalities.

Although the majority of well-controlled studies that have examined the neuropsychological implications of adolescent drug abuse do not report consistent findings of impaired functioning, long-term consequences for some drugs are clearly evident and implicated for others. Although clinicians can always recall a specific adolescent who became "burned out" on drugs and developed brain damage, these individual case studies are not conclusive. When groups of abusing individuals are studied, such dramatic findings are not as readily apparent. Severely impaired drug abusers may represent an exception rather than the rule.

In the research reported during the last decade, there has been no concerted effort to describe or to track the deficits in children who were acknowledged drug abusers who had stopped using drugs. It could be critical to our understanding of the long-term, chronic effects of drugs on children to engage in follow-up studies and participate in longitudinal research. This is important because it is during this developmental period that components of cognition, planning, evaluation, and abstracting skills are undergoing major developmental changes.

Many of the research reports have focused on global and generalized measures of cognitive functioning. Because drugs can affect specific cognitive areas of functioning, researchers need to assess motor dexterity, visual, auditory, and tactile sensory processing skills, reaction time, attention and concentration, language functioning, verbal reasoning, visual–spatial analysis and construction, verbal and nonverbal memory, planning, abstraction, problem-solving skills (Spencer, 1990), and simultaneous information processing. Because the defects may be subtle, use of computerized measures of cognitive functioning needs to be developed for child and adolescent populations. Such measures currently exist for adult populations (Kay, 1995; The Risk Management Foundation of the Harvard Medical Institutions, 1993).

This review of the studies investigating chronic effects of substance abuse on children, adolescents, and young adults does not indicate consistent neuropsychological deficits associated with the use of most substances. The substances most consistent in demonstrating chronic defects with the young include alcohol, depressants, cocaine, and multiple drug use.

Most research on both acute and chronic drug effects on neuropsychological functioning has developed from adult populations. When research is developed for children and adolescents, there are additional confounding factors that are not as important in adult research that need to be controlled. The primary factors include developmental changes involving brain functioning, emotional development, age of onset of drug use, and environmental elements. These elements suggest that there exists greater complexity in studying children and adolescents compared with adults (Tramontana, 1983).

When completing research on children, individual differences are a critical element. Issues associated with developmental delays, head injuries, attention deficits, hyperactivity, and learning disabilities need to be identified and documented. Without controlling for these factors, weaknesses in cognitive functioning may be related to cognitive process disorders rather than chronic, or even acute, effects of drugs.

Future investigations of the chronic neuropsychological sequelae of substance abuse on children, adolescents, and young adults need to address methodological issues noted earlier. The extent of drug use needs to be systematically documented and verified by an outside, objective resource. Sample sizes need to be large and matched. Longitudinal studies need to be developed that will follow large groups of drug-abusing youth before they began taking drugs and then monitor them through high school into adulthood. Lastly, the extent of alcohol use accompanying most drug abuse needs to be evaluated, documented, and reported. It is known that alcohol is usually the first substance used by most individuals who develop a history of drug abuse.

References

Aasly, J., Storsaeter, O., Nilsen, G., & Smevik, O. (1993). Minor structural brain damage changes in young drug abusers: A magnetic resonance study. *Acta Neurologica Scandinavica, 87,* 210–214.

Aitken, S., Chase, S., McCue, M., & Ratcliff, G. (1993). An American adaptation of the Multiple Errands Test: Assessment of executive abilities in everyday living. *Archives of Clinical Neuropsychology, 8*(3), 212.

Allison, W. M., & Jerrom, D. W. (1984). Glue sniffing: A pilot study of the cognitive effects of long-term use. *International Journal of the Addictions, 19,* 453–458.

American Psychiatric Association. (1980). *Diagnostic and statistical manual of mental disorders* (3rd ed.). Washington, DC: Author.

American Psychiatric Association. (1994). *Diagnostic and statistical manual of mental disorders* (4th ed.). Washington, DC: Author.

Aniline, O., & Pitts, F. N. (1982). Phencyclidine (PCP): A review and perspectives. *Critical Review of Toxicology, 10,* 1045.

Ardila, A., Rosselli, M., & Strumwasser, S. (1990). Neuropsychological deficits in chronic cocaine abusers. *International Journal of Neuroscience, 57,* 73–79.

Baldrige, E. B., & Bessen, H. A. (1990). Phencyclidine. *Emergency Medicine Clinics of North America, 8,* 541–549.

Baron, I. S., Fennell, E. B., & Voeller, K. K. S. (1995). *Pediatric neuropsychology in the medical setting.* London: Oxford University Press.

Bell, C. S. (1985, December 1). Potent pot: Today's stronger marijuana poses new dangers for adolescents. *Daily Breeze,* p. B-11.

Bergman, H., Borg, S., Engelbrecktson, K., & Vikander, B. (1989). Dependence on sedative hypnotics: Neuropsychological impact, field dependence and clinical consequences in a five year follow-up study. *British Journal of Addiction, 81,* 547–553.

Berry, G. J., Heaton, R., & Kirby, M. (1978). Neuropsychological assessment of chronic inhalant abusers: A preliminary report. In C. W. Sharp & L. T. Carroll (Eds.), *Voluntary inhalation of industrial solvents* (pp. 111–136). Rockville, MD: National Institute on Drug Abuse.

Berry, G. J., van Gorp, W. G., Herzberg, D. S., Hinkin, C., Boone, K., Steinman, L., & Wilkins, J. N. (1993). Neuropsychological deficits in abstinent cocaine abusers: Preliminary findings after two weeks of abstinence. *Drug and Alcohol Dependence, 32,* 231–237.

Bigler, E. D. (1979). Neuropsychological evaluation of adolescent patients hospitalized witih chronic inhalant abuse. *Clinical Neuropsychology, 1,* 8–12.

Blane, H. (1976). Middle-aged alcoholics and young drinkers. In H. Blane & M. Chafetz (Eds.), *Youth, alcohol and social policy* (pp. 5–38). New York: Plenum Press.

Block, R. I., & Ghoneim, M. M. (1993). Effects of chronic marijuana use on human cognition. *Psychopharmacology, 110,* 219–228.

Bower, K. J. (1992). Clinical assessment and treatment of anabolic steroid users. *Psychiatric Annuals, 22,* 35–40.

Bruhn, P., & Maage, N. (1975). Intellectual and neuropsychological functions in young men with heavy and long-term patterns of drug abuse. *American Journal of Psychiatry, 132,* 397–401.

Bukstein, O. G. (1994). Treatment of adolescent alcohol abuse and dependence. *Alcohol Health and Research World, 18,* 296–301.

Bukstein, O. G. (1995). *Adolescent substance abuse.* New York: Wiley.

Callen, D. (1984). Toluene + alcohol = danger. *ADAMHA News, 10* (Suppl., September), 211–216.

Calne, D. B. (1991). Neurotoxins and degeneration in the central nervous system. *Neurotoxicology, 12*(3), 335–339.

Campbell, A. M., Evans, M., Thompson, J. L., & Williams, M. J. (1971). Cerebral atrophy in young cannabis smokers. *Lancet, 2,* 1219–1224.

Carlin, A. (1986). Neuropsychological consequences of drug abuse. In I. Grant & K. M. Adams (Eds.), *Neuropscyhological assessment of neuropsychiatric disorders* (pp. 478–497). London: Oxford University Press.

Carlin, A. S., Grant, I., Adams, K. M., & Reed, R. (1979). Is phencyclidine (PCP) abuse associated with organic mental impairment? *American Journal of Drug and Alcohol Abuse, 6,* 273–281.

Carlin, A. S., & Trupin, E. W. (1977). The effects of long-term chronic marijuana use on neuropsychological functioning. *International Journal of the Addictions, 12,* 617–624.

Channer, K. S., & Stanley, S. (1983). Persistent visual hallucinations secondary to chronic solvent encephalopathy: Case report and review of the literature. *Journal of Neurology, Neurosurgery & Psychiatry, 46,* 83–86.

Cho, A. K. (1990). Ice: A new form of an old drug. *Science, 249,* 231–249.

Cohen, S., & Edwards, A. E. (1969). LSD and organic brain impairment. *Drug Dependence, 2,* 1–4.

Comstock, B. S. (1977). A review of psychological measures relevant to central nervous toxicity, with specific reference to solvent inhalation. *Clinical Toxicology, 11,* 317–324.

Comstock, F. G., & Comstock, B. S. (1977). Medical evaluation of inhalant abusers. In C. W. Sharp & M. L. Brehm (Eds.), *Review of inhalants: Euphoria to dysfunction* (pp. 54–80). Washington, DC: U. S. Government Printing Office.

Crane, J. A. (1984). The neurological and neuropsychological consequences of chronic, long-term phencyclidine (PCP) ingestion in adolescents. *Dissertation Abstracts International, 45,* 3-B 1010. (University Microfilms No. DA 8413715)

Culver, C. M., & King, F. W. (1974). Neuropsychological assessment of undergraduate marijuana and LSD users. *Archives of General Psychiatry, 31,* 707–711.

Eckhardt, M. J., Parker, E. S., Nobel, E. P., Feldman, D. J., & Gottschalk, L. A. (1978). Relationship between neuropsychological performance and alcohol consumption in alcoholics. *Biological Psychiatry, 13,* 551–565.

Eckhardt, M. J., Stapleton, J. M., Rawlings, R. R., Davis, E. Z., & Grodin, D. M. (1995). Neuropsychological functioning in detoxified alcoholics between 18 and 35 years of age. *American Journal of Psychiatry, 152,* 53–59.

Elliott, R. W. (1985). Aging effects and the professional pilot. *Hearings on age discrimination and the FAA age 60 rule.* Select Committment on Aging, House of Representatives, 97th Congress (Committee Publication No. 99-533, pp. 375–387). Washington, DC: U. S. Government Printing Office.

Elliott, R. W. (1987, October). *School consultation in clinical neuropsychology.* Paper presented at the meeting of the National Academy of Neuropsychologists, Chicago, Illinois.

Elliott, R. W. (1989). Neuropsychological sequelae of substance abuse by youths. In C. R. Reynolds & E. Fletcher-Janzen (Eds.), *Handbook of clinical child neuropsychology* (pp. 311–331). New York: Plenum Press.

Fals-Stewart, W., Schafer, J., Lucente, S., Rustine, T., & Brown, L. (1994). Neurobehavioral consequences of prolonged alcohol and substance abuse: A review of findings and treatment implications. *Clinical Psychology Review, 14,* 755–778.

Faucett, R. L., & Jensen, R. A. (1952). Addiction of the inhalation of gasoline fumes in a child. *Journal of Pediatrics, 41,* 364–368.

Fauman, M. A., & Fauman, B. J. (1979). Violence associated with phencyclidine abuse. *American Journal of Psychiatry, 136,* 1584–1586.

Fields, F. R., & Fullerton, J. R. (1974). The influence of heroin addiction on neuropsychological functioning. *Journal of Consulting and Clinical Psychology, 43,* 114.

Fletcher, J. M. (1987, August). *Neuropsychological and psychological correlates of chronic cannabis use in Costa Rica.* Paper presented at the annual meeting of the American Psychological Association, New York.

Foo, S. C., Jeyaratnam, J., & Koh, D. (1990). Chronic neurobehavioral effects of toluene. *British Journal of Industrial Medicine, 47,* 480–484.

Forrest, M. (1994, May/June). Adolescent drug use increases. In *NIDA notes* (Vol. 9, no. 2, pp. 11–12). Department of Health and Human Services, NIH, Rockville, MD (NIH Publication No. 94-3478).

Golden, C. J. (1985). Computer models and the human brain. *Computers in Human Behavior, 1,* 35–48.

Goldman, M. S. (1982). Reversibility of psychological deficits in alcoholics: The interactions of aging with alcohol. In A. Wilkerson (Ed.), *Symposium on cerebral deficits in alcoholism.* Toronto: Addiction Research Foundation.

Grant, I., Adams, K. M., Carlin, A. S., & Rennick, P. M. (1977). Neuropsychological deficit in polydrug users: A preliminary report of the findings of the collaborative neuropsychological study of polydrug users. *Drug and Alcohol Dependence, 2,* 91–108.

Grant, I., Adams, K. M., Carlin, A. S., Rennick, P. M., Judd, L. L., & Schott, K. (1978). The collaborative neuropsychological study of polydrug users. *Archives of General Psychiatry, 35,* 1063–1074.

Grant, I., Mohns, L., Miller, M., & Reitan, R. M. (1976). A neuropsychological study of polydrug users. *Archives of General Psychiatry, 33,* 973–978.

Grant, I., & Reed, R. (1985). Neuropsychology of alcohol and drug abuse. In A. I. Alterman (Ed.), *Substance abuse and psychopathology* (pp. 289–341). New York: Plenum Press.

Grant, I., Rochford, J., Fleming, T., & Stunkard, A. (1973). A neuropsychological assessment of the effects of moderate marijuana use. *Journal of Nervous and Mental Disease, 156,* 278–280.

Greenblatt, D. J., Sellers, E. M., & Shader, R. I. (1982). Drug disposition in old age. *Medical Intelligence, 306,* 1081–1088.

Greer, J. E. (1984). Adolescent abuse of typewriter correction fluid. *Southern Medical Journal, 77,* 297–301.

Hallagan, J. B., Hallagan, L. F., & Snyder, M. D. (1989). Anabolic steroid use by athletics. *New England Journal of Medicine, 321,* 1042–1045.

Hannon, R., Butler, C. P., Day, C. L., Kahn, S. A., Quitoriano, L. A., Butler, A. M., & Meredith, L. A. (1985). Alcohol use and cognitive functioning in men and women college students. In M. Galante (Ed.), *Recent developments in alcoholism* (Vol. 3, pp. 241–252). New York: Plenum Press.

Hannon, R., Day, C. L., Butler, A. M., Larson, A. J., & Casey, M. (1983). Alcohol consumption and cognitive functioning in college students. *Journal of Studies on Alcohol, 44,* 283–298.

Harris, L. S. (Ed.). (1994). *Problems of drug dependence, 1993: Proceedings of the 55th Annual Scientific Meeting: Vol. II. Abstracts* (NIDA Research Monograph 141). Rockville, MD: NIDA.

Hartman, D. (1995). *Neuropsychological toxicology* (2nd ed.). New York: Plenum Press.

Hastings, J. (1991, Winter). Easy to get hooked on, hard to get off. *Serenity Lane Outreach Newsletter,* p. 7.

Hill, S. Y., & Mikhad, M. A. (1979). Computerized transaxial tomographic and neuropsychological evaluations in chronic alcoholics and heroin abusers. *American Journal of Psychiatry, 136,* 598–602.

Holbrook, J. M. (1983). Hallucinogens. In G. Bennett, C. Vourakis, & D. S. Woolf (Eds.), *Substance abuse: Pharmacologic, developmental, and clinical perspectives* (pp. 86–99). New York: Wiley.

Hormes, J. T., Filley, C. M., & Rosenberg, N. L. (1986). Neurologic sequelae of chronic solvent vapor abuse. *Neurology, 36,* 698–702.

Institute for Health Policy, Brandeis University. (1993, October). *Substance abuse: The nation's number one health problem; key indicators for policy.* Princeton, NJ: Robert Wood Johnson Foundation.

Institute of Medicine, National Academy of Sciences. (1985). Research on mental illness and addictive disorders: Progress and prospects. A report of the Board of Mental Health and Behavioral Medicine, Institute of Medicine. *American Journal of Psychiatry, 142*(Suppl. 7).

Ivnik, R. J. (1986). Neuropsychological aspects of adolescent chemical abuse. *Journal of Clinical and Experimental Neuropsychology, 7,* 605.

Jernigan, T. L., Butters, N., DiTraglia, G., & Cemark, L. S. (1991). Reduced cerebral grey matter observed in alcoholics using magnetic resonance imaging. *Alcohol Clinical Experimental Research, 15,* 418–427.

Johnston, L. D., O'Malley, P., & Bachman, J. G. (1993). *National survey results on drug use from the Monitoring the Future Study, 1975–1992.* U. S. Department of Health and Human Services, National Institute on Drug Abuse. Washington, DC: U. S. Government Printing Office.

Judd, L. L., & Grant, I. (1975). Brain dysfunction in chronic sedative users. *Journal of Psychedelic Drugs, 7,* 143–149.

Kaplan, H. I., Freedman, A. M., & Sadock, B. J. (1980). *Comprehensive textbook of psychiatry III.* Baltimore: Williams & Wilkins.

Kay, G. G. (1995). *CogScreen: Aeromedical edition.* Odessa, FL: Psychological Assessment Resources.

Kissin, B. (1977). Alcoholism and drug dependence. In R. C. Simons & H. Pardes (Eds.), *Understanding human be-*

havior in health and illness (pp. 35–42). Baltimore: Williams & Wilkins.

Korman, M. (1977). Clinical evaluation of psychological factors. In C. W. Sharp & M. L. Brehm (Eds.), *Review of inhalants: Euphoria to dysfunction* (pp. 30–47). Rockville, MD: U. S. Government Printing Office.

Korman, M., Matthews, R. W., & Lovitt, R. (1981). Neuropsychological effects of abuse of inhalants. *Perceptual and Motor Skills, 53,* 547–553.

Krull, K. R., Tivis, L., Blanco, C., Hames, K., & Smith, L. T. (1994). Neurophysiological and neuropsychological functioning in adolescent alcohol abusers. *Archives of Clinical Neuropsychology (Abstracts), 9,* 109.

Levy, D. (1995, June 20). Experts fear sedative gaining favor on streets. *USA Today,* p. 1A.

Lewis, J. E., & Hordan, R. B. (1986). Neuropsychological assessment of phencyclidine abusers. In D. H. Clouet (Ed.), *Phencyclidine: An update* (NIDA Research Monograph 64, pp. 190–208). Washington, DC: Department of Health and Human Services.

Lewis, P. W., & Patterson, D. W. (1974). Acute and chronic effects of the voluntary inhalation of certain commercial volatile solvents by juveniles. *Journal of Drug Issues, 4,* 162–175.

Lezak, M. D. (1995). *Neuropsychological assessment* (3rd ed.). London: Oxford University Press.

Light, R. (1984). *Neuropsychological, intellectual, and personality functioning in phencyclidine abusing adolescents and young adults.* Unpublished doctoral dissertation, Indiana University, Bloomington.

McLellan, A. T., Woody, G. E., & O'Brien, C. P. (1979). Development of psychiatric disorders in drug abusers. *New England Journal of Medicine, 301,* 1310–1313.

Maddux, J. F., Hoppe, S. K., & Costello, R. M. (1986). Psychoactive substance use among medical students. *American Journal of Psychiatry, 143,* 187–191.

Malm, G., & Lying-Tunell, U. (1980). Cerebellar dysfunction related to toluene sniffing. *Acta Neurologica Scandinavica, 62,* 188–190.

Manning, A. (1995, March 14). '90s teens find a new high by abusing Ritalin. *USA Today,* p. 1A.

Massengale, O. N., Glaser, H. H., LeLievre, R. E., Dodds, J. B., & Klock, M. E. (1963). Physical and psychologic factors in glue sniffing. *New England Journal of Medicine, 269,* 1340–1344.

Mehrabian, A., & Straubinger, T. (1989). Patterns of drug use among adults. *Addictive Behavior, 14,* 99–104.

Millsaps, C., Azrin, R. L., Schneider, B., Burns, W., & Mittenberg, W. (1995). The neuropsychological effect of chronic marijuana abuse on the WMS-R and WAIS-R. *The Clinical Neuropsychologist, 9,* 293.

Mittenberg, W., & Motta, S. (1993). Effects of chronic cocaine abuse on memory and learning. *Archives of Clinical Neuropsychology, 8,* 477–483.

Montoya-Cabrera, M. A. (1990). Neurotoxicology in Mexico and its relation to the general and work environment. In B. L. Johnson (Ed.), *Advances in neurobehavioral toxicology: Applications in environmental and occupational health* (pp. 35–57). Chelsea, MI: Lewis Publications.

Morrison, M. A. (1990). Addiction in adolescents. *Western Journal of Medicine, 152,* 543–546.

Myers, J. A., & Earnest, M. P. (1984). Generalized seizures and cocaine abuse. *Neurology, 34,* 675–676.

National Institute on Drug Abuse. (1994). NIDA reflects on 20 years of neuroscience research. *NIDA Notes, 9*(3), SS-2.

Newcomb, M. D., & Bentler, P. M. (1991). *Adult health consequences of teen age drug use: Eight-year prospective finding.* Paper presented at the annual convention of the American Psychological Association, San Francisco.

Nightingale, S. (1991). Anabolic steroids as controlled substances. *Journal of the American Medical Association, 265,* 1129.

Oscar-Berman, M., & Hutner, N. (1993). Frontal lobe changes after chronic alcohol ingestion. In W. A. Hunt & S. J. Nixon (Eds.), *Alcohol-induced brain damage* (pp. 121–156). (National Institute on Alcohol Abuse and Alcoholism Research Monograph 22). Rockville, MD: U. S. Department of Health and Human Services.

Parry, G. J. G. (1995). Neurological complications of toxin exposure in the workplace. In M. J. Aminoff (Ed.), *Neurology and general medicine* (2nd ed., pp. 641–662). Edinburgh: Churchill Livingstone.

Parsons, O. A. (1993). Impaired neuropsychological cognitive functioning in sober alcoholics. In W. A. Hunt & S. J. Nixon (Eds.), *Alcohol-induced brain damage* (pp. 173–194). National Institute on Alcohol Abuse and Alcoholism Research Monograph 22). Rockville, MD: U. S. Department of Health and Human Services.

Parsons, O. A., & Adams, R. L. (1983). The neuropsychological examination of alcohol and drug abuse patients. In C. J. Golden & P. J. Vincenti (Eds.), *Foundations of clinical neuropsychology* (pp. 215–248). New York: Plenum Press.

Parsons, O. A., & Farr, S. P. (1981). The neuropsychology of alcohol and drug use. In S. B. Filskov & T. J. Boll (Eds.), *Handbook of clinical neuropsychology* (pp. 320–365). New York: Wiley.

Pascual-Leone, A., Dhuna, A., & Anderson, D. C. (1991a). Longterm neurological complications of chronic, habitual cocaine abuse. *NeuroToxicology, 12,* 393–400.

Pascual-Leone, A., Dhuna, A., & Anderson, D. C. (1991b). Cerebral atrophy in habitual cocaine abusers: A planimetric CT study. *Neurology, 41,* 34–38.

Perry, P. J., Andersen, K. H., & Yates, W. R. (1990). Illicit anabolic steroid use in athletics: A case series analysis. *American Journal of Sports Medicine, 18,* 422–428.

Perry, P. J., Yates, W. R., & Andersen, K. H. (1990). Psychiatric symptoms associated with anabolic steroids: A controlled retrospective study. *Annals of Clinical Psychiatry, 2,* 11–17.

Phelps, L., & Cox, D. (1993). Children with prenatal cocaine exposure: Resilient or handicapped? *School Psychology Review, 22,* 710–724.

Pogge, D. L. (1994). Lack of attention can be a red flag for substance abuse. *Clinical Psychiatry News,* 15.

Pogge, D. L., Stokes, J., & Harvey, P. D. (1992). Psychometric versus attentional correlates of early onset alcohol and substance abuse. *Journal of Abnormal Child Psychology, 20,* 151–162.

Pope, H. G., & Katz, D. L. (1988). Affective and psychotic symptoms associated with anabolic steroid use. *American Journal of Psychiatry, 145,* 487–490.

Portnoff, L. A. (1982). Halstead–Reitan impairment in chronic alcoholics as a function of age of drinking onset. *Clinical Neuropsychology, 4,* 115–119.

Post, R. M., Weiss, S. R. B., Pert, A., & Uhde, T. W. (1987). Chronic cocaine administration: Sensitization and kindling effects. In S. Fisher, A. Raskin, & E. H. Uhlenhuth (Eds.), *Cocaine: Clinical and biobehavioral aspects* (pp. 109–173). New York: Oxford University Press.

Prejean, J., & Gouvier, W. D. (1994). Neuropsychological sequelae of chronic recreational gasoline inhalation. *Archives of Clinical Neuropsychology, 9,* 173–174.

Quintanilla, M. (1994, February 16). Bad habits: Drugs. *Los Angeles Times,* p. E1.

Rainone, G. A., Deren, S., Kleinman, P. H., & Wish, E. D. (1987). Heavy marijuana users not in treatment: The continuing search for the "pure" marijuana users. *Journal of Psychoactive Drugs, 19* (4), 353–359.

Ranlett, G., Gansler, D. A., & Kodituwakku, P. (1995). *Planning deficits in cocaine addicted adults: Evidence of prefrontal dysfunction.* Paper presented at the annual meeting of the National Academy of Neuropsychology, San Francisco.

Reuhl, K. R. (1991). Delayed expression of neurotoxicity. The problem of silent damage. *Neurotoxicology, 12,* 341–346.

Ricaurte, G. A., & Langston, J. W. (1995). Neurological complications of drugs of abuse. In M. J. Aminoff (Ed.), *Neurology and general medicine* (2nd ed., pp. 631–640). Edinburgh: Churchill Livingstone.

The Risk Management Foundation of the Harvard Medical Institutions, Inc. (1993). *MicroCog: Assessment of cognitive functioning.* San Antonio, TX: The Psychological Corporation.

Ross, C. A. (1982). Gasoline sniffing and encephalopathy. *Canadian Medical Association Journal, 127,* 1195–1197.

Rylander, G. (1972). Psychoses and the punding and choreiform syndromes in addiction to central stimulant drugs. *Psychiatria, Neurologia, Neurochirurgia, 75,* 203–212.

Schroeder, S. P. (1995). Environmental toxins. In M. C. Roberts (Ed.), *Handbook of pediatric psychology* (2nd ed., pp. 774–790). New York: Guilford Press.

Schuckit, M. A. (1984). *Drug and alcohol abuse: A clinical guide to diagnosis and treatment* (2nd ed.). New York: Plenum Press.

Schuckit, M. A. (1994). MDMA (Ecstasy): An old drug with new tracks. *Drug Abuse and Alcoholism Newsletter,* Vista Hill Foundation, *23*(2).

Schuckit, M. A. (1995a). Abuse and dependence on nitrous oxide. *Drug Abuse and Alcoholism Newsletter,* Vista Hill Foundation, *24.*

Schuckit, M. A. (1995b). Is there a clinically significant marijuana withdrawal syndrome? *Drug Abuse and Alcoholism Newsletter,* Vista Hill Foundation, *24*(2).

Schwartz, R. H., Gruenewald, P. J., Klitzner, M., & Fedio, P. (1989). Short-term memory impairment in cannabis-dependent adolescents. *American Journal of Diseases of Childhood, 143,* 1214–1219.

Seshia, S. S., Rajani, K. R., Boeckx, R. L., & Chow, P. N. (1978). The neurological manifestations of chronic inhalation of leaded gasoline. *Developmental Medicine and Child Neurology, 20,* 323–334.

Sharp, C. W. (1992). Introduction to inhalant abuse. In C. W. Sharp, F. Beauvais, & R. Spence (Eds.), *Inhalant abuse: A volatile research agenda* (pp. 1–12). (NIDA Research Monograph 129). Rockville, MD: U. S. Department of Health and Human Services.

Spencer, J. W. (1990). Why evaluate for residual drug effects. In J. W. Spencer & J. J. Boren (Eds.), *Residual effects of abused drugs and behavior* (pp. 1–9). (NIDA Research Monograph 101). Rockville, MD: U. S. Department of Health and Human Services.

Spitzer, R. L., Williams, J. B. W., & Skodal, A. E. (1980). DSM-III: The major achievements and an overview. *American Journal of Psychiatry, 143,* 463–468.

Stepp, L. S. (1994, February 20). More youth sniff for high that can snuff life. *Los Angeles Times,* p. A20.

Strickland, T. L., Mena, I., Meyer, J. V., Miller, B., Mehringer, C. M., Satz, P., & Myers, H. (1991). *Cerebral perfusion and neuropsychological consequences of chronic cocaine use.* Paper presented at the annual meeting of the National Academy of Neuropsychology, Dallas.

Strickland, T. L., Mena, I., Villanueva-Meyer, J., & Miller, B. (1993). Cerebral perfusion and neuropsychological consequences of chronic cocaine use. *Journal of Neuropsychology and Clinical Neurosciences, 5,* 419–427.

Strickland, T. L., & Stein, R. A. (1995). *Neurobehavioral functioning in chronic cocaine abusers following sustained abstinence.* Paper presented at the annual meeting of the National Academy of Neuropsychology, San Francisco.

Stuss, D. T., & Cummings, J. L. (1990). Subcortical vascular dementia. In J. L. Cummings (Ed.), *Subcortical dementia* (pp. 145–163). London: Oxford University Press.

Swan, N. (1995, March/April). Marijuana, other drug use among teens continues to rise. *NIDA Notes,* p. 8.

Tarter, R. E., & Edwards, K. L. (1985). Neuropsychology of alcoholism. In R. E. Tarter & D. H. Van Thiel (Eds.), *Alcohol and the brain: Chronic effects* (pp. 217–242). New York: Plenum Press.

Tramontana, M. G. (1983). Neuropsychological evaluation of children and adolescents with psychopathological disorders. In C. J. Golden & P. J. Vincente (Eds.), *Foundations in clinical neuropsychology* (pp. 309–340). New York: Plenum Press.

Trites, R. L., Suh, M., Offord, D., Neiman, G., & Preston, D. (1974, October). *Neuropsychologic and psychosocial antecedents and chronic effects of prolonged use of solvent and methamphetamine.* Paper presented at the meeting of the International Psychiatric Research Society, Ottawa.

Tsushima, W. T., & Towne, W. S. (1977). Effects of paint sniffing on neuropsychological test performance. *Journal of Abnormal Psychology, 86,* 402–407.

Turkington, C. (1986, March). Brain damage found with designer drugs. *APA Monitor,* p. 18.

University of Michigan. (1994). *1993 Monitoring the Future Survey.* Ann Arbor, MI: Institute for Social Research.

U. S. Department of Health and Human Services, Centers for Disease Control. (1991). Alcohol and other drug use among high school students—United States, 1990. *Morbidity and Mortality Weekly Report, 777*. Washington, DC: U. S. Government Printing Office.

van Gorp, W. G., Wilkins, J. N., Hinkin, C. H., Horner, M., Plotkin, D., Welch, B., Moore, L., Marcotte, T., Boris, S., Beckson, M., & Wheatley, W. S. (1995). *Acute versus persistent effects of cocaine use on neuropsychological functioning*. Paper presented at the annual convention of the American Psychological Association, New York.

Varney, N. R., Alexander, B., & MacIndoe, J. H. (1984). Reversible steroid dementia in patients without steroid psychosis. *American Journal of Psychiatry, 141*, 369–372.

Volkow, N. D., Mullani, N., Gould, K. L., Adler, S., & Krajewski, K. (1988). Cerebral blood flow in chronic cocaine users: A study with positron emission tomography. *British Journal of Psychiatry, 152*, 641–648.

Vorhees, C. V. (1994). Developmental neurotoxicity induced by therapeutic and illicit drugs. *Environmental Health Perspectives, 102* (Suppl. 2), 145–153.

Ware, L. A. (1979). Neuropsychological functioning in users and nonusers of phencyclidine. *Dissertation Abstracts International, 39*, 5126–5127. (University Microfilms No. 7908094)

Washton, A. M., & Stone-Washton, N. (1993). Outpatient treatment of cocaine and crack addiction: A clinical perspective. In F. M. Tims & C. G. Leukefelds (Eds.), *Cocaine treatment: Research and clinical perspectives* (NIDA Research Monograph 135, pp. 15–30). Rockville, MD: U. S. Department of Health and Human Services.

Wilde, C. (1975). Aerosol metallic paints: Deliberate inhalation. A study of inhalation and/or ingestion of copper and zinc particles. *International Journal of Addiction, 10*, 127–134.

Wolkowitz, O. M., Reus, V. I., Weingartner, H., & Thompson, K. (1990). Cognitive effects of corticosteroid. *American Journal of Psychiatry, 147*, 1297–1303.

Wolkowitz, O. M., Weingartner, H., Rubinow, D. R., Jimerson, D., Kling, M., Berretini, W., Thompson, K., Breier, A., Doran, A., Reus, V. I., & Pickar, D. (1993). Steroid modulation of human memory: Biochemical correlates. *Biological Psychiatry, 33*(10), 744–746.

Woody, G. E., McLellan, A. T., & O'Brien, T. (1990). Clinical–behavioral observations of the long-term effects of drug abuse. In J. W. Spencer & J. J. Boren (Eds.), *Residual effects of abused drugs on behavior* (pp. 71–85). (NIDA Research Monograph 101). Rockville, MD: U. S. Department of Health and Human Services.

Woolf, D. S. (1983). Polypharmacy and the addict. In G. Bennett, C. Vourakis, & D. Woolf (Eds.), *Substance abuse: Pharmacologic, developmental, and clinical perspectives* (pp. 110–120). New York: Wiley.

Wright, M., & Hogan, T. P. (1972). Repeated LSD ingestion and performance on neuropsychological tests. *Journal of Nervous and Mental Disease, 154*, 432–438.

Yamaguchi, K., & Kandel, D. B. (1994). Patterns of drug use from adolescence to young adulthood. II. Sequences of progression. *American Journal of Public Health, 74*, 668–672.

Yesalis, C. E., Kennedy, N. J., Kopstein, A. N., & Bahrke, M. S. (1993). Anabolic-androgenic steroid use in the United States. *Journal of the American Medical Association, 270*, 1217–1221.

Yesavage, J. A., Leirer, V. O., Denari, M., & Hollister, L. E. (1985). Carry-over effects of marijuana intoxication on aircraft pilot performance: A preliminary report. *American Journal of Psychiatry, 142*, 1325–1329.

Young, L. A., Young, L. G., Klein, M. M., Klein, D. M., & Beyer, D. (1977). *Recreational drugs*. New York: Collier Books.

IV

Special Topics in Clinical Child Neuropsychology

Neuropsychological Aspects of Attention Deficit/Hyperactivity Disorder

CAROL A. BOLIEK AND JOHN E. OBRZUT

Introduction

According to the *Diagnostic and Statistical Manual of Mental Disorders* (4th edition) (DSM-IV) (American Psychiatric Association, 1994), major diagnostic criteria of attention deficit/hyperactivity disorder (ADHD) include persistent patterns of inattentiveness, impulsivity, and hyperactivity. In comparison with other children of the same mental age, children with ADHD exhibit these symptoms in varying degrees of excess. The prevalence of ADHD is estimated at between 3 and 5% of all school-age children. Although data on prevalence in adolescence and adulthood are limited, it is thought that the percentages remain relatively stable through early adolescence. In a majority of cases, symptoms abate during late adolescence and adulthood. However, a lesser number of individuals continue to experience the entire array of symptoms associated with ADHD into midadulthood.

Children diagnosed as experiencing ADHD often are school underachievers (Barkley, DuPaul, & McMurray, 1990), exhibit disturbed peer relationships (Pelham & Bender, 1982), and a majority demonstrate conduct problems or hostility toward adults (Loney & Milich, 1982). This behavioral disorder is one of the most common childhood psychiatric disorders (Barkley, 1990), yet criteria for

diagnosis have been quite controversial (Cantwell & Baker, 1988; Goodyear & Hynd, 1992). The confusion stems in part from the heterogeneous nature of ADHD and the associated academic, social, and emotional problems encountered in this endeavor. With the publication of DSM-IV, several distinct subtypes of ADHD have been outlined and thus should aid in diagnostic decision-making. Besides emphasis devoted to the identification of homogeneous subtypes of ADHD, researchers have addressed issues related to comorbidity. In particular, because ADHD is believed to frequently occur with learning disabilities (LD), studies have attempted to differentiate ADHD and LD on academic, social, and neuropsychological correlates of these two syndromes (Hynd, Lorys, *et al.*, 1991). In light of the foregoing, this chapter is intended to describe the diagnostic criteria for distinguishing distinct subtypes of ADHD as operationalized by DSM-IV, provide evidence for the neurobiological basis of ADHD, differentiate behavioral symptomatology in children with ADHD and LD, and present evidence related to the reading, math, and social skills of children with ADHD.

Diagnostic Features of ADHD

According to DSM-IV the essential feature of ADHD is "a persistent pattern of inattention and/or hyperactivity–impulsivity that is more frequent and severe than is typically observed in individuals at a comparable level of development" (American Psychiatric Association, 1994, p. 78). However, this feature is but one of several that must be present in

---

CAROL A. BOLIEK • National Center for Neurogenic Communication Disorders, University of Arizona, Tucson, Arizona 85721.   JOHN E. OBRZUT • Department of Educational Psychology, College of Education, University of Arizona, Tucson, Arizona 85721.

order for a diagnosis of ADHD to be given. In addition, the symptom pattern must have existed before age 7 years and the impairment from the symptoms must be observed in at least two settings (i.e., home, school, work). These essential behavioral features must be developmentally inappropriate and exhibited in varying degrees of excess by ADHD children relative to children of the same mental age. Finally, the condition of ADHD should not occur exclusively during the course of a Pervasive Developmental Disorder (e.g., schizophrenia, autism) and cannot be accounted for by another mental disorder such as mood disorders, anxiety disorders, or personality disorders.

The specific symptoms of inattention, hyperactivity, and/or impulsivity may be manifested in academic, occupational, or social situations. For example, in schoolwork, children may demonstrate *inattention* by making careless mistakes as a result of failing to pay close attention to details. These children often find it hard to persist with tasks, act as if they are not listening, shift from one uncompleted activity to another, and fail to complete their assignments, despite the fact that instructions were understood. Tasks that require sustained attention, organization, or close scrutiny, such as homework assignments, are avoided. These individuals are easily distracted and quite often show a lack of habituation to novel or irrelevant stimuli. In the home, chores may be neglected or totally forgotten. On a social level, inattention by these children is exemplified by not listening to the flow of conversations, shifting their own conversation, and/or not following the sequence of rules in games or activities.

Children who manifest *hyperactivity* are best characterized by excessive amounts of locomotion such as running or climbing when inappropriate, excess movement in one's seat in the classroom, difficulty in partaking quietly in extracurricular activities, lacking in motor system control, and/or talking indiscriminately. Hyperactivity seen in toddlers and preschoolers is similar to that of school-age children in symptomatology. However, the activity level is less frequent and less intense in school-age children than is reported for toddlers and preschoolers. In adolescents and adults, hyperactivity is expressed as feelings of restlessness and inability to participate in rather sedentary activities.

Children with symptoms of *impulsivity* may be described as exhibiting a lack of patience or difficulty in delaying responses to the external environ-

ment. For example, children with ADHD may not wait their turn to respond to teacher questions, make comments out of turn, or initiate comments at inappropriate times. These children will frequently interrupt others, fail to wait for specific instructions or directions before proceeding, may physically grab or touch objects that are off-limits, and may act as the class clown in excess. Some, if not all, of these symptoms may cause difficulties in academic, social, or employment environs.

As stated above, behavioral manifestations are likely to appear in multiple settings, such as school, home, and social contexts. Later, these behaviors may be manifested in occupational settings. To make the diagnosis of ADHD, some impairment must be exhibited in at least two of these settings. Although symptoms may be more evident in situations that require sustained attention or that lack internal appeal (e.g., engaging in classroom work), diagnostic features may be lessened or absent when the child is in a controlled situation, is in a new environment, is involved in a rewarding activity, or while engaged in a one-to-one exchange (e.g., the doctor's office). The symptoms are more likely to occur in group activities or situations.

Subtypes of ADHD

As stated above, controversy has focused on whether specific subtypes of ADHD exist. For example, previous research suggests that at least two subtypes do exist. These two subtypes have been labeled as: attention deficit disorder with hyperactivity (ADD/H) and attention deficit disorder without hyperactivity (ADD/WO) (American Psychiatric Association, 1980; Cantwell & Baker, 1988; Goodyear & Hynd, 1992). Although most individuals have symptoms of both inattention and hyperactivity–impulsivity, clinicians have found there are some individuals in whom one or the other pattern is more dominant. As a result, DSM-IV has identified three subtypes and states that, for purposes of making a current diagnosis, the appropriate subtype should be indicated based on the predominant symptom pattern for the past 6 months. The first subtype is labeled as *attention-deficit/hyperactivity disorder, combined type.* According to DSM-IV, this subtype should be used if six or more symptoms of inattention *and* six or more symptoms of hyperactivity–impulsivity have persisted during the last 6 months. The second subtype is labeled as *attention-deficit/hyperactiv-*

ity disorder, predominantly inattention type. This subtype should be applied if six or more symptoms of inattention, but *fewer* than six symptoms of hyperactivity–impulsivity, have persisted for the previous 6-month period. The third subtype is labeled as *attention-deficit/hyperactivity disorder, predominantly hyperactive-impulsive type.* This subtype is applied if six or more symptoms of hyperactivity–impulsivity, but *fewer* than six symptoms of inattention, have persisted for the previous 6-month period. Individuals may be diagnosed as having one subtype of the disorder at one period of time and may develop another predominant subtype at a later date. However, if the specific criteria are no longer met for the existing three subtypes, the diagnosis made is *attention-deficit/hyperactivity disorder, in partial remission.*

Associated Descriptive Symptoms and Disorders of ADHD

Criteria for diagnosis of ADHD continue to be somewhat controversial related in part to the heterogeneous nature of this disorder and to the existence of associated problems, such as poor academic achievement, inappropriate social skills, and disruptive and/or uncontrolled behavior (Goodyear & Hynd, 1992). Support for the validity of these findings is evident by the plethora of associated features and mental disorders provided in DSM-IV. According to DSM-IV, associated features of ADHD may include low frustration tolerance, temper outbursts, stubbornness, excessive and frequent insistence that requests be met, mood lability, demoralization, dysphoria, rejection by peers, and poor self-concept (American Psychiatric Association, 1994). In conjunction with these symptoms, academic achievement is often neglected and devalued. Poor academic achievement often results in conflict with family members and/or school authorities. Family relationships become strained and are characterized by resentment and antagonism in which parents consider the child's undesirable behavior to be voluntary. In addition, children with ADHD may drop out of school earlier than their peers and have less success in occupational situations.

Recent research has confirmed that intellectual development, in particular verbal IQ, is somewhat lower in children with this disorder (Korkman

& Personen, 1994). Children with ADHD who are referred to clinics often have superimposed disorders such as oppositional defiant disorder or conduct disorder. Furthermore, DSM-IV indicates there may be a higher prevalence of mood disorders, anxiety disorders, learning disorders, and communication disorders in children with ADHD. Tourette's syndrome often coexists with ADHD, the ADHD preceding the onset of the Tourette's condition. Case histories of children with ADHD often have indicated a likelihood of child abuse or neglect, multiple foster care placements, neurotoxin exposure, infections, drug exposure *in utero*, low birth weight, and mental retardation.

It is significant that ADHD is known to occur in various cultures. However, the variations in reported prevalence among Western societies are thought to be related to different diagnostic practices rather than to actual differences in clinical symptomatology. As with other diagnostic syndromes, it is difficult to diagnose children with this disorder below the age of 4, primarily because young children are not required to perform tasks that demand sustained attention or concentrated effort. Individuals with ADHD do exhibit clinical symptoms that vary with age. For example, young children with ADHD will tend to be in constant motion and may be difficult to contain. With maturity, symptoms usually become more discreet. During late childhood and early adolescence the random motor movements are less common and hyperactivity may take on the form of restlessness and/or inability to concentrate. In adulthood, restlessness may limit one's involvement or participation in sedentary activities or in vocational pursuits that inhibit spontaneous movement.

This disorder has been reported to be more prevalent in males, with male-to-female ratios ranging from 4:1 to 9:1 (American Psychiatric Association, 1994). However, with the introduction of DSM-IV, it is likely that more females will be diagnosed under the subtype ADHD-Predominantly Inattention Type. Heretofore, females without the feature of hyperactivity were underidentified as having the ADHD syndrome. This disorder also has been found to be more prevalent in first-degree familial relatives of children with ADHD. In order for an adequate differential diagnosis to be made, it is suggested that reports from multiple informants be obtained. These should include, but not be limited to, teachers, parents, grandparents, parents of peers, and so forth. This would allow for observations regarding the child's inattention, hyperactivity, and capacity for self-regulation in a multitude of settings.

Behavioral Symptomatology of ADHD and LD

Whereas data generally support the behavioral differentiation of subtyping ADHD into more homogeneous, clinically defined groups, some literature suggests that children with LD display similar behavioral symptomatology with children diagnosed as having ADHD, Predominately Inattention Type. Previously this subtype was identified as ADD/WO by DSM-III (American Psychiatric Association, 1980). Several authors have provided empirical evidence indicating comorbidity between ADD/WO and LD (Hynd, Lorys, *et al.*, 1991; Shaywitz & Shaywitz, 1991). Based on evidence from studies regarding differential characteristics of children with ADD/H, ADD/WO, and LD, Goodyear and Hynd (1992) suggested that children with ADD/WO are likely to be behaviorally more similar to children diagnosed as LD, thereby exhibiting more lethargy, social withdrawal, poorer organizational skills, and learning difficulties, relative to those children diagnosed as ADD/H. Children with ADD/H are often viewed as being more aggressive and behaviorally disruptive. According to Goodyear and Hynd (1992), these differences may occur despite the overall shared diagnostic characteristics of inattention and impulsivity within the two groups with attention disorder. Thus, the presumption is there are differences in the nature of these reported behaviors that differentiate the two attention groups beyond the trait of motor hyperactivity.

In order to investigate whether the behavioral characteristics of children diagnosed as ADD/WO more closely resembled the behavioral profiles of children diagnosed as LD than those children diagnosed as ADD/H, Stanford and Hynd (1994) examined the frequency and nature of symptoms (i.e., impulsivity, inattention, and social withdrawal) endorsed by parents and teachers on behavior rating scales. Their sample consisted of 77 outpatients in a university diagnostic and referral service and were divided into three groups. Group 1 ($N = 35$) included children with a primary diagnosis of ADD/H, Group 2 ($N = 25$) included children with a primary diagnosis of ADD/WO, and Group 3 ($N = 17$) included children with a primary diagnosis of LD, defined as developmental reading or mathematics disorder. Each child's mother was administered the Structured Interview for Diagnostic Assessment of Children (SIDAC) (Puig-Antich & Chambers, 1978), the Child Behavior Checklist-Parent Form (CBCL-P) (Achenbach & Edelbrock, 1983), and the SNAP Checklist (Pelham, Atkins, & Murphy, 1981). Each child's teacher completed the Achenbach Child Behavior Checklist Teacher Form (CBCL-T) (Achenbach & Edelbrock, 1983) and the SNAP Checklist. Previous research with these measures indicates their utility in discriminating children with ADD/H from those with ADD/WO on symptoms of hyperactivity, impulsivity, and inattention (e.g., Edelbrock & Rancurello, 1985; Lahey *et al.*, 1988).

It was hypothesized that there would be significant differences between the ADD/H and ADD/WO groups on items reflecting behavioral characteristics, such as poor organization skills, social withdrawal, and slow cognitive tempo, whereas there would be no significant difference on these behavioral characteristics between the ADD/WO and LD groups. In addition to the comparisons at the item level, cluster analysis was employed to examine group differences across constructs of inattention, impulsivity, and withdrawal/lethargy.

Although there was overall support found for the hypothesis that children with ADD/WO more closely resembled children with LD, there were also behavioral symptoms specific to both ADD subtypes that were not manifested to the same degree by children who were diagnosed as LD (Stanford & Hynd, 1994). Generally, the results indicated that parents and teachers characterized children with ADD/H as more disruptive than children with ADD/WO or LD. This finding is consistent with results of previous studies differentiating ADD/WO from ADD/H based on externalizing and internalizing symptoms (e.g., Barkley *et al.*, 1990; Gonzalez, 1991), and of a study that contrasted hyperactive children and children with LD (Holborow & Berry, 1986). The ADD/WO and LD groups of children were described as more underactive and shy and as daydreaming more often than their ADD/H counterparts. Whereas teachers rated children with ADD/WO and LD as being similar to each other on symptoms of withdrawal and impulsivity, both teachers and parents endorsed different symptoms of inattention for children with ADD/WO and LD.

Expected differences between the two ADD groups and similarities between the ADD/WO group and the LD group on items related to disorganization and need for supervision were not found in the study. Both parents and teachers endorsed these symptoms in the two ADD groups more frequently that in the LD group. However, both parents and teachers described the ADD/WO group as being more disorganized and needing more supervision than the ADD/H group. These results are similar to those found by Lahey *et al.* (1988) in which cluster analyses produced separate factors of inattention–disorganization associated with ADD/WO and motor hyperactivity–impulsivity associated with ADD/H.

In the Stanford and Hynd (1994) study, both parents and teachers rated the ADD/H group as more impulsive than the ADD/WO and LD groups, and the nature of the impulsivity was more overt and disruptive. As the authors point out, whereas these findings are consistent with previous studies that identified children with ADD/H as more disruptive, aggressive, and impulsive than children with ADD/WO or LD (e.g., Ackerman, Dykman, & Oglesby, 1983; Carlson, Lahey, Frame, Walker, & Hynd, 1987), this study utilized a direct comparison between a diagnostically differentiated ADD/WO group and a group of children diagnosed as LD.

Whereas some research has addressed issues related to comorbidity (Cantwell & Baker, 1991) and differentiation of behavioral symptomatology between subjects with ADHD and LD, recent research has begun to provide systematic comparison on neuropsychological measures related to aspects of functioning relevant for attention and learning. In this regard, studies have compared children with ADHD and those with LD on some variant of the Continuous Performance Test (CPT) or have utilized memory and language tests, as well as attention scales. For example, on the CPT, Van der Meere, van Baal, and Sergeant (1989) found that children with LD were impaired in memory search and decision processes, whereas children with hyperactivity were impaired in motor-decision processes. Although Kupietz (1990) found no differences between the two groups in number of correct detections and number of commission errors on initial examination, the LD group improved more than the ADHD group with increasing age. Other authors have found that subjects with both ADHD and LD were more affected by distractors to the target letters than were subjects with LD only (Richards, Samuels, Turnure, & Ysseldyke, 1990).

Impaired verbal memory and susceptibility to interference effects in verbal memory tasks have been found to differentiate ADHD and LD children (e.g., Benezra & Douglas, 1988; Siegel & Ryan, 1989). Impairment on measures of naming and phonological awareness also have been found to discriminate between these two groups (August & Garfinkel, 1990; Felton & Wood, 1989). Douglas and Benezra (1990) found that ADHD children were characterized by deficits on memory tasks requiring organized, deliberate rehearsal strategies, whereas LD children exhibited a more generalized verbal deficit. Robins (1992), however, did not find differences on tasks requiring verbal memory, verbal learning to trials, or sustained attention between ADHD and LD children, although other behavioral symptoms were noted. The children with ADHD were specifically characterized by impulsive behavior, impaired accuracy when speed of responding was required, aggressivity, and poor ability to work independently in the classroom.

As shown, there is much concordance in the findings of deficiencies in specific aspects of attention and learning that differentiate children with ADHD from those with LD. However, until recently, there has been no systematic comparison of children with ADHD and children with LD on a comprehensive set of neuropsychological measures relating to all or most aspects of functioning that have been found relevant for attention and learning. Korkman and Pesonen (1994) suggest such a comparison would provide insight not only on interindividual but also on intraindividual differences by analyzing test patterns or profiles. Thus, Korkman and Personen employed the Neuropsychological Assessment of Children (NEPSY) (Korkman, 1988) instrument consisting of 36 tests that "tap various aspects of attention, language, motor, sensory, and visual-spatial functions, and memory and learning" (p. 384) with a group of 8-year-old second graders who fulfilled the criteria of having either ADHD ($N = 21$) or specific LD ($N = 12$) or both ($N = 27$). Their aim was to compare differences that emerged as double disassociation; that is, children with ADHD, but not children with LD, having impairments in some tests, and children with LD, but not children with ADHD, having impairments in others.

Teachers' ratings of ADHD based on the DSM-III diagnostic criteria for ADD/H were used for the purpose of verifying the syndrome in the children. The dependent measures consisted of 19 subtests of the NEPSY, primarily those associated with attention, language, sensory–motor, visual–spatial, and memory functions. In addition, the academic areas of reading and spelling were assessed. The results indicated the children with ADHD were impaired in the control and inhibition of impulses, whereas the children with LD were specifically impaired in phonological awareness (as defined by the Auditory Analyses of Speech subtest), verbal memory (digit) span, storytelling, and verbal IQ. The children with both disorders exhibited all of these deficiencies and, in addition, demonstrated more pervasive attention problems along with a greater amount of visual–motor problems. Korkman and Pesonen (1994) also found that all three groups showed impaired performance in tasks of visual–motor precision and name retrieval. However, the authors attributed different mechanisms or causal factors underlying impairments in the clinical groups. Name-retrieval deficiencies in the LD group were assumed to be related to linguistic impairment and possibly contributing to reading and spelling problems. In the ADHD group, name-retrieval deficiencies were related to attention problems and poor active memorization and not causally related to specific reading and spelling problems. Thus, this study confirmed earlier findings of impaired control and inhibition of impulses as the main symptom of ADHD, and of phonological and linguistic deficiencies as symptoms of LD. In contrast, a double disassociation did not appear in the name-retrieval tasks as both groups were impaired.

Neurobiological Etiology of ADHD

Evidence from neuropharmacological investigations, from genetic studies, and from studies demonstrating that ADHD can be associated with other neuropsychiatric syndromes has generally led to the acceptance that ADHD is the result of CNS dysfunction (Zametkin & Rapoport, 1987). However, as Hynd and Willis (1988) point out, there is little evidence that can directly implicate any one neural system or brain structure. In fact there are hypotheses implicating dysfunctions at nearly every neuroanatomical level of the brain from the brain stem to the frontal lobes. As well, there are hypotheses implicating neurochemical dysfunctions as underlying causes of ADHD. The controversy regarding the neurological basis of ADHD will likely continue for some time to come. However, with advances in psychopharmacological treatments, neuroimaging methods, and increased sensitivity of clinical psychometrics, underlying neurologic etiologies related to specific ADHD subtypes will no doubt be clarified.

Psychopharmacological Evidence

Preclinical studies have shown that dextroamphetamine and methylphenidate block the reuptake of dopamine and norepinephrine at the presynaptic neuron (Calis, Grothe, & Elia, 1990). However, it appears from both animal and human studies that biochemical effects and behaviors differ between these stimulants (Elia, 1991). For example, when dextroamphetamine is administered, the resultant urinary excretion yields a reduction of norepinephrine and its metabolite 3-methoxy-4-hydroxyphenylglycol (MHPG). This result along with positive behavioral response to dextroamphetamine implicates norepinephrine as a possible neurotransmitter marker for ADHD (Calis *et al.,* 1990). In contrast, the administration of methylphenidate hydrochloride, pemoline, and tranylcypromine sulfate yields no change in urinary excretion of norepinephrine or MHPG. Consequently, dopamine is implicated as a possible neurotransmitter for ADHD. Therefore, it appears that both dopamine and norepinephrine do contribute to the pathophysiology of ADHD.

There also is evidence to suggest that subtypes of ADHD may respond differentially to stimulant medication. In a recent study, Barkley, DuPaul, and McMurray (1991) examined the clinical response to three dose levels of methylphenidate with 23 children identified as ADD/H and 17 children identified as ADD/WO. The study was a rigorous triple-blind, placebo-controlled, crossover design using three dose levels (5, 10, and 15 mg twice a day) of methylphenidate. Their results showed children with ADD/WO had either no clinical response or responded best to the low dose of methylphenidate (5 mg twice a day). Children with ADD/H responded positively to moderate and high dose levels of methylphenidate (10 and 15 mg twice a day). These findings led Barkley and his colleagues to conclude that ADD/WO is a different disorder than ADD/H as opposed to being a subtype of the same shared attention disturbance.

According to some reports, stimulant medication may induce or exacerbate tics (Stevenson & Wolraich, 1989). These investigators found that the risk for developing a tic disorder after use of stimulant medication was 1.3%. However, they posited that the risk would probably be higher in children with a family history of Gilles de la Tourette's disease or other tic syndromes.

Tricyclic antidepressants, monoamine oxidase inhibitors (MAOIs), and clonidine also have been used in the pharmacological treatment of ADHD. Tricyclic antidepressants such as imipramine (Trofanil) and disipramine (Norpramin) serve to block the reuptake of both norepinephrine and serotonin. MAOIs such as tranylcypromine sulfate and clorgiline have been effective in treating ADHD (Zametkin et al., 1985). MAOIs interact with both noradrenergic and dopaminergic neurons. MAOIs inhibit the enzyme MAO thus causing an increase in levels of dopamine and norepinephrine in the brain (Cooper, Bloom, & Roth, 1991). Clonidine hydrochloride, which is an antihypertensive drug, also has been shown to be an effective alternative in the treatment of ADHD (Hunt, Minderaa, & Cohen, 1985).

Children with ADHD appear to respond to stimulant and other medications. These findings support the hypothesis that certain subtypes of ADHD have a constitutional origin (Shaywitz & Shaywitz, 1987). However, whereas it is sometimes possible to understand the action of a drug at a molecular and cellular level, it is extremely difficult to explain the effect on behavior. This lack of explanation reflects the many intermediary reactions between the neuronal system and the ultimate behavior (Cooper et al., 1991).

Hormonal Evidence

Several investigations have been aimed at relating ADHD to thyroid abnormalities. Between 46 and 70% of children with generalized resistance to thyroid hormone (GRTH) also present with ADHD (Hauser et al., 1993; Refetoff, Weiss, & Usala, 1993). In addition, children with GRTH also have demonstrated a higher incidence of language disorders (Mixson et al., 1992). In a study of 277 children diagnosed as ADHD, Weiss and colleagues found a higher prevalence of thyroid abnormalities (5.4%) in children with ADHD as compared with that found in the normal population (<1%) (Weiss, Stein, Trommer, & Refetoff, 1993).

Thyroid hormone is necessary for brain development. However, the pathophysiology of the relation between ADHD and GRTH is not fully understood (Weiss et al., 1993). Using positron emission tomography, it has been demonstrated that patients with GRTH and ADHD have altered brain glucose uptake (Hauser et al., 1992). On the basis of the studies to date on GRTH and ADHD, it is probable that psychological disturbances in GRTH are multifactorial. As well, psychological abnormalities such as ADHD might be the result of exposure of the brain to high thyroid levels (Weiss et al., 1993).

Neuroimaging Findings

Neuroanatomical asymmetries in right-handed individuals have been reliably observed and appear to have functional or behavioral correlates (Witelsen, 1990). For example, the planum temporale is usually larger on the left than on the right side (Witelsen & Kigar, 1988). The right frontal volume has been found to be larger than the left frontal volume (Weinberger, Luchins, Morihisa, & Wyatt, 1982). Few neuroimaging studies have been done with normally developing child populations and even fewer studies have been done on clinical child populations. Of the studies conducted on child populations, several have focused on the neuroanatomical correlates of ADHD.

The caudate nucleus has been examined by several investigators as a possible brain structure where differences might occur in ADHD populations. The caudate nuclei have extensive pathways to the frontal lobes as well as the thalamus and could be implicated as one of several underlying mechanisms for motor control. Using cerebral blood flow (rCBF) neuroimaging techniques, it has been shown that a pure group of ADHD children with hyperactivity had significant hypoperfusion in the caudate–striatal region. Specifically, children with ADHD had significant hypoperfusion in the right striatum (Lou, Henriksen, Bruhn, Borner, & Neilsen, 1989). These investigators also reported that in contrast to children with ADHD only, children with mental retardation or dysphasia as a co-occurrence showed bilateral hypoperfusion in the caudate–striatal region. Further, when methylphenidate was administered to the pure ADHD group, there was a significant increase in perfusion in both right and left striatal regions, but more so in the left striatum.

Hynd and colleagues (Hynd et al., 1993) examined the caudate nucleus using magnetic resonance imaging (MRI). This investigation compared asymmetries in the head of the caudate nucleus in children with ADHD and matched normal controls. Whereas most of the normal children (72.7%) were found to have a left-larger-than-right (L > R) pattern of asymmetry, a large number of ADHD children (63.6%) had a left-smaller-than-right (L < R) pattern. The reason for the reversed pattern was a smaller left caudate nucleus. Further, the reversed asymmetrical pattern was found more often in boys than girls with ADHD.

Overall brain size did not differ between ADHD and control children. Therefore, the investigators suggested that the variation in the caudate nucleus might be related to deviations in brain development. Further, because the reversed pattern of asymmetry was more often found in boys rather than girls with ADHD, it is possible that boys may be at "additional" risk for deviations in brain development (Hynd *et al.*, 1993).

These findings and those of Lou *et al.* (1989) suggest that the smaller left caudate nucleus found in ADHD children might cause a right-sided bias in choline acetyltransferase and dopamine that, as discussed previously, has been associated with increased motor activity (Hynd *et al.*, 1993).

Another anatomical structure of interest in children with ADHD has been the corpus callosum. The corpus callosum plays a role in the transfer and facilitation of associative information between hemispheres. As well, the corpus callosum might be responsible, in part, for interhemispheric regulation (Lassonde, 1986). Hynd and colleagues (Hynd, Semrud-Clikeman, Lorys, Novey, Eliopulos, & Lyytinen, 1991) examined corpus callosum morphology using MRI on children with ADHD and matched normal controls. Two specific regions of the corpus callosum were found to differ between the two groups. First, the genu (anterior callosal area) was found to be smaller in children with ADHD than in normal controls. Second, a portion of the posterior callosal area also was found to be smaller in the children with ADHD. These two areas are of particular interest because of their projections to other parts of the brain. The genu is known to have interconnecting fibers to the premotor, orbitofrontal, and prefrontal regions of the brain. As Hynd *et al.* point out, the smaller genu in children with ADHD correlates with behavioral deficits in motor regulation, persistence, and inhibition possibly subserved by the frontal systems. The posterior callosal area interconnects the insula, superior and inferotemporal, and posterior-parietal cortex. The investigators suggested that the atypical morphology found in the ADHD children correlated with behavioral difficulties in visuospatial processes often observed in this population (Semrud-Clikeman & Hynd, 1990).

The frontal lobes also have been a targeted anatomic area of interest in children with ADHD. There have been several observations that the behaviors exhibited by ADHD children parallel those of adults with frontal lobe damage (Gualtieri & Hicks, 1985). The examination of frontal lobe morphology using MRI on children with ADHD and matched normal controls has shown that normal controls evidenced the expected frontal lobe asymmetry of L < R whereas ADHD children and children with dyslexia evidence symmetry of the frontal region (L = R) (Hynd, Semrud-Clikeman, Lorys, Novey, & Eliopulos, 1990). The symmetry of the frontal region in ADHD children was related to differences in right frontal width. These findings suggest that the atypical morphology found in the frontal regions of the brain in the ADHD population might be correlated with behavioral difficulties associated with frontal lobe functions.

Frontal Lobe Hypothesis

The frontal lobe hypothesis has been used to describe children and adults with ADHD. The hypothesis includes such constructs as inhibitory motor deficits and attention control deficits. In addition, the hypothesis considers other behavioral difficulties observed in children with ADHD. These difficulties include problem-solving, use of external feedback, and the generation and use of strategies (Mattes, 1980). The frontal lobes also have been implicated in the integration of prior learning as well as the regulation of response modulation of motivational and emotional states (Hamlett, Pellegrini, & Conners, 1987). Shue and Douglas (1992) have noted that patients with frontal lobe damage demonstrate difficulties in integration which in turn causes difficulties in problem-solving, responsiveness to reinforcement, and consistency in behavioral response.

Several investigations have examined the performance of children with ADHD on tasks that are sensitive to frontal lobe damage. For example, Boucugnani and Jones (1989) examined the performance of children with ADHD and matched controls on a series of tasks presumably tapping frontal lobe function. In their study, both groups of children were administered the Wisconsin Card Sorting Test (WCST), Trail-Making Test (Part B), the Stroop Test, and two WISC-R subtests. Children with ADHD differed on the WCST, Trail-Making (Part B), and the Color-Word (distraction) card of the Stroop. On the WCST, ADHD children were found to have more perseverative responses, perseverative errors, fewer categories completed, and fewer correct responses. This group also performed more poorly than controls on the time measure of the

Trail-Making (Part B) and made more errors on the Color-Word card of the Stroop. The investigators suggested that children with ADHD had more difficulties on tasks requiring disinhibition, attention, response planning, organization, and follow-through.

Shue and Douglas (1992) designed a study to address whether or not children with ADHD demonstrated a frontal lobe dysfunction or a more generalized dysfunction. Two test batteries were administered to 24 children with ADHD and 24 normal control subjects. The first battery included tasks sensitive to frontal lobe damage. The second battery included tasks sensitive to temporal lobe damage. The first battery included four measures of motor control as measured by a Go–No Go paradigm, Conflicting Motor Response Test, Incompatible Conditional Discrimination task, and Trail-Making Test (A and B). The first battery also included two measures of complex problem-solving skills as measured by the WCST and the Self-Ordered Pointing task. The results indicated that children with ADHD had significantly more difficulties than controls across tasks and that the patterns of performance were similar to patterns exhibited by patients with frontal lobe damage. Performance on the motor tasks indicated that children with ADHD could not inhibit motor responses as well as normal controls. In addition, ADHD children made more ecopraxic responses, had difficulty alternating responses quickly and accurately, and exhibited impulsive errors. Problem-solving tasks indicated that the ADHD children had difficulty formulating and testing hypotheses, integrating and using feedback to modify responses, and organizing and directing their responses. ADHD children also had more perseverative and nonperseverative errors on the WCST. The combination of deficits suggested that ADHD children exhibited a more comprehensive set of difficulties associated with the frontal lobes.

The second battery (tasks sensitive to temporal lobe dysfunction) included immediate and delayed recall memory tasks as measured by Logical Memory, Paired Associate Learning, and Digit Span from the Wechsler Memory Scale. In addition, this battery included a Recall of Spatial Location task. Typically, frontal lobe patients do well on these tasks. The results indicated that ADHD children did not differ significantly from normal controls on the Wechsler Memory Scale. However, ADHD children had deficient performance on tasks that required complex memory skills such as generation of organization strategies. These more complex memory tasks also are less well performed by frontal lobe patients

(Shue & Douglas, 1992). On the basis of the performances across both test batteries, the investigators concluded that performance deficits demonstrated by the ADHD children did not reflect generalized cognitive impairment, but rather are specific to those patients experiencing frontal lobe dysfunction.

Frontal lobe development and related skill acquisition warrants consideration in understanding children with ADHD. Normative studies with children aged 6–12 have demonstrated that motor control skills are well developed by age 6–7, whereas cognitive problem-solving skills show developmental changes between ages 10 and 12. As well, problem-solving becomes more efficient and the quality of strategies gradually improves (Becker, Isaac, & Hynd, 1988; Chelune & Baer, 1986; Passler, Isaac, & Hynd, 1985). Shue and Douglas (1992) found that young children (less than 8 years of age) performed like frontal lobe patients on many motor and problem-solving tasks described earlier. There is some evidence to suggest that children with ADHD perform between 2 and 4 years behind their age-matched counterparts (Chelune, Ferguson, Koon, & Dickey, 1986). However, it is not clear whether deficits associated with ADHD are the result of a maturational lag or represent a more permanent impairment (Shue & Douglas, 1992).

Reading Outcomes of ADHD

Much of the literature seems to point to the high degree of comorbidity of ADHD and LD. However, small sample sizes do not permit an adequate subdivision of the specific disabilities. In the majority of studies, although the experimental groups may be viewed as homogeneous, the LD group in particular is usually heterogeneous in nature. Thus, it is imperative that studies employ groups composed of children with specific types of LD, in order to detect possible variations in test profiles. Whereas specific reading disability (RD) and ADHD have been found to coexist, there is no clear consensus about the nature of the disorders in isolation, still less about their overlap (Felton & Wood, 1989). It has been observed that children referred for academic problems generally have a greater than normal incidence of significant attentional problems (e.g., Holborow & Berry, 1986). In contrast, children used in studies chosen for primary attentional problems commonly exhibit academic problems (e.g., Lambert & Sandoval, 1980).

However, a major issue concerns the primary and secondary causes of each disorder when they coexist.

From a neuropsychological perspective, children with ADHD are viewed as having deficits in sustained attention, caused by frontal and limbic dysfunction. In contrast, children who experience RD are viewed as having problems in selective attention, attributable to temporal lobe dysfunction (Ackerman, Anhalt, Dykman, & Holcomb, 1986). Although both groups display attentional problems, in children with RD these problems seem to express themselves only at times when their existing deficiencies in information processing are taxed (Dykman, Ackerman, & Holcomb, 1985). Given such a theoretical model, research designs have been invoked to distinguish between ADHD and RD children on a variety of cognitive or neuropsychological measures. For example, in a study that compared three experimental groups—ADHD with no RD, no ADHD with RD, ADHD with RD—to a control group, Dykman *et al.* (1985) found no group differences on measures of rapid automatized naming, and all three clinical groups were significantly impaired on arithmetic versus the control group. Significant differences among clinical groups were found only on an acoustic–semantic memory task, with the RD subjects performing more poorly on the phonological component of the task. Halperin, Gittelman, Klein, and Rudel (1984) found no significant differences on a host of intellectual and neuropsychological measures when administered to children with both ADHD and RD and those with ADHD without RD. In 1985, Bohline examined students referred for academic problems, some with ADHD and others without ADHD, and found no significant differences on any subtests of the Woodcock–Johnson Test of Cognitive Abilities. Thus, these studies did not show clear differences between ADHD children with and without RD.

Most studies conducted on ADHD use a variety of designs and heterogeneous subject groups that make it difficult to explain the literature by a single theoretical position. Felton and Wood (1989) suggested that the need is for a series of replicated studies with a variety of converging operations (i.e., cognitive processes), so that a more comprehensive and consistent theoretical understanding may become evident from the rather divergent and inconsistent data. Consequently, Felton and Wood (1989) conducted a series of three studies: a cross-sectional study of school-referred children, a test–retest study of children classified as unique subtypes of RD, and a study of a large, randomly selected group of first graders. These researchers controlled for differences in intelligence, age, and IQ, along with ADHD and RD as factors involved in the prediction of specific cognitive test performance. The primary purpose of this approach was to isolate the effects of ADHD and RD on a broad spectrum of cognitive processes. Assessment instruments were selected to reflect certain aspects of word retrieval, rapid automatized naming, verbal memory, and verbal fluency.

Specifically, Study 1 investigated verbal memory and naming deficits in RD and control children who were characterized according to the presence or absence of ADHD. Study 2 investigated cognitive deficits associated with subtypes of RD by evaluating naming and word retrieval skills in children classified according to the Boder subtypes (Boder & Jarrico, 1982) of RD as well as the presence or absence of ADHD. Study 3 addressed the methodological limitations of Study 1 (i.e., small sample size, limited number of cognitive measures, and school-referred sample) and investigated a wide variety of cognitive skills in a large sample of randomly selected schoolchildren who were characterized according to evidence of attentional deficits and beginning reading ability.

Using multivariate statistical procedures, Felton and Wood (1989) found that the cognitive deficits associated with difficulties in reading were consistent across samples (school-referred and randomly selected), developmental levels (beginning readers and upper elementary level students), and definitions of subtypes of RD. Controlling IQ, age, and sex, subjects with RD were significantly impaired on measures of confrontation naming, rapid automatized naming, and phonological awareness. However, there were no consistent RD effects found on measures of verbal learning and memory for lists of words presented over trials, memory for narrative material, or on tasks involving visual memory or visual perception. The effects of attentional deficits were more variable and complex but were independent from the RD effects.

Because external validation of these clinical groups has been less than satisfactory, Dykman and Ackerman (1991) utilized another approach aimed at obtaining divergent as well as convergent validity. These authors recruited a large, heterogeneous group of clinic-referred children with ADHD and studied them on several dimensions (cognitive, affective, physiological), in an effort to demonstrate replicable subtypes. Based on previous work (Dykman *et al.,* 1985), this study hypothesized a nonhyperactive, nonaggressive ADD subtype, as well as the hyperactive subtype. Additionally, it was hypothesized that within each ADD group there would be significant numbers of children with RD. Measures of convergent validity of ADD behavioral subtypes included parent and teacher ratings of attention, activity, and aggression. Measures of divergent validity included ratings of temperament, personality, and emotional standing. The physiological dimension was inferred by using tasks measuring sensitivity, arousal, sustained attention, and impulsivity. Finally, to assess short-term outcome as a function of subgroup, a 4-week trial of medication (i.e., methylphenidate) was administered in two dose levels.

Cluster analysis of teacher ratings applied to this large, heterogeneous group of clinic-referred children with ADD yielded three behavioral subgroups: 40% of the children had ADD with hyperactivity, 30% had ADD with hyperactivity and aggressivity, and 30% had ADD without either hyperactivity or aggressivity. Dykman and Ackerman (1991) also found that proportionally more girls were in the ADD-only (no hyperactivity or aggressivity) subgroup. In terms of RD, more than half the sample ($N = 94$) were poor readers with proportionally more boys than girls (9:1) with a diagnosis of RD according to criteria. Analyzing data from white males, the three subgroups differed on convergent validity measures (i.e., teacher and parent ratings, ratings of externalizing behavior) but did not differ on divergent measures such as IQ, achievement scores, self-ratings, and physiological tasks. Boys in the entire sample who were not classified as RD had higher IQs than those who were, but subgroups with and without RD still differed significantly on WRAT-R reading and spelling with IQ as a covariable. Both groups with and without RD were found to be different from a control group on measures of sustained attention and impulsivity. All subgroups profited from being given methylphenidate regardless of dosage.

Although Aman's (1980) review on the effects of stimulant medication on reading performance of children with hyperactivity provided little support for their use in the treatment of RD, subsequent reviews (Gadow, 1983; Gadow & Swanson, 1985) did suggest that more careful attention to diagnostic issues (e.g., type of dependent measure) and

dosage titration might yield more positive results. For example, a meta-analysis by Kavale (1982) on the use of stimulant medication demonstrated an average increase of approximately 15 percentile ranks in reading achievement across studies. However, studies on the effectiveness of stimulant medication have been difficult to interpret because of more general problems in overlap among symptoms of hyperactivity and conduct disorders (O'Brien & Obrzut, 1986; Taylor, 1988). Thus, Forness, Cantwell, Swanson, Hanna, and Youpa (1991) studied the effects of stimulant medication (i.e., methylphenidate) on reading performance of boys with hyperactivity with and without conduct disorder. Two groups of boys, ages 8 through 11, were administered methylphenidate at three levels of dosage, along with baseline and placebo conditions. One group included 27 subjects with a diagnosis of ADHD but not conduct disorder; the other group included 28 subjects with both diagnostic disorders. Only 4 boys in each group were labeled as having a learning disability. Dependent measures involved both reading recognition and reading comprehension. Whereas no significant results were found for the ADHD group in either reading measure, boys in the group with conduct disorders did improve their performance over baseline on three of four measures of reading, significantly so in reading comprehension, with no dose effect found on this variable.

Mathematics Outcomes of ADHD

The conditions of specific mathematics disabilities and ADHD also have been found to coexist. Children with these diagnostic disorders may score lower on math word problems and computations than children without disabilities. However, similar to the research in reading performance, most studies in mathematics performance have not controlled for differences between groups of LD and ADHD in IQ or reading ability when making comparisons. For example, Lee and Hudson (1981) found that seventh-grade males with LD differed from control males in errors of math reasoning. Yet, when both IQ and reading skills were partialled out of total problem-solving scores, the group with LD did not differ from the non-LD group. Cherkes-Julkowski and Stolzenberg (1991) also reported greater difficulty with math problems requiring reorganization of information for children with ADD than for children with LD. But, the ADD group also performed poorer on a reading comprehension subtest than did the LD group.

Zentall (1990) compared samples of children with ADD/WO, ADD/H, and LD on math word problems and found specific problem-solving group differences that were attributed to changes in problem action and operation (i.e., addition, subtraction, and multiplication). Although Zentall used statistical controls for IQ and reading skill, the word problems selected for study varied in length and in level of reading ability. Thus, the specific differences possibly were related to the increased attentional load placed on subjects required for reading longer problems.

Zental and colleagues (Zentall, Smith, Lee, & Wieczorek, 1994) recently have extended the previous findings on math problem-solving by assessing math independently from cognitive and task factors that can affect math functioning of ADHD children. In doing so, the authors controlled for such variables as feedback, pacing, reading comprehension, and visual–motor skill. Computer-generated math word problems were employed requiring various operations, while at the same time controlling for changes in information presented and vocabulary level. In addition, the study was designed to assess computation speed independent of number recognition and typing skill. Zentall et al. (1994) also assessed verbal, motor, and off-task responses that were parallel to attentional task performance, as failure to maintain attention has been thought to underlie this skill deficit area. In an effort to optimize the assessment of computational performance, feedback (in the form of accuracy and time) was provided in the intertrial interval and the authors made the task self-paced.

Based on the DSM-III-R and the Iowa Conner's Teaching Rating Scale, hyperactivity status was determined for a random sample of boys, aged 7.4 through 14.5 years. From a teacher-nominated sample of 339 with parental permission, 107 boys met the criteria for ADHD (98 white and 9 African American, Asian, and Hispanic). The comparison group consisted of 121 nondisabled boys (117 white and 4 African American, Asian, and Hispanic). The remaining 111 students did not meet the criteria for either group. Students completed computer-generated tasks of reading, computation, and math problem-solving. Timed arithmetic tasks, word problems, and reading were administered to each child. Two performance measures (accuracy and speed) were recorded along with three behav-

ioral measures (head movements, bottom movements, and vocalizations).

Overall, Zentall et al. (1994) found that boys with ADHD displayed significantly lower problem-solving scores in specific math concepts and exhibited slower computational performance than did their nondisabled counterparts. Specifically, when individual children's reading vocabularies were partialled out of the analysis, findings indicated that boys with ADHD produced fewer correct word problems than controls in familiar schema problems that did not require a change in the expected order of information. That is, the demands of transforming problem information were directly related to reading comprehension and only indirectly to math problem-solving. Also, multiplication problems, which involved math concepts (e.g., distance, money, and sets), contributed to the comprehension problems observed in the familiar schema problems. The finding that math concept difficulties underlie inadequate problem-solving and are not explained by IQ, reading, or computational differences, has not been previously shown for children with ADHD.

Finally, Zentall et al. (1994) have documented that there are math outcomes of ADHD that can be assessed separately from contributing factors such as reading requirements, lack of feedback, external pacing, visual–motor skill, and problem length. For example, when problems presented have been reduced in complexity and length, specific math difficulties can be addressed. Thus, Zentall et al. suggest it is important to assess and teach math concepts, perhaps by teaching children to impose order/organization on material, and use novel instructional activities to facilitate overlearning of basic calculations (p. 518).

Summary

This review has described the diagnostic criteria for distinguishing distinct subtypes of ADHD as operationalized by DSM-IV. As well, it has presented studies that focused on (1) the neurobiological basis of ADHD; (2) the differential behavioral patterns between children with ADHD and those with LD; and (3) the related reading, math, and social skill deficits associated with ADHD.

On the basis of the studies reviewed in this chapter, the following issues have emerged. First, most studies conducted on ADHD populations have used heterogeneous subject groups thus limiting the development of sound theoretical constructs and hypotheses related to etiology, assessment, and treatment of ADHD.

Second, further clarification of ADHD subtypes and co-occurring deficits must be pursued. Currently it is not clear whether ADHD-Predominantly Inattention Type is a distinctly different disorder than ADHD-Predominantly Hyperactive–Impulsive Type. If this is the case, then each disorder should have a separate diagnostic label, clinical criteria, and course of treatment (Barkley et al., 1991). Whereas the DSM-IV criteria reflect an awareness of distinct subtypes, it considers them under one diagnostic label.

Third, a more critical examination of the current criteria applied to ADHD should be employed, specifically, criteria related to motor activity and impulsivity. Outcome studies should be designed to address the impact on where various sources of information are collected (i.e., parents, teachers, clinician) and clinical diagnosis. A problem with the current state of the art relates to a lack of solid differentiation between *overactivity* and *hyperactivity*. The lack of differentiation appears to occur within and among the various information sources during the evaluation process. The potential result is an overidentification of false positives for ADHD. Clarification of ADHD subtypes and more stringent motor activity criteria may serve to minimize this problem.

ACKNOWLEDGMENT

This work was supported in part by National Multipurpose Research and Training Center Grant DC-01409 from the National Institute on Deafness and Other Communication Disorders

References

Achenbach, T. M., & Edelbrock, C. (1983). *Manual for the child behavior checklist and revised behavior profile.* Burlington: University of Vermont.

Ackerman, P. T., Anhalt, J. M., Dykman, R. A., & Holcomb, P. J. (1986). Effortful processing deficits in children with reading and/or attention disorders. *Brain and Cognition, 5,* 22–40.

Ackerman, P. T., Dykman, R. A., & Oglesby, D. M. (1983). Sex and group differences in reading and attention disordered children with and without hyperkinesis. *Journal of Learning Disabilities, 16,* 407–415.

Aman, M. G. (1980). Psychotropic drugs and learning problems—A selective review. *Journal of Learning Disabilities, 13,* 87–97.

American Psychiatric Association. (1980). *Diagnostic and statistical manual of mental disorders* (3rd ed.). Washington, DC: Author.

American Psychiatric Association. (1994). *Diagnostic and statistical manual of mental disorders* (4th ed.). Washington, DC: Author.

August, G. J., & Garfinkel, B. D. (1990). Comorbidity of ADHD and reading disability among clinic-referred children. *Journal of Abnormal Child Psychology, 18,* 29–45.

Barkley, R. A. (1990). Associated problems, subtyping, and etiologies. In R. A. Barkley (Ed.), *Attention deficit hyperactivity disorder: A handbook for diagnosis and treatment* (pp. 74–105). New York: Guilford Press.

Barkley, R. A., DuPaul, G. J., & McMurray, M. B. (1990). Comprehensive evaluation of attention deficit disorder with and without hyperactivity as defined by research criteria. *Journal of Consulting and Clinical Psychology, 58,* 775–789.

Barkley, R. A., DuPaul, G. J., & McMurray, M. B. (1991). Attention deficit disorder with and without hyperactivity: Clinical response to three dose levels of methylphenidate. *Pediatrics, 87,* 519–531.

Becker, M. G., Isaac, W., & Hynd, G. W. (1988). Neuropsychological development of non-verbal behaviors attributed to "frontal lobe" functioning. *Developmental Neuropsychology, 3,* 275–298.

Benezra, E., & Douglas, V. I. (1988). Short-term serial recall in ADD-H, normal and reading-disabled boys. *Journal of Abnormal Child Psychology, 16,* 511–525.

Boder, E., & Jarrico, S. (1982). *The Boder Test of Reading/Spelling Patterns.* New York: Grune & Stratton.

Bohline, D. S. (1985). Intellectual and affective characteristics of attention deficit disordered children. *Journal of Learning Disabilities, 18,* 604–608.

Boucugnani, L. L., & Jones, R. W. (1989). Behaviors analogous to frontal lobe dysfunction in children with attention deficit hyperactivity disorder. *Archives of Clinical Neuropsychology, 4,* 161–173.

Calis, K. A., Grothe, D. R., & Elia, J. (1990). Attention-deficit hyperactivity disorder. *Clinical Pharmacy, 9,* 632–642.

Cantwell, D. P., & Baker, L. (1988). Issues in the classification of children and adolescent psychopathology. *Journal of the American Academy of Child and Adolescent Psychiatry, 27,* 521–533.

Cantwell, D. P., & Baker, L. (1991). Association between attention deficit-hyperactivity disorders and learning disorders. *Journal of Learning Disabilities, 24,* 88–95.

Carlson, C. L., Lahey, B. B., Frame, C. L., Walker, J., & Hynd, G. W. (1987). Sociometric status of clinic-referred children with attention deficit disorders with and without hyperactivity. *Journal of Abnormal Child Psychology, 15,* 537–547.

Chelune, G. J., & Baer, R. A. (1986). Developmental norms for the Wisconsin Card Sorting Test. *Journal of Clinical and Experimental Neuropsychology, 8,* 219–228.

Chelune, G. J., Ferguson, W., Koon, R., & Dickey, T. O. (1986). Frontal lobe disinhibition in attention deficit disorder. *Child Psychiatry and Human Development, 16,* 221–234.

Cherkes-Julkowski, M., & Stolzenberg, J. (1991). The learning disability of attention deficit disorder. *Learning Disabilities: A Multidisciplinary Journal, 2,* 8–15.

Cooper, J. R., Bloom, F. E., & Roth, R. H. (1991). *The biochemical basis of neuropharmacology* (6th ed.). London: Oxford University Press.

Douglas, V. I., & Benezra, E. (1990). Supra-span verbal memory in attention deficit disorder with hyperactivity normal and reading-disabled boys. *Journal of Abnormal Child Psychology, 18,* 617–638.

Dykman, R. A., & Ackerman, P. T. (1991). Attention deficit disorder and specific reading disability: Separate but often overlapping disorders. *Journal of Learning Disabilities, 24,* 96–103.

Dykman, R. A., Ackerman, P. T., & Holcomb, P. J. (1985). Reading disabled and ADD children: Similarities and differences. In D. Gray & J. Kavanaugh (Eds.), *Biobehavioral measures of dyslexia* (pp. 47–69). Baltimore: York Press.

Edelbrock, C., & Rancurello, M. D. (1985). Childhood hyperactivity: An overview of rating scales and their applications. *Clinical Psychology Review, 5,* 429–445.

Elia, J. (1991). Stimulants and antidepressant pharmacokinetics in hyperactive children. *Psychopharmacology Bulletin, 27,* 411–415.

Felton, R. H., & Wood, F. B. (1989). Cognitive deficits in reading disability and attention deficit disorder. *Journal of Learning Disabilities, 22,* 3–13.

Forness, S. R., Cantwell, D. P., Swanson, J. M., Hanna, G. L., & Youpa, D. (1991). Differential effects of stimulant medication on reading performance of boys with hyperactivity with and without conduct disorder. *Journal of Learning Disabilities, 24,* 304–310.

Gadow, K. D. (1983). Effects of stimulant drugs on academic performance in hyperactive and learning disabled children. *Journal of Learning Disabilities, 16,* 290–299.

Gadow, K. D., & Swanson, H. L. (1985). Assessing drug effects of academic performance. *Psychopharmacology Bulletin, 21,* 877–886.

Gonzalez, J. J. (1991). *Affective symptomatology in subtypes of attention deficit disorder.* Unpublished master's thesis, University of Georgia, Athens.

Goodyear, P., & Hynd, G. W. (1992). Attention deficit disorder with (ADD/H) and without (ADD/WO) hyperactivity: Behavioral and neuropsychological differentiation. *Journal of Clinical Child Psychology, 21,* 273–305.

Gualtieri, C. T., & Hicks, R. E. (1985). Neuropharmacology of methylphenidate and a neural substrate for childhood hyperactivity. *Psychiatric Clinics of North America, 8,* 875–892.

Halperin, J. M., Gittelman, R., Klein, D. F., & Rudel, G. (1984). Reading-disabled hyperactive children: A distinct subgroup of attention deficit disorder with hyperactivity? *Journal of Abnormal Child Psychology, 21,* 1–14.

Hamlett, K. W., Pellegrini, D. S., & Conners, C. K. (1987). An investigation of executive processes in the problem-solving of attention deficit disorder hyperactive children. *Journal of Pediatric Psychology, 12,* 227–240.

Hauser, P., Zametkin, A. J., Martinez, P., Vitiello, B., Matochik, J., Mixson, A., & Weintraub, B. (1993). Attention deficit-hyperactivity disorder in people with generalized resistance to thyroid hormone. *New England Journal of Medicine, 328,* 997–1001.

Hauser, P., Zametkin, A. J., Vitiello, B., Martinex, P., Mixson, A. J., & Weintraub, B. D. (1992). Attention deficit hyperactivity disorder in 18 kindreds with generalized resistance to thyroid hormone [Abstract]. *Clinical Research, 40,* 388A.

Holborow, P. L., & Berry, P. S. (1986). Hyperactivity and learning difficulties. *Journal of Learning Disabilities, 19,* 426–431.

Hunt, R. D., Minderaa, R. B., & Cohen, D. J. (1985). Clonidine benefits children with attention-deficit disorder and hyperactivity: Report of a double-blind placebo crossover therapeutic trial. *Journal of the American Academy of Child Psychiatry, 5,* 617–629.

Hynd, G. W., Hern, K. L., Novey, E. S., Eliopulos, D., Marshall, R., Gonzalez, J. J., & Voeller, K. K. (1993). Attention deficit-hyperactivity disorder and asymmetry of the caudate nucleus. *Journal of Child Neurology, 8,* 339–347.

Hynd, G. W., Lorys, A. R., Semrud-Clikeman, M., Nieves, N., Huettner, M., & Lahey, B. (1991). Attention deficit disorder without hyperactivity (ADD/WO): A distinctive behavioral and neurocognitive syndrome. *Journal of Child Neurology, 6*(Suppl.), S37–S41.

Hynd, G. W., Semrud-Clikeman, M., Lorys, A. R., Novey, E. S., & Eliopulos, D. (1990). Brain morphology in developmental dyslexia and attention deficit disorder/hyperactivity. *Archives of Neurology, 47,* 919–926.

Hynd, G. W., Semrud-Clikeman, M., Lorys, A. R., Novey, E. S., Eliopulos, D., & Lyytinen, H. (1991). Corpus callosum morphology in attention deficit-hyperactivity disorder: Morphometric analysis of MRI. *Journal of Learning Disabilities, 24,* 141–146.

Hynd, G. W., & Willis, W. G. (1988). *Pediatric neuropsychology.* Boston: Allyn & Bacon.

Kavale, K. A. (1982). The efficacy of stimulant drug treatment for hyperactivity: A meta-analysis. *Journal of Learning Disabilities, 15,* 282–285.

Korkman, M. (1988). *NEPSY: A proposed neuropsychological test battery for young, developmentally disabled children.* Helsinki, Finland: University of Helsinki.

Korkman, M., & Pesonen, A. E. (1994). A comparison of neuropsychological test profiles of children with attention deficit-hyperactivity disorder and/or learning disorder. *Journal of Learning Disabilities, 27,* 383–392.

Kupietz, S. S. (1990). Sustained attention in normal and in reading-disabled youngsters with and without ADHD. *Journal of Abnormal Child Psychology, 18,* 357–372.

Lahey, B. B., Pelham, W. E., Schaughency, E. A., Atkins, M. S., Murphy, H. A., Hynd, G. W., Russo, M., Hartdagen, S., & Lorys-Vernon, A. (1988). Dimensions and types of attention deficit disorder/hyperactivity in children: A factor and cluster analytic approach. *Journal of the American Academy of Child and Adolescent Psychiatry, 27,* 330–335.

Lambert, N. M., & Sandoval, J. (1980). The prevalence of learning disabilities in a sample of children considered hyperactive. *Journal of Abnormal Child Psychology, 8,* 33–50.

Lassonde, M. (1986). The facilitory influence of the corpus callosum on interhemispheric processing. In F. Lepore, M. Ptito, & H. Jasper (Eds.), *Two hemispheres—one brain* (pp. 385–401). New York: Liss.

Lee, M. M., & Hudson, F. G. (1981). *A comparison of verbal problem-solving in arithmetic of learning disabled and non-learning disabled seventh grade males.* (Available from the Institute for Research in Learning Disabilities, University of Kansas, Lawrence)

Loney, J., & Milich, R. (1982). Hyperactivity, inattention, and aggression in clinical practice. In M. Wolraich & D. K. Routh (Eds.), *Advances in developmental and behavioral pediatrics* (pp. 113–147). Greenwich, CT: JAI Press.

Lou, H. C., Henriksen, L., Bruhn, P., Borner, H., & Neilsen, J. B. (1989). Striatal dysfunction in attention deficit and hyperkinetic disorder. *Archives of Neurology, 46,* 48–52.

Mattes, J. A. (1980). Role of frontal lobe dysfunction in childhood hyperkinesis. *Comprehensive Psychiatry, 21,* 358–369.

Mixson, A. J., Parrilla, R., Ransom, S. C., Wiggs, E., McClasky, J., Hauser, P., & Weintraub, B. (1992). Correlations of language abnormalities with localization of mutations in the B-thyroid hormone receptor in 13 kindreds with generalized resistance to thyroid hormone: Identification of four new mutations. *Journal of Clinical Endocrinology and Metabolism, 75,* 1039–1045.

O'Brien, M. A., & Obrzut, J. E. (1986). Attention deficit disorder with hyperactivity: A review and implications for the classroom. *Journal of Special Education, 20,* 281–297.

Passler, M. A., Isaac, W., & Hynd, G. W. (1985). Neuropsychological development of behavior attributed to frontal lobe functioning in children. *Developmental Neuropsychology, 1,* 349–370.

Pelham, W. E., Atkins, M. S., & Murphy, H. A. (1981, August). Attention deficit disorder with and without hyperactivity: Definitional issues and correlates. Paper presented at the 1981 Conference of the American Psychological Association, Los Angeles, CA.

Pelham, W. E., & Bender, M. E. (1982). Peer relationships in hyperactive children: Description and treatment. In K. D. Gadow (Ed.), *Advances in learning and behavior disabilities* (pp. 365–436). Greenwich, CT: JAI Press.

Puig-Antich, J., & Chambers, W. (1978). *The schedule for affective disorders and schizophrenia for school-aged children.* New York: New York State Psychiatric Institute.

Refetoff, S., Weiss, R. E., & Usala, S. J. (1993). The syndromes of resistance to thyroid hormone. *Endocrine Review, 14,* 348–399.

Richards, G. P., Samuels, S. J., Turnure, J. E., & Ysseldyke, J. E. (1990). Sustained and selective attention in children with learning disabilities. *Journal of Learning Disabilities, 23,* 129–136.

Robins, P. M. (1992). A comparison of behavioral and attentional functioning in children diagnosed as hyperactive or learning-disabled. *Journal of Abnormal Child Psychology, 20,* 65–82.

Semrud-Clikeman, M., & Hynd, G. W. (1990). Right hemispheric dysfunction in nonverbal learning disabilities: Social, academic, and adaptive functioning in adults and children. *Psychological Bulletin, 107,* 196–209.

Shaywitz, B. A., & Shaywitz, S. E. (1991). Comorbidity: A critical issue in attention deficit disorder. *Journal of Child Neurology, 6*(Suppl.), S13–S22.

Shaywitz, S. E., & Shaywitz, B. A. (1987). Attention deficit disorder: Current perspectives. *Pediatric Neurology, 3,* 129–135.

Shue, K. L., & Douglas, V. I. (1992). Attention deficit hyperactivity disorder and the frontal lobe syndrome. *Brain and Cognition, 20,* 104–124.

Siegel, L. S., & Ryan, E. B. (1989). The development of working memory in normally achieving and subtypes of learning disabled children. *Child Development, 60,* 973–980.

Stanford, L. D., & Hynd, G. W. (1994). Congruence of behavioral symptomatology in children with ADD/H, ADD/WO, and learning disabilities. *Journal of Learning Disabilities, 27,* 243–253.

Stevenson, R. D., & Wolraich, M. L. (1989). Stimulant medication therapy in the treatment of children with attention-deficit hyperactivity disorder. *Pediatric Clinics of North America, 36,* 1183–1197.

Taylor, E. (1988). Attention deficit and conduct disorder syndromes. In M. Rutter, A. H. Tuma, & I. S. Lann (Eds.), *Assessment and diagnosis in child psychopathology* (pp. 377–407). New York: Guilford Press.

Van der Meere, J., van Baal, M., & Sergeant, J. (1989). The additive factor method: A differential diagnostic tool in hyperactivity and learning disability. *Journal of Abnormal Child Psychology, 17,* 409–422.

Weinberger, D. R., Luchins, D. J., Morihisa, J., & Wyatt, R. J. (1982). Asymmetrical volumes of the right and left frontal and occipital regions in the human brain. *Neurology, 11,* 97–100.

Weiss, R. E., Stein, M. A., Trommer, B., & Refetoff, S. (1993). Attention-deficit hyperactivity disorder and thyroid function. *Journal of Pediatrics, 123,* 539–545.

Witelsen, S. F. (1990). Structural correlates of cognition in the human brain. In A. B. Scheibel & A. F. Wechsler (Eds.), *Neurobiology of higher cognitive function* (pp. 167–183). New York: Guilford Press.

Witelsen, S. F., & Kigar, D. L. (1988). Asymmetry in brain follows asymmetry in anatomical form: Gross, microscopic, postmortem, and imaging studies. In F. Boller & J. Grafman (Eds.), *Handbook of neuropsychology* (Vol. 1, pp. 111–142). Amsterdam: Elsevier.

Zametkin, A. J., & Rapoport, J. L. (1987). Neurobiology of attention deficit disorder with hyperactivity: Where have we come in 50 years? *Journal of the American Academy of Child and Adolescent Psychiatry, 26,* 676–686.

Zametkin, A. J., Rapoport, J. L., Murphy, D. L., Linnoila, M., Karoum, F., Potter, W., & Ismond, D. (1985). Treatment of hyperactive children with monoamine oxidase inhibitors: Clinical efficacy. *Archives of General Psychiatry, 42,* 982–986.

Zentall, S. S. (1990). Fact-retrieval automatization and math problem-solving: Learning disabled, attention disordered, and normal adolescents. *Journal of Educational Psychology, 82,* 856–865.

Zentall, S. S., Smith, Y. N., Lee, Y. B., & Wieczorek, C. (1994). Mathematical outcomes of attention-deficit hyperactivity disorder. *Journal of Learning Disabilities, 27,* 510–519.

31

Neuropsychological and Neurobehavioral Sequelae Associated with Pediatric HIV Infection

ANTOLIN M. LLORENTE, CHRISTINE M. LoPRESTI, AND PAUL SATZ

Neuropsychological and neurobehavioral dysfunctions in infancy and childhood, resulting from human immunodeficiency virus (HIV) infection, warrant distinct consideration in a handbook of this nature. This merit stems from the unique impact of this disease process on the rapidly maturing central nervous system (CNS) of the child (Epstein *et al.,* 1986; Falloon, Eddy, Wiener, & Pizzo, 1989; Pizzo & Wilfert, 1994) in conjunction with the historical scientific and clinical purview of neuropsychology as the study of brain–behavior relationships (Lezak, 1995).

Infant and childhood mortality resulting from pediatric HIV infection and AIDS recently has experienced a dramatic spiraling increase in the United States and worldwide (Mann, Tarantola, & Netter, 1992; Novello, Wise, Willoughby, & Pizzo, 1989). This exponential rise in the number of infected cases and deaths, whether the result of enhanced surveillance techniques, rapid increases in the rate of disease transmission, or greater reporting accuracy, has had enormous social and economic consequences (Mann *et al.,* 1992). Thus, neuropsychology has been called on, as part of a multidisciplinary approach, to scientifically investigate the effects of this infection on higher brain functions and to participate in the assessment and rehabilitation of the seropositive patient.

This chapter provides an overview of the neuropsychological effects of HIV-related immunosuppression and AIDS in infancy and childhood as understood in 1995. A review of basic concepts is initially presented to introduce the reader to the pediatric HIV and AIDS terminology and diagnostic nomenclature. Subsequently, epidemiological data from the United States and around the world depicting the rapid spread and staggering impact of this epidemic are examined. The chapter then briefly traces the virological and immunological effects of the virus. Next, neuropathological and other medical concomitants associated with an HIV+ state are briefly reviewed. The bulk of the remainder of the chapter is devoted to the neuropsychological and neurobehavioral sequelae associated with HIV infection and the virtually unlimited ways that this discipline can contribute and intervene from a clinical and scientific perspective. Finally, potential avenues for future research are presented.

ANTOLIN M. LLORENTE • Department of Pediatrics, Baylor College of Medicine, and Texas Children's Hospital, Houston, Texas 77030. CHRISTINE M. LoPRESTI AND PAUL SATZ • Department of Psychiatry and Biobehavioral Sciences, University of California, Los Angeles, Los Angeles, California 90024.

Basic Concepts, Terminology, and Diagnostic Nomenclature

Infants passively acquire maternal antibodies *in utero* through placental transmission, including the anti-HIV IgG antibody, which persist at least throughout the first year of life (Koup & Wilson, 1994). Virtually all infants born to HIV$^+$ mothers will test positive for the virus at birth but may in actuality not be infected. Therefore, the use of existing diagnostic assays for the presence of HIV antibodies, indirectly suggesting the presence of the HIV retrovirus, routinely employed with adults since mid-1985 (e.g., Western blotting; see Sarngadharan, Popovic, Bruch, Shupbach, & Gallo, 1984), are inadequate for diagnosing newborns of HIV$^+$ mothers (Hanson & Shearer, 1994). For this reason, pediatric diagnosis using antibody assays solely, without clinical presentations of the disease, are generally not made until infants reach the age of 15 to 18 months. At this age, it is believed that the child's own immune system is being assayed (Prober & Gershon, 1991; see below for diagnostic criteria).

Currently, the most sensitive procedures for detecting HIV infection in babies born to HIV-seropositive mothers are the polymerase chain reaction (PCR) and virus culture (Burgard, Mayaux, & Blanche, 1992; Krivine et al., 1992). Use of these assays is accurate in nearly 100% of infected newborns 3 to 6 months postdelivery, and 30–50% of infants tested at birth. The standard p24-antigen assay is less sensitive than PCR and virus cultures, especially when HIV-antibody levels are very high. However, recent modifications (Hanson & Shearer, 1994) of this assay have increased its sensitivity in diagnosing infected infants born to HIV$^+$ mothers.

Two important concepts in the pediatric HIV literature are those of vertical versus horizontal viral transmission. HIV infection can be transmitted from a seropositive mother to her child during the perinatal, delivery, and postnatal periods. Transmission has been found to occur in utero through the placental barrier (see Sprecher, Soumenkoff, Puissant, & Degueldre, 1986), during intrapartum as a result of contact with blood or other body products (Friedland & Klein, 1987), and after birth through breast-feeding (de Martino, 1994; Rogers, 1989). Regardless of the actual course of retroviral transfer, HIV$^+$ mother-to-child viral passage is considered a form of vertical transmission. In contrast, viral transmission through blood or blood-related products associated with the treatment of medical disorders (e.g., von Willebrand's disease) or other insult is considered horizontal transmission by definition. The distinction between vertical versus horizontal transmission is not only important from a pedagogical and scientific viewpoint, it also has

significant clinical importance because the disease process tends to express itself in different fashions in children afflicted through these two distinct routes of transmission (Brouwers, Moss, Wolters, & Schmitt, 1994). According to Brouwers, Moss, et al. (1994), vertical versus horizontal transmission also has significant gender- and age-related consequences. With regard to gender, males have a greater likelihood of becoming infected via horizontal transmission because they are more prone to have medical conditions necessitating treatment with blood products (males have a higher prevalence of diseases requiring the use of blood products; e.g., hemophilia A, an X-linked recessive form requiring coagulation Factor VIII). In terms of age-related differences as it applies to mode of transmission, horizontally transmitted HIV in the United States is most likely to have occurred in boys whose chronological age in 1995 was approximately 10 years. This uncanny state of affairs is the result of the advent of available and reliable procedures to detect the presence of HIV antibodies in the blood supply. Therefore, because safe blood supplies have been available since early 1985, children who acquired HIV as a result of a contaminated blood supply are at least 10 years old. In other words, children born since 1985 have primarily acquired HIV through vertical transmission because sources associated with horizontal transmission as a result of unsafe blood products have been virtually eliminated.

In addition, the rate and course of disease progression to AIDS, as well as the onset of symptoms subsequent to infection (incubation), have been found to differ as a function of transmission mode (Brouwers, Belman, & Epstein, 1994). With regard to the onset of symptomatic disease, in maternally (vertically) infected children, investigators have discovered two distinguishable subgroups (Auger et al., 1988; DePaula et al., 1991). According to Auger et al. (1988), in a study conducted in New York examining the incubation period for pediatric AIDS, one group exhibited early symptomatic disease expression in infancy marked by an approximate median age of onset of 4.1 months associated with brief survival periods, whereas a second group of children had a median incubation period of 6.1 years with lengthier periods of survival. In contrast, the time lapsed between infection and onset of symptomatology in children infected through blood transfusions is greater (Rogers et al., 1987), relative to vertically infected children. With regard to these varying periods of incubation, Oxtoby (1994) recently reported that the median age at which AIDS is diagnosed in perinatally infected children was 12 months while the distribution of age at AIDS diagnosis is negatively skewed, with the majority of children under the age of 2 and a small number who are diagnosed as late as age 13. In summary, from a prognostic viewpoint, age of onset of symptomatic disease plays a major role in predicting length of survival.

Although viral load and strain have been hypothesized to play a major role in incubation periods, the variability in onset of symptoms and course of illness is not yet understood. Nevertheless, recent research examining risk factors in maternal–fetal infection has revealed interesting results. For example, Bryson *et al*. (1993) presented the first data examining *timing* of vertical transmission (*in utero* versus intrapartum) to help explain the developmental course of the disease. In this prospective study of 74 mother-infant pairs, 22 (28%) seropositive mothers transmitted the virus to their newborns. The median time to onset of AIDS-defining symptoms was significantly earlier in the group infected *in utero* (6 weeks) compared with the group infected in the intrapartum period (86 weeks). Brouwers, Moss, *et al*. (1994) have also described in detail the abundance of environmental factors affecting the expression of HIV infection. Finally, host factors may play an important role. For example, in adults, Satz (1993) has put forward the concept of threshold theory to explain some of the individual differences observed in the expression of the disease after infection.

As the reader may have already surmised, the population of children infected with pediatric HIV is quite heterogeneous (Brouwers, Moss, *et al.*, 1994). This heterogeneity is partly the result of differences in transmission mode, coupled with the rapid developmental changes occurring in the CNS of children, age of onset of symptomatic disease, and viral load and strain(s). In addition, environmental and host-related factors are also responsible for a great deal of the individual and group differences observed in the pediatric HIV population. This lack of homogeneity is also exhibited in the profiles of patients who undergo neuropsychological evaluation.

Just as procedures and methods used to identify infected adults are ineffective with infants born to HIV+ mothers, adult diagnostic criteria are also inappropriate for children. The Centers for Disease Control and Prevention (CDC) initially published a pediatric classification scheme in 1987 to better describe the spectrum of HIV disease and updated the classification system in 1994 (CDC, 1994). Diagnosis of HIV in children is based on infection, immunologic, and clinical status. The three infection diagnostic groups are HIV infected, perinatally exposed (E), and seroreverter (SR). Children are diagnosed as HIV infected under the following conditions: A child is younger than 18 months and is born to an HIV+ mother and (1) has had positive laboratory results on two HIV detection tests or (2) has an AIDS-defining illness based on the 1987 CDC surveillance case definition. A child 18 months or older is diagnosed as infected if either born to an HIV+ mother or infected through any route of transmission and has repeatedly tested HIV+ by antibody tests. A perinatally exposed child is one who is (1) under 18 months of age and is HIV seropositive by antibody tests or (2) is born to an HIV+ mother but has unknown antibody status. A seroreverter is a child born to an HIV+ mother but who is antibody negative, has no laboratory evidence of viral infection, and has not had an AIDS-defining illness. Children who are infected or perinatally exposed based on the criteria described above are further classified according to their immunologic and clinical status. Immunologic categories are based on both age and level of immunosuppression based on CD4+ counts and percentage of total lymphocyte and range categorically from "no evidence of suppression" to "severe suppression." Clinical categories are based on the presence and severity of symptomatology ranging from asymptomatic to severe signs and symptoms (CDC, 1994).

U.S. and Worldwide Pediatric HIV Epidemiology

Since the first case of pediatric HIV was reported to the CDC in 1982, the population of HIV-infected children has grown dramatically in the United States. As of June 1995, 6611 children under the age of 13 had been diagnosed with AIDS accounting for 1.4% of the total number of reported AIDS cases in the United States. Although by 1993 infected children had been documented in all regions (e.g., rural versus metropolitan) (Oxtoby, 1990) within the 50 states (CDC, 1993), the majority (51%) of patients come from metropolitan areas in New York, Florida, and New Jersey (CDC, 1995). The total number of children with AIDS from New York as of June 1995 accounts for approximately one-quarter (26%) of all cases reported in the country (CDC, 1995).

Nevertheless, in view of the fact that pediatric HIV studies suggest that most HIV$^+$ children will eventually progress to AIDS (Scott & Hutto, 1991), coupled with the reality that children who are HIV$^+$ without meeting CDC criteria for AIDS are not reported to this agency, the figures above are probably conservative estimates. However, Oxtoby (1991) reports that many states have recently adopted broader reporting methods to include cases of HIV and AIDS providing for increased accuracy in surveillance.

Heterosexual contact is the fastest-growing mode of transmission for women in the United States. As of June 1995, 90% of children with AIDS were vertically infected. Sixty percent of these mothers acquired HIV through IV drug use or sex with an injecting drug user (CDC, 1995). The rise in the number of vertically infected cases reflects the increasing number of infected women (Scott, Hutto, Makuch, Mastruici, *et al.,* 1989) and the relative decreases in other methods of transmission including infection from blood and blood products (Andiman & Modlin, 1991). For this reason, vertical transmission can be expected to account for virtually all cases of pediatric HIV infection in the future.

Because most children are exposed to HIV through their mother, as of June 1995, the distribution of children with AIDS reflects that of their mothers demographically. Therefore, of the pediatric population of cases reported with AIDS, 57% are African American, 24% Hispanic, 18% Caucasian, <1% Asian/Pacific Islander, and, <1% American Indian/Alaskan Native (CDC, 1995). It is evident from these data that the epidemic has had a greater impact on some minority groups, especially African Americans and Hispanics, relative to other racial groups.

Although epidemiological data from the United States are informative, these figures serve as poor indicators of the magnitude of this epidemic when looked at from a broader perspective such as worldwide prevalence. This is best depicted by statistics presented by Mann *et al.* (1992). According to these investigators, as of January 1992 the prevalence of pediatric HIV had been *conservatively* estimated at 1,076,450 cases around the world. Sub-Saharan Africa had the greatest number of infected children with a population estimate of 969,500 or 90% of the total population of infected children. Latin American, Southeast Asia, North America, and the Caribbean were the next geographic areas of affinity (GAA)

with conservative estimates of 40,500, 24,000, and 16,000 children, respectively. Western Europe, the southeastern Mediterranean, Northeast Asia, Oceania, and Eastern Europe had the next highest estimated number of cases at 8000, 1000, 750, 500, and 200 children, respectively (Mann *et al.,* 1992).

Basic Virology and Immunology of HIV Infection in Children

Although a detailed description of the virology and immunology of pediatric HIV infection is beyond the scope of this chapter, a brief introduction of these topics will be presented in order to give the reader a rudimentary understanding of these biological processes (see Connor & Ho, 1994; Feigin & Cherry, 1992; Hanson & Shearer, 1992; Overall, 1981). It is important that the reader understand these basic concepts since they are interwoven with the neuropathological and neuropsychological effects of HIV infection to be covered in later sections.

Virology

The virus (e.g., HIV-1 or HIV-2) is an RNA virus belonging to the lentivirus family of retroviruses (Connor & Ho, 1994). It is referred to as a retrovirus because of the fashion in which it carries its genetic code. In contrast to other RNA viruses (e.g., proviruses), HIV reproduces itself through reverse transcription (its genetic code is inserted into the DNA genome of the host cell). Regardless of the actual mechanism of transcription, retroviruses are capable of producing, among other pathologies, profound immunosuppressed states and cancers. Specifically, HIV-1 causes immunosuppression of the T-cell lymphotropic system in children increasing the probability of occurrence of opportunistic infections associated with this state (e.g., *Pneumocystis carinii,* lymphomas). Unfortunately, the actual pathogenetic process of HIV in the CNS is not understood despite our advanced scientific knowledge of the virus itself.

Immunology

The immune system protects against pathogens following antigenic challenge through several mechanisms, including humoral, cell-mediated, and polymorphonuclear responses (Macdonald, 1984; Mills, Regelmann, & Quie, 1981). Humoral immunity occurs primarily secondary to the development of humoral circulating antibodies. This type of response assists in the reduction or elimination of foreign microorganisms from the body. In contrast, cell-mediated or cellular immunity is predominantly moderated by a set of cells labeled T cells (lymphocytes) that are responsible for protection against infectious agents.

In the uterus, the fetus depends on the immune system of the mother for protection against pathogens, a process known as maternal immunity (Mills *et al.,* 1981). In fact, the mother passively donates her immunity to her fetus through the placenta in the form of IgG. Similarly, the neonate and newborn also depend on this donated immunity. According to Koup and Wilson (1994), adult immunoglobulin levels (IgG, A, M) are not found in normal children at adult concentrations until age 5–6 or adolescence by which time the child's own immune response system begins to operate in a fashion similar to that of an adult. Although it is known that B- and T-lymphocyte differentiation can commence as early as 10 weeks during the gestational period, vertical HIV infection can occur earlier. In addition, most immune system mechanisms known to protect infected adults, and responsible for their longer survival periods, have been shown to be impaired in normal newborns. This secondary state of immunodeficiency is also partly responsible for the inception and rapid development of HIV infection in the newborn. Recently, Wilfert, Wilson, Luzuriaga, and Epstein (1994) reported that mother-to-child transmission is most likely the result of a single virus strain that evolves into related but different strains over time. These investigators also reported that increased maternal virus burden appears to enhance the probability of vertical infection. Obviously, all of these factors combined are responsible for the inability of the fetus and newborn to protect themselves against pathogens, making them highly susceptible to HIV infection and its sequelae (e.g., opportunistic infections).

Regardless of etiology, infection with HIV (HIV-1 or HIV-2) leading to AIDS is the result of disruption in T-cell-mediated coordination responses responsible for protection or safeguard specifically of CD4+ cells, secondary to the progressive disintegration of the CD4+ cell supply. As the number of CD4+ cells decreases below certain critical threshold levels (relative to adults, children's CD4+ cell concentrations have been shown to be at clinically significant higher levels), the probability substantially increases that the now immunocompromised infected child will become symptomatic.

In addition to the impact of HIV itself, stimulation of the immune system with production of local chemokines is partly responsible for the catastrophic effects upon the CNS seen in HIV-related encephalopathy. Additionally, incomplete myelination of the young CNS may increase susceptibility.

Neurological and Neuropathological Findings in Pediatric HIV-1

In children, evidence that HIV infection was actually associated with neurological complications was published (e.g., Belman *et al.,* 1984) around 1983–1984, approximately $1\frac{1}{2}$ years after the first cases of pediatric AIDS were reported to the CDC in the United States. Nevertheless, there appears to be ample evidence in 1995 (Brouwers, Belman, & Epstein, 1994; Grant *et al.,* 1987, for evidence in adults; Masliah *et al.,* 1992) from several avenues of research (e.g., neurology, neuropathology, neuroimaging) to suggest that HIV penetrates the young and maturing CNS (Koenig *et al.,* 1986; Resnick, Berger, Shapshak, & Tourtellote, 1988) causing dramatic neuropathology. These findings are now briefly reviewed.

Neurological Findings

Although neurological symptomatology experienced by children as a result of HIV infection varies substantially from child to child, with some children exhibiting mild alterations in cognition and motor skills, more severe expressions of the disease are manifested through childhood encephalopathy capable of causing substantial deviations from normal development and death. Belman *et al.* (1988) and Belman (1990) described two forms of HIV-1 encephalopathy, namely, progressive and static HIV-related encephalopathy.

Progressive encephalopathy is further subcategorized into two different types (subacute and plateau) to describe the distinct rates of disease progression observed in infants and children. Subacute progressive encephalopathy, most commonly seen in infants and young children (Belman *et al.,* 1988), is the most crippling expression of HIV infection. It is marked by a gradual but progressive decline across most domains of neurological functioning, particularly in overall cognition, expressive functions including motor and language skills, and adaptive functioning in pre-school-age children, or loss of already attained developmental milestones in infants and younger children with no further development usually leading to death (Epstein *et al.,* 1985). Subacute encephalopathy causes serious CNS debilitation including profound cerebral atrophy and microcephaly (acquired as a result of lack of continued CNS development) (Epstein *et al.,* 1985, 1986). Neurologically, it is not uncommon to see a child with a chronological age of 4 years functioning at an age level of 6–8 months during the active course of HIV-1-related subacute encephalopathy. A plateau course is often observed in infants and young children wherein they fail to acquire new developmental milestones or acquire them very slowly. Unlike youngsters experiencing progressive subacute encephalopathy, they typically do not display losses from previously acquired levels of functioning (Belman *et al.,* 1989). Belman (1990) has reported that these children suffer from motor deficits as well as declines in overall intellectual functioning.

Relative to progressive encephalopathy, the static form is less debilitating. The gradual decline or lack of gains in development observed during progressive encephalopathy is not seen in children with static encephalopathy. Instead, static encephalopathy is demarcated by continued acquisition of skills at rates below expected levels of normal development but commensurate with their initial level of functioning. Furthermore, the delays observed during static encephalopathy longitudinally remain relatively stable from initial levels of functioning (Belman *et al.,* 1985; Brouwers, Moss, *et al.,* 1994; Epstein *et al.,* 1986).

Although the American Academy of Neurology recently amalgamated the various categorizations of HIV-related encephalopathy, as identified by Belman (1990) and discussed above, under one category termed HIV-associated encephalopathy of childhood (American Academy of Neurology AIDS Task Force, 1991), Brouwers, Belman, and Epstein (1994) argue that the singular categorization scheme fails to account for the different neurological presentations associated with the various types of encephalopathy. In fact, these investigators contend that Belman and colleagues' (1988) categorization better characterizes the various course of progression observed during the three types of encephalopathy.

In addition to the encephalopathic processes described above, a host of other neurological diseases associated with an immunodeficient state secondary to HIV infection have also been observed in children (Belman, 1990). Although the actual frequency of occurrence of these disorders is not high, nonetheless, infections and other CNS complications (e.g., neoplasms) have been reported. According to Belman (1990), the majority of these children concurrently develop encephalopathy as a result of HIV-1 infection. For example, neoplasms have been documented in the literature, the most common type being primary CNS lymphoma (Belman, 1990; Epstein, Sharer, & Goudsmit, 1988). These have been observed in children between 6 months to 10 years of age but occur primarily after the first birthday (Epstein *et al.,* 1988). Their most prominent location is in the basal ganglia and areas surrounding the third ventricle (Belman, 1990). Secondary CNS lymphomas have also been noted (Dickson *et al.,* 1989) as well as cerebrovascular complications, including infarctions (Belman, 1990; Frank, Lim, & Kahn, 1989) and strokes (Park *et al.,* 1988). Although there is a great deal of consensus regarding the infrequency of CNS opportunistic infections in children (Epstein *et al.,* 1988), they have nonetheless been reported in the neurological literature (e.g., cytomegalovirus) (Belman *et al.,* 1988; Dickson *et al.,* 1989). Of these, bacterial meningitis, candida meningitis, and CMV have been the most common. In contrast, HIV-related CNS toxoplasmosis, commonly observed in adults (McArthur, 1994), has rarely been reported in children (Belman, 1990). In fact, in a recent study, only 34 cases or less than 1% of the total of 4249 "AIDS-indicator infections" (both CNS- and non-CNS-related) reported in 1992 were due to toxoplasmosis of the brain (Nicholas, 1994).

Findings from Neuroimaging Studies

Several investigators have found abnormalities in the brains of HIV-infected children using various neuroradiological procedures (see Tardieu, 1991). For example, Belman *et al.* (1985) found varying degrees of abnormality using computed tomography (CT) in an 18-month-old with AIDS, marked by cortical atrophy with dilation of the ventricular system and calcification of the basal ganglia and frontal white matter. These abnormalities were again observed longitudinally at 18 and 21 months. More recently, CT studies conducted by Belman *et al.* (1988) found cortical atrophy and white matter abnormalities [basal ganglia (bilaterally) and frontal calcification] in children with AIDS or "ARC." In addition, 16 of 17 participants who were longitudinally evaluated in the study showed progressive levels of atrophy. These results have been substantiated by DeCarli, Civitello, Brouwers, and Pizzo (1993) who found bilateral symmetrical calcification of the basal ganglia and frontal white matter calcification in 100 children with symptomatic HIV infection. Furthermore, in a recent study assessing the clinical significance of CT scan abnormalities as they relate to cognitive delays subsequent to symptomatic HIV-1, Brouwers et al. (1995) found a positive and significant relationship between these two independent procedures. In this investigation, greater delays in cognitive development were significantly associated with increasing degrees of calcification.

Studies using magnetic resonance imaging (MRI) have also detected CNS abnormalities associated with pediatric HIV infection. Belman et al. (1986) found decreased and increased signal intensities on T_1- and T_2-weighted images, respectively, in a 10-year-old as a result of white matter atrophy in the basal ganglia (bilaterally) and cerebral atrophy. Similar findings using T_2-weighted imaging were reported by other investigators (see Epstein et al., 1986).

A study examining cerebral metabolism through positron emission tomography (PET) supported the findings obtained with the structural neuroradiological methods described above. Pizzo et al. (1988), conducting a study assessing the effects of AZT pharmacotherapy, found diffuse cortical, focal right frontal, and right superior temporal hypometabolism prior to treatment in an 11-year-old male with HIV-1 infection.

Neuropathological Features

There is substantial evidence suggesting that neuropathology in the CNS of children may be caused by AIDS secondary to pediatric HIV infection (see Ho et al., 1985; Resnick et al., 1988). Evidence supporting this hypothesis comes from research revealing measurable degrees of neuropathology in microscopic and gross specimens of the brain and spinal cord in these children.

Several investigators reported abnormalities in the brains of children afflicted with HIV (HTLV-III) as early as 1985 (e.g., Sharer, Cho, & Epstein, 1985). In this study 11 children underwent autopsy, which revealed diminished gross brain weight for age, inflammatory cell infiltrates, multinucleated

cells and multinucleated giant cells, cerebrovascular calcification, vascular and perivascular calcification, and white matter changes. In addition, inflammatory and vascular lesions were most pronounced in the basal ganglia and pons (Sharer et al., 1985). Similar findings have been published by other investigators more recently (Belman et al., 1988; Epstein et al., 1988; Pang et al., 1990). Moreover, the results of the investigation by Epstein et al. (1988) revealed diminished brain weight for age under gross examination in the children who had died of AIDS-related infection and progressive encephalopathy. This research also revealed the presence of inflammatory cell infiltrates, multinucleated giant cells, white matter changes, and vascular calcification under microscopic examination as reported earlier by Sharer et al. (1985). More important, several studies have identified viral particles or HIV-related antigen in the multinucleated cells and other cells (Koenig, Gendelman, Orentstein, et al., 1986; see also Epstein et al., 1985). This finding would argue in favor of hypotheses postulating the presence of neuropathology as a direct result of HIV-related pathogens. Based on the evidence presented above, it appears that the neuropathological effects of HIV infection on the developing brain are so devastating that they can be detected under gross examination.

Within the spinal cord, corticospinal tract (CST) degeneration (Dickson et al., 1989), a disorder characterized by remarkable myelin pallor, has been the most common histopathological finding in children infected with HIV-1. In this study, CST degeneration was seen in more than two-thirds of the children with AIDS who had undergone autopsy. Furthermore, nearly half of the cases revealed axonal loss and loss of myelination in the CST.

Disproportionate pallor of myelin, relative to axonal loss, in the CST was observed in the other half of the cases. Those children who suffered from both losses in myelin and axons usually displayed the greatest amount of cerebral pathology (Belman, 1990). Finally, Sharer et al. (1990) found inflammatory cell infiltrates and multinucleated cells in 9 and 6 of the cases evaluated, respectively, as part of a study of 18 children who died as a result of HIV-1 infection and had undergone autopsy (only 16 spinal cords were evaluated). Sharer et al. (1990) also identified degenerative changes marked by myelin pallor in the CST in nearly half of the cases, consistent with previous studies (e.g., Dickson et al., 1989).

Electrophysiological Findings

Given the abnormalities observed in the CNS using other diagnostic procedures (e.g., imaging, postmortem examinations), it should not be surprising to encounter negative findings in the gross electrical activity of the brain while conducting electroencephalographic studies with HIV$^+$ children. In fact, correlative EEGs have revealed abnormal findings. For example, in the study by Belman *et al.* (1985) of six children with AIDS, five of the six displayed EEG abnormalities consistent with the imaging results. Three of the five showed mild diffuse slowing and the other two displayed moderate diffuse slowing. Four of the six also displayed abnormalities in brain stem auditory evoked potential (BAEP) marked by an abnormal rate function (one child) and prolongation of the I–V interwave latency (three children). Other studies have found similar abnormalities (Ultmann *et al.*, 1985).

Findings from Other CNS Biological Correlates

Other abnormalities have also been identified in several CNS biological markers as a result of HIV-1 infection in children (Epstein *et al.*, 1987; Ho *et al.*, 1985). Brouwers *et al.* (1993) found a high correlation between cerebrospinal fluid (CSF) levels of quinolinic acid (QUIN) and degree of encephalopathy in 40 children with HIV infection relative to 16 controls. In addition, this study revealed decreasing levels in mental abilities [Bailey Scales (MDI), McCarthy Scales (GCI), and WISC-R (FSIQ)] to be associated with increasing levels of QUIN. Similarly, in a study assessing levels of serum tumor necrosis factor (TFN-α), Mintz (1989) found elevated levels of this marker related to progressive encephalopathy in children with AIDS. Tardieu, Blanche, Duliege, Rouzioux, and Griscelli (1989), using antigen capture assays specific to HIV-1-p24, also found detectable levels of this marker in the CSF of children. In the same year, Hutto *et al.* (1989) reported abnormalities in the CSF of children infected with HIV. In summary, other CNS biological markers, including CSF abnormalities (Ho *et al.*, 1985), have been found in children with HIV infection, especially those with advanced encephalopathy. More important, these findings suggest that the CNS proper is indeed invaded during "primary HIV-1 infection" (Belman, 1990), directly implicating this infectious disease in some of the neurological (Belman, 1990) and neuropsychological deficits observed.

Neurodevelopmental and Neuropsychological Deficits Secondary to Pediatric HIV-1 Involvement

Neuropsychological sequelae associated with HIV infection have been frequently reported in the literature (Boivin *et al.*, 1995; Brouwers, Belman, & Epstein, 1994; Cohen *et al.*, 1991; Diamond *et al.*, 1987; Fowler, 1994). Therefore, the remainder of this chapter will review neuropsychological and neurobehavioral correlates of HIV infection. An attempt is made to integrate neurological, neuropathological, and other findings presented thus far with the neuropsychological literature, thereby describing the brain–behavior relationships associated with this disease process. We also plan to discuss the variety of ways that neuropsychology can contribute meaningfully to the rehabilitative process of the seropositive and immunocompromised patient. Finally, potential neuroscientific contributions through future research are also explored. In order to accomplish these tasks in a coherent and orderly fashion, neuropsychological and neurodevelopmental deficits associated with HIV infection are presented by domains. These topics are followed by a discussion examining potential contributions in rehabilitation and research.

Overall Intellectual Functioning

Several studies have reported delays in overall levels of cognitive abilities correlated with HIV infection in some children, similar to that observed in other youngsters suffering from progressive neurological and neurodevelopmental disorders. In fact, a substantial lowering in overall intellectual functioning within the Borderline and Mild Mental Retardation ranges have been reported in the literature by several researchers particularly during the symptomatic stages of the disease (Brouwers, Belman, & Epstein, 1994; Fowler, 1994). In a recently published report, consistent with previous findings of overall intellectual compromise, Boivin *et al.* (1995) showed that a group of Zairian asymptomatic HIV$^+$ children had lower K-ABC Mental Processing Composite (MPC) scores (MPC = 75.1 ± 10.9) relative to HIV$^-$ controls born to uninfected mothers (MPC = 109 ± 21.2) and a control group of HIV$^-$ children born to HIV$^+$ mothers (MPC = 89.6 ± 9.6). In contrast, although Cohen *et al.* (1991) found differences between a group of horizontally infected

HIV$^+$ (only a third of the participants were symptomatic) versus HIV$^-$ children in school achievement, motor speed, visual scanning, and cognitive flexibility, no differences were observed in overall intelligence for as long as $8\frac{1}{2}$ years after infection. Mode of disease transmission, among other factors, most likely accounts for the differences in findings between these two studies.

In summary, although it would appear that symptomatic as well as asymptomatic HIV infection is capable of causing substantial impairment in the overall cognitive abilities in children, a great deal of variability is observed when these children undergo neuropsychological evaluation (cf. Cohen *et al.*, 1991, and Boivin *et al.*, 1995). Furthermore, it is unclear what variables if any (e.g., viral strain, environmental factors) are responsible for the variability in research findings. In addition, studies investigating the effects of HIV infection in children, to date, have been primarily cross-sectional in nature. Therefore, longitudinal studies are needed to rigorously examine the spectrum of cognitive deficits across the age span and during various stages of disease progression as a function of mode of transmission. Nevertheless, in the more advanced stages of symptomatic disease (e.g., AIDS), a clearer picture emerges whereby substantial and dramatic impairment is observed in this domain. The degree of impact on overall cognitive functioning as a result of infection during more advanced disease stages is consistent with the type of neuropathological insult commonly seen in this disease process especially during symptomatic periods (e.g., AIDS). Specifically, the reader may recall the presence of neuropathological findings including cerebral atrophy and acquired microcephaly (Epstein *et al.*, 1988) in these children. These two CNS abnormalities, in and of themselves, are quite capable of accounting for the profound dampening in global intellectual functioning observed in some of these children.

Attention and Concentration

Difficulties in attention are among the most frequent problems associated with brain damage (Lezak, 1978), probably as a result of the fragile nature of these processes. In HIV infection, this domain of functioning is sometimes compromised even in seemingly asymptomatic patients. One study (Brouwers, Moss, Wolters, Eddy, & Pizzo, 1989) examined the effects of viral involvement on attentional processes by looking at the WISC-R Freedom from Distractibility factor (Kaufman, 1975). The investigation revealed that seropositive children experienced "relative weaknesses" on this marker. In another study using cluster analytic procedures, Brouwers *et al.* (1992) discovered that one subgroup of symptomatic seropositive children could be identified by a cluster comprising items loading heavily on attentional deficits. Similarly, in the study by Boivin *et al.* (1995), a review of the results reveals that HIV$^+$ children relative to HIV$^-$ controls born to seronegative mothers had lower levels of performance on tasks believed to be partly dependent on attentional skills (e.g., K-ABC Hand Movements, Number Recall, and Spatial Memory subtests). Although tentative, these data suggest that the virus may be capable of causing attentional difficulties. However, Brouwers, Moss, *et al.* (1994) appropriately caution that these deficits could very well be the result of other intervening variables not related to the infection *per se*, such as the high base rates of attention difficulties in children for this age group in the general population, acting as potential confounds.

Although behavioral assessment has also revealed that these children may indeed suffer from attentional deficits (Hittleman *et al.*, 1991), the preschoolers studied in that investigation were quite young (15 months old) and prone to suffer from the same high base rates of diminished attention as postulated by Brouwers, Moss, *et al.* (1994). Children in this developmental stage also display a great deal of variability in attention from day to day. Clearly, further studies need to be conducted with children infected with HIV to determine in a data-based fashion whether the attentional deficits observed during neuropsychological and behavioral assessment are the result of the disease process or other unrelated etiologies.

Despite the aforementioned caveats, given the fragile nature of these processes, there is a great likelihood that these mechanisms are indeed influenced by the virus, particularly during more involved expressions of the infection. During more advanced and debilitating stages of the disease, white matter involvement has been identified as a neuropathological hallmark of pediatric HIV (Sharer *et al.*, 1986). In particular, as it relates to this domain, neuropathological and electrophysiological findings have indicated the presence of calcification in the pontine nuclei (Sharer *et al.*, 1986) and BAEP abnormalities (Belman *et al.*, 1985), respectively. Therefore, it is possible that HIV compromises attention mechanisms, responsible for the deficits observed in this domain while undergoing neuropsychological evaluation, by encroaching and infringing on the ascending pathways of the reticular activating system.

Memory

Although complications in attention are sometimes accompanied by memory difficulties, in some cases as an immediate consequence of deficits in the former domain, at first glance it appears that HIV infection may also cause memory deficits (Bellman et al., 1988; Diamond, 1989; Levenson, Mellins, Zawadzki, Kairam, Stein, 1992). Boivin et al. (1995) found impairments on tasks that were presumably capable of assessing memory in young children. In their study with HIV⁺ asymptomatic youngsters, these investigators demonstrated difficulties in verbal and visual processing tasks believed to assess memory functions in children age 2 or older. Specifically, HIV⁺ participants, relative to HIV⁻ controls born to noninfected mothers and HIV⁻ children of infected mothers, had significantly lower levels of performance on the K-ABC Immediate Recall and Spatial Memory subtests (these measures attempt to assess among other functions immediate verbal and visual recall, respectively). Significant differences were also observed on yet another K-ABC subtest of visual immediate recall (Hand Movements). However, given the insufficient number of studies examining this domain with psychometrically sound procedures, in conjunction with the potential confounds as a result of the high base rates of attentional difficulties in this population, the present results are suggestive at best. The primitive nature of these functions at this developmental stage coupled with our limited ability to validly assess them in young children also place the present findings on unstable ground.

Verbal Functions and Auditory Processing

Complications in language, specifically expressive language and auditory processing difficulties associated with HIV infection, have often been reported in the literature (Bellman et al., 1985; Brouwers, Belman, & Epstein, 1991; Ultmann et al., 1987; Wolters, Brouwers, Moss, & Pizzo, 1994). Although a great deal of variability is observed, and some children, particularly HIV⁺ asymptomatic youngsters, may not show any difficulties, language-related impairments are usually present during more pernicious disease course. In addition, these deficits seem to be affected by the mode of viral transmission in conjunction with the degree of disease progression. A vertically infected infant who suffers from subacute progressive encephalopathy will display delays in acquiring and developing language while progressively losing previously attained milestones, whereas an older child who becomes infected with HIV via transfusion may develop regression or slurred speech as well as regression in other language skills from previous level of functioning. A complete loss of speech may also be observed in older children in the late stages of disease involvement.

Although both receptive and expressive language have been found to be differentially affected by the virus (Epstein et al., 1986; Wolters et al., 1994), the majority of insults occur in the expressive domain with relatively spared receptive skills (Brouwers, Moss, et al., 1994). Data-based evidence for this observation comes from research by Wolters and her associates (Wolters et al., 1994) who demonstrated, as part of a study of adaptive functioning using the Vineland Adaptive Behavior Scales (Sparrow, Balla, & Cichetti, 1984), that expressive skills underwent greater insult relative to receptive skills. However, it should be noted that this study used the caretaker's verbal report to assess difficulties in receptive and expressive functions rather than cognitive tests designed for this purpose. Despite these cautions, and in light of the scarce number of longitudinal and controlled investigations assessing this domain, it should be clear that more advanced stages of the disease are indeed associated with serious deficits in expressive language. Some of these language complications are probably caused by oral–motor difficulties as a result of basal ganglia insult. Also, expressive skills are under rapid development at this stage making them more vulnerable to insult (Ewing-Cobbs, Fletcher, Levin, & Landry, 1985).

Motor Functioning

Given the striking and profound involvement of the basal ganglia complex in children suffering from HIV infection and AIDS, specifically calcific vasculopathy and inflammatory CNS diseases thereof (Belman et al., 1988), it is not surprising to see motor deficits in these children during developmental evaluation. As a result, gross and fine motor delays are very prominent in symptomatic seropositive infants and may also be observed in older children.

Motor skills are often the most frequent aspect of functioning vulnerable to the disease process (Fowler, 1994; Hittleman *et al.,* 1990, 1991; Ultmann *et al.,* 1985). Specifically, many symptomatic infants display muscle tone abnormalities and a very slowed rate of gross–fine motor skills acquisition. Even seemingly unaffected HIV$^+$ asymptomatic infants, less than 2 years of age, have recently been observed to suffer from motor delays using a standardized developmental screening measure (Boivin *et al.,* 1995). Symptomatic preschoolers and school-age children may also display abnormalities in this domain as expected, initially marked by disturbances in gait and balance (Brouwers, Moss, *et al.,* 1994). However, Fowler (1994) reported that unlike infants and toddlers, some older children and adolescents tend not to suffer from mild neurological impairments, including motor dysfunction (e.g., fine motor tremor), until the later stages of symptomatic disease process. We have observed these deficits in gross and fine motor tasks in children in our practice (e.g., fine motor deficits on the Grooved Pegboard Test; Kløve, 1963), during the middle–late stages of symptomatic disease, similar to those observed in adults (Selnes & Miller, 1994). In more severe cases, the ability to ambulate is lost because of pronounced involvement in the lower extremities, most likely associated with neuropathological processes affecting the basal ganglia nuclei as reported earlier. Brouwers, Moss, *et al.* (1994) report that more serious deficits in this domain may be observed, including spastic quadriparesis and pyramidal tract signs, with greater levels of CNS involvement such as progressive encephalopathy (see Belman *et al.,* 1988).

In summary, pronounced delays in motor performance are frequently evidenced in symptomatic seropositive infants and older children, including motor tone abnormalities and other motor delays, with more arrest in development associated with more progressive and debilitating disease courses (e.g., subacute progressive encephalopathy). Even in seemingly unaffected HIV$^+$ asymptomatic infants, very mild delays in this domain are sometimes evident. Although less common, reflecting the low incidence of these diseases in children, opportunistic processes can sometimes cause abrupt motor complications, vastly different from the gradual and progressive course of motor difficulties described above, as a result of an immunocompromised state. These complications include, for example, abrupt motor deficits subsequent to neoplasms.

Academic Achievement

Given the degree of impairment evident in cognitive abilities and adaptive functioning that is sometimes present in selected groups of HIV-infected children, infringing on various neuropsychological domains, it is only rational to expect them to suffer from learning difficulties. Although there is a lack of investigations examining this domain systematically, difficulties in academic achievement associated with HIV infection have been reported (e.g., Cohen *et al.,* 1991). Cohen *et al.* (1991) found mathematics and reading achievement scores below the range of expectation in a group of children infected neonatally through transfusion relative to a group of uninfected controls. It is important to note that Cohen and colleagues retrospectively (parent questionnaire) examined the rates of absenteeism in this cohort of children. Their results revealed that lack of school attendance could not account for the academic achievement discrepancies observed between their groups of control and HIV$^+$ children. However, given the few investigations assessing this domain, further research would need to elucidate how these potential confounds affect academic achievement apart from the direct effects of the infection on the CNS.

Behavioral/Adaptive Considerations

Other areas of psychological functioning, such as alterations in the behavioral and adaptive repertoire of children resulting from pediatric HIV infection, are capable of producing further impact on neuropsychological performance. For example, Brouwers, Moss, *et al.* (1994) distinguished between direct and indirect effects. HIV direct impacts are those immediately associated with the disease process such as the behavioral disturbances encountered with encephalopathic states (Belman *et al.,* 1988). Indirect effects are consequences of HIV indirectly related to the disease. These effects are usually the result of environmental factors and stressors, coupled with host variables (e.g., psychological resources, coping strategies), synergistically operating with the disease process (e.g., undergoing multiple medical procedures and hospitalizations as part of radiation treatment for an opportunistic disease). These behavioral and adaptive factors may play a major role in the way that HIV-related symptoms exhibit themselves from patient to patient and must be taken into consideration when evaluating, performing research, or providing rehabilitative services to these patients.

A large number of children infected with HIV come to research protocols and/or for treatment from low-SES backgrounds. This is partly the result of the method of transmission previously discussed. For example, more than half of vertically infected children have mothers who acquired the virus via sexual contact with men who are IV drug users or are IV drug users themselves. For this reason, some families with infected children often struggle with basic necessities such as housing and nutrition. These psychosocial variables must be carefully considered when interacting with these children and their families.

The review of epidemiological data indicated that a large percentage of infected children come from metropolitan areas of states with large minority populations. Thus, a large segment of the pediatric population infected with HIV belong to ethnic minorities for which there are sometimes little normative data or for which inferences made on the data available would be invalid for the population under investigation or the patient undergoing intervention. Caution must be exercised when interpreting neuropsychological findings as abnormal, in light of these potential confounds. In the same vein, because children with HIV infection tend to display augmented behavioral disturbances (Ultmann *et al.,* 1985), similar to children who suffer from other types of medical illnesses (Routh, 1988; Tarter, Edwards, & van Thiel, 1988), careful interpretation of behavioral observations and assessment results should follow suit in order to avoid misinterpreting normal findings as aberrant. However, unlike families with infants and children who have other chronic illnesses, families with children who have been infected perinatally commonly suffer from guilt resulting from the transmission of the virus. Mothers of vertically infected children have to provide care for their own illness, while also caring for their children. These and similar factors create further stress in the immediate environment and family circle and should be seriously considered during neuropsychological assessment of these patients or research participants.

Diagnostic and Rehabilitative Issues

The contributions of neuropsychology to the scientific understanding of this disease, and the applications of these findings to the rehabilitative and diagnostic process, are potentially unlimited. The numerous opportunities for significant contributions on these two fronts stem from the number of prominent deficits observed in some infants and children across neuropsychological domains resulting from infection with HIV.

Although advances in neuroradiology diminished somewhat the role of neuropsychology as part of the diagnostic process, especially in terms of localization of insult, it can still assist a multidisciplinary team. This assistance is particularly valuable during the early stages of HIV disease involvement, where a child may not display readily observable symptomatology (unremarkable brain scans are often seen in some of these children), except for mild impairments in higher brain functions. The potential for diagnostic support also results from specific medical complications. Certain CNS opportunistic diseases, present in some immunocompromised patients, initially manifest themselves behaviorally only. Similarly, older asymptomatic HIV⁺ children sometimes appear not to have any complications from the infection. However, when these seemingly unaffected children undergo neuropsychological examination, their neuropsychological profile reveals subtle deficits in selected domains of cognitive functioning (Brouwers, Moss, *et al.,* 1994; Brouwers, Belman, & Epstein, 1994). Therefore, this discipline can contribute to the diagnostic process in several ways. For example, longitudinal assessment of children at risk can provide information associated with changes in symptomatic status early on in the disease process while furnishing the treatment team data-based information regarding cognitive status changes and possible diagnostic information. In fact, for some children neuropsychological assessment is the only diagnostic procedure available.

Treatment outcome paradigms are another area of intervention where neuropsychology could continue to play a role of considerable significance. For example, opportunistic diseases (e.g., neoplasms) as a result of immunosuppression sometimes require the use of treatments involving radiation. Radiotherapy has been shown to be positively correlated with detrimental neuropsychological effects as a result of the impact of this treatment on cerebral white matter (Filley, 1994). Thus, these procedures must be monitored in order to assess their efficacy and impact on higher-order brain functions, especially in HIV infection where white matter compromise is present prior to the administration of radiotherapy, making these structures of the brain more susceptible to further insult. Similarly, drug treatment outcome research is another source of continued involvement (see Pizzo *et al.,* 1990; Pizzo, Brouwers, & Poplack, 1989; Wolters *et al.,* 1990, 1991). In fact, treatment outcome research abounds in the literature assessing the efficacy of zidovudine and other antiretroviral treatments (e.g., Butler *et al.,* 1991; DeCarli *et al.,* 1991; Pizzo *et al.,* 1988).

In conclusion, neuropsychology can potentially play a pivotal role in rehabilitation through its ability to assess cognitive functions subsequent to therapeutic interventions and in the diagnostic process, especially during early stages of disease involvement. The examples presented above are but a few of the areas of extant and prospective contributions.

Summary and Putative Directions for Future Research

The present chapter provides an overview of the effects of pediatric HIV infection on the developing CNS. The sequelae associated with this infectious disease implicate various facets of neurological functioning as detected by multiple procedures including neuropathological, neuroimaging, and neuropsychological assays which easily account for the dramatic debilitation seen in some children. Although scarce, research findings to date tend to suggest that several neuropsychological domains may be afflicted during the course of viral infection, particularly toward the middle to later stages of the disease or while undergoing states of HIV-related immunosuppression. Specifically, difficulties in overall intellectual functioning, attention, expressive language, motor skills, and behavioral/adaptive functioning are readily observed in some children. Because of the lack of substantive research with psychometrically sound procedures and methods, coupled with the number of potential confounds capable of obscuring research findings, impairments in other domains described above should be at best considered working hypotheses for future research.

It is important that we keep in mind that a great deal of heterogeneity exists in the pediatric HIV population. In particular, it is hoped that the reader takes away a balanced view of the impact of this disease process on neuropsychological functioning. On the one hand, AIDS (advanced stage of viral infection) is capable of causing severe impairments in neuropsychological functioning across most domains. HIV-related encephalopathy and opportunistic diseases consequent to an immunosup-

pressed state as a result of HIV infection are also capable of producing similar consequences. In contrast, there are a number of children who seem not to be affected by HIV. However, detailed neuropsychological *evaluations* of these youngsters reveal a different picture marked by subtle but minor deficits across selective domains, motor skills being some of the abilities most susceptible to the disease process. A third group emerges from the population of HIV-infected children. These children remain asymptomatic for years without any type of neuropsychological difficulties or complications. The absence of difficulties is present in some of these youngsters despite the fact that they occasionally suffer from varying degrees of immunosuppression.

Unlike its rapid spread across all corners of the world as depicted by the epidemiological data presented above, it is clear through a review of the literature that pediatric HIV neuropsychological research is in its infancy as it relates to our present understanding of the impact of this disease. It is also evident that a great deal of work lies ahead. The lack of basic research employing longitudinal investigations is unfortunate because cross-sectional research can only provide us with a minute sample of the effects of the disease process at a specific point in time revealing little about its long-term impact. Therefore, a great deal of basic neuropsychological research needs to be performed examining long-term cognitive functioning throughout the disease process and across developmental stages. Research on pediatric HIV has investigated between-group differences largely ignoring the study of within-group variation. For this reason, future investigations should examine intragroup effects associated with HIV. For example, are there specific markers for long-term survival associated with particular neuropsychological variables in asymptomatic children? If so, could these markers be used to determine when to intervene on their behalf to maintain them in an asymptomatic state?

It would be advantageous to ascertain if the deficits observed in several neuropsychological domains are the direct result of infection or other etiology. Thus, future investigations should attempt to determine whether the memory difficulties observed in HIV$^+$ patients are subsequent to attentional deficits or the result of memory impairments in their own right. In other words, a programmatic program of research should be employed to investigate the origins of memory difficulties thus far evidenced in pediatric HIV. It would also be advantageous to investigate HIV-related "primary effects" (Brouwers, Moss, *et al.*, 1994) separate from "secondary" impact. This would require that future studies use as controls children who suffer from other, but similar, infectious diseases, capable of resembling the effects of HIV, while holding other variables constant. This research paradigm would allow a comparison of these two sets of infected children and other control groups in terms of stress and coping strategies. It would also be profitable to examine in greater detail the effects of infection on expressive language. This line of investigations would consist of research designs that would systematically evaluate various methods of reporting, method of viral transmission, and other putative factors responsible for the differences in findings.

ACKNOWLEDGMENTS

Portions of this chapter were supported in part by a grant from the UCLA CIRID-Fogarty AIDS International Foundation (No. TW00003-07) to A.M.L. and an NIMH training grant (No. 1-T32-MH19535-01) to P. S. The authors wish to express their sincere thanks to I. Celine Hanson, M.D., Baylor College of Medicine, Department of Pediatrics, Section of Allergy and Immunology, for her review and comments on portions of this chapter.

References

American Academy of Neurology AIDS Task Force. (1991). Nomenclature and research case definition for neurologic manifestations of human immunodeficiency virus-type 1 infection. *Annals of Neurology, 41,* 778–785.

Andiman, W. A., & Modlin, J. F. (1991). Vertical transmission. In P. A. Pizzo & C. M. Wilfert (Eds.), *Pediatric AIDS: The challenge of HIV infection in infants, children, and adolescents* (pp. 140–155). Baltimore: Williams & Wilkins.

Auger, I., Thomas, P., De Gruttola, V., Morse, D., Moore, D., Williams, R., Truman, B., & Lawrence, C. E. (1988). Incubation periods for pediatric AIDS patients. *Nature, 336,* 575–577.

Belman, A. L. (1990). AIDS and pediatric neurology. *Neurology Clinics, 8,* 571–603.

Belman, A. L., Diamond, G., Dickson, D., Horoupian, D., Liena, J., Lantos, G., & Rubinstein, A. (1988). Pediatric acquired immunodeficiency syndrome. *American Journal of Diseases of Children, 142,* 29–35.

Belman, A., Diamond, G., Park, Y., Nozyce, M., Douglas, C., Cabot, T., Bernstein, L., & Rubinstein, A. (1989). Perinatal HIV infection: A prospective longitudinal study of the initial CNS signs [Abstract]. *Neurology, 39* (Suppl. 1), 278–279.

Belman, A. L., Lantos, G., Horoupian, D., Novick, B. E., Ultmann, M. H., Dickson, D. W., & Rubinstein, A. (1986). AIDS: Calcification of the basal ganglia in infants and children. *Neurology, 36,* 1192–1199.

Belman, A. L., Novick, B., Ultmann, M. H., Spiro, A. J., Rubinstein, A., Horoupian, D. S., & Cohen, H. (1984). Neurologic complications in children with AIDS [Abstract]. *Annals of Neurology, 16,* 414.

Belman, A. L., Ultmann, M. H., Horoupian, D., Novick, B., Spiro, A. J., Rubinstein, A., Kurtzbert, D., & Cone-Wesson, B. (1985). Neurological complications in infants and children with acquired immune deficiency syndrome. *Annals of Neurology, 18,* 560–566.

Boivin, M. J., Green, S. D. R., Davies, A. G., Giordani, B., Mokili, J. K. L., & Cutting, W. A. M. (1995). A preliminary evaluation of the cognitive and motor effects of pediatric HIV infection in Zairian children. *Health Psychology, 14* (1), 13–21.

Brouwers, P., Belman, A. L., & Epstein, L. G. (1991). Central nervous system involvement: Manifestations and evaluation. In P. A. Pizzo & C. M. Wilfert (Eds.), *Pediatric AIDS: The challenge of HIV infection in infants, children, and adolescents* (pp. 318–335). Baltimore: Williams & Wilkins.

Brouwers, P., Belman, A. L., & Epstein, L. (1994). Central nervous system involvement: Manifestations, evaluation, and pathogenesis. In P. A. Pizzo & C. M. Wilfert (Eds.), *Pediatric AIDS: The challenge of HIV infection in infants, children, and adolescents* (2nd ed., pp. 433–455). Baltimore: Williams & Wilkins.

Brouwers, P., DeCarli, C., Civitello, L., Moss, H., Wolters, P., & Pizzo, P. (1995). Correlation between computed tomographic brain scan abnormalities and neuropsychological function in children with symptomatic human immunodeficiency virus disease. *Archives of Neurology, 52,* 39–44.

Brouwers, P., Heyes, M., Moss, H., Wolters, P., Poplack, D., Markey, S., & Pizzo, P. (1993). Quinolinic acid in the cerebrospinal fluid of children with symptomatic HIV-1 disease: Relationships to clinical status and therapeutic response. *Journal of Infectious Diseases, 168,* 1380–1386.

Brouwers, P., Moss, H., Wolters, P., Eddy, J., & Pizzo, P. (1989). Neuropsychological profile of children with symptomatic HIV infection prior to antiretroviral therapy [Abstract]. *Proceedings from the V International Conference on AIDS, 1,* 316.

Brouwers, P., Moss, H., Wolters, P., el-Amin, D., Tassone, E., & Pizzo, P. (1992). Neurobehavioral typology of school-age children with symptomatic HIV disease [Abstract]. *Journal of Clinical and Experimental Neuropsychology, 14,* 113.

Brouwers, P., Moss, H., Wolters, P., & Schmitt, F. A. (1994). Developmental deficits and behavioral change in pediatric AIDS. In I. Grant & A. Martin (Eds.), *Neuropsychology of HIV infection* (pp. 310–338). London: Oxford University Press.

Bryson, Y., Dillon, M., Garratty, E., Dickover, M., Keller, A., & Deveikis, A. (1993). The role of timing of HIV maternal–fetal transmission (in-utero vs. intrapartum) and HIV phenotype on onset of symptoms in vertically infected infants [Abstract WS-C10-2]. *Proceedings from the IXth International Conference on AIDS/IV STD, World Congress (Berlin).* London: Wellcome Foundation.

Burgard, M., Mayaux, J., & Blanche, S. (1992). The use of viral culture and p24 antigen testing to diagnose human immunodeficiency virus in neonates. *New England Journal of Medicine, 327,* 1192–1197.

Butler, K. M., Husson, R. N., Balis, F. M., Brouwers, P., Eddy, J., ed-Amin, D., Gress, J., Hawkins, M., Jarosinski, P., Moss, H., Poplack, D., Santacroce, S., Venzon, D., Wiener, L., Wolters, P., & Pizzo, P. A. (1991). Dideoxyinosine (ddI) in symptomatic HIV-infected children: A phase I–II study. *New England Journal of Medicine, 324,* 137–144.

Centers for Disease Control and Prevention. (1993). *HIV/AIDS Surveillance Report, 5,* 1–19.

Centers for Disease Control and Prevention. (1994). Revised classification system for human immunodeficiency virus (HIV) infection in children less than 13 years of age. *Morbidity and Mortality Weekly Report, 43,* 1–10.

Centers for Disease Control and Prevention. (1995). *HIV/AIDS Surveillance Report.*

Cohen, S., Mundy, T., Karrassik, B., Lieb, L., Ludwig, D., & Ward, J. (1991). Neuropsychological functioning in human immunodeficiency virus type 1 seropositive children infected through neonatal blood transfusion. *Pediatrics, 88,* 58–68.

Connor, R. I., & Ho, D. D. (1994). Biology and molecular biology of HIV. In P. A. Pizzo & C. M., Wilfert (Eds.), *Pediatric AIDS: The challenge of HIV infection in infants, children, and adolescents* (2nd ed., pp. 97–113). Baltimore: Williams & Wilkins.

DeCarli, C., Civitello, L. A., Brouwers, P., & Pizzo, P. A. (1993). The prevalence of computed axial tomographic abnormalities of the cerebrum in 100 consecutive children symptomatic with the HIV. *Annals of Neurology, 34,* 198–205.

DeCarli, C., Fugate, L., Falloon, J., Eddy, J., Katz, D. A., Friedland, R. P., Rapoport, S. I., Brouwers, P., & Pizzo, P. A. (1991). Brain growth and cognitive improvement in children with human immune deficiency virus-induced encephalopathy after six months of continuous infusion azidothymidine therapy. *Journal of Acquired Immune Deficiency Syndrome, 4,* 585–592.

de Martino, M. (1994). Human immunodeficiency virus type 1 infection and breast milk. *Acta Paediatrica Supplement, 400,* 51–58.

DePaula, M., Queiroz, W., Llan, Y., Rodreguez Traveras, C., Janini, J., & Soraggi, N. (1991). Pediatric AIDS: Differentials in survival [Abstract]. *Proceedings of the VII International Conference on AIDS, 2,* 190.

Diamond, G. W. (1989). Developmental problems in children with HIV infection. *Mental Retardation, 27,* 213–217.

Diamond, G. W., Kaufman, J., Belman, A. L., Cohen, L., Cohen, H. J., & Rubinstein, A. (1987). Characterization of cognitive functioning in a subgroup of children with congenital HIV infection. *Archives of Clinical Neuropsychology, 2,* 245–256.

Dickson, D. W., Belman, A. L., Park, Y. D., Wiley, C., Horoupian, D. S., Llena, J., Kure, K., Lyman, W. D., Morecki, R.,

& Mitsudo, S. (1989). Central nervous system pathology in pediatric AIDS: An autopsy study. *Acta Pathologica, Microbiologica, et Immunologica Scandinavica, 8* (Suppl.) 40–57.

Epstein, L. G., Goudsmit, J., Paul, D. S., Morrison, S. H., Connor, E. M., Oleske, J. M., & Holland B. (1987). Expression of human immunodeficiency virus in cerebrospinal fluid of children with progressive encephalopathy. *Annals of Neurology, 21,* 397–401.

Epstein, L. G., Sharer, L. R., & Goudsmit, J. (1988). Neurological and neuropathological features of human immunodeficiency virus infection in children. *Annals of Neurology, 23* (Suppl.), S19–S23.

Epstein, L. G., Sharer, L. R., Joshi, V. V., Fogas, M. M., Koenigsberger, M. R., & Oleske, J. M. (1985). Progressive encephalopathy in children with acquired immune deficiency syndrome. *Annals of Neurology, 17,* 488–496.

Epstein, L. G., Sharer, L. R., Oleske, J. M., Connor, E. M., Goudsmit, J., Bagdon, L., Robert-Guroff, M., & Koenigsberger, M. R. (1986). Neurologic manifestations of human immunodeficiency virus infection in children. *Pediatrics, 78,* 678–687.

Ewing-Cobbs, L., Fletcher, J. M., Levin, H. S., & Landry, S. H. (1985). Language disorders after pediatric head injury. In J. Darby (Ed.), *Speech and language evaluation in neurology: Childhood disorders* (pp. 97–111). Orlando, FL: Grune & Stratton, Inc.

Falloon, J., Eddy, J., Wiener, L., & Pizzo, P. A. (1989). Human immunodeficiency virus infection in children. *Journal of Pediatrics, 114,* 1–30.

Feigin, R. D., & Cherry, J. D. (Eds.). (1992). *Textbook of pediatric infectious diseases.* Philadelphia: Saunders.

Filley, C. M. (1994). Neurobehavioral aspects of cerebral white matter disorders. In B. S. Fogel, R. S. Schiffer, & S. M. Rao (Eds.), *Neuropsychiatry: A comprehensive textbook.* Baltimore: Williams & Wilkins.

Fowler, M. G. (1994). Pediatric HIV infection: Neurologic and neuropsychological findings. *Acta Paediatrica, Supplement, 400,* 59–62.

Frank, K. Y., Lim, W., & Kahn, E. (1989). Multiple ischemic infarcts in children with AIDS, varicella zoster infection and cerebral vasculitis. *Pediatric Neurology, 5,* 64–67.

Friedland, G., & Klein, R. (1987). Transmission of the human immunodeficiency virus. *New England Journal of Medicine, 317,* 1125–1135.

Grant, I., Atkinson, J. H., Hesselink, J. R., Kennedy, C. J., Richman, D. D., Spector, S. A., & McCutchan, J. A. (1987). Evidence for early central nervous system involvement in the acquired immunodeficiency syndrome (AIDS) and other human immunodeficiency virus (HIV) infections. *Annals of Internal Medicine, 107,* 828–836.

Hanson, C. G., & Shearer, W. T. (1992). Pediatric HIV infection and AIDS. In R. D. Feigin & J. D. Cherry (Eds.), *Textbook of pediatric infectious diseases* (pp. 990–1011). Philadelphia: Saunders.

Hanson, I. C., & Shearer, W. T. (1994). Diagnosis of HIV infection. *Seminars in Pediatric Infectious Diseases, 5*(4), 266–271.

Hittleman, J., Willoughby, A., Mendez, H., Nelson, N., Gong, J., Holman, S., Muez, L., Goedert, J., & Landesman, S. (1990). Neurodevelopmental outcome of perinatally-acquired HIV infection on the first 15 months of life [Abstract]. *Proceedings from the VI International Conference on AIDS, 3,* 130.

Hittleman, J., Willoughby, A., Mendez, H., Nelson, N., Gong, J., Mendez, H., Holman, S., Muez, L., Goedert, J., & Landesman, S. (1991). Neurodevelopmental outcome of perinatally-acquired HIV infection on the first 24 months of life [Abstract]. *Proceedings from the VI International Conference on AIDS, 1,* 65.

Ho, D. D., Rota, T. R., Schooley, R. T., Kaplan, J. C., Allan, J. D., Groopman, J. E., Resnick, L., Felsenstein, D., Andrews, C. A., & Hirsch, M. S. (1985). Isolation of HTLV-III from cerebrospinal fluid and neural tissues of patients with neurologic syndromes related to the acquired immunodeficiency syndrome. *New England Journal of Medicine, 313,* 1493–1497.

Hutto, C., Scott, G. B., Parks, E. S., Fischl, M., & Parks, W. P. (1989). Cerebrospinal fluid (CSF) studies in adults and pediatric HIV infections. *Third International Conference on AIDS,* Washington, DC.

Kaufman, A. S. (1975). Factor analysis of the WISC-R at 11 age levels between 6 1/2 and 16 1/2 years. *Journal of Consulting and Clinical Psychology, 43,* 135–147.

Kløve, H. (1963). Clinical neuropsychology. In F. M. Foster (Ed.), *The medical clinics of North America.* New York: Saunders.

Koenig, S., Gendelman, H. E., Orenstein, J., Dal Canto, M. C., Pezeshkpour, G. H., Yungbluth, M., Janotta, F., Aksamit, A., Martin, M. A., & Fauci, A. S. (1986). Detection of AIDS virus in macrophages in brain tissue from AIDS patients with encephalopathy. *Science, 233,* 1089–1093.

Koup, R. A., & Wilson, C. B. (1994). Clinical immunology of HIV infected children. In P. A. Pizzo & C. M. Wilfert (Eds.), *Pediatric AIDS: The challenge of HIV infection in infants, children, and adolescents* (2nd ed., pp. 129–157). Baltimore: Williams & Wilkins.

Krivine, A., Firtion, G., Cao, L., Francoual, C., Henrion, R., & Lebon, P. (1992). HIV replication during the first weeks of life. *Lancet, 339,* 1187–1189.

Levenson, R. L., Jr., Mellins, C. A., Zawadzki, R., Kairam, R., & Stein, Z. (1992). Cognitive assessment of human immunodeficiency virus-exposed children. *American Journal of Diseases of Children, 146,* 1479–1483.

Lezak, M. D. (1978). Subtle sequelae of brain damage: Perplexity, distractibility, and fatigue. *American Journal of Physical Medicine, 57,* 9–15.

Lezak, M. D. (1995). *Neuropsychological assessment* (3rd ed.). New York: Oxford University Press.

McArthur, J. C. (1994). Neurological and neuropathological manifestations of HIV infection. In I. Grant & A. Martin (Eds.), *Neuropsychology of HIV infection* (pp. 56–107). London: Oxford University Press.

Macdonald, W. B. (1984). Viral and chlamydial infections. In M. Ziai (Ed.), *Pediatrics* (pp. 505–542). Boston: Little Brown.

Mann, J. M., Tarantola, D. M., & Netter, T. W. (1992). *AIDS in the world.* Cambridge, MA: Harvard University Press.

Masliah, E., Achim, C. L., Ge, N., DeTerresa, R., Terry, R. D., & Wiley, C. A. (1992). Spectrum of human immunodeficiency virus associated neocortical damage. *Annals of Neurology, 32,* 321–329.

Mills, E. L., Regelmann, W. E., & Quie, P. G. (1981). Immunology of the newborn. In R. D. Feigin & J. D. Cherry (Eds.), *Textbook of pediatric infectious diseases* (pp. 729–746). Philadelphia: Saunders.

Mintz, M. (1989). Elevated serum levels of tumor necrosis factor associated with progressive encephalopathy in children with acquired immunodeficiency syndrome. *American Journal of Diseases of Children, 143,* 771–774.

Nicholas, S. W. (1994). The opportunistic and bacterial infections associated with pediatric human immunodeficiency virus disease. *Acta Paediatrica, Supplement, 400,* 46–50.

Novello, A. C., Wise, P. H., Willoughby, A., & Pizzo, P. A. (1989). Final report of the United States Department of Health and Human Services Secretary's Work Group on pediatric human immunodeficiency virus infection disease: Content and implications. *Pediatrics, 84,* 547–555.

Overall, J. C. (1981). Viral infections of the fetus and neonate. In R. D. Feigin & J. D. Cherry (Eds.), *Textbook of pediatric infectious diseases* (pp. 684–721). Philadelphia: Saunders.

Oxtoby, M. J. (1990). Epidemiology of pediatric AIDS in the United States. In P. Kozlowski, D. Wnider, P. Vietze, & H. Wisniewski (Eds.), *Brain in pediatric AIDS* (pp. 1–8). Basel: Karger.

Oxtoby, M. J. (1991). Perinatally acquired HIV infection. In P. A. Pizzo & C. M. Wilfert (Eds.), *Pediatric AIDS: The challenge of HIV infection in infants, children, and adolescents* (pp. 3–21). Baltimore: Williams & Wilkins.

Oxtoby, M. J. (1994). Vertically acquired HIV infection in the United States. In P. A. Pizzo & C. M. Wilfert (Eds.), *Pediatric AIDS: The challenge of HIV infection in infants, children, and adolescents* (2nd ed., pp. 3–20). Baltimore: Williams & Wilkins.

Pang, S., Koyanagi, Y., Miles, S., Wiley, C., Vinters, H., & Chen, I. (1990). High levels of unintegrated HIV-1 DNA in brain tissue of AIDS dementia patients. *Nature, 343,* 85–89.

Park, Y., Belman, A., Dickson, D., Llena, J., Josephina, F., Lantos, G., Diamond, G., Bernstein, L., & Rubinstein, A. (1988). Stroke in pediatric AIDS [Abstract]. *Annals of Neurology, 24,* 279.

Pizzo, P., Brouwers, P., & Poplack, D. (1989). Intravenous infusion of zidovudine (AZT) in children with HIV infection. *New England Journal of Medicine, 320,* 805–806.

Pizzo, P., Butler, K., Balis, F., Brouwers, P., Hawkins, M., Eddy, J., Einloth, M., Falloon, J., Husson, R., Jarosinski, P., Meer, J., Moss, H., Poplack, D., Santacroce, S., Wiener, L., & Wolters, P. (1990). Dideoxycytidine alone and in an alternating schedule with zidovudine in children with symptomatic human immunodeficiency virus infection. *Journal of Pediatrics, 117,* 799–808.

Pizzo, P., Eddy, J., Falloon, J., Balis, F., Murphy, R., Moss, H., Wolters, P., Brouwers, P., Jarosinski, P., Rubin, M., Broder, S., Yarchoan, R., Brunetti, A., Maha, M., Nusinoff-Lehrman, S., & Poplack, D. (1988). Effect of continuous intravenous infusion of zidovudine (AZT) in children with symptomatic HIV infection. *New England Journal of Medicine, 319,* 889–896.

Pizzo, P. A. & Wilfert, C. M. (Eds.). (1994). *Pediatric AIDS: The challenge of HIV infection in infants, children, and adolescents* (2nd ed.). Baltimore: Williams & Wilkins.

Prober, C., & Gershon, A. (1991). Medical management of newborns and infants born to seropositive mothers. In P. A. Pizzo & C. M. Wilfert (Eds.), *Pediatric AIDS: The challenge of HIV infection in infants, children, and adolescents* (pp. 516–530). Baltimore: Williams & Wilkins.

Resnick, L., Berger, J. R., Shapshak, P., & Tourtellote, W. W. (1988). Early penetration of blood–brain barrier by HIV. *Neurology, 38,* 9–14.

Rogers, M. F. (1989). Modes, rates, and risk factors for perinatal transmission of HIV [Abstract T.B.O. 19]. *Proceedings of the V International Conference on AIDS, 1,* 199.

Rogers, M. F., Thomas, P. A., Starcher, E. T., Noa, M. C., Bush, T. J., & Jaffe, J. W. (1987). Acquired immunodeficiency syndrome in children: Report of the Center for Disease Control National Surveillance, 1982 to 1985. *Pediatrics, 79,* 1008–1014.

Routh, D. K. (Ed.). (1988). *Handbook of pediatric psychology.* New York: Guilford Press.

Sarngadharan, M. G., Popovic, M., Bruch, L., Shupbach, J., & Gallo, R. C. (1984). Antibodies reactive with human T-lymphotropic retroviruses (HTLV-III) in the serum of patients with AIDS. *Science, 224,* 506–508.

Satz, P. (1993). Brain reserve capacity on symptom onset after brain injury: A formulation and review of evidence for threshold theory. *Neuropsychology, 7,* 273–295.

Scott, G. B., & Hutto, C. (1991). Prognosis in pediatric HIV infection. In P. A. Pizzo & C. M. Wilfert (Eds.), *Pediatric AIDS: The challenge of HIV infection in infants, children, and adolescents* (pp. 187–198). Baltimore: Williams & Wilkins.

Scott, G. B., Hutto, C., Makuch, R. W., Mastrucci, M. T., O'Connor, T., Mitchell, C. D., Trapido, E. J., & Parks, W. P. (1989). Survival in children with perinatally acquired human immunodeficiency virus type 1 infection. *New England Journal of Medicine, 321,* 1791–1796.

Selnes, O. A., & Miller, E. N. (1994). Development of a screening battery for HIV-related cognitive impairment: The MACS experience. In I. Grant & A. Martin (Eds.), *Neuropsychology of HIV infection* (pp. 176–187). London: Oxford University Press.

Sharer, L., Cho, E. S., & Epstein, L. G. (1985). Multinucleated giant cells and HTLV-III in AIDS encephalopathy. *Human Pathology, 16,* 760.

Sharer, L. R., Dowling, P., Micheals, J., Cook, S., Menonna, J., Blumberg, B., & Epstein, L. (1990). Spinal cord disease in children with HIV-1 infection: A combined biological and neuropathological study. *Neuropathology and Applied Neurobiology, 16,* 317–331.

Sharer, L. R., Epstein, L. G., Cho, E., Joshi, V. V., Meyenhofer, M. F., Rankin, L. F., & Petito, C. K. (1986). Pathologic features of AIDS encephalopathy in children: Evidence for LAV/HTLV-III infection of brain. *Human Pathology, 17,* 271–284.

Sparrow, S., Balla, D., & Cichetti, D. (1984). *Vineland Adaptive Behavior Scales.* Circle Pines, MN: American Guidance Service.

Sprecher, S., Soumenkoff, G., Puissant, F., & Degueldre, M. (1986). Vertical transmission of HIV in a 15-week fetus [Letter]. *Lancet, 2,* 288–289.

Tardieu, M. (1991). Brain imaging in pediatric HIV infection. In A. Belman & A. M. Laverda (chairs), *Pediatric HIV-1 infection: Neurological and neuropsychological aspects.* Symposium conducted at the meeting of the Neuroscience of HIV infection: Basic and Clinical Frontiers, Padva Italy.

Tardieu, M., Blanche, S., Duliege, A., Rouzioux, C., & Griscelli, C. (1989). Neurologic involvement and prognostic factors after materno-fetal infection [Abstract]. *Proceedings of the V International Conference on AIDS, 1,* 194.

Tarter, R. E., Edwards, K. L., & van Thiel, D. H. (1988). Perspective and rationale for neuropsychological assessment of medical disease. In R. E., Tarter, D. H. van Thiel, & K. L. Edwards (Eds.), *Medical neuropsychology: The impact of disease on behavior* (pp. 1–10). New York: Plenum Press.

Ultmann, M. H., Belman, A. L., Ruff, H. A., Novick, B. E., Cone-Wesson, B., Cohen, J. J., & Rubinstein, A. (1985). Developmental abnormalities in infants and children with acquired immune deficiency syndrome (AIDS) and AIDS-related complex. *Developmental Medicine and Child Neurology, 27,* 563–571.

Ultmann, M. H., Diamond, G. W., Ruff, H. A., Belman, A. L., Novick, B. E., Rubinstein, A., & Cohen, H. J. (1987). Developmental abnormalities in children with acquired immunodeficiency syndrome (AIDS): A follow up study. *International Journal of Neuroscience, 32,* 661–667.

Wilfert, C. M., Wilson, C., Luzuriaga, K., & Epstein, L. (1994). Pathogenesis of pediatric human immunodeficiency virus type 1 infection. *Journal of Infectious Diseases, 170,* 286–292.

Wolters, P., Brouwers, P., Moss, H., el-Amin, D., Eddy, J., Butler, K., Husson, R., & Pizzo, P. (1990). The effect of 2'3' dideoxyinosine (ddI) on the cognitive functioning of infants and children with symptomatic HIV infection [Abstract]. *Proceedings of the VI International Conference on AIDS, 3,* 130.

Wolters, P., Brouwers, P., Moss, H., el-Amin, D., Gress, J., Butler, K., & Pizzo, P. (1991). The effect of dideoxyinosine on the cognitive functioning of children with HIV infection after 6 and 12 months of treatment [Abstract]. *Proceedings from the VII International Conference on AIDS, 2,* 194.

Wolters, P., Brouwers, P., Moss, H., & Pizzo, P. (1994). Adaptive behavior of children with symptomatic HIV infection before and after zidovudine therapy. *Journal of Pediatric Psychology, 19,* 47–61.

32

Child Behavioral Neuropsychology

Update and Further Considerations

ARTHUR MacNEILL HORTON, JR.

For many years there has been a realization that neuropsychological functioning and learning theory overlap to a considerable degree. One of the first persons to differentiate brain and mind was the famous British neurologist, John Hughlings Jackson, who made this observation in 1872. In addition, Gaddes (1981) suggests that contemporary models and conceptualizations regarding learning disabilities have their beginnings in the research of 19th century neurologists who first began to explore the relationship of human brain structure and spoken and written language. As noted by Horton and Wedding (1984), many workers have made contributions to this effort.

In the last three decades, interest in brain–behavior relationships has expanded at an ever increasing rate. Contributing to this development is the impressive cross-cultural validity of neuropsychological research (Golden, 1981; Horton & Wedding, 1984; Luria, 1966; Reitan & Davison, 1974) as well as very successful applications of neuropsychological testing to the assessment of school-age children (Horton & Wedding, 1984; Hynd & Obrzut, 1981; Reitan & Davison, 1974). It is clear that human clinical neuropsychology is of great importance to child/school psychology.

In addition to the tremendous growth of neuropsychology, there has been dramatic development of behavior therapy programs for school-age children (Horton, 1994). Since the advent of large-scale behavioral programs following the work of Ayllon

and Azrin (Kazdin, 1978), there has been greatly increased use of behavioral methods by providers of educational and psychological services to school-age children. The extent of the empirical data base supporting the use of behavioral methods is only matched by that amassed by human neuropsychology (Wesolowski & Zencius, 1994).

Given these dual developments, a reasonable question would be the possibility of merger. Indeed, there have been significant efforts devoted to the amalgamation of neuropsychological assessment and behavioral treatment methods. A new area of research and practice that combines behavior therapy treatment approaches with neuropsychological assessment methods has been suggested (Horton, 1979) and entitled *behavioral neuropsychology.* Educational, psychological, and neurological professionals who treat children with learning and behavior problems related to impaired neuropsychological functioning could find this new area of research and clinical practice valuable.

The intent of this chapter is to review and update the research and clinical knowledge base that underlies behavioral neuropsychology since the earlier version of this chapter was published in 1989. The first step will be to describe what is meant by behavioral neuropsychology. The first use of the term was in 1978, when the Behavioral Neuropsychology Special Interest Group was formed under the administrative aegis of the Association for Advancement of Behavior Therapy (AABT). The first meeting of the group was held in Chicago at the 1978 annual AABT meeting and the Special Interest Group was active in AABT for a dozen years.

ARTHUR MacNEILL HORTON, JR. • Psych Associates, Towson, Maryland 21214.

At that time a tentative definition was suggested, as follows:

> Behavioral Neuropsychology may be defined as the application of behavior therapy techniques to problems of organically impaired individuals while using a neuropsychological assessment and intervention perspective. This treatment methodology suggests that inclusion of data from Neuropsychological assessment strategies would be helpful in the formulation of hypotheses regarding antecedent conditions (external or internal) for observed phenomena of psychopathology. That is, a neuropsychological perspective will significantly enhance the ability of the behavior therapist to make accurate discriminations as to the etiology of patient behavior. Moreover, the formulation of a cogent plan of therapeutic intervention and its skillful implementation could, in certain cases, be facilitated by an analysis of behavior deficits implicating impairment of higher cortical functioning. (Horton, 1979, p. 20)

Although the above definition is dated, it still serves to focus the discussion of behavioral neuropsychology. It may be acknowledged that alternate interpretations of behavioral neuropsychology, as a field, could be advanced, and that many researchers or clinicians in either neuropsychology or behavior therapy (or applied behavioral analysis) may have very different points of view.

The chapter will be organized into four sections related to the specific application of behavioral neuropsychology with school-age children. The first section focuses on theoretical issues and briefly describes how behavioral neuropsychology relates to radical and more contemporary conceptualizations of behaviorism. The second section deals with treatment planning issues and discusses a framework for conceptualizing therapeutic interventions. The third section briefly describes selective portions of the existing body of research on the application of behavioral methods with brain-injured children. The fourth section, a concluding statement, also advances some tentative hypotheses about possible developments in child behavioral neuropsychology.

Theoretical Issues

Behavioral Concerns

The first theoretical concern to be addressed is how radical behaviorism relates to clinical neu-

ropsychology. The second theoretical concern will be the relationship of contemporary behaviorism and clinical neuropsychology. This discussion will be fairly superficial and quite brief as more in-depth discussions have appeared (Horton, 1979, 1981, 1994; Horton & Puente, 1986; Lawson-Kerr, Smith, & Beck, 1990; Wesolowski & Zencius, 1994).

Briefly, the radical behaviorist paradigm holds that all human behavior can be explained by observed stimulus–response relationships (Watson, 1913). Radical behaviorists aver that the behavior of humans can be understood without any need to suggest the existence of unobserved factors (Skinner, 1938). In other words, variables that are not observable stimulus–response actions are not needed to predict future human behaviors (Marr, 1984). Variables that may not be observed, which are also termed *inferred variables,* are seen as of little value by radical behaviorists.

It is important to consider the proposition that there may be legitimate inferred variables in the functional analysis of human behavior (Mahoney, 1974), in order to meld neuropsychology into a radical behaviorist framework. As averred before (Horton, 1979), inferred variables are of two distinct types. These are *intervening variables* and *hypothetical constructs* (Craighead, Kazdin, & Mahoney, 1976). As suggested previously (Horton, 1979):

> an intervening variable is a theoretical creation. For instance, no one has ever observed intervening variables, such as thoughts or feelings, yet they are used by cognitive behavior therapists to explain behavior. It could be said that, at least as far as we now know it, it is unlikely one would be able to directly observe an intervening variable. (p. 21)

As others have asserted (Craighead *et al.,* 1976), intervening variables exist only in theory as they are conceptual abstractions. Hypothetical constructs, on the other hand, are generally seen as more physical or empirical than intervening variables. As observed previously (Horton, 1981):

> a hypothetical construct is an actual physical object or process which is unobservable at the present time. For instance, hypothetical constructs in neuropsychology tend to have physiological referents and can, if so desired, be verified. If a child evidences certain characteristics, it might be postulated that there is damage to the right parietal lobe. In this case, our hypothetical construct is based on our knowledge of brain–behavior relationships and can be varied through neurosurgical procedures. (p. 368)

In an earlier publication (Horton, 1979), the differences between intervening variables and hypothetical constructs were explained as follows:

> an example of this distinction would be the behavior of failing to draw a Greek cross and the explanation of this behavior by each inferred variable. An intervening variable could opt for an explaining mechanism such as an emotional state as the cause. Using a hypothetical construct, one might postulate the impairment of the right parietal lobe. While this example is grossly over-simplified, the major point should be clear. Hypothetical constructs tend to have physiological referents. The major advantage is that at some point, by some means, its existence or nonexistence can be verified. In the instance cited, neurosurgical procedures could determine the actual condition of the right parietal lobe in our subject. While in clinical practice, this is rarely done, the distinction is important. At present, methods for the direct objective verification of a thought or feeling have yet to be adequately developed. (p. 21)

Relative to neuropsychology and behavior therapy, the major point of the above quote is that neuropsychological data are hypothetical constructs. Therefore, these data, being hypothetical constructs, differ conceptually from intervening variables. Because of these differences, it might be argued that the inclusion of hypothetical constructs in the radical behavioral model has markedly different implications than the inclusion of intervening variables. It is important to recall the historical context as the neglect of intervening variables by the S-R model of behaviorism at the time of major radical behavioral thinkers, such as John M. Watson (1913) and B. F. Skinner (1938), was based on the inability of the then-contemporary human neuroscience to meaningfully add to a functional analysis of human behavior. With respect to hypothetical constructs and contemporary human neuroscience, there has been an explosive rate of development over the intervening four or five decades. As observed in an earlier publication:

> Now, however, it could be observed that the knowledge base of brain–behavior relationships has changed drastically since the days of Watson. At the time, Neuropsychology was unable to provide even rudimentary guidance for research minded behaviorists. Clearly, the most appropriate strategy has a benign neglect of the area. Today, however, is a drastically different situation. In the last 20 years, the knowledge base of brain–behavior relationships has increased geometrically (Davison, 1974). Cross-cultural research has provided such impressive validation of neuropsychological insights that it would

> appear difficult to minimize the importance (Luria, 1966; Hecaen & Ajuriaguerra, 1964; Faglioni, Spinnler, & Vignolo, 1969) of Neuropsychological factors, it would seem that the time for their inclusion in an enlarged behavioral paradigm is at hand. (Horton, 1979, p. 22)

Although the ultimate test of the above remarks is of necessity empirical, it should be clear that neuropsychological factors are accessible to measurement and therefore cannot be dismissed on the grounds that they are unscientific. Moreover, in the years since the above quote was written there have been incredible advances in neuroimaging technology (Kertesz, 1994). Techniques such as computerized tomography (CT), magnetic resonance imaging (MRI), magnetic resonance spectroscopy (MRS), single-photon emission computerized tomography (SPECT), and positron emission tomography (PET), among others, have provided windows to the brain that could not have even been imagined a quarter century before. Given the wealth of data attesting to the biological activities of the brain, earlier concerns about unobserved factors seem of less importance.

At this point the second conceptual concern mentioned earlier might be addressed. That is the blend of contemporary behaviorism and neuropsychology. To provide a context for discussion context, it is helpful to mention that when the journal *Behavioral Assessment* was launched at the end of the 1970s, the founding editor, Rosemary Nelson, in her editorial statement suggested that behavioral assessment emphasizes:

> both meaningful response units and . . . their controlling variables. Behavior is defined functionally, in relation to its present controlling variables (both environmental and organismic) and to its responsiveness to intervention strategies.

Indeed, it might be said that contemporary behavior therapy has been characterized by an evolving clinical acumen. Increased sophistication in behavior therapy also reflects improved behavioral assessment techniques. As behavior therapy has matured there has been increased focus on the assessment aspects of behavior therapy. Nelson (1983), for example, has stated that behavior therapy, to an increasing degree, is defined by the techniques used. For example, some behavior therapists would define "self-monitoring" as a behavioral technique, and at the same time hold that a standard psychological test such as the Minnesota Multiphasic Personality Inventory (MMPI) is clearly nonbehavioral (Hayes &

Zettle, 1980). The difficulty with making such statements is that they are both arbitrary and nonempirical (Horton & Puente, 1986).

A better method of classifying particular assessment and treatment techniques as behavioral or nonbehavioral can be proposed. Hayes and Zettle (1980) have suggested a conceptual model for making these judgments. Their method is premised on the valid distinctions between the conceptual (how to talk about techniques) and the technical (how to perform techniques) dimensions of contemporary behaviorism. They aver that a reasonable notion is to emphasize conceptual as opposed to technical dimensions when deciding whether or not a technique is "behavioral." For instance, if a particular technique can be discussed in behavioral terms (i.e., positive reinforcement, stimulus–response contingencies) and can be empirically assessed, it is "behavioral." Considerations such as who originated the procedure or the topographical details of the technique are not germane to the judgment as to whether the technique is "behavioral." An important consideration is that antecedents and consequences of an act must be considered in order to decide what the purpose of the action was. Physical details are less relevant than the intended purpose of the action under study. In a nutshell, if one can talk about a technique in behavioral terms, and the method yields observable outcomes that can be objectively measured, then it is "behavioral." The above discussion has clear implications for behavioral neuropsychology. For example, as stated in an earlier publication:

> If behavior therapy is defined in a conceptual sense, then clinical Neuropsychological assessment instruments such as the Halstead-Reitan Neuropsychological Test Battery or the Luria–Nebraska Neuropsychological Test Battery can be classified as "behavioral." . . . If the most appropriate goal of behavior therapy is a "clinical science based upon clinical realities" (Hayes & Zettle, 1980), then it would appear that a conceptual view would be preferable. Thus, a Neuropsychological perspective could be integrated into such an enlarged and clinically realistic behavioral paradigm. Whether or not such a blend of neuropsychology and behaviorism proves a potent addition . . . remains an empirical question, which in the best tradition of behaviorism should be objectively tested. (Horton, 1981, p. 369)

As the necessary empirical basis has been amassed (Horton, 1994; Horton & Puente, 1986; Horton & Sautter, 1986; Lawson-Kerr *et al.*, 1990; Wesolowski & Zencius, 1994), it appears clear that a neuropsychological perspective can be profitably subsumed into the contemporary behavioral model.

Neuropsychological Issues

Relative to planning behavioral treatment for brain-injured school-age children, important considerations are the stage of neurological development and the specific behavioral consequences of brain impairment. Regarding research from developmental neuropsychology, Miller (1984), after reviewing the research findings from animal studies, suggested that a specific recovery pattern should be expected and that the more basic the skills, the less impaired they should be in general, and that children show considerable recovery of neural and behavioral functions. Miller also suggested that early behavioral interventions appeared to facilitate recovery of function.

Another crucial issue concerns the behavioral sequelae of brain injury. At least one group of authors (Klonoff, Crockett, & Clark, 1984) suggested a significant relationship between environmental factors and the incidence of brain injury. Moreover, they have presented data suggesting that the sequelae of brain injury are related to age of injury with younger children showing emotional and personality changes and older children displaying learning and memory difficulties. Horton and Puente (1986) declared that:

> treatment planning should take into consideration environmental factors such as actual physical environment as well as family structure in order to minimize future occurrences of neural impairment as well as to maximize the general ability of the office or institution-based treatment program.

Also, the goals of treatment planning should be considered. Treatment programs often focus on either recovery of lost abilities or suppression of problem social behaviors. As a result, more often than not treatment programs tend to be focused on patient deficits. The value of such a focus is questionable at best. Reynolds (1981) has stated that a better approach would be to focus on the brain-injured child's strengths rather than deficits. Horton, Wedding, and Phay (1981), as well as Horton and Miller (1985), have provided discussions of this concern and these discussions will not be repeated here. Briefly, focusing on a brain-injured child's strengths is the preferred strategy to maximize clinical behavioral treatment efficacy.

Treatment Strategies

Lewinsohn's Model

Peter M. Lewinsohn has made extremely impressive research and clinical contributions to the literature on the remediation of memory deficits in brain-damaged persons (Glasgow, Zeiss, Barrera, & Lewinsohn, 1977; Lewinsohn, Danaher, & Kikel, 1977). As part of his clinical research effort, Lewinsohn developed an excellent paradigm for guiding clinical work with neuropsychologically impaired persons. The model is divided into four steps: the first two steps deal with assessment and the second two steps are concerned with treatment. Specifically, the steps are as follows:

1. General assessment of neuropsychological functioning
2. Specific assessment of neuropsychological functioning
3. Laboratory evaluation of intervention techniques
4. *In vivo* application of intervention techniques

The following paragraphs briefly describe each step in turn. Regarding the first step, traditional neuropsychological batteries are used. One could use an age-appropriate version of the Wechsler Intelligence Scales, or the Kaufman Assessment Battery for Children (K-ABC), or the age-appropriate Halstead–Reitan Neuropsychological Test Battery (HRNTB), or the age-appropriate Luria–Nebraska Neuropsychological Battery (LNNB). The first step is designed to obtain normative psychometrics. These normative data facilitate a comparison of the brain-injured patient being assessed with other brain-injured and normal patients who have been previously assessed as to descriptive neuropsychological test scores. These comparisons provide the perspective of a general understanding of the patient's problems relative to other patients and normal individuals.

The second step, by contrast, focuses on a personalized or intraindividual understanding of the patient's unique problems. The intent is to examine in great detail the precise dimensions of the patient's problem. In using a traditional psychological test such as the Wechsler Intelligence Scale for Children-Third edition (WISC-III), standard scores for Full Scale, Verbal Scale, and Performance Scale IQs can be obtained. The use of normative compar-

ison with the standard score IQs allows the brain-injured child to be viewed relative to other children in the normative population on intellectual ability with great accuracy. A more intuitive understanding of the child's neuropsychological deficits can be obtained by requesting the child to verbalize how he or she solved particular subtests and to readminister certain items with progressively more help or prompts given to the brain-injured child. This dynamic approach facilitates the development of a better understanding of the actual dimension of the child's neuropsychological deficits. A level of understanding can be reached by the use of these complementary methods which is often different and deeper than that reached by normative psychometrics alone. The emphasis in the second step is on intraindividual comparisons. The risk of this approach is that examiners will overinterpret findings on the basis of wishful thinking and preexisting cognitive biases. At the same time, the great flexibility enjoyed in investigating the actual stimulus–response dimension of the problem behaviors and conducting a functional analysis of the behavior deficit is valuable.

In the third step, the focus is on a laboratory-like setting. Under carefully controlled conditions, behavioral intervention techniques are used to address the problem behaviors assessed in the first two steps. One behavioral intervention technique might be to train the brain-injured child in using verbal self-instruction to learn social skills and apply them to a variety of predesigned social problem situations that can be simulated by role-playing. The brain-injured child is trained to the point that some treatment effectiveness in the controlled setting can be demonstrated. When efficacy in the controlled setting is clear, then the intervention must be transported to the real world. Often, it will be necessary to program specific efforts to ensure generalization of the behavioral techniques to new settings.

In the fourth step, the behavioral intervention strategy that proved effective in the laboratory is introduced to the uncontrolled conditions of the real world. As can be expected, often there are major differences between a behavioral intervention strategy that works in a controlled laboratory setting and a behavioral intervention technique that works in the real world. Multiple modifications may be necessary. These can include adjustments of techniques, alternative modality strategies, and greatly increased treatment intensity and duration. Also, reprogramming of environment stimuli and behavioral contingencies could be required. To use the verbal self-instructional techniques as an example, the technique may need to be practiced until it becomes both covert and an automatic response to aversive emotional stimuli.

Lewinsohn's model allows for a structured conceptualization of clinical behavioral neuropsychology therapy with the brain-injured child. The overall paradigm requires normative and intraindividual assessment with precise behavioral interventions attempted in controlled settings followed by modification and augmentation of the behavioral intervention to work in the uncontrolled settings of the real world. It might be stressed that the range and type of quantitative and qualitative measuring devices are only limited by ingenuity and resources of the assessment and treatment providers. Although the above example used the HRNTB and LNNB as examples of normative neuropsychological assessment tools, it would be short sighted to limit assessment tools to neuropsychological tests. Rather, assessment tools in the future might include neuroimaging devices such as CT, SPECT, MRI, and PET scans (Kertesz, 1994). Indeed, any valid test of brain functioning that allows normative and intraindividual comparisons might be used.

At this point, some classical work in behavioral assessment might be briefly described. Goldfried and Davison (1976) suggested a paradigm that is similar to steps two and three of Lewinsohn's framework. Some attention will be devoted to describing the Goldfried and Davison behavioral assessment paradigm.

Goldfried and Davison (1976) postulated that four types of important variables are crucial in conceptualizing maladaptive behaviors: (1) stimulus antecedents, (2) organismic variables, (3) response variables, and (4) consequent variables.

In a nutshell, the Gottfried and Davison model is a revision of the traditional stimulus–response paradigm of radical behaviorism. To a more traditional behavioral framework, the variables of "organismic" and "consequences" are added. The resulting model does appear to have some strengths in allowing one to more adequately conceptualize a greater number of the various domains that need to be considered in a comprehensive behavioral assessment and treatment paradigm.

Some consideration of treatment planning issues will be presented to better illustrate the points made earlier. As more elaborate discussions have been published, these comments will be abbreviated (Horton,

1994; Horton & Puente, 1986; Horton & Sautter, 1986; Horton & Wedding, 1984). Primary concerns are (1) self-efficacy, (2) personality × treatment interactions, and (3) available resources for support.

Self-Efficacy

Self-efficacy as a therapeutic concept was first advanced by Albert Bandura (1982). Briefly, Bandura proposed that how a person perceives her or his personal effectiveness is a major variable in determining if the person will undertake therapeutic behavior change activities. The proposition is that behavior change techniques work by increasing an individual's self-estimate of her or his competence in a situation and/or activity. Put another way, personal belief systems determine behaviors emitted as well as the duration, frequency, and intensity of the behaviors, particularly when difficult circumstances are present. Bandura's (1982) initial description of self-efficacy suggested that four sources of data influenced personal beliefs of competency. Briefly, these are (1) successful personal behavioral performance, (2) observing successful performances by others, (3) personal status of physiological arousal, and (4) verbal persuasion.

The data sources are not all of equal potency for successful modification of self-efficacy beliefs. Rather, Bandura (1982) postulated that some were more powerful therapeutic modalities of belief change. Interestingly, he felt that the data sources ranged on a continuum from most to least powerful. Simply put, he suggested that personal behavioral performance, or actually performing an action, is the most powerful. Modeling, or watching others perform, was next most powerful. Changing one's physiological arousal status was next most powerful and the last data source, verbal persuasion, or talking about the action is the weakest. If one considered the therapeutic task as combating the social phobia of public speaking, then performing the activity would be giving a speech in front of an audience and would be the most powerful way of reducing speech anxiety, and verbal persuasion or talking about speaking would be the least powerful way of reducing speech anxiety.

Implications of self-efficacy for treatment planning are straightforward. *In vivo* behavioral performance, or actually performing the action in question, would be the preferred therapeutic task. Children with brain injury may require special assistance devices and facilitative activities to utilize performance-based feedback but the need to successfully accomplish therapeutic activities is clear. If successful personal behavioral performances are not possible, then models of others performing successfully could be used. Only if no other possibilities are available should verbal persuasion be used by itself. It is widely assumed the motivation for change is related to the magnitude of reinforcement for performing an action times the individual's estimate of the odds of accomplishing the task successfully. Therefore, personal predictions of successful performance are crucial factors in treatment planning.

Personality × Treatment Interactions

Personality × treatment interactions are selected specific client/patient/subject factors or traits that affect the success of particular therapeutic methods. Put another way, the methods work better in a subgroup of patients/clients that share a particular trait or factor. What the trait or factor is can vary widely. Client/patient/subject's personal standards for self-reinforcement (Goldfried & Davison, 1976) might be an example. Clients/patients/subjects with high standards might be given less difficult therapeutic goals as failure experiences might reduce motivation to continue in therapy.

Availability of Resources

The type and amount of resources available for treatment activities is a key consideration. It is of little avail to prescribe an elaborate program of treatment activities if a large portion of these don't exist in the patient's geographical location or are otherwise not available. Availability of resources refers, it might be noted, to both the physical features of the treatment setting (school and/or community based) as well as individual and social aspects. For example, the personal therapeutic skills of the therapist(s) might qualify as resources. As noted by others (Diller & Gordon, 1981), significant others can serve in therapeutic roles and their availability in the patient's immediate environment can be most helpful. In addition, the therapeutic techniques chosen to be implemented depend on the ability of school personnel and/or community members to fulfill specific therapeutic roles. To plan to use techniques that are difficult to implement or are very costly in terms of time

and effort will, very often, doom an intervention to failure.

Guidelines from Behavioral Neuropsychology

Selection of behavior therapy interventions for children with brain impairment is, at this point, more of an art than a science. Nonetheless, some very oversimplified suggestions have been advanced (Horton & Wedding, 1984) and will be briefly reviewed below. It may be appropriate to mention that these suggestions are based on the behavioral/structural aspects of basic neuroanatomical dimensions. It is, of course, well known that the human brain operates on many levels. In addition to the structural/behavioral level, there are also microscopic and molecular levels of information transfer (Restak, 1994). In future years, the expectation is that additional knowledge will allow the casting of suggestions for treatment selection based on the other levels of information transfer in the brain. At present, too little is known to even advance rudimentary propositions. Therefore, these suggestions will be confined to the behavioral/structural aspects of the brain.

It is possible to use a number of methods to conceptualize brain structure (Horton & Wedding, 1984), and one of the most relevant and elegant ways of considering the behavioral organization of the neurocortex has been described by Manfred Meier (1974). In a chapter discussing challenges to clinical neuropsychology, Meier (1974) saw the brain as consisting of three major dimensions: (1) left to right, (2) front to back, and (3) top to bottom.

Horton and Wedding (1984), in discussing Meier's conceptualization of brain functioning, termed the left to right parameter as "laterality," the front to back parameter as "caudality," and the top to bottom parameter as "dorsality." In the following discussion these concepts are used in unique ways and not necessarily in the manner intended by Meier (1974). Also, the parameters are intended to describe even as yet poorly understood ideas and there is a great risk of oversimplification. It is acknowledged that others might find different ways of explaining these concepts, but in the hope of simplicity of communication, this paradigm is advanced. Moreover, these guidelines are based on cases with relatively localized brain injury and may be less valid in cases of diffuse cerebral damage. Still, the expectation is that these guidelines will serve as postulates on which to base even more accurate understandings of behavioral/structural relationships and behavioral therapeutic effectiveness.

Laterality

Laterality has generated more research in U.S. neuropsychology than any other single concept. Horton and Wedding (1984), in explaining laterality, observed:

> The two cerebral hemispheres process information in different ways. Assuming right handedness, the left hemisphere is logical and language oriented, while the right hemisphere is intuitive and concerned with spatial aspects of stimuli. (p. 216)

Similarly, Reynolds (1981) noted that:

> For the vast majority of individuals, the left cerebral hemisphere appears to be specialized for linguistic, propositional, serial, and analytic tasks, and the right hemisphere for more nonverbal, spatial, appositional, synthetic, and holistic tasks. . . . It is most important to remember that cerebral hemispheric asymmetries of function are *process-specific* and not stimulus-specific. (p. 109)

Many clinicians and researchers (Broder, 1973; Hartlage, 1975; Horton, 1994; Mattis, French, & Rabins, 1975; Pirozzolo, 1981; Rourke, Fisk, & Strang, 1986) have agreed that there are subtypes of children with learning disorders. In addition, there is widespread agreement that neuropsychological assessment is crucial to diagnosing learning disorder subtypes and in guiding treatment interventions. To take the case of reading disability, or dyslexia, as an example, the two most common reading disability subtypes have auditory-linguistic and visuospatial elements (Pirozzolo, 1981).

Hartlage (1975) has suggested a framework of considering hemispheric mental asymmetry with respect to suggested educational interventions, probable emotional correlates, and prognostic predictions for three neuropsychological subtypes. The neuropsychological profiles for subtypes of brain-damaged children have been presented elsewhere (Horton, 1989; Horton & Wedding, 1984) and will not be reproduced here. Briefly, Hartlage's (1975) paradigm connects side of localized lesion injury or neurological syndrome and a number of elements. These include the patient's neuropsychological profile, emotional correlates, educational intervention, and prognosis. It is worth noting that

Hartlage's model is a most helpful tool in explaining a child's syndrome to his or her parents and/or school personnel.

Caudality

Caudality refers to localized brain damage on the anterior–posterior axis. Horton and Wedding (1984), in describing the behavioral effects of anterior brain impairment, observed:

> There is some agreement that the frontal-lobes involve the planning, execution, and verification of behavior while the posterior sections are involved with the reception, integration, and analysis of sensory information. (p. 219)

The functions of the frontal lobes have been a puzzle in neuropsychology for decades, if not centuries (Horton & Wedding, 1984). A classic paper that reveals the behavioral effects of frontal lobe lesions (Struss & Benson, 1984) might be consulted for a description of the emotional and psychological consequences of frontal lobe impairment. In terms of clinical implications, Horton and Wedding (1984) suggested that a frontal lobe lesion is more critical for predicting overall behavioral adjustment than the overall extent of brain impairment on neuropsychological testing. Luria (1966), for example, described great difficulties in the rehabilitation of brain-injured patients with frontal lobe impairment.

With respect to therapeutic implications of frontal lobe impairment with children and adolescents, one suggestion might be to use Meichenbaum's (1978) self-instructional therapy to increase self-management skills for frontally impaired children. Developmentally appropriate versions, like the turtle technique (Schneider & Robin, 1976), are available for young children.

Dorsality

Dorsality refers to the vertical axis, or the top to bottom parameter of the brain. There has been some conceptual work (MacLean, 1973) to suggest evolutionary distinct layers of brain tissue. MacLean's (1973) theory of the triune brain suggests that there are three separate independent cognitive systems in the human brain. The layers or systems all share some common functions but each successive layer adds new higher levels of cognitive complexity (Horton & Wedding, 1984). The three layers MacLean proposed are the reptilian, limbic system, and neocortex. The reptilian layer is a relic that humans share with reptiles and is related to aggression and territoriality. The limbic system is a layer shared with lower mammals and is related to more positive emotions. The third layer, the neocortex, is shared with higher mammals, such as dolphins, and subserves anticipation of events and language.

It might also be mentioned that recent research into the chemical basis of behavior (Restak, 1994) has opened new insights into the subcortical regions of the brain. Discoveries of neurotransmitters such as dopamine, serotonin, acetylcholine, and norepinephrine, to name just a few, have given neuroscientists a whole host of new brain variables to plot and track. The neurotransmitters named, it should be mentioned, all have significant projections in the subcortical areas of the brain. Among other areas, dopamine has concentrations in the substantia nigra (the name is Latin for black substance), serotonin in the midline raphe, acetylcholine in the nucleus basalis of Meynert, and norepinephrine in the locus coeruleus (the name is Latin for blue area) (Restak, 1994).

As many are aware, dopamine has been associated with Parkinson's disease, serotonin and norepinephrine with depression, and acetylcholine with Alzheimer's disease (Restak, 1994). The current popular status of the antidepressant medication, Prozac, to cite but one instance, is based on its relationship with serotonin utilization in the brain and very beneficial effects on depressive symptoms. As can be surmised from the above comments, the neurobiology of emotion appears to be centered in subcortical areas and recent neurochemical advances appear quite exciting. As noted by Horton and Wedding (1984):

> When there are cortical lesions, there are often concomitant personality changes. It is also commonly observed the premorbidly controlled antisocial character traits of brain-damaged individuals are released after the onset of the brain injury. This syndrome might be explained by the triune brain model of Paul MacLean. (p. 220)

In addition, the wealth of recent neurochemical advances might be expected to yield treatment advances in the future. Clearly, the use of Ritalin is common in the treatment of attention deficit hyperactivity disorder (ADHD) in children (Rapport & Kelly, 1991). The concurrent usage of behavior modification programs with medication (Barkley, 1981) is the treatment of choice for children and adolescents with ADHD.

Empirical Considerations

Research on the use of behavior modification/therapy techniques for children with brain injury has been reviewed. Ince (1976) surveyed the use of behavior modification with brain-injured persons in a review that was noted by Diller and Gordon (1981). Similarly, Horton (1979, 1982) has twice surveyed the research literature regarding the application of behavior therapy with individuals with brain damage. More recently, Horton and Miller (1985) surveyed this research literature and found an increasing trend toward using behavior modification/therapy with individuals with brain damage.

In the earlier version of this chapter (Horton, 1989, Table 2) and in a recent book (Horton, 1994), a table appeared that was adapted from the review of Horton and Miller (1985) focusing exclusively on behavior modification/therapy studies with brain-damaged children, not including biofeedback studies, from 1967 to 1984. Of 19 reviewed studies in the 1985 review, only 2, Dean (1984) and Denton and Citron (1983), were control group design studies. Two were group case studies, Carlin and Armstrong (1968) and Salzinger, Feldman, and Portnoy (1970), and three were single-subject design studies (i.e., multiple baseline or ABAB design), Campbell and Stremel-Campbell (1982), Gajan, Schloss, Schloss, and Thompson (1984), and Muir and Milan (1982). The remaining papers appeared to be case studies. Varieties of brain injury treated included closed head injury, cerebral palsy, and Huntington's chorea, among others.

A recent review of the child behavioral neuropsychology literature has found a total of seven small-*N*/case studies using behavioral treatment techniques with children with brain injury. These will be briefly noted. Schoen (1986) modified noncompliant behavior of a 6-year-old by manipulation of instructional reinforcers. Denton (1987) described a number of case examples of the efficacy of behavioral interventions with children and adolescents with severe brain injury. Zencius, Wesolowski, and Burke (1989) used a reversal experimental design to compare behavioral contracting, point systems, and point systems plus response cost contingencies in increasing the attendance of two head-injured adolescents at class and therapy sessions and found all conditions were effective, but the point system plus response cost was slightly more effective for one adolescent. Silver and Stelly-Seitz (1992) used behavioral procedures to increase drinking in a child with decreased thirst resulting from a gunshot wound to the hypothalamic area at age 26 months and at 16-month follow-up showed a normal drinking pattern. Slifer *et al.* (1993) used time series, within-subject designs with one female and three male children, aged 10 to 16, to demonstrate the value of behavioral procedures in reducing disruption and increasing cooperation with medical procedures. Silver, Boake, and Cavazos (1994) used a multiple baseline design to demonstrate the value of a behavioral monetary reinforcement procedure in having a 12-year-old with anoxic brain injury perform self-case tasks and to maintain treatment gains at 6-month follow-up.

Of these seven reports, it is noteworthy that almost half used sophisticated small-*N* (or, as these are often called, single-subject research designs) experimental designs. Even when small-*N* experimental designs are used, there is some evidence of a treatment effect. The reports of Zencius *et al.* (1989) and Silver *et al.* (1994) are actually quite impressive in terms of experimental control of treatment variables. Moreover, the follow-ups of 6 and 16 months by Silver and Stelly-Seitz (1992) and Silver *et al.* (1994) suggest that treatment gains endured over considerable periods of time. At this point, a total of over two dozen research reports can be found in the literature demonstrating the value of using behavioral treatment techniques with children with brain injury.

On one hand, it is encouraging that this line of research is continuing and that there appears to be a trend for researchers to more frequently use small-*N*/single-subject research designs (for a discussion of single-subject research designs see Horton, 1994). On the other hand, there are far too few studies to support any conclusions beyond the very simple statement that behavioral procedures work quite well with children with brain injury. Additional research is very sorely needed regarding the differential effectiveness of particular procedures with varieties of brain injury, including both site of injury (localization) and cause of injury (anoxia versus traumatic brain injury). Also, parameters of effectiveness need to be studied for particular behavioral methods (Horton, 1994). One very needed development is for well-controlled and methodologically sophisticated true experimental group design research with sample cell sizes that ensure adequate statistical power to draw conclusions regarding statistical significance (Horton, 1994).

Conclusions

This chapter has very selectively reviewed the status of child behavioral neuropsychology. Some effort was devoted to assessing the ability of behavioral neuropsychology to deal with the mental, emotional, and behavioral problems of children with brain damage.

The essence of the foregoing paragraphs can be summarized as follows: (1) There is evidence that behavioral methods are effective with children with brain injury. (2) The value of neuropsychological assessment to select behavior modification/therapy techniques is an area that will require additional research. (3) There is a clear need for well-controlled and methodologically sophisticated treatment group design research.

As Horton (1982) observed,

> It is clear that much additional work must be done in order to effectively integrate behavior therapy and clinical neuropsychology. At the same time, it should be noted that the field of therapy for the brain-injured is in its infancy. Thus, it would be unrealistic to expect initial efforts on research fronts to demonstrate more than significant promise. Whether or not this promise will be fulfilled, however, is a question only the future may answer. At this point, one might reflect that Neal Miller's assertion that researchers should be bold in what they try, but cautious in what they claim is a point well taken. (p. 102)

Dr. Horton's contributions to this chapter were made in his private capacity and without support or endorsement by the federal government.

References

Bandura, A. (1982). Self-efficacy mechanism in human agency. *American Psychologist, 37,* 122–147.

Barkley, R. A. (1981). *Hyperactive children: A handbook for diagnosis and treatment.* New York: Guilford Press.

Broder, E. (1973). Developmental dyslexia: A diagnostic approach based on three atypical reading–spelling patterns. *Developmental Medicine and Child Neurology, 15,* 663–687.

Campbell, C., & Stremel-Campbell, K. (1982). Programming "loose-training" as a strategy to facilitate language generalization. *Journal of Applied Behavior Analysis, 15,* 295–301.

Carlin, A. S., & Armstrong, H. E. (1968). Rewarding social responsibility in disturbed children: A group play technique. *Psychotherapy: Theory, Research, and Practice, 5,* 169–174.

Craighead, W. E., Kazdin, A. E., & Mahoney, M. J. (1976). *Behavior modification: Principles, issues and directions.* Boston: Houghton Mifflin.

Dean, R. S. (1984, August). *Treatment of learning disorders with neuropsychological impairment: A behavioral approach.* Paper presented at the American Psychological Association meeting, Toronto, Canada.

Denton, A. (1987). Behavioral change strategies for children and adolescents with severe brain injury. *Journal of Learning Disabilities, 20*(10), 581–589.

Denton, A., & Citron, C. (1983, August). *The development of group intervention strategies for impulsive adolescents with cognitive and language deficits.* Paper presented at the annual meeting of the American Psychological Association, Anaheim, CA.

Diller, L., & Gordon, W. (1981). Interventions for cognitive deficits in brain-injured adults. *Journal of Consulting and Clinical Psychology, 49,* 822–834.

Faglioni, P., Spinnler, H., & Vignola, L. A. (1969). Contrasting behavior of right and left hemisphere-damaged patients on a discriminative and a semantic test of auditory recognition. *Cortex, 5,* 366–389.

Gaddes, W. H. (1981). Neuropsychology, fact or mythology, educational help or hindrance? *School Psychology Review, 10*(31), 322–330.

Gajan, A., Schloss, P. J., Schloss, C. N., & Thompson, C. K. (1984). Effects of feedback and self-monitoring on head trauma youths' conversational skills. *Journal of Applied Behavioral Analysis, 17*(3), 353–358.

Glasgow, R. E., Zeiss, R. A., Barrera, M., & Lewinsohn, P. M. (1977). Case studies on remediating brain damage deficits in brain damaged individuals. *Journal of Clinical Psychology, 33,* 1049–1054.

Golden, C. J. (1981). *Diagnosis and rehabilitation in clinical neuropsychology.* Springfield, IL: Thomas.

Goldfried, M. R., & Davison, G. C. (1976). *Clinical behavior therapy.* New York: Holt, Rinehart, & Winston.

Hartlage, L. C. (1975). Neuropsychological approaches to predicting outcome of remedial educational strategies for learning disabled children. *Pediatric Psychology, 3,* 23–28.

Hayes, S. C., & Zettle, R. D. (1980). On being "behavioral": The technical and conceptual dimensions of behavioral assessment and therapy. *The Behavior Therapist, 3*(3), 4–6.

Heaton, T. B., & Bigler, E. D. (1993). Neuroimaging techniques in neuropsychological research. *Bulletin of the National Academy of Neuropsychology, 9,* 14–17.

Hecaen, J., & Ajuriaguerra, J. (1964). *Left-handedness, manual superiority and cerebral dominance* (E. Ponder, trans.). New York: Grune & Stratton.

Horton, A. M., Jr. (1979). Behavioral neuropsychology: Rationale and research. *Clinical Neuropsychology, 1,* 20–23.

Horton, A. M., Jr. (1981). Behavioral neuropsychology in the schools. *School Psychology Review, 10*(33), 367–372.

Horton, A. M., Jr. (1982). Behavioral neuropsychology: A brief rationale. *The Behavior Therapist, 5,* 100–102.

Horton, A. M., Jr. (1989). Child behavioral neuropsychology. In C. R. Reynolds & E. Fletcher-Janzen (Eds.), *Handbook of clinical child neuropsychology* (pp. 521–533). New York: Plenum Press.

Horton, A. M., Jr. (Ed.). (1990). *Neuropsychology across the life-span.* New York: Springer.

Horton, A. M., Jr. (1994). *Behavioral interventions with brain-injured children.* New York: Plenum Press.

Horton, A. M., Jr., & Miller, W. G. (1985). Neuropsychology and behavior theory. In M. Hersen, R. Eisler, & R. Miller (Eds.), *Progress in behavior modification* (pp. 1–55). New York: Academic Press.

Horton, A. M., Jr., & Puente, A. E. (1986). Behavioral neuropsychology with children. In G. Hynd & J. E. Obrzut (Eds.), *Child neuropsychology* (Vol. II, pp. 299–316). New York: Grune & Stratton.

Horton, A. M., Jr., & Sautter, W. (1986). Behavioral neuropsychology. In D. Wedding, A. M. Horton, Jr., & J. S. Webster (Eds.), *Handbook of clinical and behavioral neuropsychology* (pp. 259–277). New York: Springer.

Horton, A. M., Jr., & Wedding, D. (1984). *Clinical and behavioral neuropsychology.* New York: Praeger.

Horton, A. M., Jr., Wedding, D., & Phay, A. (1981). Contemporary perspectives on assessment and therapy for the brain-damaged individual. In C. J. Golden, S. S. Alcaperres, F. Strider, M. A. Strider, & B. Graber (Eds.), *Applied techniques in behavioral medicine* (pp. 59–86). New York: Grune & Stratton.

Hynd, G. W., & Obrzut, J. E. (Eds.). (1981). *Neuropsychological assessment and the school-aged child: Issues and procedures.* New York: Grune & Stratton.

Ince, L. P. (1976). *Behavior modification in rehabilitation.* Springfield, IL: Thomas.

Kazdin, A. E. (1978). The application of operant techniques in treatment, rehabilitation, and education. In S. L. Garfield & A. E. Bergin (Eds.), *Handbook of psychotherapy and behavior change* (2nd ed, pp. 549–589). New York: Wiley.

Kertesz, A. (Ed.). (1994). *Localization and neuroimaging in neuropsychology.* New York: Academy Press.

Klonoff, A., Crockett, D. F., & Clark, G. (1984). Head trauma in children. In R. Tarter & G. Goldstein (Eds.), *Advances in clinical neuropsychology* (pp. 139–157). New York: Plenum Press.

Lawson-Kerr, K., Smith, S. S., & Beck, D. (1990). The interface between neuropsychology and behavior therapy. In A. M. Horton, Jr. (Ed.), *Neuropsychology across the life-span.* (pp. 103–131). New York: Springer.

Lewinsohn, P. M., Danaher, B. G., & Kikel, S. (1977). Visual imagery as a mnemonic aid for brain-damaged persons. *Journal of Consulting and Clinical Psychology, 45,* 717–723.

Luria, A. R. (1966). *Higher cortical function in man* (B. Haigh, Trans.). New York: Basic Books.

MacLean, P. D. (1973). *On the evolution of three mentalities.* Toronto: University of Toronto Press.

Mahoney, M. J. (1974). *Cognition and behavior modification.* Cambridge, MA: Ballinger.

Marr, M. J. (1984). Conceptual approaches and issues. *Journal of the Experimental Analysis of Behavior, 42,* 353–362.

Mattis, S., French, J. H., & Rabins, T. (1975). Dyslexia in children and adults: Three independent neuropsychological syndromes. *Developmental Medicine and Child Neurology, 17,* 150–163.

Meichenbaum, D. M. (1978). *Cognitive behavior modification.* New York: Plenum Press.

Meier, M. J. (1974). Some challenges for clinical neuropsychology. In R. M. Reitan & L. A. Davison (Eds.), *Clinical neuropsychology: Current status and application* (pp. 289–324). New York: Wiley.

Miller, E. (1984). *Recovery and management of neuropsychological impairment.* New York: Wiley.

Muir, K., & Milan, M. (1982). Parent reinforcement for child achievement: The use of a lottery to maximize parent training effects. *Journal of Applied Behavioral Analysis, 15*(3), 455–460.

Nelson, R. D. (1983). Behavioral assessment: Past, present, and future. *Behavioral Assessment, 5,* 195–206.

Pirozzolo, F. J. (1981). Language and brain: Neuropsychological aspects of developmental reading disability. *School Psychology Review, 10*(3), 350–355.

Rapport, M. D., & Kelly, K. L. (1991). Psychostimulant effects on learning and cognitive function: Findings and implications for children with attention deficit hyperactivity disorder. *Clinical Psychology Review, 11,* 61–92.

Reitan, R. M., & Davison, L. A. (Eds.). (1974). *Clinical neuropsychology: Current status and applications.* New York: Wiley.

Restak, R. M. (1994). *Receptors.* New York: Bantam Books.

Reynolds, C. R. (1981). Neuropsychological assessment and the habilitation of learning: Considerations in the search for aptitude and treatment interaction. *School Psychology Review, 10,* 343–349.

Rourke, B. P., Fisk, J. L., & Strang, J. D. (1986). *Neuropsychological assessment of children: A treatment oriented approach.* New York: Guilford Press.

Salzinger, L., Feldman, R. D., & Portnoy, S. (1970). Training parents of brain-injured children in the use of operant conditioning procedures. *Behavior Therapy, 1,* 4–32.

Schneider, M., & Robin, H. (1976). The turtle technique: A method for self-control of impulsive behavior. In J. D. Krumbolts & C. E. Thorenson (Eds.), *Counseling methods* (pp. 157–183). New York: Rinehart & Winston.

Schoen, S. F. (1986). Decreasing noncompliance in a severely multihandicapped child. *Psychology in the Schools, 23*(1), 88–94.

Silver, B. V., Boake, C., & Cavazos, D. I. (1994). Improving functional skills using behavioral procedures in a child with anoxic brain injury. *Archives of Physical Medicine & Rehabilitation, 75*(7), 742–745.

Silver, B. V., & Stelly-Seitz, C. (1992). Behavioral treatment of adipsia in a child with hypothalamic injury. *Developmental Medicine & Child Neurology, 34*(6), 539–542.

Skinner, B. F. (1938). *The behavior of organisms.* New York: Appleton–Century–Crofts.

Slifer, K. J., Cataldo, M. D., Babbitt, R. L., Kane, A. C., Harrison, K. A., & Cataldo, M. F. (1993). Behavior analysis and intervention during hospitalization for brain trauma rehabilitation. *Archives of Physical Medicine & Rehabilitation, 74*(8), 810–817.

Struss, D. T., & Benson, D. F. (1984). Neuropsychological studies of the frontal lobes. *Psychological Bulletin, 95*(1), 33–38.

Watson, J. B. (1913). Psychology from the standpoint of a behaviorist. *Psychology Review, 20,* 158–177.

Wesolowski, M. D., & Zencius, A. H. (1994). *A practical guide to head injury rehabilitation.* New York: Plenum Press.

Zencius, A., Wesolowski, M. D., & Burke, W. H. (1989). Comparing motivational systems with two non-compliant head-injured adolescents. *Brain Injury, 3*(1), 67–71.

33

Neuropsychological Sequelae of Chronic Medical Disorders in Children and Youth

RICHARD A. BERG AND JOHN C. LINTON

Introduction

Neuropsychologists have been largely concerned with the evaluation of neurologic conditions that result in impairment in intellectual functioning. The majority of both clinical work and published research has been done with adults. By comparison, clinical child neuropsychology remains in its infancy. These statements were true when this chapter was first written in 1989, and remain largely true today, 5 years later.

Clinicians and researchers who work with children tend to focus their energies on the brain itself and tend to view most problems of concern as occurring within the brain or some other portion of the central nervous system (CNS). As our knowledge base grows, child neuropsychologists continue to become increasingly involved in the evaluation of children suffering from diseases that affect any part of the body. The majority of this work is clinically based whereas the research literature is still heavily based in brain-related injury research.

Although the brain and other parts of the body are separate in terms of anatomy, they function as an integrated whole. Thus, when other organ systems are affected by a disease process, the brain in general, and cognitive functioning in particular,

also may become impaired. This impairment may result from damage to brain tissue from the disease itself, or alternatively, brain dysfunction may occur as a secondary effect of a disease process elsewhere in the body. For example, the failure of other organ systems to provide nutrients to the brain may result in diminished cognitive functioning. The notion of multiple interactive systems is primary to the discussion of the diseases and conditions presented in this chapter. As nothing in the human body functions in total independence, there can be no single causal mechanism. Easily acknowledged on one level, this concept is both pervasive and essential to the understanding of brain-body relationships.

In the assessment of a child with medical problems, however, it is important that clinicians consider multiple causes for any noted neuropsychological disturbance. Additionally, psychiatric and social problems may impact on a child's behavior and overall functioning. The determination of the presence and severity of any brain effects thus requires knowledge of the possible contribution of a variety of factors including the disease itself, those organ systems directly and indirectly affected, the specific phase of the illness, any current medical treatment, premorbid personality, the coping capacity of the child, and the child's estimated functional level prior to the illness.

In many disease conditions, the cognitive sequelae have only been assumed to clinically report mental or behavioral changes of some children with the disease. There has been comparatively little research on the neuropsychological effects of individuals suffering from a great many nonneurologic diseases. Even when CNS effects are reported as

RICHARD A. BERG • Wilmington Health Associates, Wilmington, North Carolina 28401. JOHN C. LINTON • Department of Behavioral Medicine and Psychiatry, West Virginia University, Health Sciences Center, Charleston, West Virginia 25326.

possible or frequent, there is little understanding of the type of cognitive deficits likely to occur with differing disease processes, and even less is known about recovery patterns or residual effects.

In this chapter, we will discuss the functioning of the major organ systems in the body and the ways in which its malfunction may potentially impact on brain functioning. Additionally we will attempt to pull together the comparatively little research that has been done on disease processes specific to an organ system and the neuropsychological effects that have been reported. In a number of cases, specific neuropsychological data are not available: In those instances, clinical symptomatology that implicated possible neuropsychologic dysfunction will be offered.

The Brain and CNS

The basics of brain structure and function are reviewed in other sections of this book. We are concerned with the function of the brain as it relates to other body processes. The brain has large energy requirements. Although it comprises only about 2% of total body weight, it receives as much as 15% of cardiac output and accounts for 20% of the body's oxygen consumption (Freedman, Kaplan, & Sadock, 1976). As a result of this high demand for energy, brain cells tend to be extremely sensitive to alterations in their energy supply, which is mainly oxygen and glucose. Even minimal to mild energy deficits can impair the function and integrity of brain cells (Ariel & Strider, 1983). Consequently, circumstances that can significantly alter the nutrient supplies to the CNS clearly can alter brain function.

In the normally functioning brain, energy is obtained through a process of oxidation of glucose to carbon dioxide and water. Energy resulting from this process is then expended in the transportation of various compounds across cell membranes and for the synthesis of other cell constituents. Because oxygen and glucose are transported to brain cells by blood, an adequate cerebral blood flow is essential for brain metabolism. Additionally, adequate availability of nutrients is dependent on proper functioning of the digestive system.

When portions of the brain are damaged, other organs systems can be disrupted depending on which area(s) of the brain is involved. If, for example, damage occurs to areas of the cortex, generally an individual's cognitive and sensorimotor skills are affected. Damage to the subcortex may disrupt the automatic functioning of other systems, how-

ever, such as heart rate, blood pressure regulation, breathing, hormonal balance, water regulation, or immune response. Such disruption can lead to further damage to the brain.

If portions of the peripheral nervous system are damaged, only the area subserved by those nerves typically demonstrates impairment. However, if a major organ system is involved, it may begin to function improperly, creating other imbalances in other systems that may, in turn, impact on brain functioning. Thus, it appears that all parts of the body in some way contribute to maintaining brain functioning and vice versa, as a disturbance in one system is highly likely to lead to a disruption elsewhere.

Infections of the CNS

The effects of encephalitis on the developing brain have been of interest since the outbreak of epidemic encephalitis following World War I, which resulted in high mortality among children and a high frequency of subsequent psychiatric morbidity (Graham, 1983). Ebaugh (1923), Kennedy (1924), and Strecker (1929) all reported studies of children who had been followed for a number of years after the initial acute illness. The acute phase of encephalitis was characterized by sleepiness, fever, and other signs of localized CNS involvement, and was followed by a gradual onset of a number of significant personality changes. Ebaugh (1923) reported a wide range of behavioral and emotional sequelae that involved insomnia with nocturnal agitation, affective disorders of the depressive type, hysterical reaction, and unwarranted fearfulness as well as mental retardation.

Since the 1920s, reports of epidemic encephalitis and subsequent behavioral sequelae have been sporadic and Graham (1983) notes that encephalitis is now generally considered a rare cause of childhood cognitive disturbance. Levy (1959) described 100 children with hyperkinetic and antisocial behavior disorders to whom he ascribed the cause as encephalitis. However, since that study, doubt has been raised as to the actual etiology of the disorders manifested by these children. Sabatino and Cramblett (1968) reported that 14 children who had contracted documented cases of California encephalitis between the ages of 5 and 14 demonstrated auditory perceptual deficits as well as unspecified deficits in visual perception. A variety of emotional disorders were also reported including nervousness, hyperactivity, restlessness, and disruptive behavior together with learning problems.

Hern and his colleagues (1991) report a case of a 12-year-old male who had three large right frontal lobe abscesses at 18 months of age. Recurrent seizures followed surgery and were controlled with medication. Neuropsychologic examination revealed decreased verbal and performance IQ levels as well as poor math achievement, decreased constructional praxis, impaired prosody, and poor social skills. Facial recognition also was poor. Hern discusses this case in terms of a right hemisphere syndrome. Few such cases are reported in the literature and it is hard to know if an actual right hemisphere pattern exists or if this is an anomalous finding. As additional cases of focal right hemisphere damage are identified, patterns should emerge to help better delineate right hemisphere functioning in children.

Symptomatic congenital cytomegalovirus (CMV) is frequently associated with CNS involvement including sensorineural hearing loss, microcephaly, chorioretinitis, neuromuscular disorders, and seizures. Infants born with congenital CMV clearly have increased risk for mental impairment. The reported incidence has ranged from 36 to 90% (Weber, Dolske, Pass, & Boll, 1993). Some children are reported as symptomatic at birth with severe developmental difficulties whereas others have variably mild to moderate deficits. The intellectual status of 73 of 135 children with congenital CMV infection was assessed. A bimodal distribution was found in which 29 children were classified as mentally retarded with the remainder in the borderline or higher ranges (Weber et al., 1993). These data suggest that the infectious process, although not uniformly associated with impaired mental functioning, places the children at higher risk for such problems than the noninfected population.

Childhood meningitis is a relatively common infection, occurring in children under age 2, and acting on the immature brain, possibly disrupting cerebral development. A prospective study of 80 children with bacterial meningitis documented acute and long-term recovery patterns (Anderson et al., 1992). Children were evaluated at three times: at discharge, 12 months postdischarge, and 6 years postmeningitis. On the initial evaluation, motor and behavioral deficits were noted in 20% of the children. At 1 year, language and behavior problems were identified. A complicated recovery process and convulsions were related to lowered intellectual ability. At 6 years postinfection, children were found to be of average intelligence with specific deficits in expressive language, memory, and reading (Anderson et al., 1992).

Ellsworth, Bawden, and Bortolussi (1993) compared the cognitive, academic, and behavioral profiles of 34 children who had had *Haemophilus influenzae* type b meningitis with their nearest age siblings. Significantly poorer performance was noted on tests requiring processing of symbolic information, but the effects were of comparatively small magnitude. No differences on global measures of intelligence, academic achievement, or behavior were found. These authors suggested, therefore, that neuropsychological morbidity for most children with this type of meningitis is minimal, which contrasts with the work of Anderson et al. (1992). The reason for these differences is not clear but is typical of research of the neuropsychological effects of a disease process in children.

Human Immunodeficiency Virus (HIV)

A new and emerging area of study is that of HIV infection in children. It is not yet clear if, when, and how the CNS of infants and children becomes infected with HIV. CNS infection also may vary with subsets of patients and by itself does not necessarily mean that there will be clinical symptoms of the HIV infection (Tardieu, Blanche, Duliege, Rouzioux, & Griscelli, 1989).

In children with encephalopathy, neurologic changes associated with HIV infection include impaired cranial growth resulting in acquired microcephaly, cerebral atrophy, enlargement of the ventricles, and calcification in the basal ganglia (Brouwers, Moss, Wolters, & Schmitt, 1994). Clinically, extrapyramidal and cerebellar signs, delays or regression in motor or language development, and deterioration in cognitive abilities have been described, particularly in children younger than 5 (Belman et al., 1985; Epstein et al., 1985, 1986; Falloon, Eddy, Wiener, & Pizzo, 1989).

Two main domains of cognitive functioning appear to be most susceptible to the effects of CNS HIV infection in children: attention and expressive behavior. Attention difficulties have been widely recognized in adult and pediatric patients with HIV disease (Brouwers, Wolters, Moss, & Pizzo, 1993; Brouwers et al., 1994). In children, attention deficits may be documented as a relative weakness on the "freedom from distractibility" subscales of IQ tests and on behavioral assessments (Moss et al., 1996). In adults, attention deficits are one of the clear hallmarks of AIDS dementia complex (Price et al., 1988). When working with children, however, it is not clear whether attention problems are directly attributable to HIV as other etiologies are possible. Additionally, the base rate of attention disorders for this age group tends to be comparatively high in the general population. In one study, the WISC-R subtests of children with symptomatic HIV disease were analyzed and 21% of these children had performance patterns consistent with attention deficits. In another group of children with other chronic diseases (e.g., ALL), a similar group of comparable size (25%) was identified with a similar pattern (Brouwers et al., 1994). Thus, whether attention deficits can be directly associated with HIV infection or are associated with chronic illness in general remains to be further investigated.

Expressive behavior across several modalities appears to be differentially affected in a number of pediatric HIV patients (Brouwers et al., 1994). Speech and language abilities frequently become impaired in children with symptomatic HIV disease (McCardle, Nannis, Smith, & Fischer, 1991). Language may become slurred, speech may be labored, and children who were speaking in full sentences have been found to regress to using single words. Expressive language disruption appears to be more common than receptive language difficulties.

In children and infants with HIV infection (symptomatic), motor skills are frequently one of the first, and often the most severely, affected area of functioning (Hittleman et al., 1991). Infants tend to exhibit a delay in overall motor development and abnormalities in muscle tone. Preschool or older school-age children are more likely to develop impairments in lower extremity motor skills such as disturbances in gait and balance, and in some cases, they may lose the ability to walk.

HIV-infected children also may exhibit impaired social skills and affect (Moss et al., 1996; Ultmann et al., 1987). Some children become withdrawn and apathetic, and have difficulty expressing their feelings and emotions both verbally and nonverbally. In extreme cases, some children display autistic-like characteristics (Moss, Wolters, Eddy, Weiner, & Pizzo, 1989). HIV-positive children demonstrated subtle impairments in verbal concept formation, attention, mental flexibility, and/or working memory, in the absence of any global or obvious cognitive decline (Smith et al., 1993).

It is important to note that a number of HIV-positive children are unimpaired on neuropsychological measures as well as on neurologic examinations. However, subtle effects of HIV on the CNS have been observed in a number of older children who may have had opportunistic or chronic bacterial infections (Pizzo et al., 1988). Brouwers et al. (1990) noted that some children demonstrated significant improvement with AZT therapy. It is likely that the incidence of HIV infection in children will continue to rise and new treatments will likely lead to longer-term survival for these children. The neuropsychologic problems secondary to the disease and treatment will likely provide fertile ground for research for many years to come.

Brain Tumors

After malignancies of the blood-forming tissues such as leukemia, brain tumors are the most common type of malignancy in children (Graham, 1983). It has been calculated that there are approximately 600 new cases in the United States annually (Till, 1975). About 60% of childhood brain tumors occur in the subtemporal part of the brain, and of these, most are either medulloblastomas or cerebellar astrocytomas. The remainder consist of subtentorial tumors or tumors of the brain stem. About 3% of these tumors are metastatic, in marked contrast to that found in adults. Surprisingly, it has been unusual for children with brain tumors to present with symptoms of intellectual decline or behavioral change (Graham, 1983). Headache and vomiting are the most common symptoms present, and although there may be some accompanying irritability, this typically has not led to any diagnostic confusion.

Over the past several years, a good deal of longitudinal research has revealed that brain tumors in children do lead to cognitive changes. Cerebellar lesions have been associated with significantly impaired performance on the Wechsler subtests of mathematical reasoning and digit span whereas diencephalic and cerebellar lesions are associated with deficits in verbal learning and sentence span. Additionally, attentional problems have been found with cortical and cerebellar lesions (Fennell et al., 1993). Carpentieri and Mulhern (1993) studied children who had survived temporal lobe tumors and treatment for at least 1 year. They found evidence of auditory–verbal memory dysfunction in children with left and right temporal lobe tumor. In addition, poor reading and spelling performance was found to be correlated with impaired memory functioning.

Age at diagnosis and treatment has been an area of recent investigation. Very young children who were treated aggressively with surgical intervention and chemotherapy but did not receive radiation prior to age 3 years were studied. Thirty-nine percent of the children remained stable cognitively or exhibited increases in test scores, suggesting that avoiding radiation therapy before age 3 can be associated with acceptable survival and relatively good cognitive/adaptive functioning (Seidel *et al.*, 1994).

Gliomas in the pontine area in children generally present with what have been described as personality changes (Arseni & Goldenberg, 1959; Cairns, 1950; Lassman & Arjona, 1967). Characteristically, the symptom pattern seen includes a period of withdrawal, apathy, and lethargy followed by aggression, hyperactivity, temper tantrums, and physical violence. These tumors usually occur between the ages of 3 and 13. The course of the tumor may last for several years and the outcome is generally fatal despite a variety of treatments and radiation therapy. Other types of brain stem tumor are likely to present with gait disturbance and symptoms such as squint indicating cranial nerve involvement, but behavioral changes involving lethargy, irritability, inability to concentrate, enuresis, and sleep disturbance also have been known to occur (Panitch & Berg, 1970).

The prognosis for brain malignancies in children is at best poor, despite the use of the best available treatments such as surgery and irradiation. Although research has increased dramatically over the past 5–10 years on the effects of brain malignancies in children, the clearest information available is still that concerning the most common brain tumor in children, namely, medulloblastomas. The 5-year survival rate is roughly between 40 and 75%, and 50% after 10 years (Bloom, Wallace, & Henk, 1969; Hope-Stone, 1970). In one study, 18 of 22 survivors were reported to be without serious deficit (Bloom *et al.*, 1969). Two of the children followed were found to have partial disability, and two others demonstrated significant intellectual decline. It is important to note that the two children who demonstrated intellectual deterioration were those who were diagnosed at the youngest ages (11 and 15 months). These findings are similar to those noted above in the study of children with temporal lobe tumors (Seidel *et al.*, 1994) as well as to findings reported in studies of children with leukemia comparing early and later diagnosed children. Children diagnosed at an earlier age appeared to be at greater risk for the development of cognitive dysfunction

(Eiser, 1979; Meadows *et al.*, 1981). (Further discussion concerning leukemia and its effects can be found later in this chapter.) Matson and Crigler (1969) studied children with craniopharyngioma and found no particular psychological or behavioral problems even though the survivors were frequently partially sighted and required hormone replacement therapy. More recently, children who had received treatment for craniopharyngioma via microsurgery demonstrated normal intelligence; however, 45% of these individuals were found to have moderate to severe impairment in the delayed recall of verbal and nonverbal information (Kerr, Smith, DaSilva, Hoffman, & Humphries, 1991). Although the number of investigations of a child's neuropsychological status following a brain malignancy has increased significantly in recent years, additional efforts appear to be needed. The newer literature suggests that survivors show deficits of a less obvious nature that need to be better described.

Neuromuscular Diseases

There are numerous neuromuscular diseases that afflict children. It is beyond the scope of this chapter to detail the effects of each on the cognitive status of children. One disease entity, Duchenne muscular dystrophy (DMD), will be offered as a possible model for the effects that such diseases can have on the developing brain. It is important to note that the sequelae of such diseases tend to have variable identifiable effects depending on a wide variety of factors including age at diagnosis, age at testing, and so on.

DMD is a hereditary disease causing progressive muscular weakness and degeneration of skeletal muscle tissue. Its course generally includes confinement to a wheelchair by age 11 and death in the late teens. It affects males almost exclusively. Many studies on intellectual functioning in DMD patients have reported diminished or retarded intellectual development, supporting the position of Duchenne in 1872 (Dubowitz, 1979). The group IQ scores generally average about 85, one standard deviation below the mean of the general population (Dubowitz, 1977; Karagan, 1979). Although there is some support for the notion of intellectual impairment in DMD patients, there is no common consensus in the research literature. Some have reported a decline in intellectual performance (e.g., Black, 1973; Florek & Karolak, 1977) whereas others have found no significant differences in longitudinal studies (e.g., Cohen, Molnar, & Taft, 1968; Worden & Vignos, 1962).

A somewhat more recent study attempting to clarify the picture by studying 14 younger and 11 older children with DMD was reported by Sollee, Latham, Kindlon, and Bresnan (1985). It found that younger children with DMD performed more poorly on tasks requiring some language and attentional–organizational skills, but not on visual–motor tasks. The older group generally had higher IQ levels in the average range and the younger group had low-average IQ scores. The authors noted that individuals with DMD did not appear to demonstrate fixed, global cognitive deficits. Rather, deficits appeared to vary at different ages with no specific pattern evident to date.

Other CNS Disorders

Neurofibromatosis (NF) is an autosomal dominant genetic disorder affecting 1 in 3000 persons. It is characterized by numerous physical stigmata and by intellectual and cognitive impairment that may range from mild to severe. A study (Moore, Needle, Ater, Brewer, & Copeland, 1993) of 76 children with NF, brain tumor, or both was conducted to determine patterns of cognitive function characteristic of the conditions. In this study, no patient had been treated except by surgical resection of tumor. The groups were comparable in intellectual functioning, language, memory, fine motor, and attentional functioning; all test performance scores were in the average range except for memory, which was impaired across all individuals. Children with NF did, however, demonstrate significant impairment in academic achievement, visual–spatial abilities, and ability to maintain attention and concentration. In general, children with NF appear to be at significantly greater risk for learning deficits, visual–spatial processing deficits, and attention deficits than their counterparts with undifferentiated brain tumor.

The relationship of early childhood hydrocephalus and cognitive development is poorly understood. Most children who develop hydrocephalus early are not mentally deficient, although children with hydrocephalus typically demonstrate reductions in their overall level of cognitive development (Fletcher *et al.,* 1992). An investigation of ninety 5- to 7-year-old children with hydrocephalus caused by aqueductal stenosis or prematurity–intraventricular hemorrhage or associated with spina bifida was conducted. Comparison groups of normal controls, children with spina bifida and no corrective shunt, and premature children with no hydrocephalus were evaluated as well. As a group, children with hydrocephalus demonstrated poorer nonverbal than verbal skills. No memory deficits were noted. Fletcher *et al.* (1992) note that this is likely a function of effects on white matter development. Additionally, MRI studies of these children found considerable pathology in the commissural tracts. Additional research should help to address these issues.

Leukodystrophy

There are a number of different types of leukodystrophy. Degeneration of the white matter of the brain (leukodystrophy) leads to a dementialike state in children. Shapiro (1991) attempted to identify a neuropsychological performance pattern in children with white matter disease. Decreases in visual perception, visual–spatial functioning, visual–motor skills, motor skills, and attention were noted. A study of 39 children with leukodystrophy revealed a developmental course of slowing of development in one or more areas of cognitive functioning, gradual spreading of deterioration to other cognitive domains with plateauing of development, followed by a loss of achieved developmental milestones (Shapiro, Lockman, & Krivat, 1993). Treatment (via bone marrow transplantation) was found to be more successful when done before plateauing of development occurs.

Blood and Circulatory System

The primary function of the blood system is that of a carrier and delivery service transporting oxygen from the lungs to tissues and returning carbon dioxide, conveying metabolites to tissues, and returning waste products for disposal. It has other important functions such as maintaining the water content of the tissues, harboring the body's defense cells, carrying hormones that regulate a variety of bodily functions, and helping to maintain and regulate body temperature. A disruption in either the blood or circulatory system can directly impact brain functioning.

Anemia

Anemia, or an abnormal decrease in red blood cells, can produce variable CNS effects. Erythrocytes (red blood cells) contain hemoglobin, which carries oxygen, and any unusual decrease in the number of these cells can lead to an overall lowering of brain functioning as a result of cerebral hypoxia (deficiency in oxygen supply). Convulsions, diffuse organic brain syndrome, focal vascular lesions, cerebral hemorrhage, and blindness have been reported in severe cases (Aita, 1964).

Research conducted with children having sickle-cell disease found that the overall intellectual capabilities of these children were lower than those of an age- and sex-matched group of black children (Berg & Wilimas, 1983). In this pilot project, the WISC-R and the children's revision of the Luria–Nebraska Neuropsychological Battery were administered to a group of 30 black children with the disease who had not undergone hypertransfusion of packed red cells and to a similar group of black children without the disease who had been selected on the basis of age and sex. In all cases, children with the disease performed significantly more poorly on all IQ measures. No significant differences were reported on the Luria–Nebraska tests although the results appeared to follow the same direction as those found on the WISC-R.

A study assessing 58 children with sickle-cell disease with no documented history of cerebrovascular accident (CVA) found that subtle neuropsychological deficits were present in those children of lower socioeconomic backgrounds (Goonan et al., 1992). In children who had sustained a CVA, those who had had a left hemisphere stroke demonstrated a significant global decline on intelligence testing as well as on specific tests of language, visual–spatial construction ability, memory, and academic achievement (Cohen et al., 1993). Those who had sustained a right-sided CVA demonstrated marked declines in performance IQ scores, visual–spatial construction, visual memory, and arithmetic achievement suggesting a somewhat more focal pattern of impairment (Cohen et al., 1993). In contrast, a recent investigation by Goonan, Goonan, Brown, Buchanan, and Eckman (1994) reported no generalized deficits in the absence of specific laboratory findings (hemoglobin levels, days of hospitalization, and emergency room visits). These findings suggest a lack of disease-related neurocognitive impairment for children with sickle-cell syndrome.

Polycythemia Vera

Just as an abnormal decrease in red blood cells can lead to abnormal cognitive functioning, the converse also is true. Abnormal increases in red blood cell production in the bone marrow (polycythemia vera) can cause erythrocytes to clump together, creating a situation that slows blood flow and impedes circulation. Although there is an adequate oxygen supply in this condition, there is difficulty breathing and the individual may become cyanotic. Brain functioning may become lowered as a result of insufficient circulation or blockage of a cerebral vessel. Aita (1964) discussed a number of commonly reported neurologic symptoms in diseases that result in excess erythrocytes. These include headaches, dizziness, vision and hearing difficulties, and parasthesias. Children who tend to hemorrhage easily may show more focal deficits such as aphasia and hemiparesis, or they may exhibit a progressive dementia-like condition as more and more cerebral tissue is destroyed by repeated hemorrhaging (Aita, 1964; Ariel & Strider, 1983).

Excessive Increases or Decreases in Platelets

A severe reduction in the number of platelets or defects in coagulation factors in the blood may result in spontaneous bleeding. This can be a primary disease (e.g., thrombocytopenia purpura) or it can develop secondarily to another disease process such as leukemia (discussed below), toxic chemical exposure, irradiation, infection, or massive blood transfusion. If such bleeding occurs within the brain, it may be at single or multiple sites, small or large in size, and may resemble a focal stroke (Aita, 1964). The cognitive sequelae of such an incident can be tremendously varied depending on the location and size of the hemorrhage and can range from comparatively minor to pervasive with the patient existing in a vegetative state (Walton, 1977). In the more minor circumstances of such bleeding, temporary general confusion, paresis, and convulsions can be seen (Heron, Hutchinson, Boyd, & Aber, 1974).

Matoth, Zaizov, and Frankel (1971) reported that 20 children with chronic thrombocytopenia had been found to have learning and behavioral problems when compared with patients with other medical disorders. This study, which used the WISC, Bender Visual-Motor Gestalt, and Human Figure Drawing tests, revealed no statistical differences between the two groups on any test. However, it was noted that over two-thirds of the group of children with thrombocytopenia exhibited "soft" neurological signs of minimal brain dysfunction. Over half of this group also demonstrated mild, diffuse EEG abnormalities. To date, there has been no long-term follow-up of such groups to determine if noted behavioral or cognitive abnormalities persist into adulthood.

An excessive increase in the number of platelets can result in the formation of a thrombus and subsequent blockage of a blood vessel. Tissues supplied by the blocked vessel will then receive an insufficient supply of blood, and an ischemic condition wherein the tissue starves may result. If the tissue dies or is damaged, an infarction is the result. Thrombus formation anywhere in the body can be serious because of the high tendency for the thrombus to pass through the heart and be carried to the lungs or brain. When cerebral vessels become blocked and an infarction occurs, deficits in cognitive functioning can occur (Walton, 1977). If the blocked vessel supplied a small portion of the brain, the cognitive sequelae will generally resemble those seen with a fairly discrete cerebral lesion. Where the blocked vessel supplied a larger region of the brain, pervasive deficits can result.

Leukemia

Leukemia is a disease in which there is uncontrolled multiplication of certain white blood cells resulting in their accumulation in large numbers (LODAT, 1981). An abnormal growth and division of lymphoblasts (one type of white blood cell) in the bone marrow results in acute lymphocytic leukemia (ALL). ALL is the most prevalent form of malignancy in children and the one that has been the most heavily researched with respect to the effects of the disease and its treatment. This is because the therapy for the disease has become so effective that long-term disease-free survival can be expected in at least 50% of patients (Bowman, 1981; Mauer, 1980). Survival of these children has permitted an increasing emphasis on the late sequelae of ALL and its treatment. Treatments for other childhood malignancies have not been quite so effective. Thus, research into the cognitive sequelae has been restricted. The research investigating the long-term effects of ALL and its treatment, however, may be used as a temporary model for the effects of other malignant disease processes.

A complicating factor in the study of neuropsychological functioning of children with ALL lies in the standard treatment regimen for the disease. Common treatment involves the intrathecal and intravenous administration of a neurotoxic medication, methotrexate. Coupled with this is the administration of at least 1800–2400 rad of cranial irradiation, which is done prophylactically in an attempt to destroy those leukemic cells that may have migrated to the brain. Some reports over the past several years suggest that cranial irradiation may not be necessary in the treatment of what is referred to as "standard risk" leukemia and that such prophylactic measures need only be employed with "high risk" patients whose disease is diagnosed at a more advanced stage and is more likely to have invaded the CNS (Copeland, Pfefferbaum, Fletcher, Jaffee, & Culbert, 1982). It is clear that it is very difficult, if not impossible, to assess the effects of the disease alone in such instances.

Despite all of the research that has been conducted since about 1975, our understanding of the effects of the disease process and its treatment is inconsistent. Eiser and Lansdown (1977) and Goff, Anderson, and Cooper (1980) found that leukemic children who had received irradiation demonstrated significant deficits. This was particularly true for those individuals diagnosed and treated prior to age 5. Deficits included declines in intellectual abilities as well as a pattern of distractibility and memory deficits. In contrast, other investigators found that the disease and its treatment resulted in no documented dysfunction (Ivnik, Colligan, Obetz, & Smithson, 1981; Obetz et al., 1979). A longitudinal study in which a group of leukemic children were followed for a period of at least 3 years found no specific pattern of deficits or IQ declines (Berg et al., 1983). However, almost half of the children did have performance patterns consistent with mild, specific learning dysfunction when performance patterns were analyzed individually rather than as a group.

More recently, Stehbens et al. (1991) in a review of 20 years of published research report that the majority of studies suggest that CNS prophylaxis, including both cranial irradiation and intrathecal methotrexate, results in a variety of learning problems in many children who were younger than 5 when first treated. A study of the neurocognitive status of 46 children with ALL treated with systemic chemotherapy and prophylactic CNS chemotherapy found that those children receiving a 3-year course of chemotherapy were more impaired on tasks involving right-hemisphere simultaneous processing than controls or ALL children whose diagnosis was recent and treatment was just begun (Brown et al., 1992).

These recent results point to the need for the continued follow-up of children with leukemia who are treated with newer protocols. Even if cranial irradiation is not part of the treatment regimen, it would appear that late deficits do emerge. Follow-up will allow for identification and remediation of cognitive late effects and possible academic difficulties.

Endocrine System

The endocrine or ductless gland system is primarily involved in the production of hormones for correlating and regulating bodily processes. Such glands include: the pituitary, which lies in a depression of the sphenoid bone between the roof of the mouth and the hypothalamus; the pineal, which is just posterior to the pituitary; the adrenals, which are attached to the top of each kidney; the thyroid, located in front of the trachea just below the voice box; the parathyroids, which are embedded in the thyroid; the thymus, found near the lower part of the trachea; the pancreas, found in the curvature between the stomach and small intestine; the ovaries, located near the uterus; and the testes, suspended in the scrotum.

Study of this system reveals complex interrelationships among the various endocrine glands. Hormones are exceedingly powerful agents, and in some instances their activities encompass practically the entire body. In most cases, they interact normally. Production of hormones is usually regulated by the bodily requirements for each, and when this need is met, production is decreased or antihormones are released. Uncontrolled excesses or insufficiencies of glandular secretion are responsible for a variety of disorders of development and metabolism, most of which have implications for the integrity of the brain. One such disorder, diabetes mellitus, has received a great deal of recent attention by neuropsychologists.

Diabetes Mellitus

Diabetes mellitus is a disease complex resulting from abnormalities in carbohydrate metabolism, caused by insufficient production of insulin in the pancreas. Because of this lack of insulin, diabetics have chronically high blood glucose levels (hyperglycemia), and excrete a great deal of unmetabolized sugar as well as many salts and minerals essential to health. Diabetes mellitus is a heterogeneous group of disorders rather than a single disease, and its exact cause is unknown (Miller & Sperling, 1986).

However, two general classifications of diabetes are common. Both forms have the potential to injure large and small blood vessels, leading to deterioration of peripheral and autonomic nerves, the cardiovascular system, the eyes, and the kidneys (Cirillo et al., 1984; Pfeifer et al., 1984). As such, diabetics are at increased risk for heart disease, stroke, kidney dysfunction, blindness, and peripheral neuropathy.

Adult-onset, also known as type II or non-insulin-dependent, diabetes mellitus (NIDDM) is the most common, accounting for over 90% of all diabetics, and affecting about 5 million adults in the United States. Occurring typically in overweight individuals past the age of 40, the onset is subtle, and diagnosis is often made secondary to problems with the vascular system. NIDDM is characterized by diminished but not absent secretion of insulin by the pancreas. Treatment is usually by diet change and the use of medication for the stimulation of insulin production; exogenous insulin is not necessary.

Juvenile-onset, also known as type I or insulin-dependent, diabetes mellitus (IDDM) is a common chronic disease estimated to affect 150,000 children and adolescents (Cerreto & Travis, 1984) and 400,000 adults (Carter Center, 1985) in the United States. Males and females are equally affected, and peak presentation is seen at the time of puberty, although IDDM is diagnosed from early childhood through early adulthood (Miller & Sperling, 1986). In IDDM the pancreas stops producing insulin entirely. Presentation of symptoms is usually clear and dramatic, with polyuria, polydipsia, polyphagia, and rapid weight loss over a period of about 1 month. If untreated, severe hyperglycemia can lead to ketoacidosis, diabetic coma, and death. This previously fatal disorder was converted to a manageable chronic disease after 1922 with the availability of exogenous insulin (Johnson & Rosenbloom, 1982). For the youngster with IDDM, management of near-normal metabolism involves constant monitoring of bodily systems and daily insulin injections. Insulin needs vary with nutrition, exercise, physical health, and emotional state. As mentioned, insufficient insulin can lead to dangerous hyperglycemia. Conversely, too much insulin or too little food, or an imbalance of food, exercise, and insulin can result in a marked decrease in blood sugar (hypoglycemia). Hypoglycemia can progress from an insulin reaction, with mental confusion and anxiety, to hypoglycemic seizures, to insulin coma (Miller & Sperling, 1986). This metabolic seesaw may have important implications not only for the psychological adjustment, but also for the brain of the diabetic youngster.

Investigation of neuropsychological functioning in IDDM is currently being carried out by several research teams in the United States and Canada. Excellent reviews of this area include those by Ryan and Morrow (1987a) and Ryan (1995). Discussing the history of research in this area, they point out that early on, diabetes *per se* was thought to be benign with respect to impact on brain functioning, the only connection thought to be secondary to involvement of renal or cardiovascular disease in older patients who had the disease for many years. A series of studies from the 1930s through the 1960s challenged this notion by comparing the intelligence of diabetic children with general norms, yielding results that were equivocal. Although the findings were inconclusive, two important methodological innovations were introduced in these series. These were the use of nondiabetic sibling controls to control for effect of family influences and socioeconomic status, and the attempt to experimentally relate specific diabetic characteristics such as age of onset and duration of illness to outcome (Ack, Miller, & Weil, 1961). One important global finding from such work was that age of onset seemed to be an important variable, with those diagnosed as diabetic before the age of 5 having average IQs ten points lower than their siblings. A trend was also seen suggesting an inverse relationship between number of hypoglycemic seizures experienced and measured intelligence. Thus, although no clear evidence of specific neurobehavioral dysfunction in diabetic children emerged, researchers were made aware that there may be some neurobehavioral differences between diabetic and normal children, and that the age of onset and the number of hypoglycemic seizures noted in the history may related to the extent of this difference (Ryan & Morrow, 1987a).

Because global measures of intelligence were used in that series of studies, differences between diabetics and controls could not be assigned to specific structural or operational changes in the brain. However, a series of EEG studies did find a significantly higher number of clinically abnormal EEGs in a group of diabetic children compared with age-matched normal controls, further finding that the variable most related to this EEG difference was the number of severe hypoglycemic episodes (Eeg-Olofsson & Peterson, 1966), or the number of severe episodes of both hypoglycemia and hyperglycemia (Haumont, Dorchy, & Pelc, 1979).

Ryan and Morrow (1987b) posited that this IQ and EEG evidence seemed to demonstrate that diabetic children and adolescents showed a greater tendency than their nondiabetic age mates to have mild, diffuse brain dysfunction, and that multiple episodes of severe hypoglycemia were in some fashion responsible for the development of this "diabetic encephalopathy." They noted with some surprise that although these findings firmly established a basis for further investigation of this diabetes-related organic syndrome, such research essentially dried up for no apparent reason during the 1970s, in favor of studies of the psychosocial aspects of diabetes (see Cerreto & Travis, 1984).

Given these early findings, and the fact that a medical colleague found a high incidence of school difficulty in diabetic patients, Ryan and his associates at the Children's Hospital in Pittsburgh began a series of neurobehavioral studies to reassess the degree to which diabetic youngsters are at risk to develop cognitive deficits secondary to CNS defects. The goal of their series of studies was to describe particular neuropsychological difficulties found in this population, and to relate these problems if possible to specific variables associated with each case. Based on previous findings and some preliminary work, they focused on the examination of age at onset, duration of disease, and degree of metabolic control as they related to cognitive functioning, which was measured by neuropsychological testing.

To test the notion that both age at which diabetes mellitus is diagnosed and duration of the disease are potent variables, Ryan, Vega, and Drash (1985) administered a comprehensive neuropsychological battery to 125 randomly selected diabetic adolescents, all of whom had been diabetic for at least 3 years, but ranged in age of onset from 2 months to 14 years. They divided the subjects into an "early onset" group (diagnosed before age 5, $n = 46$), a "later onset" group (diagnosed after age 5, $n = 79$), and a sibling control group ($n = 83$).

A factor analysis of the cognitive measures used in their testing battery generated five clusters of tests, namely, general intelligence, visuospatial processes, learning and memory, attention and school achievement, and mental and motor speed. Statistical analyses found significant differences between early and late-onset subjects on all five clusters. Further, cutting scores of two standard deviations below the control mean were assigned to each of the 20 tests that discriminated early from late-onset subjects, with at least three such low scores necessary to be seen as "impaired." On the basis of these rules, 24% of the early onset were seen as impaired, whereas only 6% of both the late onset and controls met impairment criteria.

Further analysis of these data suggested that age at onset and disease duration differentially affected the testing results. Age at onset appeared to predict results of tests measuring "fluid intelligence," described by the authors as adaptive abilities used to process relatively unfamiliar information in novel ways, such as scanning and identification of visual stimuli. Duration of illness seemed more able to predict performance on tests tapping "crystallized intelligence," defined as the use of well-practiced skills depending largely on stored knowledge, such as reading and spelling skills, and sequencing ability. Regarding the differential effects of duration and age at onset, there is some evidence indicating that the relationship between duration and crystallized intelligence can be accounted for by the fact that school attendance is a factor in both. Ryan, Longstreet, and Morrow (1985) found that diabetics missed significantly more school than matched controls over time, and further that cognitive and achievement test findings in this group were best predicted by measures of school attendance. Therefore, perhaps like most chronically ill youngsters, diabetics miss a significant amount of school (Gortmaker & Sappenfield, 1984), and this attendance problem may reduce their ability to master classroom-related learning, or crystallized intelligence. Thus, longer duration of diabetes would lead to greater attendance problems, and more difficulty in school. However, Fowler, Johnson, and Atkinson (1985) found diabetic children miss less school than children from most other chronic disease categories, so this issue remains unclear.

Ryan, Vega, and Drash (1985) and Ryan and Morrow (1987a), on the other hand, suggested the findings regarding age of onset and performance on tasks assessing fluid intelligence may reflect structural or functional disturbances in the brain. This mild brain damage may develop from multiple episodes of severe hypoglycemia and resultant hypoglycemic seizures early in life. There is some evidence (Ternand, Go, Gerich, & Haymond, 1982) that younger diabetics are more sensitive to the effects of insulin, and therefore have more reactive hypoglycemic seizures. This is consistent with the finding of Ryan, Vega, and Drash (1985) that early onset diabetics had more of a history of hypoglycemic seizures.

In general, the work of Ryan and colleagues suggests that cognitive deficits in diabetics can be seen as early as age 10. Rovet and her colleagues in Toronto have undertaken the study of even younger diabetic patients, in an effort to further examine neurobehavioral findings in this group. Rovet, Ehrlich, and Hoppe (1988) administered an extensive series of neuropsychological tests to a diabetic sample including children as young as 6. They divided the sample into 27 early onset (pre-age 4), 24 later onset (post-age 4), and 30 sibling controls.

In contrast to Ryan's studies, they found no differences among the three groups on intelligence or achievement, actually finding that diabetics outperformed controls on tasks measuring verbal ability. However, they found some interesting results related to gender. Early onset girls performed less well on spatial tasks and had a lower performance IQ than later-onset or control girls, but this finding did not hold for boys. These early onset girls also had more academic problems, including failed grade and special education placement, than the other groups.

A multiple regression analysis for each sex separately found that for both genders taken together, the best predictor of verbal performance was socioeconomic status; for girls only, the best predictor of spatial performance was age at onset; and again for both genders, the best predictor of spatial performance was seizures before the age of 5.

Other interesting results regarding gender and age at onset include those of Ryan and Morrow (1987b), who found that early onset diabetic adolescent girls had significantly poorer self-esteem, as measured by the Piers–Harris subscales of Physical Appearance and Anxiety, than did early onset boys, later-onset boys and girls, and controls. However, the extent to which this represents a result of greater cognitive deficit, bodily changes differentially experienced by girls over time, or a unique coping reaction in the face of chronic illness is undetermined. Ryan and Morrow (1987b) summarized this literature by stating that both their and Rovet's teams have found age of onset of diabetes to be an important risk factor for the development of significant neurological deficits in both children and adolescents. They speculated that this strong association between diabetes early in life and brain dysfunction may be accounted for by two different phenomena, namely, that the brain of a young child is very sensitive to the deleterious effects of any sort of metabolic insult, and that this sensitivity may be greater in females; or that the young child has a heightened responsivity to insulin, and thus has more hypoglycemic seizures, with resultant increase in damage to the brain.

These findings seem to be consistent with increasing evidence that the time from birth to 5 years may constitute a "critical period" for the development of serious brain dysfunction from a variety of causes with a number of outcomes. Rovet, Ehrlich, and Czuchta (1990) proposed possible critical periods of sensitivity of different functional or structural substrates in the brain to the effects of diabetes, with spatial abilities vulnerable to diabetes presenting earlier, and verbal abilities more vulnerable to diabetes presenting later. The proposed mechanism suggested is that cerebral structures seem to myelinate at different times and rates, and that chronic hyperglycemia could disrupt this myelinization.

However, in an important development, Rovet and her colleagues have found that the effects of early onset diabetes on the brain may not be as clear as previously assumed. As noted, most studies in this area are retrospective, to determine if diabetic children or specific subgroups of such children are at risk for later neurocognitive impairment. Since methodological problems exist with this approach, Rovet *et al.* (1990) began a prospective study, following a cohort of 63 newly diagnosed diabetic children through their first 3 years of illness. In this first report, they found that relative to nondiabetic siblings, there was no evidence of any neurocognitive impairment in diabetic subjects either at the outset of the disease, or on retesting 1 year after the onset of the disease. In their second report (Rovet, Ehrlich, Czuchta, & Akler, 1993) they found that after 3 years this lack of impairment among diabetic children was still seen; in fact, it was the normal siblings who were having school problems, perhaps because of the stress of being a sibling of a chronically ill child who received a great deal of family attention. In addition, there was no measured negative impact of mild or severe hypoglycemia. Their findings were clearly inconsistent with previous results, and they offered several explanations for this. Perhaps the instruments chosen were not sufficiently sensitive to measure deficits, any learning deficits are cumulative and need to be followed for greater than 3 years to be seen, or new treatment methods used with diabetic youngsters in recent years have had a positive effect on their neuropsychological outcome. They also suggest that perhaps diabetic children who are learning disabled have different CNS insulin requirements than those who are not due to dietary and activity variants, and this may lead to too much insulin and more episodes of hypoglycemia, thereby questioning the direction of causation.

Northam, Bowden, Anderson, and Court (1992) also report results inconsistent with those found earlier. Using retrospective accounts of disease history, they found no relationship between neuropsychological functioning and variables such as age of onset, chronic poor control, or major metabolic crises in 100 diabetic adolescents. They criticized the sampling of earlier studies that either used volunteers or had a small percentage of potential participants agree to be studied. They suggested families who volunteered to participate in such studies might already have concerns about the patient's cognitive status, thereby skewing findings in the direction of cognitive dysfunction in diabetic subjects. Their study used a larger sample size and had a high rate of participation, and they recommended a prospective study like that in progress by Rovet's team. Finally, Jyothi, Susheela, Kodali, Balakrishnan, and Seshaiah (1993) found no relationship between age at onset and duration and neuropsychological performance in a group of diabetic children in rural India.

It is worthy of note that even though early onset has been viewed as an important variable, diabetes appears to affect performance even in those who are diagnosed later in life (Franceschi *et al.*, 1984). Ryan, Vega, Longstreet, and Drash (1984) tested 40 diabetic adolescents (aged 12–19) who were classified as late onset (diagnosed at 5–12) and a group of 40 matched nondiabetic controls using a neuropsychological battery and critical flicker fusion. They found that all subjects performed within normal limits, but that the diabetic sample had verbal IQs lower than controls (which may be related to the duration effects and school attendance noted above), but also did less well on psychomotor tasks, performing more slowly than controls.

However, similar findings regarding psychomotor performance were presented by Ryan and Williams (1993) who tested subjects with childhood-onset IDDM an average of 26 years after diagnosis. They found that diabetic subjects performed as well as nondiabetic controls on measures of learning and memory, but performed poorly on measures of psychomotor efficiency, with degree of chronic hyperglycemia best predicting psychomotor slowing. They suggested that specific neural systems in the brain may be differentially sensitive to the toxic effects of hyperglycemia at different stages of life. It has also been hypothesized that diabetics may develop a characteristic personality style that may account for some of this psychomotor task performance difference, which will be addressed briefly later.

Another variable to receive research attention is that of degree of metabolic control. As mentioned earlier, poor metabolic control implies a tendency for hyperglycemia that is implicated in the risk for disorders of the vasculature, both large and small vessels, and hypoglycemia, which has been shown to have clearly deleterious effects on the brain. Work by Holmes and her team at Iowa suggests that a recent history of poor metabolic control may increase the risk of mild neuropsychological disturbances in young adults. Holmes (1986) compared two matched groups of diabetic men in their early 20s, one classified as in "good" and the other in "poor" control as measured by tested hemoglobin AIC levels. This test measures the relative degree of metabolic control, or avoidance of blood glucose extremes, over the preceding 3 months. Holmes found that the poor-control group had lower scores on the Information and Vocabulary subtests of the WAIS, and also performed worse on reaction time tasks. Ryan and Morrow (1987a) suggested caution in interpreting this finding, as metabolic control was only measured for the 3 months before testing. They speculated that perhaps if these subjects were out of control as children, they may have attended poorly, and now retrieve poorly as adults.

In a typical day the blood glucose level of a diabetic child may vary widely, being dependent on food, insulin dose, and exercise (Miller & Sperling, 1986). Cerebral metabolism depends on the ability of serum glucose to circulate freely in the brain. Because little glucose is stored in the brain, when its supply has been compromised there is a lag time before fatty acids are utilized as a backup source (Holmes, Koepke, Thompson, Gyves, & Weydert, 1984). Temporary change in cerebral functioning might therefore be possible at the time of testing, perhaps affecting psychomotor tasks if not global intelligence. In a series of studies (Holmes, Hayford, Gonzalez, & Weydert, 1983; Holmes et al., 1984; Holmes, Koepke, & Thompson, 1986) Holmes and her colleagues inspected the acute neuropsychological consequences of deviant blood glucose levels. By use of an automatic insulin/glucose infusion system, they were able to stabilize young individuals with diabetes for extended periods at one of three blood glucose levels: hypoglycemia (55–60 mg/dl), euglycemia (110 mg/dl), or hyperglycemia (300 mg/dl). All subjects were tested in all three conditions, using a balanced design in which neither experimenter nor subject knew in which level the subject was. They found that relative to euglycemia, subjects tended to perform more slowly in the hypoglycemic state on a variety of tasks involving simple mental calculation and word production, as well as responding in choice reaction time situations. A tendency was noted for subjects to perform in a similar fashion in the hyperglycemic state.

Ryan and Morrow (1987a) summarized such research by stating that the hypoglycemic state reduces efficiency and increases response time on brief tasks. They further speculated about the possibly more dramatic effects that this state might produce on more lengthy tasks under conditions of greater fatigue, a situation that may have occurred during previously described measurements of cognitive functioning in diabetics by use of neuropsychological testing. Ryan et al. (1990) also found that transient episodes of experimentally induced hypoglycemia were associated with reduced mental efficiency in both diabetic children and adolescents, and further noted that total recovery of cognitive function is not always achieved with the restoration of euglycemia, although there is a good deal of individual variation from subject to subject. Therefore, the school-age child with diabetes may not function optimally not only immediately after a hypoglycemic episode, but for some time after it is corrected.

Reich et al. (1990) and Puczynski, Puczynski, Reich, Kaspar, and Emanuele (1990) found similar results with naturally occurring episodes of hypoglycemia, and stressed that the delay in recovery puts especially the young child at an unrecognized disadvantage in school and social situations, because even after overt physical symptoms have subsided, the child suffers from cognitive deficits for a longer period and may return to the classroom prematurely. Gold, Deary, and Frier (1993) point out that small children have difficulty recognizing and relating the symptoms of hypoglycemia, and Bischoff, Warzak, Maguire, and Corley (1992) suggest interventions to assist such children in the classroom.

Finally, there has been some question as to the relative contribution of nonorganic variables to performance on measures of neurobehavioral functioning. A number of studies have commented on behavior and personality styles among diabetics. Some have stressed problems in the family (Lancet Editorial, 1980; Winter, 1982) and school (Weitzman, 1984), whereas others have focused on IDDM as a risk factor in certain clinical syndromes such as eating disorders appearing in adolescent females (Daneman, Johnson, & Garfinkel, 1985). Other authors have tried to conceptualize the effects of diabetes as the child and adolescent attempts to cope with normal developmental tasks at different cognitive stages (Cerreto & Travis, 1984; Johnson & Rosenbloom, 1982). Some of the self-esteem problems found in early onset diabetic females may be of interest here, although Northam *et al.* (1992) found no gender differences in the measured emotional adjustment of diabetic adolescents. Research in this area of diabetic personality functioning has been fraught with methodological problems, and at least one study (Skenazy & Bigler, 1985) found that diabetics are no more poorly adjusted than other chronic disease groups, and further that degree of psychological adjustment was not predictive of performance on a battery of neuropsychological tests. Ryan and Morrow (1987b) commented that they have observed a "cautiousness" in their young diabetic patients, perhaps reflecting the youngsters' daily need for constant attention to detail. However, they admit that this is more a matter of clinical observation than evidence.

In summary, in recent years a good deal of progress has occurred in understanding the neuropsychological correlates of insulin-dependent juvenile-onset diabetes in children and adults. Specific neurobehavioral impairments have been identified, as have several diabetes-related variables that appear to be important risk factors for the development of such impairments. Ryan and Morrow (1987a) reiterated that age at onset of IDDM is a most potent variable, with those diagnosed before the age of 5 to be much more likely to show evidence of cognitive impairment than those with onset later than age 5. They suggested that diabetic encephalopathy yields deficits in a wide selection of cognitive domains, with performance disrupted on measures of attention, learning, memory, problem-solving, visuospatial, and visuomotor efficiency.

Some early onset diabetics have lower IQs than their siblings or nondiabetic peers, but not all early onset diabetics have diminished intellectual functioning, and in fact most do not. Evidence from both electrophysiological and neuropsychological measures suggests that those who have had multiple episodes of serious hypoglycemia early in life are likely to be impaired on a wide range of tasks. These findings imply clearly that because young children are quite insulin sensitive, keeping an excessively tight metabolic control (rigidly preventing hyperglycemia) may increase the risk of starting serious and perhaps debilitating hypoglycemic episodes in these patients.

Yet with all of this evidence, several recent studies and prospective work by Rovet suggest that for a variety of reasons, this impairment related to early onset diabetes may not be a given. Such prospective studies may hold the key to the next level of knowledge in this area. Most diabetic children and adults are late onset, and show relatively subtle impairments. When detected, they tend to appear on difficult information-processing tasks requiring the subject to complete novel assignments as rapidly as possible. The slowness noted may be involuntary (reflective of a transient hypoglycemic state) or voluntary (resulting from learned caution in the face of decision-making situations). It is also possible that information-processing mechanisms in this population may be disrupted by complex biochemical disturbance, resulting from a long history of poor metabolic control. And finally, performance may be impaired as a result of increased absences from school, with related academic problems. All of these hypotheses continue to be grist for the research mill, for at this time there is no strong evidence that extensive structural damage to the brain is directly causative of the subtle deficits sometimes found in patients with late-onset IDDM.

Cardiovascular System

The primary functions of the cardiovascular system are to pump blood through the body, to pick up and deliver fluids, gases, chemicals, and nutritive substances, and to increase or decrease blood flow in response to activity levels of the body. The cardiovascular system is composed of the heart, large arteries and veins, smaller arterioles and venules, and the capillaries. The manner of blood flow and its regulation are crucial factors to be considered in discussing cardiovascular functioning and the effects of dysfunction.

Blood traveling through vessels exerts different pressures and moves at different speeds according to the size of the vessel. The cardiovascular system acts to maintain a relatively constant and limited range of pressures and blood flow velocities within the vessels. Any increase in friction, such as occurs with blockages, narrowing, or roughness along the vessel walls, increases the work load of the system and can lead to failure.

CNS Effects

Disease or malfunction anywhere in the cardiovascular system tends to initiate a vicious cycle of adjustments that cause the heart to work harder to compensate for these changes, resulting in further damage. A compromised heart eventually leads to a compromised brain. Although the brain will still receive a greater share of the materials needed by the body, prolonged cardiac function will ultimately lower the amount available to brain cells. Insufficient oxygen and nutrients are likely to produce results of diffuse neuropsychological dysfunction in children with cardiovascular disease or irregularities (Cravioto & Arrieta, 1983). The child is likely to have deficits in a wide variety of functions, although these may be mild unless damage to the heart (or reduction of blood flow) has been severe. Many of the cognitive deficits in individuals with cardiac problems may not even be noticed because of the concern over other more attention-demanding physical symptoms. Mild deficits that are noticeable are often temporary and tend to be viewed with less concern (Ariel & Strider, 1983).

When circulation to the heart itself is blocked and tissue is damaged ("heart attack"), there is often an extreme drop in blood pressure. This may produce symptoms of dizziness or massive changes in mental functioning such as delirium or dementia. The lack of oxygen to brain tissue may produce focal deficits such as aphasia, sensorimotor disturbances, or visual difficulties (Rowland, 1984). Such effects can be either temporary or permanent. A cerebral hemorrhage may occur because of the increased pressure and destruction of blood vessels, producing either diffuse or focal effects that tend to be more permanent (Rowland, 1984). As these deficits are generally more disruptive to a child's ability to function, they are more likely to lead to a concern to the child, parent(s), and/or physician, and are often the symptoms that lead to requests for evaluation. If such diseases progress slowly, then compensation usually occurs and the child may appear to have normal cognitive functioning. This is particularly true for children as the developing brain tends to be somewhat more amenable to recovery of function than is the more mature adult brain. It must be cautioned, however, that there is a growing body of literature suggesting that the developing brain may not be as "plastic" as once was thought (Golden, 1981).

Another outcome of cardiac disease may be the development of bacterial endocarditis, an infection of the cardiac tissue wherein bacteria collect in damaged valves or in the pericardial sacs. In addition to creating inflammation and edema, bacteria may spread to other parts of the body by means of blood circulation. If the brain is entered, the result is usually a septic embolism (a blockage creating infection in that area), widespread meningitis, or development of a focal brain abscess (Rowland, 1984). Neuropsychological effects can be quite variable, ranging from focal deficits that resemble an adult stroke to a diffuse encephalopathy (widespread inflammation). The variations possible make it a quite difficult condition to accurately diagnose. In such instances, it has been suggested that the evaluation be conducted on a follow-up basis to determine if additional damage has occurred or to assess the extent and severity of residual impairment (Ariel & Strider, 1983; Golden, 1981).

The development of hemorrhages in the brain from hypertensive destruction of vessels also produces variable effects. Although hypertension in children is comparatively rare, it occurs with enough frequency to merit some discussion. Hemorrhages typically result in focal deficits, but these can be singular or multiple. Mild or severe disruption of cognitive functional systems can result depending on where bleeding occurs (Walton, 1977). Acute hypertensive encephalopathy may produce massive edema and pressure effects leading to severe diffuse deficits, convulsions, decerebrate rigidity, coma, or death from cerebral hemorrhage.

Hypotension, or low blood pressure, generally has only mild or unnoticeable effects on brain functioning (Ariel & Strider, 1983); however, it can produce diffuse impairment of moderate to severe degrees as well. Children may complain of amnesia, excessive fatigue, fainting, convulsions, or loss of specific cognitive abilities, all of which indicate that ischemia to brain tissue has likely occurred (Gold, 1984). As such sequelae are variable and often fluctuating, the diagnosis of brain dysfunction or permanent injury is a difficult one to make. Cardiovascular difficulties can also modify blood constituents, producing brain ischemia because of the alteration in blood flow or inability of erythrocytes to carry oxygen. Many such problems may first be labeled as "psychiatric" or emotional disorders because the child exhibits depressive symptoms or confusion as the first signs (Taylor, 1979).

Surgery for cardiovascular problems also carries a certain risk. Circulation of blood to the brain may become impaired while the patient is connected to a heart–lung machine. Thrombosis, embolism, anoxia, or toxic/allergic reactions to anesthesia or injected medications may occur. Infections can develop that spread to the brain, or the heart may simply fail to regain normal rhythm after surgery. All of these may lead to cognitive deficits of varying degree and location (Ariel & Strider, 1983).

Brobeck (1979) reported that EEG tracings revealed more abnormalities after than before cardiac surgery. He further noted that if the patient's EEG does not return to normal within 3 to 4 weeks after surgery, the likelihood of cerebral damage having occurred is quite high. Studies using neuropsychological tests have found that signs of cerebral dysfunction prior to surgery place the child at even higher risk for the development of later cerebrovascular problems as well as at a higher risk for death during surgery (Kilpatrick, Miller, Allan, & Lee, 1975).

In the research literature on adults, there have been a number of investigations conducted on patients who have undergone surgery for occlusions or narrowing of the internal carotid arteries. Such patients are often so diagnosed because they experience transient ischemic attacks with such symptoms as dizziness, memory loss or deterioration, mild speech problems, visual changes, or mild sensorimotor deficits. If untreated, a cerebral stroke is likely (Thompson, Patman, & Talkington, 1978).

Little such work has been conducted with children, and therefore, inference must be drawn from the adult research literature. Those studies that have been done with adults to determine if surgical intervention improves or changes cognitive status have reported mixed findings. Several studies have reported significant improvement (e.g., Bornstein, Benoit, & Trites, 1981; Goldstein, Kleinknecht, & Gallo, 1970; Owens *et al.*, 1975) whereas a similar number of investigations have found either no improvement or deterioration in functions (e.g., Drake, Baker, Blumenkrantz, & Dahlgren, 1968; Murphy & Maccubbin, 1966). One study concluded that any reported performance increase was likely to be a function of test–retest practice effects and not true improvement in functioning (Matarazzo, Matarazzo, Gallo, & Weins, 1979).

Children with similar cardiovascular dysfunction, therefore, may suffer from much the same forms of dysfunction; however, there remains the caveat that one is dealing with a developing brain. As the brain appears to develop functional capacity during development, early damage may impede this development. Damage incurred at later ages may result in a loss of established functional capabilities. However, it is generally felt that the prognosis for recovery of cognitive functioning or reacquisition of lost functions depends primarily on an interactive effect of a number of variables including type, location, and extent of damage, to name a few (Rourke, Bakker, Fisk, & Strang, 1983).

Finally, in cases of cardiovascular system abnormality or malfunction that has led to cognitive impairment, personality changes such as depression, irritability, anxiety, and so on may occur with some frequency (Lishman, 1978). These changes often are noticed before actual intellectual deficits appear and may be attributed to the child's inability to adjust to the illness. In some cases, the changes may be the sequelae of damage to the brain and this possibility needs to be fully explored.

Lymphatic and Connective Tissue Systems

The lymphatic system, often referred to as the immune system, is similar to the blood and cardiovascular system in its structure, but differs greatly in function. Its primary purposes are to defend the body against invasion by injurious agents, to gather and destroy worn-out cells, and to produce antibodies. It also stores extra red blood cells and produces hormones that help to regulate the development of new red blood cells. The lymphatic system is composed of the spleen, lymph vessels and nodes, and defensive cells (Rowland, 1984).

Spleen

The spleen is the main storage center for new red blood cells and the destruction center for old ones. It also makes some types of white cells (the lymphocytes). In emergency situations, large numbers of red cells are dumped into the bloodstream to ensure adequate oxygen supply.

Lymph Vessels

The lymphatic system has its own vessel system that drains fluid from the tissue space. These vessels form into larger ducts that eventually merge into the blood. Along the vessels are lymph nodes that act to help prevent large particles or foreign bodies from entering the bloodstream. Lymph cells in the nodes are generally effective in eliminating most foreign bodies with the exception of viruses. Lymph ducts and nodes are found almost everywhere in the body except in the CNS. The lymph capillary system is laid out in such a manner so that virtually all materials that enter the body through the skin or the mucosa must first pass through the lymphatic system. As the lymph system is in essence a dumping/disposal system, any disruption of it can impact on water and electrolyte balance within the body, which in turn can increase pressure on the capillary system, shut down blood flow, and eventually result in death.

Disorders of the Connective Tissue System

Connective tissue refers to fibrous tissue that provides support for holding cells together and forms a protective covering around the body and internal organs. Connective tissue cells are found everywhere in the body, but large amounts of them are found in bones and joint tissues. The connective tissue system is composed of ligaments, tendons, cartilage, skin, blood vessels, internal membrane linings, and sheath coverings of organs and muscles. It also constitutes a large portion of organs such as the eyes, lungs, heart, kidneys, and liver (American Rheumatism Association Committee, 1973).

Disorders of the connective tissue can be inherited or acquired. The genetic maladies are comparatively rare and are beyond the scope of this chapter. Acquired conditions generally include rheumatoid arthritis, systemic lupus erythematosus, progressive systemic sclerosis, polymyositis, dermatomyositis, Sjogren's syndrome, amyloidosis, various forms of vasculitis, and rheumatic fever. Although different in terms of severity and the age group affected, these diseases all display features associated with inflammation and destruction or alteration of connective tissue. Common symptoms include fatigue, fever, muscular weakness, joint swelling and pain, skin lesions, gastrointestinal erosions with hemorrhages, peripheral vascular dysfunctions, neuropathies, and blood cell disorders such as anemia and thrombocytopenia. The course of the illness may vary greatly from individual to individual, with periods of both remission and exacerbation, a chronic mild illness, severe and rapidly progressing deterioration, or fluctuations between mild and severe episodes. Some children with these diseases may become severely disabled from crippling joint deformities or loss of function in a major organ system, such as the kidneys. Initial symptoms can mimic many other diseases because they are so variable and thus difficult to diagnose in many instances (Gilroy & Meyer, 1975).

CNS Effects

Comprehensive research on the neuropsychological effects of diseases of lymph and connective tissue systems in children remains minimal, at best. The medical literature indicates that the effects on the brain and CNS tend to be variable and generally predictable (Gilroy & Meyer, 1975; Rutter, 1983; Walton, 1977). The small vessel inflammation and destruction that can occur in many of these diseases can produce focal ischemic lesions in many organs, causing them to malfunction and reduce their support to the brain. Vessels in the brain may also be affected, although pathological studies have been inconsistent in confirming this with most disease types with the exception of giant cell arteritis, a condition rarely found in children (American Rheumatism Association Committee, 1973). Hypertension is a frequent outcome of these diseases, the effects of which were described above. Compression or ischemia may result in peripheral neuropathy, with sensory or motor losses in digits or limbs (Graham, 1983). Diffuse or focal cerebral infections may occur as a result of the suppression of immune systems from drugs taken during treatment.

Although evidence of the disease process in the brain itself has not yet been confirmed, studies have indicated the presence of immune complexes associated with connective tissue and lymphatic system disease processes in the choroid plexus of the brain (Atkins, Kondon, Quismoro, & Friou, 1972; Bresnihan et al., 1979; Winfield, Lobo, & Singer, 1978). Psychoses, depression, and mental confusions have frequently been reported as sequelae of these conditions. Reactions to corticosteroids, antihypertensives, antidiuretics, anti-inflammatory agents, and other medication used for treatment have been found to produce changes in emotional or mental state, although it is difficult to separate this from the effects of the disease itself.

CNS effects have been most often reported with systemic lupus erythematosus (Ariel & Strider, 1983). The reported sequelae include emotional disorders, convulsions, choreiform movements, and cerebrovascular accidents with focal neurologic deficits. These usually occur in children with highly active and severe disease. In the early stages of lupus, the CNS effects may be mild and transient, or may so resemble a psychiatric disorder that the patient is treated as such (Bennett, Bong, & Spargo, 1978; Hughes, 1979).

CNS Effects of Liver Dysfunction

A relatively recent area of study is that of the effects of liver disease or dysfunction. Children who have received liver transplants appear to be at significant risk for the development of neuropsychologic deficits (Stewart *et al.,* 1990). Significantly lower performance IQ scores, academic achievement, and age-adjusted z-scores in learning, abstraction, visual–spatial functioning, and motor functions were found. Alertness, sensory–perceptual, and perceptual–motor skills appear not to be affected. The children in this study demonstrated greater cognitive dysfunction than adults with end-stage liver disease.

Respiratory System

The respiratory system is composed of the upper airway, including the nose, pharynx, larynx, and epiglottis; the lower airway, including the trachea, the primary or main bronchi, the segmental bronchi, and bronchioles; and the lungs, located within the thoracic cavity on either side of the heart. The exchange of gases provided by this system is vital to the brain. The cardiovascular system's function is to supply oxygen to body tissues via circulating blood. The blood also removes carbon dioxide produced by metabolism, and transports this waste product to the lungs. Here the carbon dioxide is replaced by oxygen, and the newly oxygenated blood is recirculated to the tissues, including the brain.

A network of airways provides the pathway for the transport and exchange of oxygen and carbon dioxide. Under normal circumstances, by inhalation the upper airway provides air for the lower airway, where it is conducted through smaller and smaller pathway branches in each lung field. The final branches of bronchioles (terminal respiratory bronchioles) end in clusters of alveoli, or air-filled sacs. Thus, the working area of the lung is a network of air tubes and blood vessels, through which blood ultimately reaches the alveoli, which are the primary structures for the exchange of carbon dioxide and oxygen (Luckman & Sorenson, 1980). Given that the need for oxygen by the brain is so great, a significant disruption in the functioning of the respiratory system may have negative cerebral consequences.

Bronchial Asthma

Asthma is the most common chronic disease of childhood, estimated to occur in 5% of adults and children in the United States, over 10 million people, of whom over 2 million are under the age of 16. The onset of asthma is usually within the first 5 years, although it can occur at any age. A more favorable prognosis appears to be related to an early onset, unless significant asthma attacks begin before the age of 2 (King, 1980). Asthma accounts for nearly one-fourth of all days absent from school by children, and it ranks third among all chronic illnesses as a cause of physician visits (Sadler, 1982). It also contributes greatly to acute visits to emergency rooms, days in the hospital, and problems related to psychosocial adjustment (Rubin *et al.,* 1986).

Although the symptoms of asthma have been recognized for centuries, there is currently no commonly agreed on definition of the syndrome, nor any consensus with regard to whether asthma is primarily a medical or psychological disorder (Creer, 1982). A great deal has been written about the onset of asthma from several psychological perspectives, notably psychoanalytic and behavioral (Sadler, 1982), and a variety of psychological interventions have been presented to deal with this condition (King, 1980). Basically, asthma is a bronchial disorder characterized by airway obstruction that is intermittent, variable, and reversible. The lung pathology may occur in the central or larger airways, and the peripheral or smaller airways. Obstruction of these bronchial airways may be related to smooth muscle constriction, swelling of tissue, swelling of the mucosa, and dried mucus plugs (Chai, 1975; King, 1980). The one common denominator is a peculiar hyperreactivity of the airways, whether to physical, chemical, pharmacologic, or immunologic stimuli (Sadler, 1982).

The clinical symptoms present as spasms of difficult breathing, coughing, and wheezing, with the attacks lasting from several minutes to several hours, although in a condition known as "status asthmaticus" obstruction may last for days or weeks. Attacks can vary along a continuum of severity from very mild to very severe, the latter increasing the risk of brain damage or even death (Bierman, Pierson, Shapiro, & Simons, 1975). Although the notion that cerebral anoxia secondary to bronchial asthma attacks may lead to neurobehavioral deficits seems to be defensible and stimulating, very little solid research has been conducted in this area.

Dunleavy and Baade (1980) stated that there have been a number of studies reporting on the adaptive behaviors of asthmatic children, particularly as applied to the classroom situation. Most are speculative, whereby observed maladaptive behaviors and learning problems are assumed to be related to organic damage, which is further assumed to be a result of transient hypoxia accompanying their severe asthmatic attacks.

In an effort to make use of assessment instruments better designed to detect brain–behavior relationships, Dunleavy and Baade (1980) evaluated a sample of asthmatic children using the Halstead Neuropsychological Test Battery for Children. Their goal was to identify patterns of neurobehavioral deficit characteristic of severely asthmatic children 9 to 14 years of age. Nineteen severely asthmatic subjects and 19 matched nonasthmatic controls who had no history of organic damage were administered the Halstead Battery. Significantly poorer test performance was noted for the asthmatic group, with eight Halstead Battery tests showing most difference between the groups. Three of these tests, Trail Making, Tactual Performance, and WISC Mazes, were more sensitive than the others in discriminating asthmatic from nonasthmatic subjects. The authors concluded that the primary deficits of impaired asthmatic children are in visualizing and remembering spatial configurations, in incidental memory, and in planning and executing visual and tactile motor tasks.

Using both a classification battery, developed from four of the eight Halstead Battery tests that showed greatest discrimination between groups, and blind clinical analysis, Dunleavy and Baade (1980) identified 7 of the 19 asthmatics (37%) as impaired, whereas only 1 of the controls was so labeled. They further compared the test score means of the seven neuropsychologically impaired asthmatic children with the Halstead Battery test score means of the 9- to 14-year-old brain-damaged (cerebral tumor, traumatic injury, inflammatory disease) group studied by Boll (1974). The asthmatic sample performed better than did the Boll sample, in line with the clinical assessment of very mild to mild brain damage for the asthmatic children in their study. The authors also mentioned that five of their asthmatic subjects reported they had experienced periods of unconsciousness and had "turned blue" during their attacks. Of these five, four were classified by their Halstead scores as impaired. This finding was thought to add credence to the notion that loss of consciousness and cyanosis, which occurs during some severe asthmatic attacks, can contribute to later occurrence of organic dysfunction.

Suess and Chai (1981) suggested that the conclusions of Dunleavy and Baade were premature, because the possibility of similar performance deficits as a function of antiasthma medications was not taken into account. In essence, the treatment and not the disease may account for the obtained neurobehavioral deficits. Dunleavy (1981) responded that in their sample they found no relationship between drug use, as obtained from detailed medical history, and neuropsychological test performance. Further, he reported that of the 7 children classified as impaired, only 3 were receiving antiasthma medication, and of the 12 asthmatic children who showed no evidence of performance deficit, 7 were receiving such medication.

However, Chai (personal communication, March 21, 1986) and his research team at the National Jewish Hospital in Denver completed a 3-year study of the effects of antiasthma drugs such as steroids on information retention in asthmatic children. Their preliminary analyses suggested the use of such medications has no noticeable effect on retention in reading and writing, but quite significant effects on the automatic memory required for retention of math skills. Other investigators (Bender, Lerner, & Poland, 1991; Bender & Milgrom, 1992; Schlieper, Alcock, Beaudry, Feldman, & Leikin, 1991) suggest antiasthma medications tend only to exacerbate already existing tendencies toward behavioral or attentional difficulties in asthmatic children.

In summary, limited research has demonstrated that some severely asthmatic children exhibit very mild to mild brain-damage-like behaviors, that certain such behaviors are more likely to be seen than others, and that these deficits can be predicted to a degree by previous episodes of loss of consciousness and cyanosis. Other research has suggested that such findings are consistent not only with the assumption of underlying change in cerebral structure or function, but also as an iatrogenic effect of antiasthma drugs over time.

Cystic Fibrosis

Cystic fibrosis (CF) is the most commonly seen lethal genetic syndrome of infants, children, and young adults. It is most prevalent in Caucasian youngsters, with one case of CF in every 1500–2000 live births; it is much less common in black and Asian populations. Inheritance appears to be by an autosomal recessive gene, suggesting a specific biochemical defect, but no single, unifying hypothesis exists at this time to account for the pathogenesis of CF (Matthews & Drotar, 1984).

CF is a very complex condition affecting a wide variety of bodily functions. It causes abnormalities in the exocrine gland network, pancreas, liver, gastrointestinal tract, reproductive system, and especially in the respiratory system. Chronic obstructive pulmonary problems seem to account for the majority of morbidity and mortality in the CF patient. In the past, children with CF simply died young. But the introduction of the sweat test in 1954 permitted early diagnosis, and coupled with newer treatment regimens, children with this disease are now surviving fairly well into late adolescence, young adulthood, and in some cases into early midlife (Taussig & Landau, 1986). A tremendous adjustment to the disease is required because it requires lifetime care, a great deal of medicine, a strict diet, a mechanical apparatus to assist breathing, daily postural drainage and breathing exercises, and living in constant danger of respiratory infections.

Individuals with CF are prone to such infections, and their breathing is often altered as a result of increased airway resistance. Some of the issues discussed above with asthmatics regarding decreased cerebral oxygenation and its effect on cortical integrity may be germane here, although symptoms seem to be less severe. CF is not seen as a disease that directly affects the brain. In fact, Breslau (1985) and Breslau and Marshall (1985), in studies of psychiatric disorders in children with physical disabilities, used CF subjects as non-brain-involved chronic disease controls. They found that healthy and CF subjects, previously diagnosed as troubled, improved in their mentation and psychological adjustment over a 5-year period, whereas brain-damaged subjects showed no such improvement. Stewart *et al.* (1991) used CF patients as controls for growth retardation and chronic disease to assess the neuropsychological outcomes of pediatric liver transplantation, finding the CF patients similar to normals. However, Matthews and Drotar (1984) suggested that CF children express some of their difficulty in adjusting to this multisystem disease by the development of learning problems in school. As is seen with other chronic diseases, these learning problems may in fact be symptomatic of psychological difficulties, absenteeism, and decreased sensory stimulation; however, they may also be related to mild neurobehavioral deficits. Currently, no research specifically addresses this issue in children with CF.

References

Ack, M., Miller, I., & Weil, W. B. (1961). Intelligence of children with diabetes mellitus. *Pediatrics, 28,* 764–770.

Aita, J. A. (1964). *Neurologic manifestations of general diseases.* Springfield, IL: Thomas.

American Rheumatism Association Committee. (1973). *Primer on the rheumatic diseases* (7th ed.). Atlanta: Arthritis Foundation.

Anderson, V. A., Grimwood, K., Keir, E., Nolan, T., Hore, R., & Catroppa, C. (1992). Long-term sequelae of bacterial meningitis in childhood. Abstracts of the 14th European conference of the INS, Durham, United Kingdom. *Journal of Clinical and Experimental Neuropsychology, 14,* 387.

Ariel, R., & Strider, M. A. (1983). Neuropsychological effects of general medical disorders. In C. J. Golden & P. J. Vicente (Eds.), *Foundations of clinical neuropsychology* (pp. 273–308). New York: Plenum Press.

Arseni, C., & Goldenberg, M. (1959). Psychic disturbances in infiltration of the brainstem. *Acta Neurochirurgica, 7,* 292–300.

Atkins, C. J., Kondon, J. J., Quismoro, F. P., & Friou, G. J. (1972). The choroid plexus in systemic lupus erythematosus. *Annals of Internal Medicine, 76,* 65–72.

Belman, A. L., Ultmann, M. H., Horoupian, D., Novick, B., Spiro, A. J., Rubinstein, A., Kurtzberg, D., & Cone-Wesson, B. (1985). Neurological complications in infants and children with acquired immunodeficiency syndrome. *Annals of Neurology, 18,* 560–566.

Bender, B., Lerner, J. A., & Poland, J. E. (1991). Association between corticosteroids and psychologic change in hospitalized asthmatic children. *Annals of Allergy, 66,* 414–419.

Bender, B., & Milgrom, H. (1992). Theophylline-induced behavior change in children. *Journal of the American Medical Association, 269,* 2621–2624.

Bennett, R. M., Bong, D. M., & Spargo, B. H. (1978). Neuropsychiatric problems in mixed connective tissue disease. *American Journal of Medicine, 65,* 955–962.

Berg, R. A., Ch'ien, L. T., Bowman, W. P., Ochs, J., Lancaster, W., Goff, J. R., & Anderson, H. R. (1983). The neuropsychological effects of acute lymphocytic leukemia and its treatment—A three year report: Intellectual functioning and academic achievement. *International Journal of Clinical Neuropsychology, 5,* 9–13.

Berg, R. A., & Wilimas, J. J. (1983, May). *Sickle cell disease and neuropsychological function.* Paper presented at the Mid-South Conference on Human Neuropsychology, Memphis, TN.

Bierman, C., Pierson, W., Shapiro, G., & Simons, E. (1975). Brain damage from asthma in children. *Journal of Allergy and Clinical Immunology, 55,* 126.

Bischoff, L. G., Warzak, W. J., Maguire, K. B., & Corley, K. P. (1992, September). Acute and chronic effects of hypoglycemia on cognitive and psychomotor performance. *Nebraska Medical Journal,* pp. 253–263.

Black, F. W. (1973). Intellectual ability as related to age and stage of disease in muscular dystrophy: A brief note. *Journal of Psychology, 84,* 333–334.

Bloom, H. J. G., Wallace, E. N. K., & Henk, J. M. (1969). The treatment of prognosis of medulloblastoma in childhood. *American Journal of Roentgenology, 105,* 43–62.

Boll, T. J. (1974). Behavioral correlates of cerebral damage in children aged 9 through 14. In R. M. Reitan & L. A. Davison (Eds.), *Clinical neuropsychology: Current status and applications* (pp. 91–120). Washington, DC: Winston.

Bornstein, R. A., Benoit, B. G., & Trites, R. L. (1981). Neuropsychological changes following carotid endarterectomy. *Canadian Journal of Neurological Science, 8,* 127–132.

Bowman, W. P. (1981). Childhood acute lymphocytic leukemia: Progress and problems in treatment. *CMA Journal, 124,* 129–142.

Breslau, N. (1985). Psychiatric disorder in children with physical disabilities. *Journal of the American Academy of Child Psychiatry, 24,* 87–94.

Breslau, N., & Marshall, I. A. (1985). Psychological disturbance in children with physical disabilities: Continuity and change in a 5-year follow-up. *Journal of Abnormal Child Psychology, 13,* 199–216.

Bresnihan, B., Hohmeister, R., Cutting, J., Travers, R. L., Waldburger, M., Blacj, C., Jones, T., & Hughes, G. R. (1979). The neuropsychiatric disorder in systemic lupus erythematosus: Evidence for both vascular and immune mechanisms. *Annals of Rheumatic Diseases, 38,* 301–306.

Brobeck, J. R. (Ed.). (1979). *Best and Taylor's physiological basis of medical practice* (10th ed.). Baltimore: Williams & Wilkins.

Brouwers, P., Moss, H., Wolters, P., Eddy, J., Balis, F., Poplack, D., & Pizzo, P. (1990). Effect of continuous-infusion zidovudine therapy on neuropsychologic functioning in children with symptomatic human immunodeficiency virus infection. *Journal of Pediatrics, 117,* 980–985.

Brouwers, P., Moss, H., Wolters, P., & Schmitt, F. A. (1994). Developmental deficits and behavioral change in pediatric AIDS. In I. Grant & A. Martin (Eds.), *Neuropsychology of HIV infection* (pp. 310–338). London: Oxford University Press.

Brouwers, P., Wolters, P., Moss, H., & Pizzo, P. (1993). Encephalopathy in vertically acquired pediatric HIV disease. Abstracts of the 21st annual INS meeting, Galveston, Texas. *Journal of Clinical and Experimental Neuropsychology, 15,* 95.

Brown, R. T., Madan-Swain, A., Pais, R., Lambert, R. G., Baldwin, K., Casey, R., Frank, N., Sexson, S. B., Ragab, A., & Kamphaus, R. W. (1992). Cognitive status of children treated with central nervous system prophylactic chemotherapy for acute lymphocytic leukemia. *Archives of Clinical Neuropsychology, 7,* 481–497.

Cairns, H. (1950). Mental disorders with tumors of the pons. *Folia Psychiatrica Neurologica, Neurochirurgica Neerlandica* (English abstract), *53,* 193–203.

Carpentieri, S. C., & Mulhern, R. K. (1993). Patterns of memory dysfunction among children surviving temporal lobe tumors. *Archives of Clinical Neuropsychology, 8,* 345–357.

Carter Center. (1985). Closing the gap: The problem of diabetes mellitus in the United States. *Diabetes Care, 8,* 391–406.

Cerreto, M. C., & Travis, L. B. (1984). Implications of psychological and family factors in the treatment of diabetes. *Pediatric Clinics of North America, 31,* 689–710.

Chai, H. (1975). Management of severe chronic perennial asthma in children. *Advances in Asthma and Allergy, 2,* 1–12.

Cirillo, D., Gonfiantini, E., DeGrandis, D., Bongiovanni, L., Robert, J., & Pinelli, L. (1984). Visual evoked potentials in diabetic children and adolescents. *Diabetes Care, 7,* 273–275.

Cohen, H. J., Molnar, G. E., & Taft, L. T. (1968). The genetic relationship of progressive muscular dystrophy (Duchenne type) and mental retardation. *Developmental Medicine and Child Neurology, 10,* 754–765.

Cohen, M. J., Branch, W. B., McKie, V. C., Adams, R. C., Swift, A. V., & Riccio, C. A. (1993). Neuropsychological impairment in children with sickle cell anemia and cerebrovascular accidents. Abstracts of the 15th annual INS European meeting, Funchal, Madeira. *Journal of Clinical and Experimental Neuropsychology, 15,* 384.

Copeland, D. R., Pfefferbaum, B., Fletcher, J., Jaffee, N., & Culbert, S. (1982, April). *Neuropsychological assessment of long-term survivors of leukemia.* Paper presented at the American Society of Clinical Oncology, St. Louis, MO.

Cravioto, J., & Arrieta, R. (1983). Malnutrition in childhood. In M. Rutter (Ed.), *Developmental neuropsychiatry* (pp. 32–51). New York: Guilford Press.

Creer, L. T. (1982). Asthma. *Journal of Consulting and Clinical Psychology, 50,* 912–921.

Daneman, G. M., Johnson, L. E., & Garfinkel, P. E. (1985, May). *Is diabetes a precipitant of eating pathology?* Paper presented at the meeting of the American Pediatric Society, Washington, DC.

Drake, W., Baker, M., Blumenkrantz, J., & Dahlgren, H. (1968). The quality and duration of survival in bilateral carotid occlusive disease: A preliminary survey of the effects of thromboendarterectomy. In J. Toole, R. Siekert, & J. Whisnant (Eds.), *Cerebral vascular disease* (pp. 142–162). New York: Grune & Stratton.

Dubowitz, V. (1977). Mental retardation in Duchenne muscular dystrophy. In L. P. Rowland (Ed.), *Pathogenesis of human muscular dystrophies* (pp. 64–82). Amsterdam: Excerpta Medica.

Dubowitz, V. (1979). *Involvement of the nervous system in muscular dystrophies in man.* New York: New York Academy of Sciences.

Dunleavy, R. A. (1981). Neuropsychological correlates of asthma: Effect of hypoxia or drugs. *Journal of Consulting and Clinical Psychology, 49,* 137.

Dunleavy, R. A., & Baade, L. E. (1980). Neuropsychological correlates of severe asthma in children 9–14. *Journal of Consulting and Clinical Psychology, 48,* 214–219.

Ebaugh, F. (1923). Neuropsychiatric sequelae of acute epidemic encephalitis in children. *American Journal of Diseases of Children, 35,* 89–97.

Eeg-Olofsson, O., & Peterson, I. (1966). Childhood diabetic neuropathy: A clinical and neuropsychological study. *Acta Paediatrica Scandinavica, 55,* 163–176.

Eiser, C. (1979). Intellectual development following treatment for childhood leukaemia. In J. M. A. Whitehouse & H. E. M. Kay (Eds.), *CNS complications of malignant disease* (pp. 243–271). New York: Macmillan Co.

Eiser, C., & Lansdown, R. (1977). Retrospective study of intellectual development in children with acute lymphoblastic leukemia. *Archives of Disease in Childhood, 52,* 525–529.

Ellsworth, C. P., Bawden, H. N., & Bortolussi, R. A. (1993). Cognitive and behavioral sequelae of haemophilus influenzae meningitis in children. Abstracts of the Division of Clinical Neuropsychology, American Psychological Association Annual Meeting, Toronto. *The Clinical Neuropsychologist, 7,* 327.

Epstein, L. G., Sharer, L. R., Joshi, V. V., Fojas, M. M., Koenigsberger, M. R., & Oleske, J. M. (1985). Progressive encephalopathy in children with acquired immunodeficiency syndrome. *Annals of Neurology, 17,* 488–496.

Epstein, L. G., Sharer, L. R., Oleske, J. M., Connor, E. M., Goudsmit, J., Bagdon, L., Robert-Guroff, M., & Koenigsberger, M. R. (1986). Neurologic manifestations of human immunodeficiency virus infection in children. *Pediatrics, 78,* 678–687.

Falloon, J., Eddy, J., Wiener, L., & Pizzo, P. A. (1989). Human immunodeficiency virus infection in children. *Journal of Pediatrics, 114,* 1–30.

Fennell, E. B., Mann, L. W., Maria, B., Fiano, K., Booth, M., Mickle, J. P., & Quisling, R. (1993). Neuropsychology of posterior fossa versus other focal brain tumors in children. Abstracts of the 21st annual INS meeting, Galveston, Texas. *Journal of Clinical and Experimental Neuropsychology, 15,* 58.

Fletcher, J. M., Francis, D. J., Thompson, N. M., Brookshire, B. L., Bohan, T. P., Landry, S. H., Davidson, K. C., & Miner, M. E. (1992). Verbal and nonverbal skill discrepancies in hydrocephalic children. *Journal of Clinical and Experimental Neuropsychology, 14,* 593–609.

Florek, M., & Karolak, S. (1977). Intelligence level of patients with Duchenne type of muscular dystrophy (PMD-D). *European Journal of Pediatrics, 126,* 275–282.

Fowler, M. G., Johnson, M. P., & Atkinson, S. S. (1985). School achievement and absence in children with chronic health conditions. *Journal of Pediatrics, 106,* 683–687.

Franceschi, M., Cecchetto, R., Minicucci, F., Smizne, S., Baio, G., & Canal, N. (1984). Cognitive processes in insulin dependent diabetes. *Diabetes Care, 7,* 226–231.

Freedman, A. M., Kaplan, H. I., & Sadock, B. J. (1976). *Modern synopsis of comprehensive textbook of psychiatry* (Vol. 2). Baltimore: Williams & Wilkins.

Gilroy, J., & Meyer, J. S. (1975). *Medical neurology* (2nd ed.). New York: Macmillan Co.

Goff, J. R., Anderson, H. R., Jr., & Cooper, P. F. (1980). Distractibility and memory deficits in long-term survivors of acute lymphoblastic leukemia. *Developmental Behavioral Pediatrics, 1,* 158–163.

Gold, A. E., Deary, I. J., & Frier, B. M. (1993). Recurrent severe hypoglycaemia and cognitive function in type 1 diabetes. *Diabetic Medicine, 10,* 503–508.

Gold, A. M. (1984). Stroke in children. In P. Rowland (Ed.), *Merritt's textbook of neurology* (7th ed., pp. 172–176). Philadelphia: Lea & Febiger.

Golden, C. J. (1981). *Diagnosis and rehabilitation in clinical neuropsychology* (2nd ed.). Springfield, IL: Thomas.

Goldstein, S. G., Kleinknecht, R. A., & Gallo, A. E., Jr. (1970). Neuropsychological changes associated with carotid endarterectomy. *Cortex, 6,* 308–322.

Goonan, B. T., Brown, R. T., Baldwin, K., Schoenherr, S., Buchanan, I., & Eckman, J. (1992). Cognitive processing

and learning disabilities in children with sickle cell disease (SSD). Abstracts of the 11th Annual Meeting of the National Academy of Neuropsychology, Dallas. *Archives of Clinical Neuropsychology, 7,* 329.

Goonan, B. T., Goonan, L. J., Brown, R. T., Buchanan, I., & Eckman, J. R. (1994). Sustained attention and inhibitory control in children with sickle cell syndrome. *Archives of Clinical Neuropsychology, 9,* 89–104.

Gortmaker, S. L., & Sappenfield, W. (1984). Chronic childhood disorders: Prevalence and impact. *Pediatric Clinics of North America, 31,* 3–16.

Graham, P. J. (1983). Specific medical syndromes. In M. Rutter (Ed.), *Developmental neuropsychiatry* (pp. 68–82). New York: Guilford Press.

Haumont, D., Dorchy, H., & Pelc, S. (1979). EEG abnormalities in diabetic children: Influence of hypoglycemia and vascular complications. *Clinical Pediatrics, 18,* 750–753.

Heron, J. R., Hutchinson, E. C., Boyd, W. N., & Aber, G. M. (1974). Pregnancy, subarachnoid hemorrhage, and the intravascular coagulation syndrome. *Journal of Neurology, Neurosurgery, and Psychiatry, 37,* 521–527.

Hittleman, J., Willoughby, A., Mendez, H., Nelson, N., Gong, J., Mendez, H., Holman, S., Muez, L., Goedert, J., & Landesman, S. (1991). Neurodevelopmental outcome of perinatally-acquired HIV infection on the first 24 months of life [Abstract]. *Proceedings from the VII International Conference on AIDS, 1,* 65.

Holmes, C. S. (1986). Neuropsychological profiles in men with insulin-dependent diabetes. *Journal of Consulting and Clinical Psychology, 54,* 386–389.

Holmes, C. S., Hayford, J. T., Gonzalez, J. L., & Weydert, J. A. (1983). A survey of cognitive functioning at different glucose levels in diabetic persons. *Diabetes Care, 6,* 180–185.

Holmes, C. S., Koepke, K., & Thompson, R. G. (1986). Simple versus complex performance impairments in three blood glucose levels. *Psychoneuroendocrinology, 11,* 343–357.

Holmes, C. S., Koepke, K. M., Thompson, R. G., Gyves, P. W., & Weydert, J. A. (1984). Verbal fluency and naming performance in type I diabetics at different blood glucose concentrations. *Diabetes Care, 7,* 455–459.

Hope-Stone, H. F. (1970). Results of treatment of medulloblastomas. *Journal of Neurosurgery, 32,* 83–88.

Hughes, G. V. R. (1979). *Connective tissue diseases* (2nd ed.). Oxford: Blackwell.

Ivnik, R. H., Colligan, R. C., Obetz, S. W., & Smithson, W. A. (1981). Neuropsychologic performance among children in remission from acute lymphocytic leukemia. *Developmental and Behavioral Pediatrics, 2,* 29–34.

Johnson, S. B., & Rosenbloom, A. L. (1982). Behavioral aspects of diabetes mellitus in childhood and adolescence. *Psychiatric Clinics of North America, 5,* 357–369.

Jyothi, K., Susheela, S., Kodali, V. R. R., Balakrishnan, S., & Seshaiah, V. (1993). Poor cognitive task performance of insulin dependent diabetic children in India. *Diabetes Research and Clinical Practice, 20,* 209–213.

Karagan, N. J. (1979). Intellectual functioning in Duchenne muscular dystrophy: A review. *Psychological Bulletin, 86,* 250–259.

Kennedy, R. (1924). Prognosis of sequelae of epidemic encephalitis in children. *American Journal of Disease of Children, 29,* 158–172.

Kerr, E. N., Smith, M. L., DaSilva, M., Hoffman, H. J., & Humphries, R. P. (1991). Neuropsychological effects of craniopharyngioma treated by microsurgery. Abstracts of the 19th annual INS meeting, San Antonio, Texas. *Journal of Clinical and Experimental Neuropsychology, 13,* 57.

Kilpatrick, D. G., Miller, W. C., Allan, A. N., & Lee, W. H. (1975). The use of psychological test data to predict open-heart surgery outcome: A prospective study. *Psychosomatic Medicine, 37,* 62–73.

King, N. J. (1980). The behavioral management of asthma and asthma-related problems in children: A critical review of the literature. *Journal of Behavioral Medicine, 3,* 169–189.

Lancet Editorial. (1980). Behavioral disorders in diabetic children. *Lancet, 2,* 188–189.

Lassman, L., & Arjona, V. E. (1967). Pontine gliomas of childhood. *Lancet, 1,* 913–915.

Levy, S. (1959). Post-encephalitic behavior disorder—a forgotten entity: A report of 100 cases. *American Journal of Psychiatry, 115,* 1062–1067.

Lishman, W. A. (1978). *Organic psychiatry: The psychological consequences of cerebral disorder.* Oxford: Blackwell.

LODAT, Handbook and Information Committee. (1981). *Living one day at a time.* Milwaukee: American Cancer Society.

Luckman, J., & Sorenson, K. C. (1980). *Medical–surgical nursing.* Philadelphia: Saunders.

McCardle, P., Nannis, E., Smith, R., & Fischer, G. (1991). Patterns of perinatal HIV-related language deficit [Abstract]. *Proceedings from the VII International Conference on AIDS, 2,* 187.

Matarazzo, R. G., Matarazzo, J. D., Gallo, A. E., Jr., & Weins, A. N. (1979). IQ and neuropsychological changes following carotid endarterectomy. *Journal of Clinical Neuropsychology, 1,* 97–116.

Matoth, Y., Zaizov, R., & Frankel, J. J. (1971). Minimal cerebral dysfunction in children with chronic thrombocytopenia. *Pediatrics, 47,* 698–706.

Matson, D. D., & Crigler, J. F. (1969). Management of craniopharyngioma in childhood. *Journal of Neurosurgery, 30,* 377–390.

Matthews, L. W., & Drotar, D. (1984). Cystic fibrosis—A challenging long-term chronic disease. *Pediatric Clinics of North America, 31,* 133–152.

Mauer, A. M. (1980). Therapy of acute lymphoblastic leukemia in childhood. *Blood, 56,* 1–10.

Meadows, A. T., Gordon, J., Massari, D. J., Littman, P., Ferguson, J., & Moss, K. (1981). Declines in IQ scores and cognitive dysfunctions in children with acute lymphocytic leukemia treated with cranial irradiation. *Lancet, 2,* 1015–1018.

Miller, J. D., & Sperling, M. A. (1986). Diabetes mellitus in children. In V. C. Kelley (Ed.), *Practice of pediatrics* (Vol. 6, pp. 1–19). New York: Harper & Row.

Moore, B. D., Needle, M. N., Ater, J. C. L., Brewer, V. R., & Copeland, D. R. (1993). Cognitive profile of children with neurofibromatosis, untreated brain tumor, or both.

Abstracts of the 21st annual INS meeting, Galveston, Texas. *Journal of Clinical and Experimental Neuropsychology, 15,* 84.

Moss, H. A., Brouwers, P., Wolters, P. L., Wiener, L., Hersh, S. S., & Pizzo, P. A. (1996). The development of a Q sort behavior rating procedure for pediatric HIV patients. *Journal of Pediatric Psychology, 21,* 379–400.

Moss, H., Wolters, P., Eddy, J., Weiner, J., & Pizzo, P. (1989). The effects of encephalopathy on the social and emotional behavior of pediatric AIDS patients [Abstract]. *Proceedings of the V International Conference on AIDS, 1,* 328.

Murphy, F., & Maccubbin, D. A. (1966). Carotid endarterectomy: A long-term follow-up study. In J. Shilito (Ed.), *Clinical neurology* (Vol. 13, pp. 198–212). Baltimore: Williams & Wilkins.

Northam, E., Bowden, S., Anderson, V., & Court, J. (1992). Neuropsychological functioning in adolescents with diabetes. *Journal of Clinical and Experimental Neuropsychology, 14,* 884–900.

Obetz, S. W., Invote, R. J., Smithson, W. A., Colligan, R. C., Groover, R. V., Gilchrist, G. J., Houser, D. W., Burgert, F. O., & Klass, D. V. (1979). Neuropsychologic follow-up study of children with acute lymphocytic leukemia: A preliminary report. *The American Journal of Pediatric Hematology/Oncology, 1,* 207–213.

Owens, M., Pressman, M., Edwards, A. E., Tourtellotte, W., Rose, J. G., Stern, D., Peters, G., Stabile, B. E., & Wilson, S. E. (1975). The effect of small infarcts and carotid endarterectomy on post-operative psychological test performance. *Journal of Surgical Research, 28,* 209–261.

Panitch, H. S., & Berg, B. O. (1970). Brain stem tumors of childhood and adolescence. *American Journal of Diseases of Children, 119,* 465–472.

Pfeifer, M. A., Weinberg, C. R., Cook, D. L., Reenan, A., Halter, J. B., Ensinck, J. W., & Porte, D. (1984). Autonomic neural dysfunction in recently diagnosed diabetic patients. *Diabetes Care, 7,* 447–453.

Pizzo, P., Eddy, J., Falloon, J., Balis, F., Murphy, R., Moss, H., Wolters, P., Brouwers, P., Jarnosinski, P., Rubin, M., Broder, S., Yarchoan, R., Brunetti, A., Maha, M., Nusinoff-Lehrman, S., & Poplack, D. (1988). Effect of continuous intravenous infusion of zidovudine (AZT) in children with symptomatic HIV infection. *New England Journal of Medicine, 319,* 889–896.

Price, R., Brew, B., Siditis, J., Rosenblum, M., Scheck, A., & Cleary, P. (1988). The brain in AIDS: Central nervous system HIV-1 infection and AIDS dementia complex. *Science, 239,* 586–592.

Puczynski, M. S., Puczynski, S. S., Reich, J., Kaspar, J. C., & Emanuele, M. A. (1990). Mental efficiency and hypoglycemia. *Developmental and Behavioral Pediatrics, 11,* 170–174.

Reich, J. N., Kaspar, J. C., Puczynski, M. S., Puczynski, S., Cleland, J. W., Dell'Angela, K., & Emanuele, M. A. (1990). Effect of a hypoglycemic episode on neuropsychological functioning in diabetic children. *Journal of Clinical and Experimental Neuropsychology, 12,* 613–626.

Rourke, B. P., Bakker, D. J., Fisk, J. L., & Strang, J. D. (1983). *Child neuropsychology: An introduction to theory, research, and clinical practice.* New York: Guilford Press.

Rovet, J. F., Ehrlich, R. M., & Czuchta, D. (1990). Intellectual characteristics of diabetic children at diagnosis and one year later. *Journal of Pediatric Psychology, 15,* 775–788.

Rovet, J. F., Ehrlich, R. M., Czuchta, D., & Akler, M. (1993). Psychoeducational characteristics of children and adolescents with insulin-dependent diabetes mellitus. *Journal of Learning Disabilities, 26,* 7–22.

Rovet, J. F., Ehrlich, R. M., & Hoppe, M. G. (1988). Specific intellectual deficits in children associated with early onset insulin-dependent diabetes. *Child Development, 59,* 226–234.

Rowland, L. P. (1984). Signs and symptoms in neurological diagnosis. In L. P. Rowland (Ed.), *Merritt's textbook of neurology* (7th ed., pp. 48–50). Philadelphia: Lea & Febiger.

Rubin, D. H., Leventhal, J. M., Sadock, R. T., Letovsky, E., Schottland, P., Clementine, I., & McCarthy, P. (1986). Educational intervention by computer on childhood asthma. *Pediatrics, 77,* 1–10.

Rutter, M. (1983). Issues and prospects in developmental neuropsychiatry. In M. Rutter (Ed.), *Developmental neuropsychiatry* (pp. 577–598). New York: Guilford Press.

Ryan, C. (1995). Effects of diabetes mellitus on neuropsychological functioning: A lifespan perspective. In I. Grant & K. M. Adams (Eds.), *Neuropsychological assessment of neuromedical disorders* (pp. 64–92). London: Oxford University Press.

Ryan, C. M., Atchison, J., Puczynski, S., Puczynski, M., Arslanian, S., & Becker, D. (1990). Mild hypoglycemia associated with deterioration of mental efficiency in children with insulin-dependent diabetes mellitus. *Journal of Pediatrics, 117,* 32–38.

Ryan, C., Longstreet, C., & Morrow, L. (1985). The effects of diabetes mellitus on the school attendance and school achievement of adolescents. *Child: Care, Health and Development, 11,* 229–240.

Ryan, C., & Morrow, L. (1987a). Neuropsychological characteristics of children with diabetes. In L. M. Wolraich & D. K. Routh (Eds.), *Advances in developmental and behavioral pediatrics* (Vol. VIII, pp. 132–147). Greenwich, CT: JAI Press.

Ryan, C., & Morrow, L. A. (1987b). Self-esteem in diabetic adolescents: Relationship between age at onset and gender. *Journal of Consulting and Clinical Psychology, 54,* 730–731.

Ryan, C., Vega, A., & Drash, A. (1985). Cognitive deficits in adolescents who developed diabetes early in life. *Pediatrics, 75,* 921–927.

Ryan, C., Vega, A., Longstreet, C., & Drash, A. (1984). Neuropsychological changes in adolescents with insulin dependent diabetes. *Journal of Consulting and Clinical Psychology, 52,* 335–342.

Ryan, C. M., & Williams, T. M. (1993). Effects of insulin-dependent diabetes on learning and memory efficiency in adults. *Journal of Clinical and Experimental Neuropsychology, 15,* 685–700.

Sabatino, D., & Cramblett, H. (1968). Behavioral sequelae of Californian encephalitis virus infection in children. *Developmental Medicine and Child Neurology, 10,* 331–337.

Sadler, J. E. (1982). Childhood asthma from the point of view of the liaison child psychiatrist. *Psychiatric Clinics of North America, 5,* 333–343.

Schlieper, A., Alcock, D., Beaudry, P., Feldman, W., & Leikin, L. (1991). Effect of therapeutic plasma concentrations of theophylline on behavior, cognitive processing, and affect in children with asthma. *Journal of Pediatrics, 118,* 449–455.

Seidel, W. T., Mitchell, W. G., Bell, T. S., Epport, K. L., Fodera, C., & Zeltzer, P. M. (1994). Developmental outcome in very young children treated for brain tumors. Abstracts of the Division of Clinical Neuropsychology, American Psychological Association Annual Meeting, Boston. *The Clinical Neuropsychologist, 4,* 272.

Shapiro, E. G. (1991). Neuropsychological and MRI findings before and after bone marrow transplant in children with degenerative white matter diseases. Abstracts of the 19th annual INS meeting, San Antonio, Texas. *Journal of Clinical and Experimental Neuropsychology, 13,* 57.

Shapiro, E. G., Lockman, L. A., & Krivat, W. (1993). The leukodystrophies: Natural history, neuropsychological characteristics, and treatment. Abstracts of the 21st annual INS meeting, Galveston, Texas. *Journal of Clinical and Experimental Neuropsychology, 15,* 95.

Skenazy, J. A., & Bigler, E. D. (1985). Psychological adjustment and neuropsychological performance in diabetic patients. *Journal of Clinical Psychology, 41,* 391–396.

Smith, M. L., Minden, D., Netley, C., Wasdell, M. B., Fernandes-Penney, A., Read, S. E., King, S. M., & Blanchette, V. (1993). Neuropsychological functioning in HIV-positive children with hemophilia. Abstracts of the Division of Clinical Neuropsychology, American Psychological Association Annual Meeting, Los Angeles. *The Clinical Neuropsychologist, 8,* 332.

Sollee, N. D., Latham, E. E., Kindlon, D. J., & Bresnan, M. J. (1985). Neuropsychological impairment in Duchenne muscular dystrophy. *Journal of Clinical and Experimental Neuropsychology, 7,* 486–496.

Stehbens, J. A., Kaleita, T. A., Noll, R. B., MacLean, W. E., Jr., O'Brien, T. A., Waskerwitz, M. J., & Hammond, G. D. (1991). CNS prophylaxis of childhood leukemia: What are the long-term neurological, neuropsychological, and behavioral effects? *Neuropsychology Review, 2,* 147–178.

Stewart, S. M., Hiltebeitel, C., Nici, J., Waller, D. A., Uauy, R., & Andrews, W. S. (1991). Neuropsychological outcome of pediatric liver transplantation. *Pediatrics, 87,* 367–376.

Stewart, S. M., Nici, J., Hiltebeitel, C., Bass, C., Waller, D. A., & Andrews, W. S. (1990). Neuropsychological deficits in pediatric liver transplant patients. Abstracts of the Division of Clinical Neuropsychology, American Psychological Association Annual Meeting, Boston. *The Clinical Neuropsychologist, 4,* 272.

Strecker, E. (1929). Behaviour problems in encephalitis. *Archives of Neurology and Psychiatry, 21,* 137–144.

Suess, W. A., & Chai, H. (1981). Neuropsychological correlates of asthma: Brain damage or drug effects? *Journal of Consulting and Clinical Psychology, 49,*135–136.

Tardieu, M., Blanche, S., Duliege, A., Rouzioux, C., & Griscelli, C. (1989). Neurologic involvement and prognostic factors after materno-fetal infection [Abstract]. *Proceedings of the V International Conference on AIDS, 1,* 194.

Taussig, L. M., & Landau, L. I. (1986). Cystic fibrosis. In V. C. Kelley (Ed.), *Practice of pediatrics* (Vol. 2, pp. 1–33). New York: Harper & Row.

Taylor, J. W. (1979). Mental symptoms and electrolyte imbalance. *Australian and New Zealand Journal of Psychiatry, 13,* 159–160.

Ternand, C., Go, V. L.W., Gerich, J. E., & Haymond, M. W. (1982). Endocrine pancreatic response of children with onset of insulin-requiring diabetes before age 3 and after age 5. *Journal of Pediatrics, 101,* 36–39.

Thompson, J. E., Patman, R. F., & Talkington, C. M. (1978). Carotid surgery for cerebrovascular insufficiency. *Current Problems in Surgery, 15,* 1–68.

Till, K. (1975). *Pediatric neurosurgery.* Oxford: Blackwell.

Ultmann, M. H., Diamond, G. W., Ruff, H. A., Belman, A. L., Novick, B. E., Rubinstein, A., & Cohen, H. J. (1987). Developmental abnormalities in children with acquired immunodeficiency syndrome (AIDS): A follow up study. *International Journal of Neuroscience, 32,* 661–667.

Walton, J. N. (1977). *Brain's diseases of the nervous system* (8th ed.). London: Oxford University Press.

Weber, A. M., Dolske, M. C., Pass, R. F., & Boll, T. J. (1993). Intellectual outcome of symptomatic congenital cytomegalovirus infection. Abstracts of the 12th Annual Meeting of the National Academy of Neuropsychology, Pittsburgh. *Archives of Clinical Neuropsychology, 8,* 270.

Weitzman, M. (1984). School and peer relations. *Pediatric Clinics of North America, 31,* 59–69.

Winfield, J. B., Lobo, P. I., & Singer, A. (1978). Significance of anti-lymphocyte antibodies in systemic lupus erythematosus. *Arthritis and Rheumatism, 21,* 215–216.

Winter, R. J. (1982). Special problems of the child with diabetes. *Comprehensive Therapy, 8,* 7–13.

Worden, D. K., & Vignos, P. J. (1962). Intellectual function in childhood muscular dystrophy. *Pediatrics, 29,* 968–977.

34

Coping and Adjustment of Children with Neurological Disorder

TIMOTHY B. WHELAN AND MARIE L. WALKER

Introduction

The opportunity to test the limits of one's clinical acumen is clearly apparent in the field of clinical child neuropsychology. The explosion of related theory and research, the complexity of case material, and the growing demand for applied expertise continue to challenge us daily. Indeed, the study of developmental brain–behavior relationships can be so intrinsically fascinating, so alluring, that many of us cannot imagine being satisfied in another domain of study. Yet there may be a subtle trap in all of this, the trap of becoming so enthralled with exploring brain–behavior relationships in isolation that we lose sight of the total experience of the child.

It is the premise of this chapter that not only do children and adolescents who have sustained an insult to the brain face the likelihood of altered brain function and its attendant problems, they must also contend with the effects of neurological disorder in a social context. In other words, like children with chronic illnesses, they may face severe developmental challenges during diagnosis, hospitalization, medical intervention, rehabilitation, schooling, family development, and socialization. As a consequence, there is the risk throughout the course of the disorder for the creation of secondary deforming effects on psychosocial adjustment in addition to the primary cognitive, sensory, and motor changes commonly as-

sociated with these disorders. As with the victims of other diseases, accidents, or undesirable life events who are faced with major personal and developmental crises, the presence of neurological impairment may force children and their families to question their fundamental assumptions and expectations about themselves and their world, and to react to or "cope" with multilevel effects of the disorder. It is therefore apparent that the helping professional concerned with the psychological well-being of children must remain cognizant of the nonbiological systems with which children interface.

This chapter is concerned with multiple systems affecting the coping and adjustment of children with neurological disorder. Investigation of this topic often leads to psychological literature that is conceptually relevant but somewhat apart from traditional neurodiagnostically oriented neuropsychology. For instance, social psychologists investigating coping mechanisms have primarily been concerned with adults, and the pediatric psychology literature regarding coping with neurological disorder is not highly developed. However, despite variation in specific targets of study, "good practice" in the area of clinical child neuropsychology requires a continual integration of theoretical and applied information from the domains of clinical child, developmental, educational, social, and family psychology. A related point was made by Boll (1985) who described a "threshold" movement within the field of neuropsychology toward a more psychological emphasis:

> In addition to the utilization of behaviors for exquisite neuroanatomical appreciation which represents

TIMOTHY B. WHELAN • Department of Psychiatry, Baystate Medical Center, Springfield, Massachusetts 01199. MARIE L. WALKER • Austin Neurological Clinic, Austin, Texas 78705.

a continuing and legitimate investigational area, neuropsychologists provide, with increasing sophistication, psychological descriptions designed primarily to help in understanding the whole person, rather than being confined only to the person's neuroanatomy. (p. 474)

As detailed below, mechanisms of coping and adjustment in neurologically impaired children are perhaps best viewed globally from developmental and systems-theoretic models of child psychology. After a discussion of this conceptual framework, general considerations regarding the constructs of coping and adjustment are presented. Further topics related to the coping and adjustment of neurologically impaired children are then selectively reviewed and provide a flavor of the complexity of related theory and practice.

General Systems and Developmental Models

A conceptual framework for studying the processes of coping and adjustment in children with neurological impairment can be derived from general systems theory, a general science of "wholeness" examining sets of elements standing in interrelationship (von Bertalanffy, 1968). The systems-theoretic model posits that the human organism exists in a hierarchy of systems ranging from the biological realm, through cognitive, intrapsychic, and behavioral levels of analysis, to the family and social spheres. This is an information flow-through model in which developments at one level theoretically have ramifications throughout the systems hierarchy. Whereas von Bertalanffy has perhaps been most eloquent in expressing the systems approach, these central tenets are not unfamiliar to scientists in general and they have appeared in the writings of seminal thinkers in the history of neuropsychology. For instance, more than 50 years ago Kurt Goldstein (1939, 1940) concluded that any particular symptom displayed by a patient could not be easily understood as being uniquely the product of a specific lesion or disease, but instead had to be considered as a manifestation of the total organism that behaved as a unified whole.

General systems theory has also been cited in support of a fundamental reorientation in medical education and practice (Engle, 1977, 1980). Such a shift in thought leads to reconceptualization of disease as a biopsychosocial product, and to the study of disease and medical care as interrelated processes. The reliance on such an approach is now particularly evident in the literature on families with illness (Gochman, 1985; Kerns & Curley, 1985; Kerns & Turk, 1985; Leventhal, Leventhal, & Van Nguyen, 1985) and in the field of clinical health psychology (Millon, Green, & Meagher, 1982). Moreover, this conceptual framework will undoubtedly become increasingly central in the era of capitated medical care.

This application of a general systems approach to understanding the functioning of adults with neurological impairment seems reasonable and logical: Disorders of biological functioning are likely to affect an individual's psychosocial status. The consideration of nonbiological systems in the lives of neurologically impaired children, however, is virtually mandatory. Children do not exist in isolation from others as adults can choose to do. Rather they are enmeshed in nonself systems to a far greater extent, influencing and being influenced by family, peers, health professionals, and schools. One cannot even approximate a clear clinical description, however elegant, of a child without reference to relationships between that child and those with whom they are bound.

An additional dimension of complexity must be added to the clinical child neuropsychologist's systems-theoretic model: the process of development and change. Although the notion that the individual is an active, developing organism is a fundamental concept among child development and life-span psychologists, neuropsychological literature has historically neglected this aspect of our functioning (Parsons & Prigatano, 1978; Smith, 1979). Walter Riese (1977) captured the problem aptly:

Overpowered by the ever-increasing intricacies of anatomical arrangements, . . . yielding in this self-inflicted intellectual emergency to the always threatening danger of oversimplification, the modern student of brain lesions forgot that every functional disturbance has its natural or evolutionary history. Whether affected by neurosis, psychosis or brain injury, man must write the history of his new condition which implies the history of his whole life. Nobody, healthy or not, can escape the law of time and change. (p.77)

The need for consideration of developmental issues in child health psychology has been well described by Maddux, Roberts, Sledden, and Wright (1986), and Garrison and McQuiston (1989) provide a comprehensive review of psychological aspects of chronic illness in childhood and adolescence.

Bernstein and Waber (1990) have articulated these points with particular clarity in their model of developmental neuropsychological assessment—an approach, not a technique—in which the goal is "not to diagnose deficits in a child, but rather to construct a *Child–World System* that characterizes the reciprocal relationship of the developing children and the world in which that child functions" (p. 312). This approach is derived from the systemic tradition of Luria and Vygotsky as well as the Wernerian approach most elaborated in neuropsychology by Kaplan. More specifically, the model considers manifestations both neurological and psychologic of the structure (three neuroanatomic axes, cognitive structures), development (neurological and psychological developmental timetables), alternative mechanisms (alternative pathways, alternative strategies), and context (role of experience, environmental interactions). Consistent with this approach, attributions of difficulty are shifted from the child to the system.

This, then, is the model: The child is conceptualized on multiple levels standing in interrelationship, with the hierarchy of systems set in temporal motion. It would of course be extravagant to assert that neuropsychologists can excellently or adequately conceptualize all of our clients in this fashion, but the goal of so doing seems worthy.

Coping and Adjustment

In most theoretical models, coping is a process that is initiated when an individual perceives or experiences stressful stimuli, such as a change in the pace of life or a subjective perception of an event as negative or undesirable and beyond the competence of the coping person (Chan, 1977). For example, hospitalization, sensorimotor disability, or loss of cognitive integrity associated with neurological disorder could obviously all be considered untimely, unexpected, and undesirable life changes. Coping presumably leads to adaptation or adjustment to stressful events and perceptions, and successful coping implies successful adjustment. Generally, people cope with daily stressors by responding with habitual and automatic patterns of cognition and behavior (Folkman & Lazarus, 1980). Such coping strategies may involve the cognitive functions of perception, memory, speech, judgment and reality testing, motor activity, emotional expression, and psychological defenses (Mattsson, 1972). When these customary automatic responses become unavailable, individual attempts at coping will require that old resources be used in new ways. This may be particularly true for children whose increasing cognitive and behavioral abilities continually alter the

effectiveness of their previous automatic responses. Coping, then, can be conceptualized as purposeful behavioral and/or intrapsychic activity at either conscious or unconscious levels that serves to ameliorate the experience of stress while facilitating adjustment to stressful stimuli.

In relation to coping, the process of adjustment allows a return to effective (though not necessarily prior) automatic patterns of behavior, and implies that an individual is functioning effectively. More specifically, for the child with neurological impairment, adjustment includes acceptance and age-appropriate understanding of the disease or handicap, medical compliance, absence of severe psychopathology, age-appropriate interpersonal functioning with family, peers, and in school, and "normal" or age-appropriate personality functioning (Drotar, 1981).

Cautions

Although full treatment of the constructs of coping and adjustment is beyond the scope of this chapter, several considerations are in order. First, we have implied that coping is a process and adjustment is an outcome of this process, and this may indeed be the case. However, such a scheme may also be an unfair simplification of the relationship between coping and adjustment. It may also be true, for example, that levels of adjustment influence attempts at coping. For instance, high self-esteem may be an outcome of a child's successful attempts at coping. Similarly, it may be that children who already experience high self-esteem will be better able to cope with stressful events.

Second, coping is a uniquely individual process and its exposition depends on experiential insight and/or observer inferences; it is not a construct that can be measured directly. Currently, psychosocial science relies on personality and adjustment measures, such as levels of self-esteem, depression, anxiety, and locus of control, among others, to infer both the presence and the effectiveness of the coping process. Cognitive and behavioral components may also be evaluated (Curry & Russ, 1985). Nevertheless, though the process of coping and adjustment are well understood intuitively, they remain scientifically and empirically vague.

Interested readers are referred to a series of studies reported by Tobin, Holroyd, Reynolds, and Wigal (1989) which develop a hierarchical model with three levels of the structure of coping. Eight identified primary factors (problem-solving, cognitive restructuring, emotional expression, social support, problem avoidance, wishful thinking, self-criticism, and social withdrawal) were organized into two types of problem-focused and two types of emotion-focused coping activities, and at the tertiary level there appeared two basic approaches to stressful situations, namely, engagement and disengagement. This structure was examined by means of hierarchical factor analysis of the Coping Strategies Inventory administered to young adults, and its developmental nature has yet to be established. For a more child-specific theory, see Ryan-Wenger (1992).

Third, it should be noted that coping and adjustment are processes that occur continually; they are not discrete and isolated events. People experience multiple levels of stress simultaneously, from the trials of getting to school or work on time, to fears of being perceived as different or odd, and feelings of unworthiness. Even positive changes in life events, such as promotions, may be experienced as stressful, and the perceived intensity of a stressor at a given time will influence an individual's attempt at coping. Further, what may constitute successful coping behavior at one time may change with age and other intervening variables. Again, this is especially true for children where constant development in their abilities may render previously effective patterns of coping obsolete. When neurologically based disorganization of cognitive and affective functions are superimposed on normal developmental patterns of organization, the complexity of these processes can be magnified.

Finally, coping and adjustment are processes that reflect an interaction between individual and environment (Rutter, 1981, 1986). It has long been recognized that people perceive stressful stimuli differently and that individuals will make unique attempts to cope with stress, whether by flight, fight, or inaction, based in part on personality determinants, history with coping experiences, and environmental constraints, including peer and societal expectations (Chan, 1977). The significance of this interaction, especially for children, is reflected in increasing research on the influence of the family in children's abilities to cope with their handicaps.

Societal Influence on Coping and Adjustment

A paradoxical dilemma exists when one considers the relationship of coping and neurological disorders. Traditional definitions of coping, including those presented here, suggest that stressors such as neurological deficits are external to the individual and must be adjusted to as unwanted alien agents. This idea originates from the societal doctrine of normalcy, where certain parameters of behavior are acceptable and occurrences outside of these bounds are regarded as deviant. Deviance is then considered unacceptable, obviating the need for a return (adjustment) to normalcy.

This viewpoint can be both unfortunate and not entirely necessary. Children born with a neurological deficit, for example, have always interpreted their worlds through a unique lens, and their "deficits" are a part of their identity as surely as being physically whole is a part of most of ours. Often, however, individuals with visible physical differences are considered deviant and treated accordingly. The process of accepting one's handicap is thus made more difficult when one is continually regarded by peers and society as "different."

The problem we are suggesting, then, is that handicap is defined normatively and from an "outsider's" perspective (Shontz, 1982). "Insiders," or people who have either always experienced a particular state, such as neurological disorder, or who have come to accept their differences and/or limitations, do not necessarily view their handicap as something to overcome (Massie, 1985). Once an individual has learned to cope with a handicap, the deficit itself no longer remains the focus of attention. Handicapped individuals, like ourselves, must answer the question, how does one achieve satisfaction and happiness in life, given the uniqueness of every individual? Although this question is made no less easy by the presence of a handicapping condition, the burden might be eased if it were not necessary to feel that one had to meet the normative standards of today's society.

Making Meaning of Neurological Disorder

"Words, words, words"—*Hamlet*, Act II, Scene ii

Whether in the role of consultant or therapist, child neuropsychologists are often called on to provide information to their clients regarding the nature of the neurological disorders. The process of clear and appropriate explanation may be problematic enough with adults. We are reminded of the elderly gentleman with cerebrovascular disease who had carefully listened to his physician's explanation of regional cerebral blood flow measurement, and who had given his "informed consent" to the procedure. During a later neuropsychological examination he wanted to confirm his understanding of the procedure, and said, "This is something *nuclear,* right? Like *the bomb,* right?"

Examples of well-meant yet misjudged attempts to convey the nature of medical problems to children are also present in the literature. Whitt, Dykstra, and Taylor (1979) mentioned the potential iatrogenic harm that may come from such casual statements as "the doctor will inject some 'dye' . . ." (thus effectively raising the possibility of imminent "death") or "epilepsy is excess 'electricity' in the brain" (summoning up parental admonitions regarding wall sockets, shocks, and terminal consequences). Similarly, Perrin and Gerrity (1981) have written on the young pediatric patient's assumption that when the doctor says "there's edema in your belly," the "demon" was sent there to punish him or her for wrongdoing; the notion of a "demonic" brain could evoke even more primitive fears.

The pediatric literature advises that healthcare professionals consider the child's level of cognitive development (typically in a Piagetian sense) when conveying information regarding disease processes, medical procedures, and health maintenance (Brodie, 1974; Campbell, 1975; Mechanic, 1964; Neuhauser, Amsterdam, Hines, & Steward, 1978; Palmer & Lewis, 1976). The goals of such consideration include improved regimen compliance, reduced anxiety, and enhanced understanding and acceptance of the condition by the affected child and, if also afforded developmentally appropriate explanations, by healthy peers.

According to stage theorists, children functioning at a preoperational level of cognitive development (normally between ages 2 and 7) center on single external events, which are viewed from the child's own perspective without generalization to other situations and without the application of logical operations. Illness prevention and recovery may thus be associated with sets of rigid rules surrounding immediate perceptual experience and concrete action (avoiding the touch of sick friends; staying in bed) (Perrin & Gerrity, 1981; Whitt *et al.,* 1979). Bibace and Walsh (1979) proposed refinements to this general category of cognitive development, as well as categories described below. For instance, preoperational explanations of disease are divided into the categories of Phenomenism (illness caused by single inappropriate, external, and spatially remote sources, i.e., "people get colds from the sun") and Contagion (reliance on single causes of contagion transmitted through mere proximity and manifest in a single symptom, i.e., people get colds when someone else gets near them). Siegel (1988) has suggested that familiarity with a disease results in more advanced conceptual understanding, so that one might expect a preschooler to apply more sophisticated causal reasoning concerning a cold than a neurological illness with recent onset.

At the stage of concrete operations (normally between ages 6 or 7 and 11 or 12), the child's thought becomes less egocentric and perceptually bound, and reasoning becomes more logical. Specification of relationships among events or objects, categorical classification, and transformation comprehension become possible. Illnesses at this time may be defined by the child as a set of multiple concrete symptoms, and are often believed to be caused primarily by germs. From such a perspective, diseases may impinge on the body unless sick people are avoided, and cures may consist of passively allowing medicines to act on the body. A clear appreciation of the self-healing aspects of bodily functioning is presumably lacking in the concrete operational child. Unlike the preoperational child, the concrete operational child can more clearly distinguish between internal and external events, though the focus remains on the latter. Subdivision of this stage by Bibace and Walsh includes Contamination, in which there is recognition of multiple disease symptoms caused by concrete sources such as germs, dirt, or bad behavior. The Internalization subdivision of concrete operational thought is characterized by the ways in which illnesses are internalized: swallowing or inhaling germs or other contaminants. The body's own recuperative powers become recognized, and reversibility (the sick person can become well, and vice versa) is characteristic.

With the emergence of formal operations in late childhood and early adolescence, illness may be conceptualized as having complex, interrelated, and multiple causes that affect multiple internal systems and result in multiple external symptoms. Bibace and Walsh decompose the explanation of illness in the formal operational stage into two subdivisions: Physiological and Psychophysiological. In the former, illness is defined by the child in terms of internal organs and structures whose malfunctions are manifest in multiple external symptoms and there is a clear departure from previous reliance on concretely perceptible reality. In the psychophysiological category, psychological events are included as disease symptoms as well as causes of internal dysfunction. The etiologies of a headache, for instance, may at this developmental point include too much worry.

Based on this six-stage developmental sequence, Bibace and Walsh contend that not only do conceptions of illness shift in characteristic ways, but that there is also a corresponding developmental increase in the perceived control the child has over illness, with a concomitant decline in the sense of personal vulnerability. For example, older children in the Internalization phase may believe that there are things they can do to maintain bodily health, whereas young children in the Phenomenistic phase may believe themselves to be vulnerable to disease causes that are spatially remote and uncontrollable. These points are elaborated on by Maddux *et al.* (1986) in an article on developmental issues in child health behavior that focuses on prevention of illness and injury, and on health promotion. It would be erroneous, however, to suggest that feelings of control and reduced vulnerability are inevitable accompaniments of older age or later stages of cognitive development. Once again, children's conceptualizations of their neurological disorders are likely to evolve over time, with general stages of cognition interacting with particular informational content and numerous other cognitive and affective variables.

The suitable selection of words of explanation and due consideration of the nature of the child's beliefs about disease may still be insufficient to enable children to understand neurological disorders, if only because neuropathological processes are so often without visible referents. The use of metaphor, perhaps aided by drawings, to provide appropriate explanations of medical events may be particularly beneficial for children who have not yet attained formal operational thought and/or who are not likely to have a sense of the pathophysiology of the unseen nervous system. For example, in the case of seizure disorders the analogy of a telephone system has been suggested (Whitt *et al.,* 1979). In condensed form, a discussion with the child might refer to the notion that the brain is like a telephone that sends messages to all parts of the body, and just like a telephone, the brain sometimes gets a "wrong number" by sending messages to the _____ (substitute relevant perceptual cues, perhaps those related to the aura). In some cases it can also be pointed out that just like a telephone after a wrong number, the brain works fine again.

The same authors have also provided metaphor for other neurological conditions. For instance, the

body can be analogously described as a large city made up of many people (cells) with important jobs (e.g., telephone cells, garbageman cells, doctor cells, carpenter cells, police cells), and cancer cells may be described as outlaws in the system. Treatment may then be presented as a means of helping the body's police and medical forces to establish law and order. Built-up pressure in a garden hose with blocked outlet may serve as a metaphor for children with hydrocephalus, and the swelling and potential bursting of a balloon may foster a better understanding of aneurysms (though we personally find this last example too likely to result in fears of imminent catastrophe to be used with most children).

In considering the process of aiding children and their families to better comprehend their neurological or other medical disorder, it should be remembered that the sophistication of children's concepts of illness may differ from their concepts involving different content. Perrin and Gerrity (1981) reported that in a sample of normal children, illness-causation concepts (e.g., "How do children get sick?") were slower to develop than concepts to explain physical causality (e.g., "Why does night come?"). Moreover, older children may indeed be able to provide more sophisticated explanations of illness than younger children, but in a conditional sense: Younger children with a history of poorer health have the least sophisticated concepts, whereas older healthy children may have less sophisticated concepts than peers of the same age who have been ill more often (Campbell, 1975). In addition, the value of providing illness explanations to healthy peers in order to facilitate acceptance of children with chronic illness has been questioned (Potter & Roberts, 1984). As expected, when groups of healthy preoperational and concrete operational children were provided with either symptom descriptions or metaphorical explanations of diabetes and epilepsy, those receiving the analogous explanations demonstrated significantly more general comprehension of the illnesses, and perceptions of personal vulnerability were reduced. However, these illness explanations did not significantly facilitate ratings of acceptance of a hypothetical child with these diseases.

In some cases, the trail of misunderstanding is so confused as to be impenetrable. For instance, when one latency-aged boy was asked if he knew what might be the reason for his seizures, he speculated vaguely that it was "because something was wrong"; when pressed for a specific possibility, he could only guess "AIDS?" Note that clarity of information will probably be helpful in a case like this, but perhaps not in all instances: Brewster (1982) speculated that retention of magical beliefs in illness causality and responsibility may be an important defensive function. It has also been persistently curious to hear in interviews with caring and well-informed parents that they often have no idea what their child might believe about her or his illness at this point in the child's development. For those interested in helping communicate concepts to children with neurologically based learning and behavioral difficulties, books by Mel Levine (1990, 1993) prove especially helpful.

The presence of disease conditions may also alter the normal pattern and pace of cognitive development (Mearig, 1985). Obviously this could be the case in those with brain dysfunctions that change cognitive integrity, and it may also occur in those with chronic illnesses whose intellectual functioning is relatively intact. Myers-Vando, Steward, Folkins, and Hines (1979) reported that although children with congenital heart disease manifest lower levels of cognitive performance on conservation tasks compared with healthy peers (presumably because of the disruptive "intrusive stress" of the illness), some of the ill children were capable of thinking formally in the content domain of illness causality, possibly because of the greater affective salience of the topic or greater opportunities for direct education and experience with illness. On the other hand, Carandang, Folkins, Hines, and Steward (1979) reported that healthy siblings of diabetic children failed to perform at the expected cognitive level in conceptualizing illness causality and treatment when compared with children without ill siblings matched on demographic variables and measures of Piagetian cognitive development.

In conclusion, conflicting data in the literature suggest that children's cognitive understanding of a neurological disorder is not likely to be entirely predictable simply on the basis of their age or measures of their level of intellectual/cognitive development in nonillness content domains. Attempts should be made to integrate such information with their historical experience with the disorder.

"Facts are the enemy of truth."—
Man of La Mancha

Quite apart from the strictly cognitive aspects of comprehension, a child's construction of the personal "meaning" of neurological disorder, and thus reactions to it, is likely to involve processes that blend cognition and affect, and that incorporate both past and current experience. Perhaps a clinical anecdote can illustrate this point. A large and powerful adolescent boy with a vague history of seizures entered a children's psychiatric hospital with a diagnosis of paranoid schizophrenia. Precipitating the hospitalization were social isolation, paranoid ideation, verbal threatening, and dangerous behaviors such as jumping out of trees and leaping before slow-moving cars.

During the course of therapy, two primary themes emerged sequentially. First, he believed his seizures to be a pervasive and primitive loss of bodily and self-control, and that during these episodes he might unknowingly and unwillingly kill the small children for whom he frequently cared at home. Later a history of physical abuse by the father was revealed. After one incident during which the boy secretly wished his father dead, the father promptly *did* die of a cardiac arrest. The boy was simultaneously overwhelmed by a sense of omnipotence—he believed he had actually caused his father's death—and by his perception of an organically based lack of control necessary to prevent harming those he most loved in the future. He projected great menace onto his environment, and then attempted to prove that he himself could not be killed by engaging in (but surviving) potentially injurious behaviors. His behavioral symptoms, therefore, seemed indicative of dynamic issues influenced by the objective and subjective realities of seizures and past experience. At issue, then, are the interactions between the ways in which children and adolescents react to and understand neurological disorder, with the ultimate targets of interest being their construction of meaning and daily coping and adjustment.

Defense or Coping?

If it is assumed that the onset or diagnosis of neurological disorder represents a threat not only to cerebral integrity but also to the child's self or ego in a fundamental manner, then it can be assumed that attempts will be made to control, contain, or minimize that threat. Such actions often lead to distortion, illusion, or self-deception (inaccurate reality testing), and may thus be considered classical defense mechanisms; they may thus seem contrary to mental health. For a review of empirical studies of defense mechanisms in children, see Schibuk,

Bond, and Bouffard (1989). Yet there can be a psychologically positive side to these actions as well, and a number of early papers anticipated current trends in social psychological research in this area. Goldstein (1952) distinguished between protective and defense mechanisms, suggesting that although both may be employed to protect one from fear and anxiety, the former may arise in a neurologically impaired individual from an inability to function in a shifting environment, whereas the latter may develop in response to psychodynamic conflict. Kroeber (1964) categorized and paired ego defense mechanisms (e.g., isolation, projection, repression) with parallel coping mechanisms (e.g., objectivity, empathy, suppression).

Both coping and defense mechanisms may be rooted in common attempts to deal with painful reality, though defenses would be cast in more negative terms reflecting poor adaptability, whereas coping mechanisms may represent active, flexible, and effective attempts to deal with conflict. For instance, if an early adolescent girl hospitalized for diagnostic tests is playing with dolls, she may be employing mechanisms of time reversal by recapturing experiences, feelings, and ideas of the past. The behavior is not necessarily indicative of the defense mechanism of regression (i.e., age-inappropriate behavior to avoid responsibility, aggression, or unpleasant demands), but rather of the analogous and healthy coping mechanism of playfulness (utilizing feelings and ideas from past experience that are not directly ordered by the immediate elements of the situation). Similarly, the 9-year-old girl with little manifest anxiety during a neuropsychological evaluation on the day prior to surgery for an enormous left frontal tumor was perhaps not refusing to face painful thoughts, percepts, or feelings as in the pathological sense of denial (or exhibiting frontal lobe signs, as the evaluation itself indicated). Instead she may have been able to recognize and then set aside disturbing thoughts and feelings in order to concentrate on tasks at hand. The point, then, is that some of the behaviors and thoughts of those facing extraordinary levels of disruption in their lives may not be as psychopathological as they might superficially appear. Our evaluation of their actions to contend with severe stress needs to consider the degree (focal or pervasive, flexible or rigid, transient or chronic) of distortion as well as the temporal relationship between crisis moments and defense quality.

The role of denial in the coping process has perhaps been most clearly explicated. As Lazarus (1983)

suggested, the paradox of self-deception being both adaptationally sound and psychopathological may be resolved by asking the more sophisticated question: "What kinds of self-deceptions are damaging or constructive, and under what conditions?" Lazarus initially distinguishes between classical denial, e.g., the negation of some internal impulse, feeling, or thought, or of an external reality, and avoidance or plain ignorance of threatening events. He then describes a family of denials. Partial denial, or the temporary and tentative suspension of belief, often takes place among the seriously ill in the context of reassuring social relationships with concerned friends, family, or healthcare providers. Such a situation is quite common among healthy young children who easily suspend the reality of the moment, particularly when that reality is unpleasant. In addition, Lazarus recommends that psychologists shift their emphasis from considering denial and other coping mechanisms as static states of mind to recognizing them as ongoing processes that are often not fixed or consolidated defense mechanisms and that depend on both internal events and the social context.

Perhaps most relevant are some of the conclusions Lazarus reaches on the costs and benefits of denial. If direct action to change the relationship between person and environment is adaptationally necessary, denial and subsequent inactivity will be destructive. On the other hand, when direct action is irrelevant to the outcome, denial may reduce distress and afford the individual the possibility for good morale and hope. Note that this position to some extent contrasts with many of the cognitive or rational treatment approaches employed with clients who are neurologically impaired. An additional time-related principle is that denial may be beneficial early in disease or immediately after severe injury when individuals are actually unable to participate in their own care. Later on, during extended treatment, rehabilitation, or education, it may be more important to contend directly with the insult and to struggle in a problem-focused manner. As an aside, it should be clear that reference is being made here to secondary reactions to neurological events. The existence of neurologically based forms of inaccurate perception and reality testing is not denied, nor is their significance in case management diminished.

Perception of Competence

Forms of denial may be related to other cognitive and conative attempts to cope with neurological insult. Duchenne muscular dystrophy (DMD) is a neuromuscular disease beginning in early childhood and resulting in relentlessly progressive muscle wasting and weakness, and eventually in death by late adolescence or early adulthood. In part, an understanding of the psychological functioning of children with DMD may be derived from their performances on intellectual and neuropsychological measures (Dubowitz, 1977; Karagan, 1979; Knights, Hinton, & Drader, 1973); however, the literature in this area remains conflicting (Mearig, 1979; Sollee, Latham, Kindlon, & Bresnan, 1985; Whelan, 1987). While we are continuing to research the intricacies of brain–behavior relationships in this population, we are also exploring other aspects of their psychosocial functioning. In this context, one motivational variable, perceived control of events, appears to affect a wide variety of psychological conditions. Indeed, perceptions of personal control, especially inaccurate perceptions, have been seen as central components of problems ranging from depression to paranoia to underachievement (Weisz & Stipek, 1982).

Although the conceptualization and measurement of the control dimension have been approached from the perspectives of social learning and attribution theories, the theory and concepts of intrinsic motivation are also important. Competence motivation theory assumes that humans naturally strive for effective interactions with their environments. Successful mastery of a problem produces pleasurable feelings of efficacy or competence, which, in turn, reinforce and lead the individual to seek out and attempt to master additional tasks (Stipek & Weisz, 1981). Harter (1978) claims that in order for children to experience a feeling of efficacy, they must perceive themselves as responsible for their successful performance. Moreover, she reasons, failures perceived to be caused by a lack of competence or self-worth can lead to anxiety in mastery situations and thus decrease the child's mastery motivation. Children's expectancies and perceptions of efficacy may consequently be particularly important to consider because they may determine whether coping behavior will be initiated, how much effort will be expended, and how long it will be maintained in the face of obstacles and aversive experiences (Bandura, 1977).

Certainly, children with DMD experience a particularly acute and reality-based loss of motor control. Their perceptions of motoric, academic, and social competence, and general self-worth have been subjected to empirical investigation (Whelan, 1986). The Perceived Competence Scale for Children (Harter, 1979), which measures perceptions in the four mentioned domains, was administered to 31 boys with DMD. With regard to the central tendencies of the data, mean scores on the scales of cognitive and social competence and on the scale of general self-esteem were approximately at the normative mean. Scores on the scale of physical competence (referring primarily to athletic skills) were about one standard deviation below the mean for normal children (Whelan, 1986).

On the surface, these results might suggest that children with DMD maintain relatively accurate perceptions of their own areas of competence and disability, or that the existence of a neuromuscular disorder resulting in motor dysfunction and a reduced sense of efficacy in that domain have not substantially generalized to other measured domains. However, scores on the scale of perceived physical competence were not significantly correlated with any of the neuropsychological measures used in this study including measures of motor performance. This suggests that perceptions of physical competence or, conversely, of physical disability may vary widely in this population, with little relation to the objective reality of assessed motor performance. That is, some of the mildly physically impaired children may perceive themselves as severely limited, and others with greater actual motor disability may not perceive themselves as so seriously impaired.

Other data in this study may contribute to an understanding of the ways in which dystrophic children make sense of their condition. The magnitude of the correlations between scores on the scale of perceived physical competence and those on the scale of general self-worth (0.65) and social competence (0.39) was considerably higher than in the normative population. Together, these data may suggest reasons for the lack of a significant relationship between perceived physical competence and actual motor ability: Denial of physical disability in the service of preserving a sense of self-worth may be a prominent coping mechanism in children with neuromuscular disease.

An examination of perceptions of competence in other groups of children with suspected neurological disorder has also proved interesting. For instance, the factor pattern of the Harter scales for a sample of children with learning disability showed that the physical and social competence factors were retained as in the normal population, although cognitive and self-worth factors did not emerge as discrete entities. Instead, two cognitive–self-worth factors were obtained, the first composed of trait-like descriptions (e.g., being smart, liking yourself as a person) and the second composed of concrete and behavioral items (e.g., feeling it is easy to understand what one reads, thinking the way one does things is fine). Thus, the learning-disabled child's sense of self-worth seems directly tied to scholastic competence (Harter, 1985). Harter recommends that we treat self-concept as neither epiphenomenal nor as a static construct and concludes that "we cannot simply treat all children with intellectual deficits as a homogeneous group since clearly there are quite different processes influencing the structure and content of their self-perceptions" (p.16). With necessary modifications, the measurement of domain-specific perceptions of competence and global self-worth in the neurologically impaired population of children may yield important data in the future. For instance, we are interested in determining if the factor structure described by Harter for children with learning disability is truly representative for all those bearing that label. Certainly many investigators have recognized that such children may frequently have difficulty recognizing and interpreting social cues (Maheady & Maitland, 1982). Based on the subtyping literature (e.g., Rourke, 1985), it seems quite possible that some children with learning disability maintain accurate perceptions of their competencies and areas of disability, whereas others do not. Interventions with children who are accurately perceiving their abilities may consequently differ from those with children who are not. Moreover, the assessment of self-evaluative processes may be critically important to consider in the neurologically impaired population of children: If these processes are more amenable to change than structurally based abilities *per se,* then school and other performances might be indirectly enhanced through alternative interventions. Moreover, Luthar and Zigler (1991) have made a conceptual link between issues of vulnerability and competence, and extend these issues into the domain of resilience.

Attributions

If by definition the word *victim* applies to "anyone who suffers as the result of ruthless design or incidentally or accidentally," then the term may be broadly invoked in the context of various life crises, whether accidents, crimes, or diseases (Janoff-Bulman & Frieze, 1983). Because children with neurological impairment surely suffer physical and/or psychological alteration, they may justifiably be considered victims in this sense. Even the terms commonly associated with neurological disease or injury reflect this theme: Cerebral *trauma* with *loss* of consciousness, brain *insult,* and vascular *accident.* Considerable research on the personal and social consequences of victimization has been conducted by social psychologists, and although there are few available reports concerning those with neurological disorder, the findings are generically relevant.

One relatively well-developed domain of research on coping with victimization concerns attributions of causality of undesirable events. In part, the impetus for these investigations came from refinements of learned helplessness theory that were heavily based on attribution theory (Wortman, 1983). As part of the learned helplessness reformulation (Abramson, Seligman, & Teasdale, 1978), critical questions on the nature of coping with adverse circumstances shifted from the undesirable events themselves to individuals' interpretations of the events. For example, the type, intensity, and duration of a victim's coping responses in serious accidents may depend less on the precise physiological deficits and more on cognitions regarding the cause of the accident. One of the most relevant studies of this kind examined the relation between the attributions of causality made by adult accident victims with paralysis resulting from severe spinal cord injury and their subsequent coping patterns (Janoff-Bulman & Wortman, 1977). The findings suggested that those who tended to blame themselves for the accident were rated by medical and rehabilitation staff as coping better than those who blamed others and who felt the accident could have been avoided. Indeed, many respondents (e.g., passengers in cars, people accidentally shot) seemed to attribute more blame to themselves than might seem objectively reasonable. The authors interpreted the findings as reflecting attempts on the part of the victims to gain some control over their situations, for blaming oneself may be preferable to the conclusion that random harmful events may occur in a meaningless, chaotic world.

The results of the attribution literature concerning victims may be important in the field of clinical child neuropsychology because these and other forms of cognitive distortions may partially determine the quality of coping attempts. Moreover, "real world" findings may be counterintuitive at first glance; many psychologists might not consider, from an outsider's position, self-blame to be particularly adaptive or predictive of good progress in a rehabilitation program. The clinical utility of these forms of cognitions remains to be fully investigated, especially with children and especially over the long term.

Attribution theory has also been applied to other areas of child psychology: childhood depression and learning disabilities. According to the reformulated learned helplessness model (Abramson et al., 1978), depressed individuals make more internal, stable, and global attributions for failure and more external, unstable, and specific attributions for success than nondepressed individuals. Recent research has indicated that, like adults, depressed children have a more depressed attributional style than nondepressed children (Blumberg & Izard, 1985; Kaslow, Rehm, & Siegel, 1984), and that attributional style can be used to predict depressive symptoms 6 months later (Seligman et al., 1984).

A vignette may be illustrative here. A young man with a history of severe learning and attentional disorders was asked to make a videotape of his thoughts as he negotiated the transitions from childhood to adulthood, and he was reminiscing about past depressive experiences: "When I made pottery or anything else like that, everybody else thought it was fine. But I was my own worst enemy, thinking this is good for other people but it's not good for me. So I would go home and give it to my mother and she would say, 'Oh, thank-you!' A couple of hours after that I'd get upset because it's not good enough, and I'd break it . . . and I said 'I'm sorry mom, it's not good enough . . . *I'm* not good enough'."

With regard to learning difficulties, the attribution and learned helplessness literatures are also applicable (Thomas, 1979). It has been reported that children who attribute outcome to ability do not work as long or as hard as those who attribute outcome to effort (Dweck, 1975), and those who attribute failure to ability tend to be less persistent on learning tasks (Hiroto & Seligman, 1975). Diener and Dweck (1978) indicated that helpless children attribute failure to lack of ability, and nonhelpless children focused instead on self-monitoring and self-instructions. Compared with average and good readers, poor readers have been found to take less personal responsibility for success, and when they did make internal attributions for success, they were more likely to make effort rather than ability attributions (Butkowsky & Willows, 1980). The potential importance of research in this area is that interventions designed to alter attributional patterns (e.g., to shift attributions for failure from insufficient ability to insufficient effort) may result in improved academic performance (e.g., increased academic task persistence and achievement) (Dweck, 1975; Fowler & Peterson, 1981; Schunk, 1983).

Taken together, these lines of theory and results suggest a convergence of information. Attribution patterns affect coping in affective and cognitive domains, and they seem important in adjusting to both acute insults or accidents and long-standing developmental difficulties. Equally importantly, it is possible to modify children's attribution styles through relatively brief interventions. Future research regarding the development and alteration of attributions among children with neurological disorder may consequently prove worthwhile. It may be important, for instance, not only to investigate children's cognitive understanding of the facts of the disorder, but also to explore their perceptions of who or what is responsible for the situation, why it happened to them, and to what they attribute their present successes and failures.

Issues in Psychotherapy

During the past decade, the neuropsychological literature on professional training models (e.g., Meier, 1981) and intervention procedures (e.g., Edelstein & Couture, 1984; Miller, 1984; Trexler, 1982) generally reflected the position that intervention with individuals with neurologic disorder is most commonly cognitive–behavioral in nature. Given the forms of neurological signs and symptoms, such procedures are often warranted, efficient, and effective. In addition, however, some of the challenges to children's mental health described in this chapter might also be addressed within the context of a psychotherapeutic relationship. Moreover, there may be acute (hospitalization for diagnosis or surgery) and chronic (controlled epilepsy, minor head injury, learning disorder, neuromuscular disease) situations in which there are no major behavioral difficulties but in which clients may benefit from, and psychologists may desire, a somewhat different style of intervention. Taube and Calman (1992) have provided a model for the psychotherapy of patients with complex partial seizures that might be useful to consider in this vein.

A number of general considerations to be kept in mind by the therapist have been provided by Christ (1978), Geist (1979), and Small (1973).Therapeutic goals may include the provision of nonconfrontal understanding, support, and feedback during periods of confusion, anger, anxiety, and depression. Strengthening of reality testing, learning to select areas of success and to avoid those of failure, and the improvement of relationships with others may also be appropriate targets. Traditional psychotherapeutic emphases and processes may require modification, however. For example, the development of a therapeutic alliance may purposely be extended, allowing greater opportunities for clients to recognize and display their strengths. Primitive and fragile defenses may crumble with mild cognitive or affective stress, leading to catastrophic reactions that seem disproportionate to an outsider's appraisal of the stressor. It may thus be important to concentrate on building a defensive superstructure, using defenses that are more negotiable than frank denial or projection, such as displacement, rationalization, or intellectualization. The psychologist's concepts of client resistance must be modified in the face of slowly improving or impaired cognitive and integrative capacities, and the inability to recall may obviously reflect faulty memory and not repression of conflict. Finally, it should be remembered that those with neurological disorder do not work through a permanent disability as with a neurotic problem, nor do they "get over it" as with some normal developmental hurdles; instead, they must continually adjust to the dynamic nature of the disability itself and to its consequences at various levels in the systems hierarchy. For example, realistic limitations in adaptive abilities may prevent the adolescent from taking steps of autonomous action at the same age as most others. Indeed, true termination from therapy may not be desirable, and the option to return at developmentally stressful times may be a sensible alternative.

There is another therapeutic issue that deserves comment in order to provoke additional thought or research. A variety of sources suggest that it is important to instill a sense of realistic hope in clients with neurologic impairment. Travis (1976) recommended that those caring for children and adolescents with progressive muscular dystrophy establish a "context for security and an avenue for hope." Waddell (1983) discussed the hope that medical and familial people consign to children with life-threatening illnesses, and others considered the role of hope in the process of rehabilitation

(Boone, Roessler, & Cooper, 1978; Heinemann, Geist, & Magiera, 1983) and psychotherapy (Erickson, Post, & Paige, 1975; Frank, 1968; Green, 1977; Smith, 1983).

Although *hope* is a term used frequently in everyday conversation, and although casual introspection suggests it is a pervasive human construct, there is very little related psychological research. Classical literature provides some insight into the concept. Hope was one of the evils contained within Pandora's box, and indeed, the Greeks viewed hope as an illusion and as mankind's curse because fate was seen as unchangeable. Such sentiment is reflected in lines from Antigone: "We are of the tribe that asks questions, and asks them to the bitter end . . . we are of the tribe that hates your filthy hope, your docile, female hope; hope your whore." On the other hand, the Judeo-Christian message is essentially one of hope, and in various cultures the symbol now written in most medical charts for "female" has meant eros, fertility, and hope (Menninger, 1963).

Perhaps because of the religious nature of historic tradition and because hope is a difficult construct to operationalize, psychologists may have left the study of hope to theologians and philosophers, and concentrated instead on hopelessness. Still, hope may rightly be classified as a coping phenomenon incorporating a future orientation, optimistic affect, expectant cognition, response to external stress, and resultant motivation (Petiet, 1983). Although multidimensional, and although the cognitive and developmental prerequisites of hope remain to be specified for children, the idea that hope is a desirable state during medical recovery and rehabilitation has been investigated with adults (Boone *et al.,* 1978; Brackney & Westman, 1992; Brody, 1981; Dubree & Voge'phol, 1980; Heinemann *et al.,* 1983; Lillis & Prophit, 1991; Perley, Winget, & Placci, 1971; Rabkin, Williams, Neugebauer, Remien, & Goetz, 1990; Ruvelson, 1990), and could be explored with chronically ill children. And in something of a full circle, Gottschalk, Fronczek, and Buchsbaum (1993) have considered the neurobiology of hope and hopelessness.

Psychosocial Adjustment

Much ambiguity surrounds the issue of whether chronically ill children, including those with neuropsychological deficits, are maladjusted when compared with their "normal" peers; see Harper (1991) for historical research conceptualizations in childhood illness, disability, and rehabilitation. Findings are contradictory, and diverse methodologies make comparisons between studies difficult. It is generally accepted that children with chronic illnesses are at one and one-half to three times greater risk for behavioral, social, and psychological maladjustment than healthy peers (Perrin, 1986; Pless, 1984). Rutter, Graham, and Yule (1970) reported that the occurrence of psychiatric disorders among the general population of children and adolescents was 6.6%; for children with nonneurological chronic disease, 11.6%; those with epilepsy and no other pathology, 37.5%; and children and adolescents with epilepsy associated with organic brain disease, 58.3%.

Professionals and individuals involved with children with neurologic impairment should not be misled, however, by the temptation of such figures. For any particular child, the presence of neurological disorder does not necessarily imply lowered psychosocial adjustment. Individual reactions to disability are diverse, and specific disabilities have not been found to be related to specific personality types (Bronheim & Jacobstein, 1984; O'Dougherty, 1983; Pless & Nolan, 1991; Roessler & Bolton, 1978). Also, as Garrison and McQuiston (1989) pointed out, there are reasons to consider both individual-specific (Cadman, Boyle, Szatmari, & Offord, 1987) and disease-specific (Stein & Jessop, 1982) approaches to understanding the ways in which children adjust to their illnesses.

Psychiatric Symptomatology

The range of psychiatric symptoms displayed by children with neuropsychological disorders is similar to the behaviors of their nonhandicapped peers. Results from large-scale epidemiological studies of children with chronic illnesses suggest that these children experience lower academic achievement, greater absenteeism and truancy, and increased behavioral difficulties, nervousness, and aggression (Pless & Roghmann, 1971; Rutter, Tizard, & Whitmore, 1970). In addition, emotional dependence, poor social adjustment, low self-esteem, depression, anxiety, difficulties in sexual adjustment, embarrassment, regression, poor body image, excessive shyness, lifelong feelings of failure and inadequacy, immaturity, exaggerated self-consciousness, shame, and fearfulness have all been used to described the various experiences of chil-

dren with spina bifida, epilepsy, muscular dystrophy, cerebral palsy, cancer, and closed head injury.

A word of caution is necessary. Although it is true that discrete symptoms or symptom clusters may be manifest by individual children, it should not be construed that this laundry list of psychiatric symptoms uniformly affects ill children with neurological handicaps. All children, including those at high risk for developing psychiatric sequelae, will be individually influenced both by neurophysiological constraints of the disease and by events external to the presence of disease, such as premorbid coping style, family support, and social reaction to disease presentation. For example, social adjustment may be affected when children with spina bifida who are incontinent of bladder and bowel are avoided or teased by their peers because of their "outhouse syndrome" of smells (Bronheim & Jacobstein, 1984; Shurtleff, 1980). Similarly, the social stigma of epilepsy can increase embarrassment, feelings of shame, and a vigilant need for secrecy for some epileptic children (O'Dougherty, 1983). Depression, which is experienced by some children in all disease categories, may be exacerbated in muscular dystrophy around the time the child becomes wheelchair bound and the relentless nature of the disease becomes less deniable (Lindemann & Stranger, 1981; Pierpont, LeRoy, & Baldfinger, 1984). Expression of psychopathology, then, should be considered in context. Finally, the presence of behavioral symptoms that might be considered pathological in the healthy population may be appropriate or even adaptive in those with chronic illness (Drotar & Bush, 1985; Van-Dongen-Melman & Sanders-Woudstra, 1986), and resiliency may be more impressive than psychopathology (Stabler, 1988).

Self-Concept and Self-Esteem

As empirical studies on the effects of pathoneurological involvement on children's self-concept and self-esteem are sparse, the literature on chronically ill children suggests an equivocal response to this issue. Many studies offer findings of lowered self-esteem and poorer self-concepts (e.g., Lineberger, Hernandez, & Brantley, 1984; Tropauer, Franz, & Dilgard, 1970). In contrast, other researchers (e.g., Kellerman, Zeltzer, Ellenberg, Dash, & Rigler, 1980; Simmons et al., 1985; Tavormina, Kastner, Slater, & Watt, 1976) report no significant differences between various groups of chronically ill children and healthy peers. Anecdotal reports often emphatically suggest that impaired self-concept and self-esteem are intrinsic to the experience of chronic illness (Geist, 1979). Christ (1978), for example, suggested that children with neurologic impairment in psychotherapy view themselves as different, weird, or defective, at least from the time peer comparisons are first made in grade school or preschool. In general, greater agreement exists that children with neurological involvement or deficits are at increased risk for poorer self-concept and lowered self-esteem than their healthy peers (Lindemann & Stranger, 1981; Rutter, Graham, & Yule, 1970).

Although it is not yet clear precisely why these children may be at increased risk for poorer adjustment, perhaps an understanding can be found in the nature of the relationship of neurological deficit to the development of self-identity. The key question here may be, how does altered brain integrity affect the development of self-concept and self-esteem? For example, administration of a standard measure of perceived competence to a group of educable children with metal retardation suggested that these children did not make the same categorical distinctions of self-competence and general self-worth as children in the standardization samples evidenced (Harter, 1982).

At one extreme such a question implies that because of physiological limitations, some children do not develop self-concepts in the same manner that their normal peers do, reflecting perhaps a physiologically based lack of or unique processing of information. This notion is suggested by parents and teachers who are unsure of how much to expect from their handicapped child and wonder whether the child's behaviors reflect biological limitations. Yet, although brain integrity may indeed affect formation of self-concept, the lack of findings correlating one specific emotional or social pattern of behavior with a specific disease or deficit suggests that the relationship between brain functioning and self-concept is complex, mediated by environmental and biological variables, and cannot be subjected to unqualified reductionism.

Socialization

Although undoubtedly some people are arrantly satisfied living in relative isolation from family, friends, and community, most of us recognize the immeasurable importance of our relations with other people. Indeed, it is notable that children who are withdrawn or elect not to participate with their peers are considered by many to be maladjusted.

The relative importance of peer interactions increases with age and growing autonomy. For both normal children and those with neurologic impairment, the peer group has been described as instrumental in providing confirmation or disconfirmation of children's growing sense of competence and self-esteem, meeting dependency needs, a reference point for growing beliefs about sexuality, and a means of role rehearsal where dimensions of cooperative, competitive, and aggressive behaviors can be expressed (Battle, 1984). Additionally, peer groups are seen as a major source of communication and support, conversation and companionship, and fun and socializing for most adolescents (Resnick, 1984).

The importance of peer groups may even be greater for children with a handicap. For example, adolescent cancer patients have reported that spending time with their friends is of primary importance in their ability to cope (Zeltzer, LeBaron, & Zeltzer, 1984). Based on a study of survivors of childhood cancer, O'Malley, Koocher, Foster, and Slavin (1979) reported that a decrease in the number of social relationships during diagnosis and treatment had a negative impact on subjects' future adjustment. Minde, Hackett, Killou, and Silver (1972) reported that almost 50% of children with cerebral palsy who did not have a nonhandicapped friend were labeled psychiatrically deviant whereas less than 10% of those with nonhandicapped friends were so labeled. This finding is even more striking when one considers evidence suggesting that nonhandicapped children, especially boys, who initiate contact with a handicapped child generally have less social experience, are more isolated, and adhere less to peer values (Battle, 1984).

Although diminished interactions with one's peer group can deprive children of valuable pleasure and experience in their preparation for adulthood, for some children with neurological disorders, gaining access to and acceptance by their peer group can be a formidable task. Hospitalization and requisite medical treatments for some diseases take time away from school attendance and peer activities (Zeltzer et al., 1984). At other times, peers' superstitions and misunderstanding about the nature of the disease can result in cruel teasing and unwarranted ostracism, especially when unfounded fears of contagion are involved (Isaacs & McElroy, 1980). Children who experience a loss of mobility may also face social isolation as their opportunities to participate in the normal activities of childhood and adolescence are restricted.

In contrast to the external influences that may limit a handicapped child's full participation in peer group activities, for some children, social isolation and withdrawal are means of coping with their disease. Children who are frightened and embarrassed by a loss of control during a seizure, for example, may consciously or unconsciously remove themselves from the influences of peers in attempts to reduce feelings of being different, unattractive, or socially rejected (Ozuna, 1979). Others have noted that wheelchair-bound children and children with progressive muscular weakness can be come isolated and withdrawn, relying heavily on fantasy and imagination (Lindemann & Boyd, 1981; O'Dougherty, 1983).

Although children with obvious physical limitations can face rejection from peers because of their visible differences, visible handicaps may also at times be addressed and accepted more openly than deficits with few noticeable manifestations. Indeed, children whose disabilities are less obvious or are better controlled may suffer as much or more than their severely disabled counterparts (Hertzig, 1983; Pless, 1984). They may be teased for being slow, clumsy, or different, and often face the dilemma of trying to pass as normal peers, meeting the expectations of behavior and ability that such normalcy involves, or choosing to separate from the peer group, enduring consequent ridicule and isolation (O'Dougherty, 1983).

Independence and Autonomy

Emotional separateness and independence is recognized as a significant goal of childhood and adolescence, and a hallmark of adult adjustment. Although being special may be a plausible role for some people with a handicap, U.S. society expects individuals with a disability to strive maximally toward independence and autonomy (Parsons, 1964). The influences of neurological disorder, however, can run counter to goals of individuation, as illustrated in this case description quoted by Resnick (1984):

> While his age cohorts were arguing with parents over the length of their hair, he needed help washing his; while they were resisting doing assigned chores, he was unable to perform any; while they were battling curfew, he needed not only permission, but physical assistance in order to be out. Instead of sharing his peers' increased independence from parents and others, symbolized by mild acting out behaviors, this patient could merely fantasize his acting out, with his illness providing a constant reminder of his chronic dependent status. (p. 302)

Though not all children with neurological handicaps exhibit the same degree of physical limitation, they all share in an increased dependence on parents, medical staff, and sometimes siblings for physical, financial, and emotional support (Zeltzer et al., 1984). Although disorders that demand large amounts of time and care from parents and family might appear to encourage emotional dependence compared with other diseases, the critical issue remains how to foster developmentally appropriate independence and responsibility within the context of a child's neurological deficit. For "normal" children, autonomy invariably increases with age, and parental control usually decreases proportionally. Although the progression toward adulthood may not always be as smooth as many parents and children would prefer, in most cases autonomy and responsible adult action are considered birthrights. For children with neurological disorders, however, both the pathway to autonomy and the children's right to eventually assume traditionally adult responsibilities may be questionable (Kopelman, 1985). Physical and mental abilities that have been compromised by presence of disease may in some cases realistically limit a child's ability to assume such adult activities as driving a car or making important decisions regarding medical treatment. With adults, an assumption is made that everyone over a recognized legal age is competent to make decisions for themselves, unless proven otherwise, and implicit in this supposition is the attainment of a certain, unquantified level of maturity. For children with neurological disorders, the issue of emotional maturity becomes inextricably linked with physical disability.

The physical and other limitations that some neurological disorders impose incite some parents to become overly protective of their handicapped child. Such overprotection can be detrimental to the child's quest for autonomy and can too easily create an atmosphere that encourages children to remain overly dependent, both emotionally and physically, on others. At one extreme, children may become complacent, passively accepting the ministries of others. In contrast, overly demanding, noncompliant, acting-out, or intentionally guilt-provoking behaviors may represent attempts to separate from parental domination and establish self-responsibility, while also satisfying certain emotional needs (O'Dougherty, 1983). This secondary gain that many children experience from their dependent roles can be reinforced when parents are reluctant to expect or demand independence from their handicapped child (Resnick, 1984).

Noncompliance with medical procedures can become a difficult issue when children and adolescents are unable to assert their autonomy in appropriate ways. Similarly, changing needs during illness can also complicate the process of separation and autonomy. For example, Zeltzer *et al.* (1984) reported that immediately following diagnosis and during times of disease relapse, adolescents with cancer prefer a more passive, dependent role, being less involved with the management of their disease than parents and physicians wish them to be.

Impact on the Family

Nowhere is systems theory perhaps more useful than in investigating the family. As a unit the family is affected by the presence of chronic illness, whether the illness is of neurological origin or not (for a family systems and social-ecological model of adaptation and change in families of children with chronic illnesses, see Kazak, 1989). One is reminded of John Steinbeck's *The Pearl,* the story of a poor fisherman who found a pearl so inordinate in its beauty and consequences that the lives of the entire village were altered. The birth or diagnosis of a child with neurological disorder is not unlike Steinbeck's description that time had changed and everything hence would be either before the pearl or after the pearl. Although it is perhaps ubiquitous that a neurological disorder will alter the lives of the family and individuals close to the handicapped child, it is also the case that not all families are similarly affected. Some families report being strengthened by the continuing challenge; other families cannot withstand the stress and become dysfunctional or disintegrate. Presently, no direct cause-and-effect occurrences have been identified that would fully explicate or predict the interaction of chronic illness and family dynamics; rather, the influences are mosaic.

Stages of Family Growth

Various theorists have proposed different stages of family growth and development, including marriage, childbirth, early child rearing, child schooling and increasing independence, departure of children from home, and integration of loss as parents adjust to problems associated with being alone and growing older. This model is influenced both by family subsystems and by groups external to the nuclear family, such as extended family, friends, and community. Stage theories depicting special times of stress may inadequately portray the family of a child with a neurological disorder who must deal with burdens unlike those of their average counterparts, and additional crisis points have been suggested for families of chronically ill children: when parents first become aware of the child's handicap; when the child first becomes eligible for special educational services; when the child leaves school; and when parents are aging and can no longer assume responsibility for the care of their child (Bailey & Simeonsson, 1984).

Stage models of family development are useful in that they provide a framework with which to understand family dynamics; however, variability of family structures resulting from single parenthood, and ethnic, social, and financial differences make generalizations about the consequences of chronic childhood illness, including neurological disorders, on family life a dangerous task at best. For example, it has been suggested that the birth of a child with a handicap is more devastating for lower-socioeconomic-status families than for middle- and upper-class families; yet, little data are currently available on class-related coping characteristics of parents (Schilling, Schinke, & Kirkham, 1985). Similarly, anecdotal reports suggest the importance that a family's ethnic background can have on family coping and adjustment, and on medical compliance (Hobbs, Perrin, & Ireys, 1985). Although systematic investigation of socioeconomic–ethnic variables is sparse, such influences cannot be extricated from the daily lives of children with neurological impairment and must not be forgotten in our quest for greater understanding.

Stages of Parental Adjustment

The diagnosis of a chronic illness or neurological disorder marks the beginning of a stressful and confusing time for parents. Even when there has been some suspicion of illness, diagnosis represents an immediate confirmation of parents' fears and a removal of hope. Although each parent may not feel each of these emotions, fear, shock, horror, numbness or detachment, relief, helplessness, denial, sadness, anger or rage, anxiety, depression, and guilt are all likely to be experienced at various times (Drotar, Baskiewicz, Irvin, Kennell, & Klaus, 1975; Hobbs *et al.,* 1985; McCollum, 1981).

During the initial period of diagnosis, many parents experience shock and bewilderment and sometime feel the situation is unreal, that it must either be a dream or happening to someone else. They may discuss their child as if he or she were a textbook case rather than their own child (McCollum, 1981). Parents will often have many questions, such as: "How will my child's life be affected?" "Is there a cure?" "Will my child's life be shortened?" "What does the disease do?" "Could I have done something to avoid this?" Paradoxically, in their emotional turmoil many parents are unable to remember what professionals say and, although forgetting may be an understandable defense against emotional pain, its consequences can be exacerbated when parents view it as a sign of their own inadequacy. Embarrassed, they may turn to friends or books for information rather than repeatedly question professionals. Of course there is a healthy side to seeking information from others who have negotiated the same trials, and the blossoming "chat rooms" or "discussion groups" found on computer networks are testimony. At the least there have been ongoing supportive sessions for those with epilepsy, neuromuscular disease, pervasive developmental disorders, and trauma and psychiatric symptoms, and affected individuals may share their clinical situations and affective reactions for the very first time in the privacy of their homes. However, some sources of information, although well intentioned, may be highly inaccurate, and misconceptions about their child's disease can linger for years, at times to the detriment of effective treatment (Whitten, Waugh, & Moore, 1974). During this initial period parents may also refuse to believe the diagnosis and a period of "shopping around" for second medical opinions may ensue.

Sadness, anxiety, and grief, from its raging anger and tears to its heavy numbness and pain, frequently occur next as parents begin to fully experience the unjustness of the situation (Blacher, 1984). Parents grieve for the feared loss of their child through death, for the loss of their "normal" child, and for hopes and aspirations for their child that have been relinquished (Mattsson, 1972). The intensity of emotions experienced and the isolating effects of grief can cause some parents to wonder if their reactions are normal. Customary sources of comfort and solace, such as one's spouse, may be unavailable because they too are grieving. Anger can become a prominent emotion and parents may vent their anger at each other, at other healthy children, at hospitals, physicians, and psychologists, at their church or their God, and at times, their ill child (McCollum, 1981). Worry and anxiety may also increase as both the demands of care and the family's limitations become more evident. The stress and anxiety of this time may be associated with physical illness or symptoms in the parents and can cause parents to fear they too are sick. Inevitably, their child's illness confronts parents with their own mortality and eventual death (Isaacs & McElroy, 1980).

Progression to final stages in this coping model suggests parental acceptance of the child's handicap, an ability to emphasize positive aspects of the situation, and attenuation of the intensity of earlier feelings (Hobbs et al., 1985). The ability to master guilt, fear, and self-accusatory feelings of responsibility has been suggested as critical in determining parents' acceptance of their child's illness or handicap (Mattsson, 1972). Additionally, Mattsson suggested that the awareness of and ability to verbalize feelings indicates that parents are ready to accept the reality of the illness. Parental coping and acceptance are further facilitated through their use of various defense mechanisms, including rationalization; displacement and projection of feelings onto others such as medical professionals; intellectualization, including educating themselves about medical, physiological, and psychological aspects of the disease; identification with other parents of seriously ill children; and denial and isolation of helplessness and anxious feelings, especially during medical crises. The use of any of these defense mechanisms may at times be exasperating to people who are in contact with the ill child's parents, as is most obviously the case with angry and obstreperous parents. It is important to realize, however, that such "defense" mechanisms may be quite appropriate at different times in the course of the illness.

Although useful as a structure for understanding family adjustment, the utility of stage theories is limited in specific applications. The attendant feelings of a parent toward a chronically ill child may ebb and flow chaotically, and even without apparent crisis or problem they may experience many feelings simultaneously. Parents' grief and the need for coping may reoccur as their ill child reaches chronological and developmental milestones (Schilling et al., 1985). Some parents report that although they may have learned to live with their child's illness, they do not feel they will ever accept it (Hobbs et al., 1985).

The consequences of unresolved guilt, or the inability of parents to adequately accept and cope with their child's chronic illness, can negatively affect their relationship with their ill child and other relations within the family. At one extreme, parents may reject or severely neglect their disabled child by denying the presence of illness or the need for treatment, or by blaming abandoned careers, financial ruin, and much inconvenience on their ill child (Hobbs *et al.,* 1985). More frequently, prolonged parental overconcern leads to indulgence and overprotection. Family members become more loving toward the ill child, and normal rules and discipline are suspended. Although allowances need to be made according to the realistic limitations imposed by the disease or illness, changes in family attitude can be confusing and sick children are likely to gain a sense of their own vulnerability through the fears and reactions of their parents and siblings (Mattsson, 1972). Mattsson described four situations that may predispose parents to overprotection or rejection: the child is afflicted with a hereditary disorder found among relatives; the child was unwanted; the child was not expected to live at birth or as an infant; and emotional conflicts around the death of a close relative are aroused by the child's illness.

Parental Differences in Coping Style

There are some adaptive tasks that may be common for nearly all families with a child with a chronic illness, but allocation may vary. The coping styles of parents may differ according to gender. Findings suggest that women tend to employ interpersonal and cognitive coping strategies and men more frequently use cognitive coping patterns. Using their own health inventory, McCubbin, McCubbin, *et al.* (1983) factor analyzed the scaled responses of 100 families of children with cystic fibrosis. Mothers' coping efforts were directed at the interpersonal dimensions of family cohesiveness, support, and expressiveness; fathers placed more emphasis on maintaining the family through cooperation and minimizing conflicts in family interaction through the use of rigid rules and procedures. Similar coping profiles were reported by McCubbin, Nevin, *et al.* (1983) in a study of parents of children with cerebral palsy. Such findings are consistent with available research on developmentally disabled children that suggests that parents of handicapped children tend to be more traditional in terms of sex roles than other families.

Within traditional families the father's role is most frequently as provider first and parent second, and for mothers the reverse is true (O'Donnell, 1982). In a Colorado statewide survey by Linder and Chitwood (1984), fathers of handicapped infants and preschoolers reported that their time with their handicapped child was limited by job and other family demands, even though they desired to become more involved with their child. Mothers were found to be the primary source of information about their child for fathers, though fathers indicated that newsletters or training in working with their child would be helpful. Additionally, survey replies indicated that fathers were least interested in "someone to talk to about my child" as a means of information or source of comfort and solace. Such responses are consistent with findings in other studies, and may be partially comprehensible when one considers that husbands tend to rely on their wives for intimate support, whereas wives report turning to other women and friends for support. Women in general report more dissatisfaction with family life, less freedom and opportunity to develop self-interests, worse health, and less positive moods. This is perhaps not surprising, as wives and mothers are called on to balance the needs of their handicapped or ill child, unaffected children, and spouse, with their own needs.

Dyadic Relationships

It has already been suggested that the diagnosis of chronic illness or handicap in a young child may contribute to maternal overprotection (Mattsson, 1972). Such overprotection may result in the formation of an intense dyadic relationship, usually between mother and affected child, that isolates the dyad from other family interactions (Shapiro, 1983). This relationship then becomes an axis around which other family relations develop, especially other children's resentment of the special closeness between mother and handicapped child. Paradoxically the handicapped child may also develop feelings of being outside the family, participating primarily as an observer who is never fully accepted by other siblings or is fully a part of family life. Although such an intense relationship may represent a mother's conscious or unconscious efforts to atone for the guilt she may feel, its effects on the family can be severe. Psychodynamic theory clearly posits the insult to emergent self-identity and resultant psychopathology in response to prolonged and stage-inappropriate affective symbiosis. Spousal and sibling jealousies can also arise within the family system, and consequent emotional alliances that demarcate the family may actually only represent attempts at emotional connection and survival between members excluded from the dyad. For example, the birth of a chronically ill second child may leave the mother little time for her first child who soon may exhibit a clear preference for the father. Such alliances can readily exacerbate an already stressful family or marital situation.

Siblings

Some reports indicate that siblings of chronically ill children are more likely to have adjustment, behavioral, and academic difficulties (Allan, Townley, & Phelen, 1974; Lavigne & Ryan, 1979). Others suggest that although general mental health may remain stable, social adaptation may be compromised. Still other studies report no significant differences between comparison groups on measures of adjustment or sociability (Drotar, Crawford, & Bush, 1984). Again, although generalizations are to be made with caution as methodologies, patient groups, developmental levels, and comparison groups vary across studies, it may be reasonable to suggest that, like their siblings, brothers and sisters of neurologically impaired children are at increased risk for psychosocial maladjustment.

In some families the needs of healthy children can take second place to those of the ill sibling, especially during times of stress and crisis, and throughout the course of the illness parental adjustment and coping styles will directly influence healthy siblings. For example, depleted emotional reserves and lowered ability to communicate may make parents seem unavailable or rejecting. Younger children who are not yet cognitively able to interpret their parents' feelings or understand what is happening with their ill sibling will tend to effect individual interpretations of the family situation. They may feel guilty, or blame themselves for their sibling's illness. Children may also fear they are susceptible to the same fate, and older children may wonder if they are potential genetic carriers (McCollum, 1981). Distribution of labor may change in the family and researchers have suggested that older female siblings perform a disproportionate share of extra chores. In other comparisons, younger male siblings have been reported to be more sensitive to peers' comments about the illness (Hobbs *et al.*, 1985).

Discussion

It has been assumed in this chapter that the human organism is a complex web of interaction, with normal and pathological developments taking place at multiple levels, from the biological to the social. Under this assumption, the understanding and significance of neurologically based changes in sensorimotor functioning, in cognitive and executive capacities, or in emotion and behavior are enhanced by placing these alterations in a social and historic context. When neuropsychologists listen to their clients, they may hear expected questions about the brain and the consequences of its disorder. Yet in our experiences, these questions do not often end with anatomy and physiology, or with strict brain–behavior relationships *per se*. Instead, the concerns of clients, both children and adults, extend to attempts to make sense of their condition and to the ramifications of their neurological disorder in the context of family, school, and social settings, and in terms of past experience and future expectations. Consideration of these temporal and ecological dimensions may thus lead to a richer understanding of the implications of neurological disorder in the lives of children, and may suggest additional directions for assessment and intervention in clinical child neuropsychology. Some of the topics included here have been selected for their utility in provoking additional research. In most instances, the topics purposefully suspend the trend toward reductionism in the social sciences and advocate the application of theory and methods from other domains of psychology to the field of neuropsychology.

References

Abramson, L. Y., Seligman, M. E. P., & Teasdale, J. D. (1978). Learned helplessness in humans: Critique and reformulation. *Journal of Abnormal Psychology, 87,* 49–74.

Allan, J., Townley, R., & Phelen, P. (1974). Family response to cystic fibrosis. *Australian Pediatrics Journal, 10,* 136–146.

Bailey, D. B., & Simeonsson, R. J. (1984). Critical issues underlying research and intervention with families of young handicapped children. *Journal of the Division for Early Childhood, 8,* 38–48.

Bandura, A. (1977). Self-efficacy: Toward a unifying theory of behavioral change. *Psychological Review, 84,* 191–215.

Battle, C. U. (1984). Disruptions in the socialization of a young, severely handicapped child. In R. P. Marinelli & A. E. DelOrto (Eds.), *The psychological and social impact of physical disability.* Berlin: Springer.

Bernstein, J. H., & Waber, D. P. (1990). Developmental neuropsychological assessment: In A. A. Boulton, G. B. Baker, & M. Hiscock (Eds.), *Neuromethods: Vol. 17,*

Neuropsychology (pp. 311–371). Clifton, NJ: Humana Press.

Bibace, R., & Walsh, M. E. (1979). Developmental stages in children's conceptions of illness. In G. C. Stone, F. Cohen, & N. E. Adler (Eds.), *Health psychology* (pp. 285–301). San Francisco: Jossey–Bass.

Blacher, J. (1984). Sequential stages of parental adjustment to the birth of a child with handicaps: Fact or artifact? *Mental Retardation, 22,* 359–371.

Blumberg, S. H., & Izard, C. E. (1985). Affective and cognitive characteristics of depression in 10 and 11 year old children. *Journal of Personality and Social Psychology, 49,* 194–202.

Boll, T. (1985). Developing issues in clinical neuropsychology. *Journal of Clinical and Experimental Neuropsychology, 7,* 473–485.

Boone, S. E., Roessler, R. T., & Cooper, P. G. (1978). Hope and manifest anxiety: Motivational dynamics of acceptance of disability. *Journal of Counseling Psychology, 25,* 551–556.

Brackney, B. E., & Westman, A. S. (1992). Relationships among hope, psychosocial development, and locus of control. *Psychological Reports, 70,* 864–867.

Brewster, A. B. (1982). Chronically ill hospitalized children's concepts of their illness. *Pediatrics, 69,* 355–362.

Brodie, B. (1974). View of healthy children toward illness. *American Journal of Public Health, 64,* 1156–1159.

Brody, H. (1981). Hope. *Journal of the American Medical Association, 246,* 1411–1412.

Bronheim, S. M., & Jacobstein, D. M. (1984). Psychosocial assessment in chronic and fatal illness. In P. R. Magrab (Ed.), *Psychological and behavioral assessment: Impact on pediatric care.* New York: Plenum Press.

Butkowsky, I. S., & Willows, D. M. (1980). Cognitive–motivational characteristics of children varying in reading ability: Evidence for learned helplessness in poor readers. *Journal of Educational Psychology, 72,* 408–422.

Cadman, D., Boyle, M. H., Szatmari, P., & Offord, D. R. (1987). Chronic illness, disability, and mental and social well-being: Findings of the Ontario Child Health Study. *Pediatrics, 79,* 805–813.

Campbell, J. D. (1975) Illness is a point of view. The development of children's concepts of illness. *Child Development, 46,* 92–100.

Canan, C. (1993). Common adaptive tasks facing parents of children with chronic conditions. *Journal of Advanced Nursing, 18,* 46–53.

Carandang, M. L. A., Folkins, C. H., Hines, P. A., & Steward, M. S. (1979). The role of cognitive level and sibling illness in children's conceptualizations of illness. *American Journal of Orthopsychiatry, 49,* 474–481.

Chan, K. B. (1977). Individual differences in reactions to stress and their personality and situational determinants: Some implications for community mental health. *Social Science and Medicine, 11,* 89–103.

Christ, A. E. (1978). Therapy of the child with true brain damage. *American Journal of Orthopsychiatry, 48,* 505–515.

Curry, S. L., & Russ, S. W. (1985). Identifying coping strategies in children. *Journal of Clinical Child Psychology, 14,* 61–69.

Diener, C. I., & Dweck, C. S. (1978). An analysis of learned helplessness: Effects of aversive stimulation on subsequent performance. *Journal of Experimental Psychology: Human Perception and Performance, 1,* 411–417.

Drotar, D. (1981). Psychological perspectives in chronic childhood illness. *Journal of Pediatric Psychology, 6,* 211–228.

Drotar, D., Baskiewicz, A., Irvin, N., Kennell, J., & Klaus, M. (1975). The adaptation of parents to the birth of an infant with a congenital malformation: A hypothetical model. *Pediatrics, 56,* 710–717

Drotar, D., & Bush, M. (1985). Mental health issues and services. In N. Hobbs & J. M. Perrin (Eds.), *Issues in the care of children with chronic illness* (pp. 514–550). San Francisco: Jossey–Bass.

Drotar, D., Crawford, P., & Bush, M. (1984). The family context of chronic childhood illness: Implications for psychological intervention. In M. Eisenberg (Ed.), *Chronic illness and disability through the life span: Effects on self and family.* Berlin: Springer.

Dubowitz, V. (1977). Mental retardation in Duchenne muscular dystrophy. In L. P. Rowland (Ed.), *Pathogenesis of human muscular dystrophies.* Amsterdam: Excerpta Medica.

Dubree, M., & Voge'pohl, R. (1980). When hope dies—so might the patient. *American Journal of Nursing, 80,* 2046–2049.

Dweck, C. S. (1975). The role of expectations and attributions in the alleviation of learned helplessness. *Journal of Personality and Social Psychology, 31,* 674–685.

Edelstein, B. A., & Couture, E. T. (Eds.). (1984). *Behavioral assessment and rehabilitation of the traumatically brain-damaged.* New York: Plenum Press.

Engle, G. (1977). The clinical application of the biopsychosocial model. *American Journal of Psychiatry, 137,* 535–544.

Engle, G. (1980). The need for a new medical model: The challenge for biomedicine. *Science, 196,* 129–136.

Erickson, R. C., Post, R. D., & Paige, A. B. (1975). Hope as a psychiatric variable. *Journal of Clinical Psychology, 31,* 324–330.

Folkman, S., & Lazarus, R. S. (1980). An analysis of coping in a middle-aged community sample. *Journal of Health and Social Behavior, 21,* 219–239.

Fowler, J. W., & Peterson, P. L. (1981). Increasing reading persistence and altering attributional style of learned helpless children. *Journal of Educational Psychology, 73,* 251–260.

Frank, J. (1968). The role of hope in psychotherapy. *International Journal of Psychiatry, 5,* 383–395.

Garrison, W. T., & McQuiston, S. (1989). *Chronic illness during childhood and adolescence: Psychological aspects.* Newbury Park, CA: Sage.

Geist, R. A. (1979). Onset of chronic illness in children and adolescents: Psychotherapeutic and consultative intervention. *American Journal of Orthopsychiatry, 49,* 4–23.

Gochman, D. S. (1985). Family determinants of children's concepts of health and illness. In D. Turk & R. Kerns (Eds.), *Health, illness, and families.* New York: Wiley.

Goldstein, K. (1939). *The organism*. New York: American Book Co.

Goldstein, K. (1940). *Human nature in the light of psychopathology*. Cambridge, MA: Harvard University Press.

Goldstein, K. (1952). The effect of brain damage on personality. *Psychiatry, 15,* 245–260.

Gottschalk, L. A., Fronczek, J., & Buchsbaum, M. S. (1993). The cerebral neurobiology of hope and hopelessness. *Psychiatry: Interpersonal and Biological Processes, 56,* 270–282.

Green, M. R. (1977). Anticipation, hope, and despair. *Journal of the American Academy of Psychoanalysis, 5,* 215–232.

Harper, D. C. (1991). Paradigms for investigating rehabilitation and adaptation to childhood disability and chronic illness. *Journal of Pediatric Psychology, 16,* 533–542.

Harter, S. (1978). Effectance motivation reconsidered: Toward a developmental model. *Human Development, 1,* 34–64.

Harter, S. (1979). *Perceived Competence Scale for Children. Manual.* Boulder, CO: University of Denver.

Harter, S. (1982). The Perceived Competence Scale for Children. *Child Development, 53,* 87–97.

Harter, S. (1985). Processes underlying the construction, maintenance, and enhancement of the self-concept in children. In J. Suls & A. Greenwald (Eds.), *Psychological perspectives on the self (Vol. 3)*. Hillsdale, NJ: Erlbaum.

Heinemann, A., Geist, C., & Magiera, R. (1983). *The role of hope in spinal cord injury rehabilitation.* Paper presented at the 91st annual conference, American Psychological Association, Anaheim, CA.

Hertzig, M. E. (1983). Temperament and neurological status. In M. Rutter (Ed.), *Developmental neuropsychiatry* (pp. 164–180). New York: Guilford Press.

Hiroto, D. S., & Seligman, M. E. P. (1975). Generality of learned helplessness in man. *Journal of Personality and Social Psychology, 31,* 311–327.

Hobbs, N., Perrin, J. M., & Ireys, H. T. (1985). *Chronically ill children and their families.* San Francisco: Jossey–Bass.

Isaacs, J., & McElroy, M. R. (1980). Psychosocial aspects of chronic illness in children. *Journal of School Health, 50,* 318–321.

Janoff-Bulman, R., & Frieze, I. H. (1983). A theoretical perspective for understanding reactions to victimization. *Journal of Social Issues, 39,* 1–17.

Janoff-Bulman, R., & Wortman, C. B. (1977). Attributions of blame and coping in the "real world": Severe accident victims react to their lot. *Journal of Personality and Social Psychology, 35,* 351–363.

Karagan, N. J. (1979). Intellectual functioning in Duchenne muscular dystrophy. *Psychological Bulletin, 86,* 250–259.

Kaslow, N. J., Rehm, L. P., & Siegel, A. W. (1984). Social–cognitive correlates of depression in children. *Journal of Abnormal Child Psychology, 12,* 605–620.

Kazak, A. E. (1989). Families of chronically ill children: A systems and socio-ecological model of adaptation and challenge. *Journal of Consulting and Clinical Psychology, 57,* 25–30.

Kellerman, J., Zeltzer, L., Ellenberg, L., Dash, J., & Rigler, D. (1980). Psychological effects of illness in adolescence. *Journal of Pediatrics, 97,* 126–131.

Kerns, R., & Curley, A. (1985). A biopsychosocial approach to illness and the family: Neurological diseases across the life span. In D. Turk & R. Kerns (Eds.), *Health, illness, and families.* New York: Wiley.

Kerns, R., & Turk, D. (1985). Behavioral medicine and the family: Historical perspectives and future directions. In D. Turk & R. Kerns (Eds.), *Health, illness, and families.* New York: Wiley.

Knights, R. M., Hinton, G., & Drader, D. (1973). Changes in intellectual ability with Duchenne muscular dystrophy. *Research Bulletin #8,* Department of Psychology, Carleton University, Ottawa, Canada.

Kopelman, L. (1985). Paternalism and autonomy in the care of chronically ill children. In N. Hobbs & J. M. Perrin (Eds.), *Issues in the care of children with chronic illness* (pp. 61–86). San Francisco: Jossey–Bass.

Kroeber, T. C. (1964). The coping functions of ego mechanisms. In R. W. White (Ed.), *The study of lives.* New York: Atherton.

Lavigne, J., & Ryan, M. (1979). Psychological adjustment of siblings of children with chronic illness. *Pediatrics, 63,* 616–627.

Lazarus. R. S. (1983). The costs and benefits of denial. In S. Breznetz (Ed.), *Denial of stress.* New York: International Universities Press.

Leventhal, H., Leventhal, E., & Van Nguyen, T. (1985). Reactions of families to illness: Therapeutic models and perspectives. In D. Turk & R. Kerns (Eds.), *Health, illness, and families.* New York: Wiley.

Levine, M. D. (1990). *Keeping a head in school.* Cambridge, MA: Educators Publishing Service.

Levine, M. D. (1993). *All kinds of minds.* Cambridge, MA: Educators Publishing Service.

Lillis, P. P., & Prophit, P. (1991). Keeping hope alive. *Nursing, 21,* 65–67.

Lindemann, J. E., & Boyd, R. D. (1981). Myelomenigocele. In J. E. Lindemann (Ed.), *Psychological and behavioral aspects of physical disability.* New York: Plenum Press.

Lindemann, J. E., & Stranger, M. E. (1981). Progressive muscle disorders. In J. E. Lindemann (Ed.), *Psychological and behavioral aspects of physical disability.* New York: Plenum Press.

Linder, T. W., & Chitwood, D. G. (1984). The needs of fathers of young handicapped children. *Journal of the Division of Early Childhood, 9,* 133–139.

Lineberger, H. P., Hernandez, J. T., & Brantley, H. T. (1984). Self-concept and locus of control in hemophiliacs. *International Journal of Psychiatry in Medicine, 14,* 243–251.

Luthar, S. S., & Zigler, E. (1991). Vulnerability and competence: A review of research on resilience in childhood. *American Journal of Orthopsychiatry, 61,* 6–22.

McCollum, A. T. (1981). *The chronically ill child: A guide for parents and professionals.* New Haven: Yale University Press.

McCubbin, H. I., McCubbin, M. A., Patterson, J. M., Cauble, A. E., Wilson, L. R., & Warwick, W. (1983). CHIP—coping health inventory for parents: An assessment of parental coping patterns in the care of the chronically ill child. *Journal of Marriage and the Family, 45,* 359–370.

McCubbin, H. I., Nevin, R. S., Cauble, A. E., Larsen, A., Comeau, J., & Patterson, J. M. (1983). Family coping with chronic illness: The case of cerebral palsy. In H. I. McCubbin, A. E. Cauble, & J. M. Patterson (Eds.), *Family stress, coping, and social support.* Springfield, IL: Thomas.

Maddux, J. E., Roberts, M. C., Sledden, E. A., & Wright, L. (1986). Developmental issues in child health psychology. *American Psychologist, 41,* 25–34.

Maheady, L., & Maitland, G. E. (1982). Assessing social perception abilities in learning disabled students. *Learning Disabilities Quarterly, 5,* 363–370.

Massie, R. K. (1985). The constant shadow. Reflections on the life of a chronically ill child. In N. Hobbs & J. Perrin (Eds.), *Issues in the care of children with chronic illness* (pp. 13–23). San Francisco: Jossey–Bass.

Mattsson, A. (1972). Long-term physical illness in childhood: A challenge to psychosocial adaptation. *Pediatrics, 50,* 801–811.

Mearig, J. S. (1979). The assessment of intelligence in boys with Duchenne muscular dystrophy. *Rehabilitation Literature, 40,* 262–274.

Mearig, J. S. (1985). Cognitive development of chronically ill children. In N. Hobbs & J. M. Perrin (Eds.), *Issues in the care of children with chronic illness* (pp. 672–697). San Francisco: Jossey–Bass.

Mechanic, D. (1964). The influence of mothers on their children's health attitudes and behaviors. *Pediatrics, 33,* 444–453.

Meier, M. J. (1981). Education for competency assurance in human neuropsychology: Antecedents, models, and directions. In S. Filskov & T. Boll (Eds.), *Handbook of clinical neuropsychology* (pp. 754–781). New York: Wiley.

Menninger, K. (1963). *The vital balance.* New York: Viking Press.

Miller, E. (1984). *Recovery and management of neuropsychological impairments.* New York: Wiley.

Millon, T., Green, C., & Meagher, R. (1982). *Handbook of clinical health psychology.* New York: Plenum Press.

Minde, K. K., Hackett, J. D., Killou, D., & Silver, S. (1972). How they grow up: 41 physically handicapped children and their families. *American Journal of Psychiatry, 128,* 1554–1560.

Myers-Vando, R., Steward, M., Folkins, C. H., & Hines, P. (1979). The effects of congenital heart disease on cognitive development, illness causality concepts, and vulnerability. *American Journal of Orthopsychiatry, 49,* 617–625.

Neuhauser, C., Amsterdam, B., Hines, P., & Steward, M. (1978). Children's concepts of healing: Cognitive development and locus of control factors. *American Journal of Orthopsychiatry, 48,* 335–341.

O'Donnell, L. (1982). The social worlds of parents. *Marriage and Family Review, 5,* 9–36.

O'Dougherty, M. M. (1983). *Counseling the chronically ill child: Psychological impact and intervention.* Lexington: Lewis Publishing.

O'Malley, J. E., Koocher, G., Foster, D., & Slavin, L. (1979). Psychiatric sequelae of surviving a childhood cancer. *American Journal of Orthopsychiatry, 49,* 608–616.

Ozuna, J. (1979). Psychosocial aspects of epilepsy. *Journal of Neurosurgical Nursing, 11,* 242–246.

Palmer, B., & Lewis, C. (1976). Development of health attitudes and behaviors. *Journal of School Health, 46,* 401–402.

Parsons, O., & Prigatano, G. (1978). Methodological considerations in clinical neuropsychological research. *Journal of Consulting and Clinical Psychology, 46,* 608–619.

Parsons, T. (1964). *Social structure and personality.* Glencoe, IL: Free Press.

Perley, J., Winget, C., & Placci, C. (1971). Hope and discomfort as factors influencing treatment continuance. *Comprehensive Psychiatry, 12,* 557–563.

Perrin, J. M. (1986). Chronically ill children: An overview. *Topics in Early Childhood Special Education, 5,* 1–11.

Perrin, J. M., & Gerrity, P. S. (1981). There's a demon in your belly: Children's understanding of illness. *Pediatrics, 67,* 841–849.

Petiet, C. A. (1983). *Hope: The major predictor of positive resolution after marital loss.* Paper presented at the 91st annual conference, American Psychological Association, Anaheim, CA.

Pierpont, M. E., LeRoy, B., & Baldfinger, S. (1984). Genetic disorders. In R. W. Blum (Ed.), *Chronic illness and disability in childhood and adolescence.* New York: Grune & Stratton.

Pless, I. B. (1984). Clinical assessment: Physical and psychological functioning. *Pediatric Clinics of North America, 31,* 33–45.

Pless, I. B., & Nolan, T. (1991). Revision, replication, and neglect: Research on maladjustment in chronic illness. *Journal of Child Psychology, Psychiatry, and Allied Disciplines, 32,* 347–365.

Pless, I. B., & Roghmann, K. J. (1971). Chronic illness and its consequences: Observations based on three epidemiologic surveys. *Journal of Pediatrics, 79,* 351–359.

Potter, P. C., & Roberts, M. C. (1984). Children's perceptions of chronic illness: The roles of disease symptoms, cognitive development, and information. *Journal of Pediatric Psychology, 9,* 13–27.

Rabkin, J. G., Williams, J. B. W., Neugebauer, R., Remien, R. H., & Goetz, R. (1990). Maintenance of hope in HIV-spectrum homosexual men. *American Journal of Psychiatry, 147,* 1322–1327.

Resnick, M. (1984). The teenager with cerebral palsy. In R. W. Blum (Ed.), *Chronic illness and disability in childhood and adolescence.* New York: Grune & Stratton.

Riese, W. (1977). Dynamics in brain lesions. In Y. Lebrun & E. Buyssens (Eds.), *Selected papers on the history of aphasia.* Amsterdam: Swets & Zeitlinger.

Roessler, R., & Bolton, B. (1978). *Psychosocial adjustment to disability.* Baltimore: University Park Press.

Rourke, B. P. (1985). *Neuropsychology of learning disabilities: Essentials of subtype analysis.* New York: Guilford Press.

Rutter, M. (1981). Stress, coping, and development: Some issues and some questions. *Journal of Child Psychology and Psychiatry, 22,* 323–356.

Rutter, M. (1986). Meyerian psychobiology, personality development, and the role of life experiences. *American Journal of Psychiatry, 143,* 1077–1087.

Rutter, M., Graham, P., & Yule, W. (1970). *A neuropsychiatric study in childhood* (Clinics in Developmental Medicine Nos. 35 and 36). London: Spastics International Medical Publications/Heinemann Medical Books.

Rutter, M., Tizard, J., & Whitmore, K. (1970). *Education, health and behavior: Psychological and medical study of childhood development.* London: Longman.

Ruvelson, L. (1990). The tense tightrope: How patients and their therapists balance hope and hopelessness. *Clinical Social Work Journal, 18,* 145–155.

Ryan-Wenger, N. M. (1992). A taxonomy of children's coping strategies: A step toward theory development. *American Journal of Orthopsychiatry, 62,* 256–263.

Schibuk, M., Bond, M., & Bouffard, R. (1989). The development of defenses in childhood. *Canadian Journal of Psychiatry, 34,* 581–588.

Schilling, R. F., Schinke, S. P., & Kirkham, M. A. (1985). Coping with a handicapped child: Differences between mothers and fathers. *Social Science and Medicine, 21,* 857–863.

Schunk, D. H. (1983). Ability versus effort attributional feedback: Differential effects on self-efficacy and achievement. *Journal of Educational Psychology, 76,* 1159–1169.

Seligman, M. E. P., Peterson, C., Kaslow, N. J., Tanenbaum, R. L., Alloy, L. B., & Abramson, L. Y. (1984). Attributional style and depressive symptoms among children. *Journal of Abnormal Psychology, 93,* 235–238.

Shapiro, J. (1983). Family reactions and coping strategies in response to the physically ill or handicapped child: A review. *Social Science and Medicine, 17,* 913–931.

Shontz, F. C. (1982). Adaptation to chronic illness. In T. Millon, C. Green, & R. Meagher (Eds.), *Handbook of clinical health psychology* (pp. 153–172). New York: Plenum Press.

Shurtleff, D. B. (1980). Myelodysplasia: Management and treatment. *Current Problems in Pediatrics, 10,* 1–98.

Siegal, M. (1988). Children's knowledge of contagion and contamination as causes of illness. *Child Development, 59,* 1353–1359.

Simmons, R. J., Corey, M., Cowen, L., Keenan, N., Robertson, J., & Levison, H. (1985). Emotional adjustment of adolescents with cystic fibrosis. *Psychosomatic Medicine, 47,* 111–122.

Small, L. (1973). *Neurodiagnosis in psychotherapy.* New York: Brunner/Mazel.

Smith, A. (1979). Practices and principles of clinical neuropsychology: Focusing on the hole rather than the doughnut. *International Journal of Neuroscience, 9,* 233–238.

Smith, M. B. (1983). Hope and despair: Keys to the socio-psycho-dynamics of youth. *American Journal of Orthopsychiatry, 53,* 388–399.

Sollee, N. D., Latham, E. E., Kindlon, D. J., & Bresnan, M. J. (1985). Neuropsychological impairment in Duchenne muscular dystrophy. *Journal of Clinical and Experimental Neuropsychology, 7,* 486–496.

Stabler, B. (1988). Perspectives on chronic childhood illness. In B. G. Malamed, K. A. Mathews, D. K. Rauth, B. Stabler, & N. Schneiderman (Eds.), *Child health psychology.* Hillsdale, NJ: Erlbaum.

Stein, R. E. K., & Jessop, D. J. (1982). A noncategorical approach to chronic childhood illness. *Public Health Reports, 97,* 354–362.

Stipek, D., & Weisz, J. R. (1981). Perceived personal control and academic achievement. *Review of Educational Research, 51,* 101–137.

Taube, S. L., & Calman, N. H. (1992). The psychotherapy of patients with complex partial seizures. *American Journal of Orthopsychiatry, 62,* 35–43.

Tavormina, J. B., Kastner, L. S., Slater, P. M., & Watt, S. L. (1976). Chronically ill children: A psychologically and emotionally deviant population? *Journal of Abnormal Child Psychology, 4,* 99–110.

Thomas, A. (1979). Learned helplessness and expectancy factors: Simplifications for research in learning disabilities. *Review of Educational Research, 49,* 208–221.

Tobin, D. L., Holroyd, K. A., Reynolds, R. V., & Wigal, J. K. (1989). The hierarchical factor structure of the Coping Strategies Inventory. *Cognitive Therapy and Research, 13,* 343–361.

Travis, G. (1976). *Chronic illness in children: Its impact on child and family.* Stanford: Stanford University Press.

Trexler, L. E. (Ed.). (1982). *Cognitive rehabilitation: Conceptualization and intervention.* New York: Plenum Press.

Tropauer, A., Franz, N. M., & Dilgard, V. W. (1970). Psychological aspects of the care of children with cystic fibrosis. *American Journal of Diseases in Childhood, 119,* 424.

Van Dongen-Melman, J. E. W. M., & Sanders-Woudstra, J. A. R. (1986). Psychosocial aspects of childhood cancer: A review of the literature. *Journal of Child Psychology and Psychiatry, 27,* 145–180.

von Bertalanffy, L. (1968). *General systems theory.* New York: Braziller.

Waddell, C. (1983). *Faith, hope, and luck: A sociological study of children growing up with a life-threatening illness.* Washington, DC: University Press of America.

Weisz, J. R., & Stipek, D. J. (1982). Competence, contingency, and the development of personal control. *Human Development, 25,* 250–281.

Whelan, T. (1986). *Neuropsychological performance, reading achievement, and perceptions of competence in boys with Duchenne muscular dystrophy.* Paper presented at the 14th annual meeting, International Neuropsychological Society, Denver.

Whelan, T. (1987). Neuropsychological performance of children with Duchenne muscular dystrophy and spinal muscle atrophy. *Developmental Medicine and Child Neurology, 29,* 207–211.

Whitt, J. K., Dykstra, W., & Taylor, C. (1979). Children's conceptions of illness and cognitive development. *Clinical Pediatrics, 18,* 327–339.

Whitten, C., Waugh, D., & Moore, A. (1974). Unmet needs of parents of children with sickle cell anemia. In J. Hercules (Ed.), *Proceedings of the first national symposium on sickle cell disease.* Bethesda: National Heart, Lung, and Blood Institute.

Wortman, C. B. (1983). Coping with victimization: Conclusions and implications for future research. *Journal of Social Issues, 39,* 195–221.

Zeltzer, L., LeBaron, S., & Zeltzer, P. (1984). The adolescent with cancer. In R. W. Blum (Ed.), *Chronic illness and disability in childhood and adolescence.* New York: Grune & Stratton.

35

Psycholegal Issues for Clinical Child Neuropsychology

From a legal perspective, the specialty of clinical child neuropsychology has progressed to a new stage of professionalism. Despite a myriad of public-policy forces continuing to create countervalences for definition and placement in human services, clinical child neuropsychology has clearly established itself as a viable clinical specialty. Healthcare professionals (with a few sociopolitically motivated exceptions) have embraced neuropsychology in general and clinical child neuropsychology in particular into neurologically related services, and endorsed making the services available in a plethora of clinical settings. Important research has occurred, such as refinements in psychological tests for neuropsychological interpretations, which strengthens the specialty and provides it with distinction from adult neuropsychology. As a specialization, clinical child neuropsychology is well within the scope of common practices for clinical, counseling, and school psychologists.

This expansion and dissemination is consonant with the scientist-practitioner model and is especially true for applications in healthcare and educational settings. In asserting that there is "only one psychology, no specialties, but many applications," Matarazzo (1987) states that "the discipline-specific core content of the predoctoral curriculum of courses in university departments of psychology for students in one so-called psychology predoctoral 'special track' does not differ substantially from that for students in another specialty track" (p. 893).

Interfacing the application of clinical child neuropsychology with legal considerations, there is strong reason to maintain that: (1) allegiance to being a behavioral scientist or generalist must predicate more specialized services (such as clinical child neuropsychology) and (2) the legal arena will be open to psychologists without highly advanced training in skills in clinical neuropsychology. The foregoing two assertions introduce the possibility of both legal protection and special liability for the practitioner of clinical child neuropsychology. These two premises will be interwoven in the subsequent discussion of forensic issues.

Psycholegal Issue One: Public Policy Is in Conflict over Mental Health Services

As the dawn of the 21st century approaches, healthcare reform is one of the foremost concerns of our nation. From the federal government, there is considerable impetus to change the structure of healthcare services and the roles of healthcare providers (see DeLeon, VandenBos, & Bulato, 1991, for a history of the federal policy initiative). Although there seems little doubt that changes are needed, the political influences lead to questions about the wisdom and motives of the alternatives.

It would appear that there will be continual revision of public policy, especially as manifested in government regulations and programs, for years to come. Therefore, what may be the dominant model today may be considerably different tomorrow. At present, it is prudent to hold that all healthcare ser-

ROBERT HENLEY WOODY • Department of Psychology, University of Nebraska at Omaha, Omaha, Nebraska 68182-0272.

vices are being scrutinized and none has assured support. Regrettably, it must be acknowledged that mental health services seem to be particularly vulnerable. Despite being given inclusion in various proposed healthcare reform plans, mental health services have not, thus far, received notable priority and many wags believe mental health services will be the first services to be eliminated or diminished at budget-trimming time.

As for children, there does seem to be an emerging accommodation within public policy, albeit without a clear-cut and long-term financial commitment. Of concern, however, there is a strong movement away from specialized services, at least as would be financed under third-party payment sources. Writing as an insider with the Clinton Administration, Starr (1994) sets forth the view that healthcare reform emphasizes cost reduction, accountability by practitioners, and alternative (lesser trained) providers; note that there seems to be minimal concern about quality. As Wiggins (1990) indicates, "The message is very clear that the re-definition of the health care market is based on economics rather than patient care" (p. 51).

A concomitant of healthcare reform is a marked increase in managed healthcare systems, whereby a source other than the practitioner determines what services are needed (and commonly the criterion is financial, rather than clinical benefit). Managed healthcare strips quality control away from the healthcare professional, and places treatment decisions with the payment-source's accountant: "The health care revolution is an attempt to wrest control of the health system and its costs from professionals" (Kiesler & Morton, 1988, p. 998). At the same time, the legal liability is left with the psychologist (Appelbaum, 1993).

It should be noted that the conflict between financial and treatment sources is leading, all too often, to blundering attempts to accommodate discrepant objectives. For example, nursing homes, a primary setting for clinical neuropsychological services, are witnessing stringent third-party monitoring of the neuropsychological services provided therein. At the same time, by at least one account (Kiesler & Sibulkin, 1987), government-financed programs are, consciously or unconsciously, transforming the nursing home into a mental health facility.

Public policy is proclaiming a healthcare crisis. The crisis may, however, be caused by other than abuse of the system, excessive charges, and faulty services by professionals, as alleged by Starr

(1994)—it may be that the political forces are, in fact, attacking the quality of care via denigrating the professionalization of the healthcare services. Cerney (1994) opines that "joining managed care groups has become a racket," and believes that the contempoary scene merits application of Charles Dickens's statement, "It was the best of times; it was the worst of times."

So far, the focus herein may seem to be all "worst of times." The reason is simply that the negative dimension has received the most attention in public policy analyses and discussions. The "best of times" may emerge if the honorable intention to make healthcare services available to more people is obtained, and if psychologists are successful in educating governmental and managed healthcare systems that psychological services can accommodate both fiscal and clinical objectives. Broskowski (1991) optimistically notes that "it is clear that managed care does extend the range of treatments available to patients when case managers are given the authority to override the narrow restrictions of written benefit plans and to certify a range of alternative treatments" (p. 12). This is the sort of specific potential that must be rigorously pursued by psychologists.

If promoted and managed properly, inclusion of mental health services in regulated healthcare can bring about financial benefits to all concerned. Newman and Bricklin (1991) indicate that the advantages of managed healthcare include "increased client flow, less marketing needed by providers, added stability in an otherwise changing marketplace, and increased income-cash flow" (p. 26). No doubt with some degree of chagrin, they add: "managed health care was an economic benefit to providers at the expense of quality mental health care" (p. 26).

There is no doubt that clinical neuropsychology, be it for children or adults, is subject to the vicissitudes of public policy, and public policy relevant to all healthcare, including clinical neuropsychology, is currently ill defined and policies and programs are in disarray; indeed:

> Public policy represents society's views, preferences, expectations, and demands. Public policies are developed by governmental institutions and officials through the political process (or politics). They are distinct from other kinds of policies because they result from the actions of the legitimate authorities in a political system. (Bullock, Anderson, & Brady, 1983, p. 3)

Now, perhaps more than ever, healthcare professionals must be: (1) mindful of how public policy determines services, roles, and quality care and (2) prepared to actively attempt to shape policy determination. Unfortunately, all too often there is a complacent denial of what is happening on the public policy front. Warnings were not heeded; Kiesler and Morton (1988) said:

> We predict that public and private cost-containment efforts, in tandem with rapid restructuring of the industry and growing consensus about the limits of free marketplace competition should lead to declining provider autonomy, increasing integration of services, increasing emphasis on treatment outcomes, increasing management purview and control, changing power bases, and (eventually) more consumer control via government and administrative decree. (p. 997)

Their forecast became painfully true. As detailed elsewhere (Woody, 1985b), this is an era wherein: (1) funding for healthcare and other human services has diminished; (2) cost containment is the password to entering the domain of public policy; and (3) health policy planning is plagued by competing and conflicting objectives.

Psycholegal Issue Two: Self-Regulation Has Been Replaced by Governmental and Marketplace Regulation

There has been constant expansion of governmental regulatory responsibility and authority over all professionals: "The atmosphere within which perennial issues of access, quality, and costs are considered now involves formal public policies expressed in regulatory programs that are mandated and operated by governments" (Bice, 1981, p. 12). The control and regulation by government has been buttressed by entrepreneurial allies in the insurance industry: "New and powerful forces, particularly from the private sector, are redefining health care all the way from its overall organization to the basic relationship between provider and patient" (Kiesler & Morton, 1988, p. 1002). Consequently, all psychological practices, including (of course) those of clinical child neuropsychologists, must receive recognition, endorsement, and approval by the regulatory arm of the body of public policy relevant to healthcare.

As clinical child neuropsychology develops, there must be continued consonance with public policy. Recognition, endorsement, and approval assigned to clinical, counseling, or school psychology may not be automatically or readily applied to clinical child neuropsychology. Substantial progress toward this objective has been achieved, although the healthcare reform poses new challenges. This will be exemplified later in the chapter in the discussion of the negativism toward expert clinical neuropsychological testimony that has occurred in certain legal instances (Schwartz, 1987).

Psycholegal Issue Three: There Is Detrimental Dissonance among Clinical Neuropsychologists

As indicated already, shifts in public policy have lessened the profession's ability to self-ordain the functions, roles, or services for psychological practice. Once the profession accepts a particular type of psychological practice, clinical neuropsychology for example, there is no inalienable right to operate without continued endorsement, regulation, and monitoring by society. To date, there remains distinct doubt as to just how firm is the approval from public policy for neuropsychology generally and clinical child neuropsychology specifically.

To earn this positive reception, a profession, discipline, or specialty must have a proven track record of critiquing the would-be function, definition, or role:

> As society recognizes a profession, it imposes upon that discipline a concomitant responsibility or duty— a set of expectations as to what should and should not occur in professional practice. In other words, the quid pro quo for societal recognition of professionalism is professional accountability to society. (Woody, 1985a, p. 509)

This mandate is typically fulfilled by a code of ethics and a set of standards, as would be promulgated by a professional association.

Certainly the overall profession of psychology has accomplished justification for its position in healthcare services, albeit that its permanence and authority continue to be threatened— especially under the vicissitudes of contemporary healthcare reform. What is lacking, however, is an equally forthright movement forward for clinical neuropsychology.

This is not to say that clinical neuropsychology has not garnered public policy support. The problem centers on the fact that, among themselves, clinical neuropsychologists continue to lack the degree of professional definition that is necessary to establish and preserve a viable psychological specialty. Because of healthcare reform, intraspecialty dissonance creates a problem that is especially acute and potentially damaging.

Professional associations have created "homebases" for clinical neuropsychologists, such as the American Psychological Association's Division (40) of Clinical Neuropsychology and the National Academy of Neuropsychology; and clinical neuropsychology is recognized and supported at a secondary, but important, level by a variety of other divisions of the American Psychological Association. Also, certain methods for obtaining a specialized credential in neuropsychology have been put in place, such as from the American Board of Professional Neuropsychology and the American Board of Clinical Neuropsychology (the latter being affiliated with the prestigious American Board of Professional Psychology). This professionalization of clinical neuropsychology is providing needed standards, as prescribed by public policy. Unfortunately, there remains a lack of uniformity for and failure to reach consensus about standards.

The underlying motives for having professional associations and specialty credentials in clinical neuropsychology are not necessarily hallowed. There is a wish to gain favor from public policy, which sometimes reaches to self-serving motives. Enrichment of the practitioner has led to unfortunate dissonance among neuropsychologists, as witnessed by competing organizations, publishing negative statements about other factions, and castigating opposing expert witnesses who are not aligned with the expert's affiliations. As a legalist serving mental health professionals, it is regrettable to report that among clinical neuropsychologists working in the forensic arena, there have been innumerable incidents that can only be characterized as petty bickerings, often seemingly connected to a neurotic quest for self-aggrandizement or financial remuneration. Indeed, Putnam and Anderson (1994) provide a salary survey of neuropsychologists, and it is apparent that, even in this age of fragile economics for most mental health practitioners, clinical neuropsychology is a "growth" specialty.

Clinical neuropsychology is second to no other mental health specialty in the degree of dissonance among its practitioners. In addition to the destructive and unhealthy elements of the seemingly nefarious motives, there is the possibility that the competing politically motivated forces within clinical neuropsychology could potentially damage the specialty to the point of disarray, which could produce condemnation from the public, the overall profession of psychology, and other healthcare professions alike.

Psycholegal Issue Four: Specialization in Clinical Neuropsychology May or May Not Be Wise for the Professional Discipline

Although it might seem at first blush that specialization is a positive accomplishment, it may, in fact, be ill advised. It could well be that too much specialization could prove to be detrimental to the professionalization of clinical neuropsychology.

First, it is feasible that overspecialization could lead to faulty general underpinnings, both in academics and in practices. Sarason (1987) raised the question, "what price do the student and the field pay for specialization," and urged that this question be discussed. Also, he cautioned that such analysis and discussion may be preempted by a "marketplace mentality." Sarason sagely asserted:

> The climate that provides no forum for serious and sustained discussion is one that encourages early and undue specialization. By undue I mean a degree of specialization that phenomenologically makes a part of psychology the whole of it, that makes the student an isolationist in the world of psychology. This happens unreflectively and with the best of intentions. For me the question is not whether specialization should be a postdoctoral affair. The important question is: what should be the core of the identity of a psychologist, regardless of special interest? (p. 37)

In fairness to existing organizations and credentials relevant to clinical neuropsychology, there is allegiance to the Boulder Model for training, namely, that the neuropsychologist should be a behavioral scientist or general psychologist first and a clinician or neuropsychologist second (in other words, there are certain core areas of core psychological training that must predate training in clinical neuropsychology). Regardless, Sarason's question remains to be answered. The wrong answer could be a harbinger of rejection by public policy.

Second, it is known that clinical psychology in general has an array of new practice opportunities. Of special relevance to clinical neuropsychologists is the increased opportunity to practice in a hospital setting (Enright, Resnick, DeLeon, Sciara, & Tanney, 1990). As a concomitant of the medical scene, there is distinct movement toward psychologists' having prescription privileges (Boswell & Litwin, 1992; Chafetz & Buelow, 1994; Fox, Schwelitz, & Barclay, 1992). These and other emerging practice opportunities will surely introduce new training requirements, which may sorely tax the possibility of obtaining specialization in clinical neuropsychology (recall, as well, that the current healthcare reform movement speaks against specialists, and favors generalists). The contemporary state of affairs is leading some psychologists to advocate more science-based training (deGroot, 1994b) and a return to combining specialty training (Beutler & Fisher, 1994).

Third, it seems feasible that the profession of psychology could be damaged by too many specialty credentials: A proliferation of credentials for the wrong motive could result in a public policy condemnation of the profession overall. As (past) president of the APA Division of Clinical Psychology, Sechrest (1985) believes that the creation of specialties is occurring at a "frightful rate." He reports 30 different groups' proposing themselves as specialties (apparently aligned with clinical psychology). Sechrest acknowledges the rationale that specialization credentials can assure quality control to safeguard the public, but he notes the motives that special certificates accommodate advertising to increase income. He states:

> One suspects that just sheer ego has something to do with the problem of specialization. Most diplomas, at least in psychology, are probably of very little material value; they may serve no greater purpose than persuading their possessors that they are in some way special. Presumably some warm feeling flows through the practitioner who can gaze upon the large array of neatly framed documents decorating his or her office wall. One of my colleagues has suggested that we go into business manufacturing diploma wallpaper that would simplify the whole thing. (p. 1)

Thus, with an attribution of egotism or financial greed, a specialty credential may actually trigger a percept converse to what is preferred.

Wrongful motives could create a public policy backlash against the specialty of clinical neuropsychology (or any other specialty). Public policy usually reacts to battles within a profession as reason to disavow or deny endorsement. For example, discord between psychological specialties, such as clinical psychologists' resisting the inclusion of school psychologists in licensing laws, has historically led certain legislators to back away from any governmental support, such as "sunsetting" a licensure statute. More certainly, motives that are more self-serving for the professional than benefiting to the public could easily usher in a rejection within public policy (such as, hypothetically, having language within statutory rules of evidence that would restrict or negate courtroom testimony by a clinical neuropsychologist).

Nonetheless, efforts continue to specialize psychological practices. At present, the American Psychological Association has a Joint Interim Committee for the Identification and Recognition of Specialties and Proficiencies (deGroot, 1994a) that will explore the possibility of promoting additional specialties. It seems quite likely that consideration, and many would predict acceptance, will be given to clinical neuropsychology.

Psycholegal Issue Five: The Lack of Clear-Cut Standards for Clinical Child Neuropsychology Elevates Liability

As the practice of clinical child neuropsychology expands, there will be an increasing legal liability (Woody, 1992). That is, from justifying third-party payments (i.e., getting a patient's clinical neuropsychological services reimbursed by his or her health insurance policy) to allegations of malpractice, the clinical child neuropsychologist will be expected and required to maintain an acceptable standard of care.

The term "acceptable" is defined by both the profession and society. As will be discussed shortly, the profession of psychology and, moreover, the specialty of clinical neuropsychology (be it for children or adults) will have to decide which procedures are or are not to be endorsed. As mentioned, there is still doubt about what professional source, if any, can speak definitively to the issues of standards for the practice of clinical child neuropsychology. Society remains the final arbiter for the choice of standards.

The Legal Test

Society expresses its decision through laws. Legally, it is well established that a profession's endorsed conduct will receive the benefit of the doubt, but an entire profession could be negligent. For example, clinical child neuropsychology could, by legal principle, have a standard of care that was unacceptable to public policy. The legal test is as follows:

> It thus is fundamental that the standard of conduct which is the basis of the law of negligence is usually determined upon a risk-benefit form of analysis: by balancing the risk, in light of the social value of the interest threatened, and the probability and extent of the harm, against the value of the interest which the actor is seeking to protect, and the expedience of the course pursued. For this reason, it is usually very difficult, and often simply not possible, to reduce negligence to any definite rules; it is "relative to the need and the occasion," and conduct which would be proper under some circumstances becomes negligence under others. (Keeton, Dobbs, Keeton, & Owen, 1984, p. 173)

Stated differently, just because the entire profession does or does not do a particular procedure or service does not justify the commission or omission—the determinant is whether or not the procedure or service would (with consideration given to cost and degree of invasion of personal rights) benefit the consumer or society.

As a hypothetical example, suppose that all (or most) of the practitioners of clinical child neuropsychology did only a short form of a particular neuropsychological test battery, even though it was known that the short form reduced substantially the reliability and validity of the results. Assuming that the expenditure of professional time and the cost and invasiveness to the patient were not "excessive" (which has no predetermined definition) and the benefits were substantially greater from the long form of the test (e.g., reduced risk of diagnostic error), the practitioners of clinical child neuropsychology could potentially be negligent by using the short form of the neuropsychological test battery. Common practice within a profession does not establish the standard of care.

The Reasonable Practitioner Test

When determining the standard of care, the court applies the "reasonable person" test. In this instance, the test becomes the "reasonable clinical child neuropsychologist." There is no exact prototype to which the clinical child neuropsychologist can compare his or her qualities. Often the term "prudence" is integrated in the conceptualization of "reasonableness." "Prudence" is but a short step away from "conservative," which in turn could move to "traditional," which could lead to the notion that the standard of care is counter to innovation.

In legal reasoning, there is a certain truth to the notion that tradition is favored over innovation. Innovation cannot be foolhardy or create an unreasonable risk to the patient. In opposition, public policy holds that a scientist-practitioner should, for the welfare of society, strive for advancement in competency, and thus innovation should be encouraged and legally protected—within reason. Generally speaking, if the professional has performed an innovative technique or procedure that was predicated on a reasonably sound theoretical basis, executed it with good intentions and logic, maintained precautions and safeguards, and subjected his or her work to professional scrutiny (e.g., a research-review committee), there will be an effort to uphold the innovative dimension.

The "reasonable person" test does not require superiority *per se*: "Professional persons in general, and those who undertake any work calling for special skill, are required not only to exercise reasonable care in what they do, but also to possess a standard of minimum special knowledge and ability" (Keeton *et al.*, 1984, p. 185). If the issue is breach of the standard of care, such as in a malpractice action:

> The formula under which this is usually put to the jury is that the doctor must have and use the knowledge, skill and care ordinarily possessed and employed by members of the profession in good standing; and a doctor will be liable if harm results because he does not have them. Sometimes this is called the skill of the "average" member of the profession; but this is clearly misleading, since only those in good professional standing are to be considered; and of these it is not the middle but the minimum common skill which is to be looked to. If the defendant represents himself as having greater skill than this, as where the doctor holds himself out as a specialist, the standard is modified accordingly. (p. 187)

Perfection and/or superiority are not required, but this legal formula does require that the clinical child neuropsychologist be in the mainstream of competency for the specialty.

Psycholegal Issue Six: Clinical Neuropsychology Must Obtain Reasonable Agreement on Theories and Procedures

Public policy is tolerant of disagreements between experts, but only as long as the differing views have a reasonable semblance of being birthed by professional seeds. In clinical neuropsychology, there is rampant disagreement about: (1) the theoretical explanation of neuropsychological structures and processes and (2) the assessment and treatment techniques most suitable for particular neuropsychological conditions.

In his discussion of the development of theories of brain function, Golden (1978) provided a historical trace up to localization theory and equipotential theory, and noted: "Unable to accept either the localizationist or equipotentialist models of brain function, psychologists and neuropsychologists have searched for other models" (p. 8). When considering the diverse views expressed at the typical conference of clinical neuropsychologists, it is tempting to assert that there is a model unique to each practitioner.

Legally, although the clinical child neuropsychologist will be supported in her or his professional right to be aligned with a given theory of brain function: "This does not mean, however, that any quack, charlatan or crackpot can set himself up as a 'school,' and so apply his individual ideas without liability" (Keeton *et al.,* 1984, p. 1987). By legal prescription, a professional will only receive deference from public policy on this matter if she or he espouses a theory or "school" that has earned professional respect, has a set of definite principles, and is based on a line of thought that a reasonable number of qualified professionals would share. The latter means that any clinical child neuropsychological view must be based on research, as would be compatible with the scientist-practitioner model. Although apparently not yet subjected to litigation in the area of clinical child neuropsychology, a legal analysis of cases relevant to alleged psychotherapy malpractice supports that nontraditional approaches would likely be tested against more traditional schools of therapy (Glenn, 1974).

Going from theory to procedures, public policy requires that psychologists be qualified by, among other factors, academic training according to standards maintained for the profession. To be deemed a clinical child neuropsychologist, the principle would seemingly be having fulfilled training and practice experiences compatible with specialty. Unfortunately, "there are currently no restrictions on who may call himself a neuropsychologist, although it is quite possible that such restrictions will be developed and implemented within the next few years" (Ziskin & Faust, 1988, p. 719). While there is no definite source to date, the various relevant professional associations and credentialing groups hold the potential for delineating specific training and practice experiences that will be necessary if the clinical child neuropsychologist is to receive a protective legal framework.

Again there is professional debate about clinical neuropsychology procedures. For example, there are contradictory research evidence and clinical views about many neurological conditions (Walsh, 1978). Despite all of the discussion about the left brain versus the right brain, the research is, by far, inconclusive about numerous issues (Springer & Deutsch, 1985). Perhaps the two most famous (or infamous?) debates center around: (1) whether the clinical neuropsychologist should make use of an individualized set of tests or a standardized neuropsychological battery and (2) if preference is given to a standardized battery, whether it should be given to the Luria–Nebraska or the Halstead–Reitan. Often it seems that there is a tendency to base one's preference on the shortcomings of the alternatives, which hardly seems the most professional way of garnering support from public policy.

As for procedures, there remains uncertainty about the use of technicians for administering neuropsychological tests. There are many pitfalls, as well as benefits, from using technicians, and there must be a resolution of the uncertainty. DeLuca and Putnam (1993) offer a useful analysis of the deployment characteristics and practice issues.

In terms of forensic practice, any clinical child neuropsychologist who appears as an expert witness in a legal proceeding will be subject to examination and (usually less-than-friendly) cross-examination of the discrepancies between neuropsychological theories and the controversies surrounding neuropsychological procedures. Of course, it can also be expected that every aspect of these explorations will be considered for whether or not the expert testimony should be denigrated because of failure to document reliability and validity of judgments and opinions (Faust & Ziskin, 1988). Ziskin and Faust (1988) opine that the discrepancies and controversies support a conclusion of "no standard is the standard" (p. 741), and they assert:

> Thus, ironically, the areas in which the most research exists on neuropsychological assessment are often of the least relevance for forensic assessment, and the areas that are among the best research are often of the greatest relevance. Given the paucity of data on the use of neuropsychological batteries to predict everyday functioning, the neuropsychologist's conclusions about these matters must ultimately rely on what is

essentially guesswork and yet-to-be validated clinical judgment strategies. (p. 748)

In view of the mandate that expert testimony be predicated on a reasonable degree of psychological or behavioral science certainty, it is obvious that, if the foregoing allegation by Ziskin and Faust is true, the forensic neuropsychologist will be vulnerable to impeachment and, consequently, elevated liability, as might result in a malpractice, regulatory (licensing), and/or ethics complaint.

Psycholegal Issue Seven: Clinical Child Neuropsychology Has a Special Vulnerability to Malpractice

As evident from the foregoing discussions, the standard of care is the critical component of a malpractice legal action. This chapter is not intended to be a treatise on malpractice. An elaboration on and guidelines for avoiding malpractice in mental health services are available elsewhere (Woody, 1983, 1988a,b). What is appropriate herein is to consider four risks that are, to a large extent, idiosyncratic to clinical child neuropsychology.

First, neuropsychologists do not possess a well-defined role. Qualifications for the title "neuropsychologist" have yet to be specified in a universally accepted manner (and the same is even more true for the title "clinical child neuropsychologist"). The quality of training in clinical neuropsychology is not assured, at least as compared with certain other clinical specialties. There is considerable dispute over and contradictory results from research that addresses neuropsychological theories and procedures. Individually and in combination, these factors increase a clinical child neuropsychologist's risk of having to defend against a legal action.

Second, by being part of today's "healthcare industry," there is elevated legal liability. Whereas psychologists once enjoyed a certain kind of relationship with their patients that served to minimize legal liability, their increased identity as healthcare providers leads to greater patient willingness to file a legal action (Knapp & Vandecreek, 1981). The medical context combines with the brain-based (i.e., physiological) focus of neuropsychology to produce additional risk of legal action against the clinical neuropsychologist. There is reason to wonder whether or not dealing with children, as opposed to adults, also exacerbates the liability problem. That is, human behavior seems to lead many parents to zealously protect, perhaps even overprotect, their children. Thus, any neuropsychological problem involving a child might well be subject to exaggerated parental quest for self-righteousness, such as by pointing a finger of blame for the child's misfortune at the clinical child neuropsychologist and demanding a legal remedy.

Third, the affiliations necessary for clinical neuropsychology convey legal liability. The principle of vicarious liability holds that: "One who is free from all moral blame or legal fault is held liable for the tort of another, and this may be described as a form of liability without fault" (Keeton et al., 1984, p. 593). For the clinical child neuropsychologist, this means that being a neurological "team member" could result in being named a defendant, even though the direct cause of the injury was allegedly the negligence of, say, the neurologist or another healthcare provider. As another example of vicarious liability, the use of technicians to administer neuropsychological tests is commonplace and appropriate (DeLuca & Putnam, 1993); by relying on a technician, the neuropsychologist accrues vicarious liability for the technican's errors and omissions.

Fourth, being brain-related, neuropsychology has a possible connection to causes of legal actions greater than for other psychological specialties. Psychologists are being subjected to an increasing number of lawsuits. The causes of action are many, including (but not limited to) "involuntary servitude, false arrest, trespass, malicious infliction of emotional distress, abuse of process, loss of liberty, misrepresentation, libel, assault and battery, malicious prosecution, and false imprisonment" (Hogan, 1979, p. 7). Wilkinson (1982) categorized malpractice cases involving psychiatrists as patient-inflicted injuries and suicide, harm by the patient to third persons, errors in judgment, faulty treatment methods, drug-related liability, and sexual misconduct. Fisher (1985) indicated that "the number of claims against psychologists have risen faster in the past three years than for any other mental health profession" (p. 6). There is no reason to believe that clinical child neuropsychologists would be able to find any exemption from or exception to the increasing liability. Indeed, as discussed previously, the medical context, the severity of condition association with brain-based services, and the nebulous research basis for neuropsychological theories and procedures combine to increase the liability for clinical neuropsychologists beyond the level of liability generally attributed to psychologists.

Psycholegal Issue Eight: Expert Clinical Child Neuropsychological Testimony May Be Suspect in Legal Proceedings

Several previous sections have explored certain weaknesses in the theoretical and research bases for clinical child neuropsychology, and noted criticisms of neuropsychological assessments. The ambiguity and negativism have reached to legal proceedings. As Matarazzo (1990) summarizes: "an increasing number of attorneys recognize that even in our nation's most advanced centers for psychological assessment, the measurement of intelligence (or personality, memory, or other psychological functions) is not, even today, a totally objective, completely science-based activity" (p. 1000). Matarazzo also states: "Nevertheless, as some of our psychologist colleague-critics and federal and state legislators and judges have recently made clear, psychological assessment techniques, in common with most tools, can be used for many purposes, some harmful and some helpful, and their use cannot be separated from their validity and from the training, competence, and ethical values of the psychologist using them" (p. 1001).

The door remains open to forensic clinical child neuropsychologists, albeit that those who enter will not always find unreserved professional respect. This section presents ideas for effective forensic testimony in a somewhat suspicious framework, and the next sections follow up with guidelines for prudence and caution in forensic testimony.

To provide expert testimony, a witness must have qualifications that will allow her or him to offer special information to the trier of fact (the judge and/or jury). Although there may be slight differences between state statutes, consider the definition from Florida:

> Testimony by experts. If scientific, technical, or other special knowledge will assist the trier of fact in understanding the evidence or in determining a fact in issue, a witness qualified as an expert by knowledge, skill, experience, training, or education may testify about it in the form of an opinion; however, the opinion is admissible only as can be applied to evidence at trial. (Florida Statutes, 1993, 90.702, Vol. 1, p. 591)

At first glance, it would seem that surely the testimony of a clinical child neuropsychologist would fulfill the requirements for being "expert" in nature. Such may or may not be the case.

For many years, only a medical physician could testify about the human condition. As the behavioral sciences developed, public policy was altered to accommodate professional disciplines other than medicine. Now it is commonplace for, among others, psychologists to be qualified for rendering expert testimony (*Jenkins v. United States,* 1962). Having said this, however, the area of clinical neuropsychology has not yet received unequivocal acceptance. Part of the reservation comes from the belief of many legalists that a patient's neuropsychological condition can only be adequately evaluated, diagnosed, described, and/or treated by a neurologist. Another way of phrasing the problem is that neuropsychological tests have yet to receive adequate documentation for reliability and validity.

In point of fact, there is still a dearth of supportive research for clinical neuropsychological judgments. For example, Shordone and Rudd (1986) had psychologists examine clinical vignettes for purposes of recognizing neurological disorders, and found that one-third of the psychologists failed to recognize the underlying neurological disorder. Likewise, the use of individualized test batteries allows for personal preferences by the clinical child neuropsychologist. Consequently, the subjectivity in the choice of methods or instruments can lead to questionable validity for the decisions derived from the data, which may be compounded by the limitations (e.g., inadequate standardization) of the tests (Golden, 1986).

As another weak point, misdiagnosis can result from an overcommitment to neuropsychological strategies. As Boll (1985) stated:

> All that produces cognitive dysfunction is not necessarily, primarily, or even secondarily, neurological in nature. Antecedent factors, such as disruptive environments, poor opportunity, primary emotional pathology not tied to neurological dysfunction, all can result in compromised mental performance. These deficits may, in some circumstances, appear strikingly similar to those which are likely to be produced by neurological events themselves. (p. 480)

A clinician must be attuned to both neurologically based and nonneurologically based diagnoses.

Related to the preceding point, there is often a fine line between scientific assertions and proselytizing for a cause that will benefit the professional. With any emerging strategy, and clinical neuropsychology is no exception, self-serving motives may lead to "professional enthusiasm" that is unjustified. Legalists are aware of this tendency in professionals. One trial lawyer commented about a deposition that he had taken of a well-published neuropsychologist, saying, "It should be easy to impeach his testimony during the trial because he comes across as a 'True Believer' in the infallibility of the neuropsychological tests."

For the foregoing and other reasons, certain courts have excluded testimony by clinical neuropsychologists on neurological conditions; or if the clinical neuropsychologist has been qualified to testify, the judicial opinion points toward very little weight being accorded to the neuropsychological data. Schwartz (1987) analyzed two court decisions in the Florida Court of Appeals that negated and/or restricted the testimony proffered by a clinical neuropsychologist. As there are only limited cases that are on point (and the rulings may be idiosyncratic to the case, the judge, or the jurisdiction), a review of those cases seems premature for purposes of deriving legal principles. Suffice it to say that there has not been unreserved judicial support for clinical neuropsychological testimony.

It seems probable that childhood development, with its individual differences, and the malleability of children will result in the reservations about expert testimony on adult neuropsychology being as staunch (or more so) for expert testimony on clinical child neuropsychology. The principal message for the clinical child neuropsychologist would certainly be: "Forensic cases have demanded an increasing sophistication on the part of the neuropsychologist beyond those issues encountered with other types of psychological testimony" (Golden, 1986, p. 1).

To the contrary, there have been many instances where the testimony of the clinical neuropsychologist, be it for an adult or child, has been readily accepted by the court. Galaski (1985) described the present-day relationship between the attorney and clinical neuropsychologist and indicated: "Cases in which the neuropsychologist can be of greatest practical help to the attorney include cases of personal injury, especially when there has been head trauma caused by a fall or sustained in a motor vehicle accident" (p. 10). Incagnoli (1985) described how clinical neuropsychologists can fulfill a valuable role in litigation, and she recommended that "a clinical neuropsychologist should be called as an expert witness to evaluate any client with suspected or known brain injury" (p. 60).

Writing for attorneys, Kadushin (1990) traces the evolution of neuropsychological assessment, and explains how attorneys can make use of neuropsychological evaluation for litigation. He notes that "since neuropsychological evaluations are time-consuming, stressful, and expensive, they should be undertaken only when necessary" (p. 65); nonetheless, he urges: "In head-injury cases, lawyers should consider referring clients for neuropsychological evaluation when there has been (1) a loss of consciousness; (2) a period of post-traumatic amnesia; or (3) an acceleration/deceleration injury (for example, whiplash) followed by these symptoms: headaches, dizziness, impaired memory, alcohol intolerance, irritability, or depression" (p. 65).

Related to the previous comments about the reservation of courts to admit the testimony of clinical neuropsychologists, the ever-expanding recognition of the usefulness of clinical neuropsychological data for legal determinations creates a press for specialized research on applying neuropsychological procedures to legal issues. Lanyon (1986) emphasizes that psychological assessment, in general, for legal cases must go beyond the typical clinical procedures; and he provides a useful review of specialized procedures/instruments developed for such legal issues as competency, insanity, dangerousness, child custody evaluations, homicide, and sex offenders. Regrettably, it appears that there has been precious little research on the application of clinical child neuropsychology to legal issues *per se,* and few, if any, specialized procedures/instruments within the realm of clinical child neuropsychology that are tailored to legal issues. For example, an appropriate legal query could be: What research findings have been obtained to connect certain data from children's neuropsychological tests to a specific degree/amount of damages? The answer would seemingly have to be: None.

As for expert clinical child neuropsychological testimony being suspect in legal proceedings, recall the earlier discussion of views expressed by Ziskin and Faust (1988; also Faust & Ziskin, 1988). Their message to legalists is that neuropsychological testing, and consequently forensic testimony based thereon, had dubious reliability, validity, and worth; and they provide attorneys with a myriad of techniques for impeaching the testimony of a neuropsychologist.

Psycholegal Issue Nine: Expert Clinical Child Neuropsychological Testimony Must Be Prudent and Cautious

As discussed earlier, liability can accrue to any clinical services, and there is reason to believe that expert testimony of any sort carries a special vulnerability. There are two primary reasons for this special vulnerability. First and as detailed previously, psychological testing in general and neuropsychological assessment in particular have many critics, who rely on a highly academic psychometric argument—which is often persuasive in legal proceedings. Second, there is speculation that a person with a neuropsychological condition who has engaged in a legal action may be prone to attempt to place responsibility on someone else, and this may extend to pointing a finger of blame at an expert witness (especially if the plaintiff does not prevail in the lawsuit). In other words, there is substantial liability associated with expert testimony of any kind, and most certainly with neuropsychological testimony.

Aside from liability *per se* (e.g., for negligent testimony), prudence and caution are necessary, namely, because of the suspicion commonly leveled at neuropsychological testimony (as discussed in the previous section). As Nurcombe and Partlett (1994) put it:

> Experts are often challenged on their qualification to present expert testimony. The lawyer for the opposing party may challenge an expert's credibility and reliability in the same that he would challenge a fact witness. (p. 344)

When entering the legal arena, the clinical child neuropsychologist should accept that, no matter how solid his or her qualifications or well documented his or her opinions, there will be challenges to lessen the impact or weight of the testimony.

At an early stage of the proceeding, the clinical child neuropsychologist must be qualified to serve as an "expert." That is, her or his professional credentials are presented as a means for justifying that the testimony merits being considered expert for assisting the trier of fact, as well as setting the stage for how much weight should be given to the opinions expressed. When there is a challenge to the qualifications of a potential expert, it is referred to as impeachment, and the concept extends throughout the proceedings. The impeachment process will be especially evident in the questions posed to the clinical child neuropsychologist by the attorney representing the party to whom the testimony is least favorable. As Swenson (1993) explains:

> One purpose of the cross-examination is to force a dishonest witness to reveal the truth through pressure or to reveal inconsistencies in testimony. A second purpose is to reduce the credibility of hostile witnesses, a process called impeachment. If a witness gives answers during the cross-examination that harm his or her own side, the attorney who first questioned the witness can seek to "rehabilitate" the witness. (p. 48)

It is common for the opposing attorneys to go back and forth attempting to impeach and then rehabilitate and then impeach, and on and on, as long as the witness is testifying.

A focal point for impeachment is the potential expert witness's resume (Garrison, 1993). Stated simply, any attempt to aggrandize professional qualifications is counter to logic, as well as the prudence and caution that is urged in this section. For example, "diplomate" status purchased without examination can be problematic, and may end up being characterized as a vanity degree. It is important to accept that this demeaning–enhancing exchange is a required part of the legal process, and if attempts to diminish one's professional stature cannot be tolerated, the neuropsychologist should avoid all forensic testimony.

In keeping with prudence and caution, the clinical child neuropsychologist should be sure that the attorney asking for the testimony understands neuropsychology (e.g., as explained in Kadushin, 1990), and is prepared to conduct an effective direct examination (e.g., as explained by Lubet, 1993) and counter impeachment and attacks on psychological assessment (e.g., as orchestrated by Faust & Ziskin, 1988, and Ziskin & Faust, 1988). This requires careful planning between the attorney and the clinical child neuropsychologist prior to the legal proceedings.

Ironically, one of the weaknesses most commonly encountered with forensic psychologists is academic in nature. That is, they do not do their homework to understand adequately the behavioral science bases of their own theories, techniques, and opinions. As Matarrazo (1990) puts it:

> My experience in the courtroom, where more and more psychologists' conclusions are being vigorously challenged by attorneys, has led me to conclude that too many psychologists testifying in the courts today, whether for the plaintiff or defense, are unaware of the standard errors of measurement of the scores (and accompanying confidence intervals) produced by our batteries of tests (p. 1005)

and

> Inasmuch as increasing numbers of attorneys are becoming familiar with the psychometric properties of psychological tools, it is incumbent upon psychologist

clinicians to be at least as familiar as are they with the strengths and weaknesses of the instruments currently used in psychological assessment. (p. 1016)

To paraphrase the old saw for preparedness for forensic testimony, "an ounce of academic prevention is worth a pound of impeachment/rehabilitation cure."

Being a highly trained and skilled clinician does not assure success in legal proceedings. The courtroom is not the mental health clinic. Of special concern, there are rules of civil and criminal procedure that govern what may be contained in expert testimony, and how the expert's testimony may be presented. Further, although the well-trained neuropsychologist will be quite astute with clinical interpretation, the well-trained attorney will be quite astute with using legal procedure to control the expert's testimony. Stated bluntly, the clinical child neuropsychologist is on foreign turf, and does not speak the language.

In preparation for the role of forensic expert, prudence and caution dictate that the clinical child neuropsychologist should study the legal system and its procedures, and acquire skills tailored to the demands of the expert's role. Brodsky (1991) provides a valuable set of guidelines for the psychological expert.

Psycholegal Issue Ten: Clinical Child Neuropsychology Has the Potential to Be Received Positively in the Courtroom

As might be assumed by the discussions for the preceding psycholegal issues, the future for clinical child neuropsychology is not assuredly sunny. Certainly the present-day skepticism evident in public policy and laws about healthcare providers (e.g., the demands for increased accountability and cost containment/reduction set forth by healthcare reform, third-party payment sources, managed healthcare, and regulatory agencies) creates clouds on the horizon. Also, the critics of psychological testing in general and neuropsychological assessment in specific will find allies among the healthcare reformists, and this alliance will likely become more evident in courtroom proceedings.

Nonetheless, there is reason to believe that the turbulence on the horizon may dissipate. There is political correctness in endorsing services to children. Innumerable sources are predicting a trend toward enhanced educational and health services for children, which will pave the way for clinical child neuropsychologists. It seems probable that the school will become the site for these services, as opposed to the traditional child guidance clinic or private practitioner. Psychometric limitations of assessment tools have been identified, and research methods are available to obtain remedies. Finally, it is clear that litigation has achieved a primary role and will increase its influence on the development of our society. When all of these conditions are combined, the future for clinical child neuropsychology is highly positive, far more so than can be prognosticated for other types of psychological services (e.g., psychotherapeutic interventions).

Summary

Healthcare reform is mandating increased accountability, as well as quality assurance and cost containment. Concomitantly, governmental regulations (e.g., licensing statutes and relevant disciplinary rules) are both macromanaging and micromanaging clinical services, and laws are imposing increased liability on all healthcare providers. Although public policy has issued an invitation to clinical child neuropsychology, there are many skeptics as to the scientific status and usefulness of neuropsychology. Given the pitfalls, it would be foolhardy to plunge recklessly into clinical child neuropsychology. Rather, all neuropsychology services must be predicated on academics, research, and training, consonant with standards for being both a generalist and a specialist. At this point in time, the law determines proper professional conduct and services as much or more than the disciplinary preferences set forth in professional training programs. The psycholegal future of clinical child neuropsychology is highly positive, but only with remedy of identified limitations in assessment strategies, refinement of theory and practice by research, enhanced training (including beyond degree programs per se), and prudence and caution by practitioners.

References

Appelbaum, P. S. (1993). Legal liability and managed care. *American Psychologist, 48*(3), 251–257.

Beutler, L. E., & Fisher, D. (1994). Combined specialty training in counseling, clinical, and school psychology: An idea whose time has returned. *Professional Psychology, 25*(1), 62–69.

Bice, T. W. (1981). Social science and health services: Contributions to public policy. In J. B. McKinlay (Ed.), *Issues in health care policy* (pp. 1–28). Cambridge, MA: MIT Press.

Boll, T. J. (1985). Developing issues in clinical neuropsychology. *Journal of Clinical and Experimental Neuropsychology, 7,* 473–485.

Boswell, D. L., & Litwin, W. J. (1992). Limited prescription privileges for psychologists: A 1-year follow-up. *Professional Psychology, 23*(2), 108–113.

Brodsky, S. L. (1991). *Testifying in court: Guidelines and maxims for the expert witness.* Washington, DC: American Psychological Association.

Broskowski, A. (1991). Current mental health care environments: Why managed care is necessary. *Professional Psychology, 22*(1), 6–14.

Bullock, C. S., III, Anderson, J. E., & Brady, D. W. (1983). *Public policy in the eighties.* Belmont, CA: Wadsworth.

Cerney, M. S. (1994). Health care crisis: What is SPA's role? *Society for Personality Assessment Exchange, 4*(1), 1, 10–11.

Chafetz, M. D., & Buelow, G. (1994). A training model for psychologists with prescription privileges: Clinical pharmacopsychologists. *Professional Psychology, 25*(2), 149–153.

deGroot, G. (1994a). APA seeks to recognize expertise in selected areas. *APA Monitor, 25*(4), 48.

deGroot, G. (1994b). Clinical psychologists need more science-based training. *APA Monitor, 25*(5), 46.

DeLeon, P. H., VandenBos, G. R., & Bulato, E. Q. (1991). Managed mental health care: A history of the federal policy initiative. *Professional Psychology, 22*(1), 15–25.

DeLuca, J. W., & Putnam, S. H. (1993). The professional/technician model in clinical neuropsychology: Deployment characteristics and practice issues. *Professional Psychology, 24*(1), 100–106.

Enright, M. F., Resnick, R., DeLeon, P. H., Sciara, A. D., & Tanney, F. (1990). The practice of psychology in hospital settings. *American Psychologist, 45*(9), 1059–1065.

Faust, D., & Ziskin, J. (1988). The expert witness in psychology and psychiatry. *Science, 241*(July 1), 31–35.

Fisher, K. (1985, May). Changes catch clinicians in cycle of shame, slip ups. *APA Monitor, 16*(5), 6–7.

Florida Statutes. (1993). Chapter 90—Evidence Code. Section 702—Testimony by Experts. Vol. 1, p. 591.

Fox, R. E., Schweltz, F. D., & Barclay, A. G. (1992). A proposed curriculum for psychopharmacology training for professional psychologists. *Professional Psychology, 23*(3), 216–219.

Galaski, T. (1985). The neuropsychologist: Key member of the doctor–lawyer team. *Case & Comment, 90*(4), 10, 12–14.

Garrison, D. H., Sr. (1993). Investigating the potential expert witness' resume. *Michigan Bar Journal, 72*(12), 1320–1321.

Glenn, R. D. (1974). Standard of care in administering non-traditional psychotherapy. *University of California, Davis Law Review, 7,* 56–83.

Golden, C. J. (1978). *Diagnosis and rehabilitation in clinical neuropsychology.* Springfield, IL: Thomas.

Golden, C. J. (1986). Forensic neuropsychology: Introduction and review. In C. J. Golden & M. A. Strider (Eds.), *Forensic neuropsychology* (pp. 1–47). New York: Plenum Press.

Hogan, D. B. (1979). *The regulation of psychotherapists* (Vol. II). Cambridge, MA: Ballinger.

Incagnoli, T. (1985). Clinical neuropsychologists: Their role in litigation. *Trial, 21*(6), 60, 62–63.

Jenkins v. United States. (1962). 307 F.2d 637.

Kadushin, F. S. (1990). How to assess brain damage: Neuropsychological evaluation for litigation. *Trial, 26*(10), 64–67.

Keeton, W. P., Dobbs, D. B., Keeton, R. E., & Owen, D. G. (1984). *Prosser and Keeton on the law of torts* (5th ed.). St. Paul, MN: West.

Kiesler, C. A., & Morton, T. L. (1988). Psychology and public policy in the "health care revolution." *American Psychologist, 43*(12), 993–1003.

Kiesler, C. A., & Sibulkin, A. E. (1987). *Mental hospitalization: Myths and facts about a national crisis.* Newbury Park, CA: Sage.

Knapp, S., & Vandecreek, L. (1981). Behavioral medicine: Its malpractice risks for psychologists. *Professional Psychology, 12,* 677–683.

Lanyon, R. I. (1986). Psychological assessment procedures in court-related settings. *Professional Psychology, 17,* 260–268.

Lubet, S. (1993). Eight techniques for direct examination of experts. *Trial, 29*(12), 16, 18, 20.

Matarazzo, J. D. (1987). There is only one psychology, no specialties, but many applications. *American Psychologist, 42*(10), 893–903.

Matarazzo, J. D. (1990). Psychological assessment versus psychological testing: Validation from Binet to the school, clinic, and courtroom. *American Psychologist, 45*(9), 999–1017.

Newman, R., & Bricklin, P. M. (1991). Parameters of managed mental health care: Legal, ethical, and practical guidelines. *Professional Psychology, 23*(1), 26–35.

Nurcombe, B., & Partlett, D. F. (1994). *Child mental health and the law.* New York: Free Press/Macmillan.

Putnam, S. H., & Anderson, C. (1994). The second TCN salary survey: A survey of neuropsychologists. Part I. *Clinical Neuropsychologist, 8*(1), 3–37.

Sarason, S. B. (1987, January). Is our field an inkblot? *APA Monitor, 18*(1), 37.

Schwartz, M. L. (1987). Limitations on neuropsychological testimony by the Florida appellate decisions: Action, reaction, and counteraction. *Clinical Neuropsychologist, 1,* 51–60.

Sechrest, L. B. (1985). Specialization? Who needs it? *Clinical Psychologist, 38*(1), 1 & 3.

Shordone, R. J., & Rudd, M. (1986). Can psychologists recognize neurological disorders in their patients? *Journal of Clinical and Experimental Neuropsychology, 8,* 285–291.

Springer, S. P., & Deutsch, G. (1985). *Left brain, right brain* (rev. ed.). San Francisco: Freeman.

Starr, P. (1994). *The logic of health care reform.* New York: Whittle Books (Penguin).

Swenson, L. C. (1993). *Psychology and law for the helping professions.* Pacific Grove, CA: Brooks/Cole.

Walsh, K. W. (1978). *Neuropsychology: A clinical approach.* Edinburgh: Churchill Livingstone.

Wiggins, J. G. (1990). Re-defining clinical psychology in the changing health care market. *Clinical Psychologist, 43*(3), 51–52.

Wilkinson, A. P. (1982). Psychiatric malpractice. Identifying areas of liability. *Trial, 18*(10), 73–77, 89–90.

Woody, R. H. (1983). Avoiding malpractice in psychotherapy. In P. A. Keller & L. B. Ritt (Eds.), *Innovations in clinical practice: A sourcebook* (Vol. II, pp. 205–216). Sarasota, FL: Professional Resource Exchange.

Woody, R. H. (1985a). Public policy, malpractice law, and the mental health professional: Some legal and clinical guidelines. In C. P. Ewing (Ed.), *Psychology, psychiatry, and the law* (pp. 509–525). Sarasota, FL: Professional Resource Exchange.

Woody, R. H. (1985b). Techniques for handling psycholegal cases. In C. E. Walker (Ed.), *The handbook of clinical psychology* (Vol. II, pp. 1420–1439). Homewood, IL: Dow Jones-Irwin.

Woody, R. H. (1988a). *Fifty ways to avoid malpractice: A guidebook for mental health professionals.* Sarasota, FL: Professional Resource Exchange.

Woody, R. H. (1988b). *Protecting your mental health practice: How to minimize legal and financial risk.* San Francisco: Jossey–Bass.

Woody, R. H. (1992). Malpractice in counseling neuropsychology. *Counseling Psychologist, 20*(4), 635–639.

Ziskin, J., & Faust, D. (1988). *Coping with psychiatric and psychological testimony* (4th ed., Vol. II). Marina del Rey, CA: Law and Psychology Press.

36

Child Neuropsychology in the Private Medical Practice

ERIN D. BIGLER, NANCY L. NUSSBAUM, AND HEATHER A. FOLEY

Introduction

Utilizing a broad definition of child neuropsychological practice, the scope of such a practice would encompass all children with developmental and acquired disorders that affect cognition, behavior, and/or sensory and motor skills. Dworkin (1985) presented statistics indicating that approximately 10% of a pediatrician's practice involves children with learning disabilities (LD), attention deficit hyperactivity disorder (ADHD), speech–language disorder, mental retardation, cerebral palsy, and related disorders. Similarly, Cranston and colleagues (Cranston *et al.,* 1988) reported that 11% of pediatricians' practice involved cases of developmental disorders. Computations based on Table 1 suggest that a pediatrician will see a child with a neurobehavioral disorder once every other day. Some may not see as many, some may see more, but on average the frequency of pediatricians seeing children with neurobehavioral problems is high.

National statistics (Department of Education) indicate that for 1991 and 1992, approximately 12% of all children received some form of special education. Almost half of this number (about 6%) were identified as learning disabled (National Center for Educational Statistics, 1994). Learning disabilities are now "the most common chronic disorders managed by pediatricians" (Shapiro & Gallico, 1993). Several researchers have proposed that as many as 20% of school children are learning disabled (Roush, 1995), most of whom apparently go unrecognized by educational and medical statistics. The 1988 National Health Interview Survey–Child Health Supplement found that 17% of U. S. children were reported by their parents to have a developmental disability (Boyle, Decoufle, & Yeargin-Allsopp, 1994).

During the 1970s and early 1980s there was an increase in the percentage of children who were enrolled in federal programs for the disabled. However, Figure 1 illustrates that this increase was solely the result of the rise in the number of children identified as learning disabled (National Center for Education Statistics, 1994). In the late 1970s, Burnett and Bell (1978) reported that the greatest increase in pediatric practice, in terms of new referrals, came in the area of school and related problems. This increase in the percentage of children with developmental disabilities may be related to recent advances in medicine that increase survival rates of at-risk infants as well as infants who survive high-risk pregnancies (Parette, Hourcade, & Brimberry, 1990, in reference to Kirk & Gallagher, 1989). Those children who do survive are often likely to suffer from a developmental disability (Parette *et al.,* 1990, in reference to Drillien, Thompson, & Burgoyne, 1980). The increase could also be the result of improved awareness and recognition of certain disabilities as demonstrated by the Education for All Handicapped Children Act which enabled children with a learning disability to qualify for special education services (Purvis, 1991;

ERIN D. BIGLER • Department of Psychology, Brigham Young University, Provo, Utah 84602; and LDS Hospital, Salt Lake City, Utah 84143.   NANCY L. NUSSBAUM • Austin Neurological Clinic, Austin, Texas 78705. HEATHER A. FOLEY • Department of Psychology, Brigham Young University, Provo, Utah 84602.

TABLE 1. Pediatricians' Estimates of the Number of Children in Their Practices with Handicapping Conditions[a]

Disability	Reported no. of children	
	Mean	Range
Specific learning disability (as defined by physician or school)	50.6	0–300
Hyperactive/minimal brain dysfunction (as defined by physician)	33.3	0–400
Language/speech impairment (excluding developmental articulation problems)	29.3	0–100
Mental retardation (mild to profound)	27.0	0–250
Cerebral palsy (mild to severe)	14.1	0–150
Hearing impairment (nontransient conductive or sensorineural—mild to profound)	10.6	0–250
Serious emotional disturbance (as defined by physician)	8.2	0–100
Legally blind	2.1	0–50

[a]Modified from Shonkoff, Dworkin, & Leviton (1979).

Roush, 1995). Figure 1 also illustrates a decline in speech or language impairments as well as mental retardation perhaps because some of those problems were more accurately diagnosed as learning disabilities.

Accordingly, with such an incidence of developmental disability there is a clear indication for the need and important role that the child neuropsychologist can play in the pediatric and general med-

ical setting. The most common setting for child neuropsychology to interface with the private medical practice will be the general practice of pediatrics or in pediatric neurology. Although there are other settings (i.e., family practice) or outlets for the practice of clinical child neuropsychology, this chapter will focus on the role of the child neuropsychologist in the context of a general pediatric practice.

Identification of the Patient

In the private medical setting, the pediatrician is the individual who plays the pivotal role in identifying children with a potential neuropsychological problem. It has been recommended that pediatricians "incorporate screening in the well-child care" (Dworkin, 1989a). However, one study found that only about 40% of infants and preschool-age children were receiving routine screenings by their pediatricians (Cranston *et al.*, 1988). Screening techniques employed by pediatricians include observation, listening to concerns of parents, and/or collecting data from formal questionnaires (Glascoe, 1991; Rapin, 1995). One study found that the administration of a battery of a few easily performed neurological tests can be useful in the identification of preschool-age children for potential learning disabilities (Bax & Whitmore, 1987; Huttenlocher, Levine, Huttenlocher, & Gates, 1990). Standardized developmental screening tests may also be useful to the pediatrician in the screening process (see Glascoe, Martin, & Humphrey, 1990,

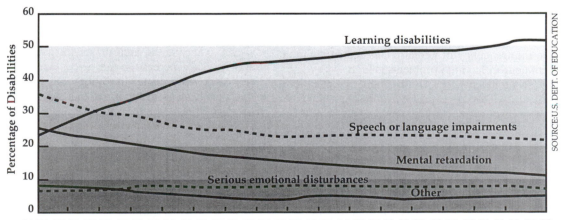

FIGURE 1. Percentage of disabilities per school year from 1976 to 1993. (Modified from Roush, 1995.)

for a review of tests). However, a recent review of the most widely used screening test (The Denver Developmental Screening Test) has found this popular test to have questionable validity as reflected by its high underreferral rate (Meisels, 1989). Therefore, it is recommended that pediatricians use screening tests with a broad developmental outlook and only in combination with other observations (Dworkin, 1989b; Meisels, 1989).

Screening tests alone are insufficient for diagnosis or remediation planning (Huttenlocher *et al.,* 1990). When a potential problem is identified, the child should then be referred for a "comprehensive multidisciplinary assessment" because considerable expertise is involved in the full evaluation of such children (Committee on Children with Disabilities, 1986, 1992; Parette *et al.,* 1990). This represents the role of the clinical child neuropsychologist.

Parents of children with developmental disability have reported complaints about their pediatricians' failure to identify their child's problems early and the lack of an effective referral system to deal with such children. Those pediatricians who gave parents more information about diagnosis and prognosis were viewed by parents to be more helpful (Fischler & Tancer, 1984; O'Sullivan, Mahoney, & Robinson, 1992). This is a role that the clinical child neuropsychologist should be particularly adept at. A recent follow-up study found that over the past 15 years, pediatricians have significantly increased their rate of referral of a suspected child for further assessment from 35% to 80% (Dobos, Dworkin, & Bernstein, 1994).

Dworkin (1985) outlined a model of an office-based approach to the child with school and developmental problems. An adaptation of this model is depicted in Figure 2. In this approach the pediatrician constitutes the first line of contact with the child, and the neuropsychologist functions as the subspecialist providing specific evaluation, assessment, and possible treatment for the referral problem. With this model, potential medical problems (e.g., thyroid dysfunction, hypoglycemia) that can influence behavior and mimic neurobehavioral disorders can be addressed directly by the pediatrician. Likewise, certain conditions, such as ADHD, which may require ongoing medical management (i.e., stimulant medication), can also be dealt with directly by the physician. In addition to a diagnostic role, the neuropsychologist is in the position (has the expertise) to assist with behavioral management, family and school intervention, as well as individual supportive psychotherapy.

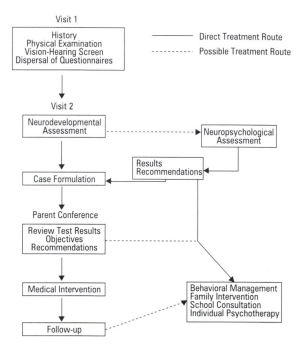

FIGURE 2. An office-based approach to children with developmental problems. (Modified from Dworkin, Woodrum, & Brooks, 1981.)

Identification of the Problem

As portrayed in Figure 3, there is a considerable overlap between the medical and the neuropsychological sphere regarding the child with developmental problems. An interdisciplinary approach to treatment of children with disabilities promotes care of the whole child (Committee on Children with Disabilities, 1992) by effectively dealing with both medical and behavioral difficulties experienced by the child in his or her day-to-day life (Fletcher & Butler, 1992). A systematic and integrated approach toward the detection, evaluation, diagnosis, and treatment of developmental disorders has been highly recommended (Committee on Children with Disabilities, 1986, 1992; Dobos *et al.,* 1994; Fletcher & Butler, 1992; Keys, 1993; Purvis, 1991).

The overlapping area in Figure 3 illustrates the type of information that the child neuropsychologist is uniquely suited to provide the medical practitioner (this topic area has been more completely addressed by Fletcher & Taylor, 1984). Information pertaining to these particular areas of functioning can be considered critical for the accurate diagnosis, definition, and prognosis of childhood problems.

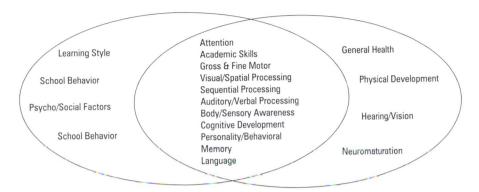

FIGURE 3. Components of the assessment of children. (Modified from Dworkin & Levine, 1980.)

Using a carefully chosen battery of assessment techniques, the neuropsychologist is able to thoroughly define the child's ability structure. The neuropsychologist can provide information regarding the child's strengths and weaknesses through the selection, administration, and proper analysis of a broad range of developmentally structured tests. It is important to emphasize that these measures should be chosen and interpreted within a developmental context; therefore, the use of normative data is essential in evaluating the individual child (Fletcher & Taylor, 1984). The neuropsychologist should consider not only what the child's abilities are now but how they may change over time. Routine assessments may be important in order to monitor development and the resultant changes in behavior and/or ability.

Next, some specific methods for obtaining this developmental information will be discussed. The battery of assessment techniques given in Table 2 has been developed at the Austin Neurological Clinic to provide a comprehensive evaluation of neuropsychological functioning in children (Nussbaum, Bigler, & Koch, 1986).

The measures included in the Comprehensive Austin Neuropsychological Assessment Battery for Children (CAN-ABC) have been found to be useful in providing the pediatrician with the data needed to accurately diagnose and plan remediation for the child with developmental problems. The measures in this battery were selected to provide comprehensive information in the areas shown in the overlapping zone in Figure 3. As shown in Table 3, information obtained from the CAN-ABC can be organized in terms of these overlapping areas. In addition, the organization of the measures into these areas can be useful when the referral question calls for a more restricted rather than a comprehensive evaluation. For example, if the child's pediatrician has a specific question regarding only the child's personality/behavioral functioning, then the battery may be modified to focus on this referral question.

The overlapping among the areas presented above is indicative of the point that very few measures of ability are pure, but are more often interdependent. This is especially true for more complex or higher-level areas of function such as cognition and memory. Thus, it is the job of the trained child neuropsychologist to interpret the results from a battery of tests in a meaningful way. For example, if a child does poorly on the Digit Span subtest of the WISC-III, is the cause an attentional problem, a memory deficit, an auditory processing problem, or some combination of these three areas? One must attempt to integrate information gathered from a wide variety of sources to provide a complete understanding of the individual child. The meaningful interpretation of information gathered through neuropsychological assessment is the truly unique capacity that the neuropsychologist brings to a private medical setting.

Communication of Assessment Results

The final stage in the process of consultation by the neuropsychologist is the communication of the assessment results. The importance of this stage cannot be overemphasized for it is at this point where it is determined whether or not the information gathered during the evaluation can be used efficaciously by the pediatrician. The clear and effective communication of assessment results is crucial for the accurate diagnosis and appropriate intervention for the child with developmental problems.

TABLE 2. The Comprehensive Austin Neuropsychological Assessment Battery for Children (CAN-ABC)[a]

General physical features

Physical measures	*Lateral dominance*	*Physical anomalies*
Height	Hand	Facial features
Weight	Foot	Epidermal features (e.g., café au lait spots)
Visual acuity	Eye	Hands
Head circumference		Other anomalies (e.g., steepled palate)

The Halstead Neuropsychological Test Battery for Children and the Reitan-Indiana Neuropsychological Test Battery for Children (selected subtests)[b]

Motor
  Strength of grip
  Finger oscillation
    Electric—5- to 8-year-olds
    Manual—9 and older
Tactual Performance Test
  6 form/horizontal—5- to 8-year olds
  6 form/vertical—9- to 14-year-olds
  10 form/vertical—14 to adult
  Sequin/Goddard (Anastasi, 1969)—poor cooperation, or under age 5
Sensory–Perceptual Examination
  Tactile
    Single, double simultaneous, ipsilateral, and contralateral
  Auditory
    Single, double simultaneous
  Visual
    Upper, middle, lower visual fields
    Single, double simultaneous
    Visual fields
  Finger recognition
  Finger graphesthesia
    5- to 8-year-old, symbols X's and O's
    9 to adult, numbers
  Form recognition
    Included if the child scores one standard deviation below the mean on tactile, finger
    recognition, and/or finger graphesthesia
Reitan–Aphasia Screening Battery (Halstead & Wepman, 1959; Selz & Reitan, 1979)
  5- to 8-year-old form
  9 and older form
Wide Range Achievement Test (Jastak & Jastak, 1965)
  Reading (primarily a test of reading recognition)
  Spelling (provides quantitative spelling level)
  Arithmetic
  Preacademic tasks as indicated
Boder Test of Reading and Spelling Patterns (Boder & Jarrico, 1982)
  Provides qualitative information on spelling/reading
Durrell Analysis of Reading Difficulty (selected subtests) (Durrell & Catterson, 1980)
  Silent reading (measure of reading comprehension)
  Oral reading (measure of visual/auditory processing and reading comprehension)
  Listening comprehension (measure of auditory/verbal comprehension)
Beery Test of Visual/Motor Integration (Beery, 1982)
  Measure of perceptual motor ability
Raven's Coloured Progressive Matrices (Raven, 1965)
  Measure of nonverbal abstract reasoning

TABLE 2. (*Continued*).

Wechsler Intelligence Scale for Children—III (Wechsler, 1991)

    Verbal IQ subscales (information, vocabulary, similarities, arithmetic, comprehension)

    Performance IQ subscales (picture completion, block design, object assembly, picture arrangement, coding)

    Digit span

Family history questionnaire

    Background information

    Pregnancy history

    Birth history

    Developmental history

    Medical history

    School history

Child Behavior Checklist—Revised (Achenbach & Edelbrock, 1983)

    Provides an easily reviewed list of possible behavior problems.

    Provides quantitative scores on such personality scales as Depression, Aggression, etc.

Personality Inventory for Children—Revised (Wirt, Lachar, Klinedinst, & Seat, 1982)

    Provides quantitative scores on such personality scales as Depression, Aggression, etc.

Projective Drawings

    House/tree/person (Buck, 1948), kinetic family drawings (Burns & Kaufman, 1972)

    —Provide qualitative information on self-concept, family dynamics, etc.

Behavioral observation inventory

    Provides a short informal assessment of behaviors observed during the evaluation

Additional measures included as needed

Benton Visual Retention Test (Benton, 1974)

—Included if:

    questionable ADHD problems

    deficient visuomotor performance (Beery) leads to questions about deficits in visual memory versus visuomotor coordination

Kaufman Assessment Battery for Children (Kaufman & Kaufman, 1983)

—Included if:

    marginal or questionable LD

    more in-depth information is needed concerning child's nonverbal intellectual abilities

    particularly useful subscales

        Hand Movements (useful attentional measure)

        Gestalt Closure (useful visual processing measure)

        Matrix Analogies (useful nonverbal reasoning measure)

        Spatial Memory (useful visual memory measure without a motor confound)

Other

    Halstead Neuropsychological Test Battery for Children subtests

    Administered to 9- to 14-year-olds as indicated

        Trails A (measure of sequential visual processing, attention)

        Trails B (measure of sequential visual processing, attention, cognitive flexibility)

        Seashore Rhythm Test (measure of sequential auditory processing, attention, auditory memory)

        Speech Sounds Perception Test (measure of auditory processing, attention, sight/sound matching)

---

[a]Measures are scored according to individual norm tables provided with each specific test or according to normative information provided by Spreen and Gaddes (1969) or Knights and Norwood (1980).

[b]Reitan and Davison (1974).

The Neuropsychological Report

The exemplary report should start with a specific presenting or identified problem. This permits focusing the results of the consultation and test findings so that the presenting questions may be answered. Sufficient background history should be reported to answer any questions concerning pregnancy, birth, and delivery, developmental milestones, psychological history, school history, and medical history that may be salient variables related to the presenting problem(s). Sources of information

TABLE 3. The Organization of Neuropsychological Test Results[a]

Motor (fine and gross)
  Strength of grip
  Finger oscillation
  Tactual Performance Test
  Grooved Pegboard
  Beery Test of Visual/Motor Integration
  WISC-R (Block Design, Object Assembly, Coding)
Visual/spatial processing
  Visual acuity
  Sensory–Perceptual Exam (visual exam)
  Beery Test of Visual/Motor Integration
  Benton Visual Retention Test
  Trails A & B
  Rey–Osterrieth Complex Figure
  Tactual Performance Test
  Reitan–Aphasia Screening Battery
    (Visual Constructional tasks)
  K-ABC (Hand Movements, Gestalt Closure)
  WISC-III (performance IQ subscales)
Body awareness
  Sensory–Perceptual Exam errors (tactile, finger recognition,
    finger graphesthesia, form recognition)
  Tactual Performance Test
Auditory verbal processing
  Sensory–Perceptual Exam errors (Auditory)
  Seashore Rhythm Test
  Speech Sounds Perception Test
  Durrell (Listening Comprehension)
  WISC-III (verbal IQ subscales)
  Peabody Picture Vocabulary Test—Revised (1981)
Sequential processing
  WISC-III (Digit Span, Picture Arrangement)
  K-ABC (Hand Movements)
  Trails A & B
  Seashore Rhythm Test
Memory
  WISC-III (Digit Span)
  Benton Visual Retention Test
  Rey–Osterrieth Complex Figure
  K-ABC (Spatial Memory, Hand Movements)
  Durrell (Silent Reading—unstructured story recall;
    Listening Comprehension—structured story recall)
  TOMAL
  WRAML
  Children's CVLT

  Tactual Performance Test (memory for objects and location)
  Seashore Rhythm Test
Cognitive development (knowledge, reasoning)
  Raven's Coloured Progressive Matrices
  WISC-III (Information, Vocabulary, Similarities, Arithmetic,
    Comprehension, Picture Arrangement)
  Children's Category Test
  K-ABC (Matrix Analogies)
Attention
  Sensory–Perceptual Exam (tactile, auditory, visual,
    finger recognition, finger graphesthesia)
  Benton Visual Retention Test
  Trails A & B
  Seashore Rhythm Test
  Speech Sounds Perception Test
  Durrell (Listening Comprehension)
  WISC-III (Arithmetic, Picture Completion, Coding, Digit
    Span)
  K-ABC (Hand Movements)
  Child Behavior Checklist
Language
  Boston Naming Test
  Peabody Picture Vocabulary Test
  Word Fluency: FAS
Academic skills
  Reitan–Aphasia Screening Battery (reading, spelling,
    arithmetic tasks)
  Wide Range Achievement Test (reading, spelling,
    arithmetic, preacademic tasks)
  Boder Test of Reading and Spelling Patterns
  Durrell (Silent Reading, Oral Reading,
    Listening Comprehension)
  WISC-III (Arithmetic)
Personality/behavioral
  Child Behavior Checklist
  Personality Inventory for Children—Revised
  Projective Drawings
  Behavioral observation inventory
Psychosocial factors
  Parent interview
  Family history questionnaire
  Child Behavior Checklist

[a]Tests from Boll (1993), Delis *et al.* (1994), Dunn & Dunn (1981), Gaddes & Crockett (1975), Kaplan *et al.* (1983), Matthews & Kløve (1964), Osterrieth (1994), Rey (1941), Reynolds & Bigler (1994), and Sheslow & Adams (1990).

should include parental interview, medical records, and school reports.

In the next selection of the neuropsychological report, a listing of the tests administered during the evaluation should be provided. This informs the reader of the specific measures that were used

to obtain information regarding the child's ability structure or behavioral characteristics.

As shown in Table 4, the section containing the assessment results has been divided into subsections dealing with the child's intellectual/cognitive functioning, academic abilities, neuropsychologi-

TABLE 4. Format of the Neuropsychological Report

Presenting problem
  Referral question (e.g., presenting seizures)
Background history
  Developmental milestones (e.g., language)
  Psychological history
  School history (e.g., special education)
  Previous test findings
  Genetic history (e.g., Down's syndrome, epilepsy)
  Pregnancy (e.g., complications—alcohol use, etc.)
  Birth and delivery (e.g., complications—forceps, etc.)
  Neonatal history (e.g., birth weight)
  Medical history (e.g., significant head injuries)
  Family history (e.g., parents' education, LD in the family)
Tests administered
Assessment results
  Intellectual/cognitive functioning
    IQ scores
    Subtest scores
    Clinical description/interpretation
Academic functioning
    Achievement scores
    Clinical description/interpretation
Neuropsychological test findings
  Physical stigmata/physical measurements
  Hand, eye, and foot dominance
  Motor functioning
    Fine motor
    Gross motor
    Praxic ability
    Visuomotor copying
Sensory–perceptual functioning
  Vision (acuity fields)
  Hearing
  Tactile (double simultaneous)

    Graphesthesia
    Stereognosis
    Finger gnosis
  Language
    Articulation
    Receptive
    Expressive
    Naming
    Spelling
    Reading
    Calculations
  Memory
    Verbal
    Visual/spatial
  General cognitive
Personality/emotional functioning
  Behavioral observations—subjective findings
  Projective test results
    Projective drawings
    Thematic testing
    Rorschach (1942)
  Objective personality scores/patterns
  Clinical summary
Clinical impression
  Summary and integration of assessment results
  DSM-III-R format followed when appropriate
Recommendations
  1. To referring doctor, including therapists
    whom the child may be seeing
  2. To school
  3. To parents
  4. When to follow up
  5. Miscellaneous

cal functioning, and personality/behavioral characteristics. We have found it useful to have the evaluation results divided into these subsections in order to provide an organized picture of the child's functioning, and to provide the reader with ready access to pertinent information.

The next section containing the evaluation summary and clinical impression is of critical importance. It is in this section that the results of the assessment are summarized and integrated in order to provide a holistic understanding of the child's functioning. In addition, this section contains the child's DSM-IV classification when such a categorization is appropriate.

Finally, appropriate recommendations should be based on the results of the assessment. These recommendations should contain general as well as specific information that may be helpful in treatment planning for the child including medical/neurological, educational, and social/psychological. The important point that must be emphasized here is that the recommendations should clearly follow from the results of the evaluation.

Follow-up Conference

The parents play a focal role in assuring that appropriate recommendations are followed; accordingly, considerable effort should be directed at providing a clear understanding on the parents' part. Typically, this will require at least an hour conference to review test results and outline potential treatment options where appropriate. Also it is most helpful to have various reading lists available to the

TABLE 5. Case Presentation for J. B.: Results of the Comprehensive Austin Neuropsychological Assessment Battery for Children

Name: J. B.   Education: 2nd grade   Date: 1/24/84
Age: 8 years, 1 month   Race: Caucasian   Examiner: M. H.
Sex: Male   Location: Austin Neurological

Motor (fine and gross)

Strength of grip
  Dominant hand = 15; Nondominant = 12.2
Finger oscillation
  Dominant hand = 39.8; Nondominant = 35.2
  SS^a = 106   SS = 106
Tactual Performance Test
  Dominant = 5.9; Nondominant =4.1; Both =1.5; Total = 11.5
  SS = 99   SS = 99   SS = 100   SS = 100
Beery Test of Visual/Motor Integration
  SS = 10; Percentile = 60; Age equivalent = 7,9
WISC-R (Block Design, Object Assembly, Coding)
        BD = 11   OA = 13   Cod = 12

Visual/spatial processing

Visual acuity
  Uncorrected: Right = 20/50; Left = 20/30
  Corrected: Right = 20/20; Left = 20/20
Sensory–Perceptual Exam (visual exam)
  Visual fields = Normal to simple confrontation
DSS errors: Right = 1; Left = 0
         SS = 76   SS = 106
Beery Test of Visual/Motor Integration
  SS = 10; Percentile = 50; Age equivalent = 7,9
Benton Visual Retention Test (normed IQ = 91, age = 8)
  Expected correct = 2; obtained correct = 5
  Expected errors = 12–13; obtained errors = 8
  Errors: Right visual field = 4; left visual field = 3
Trails A & B
  Trails A = 43 sec, 0 errors   Trails B = 52 sec, 0 errors
  (9 y.o. $\bar{X}$ = 21 sec)   (9 y.o. $\bar{X}$ = 49 sec)
Tactual Performance Test
  Memory = 3; Location = 0
  SS = 84   SS = 74
Reitan–Aphasia Screening Battery (visual constructional tasks)
  Within normal limits
K-ABC (Hand Movements, Gestalt Closure)
  HM = 8   GC = 7
WISC-R (Performance IQ = 102)
  (Picture Completion, Picture Arrangement, Block Design, Object Assembly, Coding)
  PC = 8   PA = 8   BD = 11   OA = 13   Cod = 12

Body awareness

Sensory–Perceptual Exam errors (tactile, finger recognition, finger graphesthesia, form recognition)
  Tactile: DSS, Right = 0; Left = 1
         SS = 114   SS = 95
  Finger graphesthesia: Right = 0; Left = 0
         SS = 121   SS = 119
  Finger Recognition: Right = 3; Left = 3
         SS = 70   SS = 80

TABLE 5. (*Continued*).

Tactual Performance Test
  Dominant = 5.9;   Nondominant = 4.1;   Both = 1.5;   Total = 11.5
  SS = 99   SS = 99   SS = 100   SS = 100

Auditory verbal processing

Sensory–Perceptual Exam errors (auditory)
  Right = 0;   Left = 0
  SS = 105   SS = 108
Seashore Rhythm Test
  Not applicable for this age
Speech Sounds Perception Test
  Not applicable for this age
Durrell (Listening Comprehension)
  LC = second grade level
WISC-R   (Information,   Similarities,   Arithmetic,   Vocabulary,   Comprehension)
              Info = 5   Sim = 6   Arith = 11   Voc = 7   Verbal IQ = 82
Peabody Picture Vocabulary Test—Revised (1981)
  Mental age score = 5 years, 11 months
  SS = 75

Sequential processing

WISC-R   (Digit Span,   Picture Arrangement)
              DS = 6   PA = 8
K-ABC (Hand Movements)
  HM = 8
Trails A and B
  Trails A = 43 sec, 0 errors; Trails B = 52 sec, 0 errors
  (SS, see above)
Seashore Rhythm Test
  Not applicable for this age

Memory

WISC-R   (Digit Span)
              DS = 6
Benton Visual Retention Test (normed IQ = 91, age = 8)
  Expected correct = 2; obtained correct = 5
  Expected errors = 12–13; obtained errors = 8
K-ABC (Spatial Memory,   Hand Movements)
          SM = 7   HM = 8
Durrell (Silent Reading—unstructured story recall;   Listening Comprehension—structured story recall)
          SR = Poor   LC = Fair
Tactual Performance Test (memory for objects and location)
  Memory = 3;   Location = 0
  SS = 84   SS = 74
Seashore Rhythm Test
  Not applicable for this age

Cognitive development (knowledge, reasoning)

Raven's Coloured Progressive Matrices
Percentile = 50
WISC-R   (Information,   Vocabulary,   Similarities,   Arithmetic,   Comprehension,   Picture Arrangement)
              Info = 5   Voc = 7   Sim = 6   Arith = 11   Comp = 7   PA = 8
K-ABC   (Matrix Analogies)
              MA = 11

Attention

Sensory–Perceptual Exam (tactile, auditory, visual, finger recognition, finger graphesthesia)
  Tactile: DSS, Right = 0; Left = 1

(*continued*)

TABLE 5. (*Continued*).

Auditory: Right = 0; Left = 0
Visual: DSS, Right = 1; Left = 0
Finger recognition: Right = 3; Left = 3
Finger graphesthesia: Right = 0; Left = 0
(For SS, see above)
Benton Visual Retention Test
  Expected correct = 2; obtained correct = 5
  Expected errors = 12–13; obtained errors = 8
Trails A & B
  Trails A = 43 sec, 0 errors; Trails B = 52 sec, 0 errors
  (SS, see above)
Seashore Rhythm Test
  Not applicable for this age
Durrell (Listening Comprehension)
  LC = 2nd grade level, fair structured recall
WISC-R (Arithmetic, Picture Completion, Coding, Digit Span)
  Arith = 11   PC = 8   Cod = 12   DS = 6
K-ABC (Hand Movements)
  HM = 8
Child Behavior Checklist
  Mild attentional problems noted
Behavioral observation inventory
  No attentional problems noted on informal observation

Academic skills

Reitan–Aphasia Screening Battery (reading, spelling, arithmetic tasks)
Reading errors noted

Wide Range Achievement Test

	Standard score	Grade equivalent	Percentile
Reading	89	2.4	23
Spelling	99	2.8	47
Arithmetic	105	3.1	63

Boder Test of Reading and Spelling Patterns
  Reading/Spelling Pattern = Dysphonetic type
Durrell (Silent Reading,   Oral Reading,   Listening Comprehension)
      SR = middle 1st   OR = lower 1st   LC = 2nd grade
WISC-R   (Arithmetic)
      Arith = 11

Personality/behavioral

Child Behavior Checklist (scale elevations above 70)
  Aggressive, Internalizing, Anxious, Depressed
Personality Inventory for Children—Revised (scale elevations above 70)
  Adjustment, depression, withdrawal, anxiety
Projective drawings
  House/Tree/Person: sparse, vacant, small, human stick figures
Behavioral observation inventory
  Poor eye contact, withdrawn, no spontaneous speech, brief verbal response

Psychosocial factors

Parent interview (significant points)
  Slow progress in school, father reported similar learning problems, school phobia, temper outbursts
Family history questionnaire (significant points)
  Normal pregnancy, induced labor, forceps delivery, developmental milestones within normal limits, allergies
Child Behavior Checklist
  Noted to have poor peer and family interactions

[a]SS, standard score.

parents so that they can pursue on their own further enlightenment pertaining to the nature of their child's problems.

Case Study Material

Next, a case study will be presented to illustrate the type and format of information typically obtained in a neuropsychological assessment. First, the raw data will be presented in terms of how they can be conceptually organized as outlined in Table 3. Second, the results of the evaluation will be presented in the report format shown in Table 4 in order to illustrate the communication of neuropsychological findings.

The case of J. B. presented in Tables 5 and 6 illustrate the way in which results from the neuropsychological evaluation can be communicated to the physician in report format. The goal of the neuropsychologist in writing the neuropsychological report is to: (1) address the specific referral question(s); (2) thoroughly present relevant test results; (3) provide a clinical interpretation of the data; (4) present pertinent recommendations; (5) communicate these points clearly and effectively.

Summary

The role of the child neuropsychologist in the private medical practice is that of an expert consultant. Because of the increasing identification and referral of children with developmental disorders (Dworkin, 1985) to pediatricians, there is a growing recognition of the need for better diagnostic and remediation techniques. The child neuropsychologist is uniquely suited to provide relevant information to the child's physician to aid in the delineation of problem areas and to assist in formulating an appropriate intervention strategy.

Specific information was presented earlier in this chapter outlining one test battery that has been developed to provide a comprehensive evaluation of the child's neuropsychological functioning (see Table 2). The CAN-ABC is just one battery of tests that can be used to obtain this type of information. The important feature is that a comprehensive and integrative approach be used in the assessment of the individual child.

In addition, a report format was presented to illustrate the organization and communication of the evaluation results (see Table 4). Finally, a case study was provided to exemplify the type of

---

TABLE 6. Neuropsychological Assessment Report (Based on Data in Table 5)

Child's name: J. B.
Clinic number: 99999
Assessment date: 1/24/84

Presenting problem

This child was referred by Dr. K., pediatric neurologist, for a comprehensive neuropsychological evaluation relating to questions concerning a possible learning disorder.

Background history

J. B. was an 8-year-old boy who was in the second grade at the time of assessment. He had been referred for neuropsychological evaluation because of inadequate academic progress and behavioral problems.

This child's medical history showed that he was the product of a full-term, normal pregnancy. In J. B.'s birth history, it was reported that labor was induced and he was delivered using forceps. His developmental milestones were reported to be within normal limits. He crawled at approximately 7 months, walked at 12 months, and started saying his first words at about 1 year of age.

J. B.'s parents were reported to have high school educations. His father was self-employed as a plumber and his mother was not employed outside the home. Also, J. B.'s father reported that he may have experienced similar learning problems as a child.

In addition, as part of his evaluation, J. B. received an electroencephalogram that showed sharp wave activity over the left temporal region which suggested left temporal lobe dysfunction. No electroencephalographic seizure activity was noted. There were no other significant findings in J. B.'s medical history except that he was noted to have an allergy to milk and pollens.

(continued)

TABLE 6. (*Continued*).

Test administered

Comprehensive Austin Neuropsychological Assessment Battery for Children (CAN-ABC)

- Wechsler Intelligence Scale for Children—Revised
- Kaufman Assessment Battery for Children
- Wide Range Achievement Test
- Boder Reading–Spelling Test
- Durrell Analysis of Reading Difficulty
- Peabody Picture Vocabulary Test—Revised
- Reitan–Indiana Neuropsychological Test Battery for Children
- Raven's Coloured Progressive Matrices
- Benton Visual Retention Test
- Beery Test of Visual/Motor Integration
- Behavioral observation inventory
- Personality Inventory for Children
- Child Behavior Checklist

Test results

Cognitive/intellectual functioning

WISC-R results

Full scale IQ = 91

Verbal IQ score = 82   Performance IQ score = 102

Information	5	Picture Completion	8
Similarities	6	Picture Arrangement	8
Arithmetic	11	Block Design	11
Vocabulary	7	Object Assembly	13
Comprehension	7	Coding	12
(Digit Span)	6		

K-ABC results

Mental Processing composite = 83

Sequential Processing = 74		Simultaneous Processing = 93	
Hand Movements	8	Gestalt Closure	7
Number Recall	5	Triangles	13
Word Order	4	Spatial Memory	7
		Photo Series	7

Raven's CPM Results: 50th percentile

Results of intellectual assessment indicated J. B.'s level of intellectual functioning to be in the average to low average range. On the WISC-R, J. B. was found to have severely discrepant performance between the PIQ and VIQ scales, with his VIQ score over one standard deviation below his PIQ score. He exhibited a great deal of scatter in his subtest scores, with particularly deficient performance on the Information, Similarities, and Digit Span subtests of VIQ scale. Similarly, on the K-ABC, J. B.'s score on the Sequential scale was over one standard deviation below his Simultaneous scale score. He scored especially low on the Number Recall and Word Order subtests of the Sequential scale. In addition, J. B. scored at the 50th percentile on Raven's CPM, a test of perceptual discrimination and abstract reasoning. Also, J. B. showed adequate performance on the Beery Test of Visual/Motor Integration. His score on this test showed his visual motor skills to be at age level. Likewise, J. B.'s performance on the Benton Visual Retention Test was also within normal limits.

In general, it appeared that J. B.'s overall intellectual functioning was in the normal range, but he exhibited an abnormal *pattern* of performance. His intellectual profile showed significantly more impaired verbal and sequential abilities than visual/constructional abilities.

Academic functioning

WRAT results

	Grade level equivalent	Standard score	Percentile
Reading	2.4	89	23
Spelling	2.8	99	47
Arithmetic	3.1	105	63

TABLE 6. (*Continued*).

Boder Test of Reading and Spelling Patterns
   Reading/Spelling Pattern: Dysphonetic

Durrell Analysis of Reading Difficulty
   Silent Reading = middle 1st; Oral Reading = lower 1st
   Listening Comprehension = 2nd

Peabody Picture Vocabulary Test
   Age equivalent = 5 years, 11 months; standard score = 75

On the WRAT, J. B. was found to have grade level academic skills, with slightly better arithmetic than reading and spelling abilities. However, on the Durrell, J. B.'s reading and language scores were below grade level. He was noted to have particular difficulties with sound/symbol association, and his reading comprehension was found to be quite poor. Similarly, J. B scored over one and a half standard deviations below the mean on the Peabody Picture Vocabulary Test—Revised (1981). Also, J. B. was reported to sometimes make semantic substitutions in his reading. For example, when the stimulus word was "house" he responded with "home" and "her" was read as "she," also "horse" was read as "pony." These types of reading and spelling errors have been associated with a dysphonetic type of dyslexia (Boder & Jarrico, 1982).

In general, findings from achievement testing indicated that J. B. had some basic academic skills, such as word identification skills and basic calculation skills. However, he also exhibited marked deficiencies in other academic areas, such as reading comprehension and vocabulary development.

Neuropsychological functioning

At the time of the examination, J. B. stood 50 inches in height and weighed 54 pounds. His head circumference was measured at 53 centimeters. J. B. was right hand, foot, and eye dominant. No abnormal morphological physical characteristics were noted on a brief physical examination.

Reitan–Indiana Neuropsychological Test Battery for Children

Test results for the Reitan–Indiana Battery were essentially within normal limits. His motor findings on the finger oscillation and strength of grip test were in the normal range. However, on the Sensory–Perceptual Exam, J. B. did exhibit mild, bilateral finger dysgraphesthesia, but these results in isolation were not found to be clinically significant.

Language screening

On the Reitan–Aphasia Screening Test, J. B. was found to make numerous reading errors. He also exhibited marked dysnomia on the Peabody Picture Vocabulary Test with an age equivalent score of only 5 years 11 months. (See the Intellectual and Academic sections for a review of other pertinent information.)

Visual/perceptual tests

Graphomotor ability on the Beery VMI was approximately at age level. J. B. scored at the 7 year 9 month level with a standard score of 10, which placed him at the 50th percentile.

Memory assessment

Test results from a wide variety of sources indicated that J. B. was having some difficulties with both verbal and visual/spatial memory. He exhibited deficient performance on the recall of verbal information from the WISC-R, K-ABC, and the Durrell. Similarly, he showed deficits in visual/spatial memory on the K-ABC and the Tactual Performance Test.

Summary of neuropsychological test results

Results from the neuropsychological assessment were in general agreement with other test results reviewed to this point. J. B. seemed to be showing greater problems in the area of verbal language functioning than visual/spatial functioning. He also exhibited some memory difficulties which may have been related to attentional deficits.

Personality/behavioral functioning

Objective data

J. B. was found to have significant elevations on the following scales from the Personality Inventory for Children (PIC) and the Child Behavior Checklist (CBC): Depression, Anxiety, and Aggression. Also, his scale score on PIC-Withdrawal was over one and a half standard deviations above the mean, which indicated significant problems with withdrawal.

It was reported that J. B. had apparently had some difficulty separating from his parents. He developed some form of school phobia during kindergarten, and would become physically ill prior to school. This behavior apparently abated after several weeks of school attendance. His teacher at the time of assessment noted that J. B. was a tense, shy child. He was also reported to have occasional temper tantrums with his parents and siblings.

(*continued*)

TABLE 6. (*Continued*).

During assessment, the examiner noted that J. B. was very quiet and reserved throughout the examination. He was observed to be cooperative, but in a passive way in that rapport was never established and he did not appear to become engaged during the evaluation. He was reported to initiate no spontaneous conversation, and he had poor eye contact. Similarly, his affect was noted to be somewhat flat and depressed.

Subjective data

J. B.'s projective drawings were found to be somewhat vacant and sparse. He drew a very small, simple tree. Likewise, his human figure drawings were sticklike. They were also quite small and placed at the bottom edge of the page. These findings may have indicated significant self-esteem and adjustment problems.

Summary of personality/behavioral findings

In summary, J. B. appeared to have been experiencing general problems in the area of social interaction. Specifically, he seemed to be showing internalizing-type problems with features of depression, anxiety, and withdrawal.

Clinical impression

In summary, this child performed poorly on a number of verbal/language/sequential tasks typically thought to be dependent on left hemisphere functioning, whereas he exhibited relatively intact visual–spatial functioning. Such findings suggested a probable left-hemisphere-based learning disorder. This interpretation was supported further by abnormal EEG findings in the left temporal region.

In addition, at the time of the evaluation, J. B. appeared to be experiencing a number of significant emotional and adjustment problems related to depression and impaired socialization.

DSM-IV classification

Axis I: 309.28 possible childhood adjustment disorder with mixed anxiety and depressed mood
Axis II: 315.9 learning disorder not otherwise specified
Axis III: abnormal EEG (left temporal, sharp wave activity)

Recommendations

Given the results of J. B.'s neuropsychological assessment, it is recommended that he receive special education services. With respect to the special education curriculum, this child would probably benefit from a remediation program that focused on verbal/language training.

Some of J. B.'s verbal expression problems may be related to anxiety and a lack of spontaneity in social discourse. Thus, there may be some improvement in his level of functioning as he becomes more relaxed and comfortable in communicating with others. In addition, because of his verbal/language difficulties, J. B. may not have acquired the necessary interpersonal skills for good social interaction, which may have led to depression and withdrawal. Compounding these problems were also left-hemisphere-based academic difficulties, which may have aggravated self-esteem and adjustment problems. It is therefore recommended that he participate in a language enrichment program with a qualified speech/language therapist in order to increase his confidence and social appropriateness in communication.

In addition, J. B. appeared to show some significant problems with emotional adjustment. These findings indicated that he may benefit from some supportive counseling that would focus on social skills training to improve the quality of his peer and family relationships. This intervention should also take advantage of the strengths J. B. has in some nonverbal areas. Furthermore, his parents should encourage his participation in other nonacademic activities that would help promote positive self-esteem.

Finally, J. B.'s progress should be closely monitored, and he should return for follow-up testing on an annual basis for the next 2 to 3 years.

---

information gathered and the way in which it can be communicated to the child's physician.

References

Achenbach, T., & Edelbrock, C. S. (1983). *The Child Behavior Checklist-Revised*. Burlington: University of Vermont.

Anastasi, A. (1969). *Psychological testing* (3rd ed.). London: Macmillan & Co.

Bax, M., & Whitmore, K. (1987). The medical examination of children on entry to school. The results and use of neurodevelopmental assessment. *Developmental Medicine and Child Neurology, 29*, 40–55.

Beery, K. (1982). *Revised administration, scoring and teaching manual for the developmental test of visual–motor integration*. Cleveland: Modern Curriculum Press.

Benton, A. (1974). *The Revised Visual Retention Test* (4th ed.). New York: Psychological Corporation.

Boder, E., & Jarrico, S. (1982). *The Boder Test of Reading–Spelling Patterns: A diagnostic screening test for subtypes of reading disability.* New York: Grune & Stratton.

Boll, T. (1993). *The Children's Category Test Manual.* San Antonio, TX: The Psychological Corporation.

Boyle, C. A., Decoufle, P., & Yeargin-Allsopp, M. (1994). Prevalence and health impact of developmental disabilities in US children. *Pediatrics, 93*(3), 399–403.

Buck, J. (1948). House–tree–person test. *Journal of Clinical Psychology, 4,* 151–159.

Burnett, R., & Bell, L. (1978). Projecting practice patterns. *Pediatrics, 62*(Suppl.), 625–680.

Burns, R., & Kaufman, S. (1972). *Actions, styles and symbols in kinetic family drawings.* New York: Brunner/Mazel.

Committee on Children with Disabilities. (1986). Screening for developmental disabilities. *Pediatrics, 78*(3), 526–528.

Committee on Children with Disabilities. (1992). Pediatrician's role in the development and implementation of an individual education plan (IEP) and/or an individual family service plan (IFSP). *Pediatrics, 89*(2), 340–342.

Cranston, C. S., Ulrey, G., Hansen, R., Hudler, M., Marshall, R., & Wuori, D. (1988). Interprofessional collaboration: Who is doing it? Who isn't? *Developmental and Behavioral Pediatrics, 9*(3), 134–139.

Delis, D. C., Kramer, J. H., Kaplan, E., & Ober, B. A. (1994). *The California Verbal Learning Test-Children Manual.* San Antonio, TX: The Psychological Corporation.

Dobos, A. E., Dworkin, P. H., & Bernstein, B. A. (1994). Pediatricians' approaches to developmental problems: Has the gap been narrowed? *Developmental and Behavioral Pediatrics, 15*(1), 34–38.

Drillien, D., Thompson, A., & Burgoyne, K. (1980). Low birthweight children at early school age: A longitudinal study. *Developmental Medicine and Child Neurology, 22,* 26–47.

Dunn, L. M., & Dunn, L. M. (1981). *Peabody Picture Vocabulary Test-Revised.* Circle Pines, MN: American Guidance Service.

Durrell, D., & Catterson, J. (1980). *Durrell analysis of reading difficulty.* New York: Psychological Corporation.

Dworkin, P. H. (1985). *Learning and behavior problems of school-children.* Philadelphia: Saunders.

Dworkin, P. H. (1989a). British and American recommendation for developmental monitoring: The role of surveillance. *Pediatrics, 84*(6), 1000–1010.

Dworkin, P. H. (1989b). Developmental screening—Expecting the impossible? *Pediatrics*(commentaries), *83*(4), 619–622.

Dworkin, P., & Levine, M. (1980). The preschool child: Prediction and prescription. In A. Scheiner & I. Abrams (Eds.), *The practical management of the developmentally disabled child.* St. Louis: Mosby.

Dworkin, P., Woodrum, D., & Brooks, K. (1981). Pediatric-based assessment: Children with school problems. *Journal of School Health, 51,* 325–329.

Fischler, R., & Tancer, M. (1984). The primary physician's role in care for developmentally handicapped children. *The Journal of Family Practice, 18*(1), 85–88.

Fletcher, J. M., & Butler, I. J. (1992). The behavioral sciences and issues in child neurology and developmental pediatrics. *Journal of Child Neurology, 7,* 131–134.

Fletcher, J., & Taylor, H. (1984). Neurological assessment of children: A developmental approach. *Texas Psychologist, 36*(3), 14–20.

Gaddes & Crockett. (1975). Word Fluency Test norms for children.

Glascoe, F. P. (1991). Can clinical judgment detect children with speech–language problems? *Pediatrics, 87*(3), 317–322.

Glascoe, F. P., Martin, E. D., & Humphrey, S. (1990). A comparative review of developmental screening tests. *Pediatrics, 86*(4), 547–554.

Halstead, W., & Wepman, J. (1959). The Halstead–Wepman Aphasia Screening Test. *Journal of Speech and Hearing Disorders, 14,* 9–15.

Huttenlocher, P. R., Levine, S. C., Huttenlocher, J., & Gates, J. (1990). Discrimination of normal and at-risk preschool children on the basis of neurological tests. *Developmental Medicine and Child Neurology, 32,* 394–402.

Jastak, J., & Jastak, S. (1965). *The Wide Range Achievement Test manual.* Wilmington, DE: Guidance Service.

Kaplan, E. F., Goodglass, H., & Weintraub, S. (1983). *The Boston Naming Test.* Philadelphia: Lea & Febiger.

Kaufman, A., & Kaufman, N. (1983). *Kaufman Assessment Battery for Children: Administration and interpretative manual.* Circle Pines, MN: American Guidance Service.

Keys, M. P. (1993). The pediatrician's role in reading disorders. *Pediatric Clinics of North America, 40*(4), 869–879.

Kirk, S. A., & Gallagher, J. J. (1989). *Educating exceptional children* (6th ed.). Boston: Houghton Mifflin.

Knights, R., & Norwood, J. (1980). *Revised smoothed normative data on the neuropsychological test battery for children.* Ottawa, Canada: Robert M. Knights Psychological Consultants.

Matthews, C. G., & Kløve, H. (1964). *Instruction manual for the Adult Neuropsychology Test Battery.* Madison: University of Wisconsin Medical School.

Meisels, S. J. (1989). Can developmental screening tests identify children who are developmentally at risk? *Pediatrics, 83*(4), 578–585.

National Center for Educational Statistics. (1994). *Mini-Digest of Education Statistics 1994.* U. S. Department of Education.

Nussbaum, N., Bigler, E., & Koch, W. (1986). Neuropsychologically derived subgroups of learning disabled children: Personality/behavioral dimensions. *Journal of Research and Development in Education, 19,* 57–67.

Osterrieth, P. A. (1944). Le test de copie d'une figure complexe. *Archives de Psychologie, 30,* 206–356.

O'Sullivan, P., Mahoney, G., & Robinson, C. (1992). Perceptions of pediatricians' helpfulness: A national study of mothers of young disabled children. *Developmental Medicine and Child Neurology, 34,* 1064–1071.

Parette, H. P., Hourcade, J. J., & Brimberry, R. K. (1990). The family physician's role with parents of young children with developmental disabilities. *The Journal of Family Practice, 31*(3), 288–296.

Purvis, P. (1991). The public laws for education of the disabled—The pediatrician's role. *Developmental and Behavioral Pediatrics, 12*(5), 327–339.

Rapin, I. (1995). Physician's testing of children with developmental disabilities. *Journal of Child Neurology, 10* (Suppl.), S2121–S15.

Ravens, J. C. (1965). *Guide to using the colored progressive matrices.* London: H. K. Lewis.

Reitan, R., & Davison, L. (1974). *Clinical neuropsychology: Current status and application.* New York: Hemisphere.

Rey, A. (1941). L'examen psychologique dans le cas l'encephalopathie traumatique. *Archives de Psychologie, 28,* 286–340.

Reynolds, C. R., & Bigler, E. D. (1994). *Test of Memory and Learning.* Austin, TX: PRO-ED.

Rorschach, H. (1942). *Psychodiagnostics: A diagnostic test based on perception* (P. Lemkau & B. Kronenburg, Trans.). Bern: Huber (U.S. distributor: Grune & Stratton).

Roush, W. (1995). Arguing over why Johnny can't read. *Science, 267,* 1896–1898.

Selz, M., & Reitan, R. (1979). Rules for neuropsychological diagnosis: Classification of brain function in older children.
Journal of Consulting and Clinical Psychology, 47, 258–264.

Shapiro, B. K., & Gallico, R. P. (1993). Learning disabilities. *Pediatric Clinics of North America, 40*(3), 491–505.

Sheslow, D., & Adams, W. (1990). *Wide Range Assessment of Memory and Learning.* Wilmington, DE: Jastak Associates, Inc.

Shonkoff, J., Dworkin, P., & Leviton, A. (1979). Primary care approaches to developmental disabilities. *Pediatrics, 64,* 505–514.

Spreen, O., & Gaddes, W. (1969). Developmental norms for fifteen neuropsychological tests for ages 6 to 15. *Cortex, 5,* 171–191.

Wechsler, D. (1991). *Wechsler Intelligence Scale for Children-Third Edition.* New York: Psychological Corporation.

Wirt, R., Lachar, D., Klinedinst, J., & Seat, P. (1982). *The Personality Inventory for Children, Revised.* Los Angeles: Western Psychological Services.

Index

ISBN 0-306-45257-X

90000